KAPLAN & SADOCK'S

STUDY GUIDE AND
SELF-EXAMINATION
REVIEW IN PSYCHIATRY

SEVENTH EDITION

KAPLAN & SADOCK'S

Study Guide and Self-Examination Review in Psychiatry

SEVENTH EDITION

Benjamin James Sadock, M.D.

Menas S. Gregory Professor of Psychiatry and Vice Chairman,
Department of Psychiatry, New York University School of Medicine;
Attending Psychiatrist, Tisch Hospital;
Attending Psychiatrist, Bellevue Hospital Center;
Consulting Psychiatrist, Lenox Hill Hospital,
New York, New York

Virginia Alcott Sadock, M.D.

Professor of Psychiatry, Department of Psychiatry,
New York University School of Medicine;
Attending Psychiatrist, Tisch Hospital;
Attending Psychiatrist, Bellevue Hospital Center,
New York, New York

Rebecca Marie Jones, M.D.

Clinical Assistant Professor of Psychiatry,
New York University School of Medicine,
New York, New York

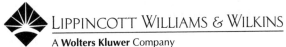

LIPPINCOTT WILLIAMS & WILKINS
A **Wolters Kluwer** Company
Philadelphia • Baltimore • New York • London
Buenos Aires • Hong Kong • Sydney • Tokyo

Acquisitions Editor: Charles W. Mitchell
Managing Editor: Joyce A. Murphy
Developmental Editor: Lisa R. Kairis
Supervising Editor: Melanie Bennitt
Production Editor: Alyson Langlois, Silverchair Science + Communications
Compositor: Silverchair Science + Communications
Manufacturing Manager: Colin J. Warnock
Printer: Quebecor World, Taunton

© 2003 by LIPPINCOTT WILLIAMS & WILKINS
530 Walnut Street
Philadelphia, PA 19106 USA
LWW.com

"Kaplan Sadock Psychiatry" with the pyramid logo is a trademark of Lippincott Williams & Wilkins.

Printed in the USA

Library of Congress Cataloging-in-Publication Data
Sadock, Benjamin J., 1933-
  Kaplan & Sadock's study guide and self-examination review in psychiatry.-- 7th ed. /
Benjamin James Sadock, Virginia Alcott Sadock, Rebecca Marie Jones.
    p. ; cm.
  Rev ed. of: Study guide and self-examination review for Kaplan and Sadock's synopsis of psychiatry.
  "Complements the 9th edition of Kaplan and Sadock's synopsis of psychiatry"--Pref.
  Includes index.
  ISBN 0-7817-3359-6
    1. Mental illness--Examinations, questions, etc. 2. Psychiatry--Examinations, questions,
etc. I. Title: Kaplan and Sadock's study guide and self-examination review in psychiatry.
II. Title: Study guide and self-examination review in psychiatry. III. Sadock, Benjamin J.
IV. Kaplan, Harold I., 1927-1998 Study guide and self-examination review for Kaplan
and Sadock's synopsis of psychiatry. V. Sadock, Benjamin J. Kaplan & Sadock's
synopsis of psychiatry. VI. Title.
    [DNLM: 1. Mental Disorders--Examination Questions. 2. Psychiatry--Examination
Questions. WM 140 S126k 2003 Suppl.]
  RC454.K35 2003 Suppl.
  616.89'0076--dc21

                                                            2003040042

10 9 8 7 6 5 4 3 2 1

Preface

This edition of *Study Guide and Self-Examination Review in Psychiatry* is designed to complement the 9th edition of *Kaplan & Sadock's Synopsis of Psychiatry* published in 2003. It is written to meet the needs of medical students, psychiatrists, neurologists, primary care and other nonpsychiatric physicians, and mental health professionals from all fields who require a review of the behavioral sciences and clinical psychiatry. *Study Guide* is designed especially to help those preparing for examinations, such as the United States Medical Licensing Examination (USMLE) and the examination in psychiatry of the American Board of Psychiatry and Neurology (ABPN). It also stands alone as a separate book to provide a unique learning experience in all areas of psychiatry.

The first *Study Guide* was published over 20 years ago and to each subsequent edition, including this one, the authors added new and different questions and modified and updated material from earlier editions. This *Study Guide* contains over 1,000 questions, including a specially prepared section on case studies. Questions are consistent with the format used by the USMLE, and their allocation has been carefully weighted with attention to both clinical and theoretical issues.

The authors of the last edition of *Study Guide* are particularly pleased that Rebecca Jones, M.D., a close personal and professional associate and outstanding academician, has joined them as third author. Her participation has immeasurably facilitated and enhanced the preparation of this work.

Case Studies

A new section of never-before-published accounts of actual patients has been added to this edition. Each case history includes questions and a discussion of diagnosis, differential diagnosis, treatment strategies, and other related topics. The cases are from the authors' and other clinicians' experiences, including many derived from the medical student and psychiatric resident teaching services of the NYU Medical Center and Bellevue Hospital. In keeping with the *Principles of Medical Ethics with Annotation Especially Applicable to Psychiatry,* published by the American Psychiatric Association, each case history has been suitably disguised to safeguard patient confidentiality without altering material to provide less than a complete portrayal of the patient's actual condition.

This section of case studies will be of value to students preparing for examinations that increasingly use case examples

(such as the USMLE); to those mental health professionals who may not be exposed to similar cases in their day-to-day work; to primary care physicians, who are often on the front lines of psychiatry; and to psychiatrists who wish to test their clinical acumen or who wish to learn more about complex diagnostic and treatment decisions.

COMPREHENSIVE TEACHING SYSTEM

Study Guide forms one part of a comprehensive system developed by the authors to facilitate the teaching of psychiatry and the behavioral sciences. At the head of the system is *Comprehensive Textbook of Psychiatry,* which is global in depth and scope; it is designed for and used by psychiatrists, behavioral scientists, and all other workers in the mental health field. *Kaplan & Sadock's Synopsis of Psychiatry* is a relatively brief, highly modified, original, and current version useful for medical students, psychiatric residents, practicing psychiatrists, and other mental health professionals. Other parts of the system are the pocket handbooks: *Pocket Handbook of Clinical Psychiatry, Pocket Handbook of Psychiatric Drug Treatment, Pocket Handbook of Emergency Psychiatric Medicine,* and *Pocket Handbook of Primary Care Psychiatry.* Those books cover the diagnosis and the treatment of mental disorders, psychopharmacology, psychiatric emergencies, and primary care psychiatry, respectively, and are compactly designed and concisely written to be carried in the pocket by clinical clerks and practicing physicians, whatever their specialty, to provide a quick reference. Finally, *Comprehensive Glossary of Psychiatry and Psychology* provides simply written definitions for psychiatrists and other physicians, psychologists, students, other mental health professionals, and the general public. Taken together, these books create a multiple approach to the teaching, studying, and learning of psychiatry.

HOW TO USE THIS BOOK

Because this is a study guide, each chapter begins with an introduction that can be used as an outline that directs students to areas of special significance used in their studying. The authors have prepared lists of helpful hints—now expanded and also in alphabetical order—that present key terms and concepts essential to a basic knowledge of psychiatry. Students should be able to define and discuss each of the terms in depth as preparation for examinations.

The section "Objective Examinations in Psychiatry" will provide the student with helpful hints on how to take examinations. If the student understands how questions are constructed, his or her chances of answering correctly are greatly improved. This book defines distractors (wrong answers) as well as correct answers in each discussion.

To use this book most effectively, the student should attempt to answer all the questions in a particular chapter. By allowing about 1 minute for each answer, the student can approximate the time constraints of an actual written examination. The answers should then be verified by referring to the corresponding answer section in each chapter. Pay particular attention to the discussion of the wrong answers, a feature unique to this book. If further information is needed, the reader is referred to the current editions of either the *Synopsis of Psychiatry* or the *Comprehensive Textbook of Psychiatry*.

ACKNOWLEDGMENTS

Several persons helped in the preparation of this book. We especially thank Carole Jo Sharin for her excellent editorial skills. She was of immense help in the preparation of this edition.

Myrl Manley, M.D., Professor and Director of Medical Student Education in Psychiatry at NYU School of Medicine, served as contributing editor, along with James C. Edmondson, M.D., Ph.D., Caroly S. Pataki, M.D., and Norman Sussman, M.D., all of whom were also contributing editors to the 9th edition of *Kaplan & Sadock's Synopsis of Psychiatry*.

Yande McMillan played a key role in the preparation of the manuscript ably assisted by Nitza Jones and Peggy Cuzzolino. They worked with alacrity and their help was invaluable.

We especially acknowledge James Sadock, M.D., and Victoria Sadock, M.D., for help in their areas of expertise, emergency adult and emergency pediatric medicine, respectively. We thank Melanie Bennitt and the staff at Lippincott Williams & Wilkins who were most efficient. Alyson Langlois was also of great help in the preparation of this book.

Finally, we want to express our deepest thanks to Robert Cancro, M.D., Med.D.Sc., Professor and Chairman of the Department of Psychiatry at New York University School of Medicine. Dr. Cancro's commitment to psychiatric education and psychiatric research is recognized throughout the world. He is a much valued and highly esteemed colleague and friend. Our collaboration and association with this outstanding American educator has been a source of great inspiration.

B.J.S.
V.A.S.
R.M.J.

Contents

KAPLAN & SADOCK'S

STUDY GUIDE AND SELF-EXAMINATION REVIEW IN PSYCHIATRY

SEVENTH EDITION

The Doctor–Patient Relationship and Interviewing Techniques

To be an effective clinician in any field, a physician must understand both the science and the art of medicine. With all of the technological advances in medicine, successful caregiving still relies on the very basic, and deceptively simple, relationship between doctor and patient. Without good communication between practitioner and patient, it may not matter how sophisticated the available treatments are.

It is often debated whether or not the art of medicine can be taught alongside the science. Some would argue that an individual practitioner either has or lacks an innate ability for empathy and rapport. Is it possible to learn how to listen to (and to really hear) someone, to empathize and to recognize when a patient has questions or resistances that are unspoken and if not addressed can lead to a failure of care?

While some clinicians are naturally better at these skills than others, if these capabilities are not required of students, they may be seen as peripheral or tangential to the practice of quality care; but if learning how to establish and sustain rapport becomes part of learning how to be a doctor, then these skills are deepened in those who are naturally gifted, and modeled for those who are less so. The key is to underscore how these interpersonal and cognitive abilities translate into real advantages in the day-to-day management of patients.

Today's physicians care for people of all races, ethnicities, and economic levels. Without sensitivity to the nuances and potential pitfalls inherent in providing care to people of different backgrounds, the clinician's knowledge may become useless. The ability to remain flexible, curious, and self-aware is part of the larger whole of a successful and satisfying lifelong practice. Caring for the difficult patient can be frustrating and demoralizing; however, it will be challenging, and even gratifying, if the appropriate approaches, questions, and skills are employed. "The secret of care of the patient is in caring for the patient," remarked Francis Peabody, a talented teacher and clinician. All physicians must understand the critical factors that shape the physician–patient relationship and the importance of this relationship in "caring for the patient."

This chapter encompasses such topics as rapport, transference and countertransference, compliance, interviewing skills, and working with a range of patient populations. Students can reinforce their knowledge of these topics by reflecting on the questions and answers provided below.

HELPFUL HINTS

The key terms listed below should be understood by the student.

- active versus passive patients
- aggression and counteraggression
- authority figures
- belligerent patients
- biopsychosocial
- biopsychosocial model
- burnout
- closed-ended questions
- compliance
- compliance versus noncompliance
- confrontation
- content versus process
- countertransference
- cultural attitudes
- defensive attitudes
- distortion
- doctor–patient models
- early social pressures
- emotional reactions
- emotionally charged statements
- empathy
- George Engel
- "good patients"
- humor
- identification
- illness behavior
- individual experience
- insight
- interpretation
- listening
- misperception
- misrepresentation
- mutual participation
- need–fear dilemma
- open-ended questions
- overcompensatory anger
- personality
- psychodynamics
- rapport
- reflection
- self-monitoring
- sick role
- socioeconomic background
- sublimation
- therapeutic limitations
- transference
- unconscious guilt
- unresolved conflicts

▲ QUESTIONS

DIRECTIONS: Each of the incomplete statements or questions below is followed by five suggested completions or responses. Select the *one* that is *best* in each case.

1.1 The biopsychosocial model of disease

A. is derived from general systems theory
B. is associated prominently with George Engel
C. does not view medical illness as a direct result of one's psychological and sociocultural makeup
D. postulates that illness or even death may be associated with psychological stress or trauma
E. all of the above

1.2 Which of the following statements describes a symptom-oriented approach to psychiatric interviewing?

A. Identifying a patient's course of illness is of primary interest.
B. A clinician can help a patient confront his or her innermost fears.
C. A patient's behavioral pattern can be clarified by interpreting unconscious anxieties.
D. Identifying symptoms helps psychiatrists understand a patient's unconscious conflicts.
E. Symptoms are usually seen as symbolic.

1.3 Of the following interview techniques, which is the *most* helpful for establishing good rapport?

A. taking in-session notes
B. using a private office
C. maintaining eye contact
D. listening to the patient without interrupting
E. pursuing, understanding, and responding to the patient's emotional concerns

1.4 All of the following statements about confidentiality are correct *except*

A. Medical students may have access to a patient's record.
B. A physician should clarify confidentiality issues with a patient.
C. A clinician must warn a person toward whom a patient has violent fantasies.
D. Family members are sometimes informed about a patient's problem.
E. Information cannot be released to an insurance company without the patient's written consent.

1.5 Countertransference feelings

A. are rarely based on a physician's expectations of what constitutes a good patient
B. do not occur if the patient is emotionally controlled and compliant
C. are always detrimental to the doctor–patient relationship
D. can accentuate a patient's hostility
E. are unrelated to a physician's wish to rescue a patient from imminent death

1.6 If a patient threatens to sue a clinician unless the clinician provides an immediate solution to the patient's presenting problem, the clinician's best response would be to

A. ask a colleague to join the clinician in the interview
B. attempt to turn the patient's attention to another subject
C. assure the patient that the clinician will provide a cure
D. discuss with the patient the inherent uncertainty of treating any clinical disorder
E. inform the patient that the clinician finds it necessary to transfer the patient to another practitioner's care

1.7 With paranoid patients a physician

A. should be as relaxed and friendly as possible
B. should be prepared to explain in detail every decision
C. should not take seriously a patient's hostile or conspiratorial misperception of a neutral event
D. must react defensively to a patient's suspicions
E. should not allow a patient to remain evasive

1.8 Antisocial patients

A. rarely malinger
B. must be approached with a heightened sense of vigilance
C. rarely present as socially adept or intelligent
D. should never be confronted directly about inappropriate behavior
E. seldom cause physicians to feel threatened

1.9 At the beginning of an appointment, a patient wants to discuss her perception of why she fell ill, but the physician wants to know the chronology of her symptoms. The physician should

A. allow the patient to complete her thoughts
B. politely interrupt the patient and continue with closed-ended questions
C. inform her that time is of the essence
D. inform her that an extra charge will be made if more time is needed for the appointment
E. immediately discuss how compliance will be affected by her perceptions and responses

DIRECTIONS: Each set of lettered headings below is followed by a list of numbered statements. For each numbered statement, select the *best* lettered heading. Each heading may be used once, more than once, or not at all.

Questions 1.10–1.14

A. More associated with compliance
B. More associated with noncompliance
C. No correlation with compliance or noncompliance

1.10 Psychiatric patients when compared to medical patients
1.11 Female patients when compared to male patients
1.12 Younger patients when compared to older patients
1.13 High school dropouts when compared to college graduates
1.14 Economically disadvantaged patients when compared to wealthier patients

Questions 1.15–1.19

    A. Interpretation
    B. Clarification
    C. Reflection
    D. Reassurance
    E. Advice

1.15 A doctor repeats to a patient in a supportive manner something that the patient has said

1.16 A sophisticated technique, meant to help make explicit inter-relationships that the patient may understand only implicitly

1.17 An attempt to elicit details from a patient about what he or she has already said

1.18 A physician making suggestions to a patient, ideally based on adequate information obtained by careful listening to the patient

1.19 Can be experienced (positively) as an empathic response from a concerned physician or (negatively) as a false attempt to make a patient feel better

Questions 1.20–1.24

    A. Content of interview
    B. Process of interview

1.20 Nonverbal communication
1.21 Body language
1.22 Shifting the interview away from an anxiety-provoking subject onto a neutral topic
1.23 Discussion of symptoms
1.24 Social history

Questions 1.25–1.28

    A. Open-ended questions
    B. Closed-ended questions

1.25 Intent of question is vague
1.26 May invite yes or no answers
1.27 Low time efficiency
1.28 Patient selects topic

Questions 1.29–1.32

    A. Depressed patients
    B. Dependent patients
    C. Impulsive patients
    D. Obsessive patients

1.29 Most important factor is assessing risk of suicide
1.30 Have a condition that can be curable in 95 percent of cases
1.31 Often act in overly aggressive ways out of a fear that they will never get what they need or want from others
1.32 Often appear unemotional and aloof

Questions 1.33–1.37

    A. Active–passive model
    B. Teacher–student model
    C. Mutual participation model
    D. "Friendship" model

1.33 A patient is admitted to the hospital with a sudden onset of altered mental status when found thrashing about in bed. After a workup, a physician restrains him to perform a lumbar puncture.

1.34 A 64-year-old woman with diabetes mellitus visits her physician after repeatedly drawing high blood glucose levels during home monitoring.

1.35 After a patient's complete recovery from illness, her physician continues to phone and visit her—and declares his love for her.

1.36 Three days after abdominal surgery, a 32-year-old man has mild basal rales by auscultation. His surgeon tells him to ambulate.

1.37 The doctor of a 16-year-old girl with persistent abdominal problems tells her that she must go for a lower gastrointestinal (GI) series.

ANSWERS

The Doctor–Patient Relationship and Interviewing Techniques

1.1 The answer is E (all)

The most prominent proponent of the *biopsychosocial model of disease* was *George Engel,* who stressed an integrated systems approach to human behavior and to disease. The biopsychosocial model *is derived from general systems theory:* The *biological* system deals with the anatomical, structural, and molecular substrates of disease and the effects on patients' functioning; the *psychological* system treats the effects of psychodynamic factors, motivation, and personality on the experience of, and reaction to, illness; and the *social* system examines cultural, environmental, and familial influences on the experience and expression of illness.

Engel postulated that each system affects and is affected by the others. Engel's model *does not view medical illness as a direct result of one's psychological and sociocultural makeup* but, rather, promotes a comprehensive understanding of disease and treatment.

A dramatic example of Engel's concept of the biopsychosocial model was his study of the relationship between psychological factors and sudden death. After investigating episodes of sudden death, Engel concluded that serious *illness and death may be associated with psychological stress or trauma.* Among potential triggering events are the death of a close friend, grief, anniversary reactions, loss of self-esteem, personal danger or threat, the letdown after the threat has passed, and reunions or triumphs.

The doctor–patient relationship is a critical component of the biopsychosocial model. All physicians must not only have a working knowledge of patients' medical status but also be familiar with how patients' individual psychology and sociocultural milieu affect the medical condition, and be aware of the emotional responses to the condition.

1.2 The answer is A

Identifying *a patient's course of illness* is a symptom-oriented approach. There are two major goals of psychiatric interviewing: to recognize the psychological components of behavior and to clarify symptoms. Insight-oriented approaches emphasize eliciting and interpreting unconscious conflicts, anxieties, and defenses, whereas symptom-oriented approaches emphasize classifying patients' dysfunctions according to specific diagnostic categories.

In fact, psychiatrists would probably use both approaches, switching back and forth or combining the two, rather than applying only one or the other. Both ways of understanding patients are necessary for gathering information about the complexities of psychiatric disorders. Identifying a patient's *course of illness, behavioral patterns, and identifying symptoms* comprise a symptom-oriented approach. In insight-oriented psychiatry, the study of *unconscious conflicts, anxiety, symbols, and fears* is the major focus.

1.3 The answer is E

An important feature of establishing a good doctor–patient relationship is the ability to make the patient aware that the clinician is genuinely interested in and empathic with the patient's unspoken anxieties: an experienced interviewer can sense and elicit a *patient's emotional concerns*. Although early in the interview the clinician hopes to elicit as much information as possible and thus allows the patient to talk at length, it may sometimes be necessary to interrupt so as to focus the patient on another area or to obtain more specific information about the patient's problem. Therefore, a clinician would not always listen *without interrupting*. A comfortable *private office* is an ideal setting for a first interview, but when such an office is unavailable, the interview need not be canceled. An experienced clinician can establish a good relationship with a patient almost anywhere; the clinician's ability to communicate respect, interest, and genuine concern is more important than the setting.

During the first interview, a clinician usually takes notes for the patient's record, but not so obsessively that rapport is disturbed; in addition to acquiring needed information, a clinician who *takes notes* demonstrates that what the patient says is worth paying attention to. Nevertheless, note-taking is not essential for establishing a good doctor–patient relationship, and a clinician may refrain for good reason, such as the patient's discomfort with the procedure.

Although *maintaining eye contact* (without forcing the issue) is an important tool to show patients that the clinician is paying attention and taking them seriously, the technique is less important than establishing empathy with the patient's concerns.

1.4 The answer is C

A clinician must warn a person who is likely to be harmed violently by a patient. Clinicians, however, do not warn anyone about whom a patient speaks disparagingly or has violent fantasies, unless the clinician is convinced that the patient intends to do physical harm to that person.

Physicians should explain to patients the nature of doctor–patient confidentiality, point out the instances in which the doctor must disclose information about the patient, and *clarify confidentiality issues* that a patient may raise. As part of discussing confidentiality, the clinician should inform the patient that *no information will be released to an insurance company without the patient's consent* and that, in teaching hospitals and other institutions, *medical students* and other medical staff *may have*

access to a patient's record, although again only with the patient's consent. A clinician may inform *family members about a patient's problems* if the clinician thinks they can help alleviate the problem or if informing the family is otherwise in the patient's best interests.

1.5 The answer is D

Countertransference can accentuate a patient's *hostility* and may take the form of negative feelings that are *disruptive to the doctor–patient relationship*. Countertransference may also encompass disproportionately positive, idealizing, or even eroticized reactions. Just as patients have expectations—such as competence, lack of exploitation, objectivity, comfort, and relief—*physicians often have unconscious or unspoken expectations of patients*. Most commonly, physicians think of patients as good when (1) their expressed severity of symptoms correlates with an overtly diagnosable biological disorder, (2) *they are compliant* and generally do not challenge the treatment, (3) they are emotionally controlled, and (4) they are grateful. If these expectations are not met, physicians may blame patients and experience them as unlikable, untreatable, or bad.

A psychiatrist who actively dislikes a patient is apt to be ineffective in dealing with him or her. Emotion breeds counteremotion. For example, if a physician is hostile, the patient may react with hostility; the physician then becomes even angrier than before, and the relationship deteriorates rapidly. If a physician can rise above negative emotions and handle a resentful patient with equanimity, the interpersonal relationship may shift from one of mutual overt antagonism to one of at least increased acceptance and grudging respect. Transcending such emotions involves being able to recognize and step back from the intense countertransferential reactions and to dispassionately explore why a patient reacts to the doctor in such an apparently self-defeating way.

Psychiatrists with strong unconscious needs to be all-knowing and all-powerful may have particular problems with certain types of patient: those who appear to repeatedly defeat attempts to help them (for example, patients with severe heart disease who continue to smoke or drink); those perceived as uncooperative (for example, patients who question or refuse treatment); those who request a second opinion; those who fail to recover in response to treatment; those who use physical or somatic complaints to mask emotional problems (for example, patients with somatization disorder, pain disorder, hypochondriasis, or factitious disorders); those with chronic cognitive disorders (for example, patients with dementia of the Alzheimer's type); and *those who are dying* or in chronic pain (for example, patients who represent a professional failure and are thus a threat to a physician's identity and self-esteem). These patients may be difficult for most physicians to deal with, but if a physician is as aware as possible of his or her own needs, capabilities, and limitations, such patients will pose no threat.

1.6 The answer is D

The clinician's best approach would be to honestly discuss *the uncertainty of treating any clinical disorder* with the patient and to assure the patient that the clinician will do everything possible to help the patient but that life has no guarantees. The patient will probably find this answer more helpful than *a false promise that the clinician can provide a cure.* Turning *the patient's attention to another subject* can suggest to the patient that the clinician does not take him or her seriously.

If the clinician tries to understand the patient's intended threat and to interpret the unsaid feelings behind it—usually anxiety—their discussion may have satisfactory results. If, however, the doctor senses that this is not the case, transferring *the patient to another clinician's care* should be considered.

The clinician would not *ask a colleague to join* the interview unless the clinician thought that the patient was dangerous.

1.7 The answer is B

Paranoid patients fear that people want to hurt them and intend to do them harm. Doctors *should be able to explain in detail every decision* and planned procedure to paranoid patients and should react nondefensively to patients' suspicions. Patients may misperceive cues in their environment to the degree that they see *conspiracies in neutral events.* They are critical, *evasive,* and suspicious. They are often called grievance seekers because they tend to blame others for everything bad that happens in their lives. They are extremely mistrustful and may question everything that doctors advise doing. Physicians must remain somewhat formal, albeit always respectful and courteous, with these patients, as they often view expressions of warmth and empathy with suspicion ("What does he want from me?").

1.8 The answer is B

Doctors must *treat* antisocial patients with respect but also *with a heightened sense of vigilance.* These patients can inspire fear in others, often legitimately so, as many have violent histories. Doctors who *feel threatened by patients* should unashamedly seek assistance and not feel compelled to see the patients alone. Firm limits must be set on behavior (for example, no drugs in the hospital and no sexual activity with other patients), and the consequences of transgressing must be stated firmly and adhered to (for example, discharge from the hospital if the patient is medically stable, isolation if not). If inappropriate behavior is discovered, patients *must be confronted directly* and nonangrily, and they must be held responsible for their actions. On the surface these patients may appear charming, socially adept, and intelligent, since over many years they have perfected the behaviors they know to be appropriate, and they perform almost as actors. Antisocial patients often malinger, the term for willfully feigning illness for a clear secondary gain (for example, to obtain drugs, get a bed for the night, or hide from people pursuing them). They obviously get sick, as nonantisocial people do, and when they are sick they need to be cared for in the same ways as others.

1.9 The answer is A

The early part of the interview is generally the most open-ended, in that the physician allows patients to speak as much as possible in their own words by asking open-ended questions and also permits them to *finish.* An example of an open-ended question is, "Can you tell me more about that?" That type of questioning is important to establish rapport, which is the first step in an interview. In one survey of 700 patients, the patients substantially agreed that physicians do not have the time or the inclination to listen and to consider the patient's feelings, that physicians do not have enough knowledge of the emotional problems and socioeconomic background of the patient's family, and that physicians increase the patient's fear by giving explanations in technical language. Psychosocial and economic factors exert a profound influence on human relationships, so the physician should have as much understanding as possible of the patient's environment and subculture.

Ekkehard Othmer and Sieglinde Othmer defined the development of rapport as encompassing six strategies: (1) putting the patient and the interviewer at ease; (2) finding the pain and expressing compassion; (3) evaluating the patient's insight and becoming an ally; (4) showing expertise; (5) establishing authority as a physician and a therapist; and (6) balancing the roles of empathic listener, expert, and authority. Interviewing any patient involves a fine balance between allowing the patient's story to unfold and obtaining the data necessary for diagnosis and treatment. Most experts on interviewing agree that the ideal interview is one in which the interviewer begins with broad, open-ended questions, continues by becoming increasingly specific, and closes with detailed and direct questions. Although closed-ended questions are valuable during the interview, they are generally not used at the start of the interview. A *closed-ended* or directive question is one that asks for specific information and that allows the patient limited options in answering. Too many closed-ended questions, especially in the early part of the interview, can lead to an unwanted restriction of the patient's responses.

If the patient states that he or she has been feeling depressed, a closed-ended question might be, "Your mother died recently, didn't she?" That question can be answered only by a "yes" or a "no," and the mother's death may or may not be the reason the patient is depressed. More information is likely to be obtained if the physician responds with, "Can you tell me more about what you're feeling and what you think may be causing your depression?" That is an open-ended question. Sometimes directive questions are necessary to obtain important data, but, when used too often, the patient may think that information is to be given only in response to direct questioning by the physician.

As for *time* and *charges,* physicians should inform patients about their fee policies but should not interrupt patients to do so. Instead, those areas of business should be dealt with before the initial visit, so that an ongoing relationship with a patient can be established. The matter of fees must be discussed openly from the outset: the physician's charges, whether the physician is willing to accept insurance payments directly (known as assignments), the policy concerning payment for missed appointments, and whether the physician is part of a managed care plan. Discussing those questions and any other questions about fees at the beginning of the relationship can minimize misunderstandings later.

A discussion of compliance with a medical plan is important, but premature early in the interview. Furthermore, *compliance,* which is the degree to which the patient carries out clinical recommendations by the treating physician, is a two-way street. Studies have shown that noncompliance is associated with physicians perceived as rejecting and unfriendly. Noncompliance is also associated with asking a patient for information without giving any feedback and with failing to explain a diagnosis or the cause of the presenting symptoms. A physician who is aware of the patient's belief system, feelings, and habits and who enlists the patient in establishing a treatment regimen increases compliant behavior.

Answers 1.10–1.14

1.10 The answer is B

1.11 The answer is C

1.12 The answer is C

1.13 The answer is C

1.14 The answer is C

Compliance, also known as adherence, is the degree to which a patient carries out the clinical recommendation of a treating physician. Examples of compliance include keeping appointments, entering into and completing a treatment program, taking medications correctly, and following recommended changes in behavior or diet. Compliant behavior depends on the specific clinical situation, the nature of the illness, and the treatment program. In general, about one-third of all patients comply with treatment, one-third sometimes comply with certain aspects of treatment, and one-third never comply with treatment.

An increased complexity of regimen, along with an increased number of required behavioral changes, appears to be associated with noncompliance. *Psychiatric patients exhibit a higher degree of noncompliant behavior than do medical patients.* There is *no clear association,* however, between compliance and a patient's *age, sex,* marital status, race, religion, *socioeconomic status,* intelligence, or *education level.*

The doctor–patient relationship, or doctor–patient match, is the most important factor in compliance issues. When doctor and patient have different priorities and beliefs, different styles of communication (including a different understanding of medical advice), and different medical expectations, patients' compliance diminishes. Compliance can increase when physicians explain to a patient the value of a particular treatment as desirable and also emphasize that following the recommendation will produce a positive outcome. Compliance can also increase if patients know the names and effects of each drug they are taking.

A highly significant factor in compliance seems to be patients' subjective feelings of distress or illness, as opposed to doctors' often objective medical estimates of the disease and required therapy. Patients must believe that they are ill. Thus, asymptomatic patients, such as those with hypertension, are at greater risk for noncompliance than are patients with symptoms.

Answers 1.15–1.19

1.15 The answer is C

1.16 The answer is A

1.17 The answer is B

1.18 The answer is E

1.19 The answer is D

In the techniques of *reflection* a doctor repeats to a patient in a supportive manner something that the patient has said. The purpose of reflection is twofold: to assure the doctor that he or she correctly understood what the patient is trying to say and to let the patient know that the doctor is following what is being said. It is an empathic response meant to show the patient that the doctor is both listening to the patient's concerns and comprehending them. For example, if a patient is speaking about fears of dying and the effects of talking about these fears with his or her family, the doctor may say, "It seems that you are concerned with becoming a burden to your family." This reflection is not an exact repetition of what the patient has said but, rather, a paraphrase that indicates that the doctor has grasped what the patient is trying to say.

The technique of *interpretation* is most often used when a doctor states something about a patient's behavior or thinking that a patient may not be aware of. The technique follows from the doctor's attentive listening to the underlying themes and patterns in the patient's story. Interpretations usually help to clarify interrelationships that the patient may not see. The technique is a sophisticated one and should generally be used only after the doctor has established some rapport with the patient and has a reasonably *good idea of what some interrelationships are.* For example, a doctor may say, "When you talk about how angry you are that your family has not been supportive, I think you're also telling me how worried you are that I won't be there for you either. What do you think?"

In *clarification,* doctors attempt to draw out details from patients about what they have already said. For example, a doctor may say, "You are feeling depressed. When is it that you feel most depressed?"

In many situations it is not only acceptable but desirable for physicians to give patients *advice.* To be effective and to be perceived as empathic rather than inappropriate or intrusive, the advice should be given only after patients are allowed to talk freely about their problems, so that physicians have an adequate information base from which to make suggestions. At times, after a doctor has listened carefully to a patient, it becomes clear the patient does not, in fact, want advice as much as an objective, caring, nonjudgmental listener. Giving advice too quickly can lead a patient to feel that the doctor is not really hearing but responding from either anxiety or the belief that the doctor inherently knows better than the patient what should be done in a particular situation. In an example of advice given too quickly, a patient says, "I cannot take this medication; it's bothering me," and the physician responds, "Fine. I think you should stop taking it, and I'll start you on something new." A more appropriate response is the following: "I'm sorry to hear that. Tell me what about the medication is bothering you, so that I have a better idea of what we may do to make you feel more comfortable." In another example the patient says, "I've really been feeling down lately," and the doctor responds, "Well, I think in that case it would be a good idea for you to go out and do some things that are fun, like going to the movies or walking in the park." In this case a more appropriate and helpful response is the following: "Tell me what you mean by 'feeling down.' The more I know about how you're feeling, the more likely I can help."

Truthful *reassurance* to a patient can lead to increased trust and compliance and can be experienced as an empathic response of a concerned physician. False reassurance, however, is essentially lying to a patient and can badly impair the patient's trust and compliance. False reassurance is often given

Table 1.1
Pros and Cons of Open-Ended and Closed-Ended Questions

Aspect	Broad, Open-Ended Questions	Narrow, Closed-Ended Questions
Genuineness	High They produce spontaneous formulations.	Low They lead the patient.
Reliability	Low They may lead to nonreproducible answers.	High Narrow focus, but they may suggest answers.
Precision	Low *Intent of question is vague.*	High Intent of question is clear.
Time efficiency	Low Circumstantial elaborations.	High *May invite yes or no answers.*
Completeness of diagnostic coverage	Low *Patient selects topic.*	High Interviewer selects topic.
Acceptance by patient	Varies Most patients prefer expressing themselves freely; others feel guarded and insecure.	Varies Some patients enjoy clear-cut checks; others hate to be pressed into a yes or no format.

Reprinted with permission from Othmer E, Othmer SC. *The Clinical Interview Using DSM-IV-TR.* Washington, DC: American Psychiatric Press; 1994.

from a desire to make a patient feel better, but once a patient knows that a doctor has not told the truth, the patient is unlikely to accept or believe truthful reassurance. In an example of false reassurance a patient with a terminal illness asks, "Am I going to be all right, Doctor?" and the doctor responds, "Of course you'll be all right; everything is fine." In an example of truthful reassurance, the doctor responds, "I am going to do everything to make you as comfortable as possible, and part of being comfortable is for you to know as much as I know about what is going on with you. We both know that what you have is serious. I'd like to know exactly what you think is happening to you and to clarify any questions or confusion you have."

Answers 1.20–1.24

1.20 The answer is B

1.21 The answer is B

1.22 The answer is B

1.23 The answer is A

1.24 The answer is A

The content of an interview is literally what is said between doctor and patient: for instance, *the discussion of symptoms*, or obtaining a *social history*. The *process of the interview is what occurs nonverbally* between doctor and patient: what is happening in the interview beneath the surface. Process involves feelings and reactions that are unacknowledged, or unconscious. For example, a patient may use *body language* to express feelings he or she cannot convey verbally—a clenched fist or nervous tearing at a tissue by a patient with an otherwise calm demeanor. A patient may *shift the interview away from an anxiety-provoking subject onto a neutral topic* without realizing that he or she is doing so. A patient may return repeatedly to a particular topic, regardless of the direction the interview appears to be taking. Trivial remarks and apparently casual asides may reveal serious underlying concerns as, for example, "Oh, by the way, a neighbor of mine tells me that he knows someone with the same symptoms as my son, and that person has cancer."

Answers 1.25–1.28

1.25 The answer is A

1.26 The answer is B

1.27 The answer is A

1.28 The answer is A

Interviewing any patient involves a fine balance between allowing the patient's story to unfold at will and obtaining the necessary data for diagnosis and treatment. Most experts on interviewing agree that the ideal interview is one in which an interviewer begins with broad, open-ended questioning, continues by becoming more specific, and closes with detailed direct questioning.

The early part of the interview is generally the most open ended, in that physicians allow patients to speak as much as possible in their own words. A closed-ended, or directive, question is one that asks for specific information and that allows a patient few options in answering. Too many closed-ended questions, especially in the early part of an interview, can lead to a restriction of patients' responses. Sometimes, directive questions are necessary to obtain important data, but when used too often, a patient may think that information is to be given only in response to direct questioning by the doctor. An example of an open-ended question is, "Can you tell me more about that?" Closed-ended questions, however, can be effective in generating quick responses about a clearly delineated topic. Closed-ended questions have been shown to be useful in eliciting information about the absence of certain symptoms (for example, auditory hallucinations and suicidal ideation). Closed-ended questions have also been found to be effective in assessing such factors as frequency, severity, and duration of symptoms. With open-ended questions, *the intent is purposefully vague*, the patient is allowed to *select the topic*, and they tend by their nature to be of *lower time efficiency* than closed-ended questions. Table 1.1 summarizes some of the pros and cons of open-ended and closed-ended questions.

Answers 1.29–1.32

1.29 The answer is A

1.30 The answer is A

1.31 The answer is C

1.32 The answer is D

The *most important factor in interviewing depressed patients is assessing the risk of suicide.* Clinicians should pose questions geared to determining feelings of pessimism, worthlessness, and despair. A profound feeling of hopelessness is an ominous sign that many psychiatrists consider pathognomonic of suicidal risk. A history of suicide attempts, the presence of chronic illness, especially if associated with pain, a recent life stressor, such as the loss of a loved one, and a family history of suicide are signs of increased risk. It is a myth that asking about suicidal ideation plants the seed for a suicide attempt, and this should not stop physicians from questioning patients as to whether they have thoughts that life is no longer worth living, that they might want to harm themselves, or that they would wish to die.

Depressed patients often demand reassurance from an interviewer but often do not respond to a physician's attempts to meet this need. Physicians should offer patients a realistic appraisal. When depression is present, doctors should tell patients so, and should explain that therapeutic intervention, such as psychotherapy, drug therapy, or hospitalization (especially if a patient is suicidal), is necessary. Depression can be a *curable condition in 95 percent of cases,* and patients and their families often respond positively and gratefully to this fact.

Dependent patients need a great amount of reassurance and encouragement, and yet are often resistant to any and all such offers. They are the patients most likely to make repeated, even urgent, calls between scheduled appointments and to demand that doctors provide special attention. They often become angry or frightened when they perceive that doctors are not taking their concerns seriously. Doctors must be prepared to set necessary limits within the context of an expressed willingness to listen and to care for patients.

Impulsive patients have a difficult time delaying gratification and may demand that their discomfort be eliminated immediately. They are frustrated easily and may become petulant or even angry and *aggressive* when they do not get what they want as soon as they want it. They may impulsively do something self-destructive if they feel thwarted by the doctor, and they may appear manipulative and attention seeking. Underneath the surface manifestations, they may *fear that they will never get what they need from others* and thus must act in this inappropriately aggressive way.

Obsessive and controlling *patients* are orderly, punctual, and overconcerned with detail. They *often appear unemotional, even aloof,* especially with regard to anything potentially disturbing or frightening. They may be resistant to any perceived control on the doctor's part because of their strong needs to be in control of everything in their environment. Underneath, these patients are often frightened of losing control and of being dependent and helpless. Physicians must be prepared to strengthen the patients' sense of control by including them as much as possible in their own care and treatment. Doctors should explain in ongoing detail what is happening and what is being planned.

Answers 1.33–1.37

1.33 The answer is A

1.34 The answer is C

1.35 The answer is D

1.36 The answer is B

1.37 The answer is B

The doctor–patient relationship has a number of potential models. Often, neither the physician nor the patient is fully conscious of choosing one or another model. The models derive most often from the personalities, expectations, and needs of both the physician and the patient. The fact that their personalities, expectations, and needs are largely unspoken and may differ can lead to miscommunication and disappointment for both participants, physician and patient, in the relationship. The physician must be consciously aware of which model is operating with which patient and should be able to shift models, depending on the particular needs of specific patients and on the treatment requirements of varying clinical situations. Models of the doctor–patient relationship include the active–passive model, the teacher–student (or parent–child or guidance–cooperation) model, the mutual participation model, and the "friendship" (or socially intimate) model.

The *active–passive model* implies passivity on the part of the patient and the taking over by the physician that necessarily results. In this model, patients assume no responsibility for their own care and play no active role in treatment. The model is appropriate when a patient is unconscious, immobilized, or delirious. The sudden onset of the patient's altered mental status can be a potentially life-threatening situation. Possible causes of the profoundly changed mental status are trauma, vascular disorders, brain tumors, meningitis, encephalitis, and toxicological, metabolic, endocrine, and psychiatric disorders. For some patients with an altered mental status, *a lumbar puncture* is necessary and should be performed, as long as increased intracranial pressure, which can cause brainstem herniation, is not suspected. A computed tomographic (CT) scan or an eye examination that checks for papilledema may aid in the assessment before a lumbar puncture is performed.

In the *teacher–student model* the physician's dominance is assumed and emphasized. The physician is paternalistic; the patient is essentially dependent and accepting. The model is often observed *after surgery* and before such diagnostic tests as a *GI series.*

The *mutual participant model* implies equality between the physician and the patient: both participants in the relationship require and depend on each other's input. The need for a doctor–patient relationship based on a model of mutual, active participation is most obvious in the treatment of such chronic illnesses as renal failure and *diabetes,* in which a patient's knowledge and acceptance of treatment is critical to success. The model may also be effective in more subtle situations—for example, in pneumonia.

The *"friendship" model* of the doctor–patient relationship is generally considered dysfunctional, and can lead to unethical behavior. It is most often prompted by an underlying psychological problem in the physician, who may have an emotional need to turn the care of the patient into a relationship of mutual sharing of personal information and *love.* The model often involves a blurring of boundaries between professionalism and intimacy and an indeterminate perpetuation of the relationship, rather than an appropriate ending and termination of treatment.

Human Development Throughout the Life Cycle

Developmental theory, when applied to real-life milestones and challenges, has the potential to dramatically deepen our understanding and appreciation of the complex and interrelated aspects of being human. To understand how a human being develops biologically, cognitively, psychosexually, psychosocially, and in terms of attachment, is to understand how behavior evolves, from infancy to old age. To comprehend this is to appreciate the many factors contributing to happiness, unhappiness, function, and dysfunction.

The theorists discussed in Chapter 2 of *Synopsis IX* approach the life cycle from very different perspectives. Viewed as a whole they provide a picture of what it means to be human. Each theorist postulates that later stages in development are predicated on earlier stages, and that the early stages build progressively to create a personality that may be stable or unstable.

Jean Piaget studied the cognitive and intellectual development of children, from birth to adolescence. Not all contemporary theorists agree with his findings or observations, but his work is evocative and seminal, and offers a striking theory of cognitive development through different ages. Sigmund Freud's observations and theories about psychosexual development are provocative and challenging. No one can argue with the profound and lasting effect his thinking had on 20th-century culture, nor on the increased understanding of psychodynamic forces that shape behavior. A new psychology is evolving for the current century that will rely on many of Freud's observations but which will differ in concepts still to be defined.

Erik Erikson formulated age-specific crises that he observed to occur in correlation with specific psychosocial phases. The student should understand each of these crises in depth. Margaret Mahler viewed development through a perspective of attachment, and defined what she felt was the challenge of the first 3 years of life, in terms of separation-individuation. Her theories concerning the development of object constancy as well as her descriptions of various forces interfering with the development of both attachment and autonomy are helpful in understanding the dynamics and disturbances of behavior, especially those underlying the personality disorders. More recent theorists, such as Daniel Levinson and Carol Gilligan, have continued to expand and clarify different aspects of development and life stresses.

As part of an overview of the life cycle, Chapter 2 of the text also includes a discussion of death, grief, mourning, and bereavement. End-of-life issues have emerged as crucial areas in the practice of psychiatry and medicine and inform every stage of the life cycle. The skilled physician must be able to deal with all the complexities associated with end-of-life care issues. This requires a thorough understanding of the stages of grief and mourning as outlined by such workers as Elisabeth Kübler-Ross, among others.

The student should study the questions and answers below for a useful review of all of these topics.

HELPFUL HINTS

Readers should be aware of the following theories, theorists, and developmental stages as they relate to human development throughout the life cycle.

- adolescent homosexuality
- adoption
- adultery
- affectional bond
- age-30 transition
- age-related cell changes
- ageism
- Mary Ainsworth
- alimony

- anal personality
- attachment
- autonomous ego functions
- John Bowlby's stages of bereavement
- castration anxiety
- characteristics of thought:
  concrete operations
  formal operations

  preoperational phase
  sensorimotor phase
  (object permanence)
- climacterium
- cognitive decline
- concepts of normality
- core identity
- crushes
- cults
- death and children
- death criteria

- delayed, inhibited, and denied grief
- dependence
- developmental landmarks
- developmental tasks
- divorce
- dreams in children
- dual-career families
- effects of divorce
- egocentrism

- ► Electra complex
- ► empty-nest syndrome
- ► epigenetic principle
- ► Erik Erikson: eight psychosocial stages
- ► failure to thrive
- ► family planning
- ► family size
- ► fathers and attachment
- ► feeding and infant care
- ► fetal development
- ► formal operations and morality
- ► foster parents
- ► Anna Freud
- ► gender expectations
- ► gender identity
- ► generativity
- ► genetic counseling
- ► geriatric period
- ► Arnold Gesell
- ► goodness of fit
- ► grief
- ► Roy Grinker
- ► Heinz Hartmann
- ► hormones
- ► identification
- ► identity
- ► identity diffusion
- ► imagery and drawings
- ► imaginary companions
- ► imprinting
- ► inborn errors of metabolism

- ► integrity
- ► intimacy
- ► Carl Jung
- ► Melanie Klein
- ► Elisabeth Kübler-Ross
- ► language development
- ► learning problems
- ► Daniel Levinson
- ► linkage objects
- ► Madonna complex
- ► Margaret Mahler: infant-developmental stages
- ► marriage
- ► Masters and Johnson
- ► masturbation
- ► maternal behavior
- ► maternal neglect
- ► menarche
- ► midlife crisis
- ► mourning
- ► "Mourning and Melancholia"
- ► mutuality
- ► negativism
- ► neural organization of infancy
- ► normal autistic and normal symbiotic phases
- ► normality
- ► Daniel Offer
- ► perinatal complications
- ► Jean Piaget
- ► plasticity

- ► play and pretend
- ► postpartum mood disorders and psychosis
- ► pregnancy: marriage and alternative lifestyle sexuality and prenatal diagnosis teenage
- ► pregnancy and childbirth
- ► primary and secondary sex characteristics
- ► pseudodementia
- ► psychosexual moratorium
- ► puberty
- ► racism, prejudice
- ► reactions to authority
- ► reflexes (i.e., rooting, grasp, Babinski, Moro)
- ► religious behavior
- ► remarriage
- ► retirement
- ► Dame Cicely Saunders
- ► school adjustment, behavior, refusal
- ► self-blame
- ► senility
- ► separation
- ► separation-individuation process: differentiation practicing

- rapprochement consolidation
- ► sex in the aged
- ► sibling and parental death
- ► sibling rivalry
- ► single-parent home
- ► smiling
- ► social deprivation syndromes (anaclitic depression-hospitalism)
- ► somnambulism
- ► spacing of children
- ► René Spitz
- ► spouse and child abuse
- ► stepparents and siblings
- ► stranger and separation anxiety
- ► stress reaction
- ► suicide in the aged
- ► Harry Stack Sullivan
- ► superego
- ► surrogate mother
- ► survivor guilt
- ► Thomas Szasz
- ► temperament
- ► thanatology
- ► toilet training
- ► uncomplicated bereavement
- ► George Vaillant
- ► vasomotor instability
- ► vocation and unemployment

▲ QUESTIONS

DIRECTIONS: Each of the statements or questions below is followed by five suggested responses or completions. Select the *one* that is *best* in each case.

2.1 True statements about CNS maturation and perceptual development include

   A. in utero, a fetus can hear sounds
   B. 3-day-old infants can recognize their mothers' voices
   C. by age 2, auditory perception has reached adult levels
   D. visual perception is not well developed at birth
   E. all of the above

2.2 Principles of temperamental development include

   A. each child is born with specific temperamental patterns of behavioral response
   B. temperamental traits are rarely stimulated or inhibited by external factors
   C. temperamental development does not significantly affect other areas of growth
   D. culture is the primary contributor to temperament
   E. "goodness of fit" is defined as the child acting like the parent

2.3 Terms associated with Piaget's theory of development include all of the following *except*

   A. sensorimotor state
   B. concrete operational stage
   C. object permanence
   D. schemas
   E. object constancy

2.4 True statements about the development of gender identity include all of the following *except*

A. gender identity generally appears earlier in boys than girls
B. by the age of 2 to 3 years, almost everyone has a firm sense of gender identity
C. formation of gender identity arises in part from parental and cultural attitudes
D. changing gender identity is very difficult after age 4
E. behaviors that are labeled masculine or feminine are relatively fixed by ages 4 to 5

2.5 Erik Erikson's description of adolescent development includes which of the following concepts?

A. the developmental period of identity versus identity diffusion
B. normal adolescence may involve discomfort, confusion, anxiety, and unhappiness
C. early adolescence is marked by potentially negative emotions
D. pathological outcomes in identity formation can lead to delinquent behaviors
E. all of the above

2.6 Elisabeth Kübler-Ross's five stages of death and dying include all the following *except*

A. denial
B. protest
C. bargaining
D. depression
E. acceptance

2.7 Dying children

A. are rarely aware of their condition or want to discuss it
B. often have less sophisticated views about dying than their healthy counterparts
C. in the preoperational stage of cognitive development see death as a temporary absence
D. seldom feel a sense of guilt about dying
E. usually have no increase in aggressive play

2.8 The clinician working with the aged

A. should expect age to be a risk factor for poor outcome
B. generally finds that depression is a normal response to aging
C. rarely finds resilience to be present
D. will find little difference between older adults above the age of 85 and those between the ages of 65 and 85
E. none of the above

2.9 True statements about age-specific bereavement behavior include

A. Children under the age of 2 do not display bereavement behaviors.
B. Children ages 2 to 5 most often display strong, persistent feelings of sadness, fear, and anxiety.
C. School-aged children may become phobic, hypochondriacal, or withdrawn.
D. Children and adolescents typically have lower rates of depressive episodes than adults.
E. Bereavement in children and adolescents does not result in a long-term vulnerability to depressive disorders.

2.10 Age-related CNS changes include

A. gross brain atrophy
B. selective regional neuronal loss
C. appearance of senile plaques and neurofibrillary tangles
D. remodeling of dendrites, axons, and synapses
E. all of the above

2.11 True statements about mental health and the life span include

A. Delirium is more common in elderly adults than in younger age groups.
B. The prevalence of major depressive and anxiety disorders is generally higher in those over age 65 than for younger age cohorts.
C. Older adults feel less control over their emotions than younger adults.
D. Older adults report more negative emotional experiences than younger adults.
E. None of the above

2.12 George Vaillant's work on defensive processes and aging

A. suggested that coping abilities become more regressive over the life span
B. found increased use of mature defenses as individuals age
C. found decreased use of mature defenses as psychopathology decreased
D. found that individuals receiving the highest life-adjustment ratings were those who used immature defenses
E. considered humor to be an immature defense

2.13 Some defense mechanisms used by the average 50-year-old man or woman include all of the following *except*

A. dissociation
B. repression
C. sublimation
D. altruism
E. splitting

2.14 The stage of formal operations, according to the theories of Jean Piaget, is characterized by the ability

A. to think abstractly
B. to reason deductively
C. to define concepts
D. to understand symbols
E. all of the above

2.15 Good adult adjustment despite a high-risk childhood is associated with

A. social support
B. high intelligence
C. structured upbringing
D. ability to bounce back
E. all of the above

2.16 Infancy is generally said to end when a child is able to

A. creep
B. stand without assistance
C. control his or her anal sphincter completely
D. climb stairs
E. speak

2.17 In an infant, social smiling is elicited preferentially by the mother at

A. under 4 weeks of age
B. 4 to 8 weeks
C. 8 to 12 weeks
D. 3 to 4 months
E. more than 4 months

2.18 The main characteristic of Margaret Mahler's differentiation subphase is

A. separation anxiety
B. stranger anxiety
C. rapprochement
D. castration anxiety
E. none of the above

2.19 Infants are born with

A. the Moro reflex
B. the rooting reflex
C. the Babinski reflex
D. endogenous smiling
E. all of the above

2.20 An infant can differentiate

A. sweet-tasting sugar
B. the sour taste of lemon
C. the smell of bananas
D. the smell of rotten eggs
E. all of the above

2.21 Normal adolescence is marked by

A. episodes of depression
B. occasional delinquent acts
C. the dissolution of intense ties to parents
D. vulnerability to crisis
E. all of the above

2.22 A child is generally able to conceptualize the true meaning of death by age

A. 3 years
B. 5 years
C. 7 years
D. 10 years
E. 13 years

2.23 People more prone to midlife crises tend to come from families characterized by which of the following during their adolescence

A. parental discord
B. withdrawal by same-sex parent
C. anxious parents
D. impulsive and irresponsible parents
E. all of the above

2.24 True statements about sexual activity and aging include

A. Longitudinal studies have found that sex drive decreases with age.
B. There is no correlation between how active one's sexual life was in early adulthood and how active it is in old age.
C. An estimated 40–50 percent of men and women over age 60 are sexually active.
D. Sexual activity in men and women is usually limited by the absence of an available partner.
E. All of the above

DIRECTIONS: Each group of questions below consists of five lettered headings followed by a list of numbered words or statements. For each numbered word or statement, select the *one* lettered heading that is most closely associated with it. Each lettered heading may be selected once, more than once, or not at all.

Questions 2.25–2.29

A. 18 months
B. 2 years
C. 3 years
D. 4 years
E. 6 years

2.25 Copies a triangle
2.26 Copies a cross
2.27 Walks up stairs with one hand held
2.28 Puts on shoes
2.29 Refers to self by name

Questions 2.30–2.34

A. Birth to 6 months
B. 7 to 11 months
C. 12 to 18 months
D. 54 months on
E. None of the above

2.30 Plays at making sounds and babbles
2.31 Plays language games (pat-a-cake, peekaboo)
2.32 Understands up to 150 words and uses up to 20 words
2.33 Speech is 100 percent intelligible
2.34 Uses language to tell stories and share ideas

Questions 2.35–2.39

A. 4 weeks
B. 16 weeks
C. 28 weeks
D. 40 weeks
E. 12 months

2.35 Grasping and manipulation
2.36 Ocular control
2.37 Verbalization of two or more words
2.38 Standing with slight support
2.39 Sitting alone

Questions 2.40–2.44

    A. Secure base effect
    B. Chum periods
    C. "Good enough" mothering
    D. Separation-individuation
    E. "Goodness of fit"

2.40 Margaret Mahler
2.41 Mary Ainsworth
2.42 Harry Stack Sullivan
2.43 D. W. Winnicott
2.44 Stella Chess and Alexander Thomas

Questions 2.45–2.47

    A. Superego is a result of resolution of Oedipal complex
    B. Heteronomous and autonomous stages of morality
    C. Three levels and six stages of moral maturation
    D. Female moral development ends in an ethics of caring
    E. None of the above

2.45 Lawrence Kohlberg
2.46 Carol Gilligan
2.47 Sigmund Freud

ANSWERS

Human Development Throughout the Life Cycle

2.1 The answer is E

To process their world, infants and children use their perceptions. Theorists who endorse nature over nurture point to the presence of well-developed perceptions, except for vision, in newborns. Even *in utero, a fetus can hear sounds, and 3-day-old infants can recognize their mothers' voices. By age 2, auditory perception has reached adult levels.* Taste and odor are perceived by newborns, who show a preference for sweet milk and can identify their mothers by odor. Neonates have a well-developed sense of touch and can discriminate between reassuring and threatening sensations.

Visual perception, however, is not well developed at birth and confirms the developmental principle that nature and nurture must operate together for optimal maturation. At birth an infant's visual acuity is only 20/800, but at 8 months it ranges from 20/200 to 20/70. In the 6 months after birth, an infant's visual cortex changes enormously. As many as 1,800 new visual synapses can potentially form in that time. The number of synapses is predicated not only on genetic priming of electrical impulses, but also on environmental visual feedback that stimulates certain synapses and prevents the atrophy of others. Functionally, the new synapses are responsible for depth perception, better visual acuity, perceptual organization, and eye–hand coordination. In addition, visual acuity is affected significantly by environmental factors such as diet. In one recent study prompted by current cultural concerns with fat content of foods, researchers determined that infants who received breast milk, which contains higher levels of certain fatty acids, had acquired better visual acuity at both 3 months and 6 months of age than those given milk with lower fatty acid compositions (i.e., commercial formula milk or evaporated milk).

2.2 The answer is A

Each child is born with specific temperamental patterns of behavioral response. These traits can be discerned throughout the span of childhood and adolescence. As with other developmental areas, *temperamental traits can be stimulated* or *inhibited by external factors,* including family interactions, cultural and environmental influences, and social interactions. Jerome Kagan demonstrated that certain children are irritable and fearful in new situations regardless of a parent's sensitivity and support. Kagan's work also demonstrated that temperament remained the same until a child reached 5½ years. Sometime near the 7½ year mark, however, environment begins to shape such traits.

Temperamental development can significantly affect other areas of growth. In the parent–child relationship, temperamental traits are particularly relevant for emotional growth. The compatibility of traits between children and their parents is termed *goodness of fit.* A good fit results in parents behaving with more sensitivity and positive interactions. It does not refer to the child acting like the parent.

Stella Chess and Alexander Thomas found that temperamental traits in children could be identified from infancy and at least through adolescence. The results strongly indicate that *temperament has a genetic base* and that culture is *not the primary contributor to temperament.* However, temperament can be altered by environmental factors, including family and sociocultural status. Successful attempts to identify specific genetic markers involving temperament have bolstered both the genetic foundations as well as transactional aspects of temperamental development.

2.3 The answer is E

Object constancy is Margaret Mahler's term for the capacity developed by a socially successful child after the age of 2 to maintain an internal sense of the parent as constant, consistent, and safe.

Piaget developed a theory to explain cognitive maturation using a biological model that focuses upon *schemas* (i.e., organized ways for children's developing brains to make sense of their experiences). According to Piaget, cognitive growth occurs in stages, which are always in fixed order (invariant). Overall, cognitive maturity is defined by a child's increasingly refined ability to conceptualize space, both internally and externally. In the first stage, the *sensorimotor stage,* from birth to 2 years, infants use body senses and activity to explore their environment. In the process of exploration, infants learn to anticipate an experience by internally constructing a model of each of their own experiences. Cognitive growth results in forming new skills, such as *object permanence* (i.e., the ability to remember an object once it is out of sight). Children discover that objects can be assimilated into an experience they have already encountered: a top spins, a mobile makes music, apple juice tastes sweet, hot food burns.

Piaget asserts that infants and children have the cognitive challenge of internally constructing new schemas to fit old and new experiences into a universally uniform reality. Piaget's schemas are thought of in absolute terms. During the second stage, the preoperational stage, from ages 2 to 7, children become intuitive, anticipating experiences with consequences. Children in the preoperational phase think symbolically but illogically and with egocentricity and a distinct inability to distinguish self from others in their environment. Preoperational processes combine to create a child's inner world populated with the creations of magical thinking. A stuffed kitty becomes a ferocious tiger, a darkened room is transformed into a dungeon, and the shadow of a swaying tree's bough conjures up monsters with unlimited powers. From ages 7 to 11, children enter a *concrete operational stage* that involves an ability to think logically and in an organized fashion. The magical woes of the younger child are replaced by a more realistic set of concerns that

are stimulated by a new-found conception of cause and effect. Between the ages of 7 and 11, children normally spend some of their time worrying about such issues as school success, health and dying, and social relationships. At the end of this stage at age 11, children begin the process of developing the capacity to think abstractly. By adolescence, formal operations appear as abstract thought and the interesting imaginary-audience phenomenon, which joins egocentrism and the capacity to abstract to then torment adolescents into thinking that the entire world is looking at them and watching them. Table 2.1 outlines Piaget's stages of cognitive development in infants and children.

2.4 The answer is A

There is a large range of individual difference in the timing of gender identity. *Gender identity generally appears earlier in girls than in boys (not the reverse)*. From infancy onward most

Table 2.1
Theories and Skills of Cognitive Development in Infants and Children

Period of Development	Piaget's Cognitive Spatial Stages
Gestational	
Infancy: birth–2 years	Sensorimotor
	Includes concepts:
Birth–1 month	Reflective; egocentric (newer research refutes this)
1–4 months	Primary circular: imitation, smiles, playful
4–8 months	Secondary circular: looks for objects partially hidden
8–12 months	Secondary circulation coordinated: peek-a-boo, finds hidden objects
12–18 months	Tertiary circular: explores properties and drops objects
18 months–2 years	Mental representation, make-believe play; memory of objects
Early childhood: 2–5 years	
2–7 years	Preoperational
	Includes concepts:
	Egocentrism: "I want you to eat this too"
	Animistic: "I'm afraid of the moon"
	Lack of hierarchy: "Where do these blocks go?"
	Centration: "I want it now, not after dinner"
	Irreversibility: "I don't know how to go back to that room"
2–5 years	*Transductive reasoning:* "We have to go this way because that's the way Daddy goes"
Middle childhood: 6–11 years	
6 years onward	
7–11 years	Concrete operational
	Includes concepts:
	Hierarchical classification: arranges cars by types
	Reversibility: can play games backward and forward, checkers triple kings
	Conservation: lose two dimes can look for same
	Decentration: worry about small details, obsessive
	Spatial operations: likes models for directions
	Horizontal decalage: conservation of weight, logic
	Transitive inference: syllogisms; compare everything, brand names important
Adolescence: 11–19 years	
11 years onward	Formal operational
	Includes concepts:
	Hypothetic-deductive reasoning; adolescent quick thinking or excuses
	Imaginary audience: everyone is looking at them
	Personal fable: inflated opinion of themselves
	Propositional thinking: logic

psychosexual maturation focuses upon the psychological stages of sexual development. *Gender identity—a child's perception of the self as either male or female—is generally firm by the age of 2 to 3 years. Formation of gender identity arises from parental and cultural attitudes, the infant's external genitalia, and genetic influences. Changing gender identity is very difficult after age 4.*

By ages 3 to 4 years, most boys show masculine preferences in choices of activities, toys, and peers. Studies show that gender role appears, especially in boys, as early as age 2, even before gender identity, with gender-labeling. A 2-year-old can say, "He is a boy." A 3-year-old can identify herself: "I am a girl." Gender role is refined through early childhood so that by early school years a child has a sense of gender stability as well: "I will always be a girl." From the early school years to adolescence, gender role is further developed to include gender consistency: "I know I'm a girl even if my haircut looks like my brother's." *Behaviors that are labeled clearly masculine or feminine are relatively fixed by ages 4 to 5.* Gender relationships have certain patterns. Infant boys and girls can engage in genital manipulation, but between ages 2 to 5 years, genital interest and sex play increases markedly. In spite of the use of the term "latency," children between the ages of 5 and puberty have an ongoing interest in genital play. Masturbation normally increases during this period. The cause of gender preference in relationships is currently quite controversial. Homosexual play in early childhood is considered transient and generally does not predict adult sexual orientation.

2.5 The answer is E (all)

Erik Erikson has called adolescence the *developmental period of identity versus identity diffusion* as the teenager works through issues of being or not being oneself. Even in normal adolescence, self-discovery may involve discomfort, confusion, anxiety, and unhappiness in the short run. *Early adolescence is particularly marked by potentially negative emotions caused by the inner reworking of the self.* The positive outcome of this process, in later adolescence, is the development of "the real me" or a clear, integrated, realistic, internalized sense of an acceptable self (positive self-esteem). *The healthy adolescent identity is not the final self,* but the basis for the continued search for meaningful identity in the future.

Erikson describes the normative process of identity formation as moving through a period of exploration of alternative selves (identity diffusion) toward a period of choice, commitment, and consolidation. Maladaptive attempts at identity formation can result in premature commitment (foreclosure) or *failure to commit (identity diffusion).* Teenagers who foreclose the process adopt identities prescribed by parents or other authority figures without ever experiencing tension or exploring options. Although diffusion is developmentally appropriate in early adolescence, in later adolescence and young adulthood it represents a maladaptive inability to make decisions and commitments. *Pathological outcomes in identity formation lead to turning against the self* (e.g., depression, eating disorders, and suicidality) *or turning against others or society (e.g., delinquent behaviors).*

2.6 The answer is B

Kübler-Ross postulates five stages that many dying patients pass through from the time they first become aware of their fatal prognosis to their actual death:

1. *Denial.* "No, not me!" is the dying patient's common first response. If it does not interfere with treatment, denial can mitigate the initial overwhelming anxiety.

2. *Anger.* "Why me?" Indignation may surface when denial subsides. Patients are irritable, demanding, and critical; anger may be directed at themselves, caretakers, family, friends, or God.

3. *Bargaining.* "Yes, me, but . . ." This stage entails promises in order to buy additional time. Patients may promise to donate their organs to research or they may reaffirm an earlier faith in God.

4. *Depression.* "Yes, me." The patient comes to a full realization of what is going to happen and to whom. With the impending loss of life, a pervasive despondency may set in.

5. *Acceptance.* The patient begins to accept the inevitable. This stage need not constitute defeat or total surrender: "Yes, me, and I'm ready."

These five stages are not all-encompassing or prescriptive. Not everyone will reach these stages; perhaps only a small minority will reach acceptance. A patient may demonstrate aspects of all five stages in one interview or may fluctuate from one stage to another. Moreover, patients may exhibit other coping methods—from terror to humor to compassion—to offset each stage.

John Bowlby used the term protest. He described three phases of the bereavement process in children: the *protest, despair,* and *detachment* phases.

2.7 The answer is C

What is known about children's attitudes toward death comes from surveying healthy children, relying on adult memories of childhood, and exploring the fantasies and beliefs that children express during bereavement. Systematic studies of dying children have been few because children generally experience sudden, violent deaths rather than lingering illnesses. Most late-childhood and adolescent deaths are unnatural (accident, homicide, suicide); natural causes are generally malignancies or congenital abnormalities.

The affective and cognitive development of children colors their understanding of death and their subsequent fears about dying. *For example, at the preschool, preoperational stage of cognitive development, death is seen as a temporary absence, incomplete and reversible,* like departure or sleep. Separation from the primary caretakers is the main fear of preschoolers. This fear surfaces as an increase in nightmares, *more aggressive play,* or concern about the deaths of others. Regression to more infantile behaviors signals increasing dependence on parents. Dying children may assume responsibility for their death, *feeling guilty for dying.* Hospitalizations, separations from parents, and being subjected to painful procedures may reinforce their guilt and their belief that they are being punished. They may be unable to relate the treatment to the illness, and may instead view treatment as punishment. Dying preschoolers need reassurance from their parents that they are loved, that they have done nothing wrong, that they are not responsible for their illness, and that they will not be abandoned.

School-aged children manifest concrete operational thinking and recognize death as a final reality. However, they view death as something that happens to old people, not to them. Between the ages of 6 and 12 years children have active fantasy lives of violence and aggression, often dominated by themes of death and killing.

Dying children often are aware of their condition and want to discuss it. Research suggests that terminal and preterminal children 3 years of age and older are aware that they are dying without being told. *They often have more sophisticated views about dying than their healthy counterparts,* probably because of their own failing health, separations from parents, subjection to painful procedures, and deaths of hospital friends. Attendant fears and anxieties may be unexpressed or channeled in maladaptive directions.

Often unable to meet dying children's needs or to face their own feelings, parents and caretakers may tend to avoid afflicted children, even though human contact and communication are crucial. Perplexed parents may go to extremes—overindulging their dying children, withdrawing from them, or insisting that nothing is wrong. In such instances the child receives little help with the anxieties and fears of separation and abandonment or in developing the requisite hope and courage. Eventually sensing that they are dying, such children become more terrified that those who receive guidance and support from empathic family members.

2.8 The answer is E (none)

Older adults usually cope well with adversities and challenges, often despite facing chronic and accumulating risks. The concept of *resilience* is defined as the process of both maintaining adaptive behavior in the face of stress and recovering from adversity. Rather than viewing the last epoch of life as a period of multiple losses that deplete the individual, resilience theory suggests that maintenance of adaptive behavior despite these losses is an example of the resilience of the aging self.

The clinician working with older adults should not expect age to be a risk factor for poor outcome. There has been a tendency to underdiagnose depression in elderly cohorts because *many clinicians used to believe that depression was a normal response to aging.* Older adults struggle with life themes that differ from those of younger adults, and the clinician should be prepared to deal with issues of loss, increasing dependency, and the struggle to come to terms with the past.

The important exception to some assumptions stated above may be individuals in the oldest-old category (*those over the age of 85*). Research has shown that *these individuals may be at higher risk for social isolation than younger age groups, especially those without living children.* Clinicians should be alert to the unique life situations faced by individuals in this age group, who may be especially vulnerable not only to isolation but also to increasing frailty and the cumulative deleterious effects of chronic medical conditions. Interventions that both provide social support and encourage alternative sources of social support such as senior centers may be particularly helpful for persons in this age group.

In terms of cognitive processes, decrements exist in some, but not all, cognitive functions as one ages. However, with the exception of processing speed, these changes are generally small.

2.9 The answer is C

About 4 percent of North American children lose one or both parents by age 15; sibling death is the second most commonly experienced bereavement. Grief reactions are colored by developmental levels and concepts of death, and may not resemble adult reactions. Children may display minimal grief at the time of death and experience the full effect of the loss later. Indifference, anger, or misbehavior may be displayed rather than sadness; behaviors may be erratic and labile. Even older children frequently feel abandoned or rejected when a parent dies, and may show hostility toward the deceased or the surviving parent, now perceived as one who might also abandon them. They may feel responsible for the parent's death because of their own past misbehavior or because they said or wished that the parent would die at some time. Psychological tasks particularly relevant to bereaved children and adolescents have to do with their capacity to accept the tragedy of death, and to tolerate the anguish that ordinarily accompanies grief.

School-aged children may become phobic or hypochondriacal, withdrawn, or pseudomature, and school performance and peer relations often suffer. Children *under the age of 2* may show bereavement behavior through loss of speech or diffuse distress. Children *under the age of 5* may respond by developing eating, sleeping, bowel, and bladder dysfunction. *Strong feelings of sadness, fear, and anxiety can occur, but these feelings are not persistent and tend to alternate with longer-lasting normative states.* Like adults, adolescents run the gamut of bereavement reactions, ranging from behavioral problems, to somatic symptoms, to erratic moods, to stoicism. Adolescents losing a parent may become delinquent or may turn to a sexual partner for comfort and reassurance. Behavioral disturbances and depressions are common at all ages. *Although the surviving parents may underestimate their children's dysphoria, interviews of children and adolescents themselves reveal rates of depressive episodes that are at least as high as those of bereaved adults.* Severely bereaved children and adolescents have long-term *vulnerability to a variety of physical and mental illness,* especially depression.

2.10 The answer is E (all)

An understanding of the expected impact of aging on the central nervous system (CNS) is important to geriatric psychiatry. Changes in neurological and neurochemical functioning alter senescent vulnerability to psychiatric disorders and response to medication.

Table 2.2 outlines aging-related CNS changes. These include *brain atrophy, regional neuronal loss, senile plaques, and remodeling of dendrites, axons, and synapses.*

2.11 The answer is A

With the exception of dementing disorders and delirium, mental disorders are no more common in elderly adults than in younger age groups. Delirium is more common in the elderly. The prevalence of common disorders such as major depression, anxiety disorders, substance abuse, and psychotic disorders *are generally lower, not higher, for those over the age of 65 than for younger age cohorts. Furthermore, longitudinal studies find no evidence that rates of emotional distress increase with age.*

The experience and expression of both positive and negative emotions have been studied to determine if older adults report more negative emotional experience than younger adults. In a series of large ethnically diverse samples, *older adults reported experiencing fewer negative emotions such as sadness, anger, and fear but more positive emotions such as happiness than those in the younger age cohorts.* In addition, *older adults reported a greater sense of emotional control over negative internal emotional states than younger subjects.* To explain their data, the authors proposed an emotional control model suggesting that *aging is associated with an increased ability to inhibit negative emotional states and maintain positive emotional ones.*

Table 2.2
Summary of Age-Related Changes in the CNS

Gross brain atrophy
Ventricular enlargement
Selective regional neuronal loss
Remodeling of dendrites, axons, and synapses
Appearance of intraneuronal lipofuscin
Selective regional decrease in neurotransmitters and neuropeptides
Selective modification of neurotransmitter metabolism
Possible dysregulation of gaseous neurotransmitters
Glucocorticoid neurotoxicity
Changes in receptors
Changes in neurotrophins
Changes in signal transduction
Impairment of calcium homeostasis
Possible changes in cell cycle regulators (e.g., cyclins)
Possible changes in extracellular matrix proteins (e.g., laminins, proteoglycans)
Probable regional decline in cerebral blood flow
Probable regional decline in cerebral metabolic rate
Appearance of senile plaques and neurofibrillary tangles

2.12 The answer is B

George Vaillant outlined a hierarchy of defensive processes and found that individuals who received the highest life-adjustment ratings were those who used *primarily mature defenses* (e.g., humor). Low life-adjustment scores were correlated with the use of *immature defenses* (e.g., projection). Vaillant also found *increased use of mature defensive processes as individuals age*, as well as increased use of mature defenses as psychopathology decreased. His work suggests that coping abilities *become more adaptive (rather than more regressive)* over the life span. See Table 2.3 for Vaillant's description of mature defenses.

2.13 The answer is E

Splitting is a mental mechanism in which the object is perceived as either all good or all bad and is characterized by ambivalent feelings toward the object. It is common in borderline personality disorder. Some defenses used during middle age are *dissociation, repression, sublimation,* and *altruism.*

Dissociation is an unconscious defense mechanism involving the segregation of any group of mental or behavioral processes from the rest of the person's psychic activity. It may entail the separation of an idea from its accompanying emotional tone, as seen in dissociative disorders. *Repression* is an unconscious defense mechanism in which unacceptable mental contents are kept out of consciousness. A term introduced by Sigmund Freud, it is important in both normal psychological development and in neurotic and psychotic symptom formation. *Sublimation* is an unconscious defense mechanism in which the energy associated with unacceptable impulses or drives is diverted into personally and socially acceptable channels. Unlike other defense mechanisms, sublimation offers some minimal gratification of the instinctual drive or impulse. *Altruism* is a regard for and dedication to the welfare of others. In psychiatry the term is closely linked with ethics and morals. Freud described altruism as the only basis for the development of community interest and Eugen Bleuler equated it with morality.

Table 2.3
The Mature Defenses

Altruism. The vicarious but constructive and instinctually gratifying service to others. This must be distinguished from altruistic surrender, which involves a surrender of direct gratification or of instinctual needs in favor of fulfilling the needs of others to the detriment of the self, with vicarious satisfaction only being gained through introjection.

Anticipation. The realistic anticipation of, or planning for, future inner discomfort; implies overly concerned planning, worrying, and anticipation of dire and dreadful possible outcomes.

Asceticism. The elimination of directly pleasurable affects attributable to an experience. The moral element is implicit in setting values on specific pleasures. Asceticism is directed against all "base" pleasures perceived consciously, and gratification is derived from the renunciation.

Humor. The overt expression of feelings without personal discomfort or immobilization and without unpleasant effect on others. Humor allows one to bear, and yet focus on, what is too terrible to be borne, in contrast to wit, which always involves distraction or displacement away from the affective issue.

Sublimation. The gratification of an impulse whose goal is retained, but whose aim or object is changed from a socially objectionable one to a socially valued one. Libidinal sublimation involves desexualization of drive impulses and placing a value judgment that substitutes what is valued by the superego or society. Sublimation of aggressive impulses takes place through pleasurable games and sports. Unlike neurotic defenses, sublimation allows instincts to be channeled rather than to be dammed up or diverted. Thus, in sublimation, feelings are acknowledged, modified, and directed toward a relatively significant person or goal so that modest instinctual satisfaction results.

Suppression. The conscious or semiconscious decision to postpone attention to a conscious impulse or conflict.

Courtesy of William W. Meissner, M.D.

2.14 The answer is E (all)

The stage of formal operations is characterized by the young (11 years through adolescence) person's ability to think *abstractly,* to reason *deductively,* and to *define concepts.* This stage is so named because the person's thinking ideally operates in a formal, highly logical, systematic, and *symbolic* manner. This stage is also characterized by skills in dealing with permutations and combinations; the young person can grasp the concept of probabilities. The adolescent attempts to deal with all possible relations and hypotheses to explain data and events. During this stage, language use is complex, follows formal rules of logic, and is grammatically correct. Abstract thinking is shown by the adolescent's interest in a variety of issues: philosophy, religion, ethics, and politics.

2.15 The answer is E (all)

Many adults who have undergone high-risk or traumatic childhood experiences have shown good adjustment in maturity. These adults were able to overcome their earlier problems because of several factors including *social support, high intelligence, structured upbringing,* and *the ability to bounce back (resiliency).* A strong network of friends, siblings, and coworkers offers support and security that encourages high-risk children to work on their difficulties in life. A family that offers a person a sense of structure and a set of standards accustoms the person to see life as orderly and rational, and helps him or her overcome a chaotic episode or traumatic event. Children who meet adversities resiliently and struggle to overcome them are more likely to be well-adjusted adults.

2.16 The answer is E

Infancy is generally considered to end when the child is able to *speak.* It is the period from birth until about 18 months to 2 years of age. During the first month of life, the infant is termed a neonate or newborn. The child *creeps* at 40 weeks, *stands without assistance* at 52 weeks, develops meaningful speech and language at 15 months, *climbs stairs* at 2 years, and *controls his or her anal sphincter completely* at three years. There are normal variations in these figures among children.

2.17 The answer is B

Arnold Gesell, a developmental psychologist and physician, described developmental schedules that outline the qualitative sequence of motor, adaptive, language, and personal-social behavior of the child from the age of 4 weeks to 6 years. Gesell's approach is normative; he viewed development as the unfolding of a genetically determined sequence. According to his schedules, at birth all infants have a repertoire of reflex behaviors—breathing, crying, and swallowing. By 1 to 2 weeks of age, the infant smiles. The response is endogenously determined, as evidenced by smiling in blind infants. By 2 to 4 weeks of age, visual fixation and following are evident. *By 4 to 8 weeks,* social smiling is elicited preferentially by the face or the voice of the caretaker.

2.18 The answer is B

Margaret S. Mahler (1897–1985) was a Hungarian-born psychoanalyst who practiced in the United States and who studied early childhood object relations. She described the separation-individuation process, resulting in a person's subjective sense of separateness and the development of an inner object constancy. The separation-individuation phase of development begins in the fourth or fifth month of life and is completed by the age of 3 years.

As described by Mahler, the characteristic anxiety during the differentiation subphase of separation-individuation is *stranger anxiety.* The infant has begun to develop an alert sensorium and has begun to compare what is and what is not a mother. The subphase occurs between 5 and 10 months of age. A fear of strangers is first noted in infants at 26 weeks of age but does not fully develop until about 8 months. Unlike babies exposed to a variety of caretakers, babies who have only one caretaker are likely to have stranger anxiety. But, unlike stranger anxiety, which can occur even when the infant is in its mother's arms, *separation anxiety*—which is seen between 10 and 16 months, during the practicing subphase—is precipitated by the separation from the person to whom the infant is attached. The practicing subphase marks the beginning of upright locomotion, which gives the child a new perspective and a mood of elation, the "love affair with the world." The infant learns to separate as it begins to crawl and to move away from its mother but continues to look back and to return frequently to its mother as home base. Between the ages of 16 and 24 months, the *rapprochement* subphase occurs, with the characteristic event being the rapprochement crisis, during which the infant's struggle becomes one between wanting to be soothed by its mother and not wanting to accept her help. The visual symbol of rapprochement is the child standing on the threshold of a door in helpless frustration, not knowing which way to turn.

Castration anxiety, as described by Sigmund Freud, is a characteristic anxiety that arises during the Oedipal phase of development, ages 3 to 5 years, concerning a fantasized loss of or an injury to the genitalia.

2.19 The answer is E (all)

Infants are born with a number of reflexes, many of which were once needed for survival. Experts assume that the genes carry messages for those reflexes. Among the reflexes are the *Moro reflex,* flexion of the extremities when startled; the *rooting reflex,* turning toward the touch when the cheek is stroked; and the Babinski reflex, spreading of the toes with an up-going big toe when the sole is stroked.

Infants are also born with the innate reflex pattern, *endogenous smiling,* which is unintentional and is unrelated to outside stimuli.

2.20 The answer is E (all)

Infants are able to differentiate among various sensations. Babies as young as 12 hours old gurgle with satisfaction when *sweet-tasting sugar* water is placed on the tongue, and they grimace at *the sour taste of lemon* juice. Infants smile at *the smell of bananas* and protest at *the smell of rotten eggs.* At 8 weeks of age, they can differentiate between the shapes of objects and colors. Stereoscopic vision begins to develop at 3 months of age.

2.21 The answer is E (all)

Early adolescence (12 to 15 years) is marked by increased anxiety and *episodes of depression,* acting-out behavior, and *occasional delinquent acts.* Teenagers, for example, obtain about 300,000 legal abortions and give birth to about 600,000 babies each year. They have a diminution in sustained interest and creativity; there is also *a dissolution of intense ties* to siblings, parents, and parental surrogates. Middle adolescence (14 to 18 years) is marked by efforts to master simple issues concerned with object relationships. The late adolescent phase (17 to 21 years), which is marked by the resolution of the separation-individuation tasks of adolescence, is characterized by *vulnerability to crisis,* particularly with respect to personal identity.

If adolescence does not proceed normally, the teenager may have an identity problem that is characterized by a chaotic sense of self, usually involving a social role conflict as perceived by the person. Such conflict occurs when adolescents feel unwilling or unable to accept or adopt the roles they believe are expected of them by society. The identity problem is often manifested by isolation, withdrawal, rebelliousness, negativism, and extremism.

2.22 The answer is D

By the age of *10 years,* a child is able to conceptualize the true meaning of death—something that may happen to the child and to the parent. At that time, the child shows a greater tendency for logical exploration to dominate fantasy and shows an increased understanding of feelings and interactions in relationships. The child has well-developed capacities for empathy, love, and compassion, as well as emerging capacities for sadness and love in the context of concrete rules. As opposed to parents in some other parts of the world, middle-class adults in the United States tend to shield children from a knowledge of death. The air of mystery with which death is surrounded in such instances may unintentionally create irrational fears in children. Attending funerals is recommended for children if the adults present are trustworthy and reasonably composed. A funeral may act as an introduction to the adult world of crises and tribulations, on the way to a full transition to other phases of development.

The preschool child under age 5 years is beginning to be aware of death not in the abstract sense but as a separation similar to sleep. Between the ages of 5 and 10 years, the child shows a developing sense of inevitable human mortality; the child first fears that the parents may die and that the child will be abandoned. Discussing death with an inquiring child requires simplicity and candor. Adults are cautioned not to invent answers when they have none. Basically, death must be conveyed as a natural event that cannot be avoided but that causes pain because it separates people who love each other.

2.23 The answer is E (all)

Normal turning points during middle age are usually mastered without distress. Only when life events are severe or unexpected—such as the death of a spouse, the loss of a job, or a serious illness—does a person experience an emotional disorder serious enough to warrant the term *midlife crisis*. Men and women who are most prone to midlife crises tend to come from families characterized by one or more of the following during their adolescence: *parental discord, withdrawal by the same-sex parent, anxious parents, and impulsive parents with a low sense of responsibility.*

2.24 The answer is D

An *estimated 70 percent of men and 20 percent of women over age 60 are sexually active; sexual activity is usually limited by the absence of an available partner.* Longitudinal studies have found that the *sex drive does not decrease as men and women*

age; in fact, some report an increase in sex drive. William Masters and Virginia Johnson reported sexual functioning among those in their 80s. Expected physiological changes in men include a longer time for erection to occur, decreased penile turgidity, and ejaculatory seepage; in women, decreased vaginal lubrication and vaginal atrophy are associated with lowered estrogen levels. Medications can also adversely affect sexual behavior. A significant finding was that *the more active a person's sex life was in early adulthood, the more likely it is to be active in old age.*

Answers 2.25–2.29

2.25 The answer is E

2.26 The answer is D

2.27 The answer is A

2.28 The answer is C

2.29 The answer is B

To understand normal development, one must take a comprehensive approach and have an internal map of the age-expected norms for various aspects of human development. The areas of neuromotor, cognitive, and language milestones have many empirical normative data. The normal child is able to accomplish specific tasks at certain ages. For example, *a cross can be copied at 4 years,* a square can be copied at 5 years, and a *triangle can be copied at 6 years. By 18 months,* children can *walk up the stairs with one hand held;* at *2 years,* they can *refer to themselves by name;* and at 3 years, they can *put on their shoes.* Some children may be able to perform a task at an earlier or later age and still fall within the normal range. Other landmarks of normal behavioral development are listed in Table 2.4.

Table 2.4
Landmarks of Normal Behavioral Development

Age	Motor and Sensory Behavior	Adaptive Behavior	Personal and Social Behavior
Under 4 weeks	Makes alternating crawling movements Moves head laterally when placed in prone position	Responds to sound of rattle and bell Regards moving objects momentarily	Quiets when picked up Impassive face
16 weeks	Symmetrical postures predominate Holds head balanced Head lifted 90 degrees when prone on forearm Visual accommodation	Follows a slowly moving object well Arms activate on sight of dangling object	Spontaneous social smile (exogenous) Aware of strange situations
28 weeks	Sits steadily, leaning forward on hands Bounces actively when placed in standing position	One-hand approach and grasp of toy Bangs and shakes rattle Transfers toys	Takes feet to mouth Pats mirror image Starts to imitate mother's sounds and actions
40 weeks	Sits alone with good coordination Creeps Pulls self to standing position Points with index finger	Matches two objects at midline Attempts to imitate scribble	Separation anxiety manifest when taken away from mother Responds to social play, such as pat-a-cake and peekaboo Feeds self cracker and holds own bottle
52 weeks	Walks with one hand held Stands alone briefly	Seeks novelty	Cooperates in dressing

Adapted from Stella Chess, M.D.

Answers 2.30–2.34

2.30 The answer is A

2.31 The answer is B

2.32 The answer is C

2.33 The answer is D

2.34 The answer is D

Language development occurs in well-delineated stages. At *birth to 6 months*, the child *plays at making sounds and babbles;* at *7 to 11 months*, the child *plays language games (pat-a-cake and peekaboo);* at *12 to 18 months*, the child *understands up to 150 words and uses up to 20 words;* and from *54 months on*, the child's *speech is 100 percent intelligible,* and the child *uses language to tell stories and share ideas.*

Answers 2.35–2.39

2.35 The answer is B

2.36 The answer is A

2.37 The answer is E

2.38 The answer is E

2.39 The answer is C

Most of the developmental landmarks are readily observed. Growth is so rapid during infancy that developmental landmarks are measured in terms of weeks. Examples of some major developmental events and their approximate time of appearance are *ocular control, 4 weeks; grasping and manipulation, 16 weeks; sitting alone, 28 weeks;* creeping, poking, and ability to say one word, 40 weeks; *standing with slight support,* cooperation in dressing, and *verbalization of two or more words, 12 months;* and the use of words in phrases, 18 months.

Answers 2.40–2.44

2.40 The answer is D

2.41 The answer is A

2.42 The answer is B

2.43 The answer is C

2.44 The answer is E

Margaret Mahler (1897–1985) proposed a theory to describe how young children acquire a sense of identity separate from their mothers. The theory of *separation-individuation* was based on her observations of the interactions of children and their mothers. The theory is outlined in Table 2.5.

Mary Ainsworth found that the interaction between the mother and her baby during the early attachment period significantly influences the baby's current and future behavior. Many observers believe that patterns of infant attachment affect future adult emotional relationships.

Ainsworth confirmed that attachment serves the purpose of reducing anxiety. What she called the *secure base effect* enables a child to move away from the attachment figure and to explore the environment. Inanimate objects, such as a teddy bear or a blanket (called the transitional object by D. W. Winnicott), also

Table 2.5
Stages of Separation-Individuation Proposed by Mahler

1. Normal autism (birth to 2 months)
   Periods of sleep outweigh periods of arousal in a state reminiscent of intrauterine life.

2. Symbiosis (2 to 5 months)
   Developing perceptual abilities gradually enable infants to distinguish the inner from the outer world; mother–infant is perceived as a single fused entity.

3. Differentiation (5 to 10 months)
   Progressive neurological development and increased alertness draw infants' attention away from self to the outer world. Physical and psychological distinctiveness from the mother is gradually appreciated.

4. Practicing (10 to 18 months)
   The ability to move autonomously increases children's exploration of the outer world.

5. Rapprochement (18 to 24 months)
   As children slowly realize their helplessness and dependence, the need for independence alternates with the need for closeness. Children move away from their mothers and come back for reassurance.

6. Object constancy (2 to 5 years)
   Children gradually comprehend and are reassured by the permanence of mother and other important people, even when not in their presence.

serve as a secure base, one that often accompanies children as they investigate the world.

Harry Stack Sullivan postulated that a *chum* or buddy is an important phenomenon during the school years. By about 10 years of age, children develop a close same-sex relationship, which Sullivan believed is necessary for further healthy psychological growth. Moreover, Sullivan believed that an early harbinger of schizophrenia is the absence of a chum during the middle years of childhood.

D. W. Winnicott believed that infants begin life in a state of nonintegration, with unconnected and diffuse experiences, and that mothers provide the relationship that enables infants' incipient selves to emerge. Mothers supply a holding environment in which infants are contained and experienced. During the last trimester of pregnancy and for the first few months of a baby's life, the mother is in a state of primary maternal preoccupation, absorbed in fantasies about experiences with her baby. The mother need not be perfect, but she must provide *"good-enough" mothering.* She plays a vital role in bringing the world to the child and in offering empathic anticipations of the infant's needs. If the mother is able to resonate with the infant's needs, the baby can become attuned to its own bodily functions and drives that afford the basis for the gradually evolving sense of self.

Parental fit describes how well the mother or father relates to the newborn or developing infant; the idea takes into account temperamental characteristics of both parent and child. Each newborn has innate psychophysiological characteristics, which are known collectively as temperament. *Stella Chess and Alexander Thomas* identified a range of normal temperamental patterns, from the difficult child at one end of the spectrum to the easy child at the other end.

Table 2.6
Moral Developmental Theories and Achievements[a]

		Theories of Moral Development			
Piaget's Stages of Moral Behavior Related to Cognitive Phases	Piaget's Two-Stage Theory of Moral Judgment (cognitively based)	Kohlberg's Six-Stage Theory of Moral Reasoning (cognitively, socially, and emotionally influenced)	Freud's Concept of Superego as Conscience (psychosexually influenced)	Gilligan's Sex Theory of Morals Development (cognitively and psychosexually influenced)	Moral-Skills
0–4 years					Child makes first observations of behavior Gratification delay begins
Egocentric stage (4–7 years) (preoperational cognitive)	Heteronomous Morality (morality of constraint) Morality based upon authority's rules Rules are fixed No concept of motive; concept of permanence "You can't play because you cheat" Board games chosen because of clear, objective rules Rigidity	Preconventional level (morality due to external controls) Stage 1—Punishment and obedience; child's limited thinking bases moral decisions upon fear or self-interest Stage 2—Relativistic orientation; child moves from fear of punishment to concern for fairness; rewards obtained by bartering Conventional level of morality (morality as rules for society's order)	Resolution of Oedipal complex results in formation of superego with guilt and shame as boundaries Conscience		Self-control develops Ability to relate behavior to moral ideas takes shape Guilt appears
Incipient cooperation (7–11 years) (concrete operational)	Autonomous morality (morality of negotiation) Child can accept respect for rules negotiated with peers—concept of reciprocity Child capable of evaluating own behavior based on motives Children argue about punishment because they view it as relative "I think he should get less allowance because he didn't finish his chores" Punishment adjusted to crime Flexibility and cooperation	Stage 3—Social approval level Stage 4—Maintains laws of system; teen and adult move from preoccupation with what is "fair" for individuals to factor in conformity to society's needs; social conscience		Agrees with Kohlberg until here Ethics of caring in girls Girl's goal focuses upon compassion, relationships and responsibilities; Not better, but different from boys Ethics of justice in boys Boy's goal is rationally committing to moral ideals of justice	Better self-control Child understands motives Principles of parents internalized Empathy Moral principles more refined Morality abstractly formulated Moral self-monitoring better Empathy and more cognitive moral integration occur Altruism Peers considered in principles
Early teens to adulthood		Postconventional principled level (morality as value defined) Stage 5—Society's good paramount Stage 6—Universal ethics; focus on justice, fairness; recognition of others' moral standards			Individual rights count Laws are changeable Goal to be fair to self and others

[a]Development and achievement levels may overlap ages.

Chess and Thomas use the term *goodness of fit* to characterize the harmonious and consonant interaction between a mother and a child in their motivations, capacities, and styles of behavior. Poorness of fit is likely to lead to distorted development and maladaptive functioning. A difficult child must be recognized because parents of such infants often have feelings of inadequacy and believe that something they are doing accounts for the child's difficulty in sleeping and eating and the problems in comforting the child. In addition, a majority of difficult children have emotional disturbances later in life.

Answers 2.45–2.47

2.45 The answer is C

2.46 The answer is D

2.47 The answer is A

In developmental terms, moral maturation refers to children's acquisition of internal standards that guide their observable actions or behavior. Infants have only a rudimentary awareness of the effects of their response on others. They know that smiling makes their parents hug them. Small children can understand that sometimes they do things that make their parents concerned. A 3-year-old can say, "My daddy gets upset when I say yucky words." However, by the time children enter adolescence, they should have acquired enough moral skills to be able to make decisions on the basis of something other than fear of punishment. They are already able to understand rules in terms of a sense of fairness. At this point, external restrictions are replaced by *conscience,* a person's inner ability to make decisions regarding concepts of right and wrong. In certain cultures elaborate rituals mark the acquisition of conscience. As with other areas, various explanations are offered to help understand the moral developmental process.

Cognitive developmentalists, such as Piaget and Lawrence Kohlberg, suggest that moral maturation is an active process of acquiring a moral sense through a set of cognitively derived constructions that operate in conflictual situations. In *Piaget's schema, morality is formed in two stages: Heteronomous morality* develops as children are able to see rules as being fixed and dictated by authority, a period also called "the morality of constraint." A child's behavior is determined by physical consequences, and rules are considered unchangeable; motives are not related to intention, actual consequences rule intention. Justice is a concept that is meted out as punishment by some super-

natural agent in response to the child's misbehavior. *Autonomous morality,* or the morality of cooperation, forms as children see rules as flexible and people-dictated rather than absolute. In this second stage, children are able to see morality as linked to intentions, not consequences, and are able to see that moral punishment can be modified by circumstances. In the latter stage, incidents such as illness are no longer connected to punishment for bad behavior in the child's mind. Justice becomes a more abstract consequence and goal. *Kohlberg elaborates upon piagetian views by dividing the moral maturation of children into three levels with six stages.* At the preschool and early childhood level, morality is based on a system of rewards and punishment meted out by authority figures. In a later phase, beginning after age 6, relativism and social approval are important enforcers. In the middle-childhood to preteen years, morality is based on a system of laws that overrides simple approval. The framework for both piagetian moral development and Kohlberg's form lies in cognitive growth and understanding.

Social theorists, on the other hand, stress that a child's morality is learned when adult models offer instructive examples in their interactions with children. Helpfulness, generosity, and altruism are learned and reinforced by positive feedback. Punishment tends to preclude the development of a conscience. Social theorists explain that negative experiences make the child more stressed and less amenable to adopting any part of the parental directive.

Psychoanalytic theories also stress the importance of the environment on the child. *Classical psychoanalytic theory suggests that the conscience is actually a superego that arises from repressed hostility held toward a parent following the resolution of the Oedipal and Electra issues.* Guilt and self-punishment occur when a child behaves in a way that is contradictory to internalized parental values. More modern psychoanalytic theory stresses conscience development as the growth of a superego—arising out of a positive identification with parental values rather than over guilt.

More recent approaches to explain moral development include gender-based theories. *Carol Gilligan asserts that male and female morality develops along different tracks. Women's moral development ends in compassion and an ethics of caring,* whereas men's morality culminates in a moral system dominated by the ethics of justice and the assertion of rights. Table 2.6 outlines moral development from birth through adulthood as conceptualized by various theorists.

3 ▲

The Brain and Behavior

Psychiatry is one of the most exciting fields of medicine because of the explosion of data derived from psychopharmacology, functional neuroimaging, and human neurogenetics. Knowledge of the brain and its correlates in behavior becomes more subtle, specific, and complex every day. Students of clinical psychiatry now must have intimate knowledge of, and be comfortable with, the gross and fine structure of the brain, the principles of chemical neurotransmission, the major classes of neurotransmitters, and the premises and possibilities of a molecular genetic analysis of behavior. The psychiatrist must be able to critically review new data and research and to apply knowledge to evaluating new drugs, new treatments, and new diagnostic techniques.

A basic understanding of behavioral neuroanatomy informs a knowledge of classical syndromes, such as those of lobar dysfunction. The basal ganglia, limbic structures, hypothalamus, and lobes of the cerebral cortex are of special relevance. For instance, cerebral cortical lesions can lead to aphasias, apraxias, and visuoperceptual disorders; damage to the limbic system can lead to disruptive behavior and memory dysfunction; and disturbance of the basal ganglia can produce movement disorders. The subdivisions of the prefrontal cortex are particularly important, since these regions are increasingly implicated in production of both normal and abnormal behavior that may be detected by neuroimaging techniques.

It is also crucial to understand the ultrastructure of individual brain cells, the details of synaptic connectivity, the functional organization of the brain, and the behavioral consequences of pathological processes in the central nervous system. Students should be knowledgeable about the vast functional diversity of brain cells and their organization. These can include basic multicellular units of highly repetitive structures such as the olfactory bulb, cerebellum, hippocampus, and Brodmann's cytoarchitectural classification, as well as many other divisions that relate to arousal and attention (the brainstem and diencephalon), sensory processing and associations (the posterior cortex), and executive functions (the frontal cortex).

Students need to be aware of the neuroanatomy of the sensory and motor systems, and to understand that most behaviors are the result of complex activation of various brain regions. The concept that synaptic connectivity may be modified during development and in adulthood must be appreciated clinically. Students need to know about the stages of brain development, including cell birth, migration, elaboration of dendrites and axons, and onset of synaptic activity.

Of central importance to clinical psychopharmacology is a thorough knowledge of the neurotransmitters, including the brainstem location of the biogenic amine neurotransmitter nuclei and the widespread distribution of their axonal projections. Excitatory neurotransmitters (e.g., glutamate), inhibitory neurotransmitters (e.g., GABA), the monoamine neurotransmitters (e.g., serotonin, dopamine, norepinephrine, epinephrine, histamine, and acetylcholine), and the peptide neurotransmitters (e.g., endorphins and enkephalins) are crucial to an understanding of current psychotherapeutic medications. Students should be able to associate specific drugs with one or more of the major neurotransmitter systems. They should be able to discuss critically both the evidence for and against the dopamine hypothesis of schizophrenia, the biogenic amine hypothesis of mood and anxiety disorders, and the role of GABA in psychiatric disorders.

Presynaptic, synaptic, and postsynaptic mechanisms mediate the finest gradations of thought, and the student must have a detailed understanding of the structure and function of neurotransmission. Part of this is an understanding of how chemical and electrical signals interact in neurons, and as such the student must have some basic knowledge of action potentials, voltage- and ligand-gated ion channels, and second messengers. Newer avenues of research having clinical relevance include study of the interactions between the nervous system and the endocrine and immune systems, and study of biorhythms.

Students must have a thorough grasp of the role of genetics in psychiatric disorders, including levels of regulation of gene expression, DNA replication, messenger RNA synthesis and translation into protein, and the consequences of mutations at each of these stages. They should understand the importance of assembling a complete family pedigree, and of twin and adoption studies. The relative degree of nature (genetic factors) and nurture (environmental influences) in any behavior or disorder should be appreciated, and methods of distinguishing between the two should be learned.

Finally, a knowledge of the major neuroimaging techniques, including clinical and research indications, and the limitations of each technique, is essential. These methods include magnetic resonance imaging (MRI), computed tomography (CT), magnetic resonance spectroscopy (MRS), single photon emission computed tomography (SPECT), proton emission tomography (PET), electroencephalography (EEG), and magnetoencephalography (MEG), among others. Examples of provocative findings from imaging studies include decreased frontal metabolism in patients with schizophrenia and complementary influences of the right and left prefrontal cortices on mood.

Students should test their knowledge by addressing the following questions and answers.

HELPFUL HINTS

▶ aphasia: Broca's, Wernicke's, conduction, global, transcortical motor, transcortical sensory, anomic, mixed transcortical
▶ apraxias: limb-kinetic, ideomotor, ideational
▶ autonomic sensory and motor systems
▶ basal ganglia and cerebellum and clinical syndromes
▶ behavioral neuroanatomy: arousal and attention, memory, language, emotions
▶ biological rhythms
▶ cerebral cortex
▶ chronobiology
▶ cytoarchitectonics and cortical columns
▶ development of cortical networks; plasticity
▶ dopamine and serotonin hypothesis of schizophrenia

▶ electrophysiology: membranes and charge; ion channels, action potentials, chemical neurotransmission
▶ epilepsy: complex partial seizures, temporal lobe epilepsy, TLE personality, déjà vu
▶ five primary senses (somatosensory, visual, auditory, olfaction, taste)
▶ frontal, parietal, temporal and occipital lobes and clinical syndromes
▶ GABA and serotonin hypothesis of anxiety disorders
▶ glutamate, GABA, glycine, dopamine, norepinephrine, epinephrine, serotonin, acetylcholine, histamine, opioids, substance P, neurotensin, cholecystokinin, somatostatin, vasopressin, oxytocin, neuropeptide Y

▶ gray matter and white matter
▶ inheritance patterns: autosomal dominant, autosomal recessive, sex-linked
▶ ligand-gated ion channel; G protein-coupled receptor; second messenger
▶ limbic system: amygdala, hippocampus, Papez circuit
▶ molecular genetics: pedigree, positional cloning, candidate gene, mutations
▶ neuroimaging: CT, MRI, MRS, fMRI, SPECT, PET, EEG, MEG, TMS, EP, ERP
▶ neurons and glial cells
▶ neurotransmitters: biogenic amines, amino acids, peptides, nucleotides, gases, eicosanoids, anandamides

▶ norepinephrine and serotonin hypothesis of mood disorders
▶ organization of sensory and motor systems; hemispheric lateralization
▶ prefrontal lobe syndromes
▶ psychoneuroendocrinology: hormones and hormone receptors, adrenal axis, thyroid axis, growth hormone, estrogens
▶ psychoneuroimmunology: placebo effect, cancer, infection, AIDS
▶ synapses: presynaptic membrane, synaptic compartment, postsynaptic membrane

▲ QUESTIONS

DIRECTIONS: Each of the following questions or incomplete statements is followed by five suggested responses or completions. Select the *one* that is *best* in each case.

3.1 Enkephalins are which of the following?

A. opioid-like peptides
B. cholinergic agents
C. dopamine-receptor antagonists
D. selective serotonin reuptake inhibitors
E. tricyclic drugs

3.2 All of the following statements about neuronal connections are true *except*

A. Many connections between brain regions are reciprocal.
B. The locus ceruleus is an example of a convergent neuronal system.
C. Visual input is conveyed in a serial or hierarchical fashion.
D. Regions of the brain are specialized for different functions.
E. The role of any specific brain region in the production of specific behaviors must be viewed in the context of neural connections with other brain regions.

3.3 The basal ganglia include

A. the lentiform nucleus
B. the substantia nigra
C. the subthalamic nucleus
D. the caudate nucleus
E. all of the above

3.4 Disruption of the input pathways of the basal ganglia has been associated with

A. bradykinesia
B. muscular rigidity
C. fine tremor
D. shuffling gait
E. all of the above

3.5 In schizophrenia

A. No abnormalities in neural migration have been hypothesized.
B. Reductions of 50 to 60 percent are reported in overall temporal lobe size.
C. There is decreased prefrontal cerebral blood flow on PET scans during certain tasks (when compared to healthy controls).
D. There is a proliferation of glial cells.
E. There is an associated increase in the size of the amygdala.

3.6 The velocity of conduction of the nerve action potential is increased because of the

A. axon hillock
B. myelin sheath
C. voltage-sensitive potassium channels
D. sodium-potassium ATPase
E. chloride conductance

3.7 The one advantage of computed tomography (CT) over magnetic resonance imaging (MRI) in psychiatric clinical practice is

A. CT has superior resolution.
B. CT can distinguish between white matter and gray matter.
C. CT has the ability to take thinner slices through the brain than does MRI.
D. CT is superior in detecting calcified brain lesions.
E. CT avoids exposing patients to radiation.

3.8 True statements about the relationship of GABA (γ-aminobutyric acid) to seizure activity include all of the following *except*

A. Blockage of GABA inhibition can result in seizures.
B. Benzodiazepines and barbiturates act at GABA receptors.
C. Manipulation of GABA-receptor function has little effect on seizure activity.
D. Enhancement of GABA-receptor function raises the seizure threshold.
E. Reduction of GABA clearance by inhibition of GABA uptake is clinically effective.

3.9 All of the following are true about tardive dyskinesia *except*

A. It involves a hypermotility of the facial muscles.
B. It follows prolonged phenothiazine treatment.
C. It may result from tricyclic antidepressant treatment.
D. It does not involve the extremities.
E. It affects the tongue.

3.10 Which of the following features is *least* likely to represent isolated injury to the dorsolateral prefrontal cortex?

A. deficiencies in planning and monitoring
B. inability to use foresight and feedback
C. echolalia
D. mood disorders
E. akinetic mutism

3.11 PET and SPECT scans

A. entail the injection of radioactively labeled drugs
B. provide exquisitely detailed images of brain structure
C. produce two-dimensional information
D. are similar to MRI in creating fine visual detail
E. are commonly used in clinical practice

3.12 MRI studies

A. prove that there are specific, structural brain changes in a significant number of schizophrenic patients
B. provide some evidence that there may be structural brain changes in major depressive disorder
C. prove that caudate enlargement occurs early in the course of schizophrenia
D. are inferior to CT with regard to visualizing gray versus white matter in the brain
E. suggest no brain changes secondary to alcohol dependence

3.13 Serotonin is

A. primarily located in the CNS
B. able to cross the blood–brain barrier
C. not dependent on tryptophan concentration for its synthesis
D. affected by carbohydrate intake in its synthesis
E. synthesized from the amino acid tryptophan

3.14 Pathological alterations in hypothalamic-pituitary adrenal function have been associated with

A. mood disorders
B. PTSD
C. Alzheimer's disease
D. substance use disorders
E. all of the above

3.15 Techniques that reflect regional brain activity by measuring neuronal activity rather than blood flow include

A. xenon-133 (^{133}Xe) single proton emission computed tomography (SPECT)
B. fluorine-18 [^{18}F]-fluorodeoxyglucose (FDG) positron emission tomography (PET)
C. technetium-99 (^{99}Tc) hexamethylpropyleneamine oxime (HMPAO) SPECT
D. nitrogen-13 (^{13}N) PET
E. functional magnetic resonance imaging (fMRI)

3.16 The search for the genetic basis of bipolar I disorder

A. has been more successful than that for Alzheimer's disease
B. has shown that there is a single major gene with incomplete penetrance responsible for the disorder in some families
C. has provided evidence of genetic heterogeneity and multifactorial inheritance
D. has had few difficulties with phenotype definition
E. has found strong evidence for genetic linkage of bipolar disorder in the Amish population

3.17 All of the following are true about the motor system *except*

A. The firing of the lower motor neurons is regulated by the summation of upper motor neuron activity.
B. Activation of the vestibulospinal tract causes the limbs to extend.
C. The corticospinal tract controls fine movements.
D. After a stroke, spasticity results following the release of the cortex from brainstem modulation.
E. Limb flexion occurs equally in both normal and anencephalic newborns.

3.18 All of the following associations between aspects of the basal ganglia and their respective disorders are correct *except*

A. subthalamic nucleus—hemiballismus
B. caudate nucleus—obsessive-compulsive disorder
C. caudate nucleus—Huntington's disease
D. globus pallidus—Wilson's disease
E. substantia nigra—Alzheimer's disease

3.19 True statements regarding arousal include

A. The ascending reticular activating system (ARAS) sets the level of consciousness.
B. Both the thalamus and the cortex fire rhythmic bursts of neuronal activity.
C. During wakefulness, the ARAS stimulates the thalamic interlaminar nuclei.
D. Small discrete lesions of the ARAS may produce a stuporous state.
E. All of the above

3.20 A patient is brought to your office for cognitive testing. The patient is given the task of scanning a long list of random letters and is told to identify only the letter "A." She is unable to continue this task for more than a minute. What is the most likely location of her lesion?

A. thalamus
B. lateral corticospinal tract
C. basal ganglia
D. frontal lobe
E. substantia nigra

3.21 All of the following structures are critical to memory *except*

A. medial temporal lobe
B. hippocampus
C. amygdala
D. mammilary body
E. substantia nigra

3.22 A patient with intractable epilepsy undergoes surgical removal of both hippocampi and amygdalae. Which of the following is the most likely side effect of this procedure?

A. impaired learning ability
B. impaired skill-related memory
C. impaired factual memory
D. ataxia
E. loss of vision

3.23 A chronic alcoholic presents to the emergency room with confusion and confabulation. He is not able to form new memories and is also unable to recall remote memories from the past. What is the most likely location of his lesion?

A. mamillary body
B. amygdala
C. hippocampus
D. substantia nigra
E. caudate nucleus

3.24 A patient suffers a stroke of the left hemisphere. Which of the following is the most likely sequela?

A. denial of illness
B. inability to move the left hand
C. loss of narrative aspects of dreams
D. failure to respond to humor
E. depression

3.25 A patient is diagnosed with temporal lobe epilepsy (TLE) but does not experience the classic grand mal seizures. Which of the following behaviors is the patient likely to exhibit?

A. hyposexuality
B. hypersexuality
C. placidity
D. hypermetamorphosis
E. lack of emotion to visual stimuli

3.26 All of the following are common causes of frontal lobe syndrome *except*

A. trauma
B. infarcts
C. tumors
D. Parkinson's disease
E. multiple sclerosis

DIRECTIONS: Each set of lettered headings below is followed by a list of numbered words or statements. For each numbered word or statement, select the *one* lettered heading most closely associated with it. Each lettered heading may be selected once, more than once, or not at all.

Questions 3.27–3.31

A. Serotonin
B. Glycine
C. Norepinephrine
D. Acetylcholine
E. Dopamine

3.27 Median and dorsal raphe nuclei
3.28 Locus ceruleus
3.29 Nucleus basalis of Meynert
3.30 Substantia nigra
3.31 Spinal cord

Questions 3.32–3.34

A. Orbitofrontal region of prefrontal cortex
B. Dorsolateral region of prefrontal cortex
C. Medial region of prefrontal cortex

3.32 Lesions lead to deficiencies of planning and motivation
3.33 Lesions lead to disinhibition and lack of remorse
3.34 Lesions lead to profound apathy and limited spontaneous movement, gesture, and speech

Questions 3.35–3.38

    A. Left brain localization
    B. Right brain localization

3.35 Recognition of faces
3.36 Language functions
3.37 Prosody
3.38 Maintenance of attention

Questions 3.39–3.43

    A. Dopamine
    B. Serotonin
    C. Melatonin
    D. Anticholinergic drugs
    E. Growth hormone

3.39 Cause(s) dry mouth, constipation, blurred vision, urinary retention
3.40 Synthesized by serotonin, released by pineal body
3.41 Amphetamines cause release, cocaine blocks uptake
3.42 Dietary variations in tryptophan can affect brain levels
3.43 Released in pulses

ANSWERS

The Brain and Behavior

3.1 The answer is A

Enkephalins are *opioid-like peptides* that are found in many parts of the brain and that bind to specific receptor sites. They are opioid-like because they decrease pain perception. They also serve as neurotransmitters.

Cholinergic agents are drugs that cause the liberation of acetylcholine. *Dopamine-receptor antagonists* are drugs, such as the antipsychotic haloperidol (Haldol), that block dopamine receptors on postsynaptic neurons; thus, they effectively decrease the functional levels of the neurotransmitter dopamine. Dopamine antagonists are most often used to treat psychotic patients whose psychosis is related to a hyperdopaminergic state.

The two major classes of antidepressant drugs are the *selective serotonin reuptake inhibitors (SSRIs)* and the *tricyclic drugs.* SSRIs increase synaptic serotonin activity by inhibiting the reuptake of serotonin into the presynaptic terminal through the serotonin transporter. The tricyclic drugs are potent inhibitors of the reuptake inactivation mechanism of catecholamine and serotonin neurons. The ability of tricyclic drugs to inhibit the reuptake process results in a functional increase of such neurotransmitters as norepinephrine and serotonin and leads to the medications' antidepressant activity.

3.2 The answer is B

Many neuronal connections are either divergent or convergent in nature. A divergent system involves the conduction of information from one neuron or a discrete group of neurons to a much larger number of neurons that may be located in diverse portions of the brain. *The locus ceruleus, a small group of norepinephrine-containing neurons in the brainstem that sends axonal projections to the entire cerebral cortex and other brain regions, is an example of a divergent neuronal system, not a convergent system.* In contrast, the output of multiple brain regions may be directed toward a single area, forming a convergent system.

Many, but not all, connections between brain regions are reciprocal; that is, each region tends to receive input from those regions to which it sends axonal projections. In some cases, the axons arising from one region may directly innervate the recip- rocating projection neurons in another region; in other cases, local circuit interneurons are interposed between the incoming axons and the projection neurons that furnish the reciprocal connections. For some projections, the reciprocating connection is indirect, passing through one or more additional brain regions and synapses before innervating the initial brain region.

The connections among regions may be organized in a hierarchical or parallel fashion, or both. For example, *visual input is conveyed in a serial or hierarchical fashion* through several populations of neurons in the retina to the lateral geniculate nucleus, to the primary visual cortex, and then progressively to the multiple visual association areas of the cerebral cortex. Within the hierarchical scheme, different types of visual information (e.g., motion, form) may be processed in a parallel fashion through different portions of the visual system.

Regions of the brain are specialized for different functions. For example, lesions of the left inferior frontal gyrus (Broca's area) produce a characteristic impairment in speech production. However, speech is a complex faculty that depends not only on the integrity of Broca's area but also on the processing of information across a number of brain regions through divergent and convergent, serial and parallel interconnections. Thus, the role of any specific brain region in the production of specific behaviors cannot be viewed in isolation but *must be viewed within the context of the neural circuits connecting those neurons with other brain regions.*

3.3 The answer is E (all)

The basal ganglia are a collection of nuclei that have been grouped together on the basis of their interconnections. These nuclei play an important role in regulating movement and in certain disorders of movement (dyskinesias), which include jerky movements (chorea), writhing movements (athetosis), and rhythmic movements (tremors). In addition, recent studies have shown that certain components of the basal ganglia play an important role in many cognitive functions.

The basal ganglia are generally considered to include the *caudate nucleus,* the putamen, the globus pallidus (referred to as the paleostriatum or pallidum), the *subthalamic nucleus,* and the *substantia nigra.* The term *striatum* refers to the *caudate nucleus* and the *putamen* together; the term corpus striatum refers to the caudate nucleus, the putamen, and the globus pallidus; and the term *lentiform nucleus* refers to the putamen and the globus pallidus together (see Figure 3.1).

3.4 The answer is E (all)
Disruption of the input pathways of the basal ganglia has been associated with some movement disorders, such as *Parkinson's disease, which is characterized by muscular rigidity, fine tremor, shuffling gait,* and *bradykinesia.* The most consistent neuropathological feature of Parkinson's disease is a degeneration of the dopamine neurons in the substantia nigra pars compacta, accompanied by a loss of dopamine terminals in the striatum. Levodopa (Larodopa, Dopar), a precursor in the biosynthesis of dopamine, is used as a treatment for Parkinson's disease because of its ability to augment the release of dopamine from the remaining terminals. Conversely, the administration of dopamine receptor antagonists (so-called typical antipsychotics) in the treatment of schizophrenia is frequently associated with parkinsonian features and other motor-system abnormalities; the fact that these agents are D_2-receptor antagonists is thought to explain their movement-related adverse effects.

3.5 The answer is C
Neuroimaging with single photon emission computed tomography (SPECT) and positron emission tomography (PET) can investigate the functioning of brain regions in vivo. By imaging subjects during tasks, cerebral activity patterns reflect the functioning of neural networks necessary to perform the tasks. In numerous studies, individuals with schizophrenia show dysfunction within frontal-parietal-temporal networks, even during different tasks that utilize these cerebral areas. *There is decreased prefrontal cerebral blood flow on PET blood flow scans during certain tasks (when compared to healthy controls).* An example is the Wisconsin Card Sorting Test, an abstract problem-solving test requiring attention and working memory. Monozygotic twins discordant for schizophrenia underwent PET blood flow scans while performing this test. In all but one pair the ill twin had relatively decreased prefrontal cerebral blood flow; the area of temporal lobe limbic region in the ill twin was invariably hyperactive. In vivo studies do not speak to when or how the functional abnormality arose. However, finding functional consequences as the result of cerebral areas defined as abnormal in neuropathological investigations is essential in correlating neurodevelopmental abnormalities with the clinical symptoms of schizophrenia.

Imaging the brain with magnetic resonance imaging (MRI) allows for volumetric measurements of brain structure. In schizophrenia, *reductions on the order of 10 to 15 percent, not 50 to 60 percent, are reported in overall temporal lobe size,* in temporal lobe gray matter, and in specific temporal lobe structures. Recent MRI studies suggest subtle volumetric reductions in widespread cortical areas, including the frontal and parietal secondary association areas, and in the thalamus.

Schizophrenia is associated with enlarged ventricles and a *decrease (not increase) in the size of the amygdala,* hippocampus, and parahippocampal gyrus. There is a *lack, not a proliferation, of glial cells in schizophrenia.* A proliferation of glial cells is seen in degenerative brain conditions and encephalopathies that arise after birth. This does not occur in schizophrenia and suggests that whatever causes the brain abnormalities in schizophrenia does so before the third trimester of gestation because glial cells become responsive to injury only after the third trimester.

Of considerable interest in understanding the developmental neurobiology of schizophrenia are studies exploring cortical cytoarchitecture, particularly in the networks showing in vivo dysfunction. In the cortex of individuals with schizophrenia, heterotopic groups of neurons belonging to layer II are found displaced into layer III. *This may indicate abnormal neuronal migration* that results in heterotopic neuronal islands and abnormal cytoarchitecture. Layer II of the prefrontal cortex of persons with schizophrenia shows reduced numbers of small neurons and higher densities of pyramidal neurons in layer V.

3.6 The answer is B
The increase in nerve conduction velocity that accounts for the rapid processing capabilities of the brain is due to the presence of *myelin sheaths,* which encircle larger axons. Myelin is a highly hydrophobic substance that prevents the passage of ions. It is laid down along the axon in segments that are separated by gaps of bare axonal membrane, called nodes of Ranvier. The local changes in membrane charge constituting the action potential occur at the nodes of Ranvier and then jump over the myelin segment to the next node of Ranvier. For a given distance of axon, for example, the presence of myelin segments reduces the number of times the action potential must trigger neighboring voltage-gated ion channels to conduct an impulse along this distance of axon. The nerve conduction velocity may therefore increase to as high as 65 meters per second in large, myelinated fibers. The *axon hillock* is the segment of the axon located immediately adjacent to the cell body. When the membrane potential rises above the firing threshold, typically –55 to –50 mV, because of the actions of the dendritic ion channels, an action potential is generated. The axon hillock thus initiates but does not influence the rate of conduction of the action potential. During the action potential, the polarity of the membrane goes from negative to positive because of the actions of sodium and calcium channels. Calcium ion entry activates *voltage-sensitive potassium channels* that carry an outgoing flow of potassium ions involved in arresting the action potential. The activation of these potassium channels results in the afterhyperpolarization of the membrane following an action potential. During the afterhyperpolarization, the inside of the membrane is even more negatively charged than it was at baseline. The afterhyperpolarization contributes to the refractory period of a neuron after an action potential; during this period, another action potential cannot be generated. The principal ion pump, which generates the resting potential of the membrane, is the energy-requiring *sodium potassium adenosine triphosphatase (ATPase)* ion exchange pump. Ion pumps and ion channels maintain a gradient of cations: Potassium ions are 15 to 20 times more concentrated inside neurons, and sodium ions are 8 to 15 times less concentrated inside neurons with respect to the extracellular space. Inhibitory neurotransmitters open chloride channels to allow *chloride conductance,* which hyperpolarizes the membrane and decreases the likelihood of the generation of an action potential.

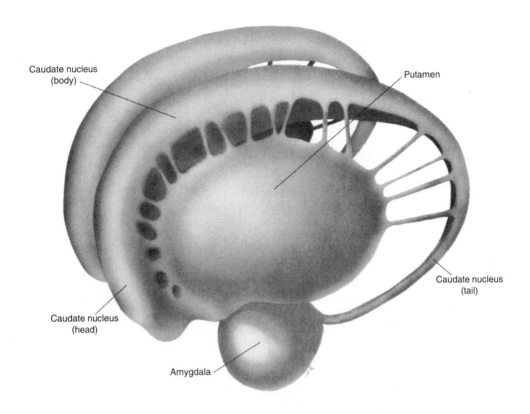

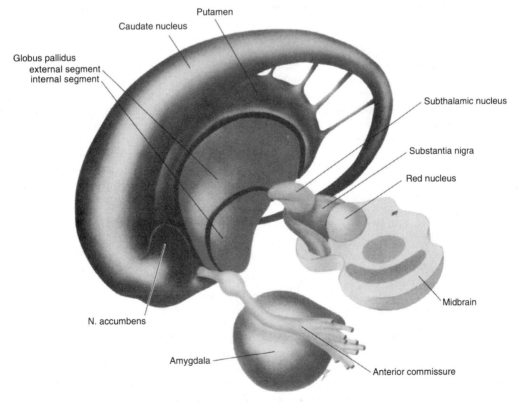

FIGURE 3.1

Schematic drawing of the isolated basal ganglia as seen from the dorsolateral perspective, so that the caudate nucleus is apparent bilaterally. In the bottom panel, the basal ganglia from the left hemisphere has been removed, exposing the medial surface of the right putamen and globus pallidus, as well as the subthalamic nucleus and substantia nigra. (Adapted from Hendelman WJ. *Student's Atlas of Neuroanatomy.* Philadelphia: Saunders; 1994.)

3.7 The answer is D

One reason to order a computed tomography (CT) scan in preference to a magnetic resonance imaging (MRI) scan is that *CT is superior in detecting calcified brain lesions.* Whether to order a CT or a more expensive MRI is one of the common clinical questions in psychiatric practice. The resolution of both techniques is under 1 mm, but *MRI has the capability of taking thinner slices through the brain, does have superior resolution,* and *can better distinguish between white matter and gray matter.* CT is based on X-ray technology; MRI utilizes magnetic fields. Therefore, *MRI, not CT, avoids exposing patients to radiation.*

3.8 The answer is C

GABA (γ-aminobutyric acid) and GABA receptor subtypes play a central role in the expression of seizures. GABA, as the major inhibitory neurotransmitter in the CNS, can be found in up to 30 percent of CNS synapses. In general, for the mature brain, loss or *blockade of GABA inhibition can result in increased hyperexcitability that results in seizures.* Several GABAergic drugs are widely used in the treatment of epilepsy. *Benzodiazepines and barbiturates act at GABA receptors* to enhance inhibition. Both have been shown to be effective in the control of partial, complex partial, and generalized tonic–clonic seizures. Benzodiazepines are also effective in the short-term treatment of generalized absence seizures, but a functional tolerance tends to develop, thereby reducing their efficacy. Barbiturates may exacerbate generalized absence seizures. Benzodiazepines are also effective in the treatment of atypical absence and myoclonic seizures. Anticonvulsant benzodiazepines and barbiturates are highly sedating, which limits their use.

Other evidence that the GABAergic system is important in the expression of seizures is that *manipulation of GABA has major effects on seizures.* It *can cause, exacerbate, or reduce seizure activity.* The mushroom poison picrotoxin antagonizes GABA receptors and can elicit seizures. Penicillin given at high doses (especially in renal failure patients or intrathecally) can also result in partial or generalized seizures. Penicillin reduces GABA-induced chloride current flow by blocking the ion channel pore.

In the mature or adult brain, *enhancement of GABA receptor function raises the seizure threshold.* Certain naturally occurring and synthetic steroids are potent modulators of GABA that may be associated with menstrually related epilepsy. *Reduction of GABA clearance, or raising the GABA level, is clinically effective.* Several of the pharmacological effects of ethanol are mediated through effects on GABA in chronic alcoholism, thus accounting for seizure activity.

3.9 The answer is D

Tardive dyskinesia is a late-appearing extra-pyramidal syndrome associated with antipsychotic drug use. It consists of slow, rhythmic, automatic stereotyped movements in one or more muscle groups *anywhere in the body.* It is most often characterized by repetitive *involuntary movements of the tongue, lips, and mouth* [buccolingual masticatory dyskinesia (BLM syndrome)]. In younger patients in particular, choreoathetoid movements of the trunk and limbs are also a part of the clinical picture. The mechanism of neuroleptic-induced dyskinesias appears to be related to a defect in the dopamine system secondary to prolonged phenothiazine use. Even though tardive

dyskinesia *follows prolonged phenothiazine use,* use of a different phenothiazine or the same phenothiazine in increased dosage and butyrophenones may relieve the associated symptoms. Because phenothiazines and butyrophenones appear to block dopamine receptors, this outcome seems to suggest that the mechanism responsible for tardive dyskinesia is an overcompensation of dopamine systems to the dopamine receptor blockade. It appears that after prolonged exposure to phenothiazines, dopamine receptors may become supersensitive to the effects of dopamine. Although neuroleptic agents may be the most likely drugs to be associated with the syndrome, it is known to be *induced also by the tricyclic antidepressants.*

3.10 The answer is C

Echolalia is one of the least likely signs of injury to the dorsolateral region, which appears to be the executive headquarters of the brain. Lesions in the dorsolateral region lead to *deficiencies* of *planning and monitoring.* There may be an *inability to use foresight and feedback.* Patients are unable to maintain goal directness, focus, and to sustain effort, and they appear inattentive and undermotivated. They cannot plan novel cognitive activity, and exhibit a tendency to linger on a trivial thought. They may react only to the details of environmental stimuli. In other words, they "miss the forest for the trees." On formal neuropsychological testing, however, they may exhibit intact memory, language, and visuospatial skills, which are functions of the occipital, temporal, and parietal lobes, respectively. Dorsolateral frontal lobe injury may also produce *mood disorders.*

The frontal lobes constitute a category unto themselves, the region that determines how the brain acts on its knowledge. There are four subdivisions of the frontal lobes. The first three, the motor strip, the supplemental motor area, and Broca's area, are components of the motor and language systems. The fourth, the most anterior division, is the prefrontal cortex. In the prefrontal cortex there are three regions—the orbitofrontal, the dorsolateral, and the medial—lesions of which produce distinct syndromes. *Akinetic mutism is characteristic of injury to the medial region,* especially the anterior cingulate gyrus, which normally appears to initiate a wide range of activities. Ablation of the medial region may produce a profound apathy characterized by limited spontaneous movement, gesture, and speech. Figure 3.2 illustrates language areas of the left hemisphere.

3.11 The answer is A

The two radiotracer methods of neuroimaging, positron emission tomography (PET) and single photon emission computed tomography (SPECT), *entail the injection of radioactively labeled drugs.* The imaging and measurement over time of the distribution of these radiotracers is used to assess the neurochemistry, blood flow, or metabolism of the brain. The three methods based on nuclear magnetic resonance are MRI, functional MRI (fMRI), and magnetic resonance spectroscopy (MRS). In general terms, MRI provides *exquisitely detailed images of brain structure*; fMRI provides images of local neuronal activity with high spatial and temporal resolution; and MRS provides measurements of the concentrations of numerous chemicals in the brain without the radiation exposure of PET and SPECT but with much lower sensitivity.

In PET and SPECT a biological process of interest is studied by synthetically incorporating a radionuclide into a mole-

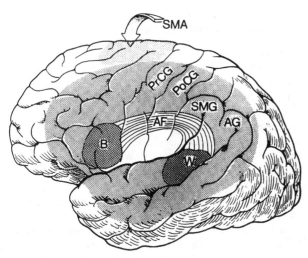

FIGURE 3.2

Language areas of the left hemisphere: *B*, Broca's area; *W*, Wernicke's area; *AF*, arcuate fasciculus; *SMA*, supplementary motor area; *PrCG*, precentral gyrus; *PoCG*, postcentral gyrus; *SMG*, supramarginal gyrus; and *AG*, angular gyrus. Language comprehension occurs in Wernicke's area, which is connected to Broca's area by the arcuate fasciculus. Generation of speech occurs in Broca's area. (Reprinted with permission from Filley CM. *Neurobehavioral Anatomy*. Niwot, CO: University Press of Colorado; 1995:76.)

cule of known physiological relevance. The so-called radiopharmaceutical is then administered to a patient either by inhalation, ingestion, or most commonly by intravenous injection. As radioactivity distributes within the subject, the radiotracer's uptake into the brain is measured over time and is used to obtain information about the physiological process of interest. *PET and SPECT rely on sophisticated principles to produce three-, not two-, dimensional information* (as in a chest X-ray). In order to understand this process, a basic understanding of the physics of photon emission is required.

Although some of the methods, such as structural magnetic resonance imaging (MRI), have been a standard component of the clinical assessment of patients with neurological disorders for more than a decade, similar *clinical applications have not yet been found for patients with psychiatric disorders*. These methods are largely restricted to research studies. Neuroimaging is also attractive to the field of psychiatry because it provides direct measurements of the brain and therefore passes the limitations of peripheral measures (e.g., concentrations of plasma hormones or urinary catecholamine metabolites), which generate only indirect assessments of central nervous system function.

3.12 The answer is B

MRI *has provided some evidence that there may be structural brain changes in major depressive disorder.* Although there have been fewer studies of mood disorders than of schizophrenia, some consistent findings have emerged. In major depressive disorder, smaller volumes of the frontal lobe, the cerebellum, the caudate, and the putamen have been reported. On the basis of these observations, neuroanatomic models of mood regulation involving specific frontosubcortical circuits have been proposed.

In patients with bipolar I disorder, the most commonly reported finding is the presence of an enlarged third ventricle. As the third ventricle lies adjacent to the hypothalamus, some researchers have suggested that hypothalamic dysfunction may play a role in the pathogenesis of bipolar I disorder. Less commonly, decreased volumes of the cerebellum and temporal lobes have also been noted.

In terms of pathological findings, several groups have reported an increased incidence of white matter hyperintensities in individuals with bipolar I disorder; unfortunately, neither the cause nor the clinical significance of these hyperintensities has been clearly established.

Even with the increased resolution provided by MRI scanning, it remains *as yet unproved (not proved) whether there are relatively specific structural brain changes in patients with schizophrenia or if cerebral mass reduction is nonspecific.* Several studies have provided convincing data regarding reduced volume in specific cortical regions, including prefrontal cortex and temporal cortical regions. Such changes have even been found in patients early in the course of illness, suggesting that the structural changes observed in the cortex are present at the onset of the illness and do not stem from progression of the illness or from iatrogenic factors. *Enlargement of caudate volume has also been reported early in the course of the illness, but multiple studies suggest that caudate enlargement may be secondary to treatment with typical dopamine-receptor antagonist agents. More recently it has been suggested that this enlargement recedes with clozapine (Clozaril) treatment.

Of the substance abuse disorders, alcohol dependence has been the most thoroughly studied using MRI. *Current evidence suggests that alcohol dependence leads to generalized reductions in brain mass* as reflected by decreases in cortical gray and white matter and increased cerebrospinal fluid volume of the cerebral ventricles, particularly the lateral ventricles. Many of the changes may be at least partially reversed during sustained periods of abstinence. *MRI is superior (not inferior) to CT in visualizing gray versus white matter.*

3.13 The answer is E

Peripheral serotonin is located in platelets, mast cells, and enterochromaffin cells of the gastrointestinal system. The *CNS contains less than 2 percent of the serotonin in the body;* despite the abundance of peripheral serotonin, it is *unable to cross the blood–brain barrier,* necessitating the synthesis of serotonin within the brain. *Serotonin is synthesized from the amino acid tryptophan,* which is derived from the diet. The rate-limiting step in serotonin synthesis is the hydroxylation of tryptophan by the enzyme tryptophan hydroxylase to form 5-hydroxytryptophan (5-HTP). Under normal circumstances this enzyme is not saturated by substrate, *so tryptophan concentration can affect the rate of serotonin synthesis.* Because tryptophan competes with other large neutral amino acids for transport, brain uptake of this amino acid is determined both by the amount of circulating tryptophan and by the ratio of tryptophan to other large neutral amino acids. This ratio *may be elevated by carbohydrate intake,* which induces insulin release and the uptake of many large-chain amino acids into peripheral tissues. Conversely, high-protein foods tend to be relatively low in tryptophan, thus lowering this ratio. The administration of specialized low-tryptophan diets has been found to produce significant declines in brain serotonin levels. Following tryptophan hydroxylation, 5-HTP is rapidly decarboxylated by aromatic amino acid decarboxylase to form serotonin.

3.14 The answer is E (all)

Pathological alterations in hypothalamic-pituitary-adrenal function have been associated primarily with *mood disorders, posttraumatic stress disorder,* and *dementia of the Alzheimer's type,* and in *substance use disorders.* Hypothalamic-pituitary-adrenal abnormalities are reversed in individuals who are successfully treated with antidepressant medications, and failure to normalize hypothalamic-pituitary-adrenal abnormalities is a poor prognostic sign.

Exposure to chronic stress produces increased concentrations of corticotropin-releasing factor (CRF) in the paraventricular nucleus of the hypothalamus. Release of CRF results in a simultaneous activation of the locus-ceruleus noradrenergic circuit, which functionally increases arousal and selective attention, and decreases vegetative functions such as appetite and sex drive. ACTH concentrations are increased in acute stress, but diminish over time in sustained stress, suggesting that corticosteroid receptor downregulation at the level of the hippocampus leads to an inhibition of negative feedback on CRF.

3.15 The answer is B

Fluorine-18 [^{18}F]-fluorodeoxyglucose (FDG) is an analogue that the brain cannot metabolize. Glucose is by far the predominant energy source available to brain cells, and its utilization is therefore a highly sensitive indicator of the rate of brain metabolism. Thus, the brain regions with the highest metabolic rate and the highest blood flow take up the most FDG but are unable to metabolize and excrete the usual metabolic products. The concentration of ^{18}F builds up in these neurons and is detected by the PET camera. FDG PET therefore measures glucose metabolism.

Each of the other choices measures blood flow rather than metabolism. Blood flow generally is proportional to brain metabolism and may be measured by a wider variety of clinical techniques. *Xenon-133* is a noble gas that is inhaled directly and is detected by SPECT scanners. The xenon quickly enters the blood and is distributed to areas of the brain as a function of regional blood flow. It may therefore be referred to as the regional cerebral blood flow (rCBF) technique. Because of technical factors, xenon SPECT can measure blood flow only on the surface of the brain. This limitation is important because many mental tasks require communication between the cortex and subcortical structures, and the latter activity is missed by xenon SPECT. Assessment of blood flow over the whole brain with SPECT requires the injectable tracers, *technetium-99* (^{99}Tc) *d,l-hexamethylpropyleneamine oxime* [*HMPAO* (Ceretec)] or iodoamphetamine (Spectamine).

These radiotracers are highly lipophilic, cross the blood–brain barrier rapidly, and enter cells. Once inside a cell, the ligands are enzymatically converted to charged ions, which remain trapped in the cell. Thus, over time, the tracers are concentrated in areas of relatively higher blood flow. Although blood flow is usually assumed to be the major variable tested in HMPAO SPECT, local variations in the permeability of the blood–brain barrier and in the enzymatic conversion of the ligands in cells also contribute to regional differences in signal levels. In *nitrogen-13* (^{13}N) PET, the radioactive nitrogen isotope (^{13}N) is usually linked to another molecule that is distributed into cells as a function of blood flow.

3.16 The answer is C

The search for the genetic basis of bipolar I disorder *has been less (not more) successful than* that for Alzheimer's disease. Bipolar I disorder is an episodic illness characterized by recurrent periods of both mania and depression; psychotic symptoms are often a part of the clinical picture, particularly in more severely affected individuals. Some epidemiological studies have indicated that there may be *a single major gene with incomplete penetrance responsible for the disorder* in some families; however, the mode of inheritance in these studies is inconsistent—some have indicated autosomal dominant inheritance whereas others have suggested X-linked or recessive inheritance. Recent studies indicate that the genetics of bipolar I disorder provide *evidence for genetic heterogeneity, multifactorial inheritance,* or both. Problems with linkage studies of bipolar I disorder have included many (not few) difficulties with *phenotype definition.* Using a narrowly defined phenotype often means using fewer individuals with less accurate results.

The genetic studies of bipolar disorders in the Amish illustrate many of the difficulties of doing genetic analysis on complex disorders. The Amish appear to be a perfect population for such investigations; they are an isolated population with known genealogies, clean phenotypes with little comorbidity, and large extended families. However, the findings for bipolar disorders in this group have so far been inconsistent or contradictory, and even in this ideal population there has been *no strong evidence for genetic linkage.*

3.17 The answer is D

The movements of the body muscles are controlled by the lower motor neurons, which extend axons, some as long as 1 meter in length, to the muscle fibers. *The firing of the lower motor neurons is regulated by the summation of upper motor neuron activity.* In the brainstem, primitive systems produce gross coordinated movements of the entire body. Activation of the rubrospinal tract stimulates flexion of all limbs, *whereas activation of the vestibulospinal tract causes all limbs to extend. In newborn infants, for example, all limbs are held tightly flexed, presumably through the dominance of the rubrospinal system. In fact, the movements of an anencephalic infant, who completely lacks a cerebral cortex, may be indistinguishable from the movements of a normal newborn.* In the first few months of life, the flexor spasticity is mitigated gradually by the opposite actions of the vestibulospinal fibers, and more limb mobility occurs.

At the top of the motor hierarchy is the *corticospinal tract, which controls fine movements* and eventually dominates the brainstem system during the first years of life. The upper motor neurons of the corticospinal tract reside in the posterior frontal lobe, in a section of cortex known as the motor strip. Planned movements are conceived in the association areas of the brain, and, in consultation with the basal ganglia and cerebellum, the motor cortex directs their smooth execution. *The importance of the corticospinal system becomes immediately evident in strokes, where spasticity results as the cortical influence is ablated and the actions of the brainstem motor systems are released from cortical modulation.*

3.18 The answer is E

The *basal ganglia,* a subcortical group of gray matter nuclei, appear to mediate postural tone. There are four functionally distinct ganglia: the striatum, the pallidum, the substantia nigra, and the subthalamic nucleus. The caudate nucleus plays an important role in the modulation of motor acts. When functioning properly, it acts as a gatekeeper to allow the motor system to perform only those acts that are goal directed. *Anatomic and functional neuroimaging studies have correlated decreased activation of the caudate with obsessive-compulsive behavior. The caudate also shrinks dramatically in Huntington's disease.* This disorder is characterized by rigidity, on which is gradually superimposed choreiform or "dancing" movements. Psychosis may be a prominent feature of Huntington's disease, and suicide is not uncommon.

The globus pallidus contains two parts. The internal and external parts of the globus pallidus are nested within the concavity of the putamen. The globus pallidus receives input from the corpus striatum and projects fibers to the thalamus. *This structure may be severely damaged in Wilson's disease* and in carbon monoxide poisoning, which are characterized by dystonic posturing and flapping movements of the arms and legs.

The substantia nigra is named the black substance because the presence of melanin pigment causes it to appear black to the naked eye. It *degenerates in Parkinson's disease. Parkinsonism* is characterized by rigidity and tremor and is associated with depression in over 30 percent of cases.

Lesions in the subthalamic nucleus yield ballistic movements, which are sudden limb jerks of such velocity that they are compared to projectile movement (hemiballismus).

3.19 The answer is E (all)

Arousal, or the establishment and maintenance of an awake state, appears to require at least three brain regions. Within the brainstem, *the ascending reticular activating system (ARAS), a diffuse set of neurons, appears to set the level of consciousness.* The ARAS projects to the intralaminar nuclei of the thalamus, and these nuclei in turn project widely throughout the cortex. Electrophysiological studies show that *both the thalamus and the cortex fire rhythmic bursts of neuronal activity at the rates of 20 to 40 cycles per second.* During sleep, these bursts are not synchronized. *During wakefulness, the ARAS stimulates the thalamic intralaminar nuclei, which in turn coordinate the oscillations of different cortical regions.* The greater the synchronization, the higher the level of wakefulness. The absence of arousal produces stupor and coma. In general, *small discrete lesions of the ARAS may produce a stuporous state, whereas at the hemispheric level, large bilateral lesions are required to cause the same depression in alertness.* One particularly unfortunate but instructive condition involving extensive, permanent bilateral cortical dysfunction is the persistent vegetative state. Sleep–wake cycles may be preserved, and the eyes may appear to gaze, but there is no registering of the external world and no evidence of conscious thought.

3.20 The answer is D

The maintenance of attention appears to require an intact right *frontal lobe. For example, a widely used test of persistence requires scanning and identifying only the letter "A" from a long list of random letters. Normal individuals can usually*

Table 3.1
Major Causes of Acute Confusion

Toxic
  Prescription drugs
  Nonprescription drugs
  Drug withdrawal
Metabolic
  Hypoxia
  Hypoglycemia
  Uremia
  Hepatic disease
  Thiamine deficiency
  Electrolyte disturbances
  Endocrinopathies
Infectious and inflammatory
  Meningitis
  Encephalitis
  Vasculitis
  Abscess
Epileptic
  Postictal state
  Complex partial status epilepticus
  Absence status epilepticus
Vascular
  Stroke
  Subarachnoid hemorrhage
Traumatic
  Concussion
  Severe traumatic brain injury
Neoplastic
  Deep midline tumors
  Increased intracranial pressure
Postsurgical
  Preoperative atropine
  Hypoxia
  Analgesics
  Electrolyte imbalance
  Fever

Reprinted with permission from Filley CM. *Neurobehavioral Anatomy.* Niwot, CO: University Press of Colorado; 1995:52.

maintain performance of such a task for several minutes, but in patients with right frontal lobe dysfunction, this capacity is curtailed severely. Lesions of similar size in other regions of the cortex usually do not affect persistence tasks. In contrast, the more generally adaptive skill of maintaining a coherent line of thought is distributed diffusely throughout the cortex. Major causes of confusion are listed in Table 3.1.

3.21 The answer is E

The *substantia nigra* is involved with metabolic disturbances associated with Parkinson's and Huntington's diseases.

Three brain structures are critical to the formation of memories: the *medial temporal lobe,* certain diencephalic nuclei, and the basal forebrain. The *medial temporal lobe* houses the *hippocampus. The amygdala,* which is adjacent to the anterior end of the hippocampus, assesses the emotional importance of an experience and activates the level of hippocampal activity accordingly. Thus, an emotionally intense experience is etched in memory. Within the diencephalon, the dorsal medial nucleus of the thalamus and *the mamillary bodies* appear necessary for memory formation.

3.22 The answer is C

The most famous human subject in the study of memory is H. M., a man with intractable epilepsy, whose entire hippocampus and amygdala were surgically removed. The epilepsy was thus controlled, but he was left with *a complete inability to form and recall memories of facts.* The finding that H. M.'s *learning and memory skills were relatively preserved* has led to the suggestion that factual memory may be separate within the brain from skill-related memory. A complementary deficit in skill-related memory with preservation of factual memory may be seen in individuals with Parkinson's disease, in whom dopaminergic neurons of the nigrostriatal tract degenerate. Because this deficit in skill-related memory can be ameliorated with levodopa, which is thought to potentiate dopaminergic neurotransmission in the nigrostriatal pathway, a role has been postulated for dopamine in skill-related memory. Additional case reports have implicated the amygdala and the afferent and efferent fiber tracts of the hippocampus as being essential to the formation of memories. Lesional studies have also suggested a mild lateralization of hippocampal function in which the left hippocampus is more efficient at forming verbal memories and the right hippocampus tends to form nonverbal memories. After unilateral lesions in humans, however, the remaining hippocampus may compensate to a large extent. Medical causes of amnesia include alcoholism, seizures, migraine, drugs, vitamin deficiencies, trauma, strokes, tumors, infections, and degenerative diseases. *Ataxia and loss of vision are unrelated to the hippocampus and amygdalae.*

3.23 The answer is A

The dorsal medial nucleus of the thalamus and *the mamillary bodies appear necessary for memory formation.* These two structures are damaged in thiamine deficiency states usually seen in chronic alcoholics, and their inactivation is associated with Korsakoff's syndrome. This syndrome is characterized by severe inability to form new memories and a variable inability to recall remote memories. Patients may confabulate to resolve gaps in memory.

The *substantia nigra* is involved with metabolic disturbances associated with Parkinson's disease.

The medial temporal lobe houses the *hippocampus,* an elongated, highly repetitive network. The *amygdala* is adjacent to the anterior end of the hippocampus. These structures attach emotional importance to memories.

The *caudate nucleus* has been implicated in the pathophysiology of Huntington's disease.

3.24 The answer is C

Several studies have suggested a hemispheric dichotomy within the cortex of emotional representation. The left hemisphere houses the analytical mind but may have a limited emotional repertoire. Lesions to the right hemisphere, which cause profound functional deficits, may be noted with indifference by the intact left hemisphere. *The denial of illness (called anosognosia) and inability to move the left hand are associated with injury to the right hemisphere.*

In contrast, *left hemisphere lesions, which cause profound aphasia, may trigger a catastrophic depression, as the intact right hemisphere struggles with the realization of the loss.* The right hemisphere appears dominant for affect, socialization, and body image.

Damage to the left hemisphere produces intellectual disorder and a loss of the narrative aspect of dreams. Damage to the right hemisphere produces affective disorders, loss of the visual aspects of dreams, and a failure to respond to humor, shadings of metaphor, and connotations.

3.25 The answer is A

Within the hemispheres, the temporal and frontal lobes play a prominent role in emotion. The temporal lobe exhibits a high frequency of epileptic foci. *TLE is of particular interest in psychiatry because temporal lobe seizures may often manifest bizarre behavior without the classic grand mal shaking movements caused by seizures in the motor cortex. A proposed TLE personality is characterized by hyposexuality, emotional intensity, and a perseverative approach to interactions, termed viscosity.* Patients with left TLE may generate references to personal destiny and philosophical themes and may display a humorless approach to life. In contrast, patients with right TLE may display excessive emotionality, ranging from elation to sadness. Although TLE patients may display excessive aggression between seizures, the seizure itself may evoke fear.

The inverse of a TLE personality appears in people with bilateral injury to the temporal lobes after head trauma, cardiac arrest, herpes simplex encephalitis, or in Pick's disease. *This lesion resembles the one described in the Kluver-Bucy syndrome, an experimental model of temporal lobe ablation in monkeys. Behavior in this syndrome is characterized by hypersexuality, placidity, a tendency to explore the environment with the mouth, inability to recognize the emotional significance of visual stimuli, and constantly shifting attention, called hypermetamorphosis.*

3.26 The answer is D

Bilateral lesions of the frontal lobes are characterized by changes in personality and how people interact with the world. The *frontal lobe syndrome,* which is *most commonly produced by trauma, infarcts, tumors, lobotomy, multiple sclerosis, or Pick's disease,* consists of slowed thinking, poor judgment, decreased curiosity, social withdrawal, and irritability. Patients typically manifest an apathetic indifference to experience that can suddenly explode into impulsive disinhibition. Unilateral frontal lobe lesions may be largely unnoticed because the intact lobe can compensate with high efficiency. *Parkinson's disease* is caused by lesions to the substantia nigra.

Answers 3.27–3.31

3.27 The answer is A

3.28 The answer is C

3.29 The answer is D

3.30 The answer is E

3.31 The answer is B

The major site of serotonergic cell bodies is in the upper pons and the midbrain—specifically, the *median and dorsal raphe nuclei.* These neurons project to the basal ganglia, the limbic system, and the cerebral cortex.

The major concentration of norepinephrine in the cell bodies that project upward in the brain is in the *locus ceruleus* in the pons. The axons of these neurons project through the medial forebrain bundle to the cerebral cortex, the limbic system, the thalamus, and the hypothalamus.

A group of acetylcholine producing neurons in the *nucleus basalis of Meynert* project to the cerebral cortex, the limbic system, the hypothalamus, and the thalamus. Some patients with dementia of the Alzheimer's type or Down's syndrome appear to have degeneration of the neurons in the nucleus basalis of Meynert.

The three most important dopaminergic producing tracts for psychiatry are the nigrostriatal tract, the mesolimbic-mesocortical tract, and the tuberoinfundibular tract. The nigrostriatal tract projects from its cell bodies in the *substantia nigra* to the corpus striatum. When the dopamine (D_2) receptors at the end of this tract are blocked by classic antipsychotic drugs, parkinsonian side effects emerge. In Parkinson's disease the nigrostriatal tract degenerates and results in the rotor symptoms of the disease. Because of the significant association between Parkinson's disease and depression, the nigrostriatal tract may also be involved with the control of mood, in addition to its classic role in motor control.

The receptor for the inhibitory amino acid neurotransmitter glycine is present in highest quantities in the *spinal cord.* Mutations in the glycine receptor cause a rare neurological condition called hyperekplexia, which is characterized by an exaggerated startle response.

Answers 3.32–3.34

3.32 The answer is B

3.33 The answer is A

3.34 The answer is C

The *frontal lobes,* the region that determines how the brain acts on its knowledge, constitute a category unto themselves. In comparative neuroanatomical studies, the massive size of the frontal lobes is the main feature that distinguishes the human brain from that of other primates and that lends it uniquely human qualities. Within the prefrontal cortex, there are three regions, lesions of which produce distinct syndromes: the *orbitofrontal,* the *dorsolateral,* and the *medial.*

Dysfunction of the orbitofrontal area causes *disinhibition and lack of remorse.* Insight and judgment are impaired. The dorsolateral area appears to be the executive headquarters of the brain. Lesions in this region lead to *deficiencies of planning and motivation.* Patients may be unable to use foresight and feedback and to maintain goal directedness, focus, and sustained effort. Dorsolateral frontal lobe injury may also produce mood disorders. On formal neuropsychological testing, however, patients may exhibit intact memory, language, and visuospatial skills, which are functions of the occipital, temporal, and parietal lobes.

The medial area appears to initiate a wide range of activities. Ablation of this region may produce a *profound apathy characterized by limited spontaneous movement, gesture, and speech.* In the extreme, there may be a state of akinetic mutism, without any initiation of activity at all.

Answers 3.35–3.38

3.35 The answer is A

3.36 The answer is A

3.37 The answer is B

3.38 The answer is B

Hemispheric lateralization of function is a key feature of higher cortical processing. The primary sensory cortices for touch, vision, hearing, smell, and taste are represented bilaterally. However, *recognition of faces* appears localized to the left brain. The clearest known example of hemispheric lateralization is the localization *of language functions* to the left hemisphere. *Prosody,* the emotional components of language, appears to be localized in the right brain.

The maintenance of attention appears to require an intact right frontal lobe. One widely diagnosed disorder of attention is attention-deficit/hyperactivity disorder (ADHD). No pathological findings have been associated consistently with this disorder. Functional neuroimaging studies have variously documented either frontal lobe or right hemisphere hypometabolism in ADHD patients.

Answers 3.39–3.43

3.39 The answer is D

3.40 The answer is C

3.41 The answer is A

3.42 The answer is B

3.43 The answer is E

Blockade of *anticholinergic and cholinergic* receptors is a common pharmacodynamic effect of many psychotropic drugs. Blockage of these receptors leads to the commonly seen side effects of blurred vision, dry mouth, constipation, and difficulty in initiating urination. Excessive blockage of cholinergic receptors causes confusion and delirium. Melatonin is released by the pineal body, which also contains many other peptides and hormones.

Melatonin is secreted when the eye perceives darkness, and its release is inhibited when the eye perceives light. Melatonin is synthesized from serotonin by the action of two enzymes: serotonin-*N*-acetylase anal 5-hydroxyindole-*O*-methyltransferase. Melatonin is involved in the regulation of circadian rhythms and has been implicated in the pathophysiology of depression.

Substances that affect the dopamine system include amphetamine and cocaine. Amphetamines cause the release of *dopamine* and cocaine blocks the uptake of dopamine. Thus, both substances increase the amount of dopamine present in the synapse. Cocaine and methamphetamine (Desoxyn) are among the most addicting substances. Their use may permanently deplete the brain's stores of dopamine. The dopaminergic systems may be particularly involved in the brain's so-called reward system, and this involvement may explain the high addiction potential of cocaine. Mutant "knockout mice," in which the dopamine transport gene has been experimentally deleted, do not respond biochemically or behaviorally to cocaine. This suggests that the dopamine transporter is necessary for the pharmacological effects of cocaine.

The precursor amino acid to *serotonin* is tryptophan. Dietary variations in tryptophan can measurably affect serotonin levels in the brain. Tryptophan depletion causes irritability and hunger, whereas tryptophan supplementation may induce sleep, relieve anxiety, and increase a sense of well-being. Once synthesized, serotonin is packaged into vesicles for release upon the arrival of an action potential. The synaptic action of serotonin concludes by reuptake into the presynaptic terminal by the plasma.

The components of the *growth hormone* axis are growth hormone–releasing hormone (GHRH) and growth hormone–release-inhibiting factor (GHRIF), also known as somatostatin, from the hypothalamus, and growth hormone itself from the anterior pituitary. Growth hormone is released in pulses throughout the day. The pulses are closer together during the first hours of sleep than at other times. Growth hormone regulation has been studied particularly in schizophrenia and mood disorders, in which some data suggest a disordered regulation of the growth hormone axis.

4

Contributions of the Psychosocial Sciences to Human Behavior

The psychosocial sciences include psychology, anthropology, sociology, ethology, and epidemiology, among others. Our understanding of human behavior has been enriched by the work of professionals in each of these fields.

Students should be able to define these disciplines, and a brief description of each follows: Psychology is concerned with behavior and its related mental and physiological processes. There are several types, ranging from clinical psychology that specializes in applying psychological theory to persons with emotional or behavioral disorders to *educational psychology,* which is the application of psychological principles to problems of teaching and learning. *Anthropology* is that branch of science concerned with the origin and development of humans in all their physical, social, and cultural relationships. *Sociology* is the study of the collective behaviors of human beings, including the developmental structure and interactions of their social institutions. *Ethology* is the study of animal behaviors and *epidemiology* is the study of the various factors that determine the frequency and distribution of diseases.

Jean Piaget (1896–1980) focused on the ways that children think and develop cognitive abilities, describing four major stages leading to more adult organizations of thought. John Bowlby (1907–1990) focused on the development of attachment and the belief that normal attachment in infancy is essential to ongoing healthy development. René Spitz (1887–1974) described anaclitic depression, or hospitalism, in which normal children who were separated for long periods from adequate caregiving in institutions failed to thrive, becoming depressed and nonresponsive. Ethologists such as Konrad Lorenz (1903–1988) and Harry Harlow (1905–1981) studied bonding and attachment behaviors in animals, and showed how studying animal behavior could help to illuminate human behavior.

Learning theory was developed by such behavioral researchers as Ivan Pavlov (1849–1936), John B. Watson (1878–1958), and B. F. Skinner (1904–1990). Tenets of learning theory, including operant and classical conditioning, underlie behavioral treatments of various mental disorders.

The questions and answers below will help students test their knowledge of the subjects highlighted.

HELPFUL HINTS

The student should know the following terms, theoreticians, and concepts.

- abstract thinking
- accommodation
- acculturation
- adaptation
- aggression
- Mary Ainsworth
- anaclitic depression
- animistic thinking
- anxiety hierarchy
- *Aplysia*
- assimilation
- attachment
- attachment phases
- attribution theory
- aversive stimuli
- basic study design
- behavior disorders
- Ruth Benedict

- bias
- biostatistics
- bonding
- John Bowlby
- catharsis
- chronic stress
- cognitive dissonance
- cognitive organization
- cognitive strategies
- cognitive triad
- concrete operations
- contact comfort
- cross-cultural studies and syndromes: amok, *latah, windigo, piblokto, curandero, esperitismo,* voodoo
- culture-bound syndromes
- deductive reasoning

- deviation, significance
- double-blind method
- drift hypothesis
- egocentric
- epidemiology
- epigenesis
- escape and avoidance conditioning
- ethology
- experimental neurosis
- extinction
- family types, studies
- Faris and Dunham
- fixed and variable ratios
- formal operations
- frequency
- frustration-aggression hypothesis

- genetic epistemology
- Harry Harlow
- Hollingshead and Redlich
- Holmes and Rahe
- hospitalism
- Clark L. Hull
- illness behavior
- imprinting
- incidence
- indirect surveys
- inductive reasoning
- information processing
- inhibition
- Eric Kandel
- learned helplessness
- learning theory
- Alexander Leighton

- ▶ H. S. Liddell
- ▶ lifetime expectancy
- ▶ Konrad Lorenz
- ▶ Margaret Mead
- ▶ Midtown Manhattan study
- ▶ monotropic
- ▶ Monroe County study
- ▶ motivation
- ▶ New Haven study
- ▶ normative
- ▶ object permanence
- ▶ operant and classical conditioning
- ▶ operant behavior
- ▶ organization
- ▶ Ivan Petrovich Pavlov
- ▶ phenomenalistic causality

- ▶ Jean Piaget
- ▶ positive and negative reinforcement
- ▶ preattachment stage
- ▶ preoperational stage
- ▶ prevalence
- ▶ protest-despair-detachment
- ▶ punishment
- ▶ randomization
- ▶ reciprocal determinism
- ▶ reciprocal inhibition
- ▶ reliability
- ▶ respondent behavior
- ▶ risk factors
- ▶ schema
- ▶ segregation hypothesis
- ▶ Hans Selye

- ▶ semiotic function
- ▶ sensorimotor stage
- ▶ sensory deprivation
- ▶ separation anxiety
- ▶ signal indicators
- ▶ B. F. Skinner
- ▶ social causation and selection theory
- ▶ social class and mental disorders
- ▶ social isolation and separation
- ▶ social learning
- ▶ sociobiology
- ▶ René Spitz
- ▶ stimulus generalization
- ▶ Stirling County study

- ▶ strange situation
- ▶ stranger anxiety
- ▶ surrogate mother
- ▶ syllogistic reasoning
- ▶ symbolization
- ▶ systematic desensitization
- ▶ tension-reduction theory
- ▶ therapist monkeys
- ▶ Nikolaas Tinbergen
- ▶ type I and type II errors
- ▶ use of controls
- ▶ validity
- ▶ variation, average
- ▶ vulnerability theory
- ▶ John B. Watson
- ▶ Joseph Wolpe

▲ QUESTIONS

DIRECTIONS: Each of the questions or incomplete statements below is followed by five suggested responses or completions. Select the *one* that is *best* in each case.

4.1 True statements about violence and aggression include all of the following *except*

- A. In the United States, homicide is the second leading cause of death among people 15 to 25 years of age.
- B. A young black man is 8 times more likely to be murdered than is a white man of the same age.
- C. Less than 50 percent of people who commit homicides or assaultive behavior have imbibed significant amounts of alcohol immediately beforehand.
- D. The best predictor of violent acts is a previous violent act.
- E. More than 70 percent of homicides are committed with handguns.

4.2 Attachment theory states

- A. Infants are generally polytropic in their attachments.
- B. Attachment occurs instantaneously between the mother and the child.
- C. Attachment is synonymous with bonding.
- D. Attachment disorders may lead to a failure to thrive.
- E. Separation anxiety is most common when an infant is 5 months old.

4.3 In operant conditioning

- A. Continuous reinforcement is the reinforcement schedule least susceptible to extinction.
- B. Negative reinforcement is a type of punishment.
- C. The process is related to trial-and-error learning.
- D. Shaping occurs when responses are coincidentally paired to a reinforcer.
- E. Respondent behavior is independent of a stimulus.

4.4 The increased frequency of aggressive behavior in certain children defined as abnormal has been correlated with all of the following *except*

- A. brain injury
- B. faulty identification models
- C. cultural environment
- D. violence in movies
- E. curiosity

4.5 Cross-cultural studies

- A. are free from experimental bias
- B. show that depression is not a universally expressed symptom
- C. show that incest is not a universal taboo
- D. show that schizophrenic persons are universally stigmatized as social outcasts
- E. show that the nuclear family of mother, father, and children is a universal unit

4.6 Prevalence is the

- A. proportion of a population that has a condition at one moment in time
- B. ratio of persons who acquire a disorder during a year's time
- C. risk of acquiring a condition at some time
- D. standard deviation
- E. rate of first admissions to a hospital for a disorder

4.7 Cross-cultural misinterpretation during the mental status exam may affect the assessment of

- A. motor behavior
- B. affect
- C. relationship to the evaluator
- D. appearance
- E. all of the above

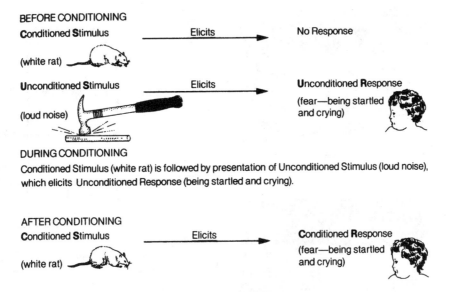

FIGURE 4.1
Reprinted with permission from Dworetzky JP. *Psychology.* 3rd ed. St. Paul, MN: West Publishing Company; 1988:195.

4.8 The child in the paradigm of classical conditioning shown in Figure 4.1 is conditioned to respond fearfully to a rat and subsequently responds fearfully to similar furry objects (a rabbit or a dog) but not to other dissimilar objects. This behavior is an example of

A. sensitization
B. stimulus generalization
C. discrimination
D. extinction
E. reinforcement

4.9 Which of the following statements best describes the long-term effects of 6 months of total social isolation in monkeys?

A. They rarely exhibit aggression against agemates who are more physically adept than they.
B. They are able to make a remarkable social adjustment through the development of play.
C. They are unresponsive to the new physical and social world with which they are presented.
D. They are both abnormally aggressive and abnormally fearful.
E. They assume postures that are bizarre, as opposed to depressive-type postures.

4.10 Asian patients seem to achieve a clinical response comparable to those of non-Asian patients, even though they require a significantly lower dose of

A. lithium
B. antipsychotics
C. tricyclics
D. benzodiazepines
E. all of the above

4.11 Recent studies seem to indicate that women are no more distressed than men by all the following major life crises *except*

A. job loss
B. divorce
C. widowhood
D. death of a loved one other than a spouse
E. financial difficulties

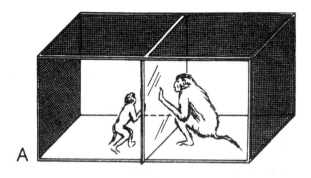

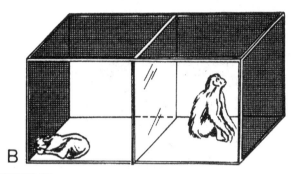

FIGURE 4.2

Two stages that occur when the infant is separated from its mother.

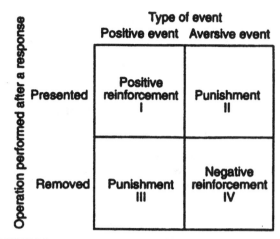

FIGURE 4.3

Reprinted with permission from Kazdin AE: *Behavior Modification in Applied Settings.* 2nd ed. Dorsey Press, Homewood, IL; 1983.

4.12 Figure 4.2 depicts an experiment that interferes with normal social interactions among monkeys. *A and B* represent the two sequential stages that occur when the infant is separated from its mother. The stages are protest (A) and

A. yearning
B. denial
C. despair
D. agitation
E. acceptance

4.13 Learned helplessness studies

A. used Rhesus monkeys as experimental animals
B. are used as paradigms for clinical depression in humans
C. demonstrated that outcomes were contingent on behavior
D. suggest that cortisol may be specifically decreased in helpless animals
E. involved peer separations

4.14 With regard to Figure 4.3, which of the following statements is *true?*

A. A teenager mowing the lawn to avoid parental complaints is an example of negative reinforcement.
B. A patient with anorexia nervosa eating and gaining weight to be discharged from the hospital is an example of positive reinforcement.
C. An animal jumping off a grid to escape a painful shock is an example of punishment.
D. The figure illustrates the principles of classical conditioning.
E. All of the above

DIRECTIONS: Each set of lettered headings below is followed by a list of numbered words or phrases. For each numbered word or phrase, select the *one* lettered heading that is closely associated with it: Each lettered heading may be selected once, more than once, or not at all.

Questions 4.15–4.17

A. Hollingshead and Redlich
B. Stirling County Study
C. Midtown Manhattan Study

4.15 Treated prevalence rate was highest in the lowest social class

4.16 About 82 percent of the population were found to have at least mild psychological impairment, whereas about 24 percent had significant impairment

4.17 Estimates of lifetime prevalence include a rate of 20 per 100 for conditions in need of psychiatric attention

Questions 4.18–4.19

A. Type I error
B. Type II error

4.18 When the null hypothesis is retained where it should have been rejected

4.19 When the null hypothesis is rejected where it should have been retained

Questions 4.20–4.23

A. Ivan Petrovich Pavlov
B. Eric Kandel
C. Konrad Lorenz
D. Harry Harlow

4.20 Imprinting

4.21 Surrogate mother

4.22 Experimental neurosis

4.23 *Aplysia*

Questions 4.24–4.28

    A. Magical thinking
    B. Thinking about thoughts
    C. Object permanence
    D. Symbolic thought
    E. Cause and effect

4.24 9 to 18 months
4.25 18 to 24 months
4.26 2 to 7 years
4.27 7 to 11 years
4.28 11 years through adolescence

DIRECTIONS: Match the items in Figure 4.4 with the correct lettered heading below.

Questions 4.29–4.33

    A. Conservation of substance
    B. Conservation of length
    C. Conservation of numbers
    D. Conservation of space
    E. Conservation of liquid

4.29 Item I
4.30 Item II
4.31 Item III
4.32 Item IV
4.33 Item V

Questions 4.34–4.38

    A. John Bowlby
    B. Harry Harlow
    C. Mary Ainsworth
    D. René Spitz

4.34 Surrogate mother
4.35 "Secure base" effect
4.36 Protest, despair, detachment
4.37 First described anaclitic depression
4.38 Primarily associated with ethological studies

DIRECTIONS: Each set of lettered headings below is followed by a list of numbered phrases. For each numbered phrase, select
    A. if the item is associated with *A only*
    B. if the item is associated with *B only*
    C. if the item is associated with *both A and B*
    D. if the item is associated with *neither A nor B*

Questions 4.39–4.44

    A. Classical conditioning
    B. Operant conditioning
    C. Both
    D. Neither

4.39 Instrumental conditioning
4.40 Learning takes place as a result of the contiguity of environmental events
4.41 Learning occurs as the consequence of action
4.42 Repeated pairing of a neutral stimulus with one that evokes a response
4.43 Ivan Petrovich Pavlov
4.44 B. F. Skinner

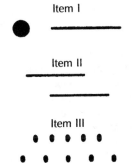

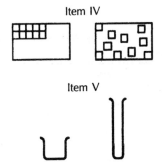

FIGURE 4.4
Tests for Piaget's theory of conservation. (Reprinted with permission from Lefrancois GR. *Of Children: An Introduction to Child Development.* Belmont, CA: Wadsworth; 1973.)

ANSWERS

Contributions of the Psychosocial Sciences to Human Behavior

4.1 The answer is C

People may have violent thoughts or fantasies but unless they lose control, thoughts do not become acts. Any set of conditions that produces increased aggressive impulses in the context of diminished control may produce violent acts. Situations with combinations of factors include toxic and organic states, developmental disabilities, florid psychosis, conduct disorder, and overwhelming psychological and environmental stress.

Table 4.1 summarizes some of the best-known concepts of violence predictors. *One of the best predictors of violent acts is a previous violent act.* Any predictor, however, is merely a guideline for the possibility of an increased risk for violence, and many potentially violent people do not fit any particular profile.

Violent acts are most often committed by persons who know or knew each other. Homicides are most prevalent among strangers (55 percent); *more than 70 percent of homicides are committed with handguns.* In the United States, *homicide is the second leading cause of death among people 15 to 25 years of age. Furthermore, a young black man is 8 times more likely to be murdered than is a white man of the same age.*

Generally, the probability of aggressive behavior increases when people become psychologically decompensated, perhaps also when the onset of a mental disorder is rapid. Otherwise, little is known about the relationship between the course of illness and aggression. Episodic decompensation may occur in those who ingest large quantities of alcohol; *more than 50 percent (not less than 50 percent) of people who commit criminal homicides or assaultive behavior* are reported to have imbibed significant amounts of alcohol immediately beforehand.

Table 4.1
Commonly Cited Predictors of Dangerousness to Others

High degree of intent to harm
Presence of a victim
Frequent and open threats
Concrete plan
Access to instruments of violence
History of loss of control
Chronic anger, hostility, or resentment
Enjoyment in watching or inflicting harm
Lack of compassion
Self-view as victim
Resentful of authority
Childhood brutality or deprivation
Decreased warmth and affection in home
Early loss of parent
Fire setting, bed-wetting, and cruelty to animals
Prior violent acts
Reckless driving

4.2 The answer is D

Attachment disorders are characterized by biopsychosocial pathology that results from maternal deprivation, a lack of care by and interaction with the infant's mother or caretaker. Psychosocial dwarfism, separation anxiety disorder, avoidant personality disorder, depressive disorders, delinquency, learning disorders, borderline intelligence, and *failure to thrive* have been traced to negative attachment experiences. Failure to thrive results in the infant's being unable to maintain viability outside a hospital setting. When maternal care is deficient because the mother is mentally ill, because the child is institutionalized for a long time, or because the primary object of attachment dies, the child suffers emotional damage.

John Bowlby formulated a theory that normal attachment is crucial to healthy development. According to Bowlby, attachment occurs when the infant has a warm, intimate, and continuous relationship with its mother, and both mother and infant find satisfaction and enjoyment. *Infants are generally monotropic, not polytropic, in their attachments,* but multiple attachments may also occur; attachment may be directed toward the father or a surrogate. *Attachment does not occur spontaneously between the mother and the child;* it is a gradually developing phenomenon. Attachment results in one person's wanting to be with a preferred person who is perceived as stronger, wiser, and able to reduce anxiety or distress. Attachment produces a feeling of security in the infant. It is a process that is facilitated by interaction between the mother and the infant. The amount of time together is less important than the quality of activity between the two.

Attachment is not synonymous with bonding; they are different phenomena. Bonding concerns the mother's feelings for her infant. It differs from attachment in that a mother does not normally rely on her infant as a source of security, a requirement of attachment behavior. A great deal of research on the bonding of a mother to her infant reveals that it occurs when they have skin-to-skin contact or other types of contact, such as voice and eye contact.

Separation from the attachment person may or may not produce intense anxiety, depending on the child's developmental level and the current phase of attachment. Separation anxiety is an anxiety response, expressed as tearfulness or irritability, in a child who is isolated or separated from its mother or caretaker. *Separation anxiety is most common when an infant is 10 to 18 months of age (not 5 months),* and it disappears generally by the end of the third year. Table 4.2 delineates aspects of normal attachment at different ages.

4.3 The answer is C

B. F. Skinner (1904–1990) proposed a theory of learning and behavior known as operant or instrumental conditioning. In operant conditioning the subject is active and behaves in a way that produces a reward; that is, learning occurs as a consequence of action.

The process is related to trial-and-error learning, as described by the American psychologist Edward L. Thorndike (1874–1949). In trial-and-error learning, one attempts to solve

Table 4.2
Normal Attachment

Birth to 30 days
  Reflexes at birth
    Rooting
    Head turning
    Sucking
    Swallowing
    Hand-mouth
    Grasp
    Digital extension
    Crying—signal for particular kind of distress
    Responsiveness and orientation to mother's face, eyes, and
      voice
  4 days—anticipatory approach behavior at feeding
  3 to 4 weeks—infant smiles preferentially to mother's voice
Age 30 days through 3 months
  Vocalization and gaze reciprocity further elaborated from 1 to 3
    months; babbling at 2 months, more with the mother than
    with a stranger
  Social smile
  In strange situation, increased clinging response to mother
Age 4 through 6 months
  Briefly soothed and comforted by sound of mother's voice
  Spontaneous, voluntary reaching for mother
  Anticipatory posturing to be picked up
  Differential preference for mother intensifies
  Subtle integration of responses to mother
Age 7 through 9 months
  Attachment behaviors further differentiated and focused specifi-
    cally on mother
  Separation distress, stranger distress, strange-place distress
Age 10 through 15 months
  Crawls or walks toward mother
  Subtle facial expressions (coyness, attentiveness)
  Responsive dialogue with mother clearly established
  Early imitation of mother (vocal inflections, facial expression)
  More fully developed separation distress and mother preference
  Pointing gesture
  Walking to and from mother
  Affectively positive reunion responses to mother after separation or,
    paradoxically, short-lived, active avoidance or delayed protest
Age 16 months through 2 years
  Involvement in imitative jargon with mother (12 to 14 months)
  Head-shaking "no" (15 to 16 months)
  Transitional object used during the absence of mother
  Separation anxiety diminishes
  Mastery of strange situations and persons when mother is near
  Evidence of delayed imitation
  Object permanence
  Microcosmic symbolic play
Age 25 months through 3 years
  Able to tolerate separations from mother without distress when
    familiar with surroundings and given reassurances about
    mother's return
  Two- and three-word speech
  Stranger anxiety much reduced
  Object consistency achieved—maintains composure and psycho-
    social functioning without regression in absence of mother
  Microcosmic play and social play; cooperation with others begins

Based on material by Justin Call, M.D.

a problem by trying out a variety of actions until one action proves successful; a freely moving organism behaves in a way that is instrumental in producing a reward. For example, a cat in a Thorndike puzzle box must learn to lift a latch to escape from the box. For that reason, operant conditioning is sometimes called instrumental conditioning. Thorndike's law of effect states that certain responses are reinforced by reward, and the organism learns from those experiences.

In operant conditioning, the experimenter can vary the schedule of reward or reinforcement given to a behavioral pattern—a process known as programming. The intervals between reinforcements may be fixed (for example, every third response is rewarded) or variable (sometimes the third response is rewarded and at other times, the sixth response is rewarded). A continuous reinforcement (also known as contingency reinforcement or management) schedule, in which every response is reinforced, leads to the most rapid acquisition of a behavior. However, *continuous reinforcement is the reinforcement schedule most, not least, susceptible to extinction.* Extinction occurs when a desired response no longer occurs. Table 4.3 lists reinforcement schedules in operant conditioning.

Negative reinforcement is not punishment. Punishment is an aversive stimulus (for example, a slap) that is presented specifically to weaken or suppress an undesired response. Punishment, theoretically, reduces the probability that a response will recur. In learning theory, the punishment delivered is always contingent on performance, and its use reduces the frequency of the behavior being punished. Negative reinforcement is the process by which a response that leads to the removal of an aversive event increases that response. For example, a teenager mows the lawn to avoid parental complaints, and an animal jumps off a grid to escape a painful shock. Any behavior that enables one to avoid or escape a punishing consequence is strengthened.

Shaping involves changing behavior in a deliberate and predetermined way. By reinforcing those responses that are in the desired direction, the experimenter shapes the subject's behavior. If the experimenter wants to train a seal to ring a bell with its nose, he or she can give a food reinforcement as the animal's random behavior brings its nose near the bell. *Shaping does not occur when responses are coincidentally paired to a reinforcer.* When that occurs, it is called adventitious reinforcement. Adventitious reinforcement may have clinical implications in the development of phobias and other behaviors.

In formulating his theory of operant conditioning, Skinner described two types of behavior: (1) respondent behavior, which results from known stimuli (for example, the knee jerk reflex to patellar stimulation) and (2) operant behavior, which is independent of a stimulus (for example, the random movements of an infant or the aimless movements of a laboratory rat in a cage). Thus, *operant behavior, not respondent behavior, is independent of a stimulus.*

4.4 The answer is E

Curiosity and aggression show no correlation. In the normal child, aggression can be effectively understood in terms of the motives (for example, defense and mastery) for which aggressiveness is a suitable mediator. Its increased frequency in abnormal children can be correlated with defects in the organism, as in the case of *brain injury,* or with distortions in the

Table 4.3
Reinforcement Schedules in Operant Conditioning

Reinforcement Schedule	Example	Behavioral Effect
Fixed-ratio (FR) schedule	Reinforcement occurs after every 10 responses (10:1 ratio); 10 bar presses release a food pellet; workers are paid for every 10 items they make.	Rapid rate of response to obtain the greatest number of rewards. Animal knows that the next reinforcement depends on a certain number of responses being made.
Variable-ratio (VR) schedule	Variable reinforcement occurs (e.g., after the third, sixth, then second response, and so on).	Generates a fairly constant rate of response because the probability of reinforcement at any given time remains relatively stable.
Fixed-interval (FI) schedule	Reinforcement occurs at regular intervals (e.g., every 10 minutes or every third hour).	Animal keeps track of time. Rate of responding drops to near 0 after reinforcement and then increases at about the expected time of reward.
Variable-interval (VI) schedule	Reinforcement occurs after variable intervals (e.g., every 3, 6, and then 2 hours), similar to VR schedule.	Response rate does not change between reinforcements. Animal responds at a steady rate to get the reward when it is available; common in trout fishing, use of slot machines, checking mailbox.

child's environment, as in the case of *faulty identification models.* Moreover, the frequency of the display of aggressive behavior is a function of the child's *cultural environment.* Aggressive fantasy materials (*violence in movies,* crime comics, and television) rather than affording catharsis for instinctual aggressiveness generate the very tensions they profess to release.

A central issue is the meaning to be ascribed to the term "aggression." If a boy is observed taking apart a watch, that behavior may be aggressive if, for example, the watch belongs to the child's father, and the father has just punished him. However, if the watch is an old one in his stock of toys, the boy's motive may be curiosity about its mechanism, especially if he takes delight in reassembling it. If he strikes another child, that act may be motivated by aggression if the victim is the baby sister his parents have just embraced. Or the blow may be defensive if the victim has made a threatening gesture or has tried to seize the boy's favorite toy. Anecdotes make the point, but documented experimental examples of aggressive children are also available: children emulating adult models, children systematically subjected to frustration, and children watching films or television of aggressive behavior, all of whom show predictable increases in aggressiveness.

4.5 The answer is E
Cross-cultural studies examine and compare various cultures along a number of parameters: attitudes, beliefs, expectations, memories, opinions, roles, stereotypes, prejudices, and values. Usually, the cultures studied have differing languages and political organizations.

The nuclear family of mother, father, and children is a universal unit in all cultures. The extended family—in which grandparents, parents, children, and other relatives all live under the same roof—is no longer as common in the United States, but it is still prevalent in less industrialized cultures. In the United States, more than 85 percent of the men and women between the ages of 35 and 45 are husbands or wives in a nuclear family.

Cross-cultural studies *are not free from experimental bias;* in fact, they are subject to extreme bias because of problems in translation and other areas of information gathering. Questions have to be asked in ways that are clearly understood by the group under study. One of the best-known cross-cultural studies, *Psychiatric Disorder among the Yoruba* by Alexander Leighton, was his attempt to replicate in Nigeria the Stirling County study he had conducted in Canada. The study was criticized because not only did it fail to distinguish psychophysiological symptoms from those associated with infections, parasites, and nutritional diseases, but also it assumed that the indicators of sociocultural disintegration in Stirling County could be used among the Yoruba. All cultures are relative; that is, each must be examined within the context of its own language, customs, and beliefs.

4.6 The answer is A
Prevalence is the *proportion of a population that has a condition at one moment in time.* The *ratio of persons who acquire a disorder during a year's time* (new cases) is called the annual incidence. In a stable situation, the prevalence is approximately equal to the annual incidence times the average duration, measured in years, of the condition. The *risk of acquiring a condition at some time* in the future is the accumulation of age-specific annual incidence rates over a period of time.

Standard deviation (SD) is a statistical measure of variability within a set of values so defined that, for a normal distribution, about 68 percent of the values fall within one SD of the mean, and about 95 percent lie within two SDs of the mean. It is sometimes presented by Σ, the Greek letter sigma.

The rate of first admissions to a hospital for a disorder is the ratio of all first admissions to an average general hospital during a particular time.

4.7 The answer is E (all)
The mental status examination, the key component of a psychiatric diagnostic interview, is subject to many distortions when conducted across a language and cultural barrier. The central process of the mental status examination requires observation and interpretation of the patient's appearance, behavior, language, and mental activity, both spontaneous and as elicited by the clinician's questions. The following items of the mental status examination are most sensitive to cross-cultural misinterpretation.

Appearance. The mental status sections of psychiatric case reports are often replete with such expressions as "normal," "attractive," and "appropriate" and others that are subject to significant cultural variation and must be carefully evaluated by the clinician, with the patient's own development and culturally determined normative framework as a referent.

Relationship to the Evaluator. The assessment of a patient's relationship to the clinician who is performing a psychiatric evaluation is affected by many psychosocial variables, including whether the interview is voluntary and the relative emergency of the clinical situation. Key factors of such an assessment (e.g., maintenance or avoidance of eye contact, deference, reserve, physical proximity, and physical contact) are subject to cultural prescriptions that the clinician should strive to decode.

Motor Behavior. The assessment of motor activity is considered a fundamental part of the mental status assessment. Patients who communicate in a nondominant language may use extra nonverbal activity to facilitate verbalization across the language barrier. This extra activity needs to be carefully evaluated, lest it be attributed to tension, hyperactivity, or other forms of motor psychopathology.

Affect. Both the spontaneous and the elicited expressions of affect are deeply patterned by cultural norms and expectations. Culturally sanctioned impassiveness should not be misinterpreted as poverty of affect any more than the ebullience attributed to persons of Mediterranean origin should be evaluated as excessively intense affect. Clinicians need to be equally sensitive to the significance of linguistic factors that may cloud the interpretation of affect.

When a mental status evaluation is performed across language and cultural barriers, certain linguistic problems may be misinterpreted as psychopathology, and clinicians should guard against this error by repeating critical questions, introducing redundancies to facilitate communication, and identifying paralinguistic cues that may color their evaluation of mood and emotional expression, and when in doubt they should use trained translators, cultural consultants, or structured, validated interviews.

4.8 The answer is B
All of the terms (A–E) are concepts used in learning theory. *Stimulus generalization* is the process whereby a conditioned response is transferred from one stimulus to another similar stimulus, such as from a rat (in this example) to a rabbit or a dog.

Sensitization is the process by which pairing the eliciting stimulus with a painful stimulus results in a stronger, more sensitive response. After sensitization to a sound, for example, one startles more easily upon hearing that sound than before being sensitized.

Discrimination is the process of recognizing and responding to the difference between similar stimuli. A child, for example, learns to discriminate four-legged animals (the common stimulus) into dogs, cats, cows, and other quadrupeds.

Extinction occurs when the conditioned stimulus is repeated constantly without the unconditioned stimulus and the response weakens gradually and eventually disappears.

Reinforcement is a term used in operant conditioning. Positive reinforcement refers to the process by which certain consequences of behavior increase the probability that the behavior will occur again. Negative reinforcement describes the process by which behavior that leads to the removal of an unpleasant event strengthens that behavior.

4.9 The answer is D
The long-term effects of 6 months of total social isolation produce adolescent monkeys that are *both abnormally aggressive and abnormally fearful.* The isolates *exhibit aggression against agemates who are more physically adept than they.*

Infant monkeys that survive a 3-month, rather than a 6-month, total social isolation can *make a remarkable social adjustment through the development of play.* When allowed to interact with equally aged normally reared monkeys, the isolates play effectively within a week.

Monkeys totally isolated for a 12-month period (not a 6-month period) *are totally unresponsive to the new physical and social world with which they are presented.* Those isolates are devoid of social play and strong emotion. Totally isolated monkeys exhibit a depressive-type posture, including self-clutching, rocking, and depressive huddling. Partially isolated monkeys assume, with increasing frequency, *postures that are bizarre;* such as extreme stereotypy and sitting at the front of the cage and staring vacantly into space.

4.10 The answer is E (all)
Asian patients require lower dosages of dopamine receptor antagonist (typical antipsychotic) medications than comparable non-Asian patients to achieve a desirable clinical outcome. Also, when treated on a fixed-dosage schedule, Asians seem to develop significantly greater extrapyramidal adverse effects. One study found a 52 percent higher plasma concentration of haloperidol (Haldol) in Chinese schizophrenic patients living in China than in non-Asian schizophrenic patients residing in the United States when both groups received treatment on a fixed-dosage schedule. Another study demonstrated that Chinese schizophrenic patients residing in Taiwan and Taipei achieved haloperidol plasma concentrations comparable to those of white, African-American, and Hispanic patients hospitalized in San Antonio while using significantly lower daily dosages of haloperidol.

As is the case with neuroleptics, studies with *tricyclic drugs have shown that average dosages prescribed for Asians are significantly lower* (up to 50 percent lower) than dosages prescribed in the United States for non-Asians. The reasons for this responsiveness have not been clearly established, although preliminary evidence suggests differential responsiveness of relevant receptors, differences in resulting plasma concentrations, or both.

Similar conclusions have been reached for depressed Hispanic women and African-American patients, both of whom are reported to respond faster and more completely to tricyclics than white patients, albeit with higher rates of adverse effects. Sensitivity to development of anticholinergic adverse effects is important to compliance as well as morbidity in accidental or intentional overdoses. Researchers have reported that delirium as a complication of tricyclic drugs appears more frequently among African-Americans than among other ethnic groups.

Studies of prescription patterns as well as those comparing the pharmacokinetics and pharmacodynamics of benzodiazepines across ethnic groups have established the *enhanced sensitivity of Asians to the effects of benzodiazepines.* Typically prescribed doses are one-half to two-thirds those of similar non-minority populations. The ethnic differences in benzodiazepine metabolism are most often linked to polymorphisms in the (S)-

mephenytoin phenotype, yielding a higher percentage of poor metabolizers in the Chinese ethnic group. Additional mechanisms, both genetic and environmental, have been invoked by other investigators.

As with tricyclic drugs, antipsychotics, and benzodiazepines, *Asians seem to achieve clinical responses comparable to those of non-Asian patients using significantly lower dosages and with serum concentrations of lithium 0.5 to 0.7 mEq/L versus the 0.8 to 1.2 mEq/L generally required by white populations.*

4.11 The answer is D

Aggregate analyses of life event inventories show that women are on average more vulnerable than men to stressful life events; however, there are some stresses for which this is not true. For example, *women adjust to spousal death better than men; women also adjust as well as or better than men to divorce. Furthermore, women cope with financial difficulties better than do men.*

A meta-analysis of several large-scale community surveys, in which the effects of different types of events were assessed separately, *found no evidence that women are more distressed than men by such major life crises as job loss, divorce, or widowhood.* Women's greater vulnerability was primarily associated with events that happen to people close to them—*death of a loved one other than a spouse being the most commonly reported event in this regard.*

4.12 The answer is C

The initial reaction of the infant monkey to separation from its mother is the strongly emotional protest stage, which is characterized by upset and continuous agitation on the part of the infant. When the separation is prolonged beyond 2 or 3 weeks, the infant's behavior changes to reflect the onset of the *despair* stage, in which the deprived monkey engages in less than usual activity, little or no play, and occasional crying. There is a parallel here to separation among humans and the occurrence of grief that is sometimes reflected in initial protest and later in despair.

Yearning is an urgent longing that is sometimes felt toward the missing. *Resolution* is similar to C. M. Parkes' stage of reorganization in which a person comes to accept the loss of a loved one.

Acceptance is the final stage to impending death described by Elisabeth Kübler-Ross and is the recognition that death is universal.

4.13 The answer is B

The animal model of learned helplessness relates closely to some important aspects of *clinical depression,* particularly cognitive aspects. Those cognitive aspects are reflected in feelings of helplessness and hopelessness. Etiological theories, as well as therapeutic approaches, have developed from that cognitive view of depression.

In the original experimental study with animals, *dogs (not monkeys) were observed in one of three situations.* In the first situation they were put in harnesses and subjected to electric shock that they could terminate by touching a panel; not surprisingly, they learned to escape the shock rather quickly. In the second situation the dogs were prepared as in the preceding situation, but when the shock was given, they were unable to terminate it. Finally, to control for the effect of the shock itself, dogs were put in harnesses but were not subjected to shock at all. In Phase 2 of the study, dogs were given electric shock while unharnessed in a shuttle box. Normally, dogs have no difficulty learning to avoid the shock by going to the other side of the box, which proved to be true for the dogs that had been exposed to escapable shock while in the harness. However, the dogs that had been exposed to inescapable shock failed to learn that they could escape from the electric shock in Phase 2 by jumping over a barrier that separated the two sides of the shuttle box. They were described as being initially agitated in reaction to the shock, but instead of running around frantically until they discovered that they could escape the shock by crossing the barrier, they would sit or lie down, whining quietly—that is, they acted as if they were helpless and incapable of escaping. The interpretation was that the inescapable shock they had experienced earlier made them unable to cope with the present situation. One explanation was that they had learned during their initial experience *that outcomes were not contingent on their behavior.* No matter what they did, it did no good; they learned to be helpless.

Studies suggest that *cortisol may be specifically elevated (not decreased) in helpless animals.* Norepinephrine depletions in the locus ceruleus also have been found. Some investigators have suggested alterations in the hippocampal β-receptors (related to memory), occurring with the development of helpless behaviors, and that those changes can be reversed by antidepressant drug treatments since serotonin appears to regulate β-adrenergic receptor concentrations in the hippocampus.

Peer separation studies have been used with *Rhesus monkeys.* In general, the behavioral reaction to *peer separation is quite similar to that following maternal separation in terms of the classic protest-despair response.* Furthermore, when peer groups are formed and separations are repeated, the response is seen with each separation. Not surprisingly, a number of variables can influence the nature of the response, including age; rearing conditions; housing conditions before, during, and after each separation; and treatment with pharmacological agents.

4.14 The answer is A

The figure illustrates the principal procedures of operant conditioning (not classical conditioning). In the case of *operant conditioning,* learning is thought to occur as a result of the consequences of one's actions and the resultant effect on the environment. In *classical conditioning,* in contrast, learning is thought to take place as the result of the contiguity of environmental events; when events occur closely together in time, persons will probably come to associate the two.

In operant conditioning, *positive reinforcement* is the process by which certain consequences of a response increase the probability that the response will occur again. Food, water, praise, and money, as well as substances such as opium, cocaine, and nicotine, all may serve as positive reinforcers.

Negative reinforcement is the process by which a response that leads to the removal of an aversive event increases that response. A teenager mowing the lawn to avoid parental complaints or an animal jumping off a grid to escape painful shock are both examples of negative reinforcement. Any behavior that enables one to avoid or escape a punishing consequence is strengthened; therefore, a patient with anorexia nervosa eating and gaining weight in order to get out of the hospital (presuming she prefers going home to a prolonged hospitalization) is also an example of negative reinforcement.

Negative reinforcement is not punishment. *Punishment* is an aversive stimulus (for example, a slap) that is presented explicitly to weaken or suppress an undesired response. Punishment reduces the probability that a response will occur.

4.15 The answer is A

4.16 The answer is C

4.17 The answer is B
In the early 1950s August de Belmont Hollingshead and Fredrick Carl Redlich conducted a survey of every mental health facility and private office practice psychiatrist who treated any patient in the New Haven area. The authors could define an overall mental disorder 6-month treated prevalence rate of 8 per 1,000 population in the community. The rates varied by socioeconomic status. *Treated prevalence rates were highest in the lowest social class.* Social class was a principal descriptive variable used to stratify frequency of diagnoses and the frequency of treatment setting use. Although careful attention was given to controlling for potential confounding variables of age, sex, or mental disorder type, a strong association was found between higher social class, less severe disorders, and private office treatment settings. This association contrasted with the concentration of severe disorders in both the lower social classes and in the long-stay public mental hospitals.

The study of Stirling County, directed by Alexander Leighton and continued by Jane Murphy, sampled 1,010 adults from the 20,000 residents of a rural county in Canada. Mental disorders were defined in accordance with the newly developed DSM, using structured psychiatric interviews.

Estimates of the lifetime prevalence of *conditions in need* of *psychiatric attention was 20 percent.* The Stirling County study also found that women showed more mental disorders than did men and that only 20 percent of the population were free of psychiatric symptoms. Age was found to be a factor; mental disorders increased with age. The study also disclosed that mental health was related to economic status.

The Midtown Manhattan study of Thomas Rennie, Leo Srole, and colleagues selected a sample of 1,660 adult residents from an area of midtown Manhattan that had a population of 110,000 adults. The independent variables included measures of stress, immigration status, social class, occupation, and marital status; the dependent variables measured impairment in adult life function on a 6-point gradient scale from "none" to "incapacitated."

Psychologists and social workers used a structured psychiatric interview to obtain information from respondents, which was subsequently rated by two psychiatrists. The most celebrated findings were that about 82 *percent of the population had at least mild impairment from psychological symptoms, whereas about 24 percent had significant impairment.* Correlations were found between sociodemographic and social stress variables and levels of impairment.

Answers 4.18–4.19

4.18 The answer is B

4.19 The answer is A
The null hypothesis states that observed differences or variation in scores can be attributed to random sources. When the null hypothesis is rejected, observed differences between groups are deemed to be improbable by chance alone. For example, if drug A is compared to a placebo for its effects on depression and the null hypothesis is rejected, the investigator concludes that the observed differences most likely are not explainable simply by sampling error. When offering this conclusion, the investigator has the odds on his or her side. However, what are the chances of the statement being incorrect?

In statistical inference there is no way to say with certainty that rejection or retention of the null hypothesis was correct. There are two types of potential errors.

Type I errors occur when the null hypothesis is rejected but should have been retained, such as when a researcher decides that two means are different. He or she might conclude that the treatment works or that groups are not sampled from the same population, whereas in reality the observed differences are attributable only to sampling error. In a conservative scientific setting, type I errors should be made rarely. There is a great disadvantage to advocating treatments that really do not work. The probability of a type I error is denoted with the Greek letter alpha (α). Because of the desire to avoid type I errors, statistical models have been created so that the investigator has control over the probability of a type I error. At the .05 significance or alpha level, a type I error is expected to occur in 5 percent of all cases. At the .01 level, it may occur in 1 percent of all cases. Thus, at the .05 a level, one type I error is expected to be made in each of 20 independent tests. At the .01 a level, one type I error is expected to be made in each 100 independent tests.

In a type II error the null hypothesis is retained when it really was wrong and should have been rejected. For example, an investigator may reach the conclusion that a treatment does not work when in fact it is efficacious. The probability of a type II error is symbolized by the Greek letter beta (β).

Answers 4.20–4.23

4.20 The answer is C

4.21 The answer is D

4.22 The answer is A

4.23 The answer is B
Imprinting has been described as the process by which certain stimuli become capable of eliciting certain innate behavior patterns during a critical period of an animal's behavioral development. The phenomenon is associated with *Konrad Lorenz,* who in 1935 demonstrated that the first moving object (in that case, Lorenz himself) a duckling sees during a critical period shortly after hatching is regarded and reacted to thereafter as the mother duck.

Harry Harlow is associated with the concept of the *surrogate mother* from his experiments in the 1950s with Rhesus monkeys. Harlow designed a series of experiments in which infant monkeys were separated from their mothers during the earliest weeks of life. He found that the infant monkeys, if given the choice between a wire surrogate mother and a cloth-covered surrogate mother, chose the cloth-covered surrogates even if the wire surrogate provided food.

Ivan Petrovich Pavlov coined the terms *"experimental neurosis"* to describe disorganized behavior that appears in the experimental subject (in Pavlov's case, dogs) in response to an inability to master the experimental situation. Pavlov described extremely agitated behavior in his dogs when they were unable to discriminate between sounds of similar pitch or test objects of similar shapes.

Eric Kandel contributed to the knowledge of the neurophysiology of learning. He demonstrated in the study of the snail *Aplysia* that synaptic connections are altered as a result of learning. His work earned him the Nobel Prize in Medicine in 2001.

Answers 4.24–4.28

4.24 The answer is C

4.25 The answer is D

4.26 The answer is A

4.27 The answer is E

4.28 The answer is B
During Piaget's sensorimotor stage of development, the child shows *the preliminary signs of object permanence.* By *9 to 12 months,* the child comprehends the vague concept that objects *continue to exist when the object is no longer in view.* Object permanence is not fully obtained until *18 months to 2 years.* At that time, peekaboo becomes a game joyfully played with the child.

The end of the sensorimotor stage is marked by the attainment of *symbolic thought* by the child of *18 to 24 months.* With the acquisition of symbolic thought, the whole world of symbolic play opens to the child.

Ages *2 through 7* years mark the years of preoperational thought, the stage of prelogical thinking. The child believes in imminent justice—that a bad deed will inevitably be punished. The child also believes in *magical thinking,* the idea that thoughts or wishes—good or bad—can come true. Magical thinking has positive and negative repercussions. After some ill has befallen a loved one, for example, the child may blame himself or herself because of "bad" wishes. Happily, some children believe they are gaining a new sibling because they have wished for it, and they can view a new baby as a present.

Ages 7 to 11 years are the years of concrete operations. The child is able to understand classifications and *cause and effect.* At that time the child is also able to take another's point of view and in games, children can take turns and follow rules.

The stage of formal operations is entered at about age *11 years through adolescence.* It is the time of the acquisition of abstract logic. In addition to being able to hypothesize and make deductions, the young person can comprehend probabilities and can now *think about thoughts.*

Answers 4.29–4.33

4.29 The answer is A

4.30 The answer is B

4.31 The answer is C

4.32 The answer is D

4.33 The answer is E
Conservation is the ability to recognize that, even though the shape and the form of objects may change, the objects still maintain or conserve other characteristics that enable them to be recognized as the same. It occurs between 7 and 11 years of age. In Figure 4.4 Item I is conservation of substance. One of the balls is deformed, and the subject is asked whether the balls still contain equal amounts. Item II is conservation of length. One of the sticks is to the right of the other, and the subject is asked whether they are the same length. Item III is conservation of numbers. The elongated line has the same numbers as the contracted row. Item IV is conservation of space. The experimenter scatters the blocks over one of the sheets and is asked if they are the same amount. Item V is conservation of liquid. Both containers can contain the same amount of liquid.

Answers 4.34–4.38

4.34 The answer is B

4.35 The answer is C

4.36 The answer is A

4.37 The answer is D

4.38 The answer is B
Attachment can be defined as the emotional tone between children and their caregivers and is evidenced by an infant's seeking and clinging to the caregiving person, usually the mother. By their first month, infants usually have begun to show such behavior, which is designed to promote proximity to the desired person.

John Bowlby, a British psychoanalyst (1907–1990), formulated the theory that normal attachment in infancy is crucial to healthy development.

Bowlby described a predictable set and sequence of behavior patterns in children who are separated from their mothers for long periods (more than 3 months): *protest,* in which the child protests against the separations by crying, calling out, and searching for the lost person; *despair,* in which the child appears to lose hope that the mother will return; and *detachment,* in which the child emotionally separates himself or herself from the mother. Bowlby believed that this sequence involves ambivalent feelings towards the mother; the child both wants her and is angry at her for her desertion.

Mary Ainsworth built on Bowlby's observations and found that the interaction between the mother and her baby during the attachment period influences the baby's current and future behavior significantly. Many observers believe that patterns of infant attachment affect future adult emotional relationships. Patterns of attachment vary among babies; for example, some babies signal or cry less than others. Sensitive responsiveness to infant signals, such as cuddling the baby when it cries, causes infants to cry less in later months. Close bodily contact with the mother when the baby signals for her is also associated with the growth of self-reliance, rather than with a clinging dependence, as the baby grows older. Unresponsive mothers produce anxious babies; these mothers often have lower intelligence quotients (IQs) and are emotionally more immature and younger than responsive mothers.

Ainsworth also confirmed that attachment serves the purpose of reducing anxiety. What she called the *secure base effect* enables a child to move away from the attachment figures and to explore the environment. Inanimate objects, such as a teddy bear or a blanket (called the transitional object by Donald Winnicott), also serve as a secure base, one that often accompanies children as they navigate the world.

Harry Harlow's *ethological studies* with monkeys are relevant to attachment theory. Harlow demonstrated the emotional and behavioral effects of isolating monkeys from birth and keeping them from forming attachments. The isolates were withdrawn, unable to relate to peers, unable to mate, and incapable of caring for their offspring.

Anaclitic depression, also known as hospitalism, was first described by René Spitz in infants who had made normal attachments but were then separated suddenly from their mothers for varying times and placed in institutions or hospitals. The children became depressed, withdrawn, nonresponsive, and vulnerable to physical illness but recovered when their mothers returned or when surrogate mothering was available. Attachment theory is summarized in Table 4.2.

Answers 4.39–4.44

4.39 The answer is B

4.40 The answer is A

4.41 The answer is B

4.42 The answer is A

4.43 The answer is A

4.44 The answer is B

Among the building blocks of learning theory are classical and operant conditioning. In *classical conditioning,* learning is thought to take place as a result of the *contiguity of environmental events*: When events occur closely together in time, people will probably come to associate the two. In the case of *operant conditioning,* learning is thought to occur as a result of the *consequences of a person's actions* and the resultant effect on the environment. As *B. F. Skinner* (1904–1990) stated, "A person does not act upon the world, the world acts upon him."

Classical or respondent conditioning results from the repeated *pairing of a neutral (conditioned) stimulus with one that evokes a response* (unconditioned stimulus), such that the neutral stimulus eventually comes to evoke the response. The time relation between the presentation of the conditioned and unconditioned stimuli is important and varies for optimal learning from a fraction of a second to several seconds.

The Russian physiologist and Nobel prize winner, *Ivan Petrovich Pavlov* (1849–1936), observed in his work on gastric secretion that a dog salivated not only when food was placed in its mouth but also at the sound of the footsteps of the person coming to feed the dog, even though the dog could not see or smell the food. Pavlov analyzed these events and called the saliva flow that occurred with the sound of footsteps a *conditioned response* (CR)—a response elicited under certain conditions by a particular stimulus.

In a typical pavlovian experiment, a *stimulus* (S) that had no capacity to evoke a particular response before training did so after consistent association with another stimulus. For example, under normal circumstances, a dog does not salivate at the sound of a bell, but when the bell sound is always followed by the presentation of food, the dog ultimately pairs the bell and the food. Eventually, the bell sound alone elicits salivation (CR).

Skinner's theory of learning and behavior is known as operant or *instrumental conditioning*. Whereas in classical conditioning an animal is passive or restrained and behavior is reinforced by the experimenter, in operant conditioning the animal is active and behaves in a way that produces a reward; thus *learning occurs as a consequence of action*. For example, a rat receives a reinforcing stimulus (food) only when it responds correctly by pressing a lever. Food, approval, praise, good grades, or any other response that satisfies a need in an animal or a person can serve as a reward.

Operant conditioning is related to trial-and-error learning, as described by the American psychologist Edward L. Thorndike (1874–1949). In trial-and-error learning, a person or an animal attempts to solve a problem by trying different actions until one proves successful: A freely moving organism behaves in a way that is instrumental in producing a reward. For example, a cat in a Thorndike puzzle box must learn to lift a latch to escape from the box. For this reason, operant conditioning is sometimes called *instrumental conditioning*. Thorndike's law of effect states that certain responses are reinforced by reward and the organism learns from these experiences.

Four kinds of instrumental or operant conditioning are described in Table 4.3.

5 ▲

Clinical Neuropsychological Testing

For the most part, psychiatrists depend on clinical psychologists to perform the different batteries of psychometric and neuropsychological tests on their patients. However, the psychiatrist must be aware of which tests are available and their indications and limitations. How to interpret the results and how to discuss those results are crucial skills to be mastered.

Tests are both objective and projective, and can be administered individually or in a group. Tests can evaluate intellectual and psychological functioning, can assess cognitive functioning, and can hypothesize personality dynamics and conflicts. They can be overread and underused; they can also be underread and overused. They are helpful aids in diagnosis and treatment, yet they must be interpreted with care and skill.

A significant area of neuropsychological testing concentrates on neuroanatomical localization of mental deficits. Both clinicians and researchers can use such tests to learn, for instance, the area of a patient's brain associated with the ability to speak words correctly or to understand a spoken word. In addition to its use in cognitive and amnestic disorders, neuropsychological testing is important in mood disorders associated with insults to the brain—for example, tumors and strokes—and in schizophrenia. As this area expands and grows, neuropsychiatric testing can produce even more spectacular results.

This chapter covers both psychological and neuropsychiatric testing. Students should study the questions and answers below to test their knowledge of the field.

The psychological terms and tests listed here should be defined and distinguished.

HELPFUL HINTS

- abstract reasoning
- accurate profile
- attention
- attention-deficit/ hyperactivity disorder
- average IQ
- battery tests
- behavioral flexibility
- bell-shaped curve
- Bender Visual Motor Gestalt test
- Alfred Binet
- catastrophic reaction
- clang association
- classification of intelligence
- coping phase
- dementia
- dressing apraxia
- dysgraphia
- dyslexia
- EEG abnormalities

- Eysenck personality inventory
- fluency
- full-scale IQ
- Gestalt psychology
- Halstead-Reitan
- House-Tree-Person test
- individual and group tests
- intelligence quotient (IQ)
- learning disability
- left versus right hemisphere disease
- Luria-Nebraska Neuropsychological Battery (LNNB)
- manual dexterity
- maturational levels
- memory: immediate, recent, recent past, remote

- mental age
- mental status cognitive tasks
- MMPI
- motivational aspects of behavior
- neuropsychiatric tests
- objective tests
- organic dysfunction
- orientation
- performance subtests
- perseveration
- personality functioning
- personality testing
- primary assets and weaknesses
- prognosis
- projective tests
- prosody
- psychodynamic formulations

- Raven's Progressive Matrices
- reaction times
- recall phase
- reliability
- response sets
- Rorschach test
- scatter pattern
- Shipley Abstraction test
- standardization
- Stanford-Binet
- stimulus words
- TAT
- temporal orientation
- test behavior
- validity
- verbal subtests
- visual-object agnosia
- WAIS
- WISC
- word-association technique

▲ QUESTIONS

DIRECTIONS: Each of the incomplete statements below is followed by five suggested completions. Select the *one* that is *best* in each case.

5.1 Neuropsychological deficits associated with left hemisphere damage include all of the following *except*

    A. aphasia
    B. right-left disorientation
    C. finger agnosia
    D. visuospatial deficits
    E. limb apraxia

5.2 A right hemispheric stroke is most often associated with

    A. inability to appreciate the gestalt or global features of a design
    B. inaccurate reproduction of internal details of a design
    C. inability to draw isolated details of a model design
    D. maintaining the global framework of a design but losing the details
    E. decreased analysis of local features and details

5.3 Neuropsychological referrals are made for

    A. establishing a baseline of performance for assessing future change
    B. diagnostic purposes
    C. ascertaining if brain impairment is present
    D. planning for rehabilitation
    E. all of the above

5.4 Neuropsychological testing is used to assess

    A. normal aging
    B. early dementia
    C. competence
    D. a diagnosis of pseudodementia
    E. all of the above

5.5 True statements about projective personality tests include

    A. They tend to be more direct and structural than objective personality instruments.
    B. The variety of responses is limited.
    C. Instructions are usually specific.
    D. They often focus on latent or unconscious aspects of personality.
    E. None of the above

5.6 In the field of memory

    A. A nonverbal visual task is a poor assessor of immediate memory.
    B. Recent memory can be tested by digit-span tasks.
    C. Episodic memory is memory for knowledge and facts.
    D. The Wechsler Memory Scale yields a memory quotient.
    E. Semantic memory and implicit memory decline with age.

5.7 An intelligence quotient (IQ) of 100 corresponds to intellectual ability for the general population in the

    A. 20th percentile
    B. 25th percentile
    C. 40th percentile
    D. 50th percentile
    E. 65th percentile

5.8 In the assessment of intelligence

    A. The highest divisor in the IQ formula is 25.
    B. The IQ is a measure of future potential.
    C. The Stanford-Binet test is the most widely used intelligence test.
    D. The average or normal range of IQ is 70 to 100.
    E. Intelligence levels are based on the assumption that intellectual abilities are distributed normally.

5.9 After taking the Wechsler Adult Intelligence Scale (WAIS), a patient showed that poor concentration and attention had adversely influenced the answers on one of the subtests. Select the letter of the WAIS subtest that most likely screened the patient for these symptoms.

    A. arithmetic
    B. block design
    C. digit symbol
    D. comprehension
    E. picture completion

5.10 The Bender Visual Motor Gestalt test is administered to test

    A. maturation levels in children
    B. organic dysfunction
    C. loss of function
    D. visual and motor coordination
    E. all of the above

5.11 The Minnesota Multiphasic Personality Inventory (MMPI) is most correctly described as

    A. composed of 200 questions
    B. generally used as a good diagnostic tool
    C. the most widely used personality assessment instrument
    D. a good indication of a subject's disorder when the person scores high on one particular clinical scale
    E. in the form of ten clinical scales, each of which was derived empirically from heterogeneous groups

DIRECTIONS: Each group of questions below consists of lettered headings followed by a list of numbered words or statements. For each numbered word or statement, select the *one* lettered heading most closely associated with it. Each lettered heading may be selected once, more than once, or not at all.

Questions 5.12–5.16

   A. Frontal lobes
   B. Dominant temporal lobe
   C. Nondominant parietal lobe
   D. Dominant parietal lobe
   E. Occipital lobe

5.12 The loss of gestalt, loss of symmetry, and distortion of figures

5.13 Patient not able to name a camouflaged object but able to name it when it is not camouflaged

5.14 Two or more errors or two or more 7-second delays in carrying out tasks of right-left orientation

5.15 Any improper letter sequence in spelling "earth" backward

5.16 Patient not able to name common objects

Questions 5.17–5.21

   A. Rorschach test
   B. Luria-Nebraska Neuropsychological Battery
   C. Halstead-Reitan Battery of Neuropsychological Tests
   D. Stanford-Binet Intelligence Scale
   E. None of the above

5.17 Consists of ten tests, including the trail-making test and the critical flicker frequency test

5.18 Is extremely sensitive in identifying discrete forms of brain damage, such as dyslexia

5.19 Consists of 120 items, plus several alternative tests, applicable to the ages between 2 years and adulthood

5.20 Furnishes a description of the dynamic forces of personality through an analysis of the person's responses

5.21 A test of diffuse cerebral dysfunction to which normal children by the age of 7 years respond negatively

Questions 5.22–5.24

   A. Short-term memory loss
   B. Signs of organic dysfunction
   C. Korsakoff's syndrome
   D. Posterior right hemisphere lesion
   E. Damage to frontal lobes or caudate

5.22 Wechsler Memory Scale
5.23 Wisconsin Card Sorting Test
5.24 Benton Visual Retention Test

Questions 5.25–5.29

   A. Wechsler Adult Intelligence Scale (WAIS)
   B. Thematic Apperception Test (TAT)
   C. Shipley Abstraction Test
   D. Sentence Completion Test
   E. Raven's Progressive Matrices

5.25 A broad set of complex verbal and visuospatial tasks that are normatively summarized by three scales

5.26 Impaired performance is associated with posterior lesions of either cerebral hemisphere

5.27 Series of 20 black-and-white pictures depicting individuals of different ages and sexes involved in a variety of settings

5.28 More direct than most projective tests in soliciting responses from the patient

5.29 Requires the patient to complete logical sequences

Questions 5.30–5.34

   A. Executive functions
   B. Attention and concentration
   C. Visuospatial–constructional
   D. Motor
   E. None of the above

5.30 Clock drawing and facial recognition
5.31 Finger tapping
5.32 Trail-making test
5.33 Digit span
5.34 Wisconsin Card Sorting Test

Questions 5.35–5.37

   A. Stanford-Binet Intelligence Scale
   B. Wechsler Preschool and Primary Scale of Intelligence (WPPSI)
   C. Wechsler Intelligence Scale for Children (WISC)—Third Edition
   D. All of the above
   E. None of the above

5.35 Appropriate for children at least 6 years of age to 16 years

5.36 Appropriate for children beginning at 2½ years of age

5.37 Yields a composite IQ score, and scores for verbal reasoning, abstract visual reasoning, quantitative reasoning, and short-term memory

Questions 5.38–5.39

   A. Brief Psychiatric Rating Scale (BPRS)
   B. Schedule for Affective Disorders and Schizophrenia (SADS)
   C. Both
   D. Neither

5.38 Ratings are made on the basis of mental status interview and do not require that the examiner ask any specific questions

5.39 Highly structured interview instrument

ANSWERS

Clinical Neuropsychological Testing

5.1 The answer is D

Many functions are mediated by both the right and left cerebral hemispheres. However, important qualitative differences between the two hemispheres can be demonstrated in the presence of lateralized brain injury. Various cognitive skills that have been linked to the left or right hemisphere in right-handed people are listed in Table 5.1. Although *language* is the most obvious area that is largely controlled by the left hemisphere (with injuries leading to aphasias), the left hemisphere is also generally considered to be dominant for *limb praxis* (i.e., performing complex movements, such as brushing teeth, commanding, or imitation) and has been associated with a cluster of deficits identified as Gerstmann syndrome (i.e., *finger agnosia,* dyscalculia, dysgraphia, and *right-left disorientation*). In contrast, the right hemisphere is thought to play a more important role in controlling *visuospatial abilities and hemispatial attention,* which are associated with the clinical presentations of constructional apraxia and neglect, respectively.

Although lateralized deficits such as these are typically characterized in terms of damage to the right or left hemisphere, it is important to keep in mind that the patient's performance can also be characterized in terms of preserved brain functions. In other words, it is the remaining intact brain tissue that drives many behavioral responses following injury to the brain and not only the absence of critical brain tissue.

5.2 The answer is A

Right hemispheric damage in right-handers is frequently associated with deficits in visuospatial skills. Common assessment techniques include drawings and constructional or spatial assembly tasks. Distinctive qualitative errors in constructing block designs and in drawing a complex geometric configuration can be seen with either right or left hemisphere damage. In the presence of *lateralized damage to the right hemisphere,* impaired performances often reflect the patient's inability to appreciate the gestalt or global features of a design. In the example shown in Figure 5.1, this is seen in the patient's failure to maintain the 2 × 2 matrix of blocks, which was instead converted into a column of four blocks. In contrast, damage to the left hemisphere commonly results in inaccurate reproduction of internal details of the design, including improper orientation of

individual blocks, but the 2 × 2 matrix (i.e., the gestalt) is more likely to be preserved. Similar differences can be seen with drawings, as in the example of the Rey-Osterreith Complex Figure shown in Figure 5.2. The patient with right parietal damage draws isolated details of the design, while failing to convey the interrelationship of the details in the overall design configuration. In contrast, the patient with left hemisphere damage tends to maintain the global framework of the design but to lose the details. Therefore, many neuropsychologists emphasize that a neuropsychological understanding of the impairment depends not just on a set of test scores but also on a qualitative description of the type of error. This often allows the impairment to be linked to a specific neuroanatomical region and also enables a better understanding of the mechanisms of the deficit for rehabilitation purposes.

In another example, damage to the right hemisphere tends to be associated with decreased appreciation of global features of visual stimuli while left hemispheric damage tends to be associated with decreased analysis of local features and detail. This notion is illustrated in Figure 5.3, where a left hemisphere–damaged patient reproduces ambiguous figures as a simple triangle or letter "M" with no regard for the internal characters that actually make up the designs. In contrast, the local approach of a patient with right hemispheric damage emphasizes the internal details (small rectangles of letter "Z") without appreciation for the gestalt that is formed by the internal details. This example also illustrates the important point that behavioral responses (including errors) are driven as much by preserved regions of intact brain functioning as by the loss of other regions of brain functioning.

5.3 The answer is E (all)

Most neuropsychological referrals are made for diagnostic purposes, to ascertain if brain impairment is present, or to differentiate among neurological or psychiatric disorders. Other important uses of testing include establishing a baseline of performance for assessing future change and planning for rehabilitation or management of behaviors affected by brain

Table 5.1
Selected Neuropsychological Deficits Associated with Left or Right Hemisphere Damage

Left Hemisphere	Right Hemisphere
Aphasia	Visuospatial deficits
Right-left disorientation	Impaired visual perception
Finger agnosia	Neglect
Dysgraphia (aphasic)	Dysgraphia (spatial, neglect)
Dyscalculia (number alexia)	Dyscalculia (spatial)
Constructional apraxia (details)	Constructional apraxia (Gestalt)
Limb apraxia	Dressing apraxia
	Anosognosia

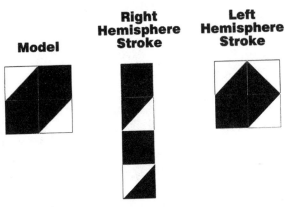

FIGURE 5.1

Examples of Block Design constructions seen in a right hemispheric stroke patient and a left hemispheric stroke patient.

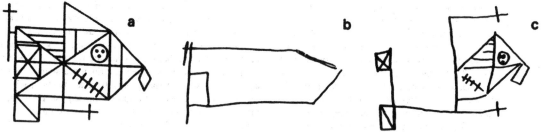

FIGURE 5.2

Rey-Osterreith Complex Figure **(a)** model, and drawings from memory by **(b)** a patient with left hemispheric injury and **(c)** a patient with right hemispheric injury. (Courtesy of Academic Press.)

impairment. The specific methods of neuropsychological assessment reflect the individual's unique presentation of symptoms and complaints, history and development, the perspective of the neuropsychologist, and the referral question.

A common referral issue involves documentation of level of functioning for a variety of purposes, including assessment of change or competence, especially in the presence of diagnoses such as dementia, stroke, and head injury.

5.4 The answer is E (all)

Neuropsychological testing provides a detailed, objective picture of different aspects of memory and attention, which can be helpful in *reassuring healthy persons about their abilities.* It also provides an opportunity for assessing undetected mood or anxiety disorders that may be reflected in cognitive concerns, and for offering suggestions about mnemonic strategies that can sharpen everyday function.

When concerns about a person's memory functioning are expressed by relatives instead of the patient, there is a higher probability of a neurological basis for the functional problems. Neuropsychological testing combined with a good clinical history and other medical screening tests is highly effective in distinguishing early dementia from the milder forms of *declining memory that can be seen with normal aging.* Neuropsychological evaluation is particularly helpful in documenting cognitive deterioration and differentiating among forms of *dementia,* such as Alzheimer's disease and frontal lobe dementia.

Neuropsychologists are often asked to consult in *determining individuals' competence* to make decisions or to manage personal affairs. Neuropsychological testing can be useful in these cases by documenting areas of clear and significant impairment and identifying areas of strength and well-preserved skill. However, opinions about competence should not be based on test findings alone but must include other, more indirect

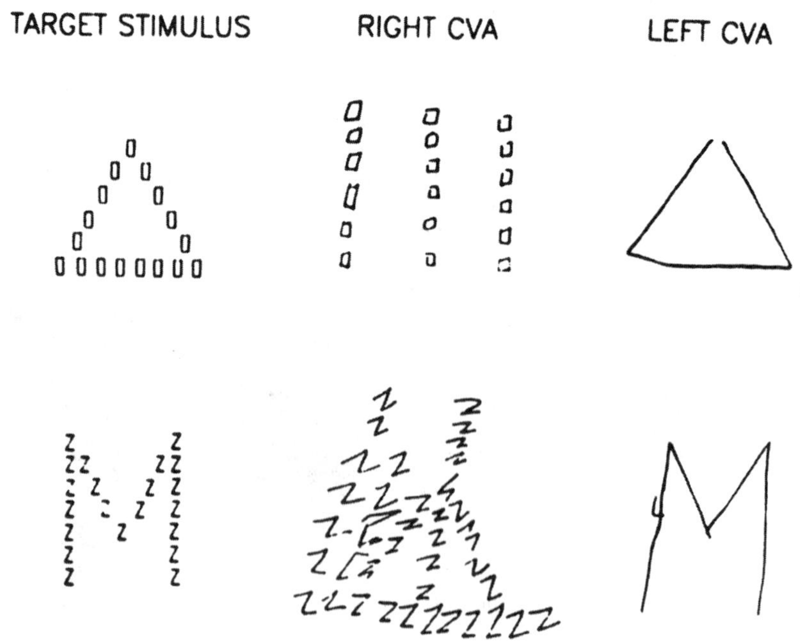

TARGET STIMULUS   RIGHT CVA   LEFT CVA

FIGURE 5.3

Global local target stimuli with drawings from memory by a patient with right hemispheric cerebrovascular accident (CVA) and by a patient with left hemispheric CVA. (Courtesy of Academic Press.)

observations (e.g., in-home assessment, collateral interviews) of everyday functioning.

A substantial minority of patients with severe depression exhibit serious generalized impairment of cognitive functioning. In addition to problems with attention and slowing of thought and action, there may be significant forgetfulness and difficulties with reasoning. By examining the pattern of cognitive impairments, neuropsychological testing can help to identify *pseudodementia,* a dementia-like condition seen in elderly patients with depressive disorders. Perhaps more common is a mixed presentation, in which depression coexists with various forms of cognitive decline, increasing the severity of cognitive dysfunction beyond what would be expected from the neurological impairment alone. Neuropsychological testing can provide a baseline for measuring the effectiveness of antidepressant therapy in alleviating cognitive and mood symptoms.

5.5 The answer is D

Projective personality tests, in contrast to objective personality instruments, are more indirect and unstructured. Unlike objective tests, in which the patient may simply mark "true" or "false" to given questions, the variety of responses to projective personality tests is almost unlimited. Instructions are usually general, allowing the patient's fantasies to be expressed. Patients generally do not know how their responses will be scored or analyzed, making it difficult to obtain a desired result. Projective tests typically do not measure one particular personality characteristic such as type A personality (i.e., narrow-band measurement) but instead are designed to assess a personality as a whole (i.e., broad-band measurement).

Projective tests often focus on latent or unconscious aspects of personality. Obviously, psychologists and others differ in the degree to which they rely on unconscious information. In many projective techniques, patients are simply shown a picture of something and asked to tell what the picture reminds them of. Projective techniques assume that when presented with an ambiguous stimulus such as an inkblot, for which there are an almost unlimited number of responses, the patients' responses will reflect fundamental aspects of their personalities. The ambiguous stimulus is a sort of screen on which individuals project their own needs, thoughts, or conflicts. Different persons have different thoughts, needs, and conflicts and hence will have different responses. In particular, a schizophrenic patient's responses will often reflect a rather bizarre, idiosyncratic view of the world.

Hundreds of different projective techniques have been developed—most of which are not used widely today. Table 5.2 lists commonly used projective tests, gives brief descriptions, and summarizes the strengths and weaknesses of each.

5.6 The answer is D

Memory is a comprehensive term that covers the retention of all types of material over various periods of time and that involves diverse forms of response. The Wechsler Memory Scale (WMS) is the most widely used memory test battery for adults. It is a composite of verbal paired-associate retention, paragraph retention, visual memory for designs, orientation, digit span, rote recall of the alphabet, and counting backward. *The Wechsler Memory Scale yields a memory quotient* (MQ), *which is corrected for age and generally approximates the Wechsler Adult Intelligence Scale* (WAIS) IQ.

Immediate (or short-term) memory is the reproduction, recognition, or recall of perceived material within 30 seconds of presentation. It is most often assessed by digit repetition and reversal (auditory) tests and memory-for-designs (visual) tests. *Both an auditory-verbal task, such as digit span or memory for words or sentences, and a nonverbal visual task, such as mem-*

Table 5.2
Projective Measures of Personality

Name	Description	Strengths	Weaknesses
Rorschach test	10 stimulus cards of inkblots, some colored, others achromatic	Most widely used projective device and certainly the best researched; considerable interpretative data available	Some Rorschach interpretive systems have unproved validity
Thematic Apperception Test (TAT)	20 stimulus cards depicting a number of scenes of varying ambiguity	A widely used method that, in the hands of a well-trained person, provides valuable information	No generally accepted scoring system results in poor consistency in interpretation; time-consuming administration
Sentence completion test	A number of different devices available, all sharing the same format with more similarities than differences	Brief administration time; can be a useful adjunct to clinical interviews if supplied beforehand	Stimuli are obvious in intent and subject to easy falsification
Holtzman Inkblot Technique (HIT)	Two parallel forms of inkblot cards with 45 cards per form	Only one response is allowed per card, making research less troublesome	Not widely accepted and rarely used; not directly comparable to Rorschach interpretive strategies
Figure drawing	Typically human forms but can involve houses or other forms	Quick administration	Interpretive strategies have typically been unsupported by research
Make-a-Picture Story (MAPS)	Similar to TAT; however, stimuli can be manipulated by the patient	Provides idiographic personality information through thematic analysis	Minimal research support; not widely used

Courtesy of Robert W. Butler, Ph.D., and Paul Satz, Ph.D.

ory for designs or for objects or faces, should be given to assess a patient's immediate memory. Patients can also be asked to listen to a standardized story and then to repeat it as accurately as possible. Patients with lesions of the right hemisphere are likely to show more severe defects on visual nonverbal tasks than on auditory verbal tasks. Conversely, patients with left hemisphere disease, including those who are not aphasic, are likely to show severe deficits on the auditory verbal tests, with variable performance on the visual nonverbal tasks.

Recent memory cannot be tested by digit-span tasks, as can immediate memory. Recent memory concerns events over the past few hours or days; it can be tested by asking patients what they had for breakfast and who visited them in the hospital.

Other types of memory that theorists have described include episodic memory, semantic memory, and implicit memory. Episodic memory is memory for specific events, such as a telephone message. *Episodic memory is not memory for knowledge and facts;* that is semantic memory. An example of semantic memory is knowing who was the first President of the United States. *Semantic memory and implicit memory do not decline with age;* persons continue to accumulate information over a lifetime. Episodic memory shows a minimal decline with aging that may relate to impaired frontal lobe functioning. *Implicit memory* is for automatic skills (e.g., driving a car).

5.7 The answer is D

An intelligence quotient (IQ) of 100 corresponds to the *50th percentile* in intellectual ability for the general population. Modern psychological testing began in the first decade of the 20th century when Alfred Binet (1857–1911), a French psychologist, developed the first intelligence scale to separate the mentally defective youngsters (who were to be given special education) from the rest of the children (whose school progress was to be accelerated).

5.8 The answer is E

Intelligence levels are based on the assumption that intellectual abilities are distributed normally (in a bell-shaped curve) throughout the population. Intelligence can be defined as a person's ability to assimilate factual knowledge, recall either recent or remote events, reason logically, manipulate concepts (either numbers or words), translate the abstract to the literal and the literal to the abstract, analyze and synthesize forms, and deal meaningfully and accurately with problems and priorities deemed important in a particular setting. In 1905 Alfred Binet introduced the concept of the mental age (MA), which is the average intellectual level at a particular age. The intelligence quotient (IQ) is the ratio of MA over CA (chronological age) multiplied by 100 to do away with the decimal point; it is represented by the following equation:

$$\frac{MA}{CA} \times 100 = IQ$$

When the chronological age and the mental age are equal, the IQ is 100—that is, average. Because it is impossible to measure increments of intellectual power past the age of 15 by available intelligence tests, *the highest divisor in the IQ formula is 15, not 25.*

As measured by most intelligence tests, IQ is an interpretation or a classification of a total test score in relation to norms established by a group. *IQ is a measure of present functioning*

ability, not of future potential. Under ordinary circumstances, the IQ is stable throughout life, but there is no certainty about its predictive properties.

The Wechsler Adult Intelligence Scale (WAIS), not the Stanford-Binet test, is the most widely used intelligence test in clinical practice today. The WAIS was constructed by David Wechsler at the New York University Medical Center and Bellevue Psychiatric Hospital. It comprises 11 subtests—six verbal subtests and five performance subtests—yielding a verbal IQ, a performance IQ, and a combined or full-scale IQ. The verbal IQ, the performance IQ, and the full-scale IQ are determined by the use of separate tables for each of the seven age groups (from 16 to 64 years) on which the test was standardized.

The average or normal range of IQ is 90 to 110, not 70 to 100. IQ scores of 120 and higher are considered superior. According to the American Association of Mental Deficiency (AAMD) and the fourth edition of *Diagnostic and Statistical Manual of Mental Disorders* (DSM-IV), mental retardation is defined as an IQ of 70 or below, which is found in the lowest 2.2 percent of the population. Consequently, two of every 100 persons have IQ scores consistent with mental retardation, which can range from mild to profound.

Table 5.3 presents the DSM-IV-TR classification of intelligence by IQ range.

5.9 The answer is A

The *arithmetic* subtest showed that the patient's ability to do simple arithmetic was influenced adversely by poor attention and concentration. The *block design* subtest requires a subject to arrange a series of pictures to tell a story. This process tests performance and cognitive styles. The *digit symbol* subtest requires a subject to match digits and symbols in as little time as possible, as a test of performance. The *comprehension* subtest reveals a subject's ability to adhere to social consequences and to understand social judgments when the subject answers questions about how people should behave. On the *picture completion* subtest a subject must complete a picture with a missing part. Visuospatial defects appear when errors are made on this procedure.

5.10 The answer is E (all)

The Bender Visual Motor Gestalt test, devised by the American neuropsychiatrist Lauretta Bender in 1938, is a technique that

Table 5.3
Classification of Intelligence by IQ Range

Classification	IQ Range
Profound mental retardation (MR)[a]	Below 20 or 25
Severe MR[a]	20–25 to 35–40
Moderate MR[a]	35–40 to 50–55
Mild MR[a]	50–55 to about 70
Borderline	70–79
Dull normal	80 to 90
Normal	90 to 110
Bright normal	110 to 120
Superior	120 to 130
Very superior	130 and above

[a]According to the text revision of the fourth edition of *Diagnostic and Statistical Manual of Mental Disorders* (DSM-IV-TR).

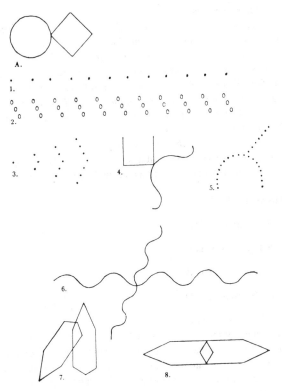

FIGURE 5.4

Test figures from the Bender Visual Motor Gestalt test, adapted from Max Wertheimer. (Reprinted with permission from Bender L. *A Visual Motor Gestalt Test and Its Clinical Use*. New York: American Orthopsychiatric Association; 1938:33.)

consists of nine figures that are copied by the subject (Fig. 5.4). It is administered as a means of evaluating *maturation levels in children* and *organic dysfunction*. Its chief applications are to determine retardation, *loss of function*, and organic brain defects in children and adults. The designs are presented one at a time to the subject, who is asked to copy them onto a sheet of paper. The subject then is asked to copy the designs from memory (Figs. 5.5 and 5.6); thus, the Bender designs can be used as a test of both *visual and motor coordination* and immediate visual memory.

5.11 The answer is C

The MMPI is composed of over 500 *statements, not* 200 *questions*. It is the *most widely used* test. Although the test was initially thought to be a *diagnostic tool*, workers now use the inventory to interpret the patterning of the entire profile obtained from the clinical scales. Researchers have identified personality correlates of various configurations produced on the inventory, which can serve as diagnostic aids. Therefore, a *good indication of a subject's disorder is not a single high score on one scale;* the complete results are examined for an interpretation, and at least two of the highest scores are used to arrive at a diagnosis. The inventory is in the form of clinical scales, but these scales were derived from *homogeneous* groups of psychiatric patients, not from heterogenous groups of people.

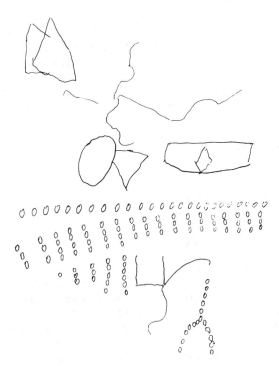

FIGURE 5.5

Bender Visual Motor Gesalt test drawings of a 57-year-old brain-damaged woman.

Answers 5.12–5.16

5.12 The answer is C

5.13 The answer is E

5.14 The answer is D

5.15 The answer is A

5.16 The answer is B

Numerous mental status cognitive tasks are available to test and localize various brain dysfunctions. Construction apraxia—*the loss of gestalt, loss of symmetry, and distortion of figures*—seen in the task of copying the outline of simple objects, is localized to the *nondominant parietal lobe*. Dysfunction of the *occipital lobes* is suggested when a *patient cannot name a camouflaged object but can name it when it is not camouflaged. Two or more errors or two or more 7-second delays in carrying out tasks of*

FIGURE 5.6

Bender Visual Motor Gesalt test recall by the 57-year-old brain-damaged patient who drew Figure 5.5.

right-left orientation (for example, place left hand to right ear, right elbow to right knee) are localized to dysfunction of the *dominant parietal lobe.* A dysfunction in concentration is thought to be localized to the *frontal lobes* and can be tested by eliciting *any improper letter sequence in spelling "earth" backward.* In anomia the *patient cannot name common objects* (for example, watch, key); the impairment is localized to the *dominant temporal lobe.*

Answers 5.17–5.21

5.17 The answer is C

5.18 The answer is B

5.19 The answer is D

5.20 The answer is A

5.21 The answer is E

Various neuropsychiatric tests, including the Halstead-Reitan and the Luria-Nebraska batteries, are sometimes useful in bringing to light subtle organic dysfunctions that are undetected in standard psychiatric, psychological, and even neurological assessments. The *Halstead-Reitan Battery of Neuropsychological Tests consists of ten tests, including the trail-making test and the critical flicker frequency test.* It was developed in an attempt to improve the reliability of the criteria used to diagnose brain damage. Assessment data were gathered on a group of patients with left hemisphere injury, right hemisphere injury, and global involvement. The trail-making test is a test of visuomotor perception and motor speed, and the critical flicker frequency test (noting when a flicker light becomes steady) tests visual perception.

The *Luria-Nebraska Neuropsychological Battery* (LNNB) *is extremely sensitive in identifying discrete forms of brain damage, such as dyslexia* (an impairment in the ability to read) and *dyscalculia* (an inability to perform arithmetical operations), rather than more global forms.

The *Stanford-Binet Intelligence Scale* is one of the tests most frequently used in the individual examination of children. It *consists of 120 items, plus several alternative tests, applicable to the ages between 2 years and adulthood.* The tests have a variety of graded difficulties, both verbal and performance, designed to assess such functions as memory, free association, orientation, language comprehension, knowledge of common objects, abstract thinking, and the use of judgment and reasoning.

The *Rorschach test* is a psychological test consisting of ten inkblots that the person is asked to look at and interpret. It *furnishes a description of the dynamic forces of personality through an analysis of the person's responses.*

The face-hand test, devised by Lauretta Bender, is *a test of diffuse cerebral dysfunction to which normal children by the age of 7 years respond negatively.* The person, whose eyes are closed, is touched simultaneously on the cheek and the hand; retesting is done with the person's eyes open. The results are considered positive if the person fails consistently to identify both stimuli within ten trials.

Answers 5.22–5.24

5.22 The answer is C

5.23 The answer is E

5.24 The answer is A

The *Wechsler Memory Scale* screens for verbal and visual memory and yields a memory quotient. The results can reveal whether a subject has *amnestic Korsakoff's syndrome. The Wisconsin Card Sorting Test* assesses a person's abstract reasoning ability and flexibility in problem solving. The results can reveal whether a person has *damage to the frontal lobes or to the caudate.*

The *Benton Visual Retention Test* screens for *short-term memory loss.*

Signs of organic dysfunction may be screened for by the Bender Visual Motor Gestalt test. *Posterior right-hemisphere lesions* can be revealed through a Facial Recognition Test.

Answers 5.25–5.29

5.25 The answer is A

5.26 The answer is E

5.27 The answer is B

5.28 The answer is D

5.29 The answer is C

Assessment of intellectual functioning serves as the cornerstone of the neuropsychological examination. The Wechsler intelligence scales, based on carefully developed normative standards, have represented the traditional gold standard in intellectual assessment for many years. The scope and variety of subtests on which the summary intelligence quotient (IQ) values are based also provide useful benchmarks against which to compare performances on other tests of specific abilities. The latest revision of this instrument is the Wechsler Memory Scale-III. In general, *the Wechsler intelligence scales use a broad set of complex verbal and visuospatial tasks that are normatively summarized as a Verbal IQ, a Performance IQ, and Full Scale IQ.* In the context of a neuropsychological examination, the patient's performance across the procedures provides useful information regarding longstanding abilities as well as current functioning. Most neuropsychologists recognize that the summary IQ values provide only a ball-park range for characterizing an individual's general level of functioning. Therefore, it is usually more appropriate and meaningful to characterize an individual's intellectual functioning in terms of the range of functioning (e.g., borderline, low average, average, high average, superior) represented by the IQ value rather than the specific value itself. Table 5.3 lists the classification of intelligence by IQ range.

Raven's Progressive Matrices require the patient to complete a design by selecting from a multiple-choice pictorial display the stimulus that completes a design in which a part is omitted. The difficulty of the discrimination increases over trials in the lengthy test. A briefer, less difficult version (Color Matrices) is especially useful for patients who are unable to complete the standard test, which can require 30 to 45 minutes. *Impaired performance is associated with poor visuoconstructive ability and with posterior lesions of either cerebral hemisphere,* but receptive language deficit may contribute to poor performance in patients with dominant hemisphere damage.

Although the Rorschach test is clearly the most frequently used projective personality test, the *Thematic Apperception Test* (TAT) is probably in second place. Many clinicians include both the TAT and the Rorschach test in a battery of tests for personality assessment. *The TAT consists of a series of 20 black-and-white pictures that*

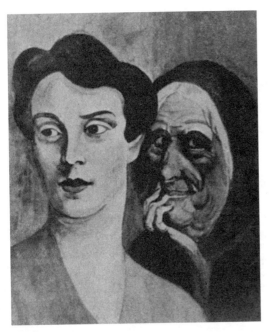

FIGURE 5.7
Card 12F of the Thematic Apperception Test. (Reprinted with permission from Henry A. Murray, Thematic Apperception Test, Harvard University Press, Cambridge, MA. Copyright © 1943 President and Fellows of Harvard College, © 1971 Henry A. Murray.)

Table 5.4
Sample Thematic Apperception Test Responses to TAT Card 12F

Diagnostic Category	Indicated Response
Nonpatient	This lady has a serious look on her face. She had been talking with the older woman in the background. The older woman had been trying to persuade her to do something that she did not feel was quite right. The younger lady is thinking "I can't do what she wants." She is feeling somewhat put upon by this woman. The young lady is frustrated by the request. She is trying to think of a response to the request. What happens in the future is she ignores the old woman's request.
Schizo-phrenic patient	This young lady is about to be killed by that witch in the background. The witch is getting ready to poison her. You have to be careful nowadays, the witch wants all of her money and her car. I know I have to watch out. Everybody will get you if they can. I don't trust anyone. Better safe than sorry . . . I'm not sorry for what I've done, sorry is not something a person should be. Love means you don't have to say you are sorry.
Depression	I hate pictures like this, I am not really good at it anyway. The lady in front is thinking about her mother. Her mother was not an evil lady but the young lady feels like her mother didn't care about her, didn't love her, and was very selfish. Her mother didn't provide support. The young woman is thinking that she has been deprived and emotionally abused. The young lady will think for a few minutes and will then go into the bedroom to be by herself.
Anxiety	The young lady is getting ready to go to work but she doesn't want to go. She rented a room from the old lady in the background. The young lady is about to get fired at work. She does not like her job but she needs the money. She doesn't know how she is going to support herself when she loses her job. She goes on to work but has a miserable day. She eventually loses her job and the old landlady kicks her out of her room.

depict individuals of both sexes and of different age groups involved in a variety of different settings. For example, on Card 1, a young boy is shown sitting at a table, looking at a violin. Card 2 depicts a farm scene in which a young woman in the foreground is carrying books in her hands; a man is working in the fields nearby, and an older woman is seen in the background. Typically, a patient is shown ten TAT cards and asked to make up stories about them. The patient is asked to tell what is going on in the picture, what was going on before the picture was taken, what the individuals in the picture are thinking and feeling, and what is likely to happen in the future. An example of a TAT card is presented in Figure 5.7. Some examples of typical responses to the TAT appear in Table 5.4.

Henry Murray developed the TAT at the Harvard Psychological Clinic in 1943. The stories the patient make up concerning the pictures, according to the projective hypothesis, reflect the patient's own needs, thoughts, feelings, stresses, wishes, desires, and view of the future.

Although a projective instrument, the Sentence Completion Test is much more direct in soliciting responses from the patient. The patient is simply presented with a series of incomplete sentences and asked to complete each sentence stem with the first response that comes to mind. Examples of possible incomplete sentences are as follows:

My father seldom . . .
Most people don't know that I'm afraid of . . .
When I was a child, I . . .
When encountering frustration, I usually . . .

The purpose of the test is to elicit, somewhat indirectly, information about the patient that cannot be elicited by other measures. Since the patient responds in writing, the examiner's time is limited. The length of time it takes to complete this test varies greatly, depending on the number of incomplete sentences. Tests can range from fewer than ten sentences to more than 75.

There are many variations of sentence completion tests. Some clinicians have developed their own. One form developed by Julian Rotter has some established validity and reliability, but most sentence completion tests do not. Special-purpose sentence completion tests have been developed to measure different problem areas. For example, one sentence completion test is used with patients who have chronic pain, and another to assess issues concerning transsexual patients. The sentence completion test is seldom, if ever, used alone but is combined with other appropriate instruments.

Advantages of the sentence completion are short administration time, ease of administration, variety of instruments, and ease of construction. Disadvantages are lack of reliability and validity studies and ease of fabrication and deception.

The *Shipley Abstraction Test requires the patient to complete logical sequences;* it assesses the patient's capacity to think abstractly. Because performance on a test of this type is related to educational background, an accompanying vocabulary test is also given to the patient, and a comparison is made between the patient's performances on the two tests. A low abstraction score

Table 5.5
Selected Tests of Neuropsychological Functioning

Area of Function	Comment
INTELLECTUAL FUNCTIONING	
Wechsler Intelligence Scales	Age-stratified normative references; appropriate for adults up to age 89, adolescents, and young children
Shipley Scale	Brief (20-minute) paper-and-pencil measure of multiple-choice vocabulary and open-ended verbal abstraction
ATTENTION AND CONCENTRATION	
Digit Span	Auditory-verbal measure of simple span of attention (*Digits Forward*) and cognitive manipulation of increasingly longer strings of digits (*Digits Backward*)
Visual Memory Span	Visual-spatial measure of ability to reproduce a spatial sequence in forward and reverse order
Paced Auditory Serial Addition Test	Requires double tracking to add pairs of digits at increasing rates; particularly sensitive to subtle simultaneous processing deficits, especially in head injury
MEMORY	
Wechsler Memory Scale—III	Comprehensive set of subtests measuring attention and encoding, retrieval, and recognition of various types of verbal and visual material with both immediate recall and delayed retention; excellent age-stratified normative comparisons for adults up to age 89, with intellectual data for direct comparison
California Verbal Learning Test	Documents encoding, recognition, and both immediate and 30-minute recall; also affords examination of possible learning strategies as well as susceptibility to semantic interference
Fuld Object Memory Evaluation	Selective reminding format requires that patient identify objects tactually, then assesses consistency of retrieval and storage as well as ability to benefit from cues; normative reference group is designed for use with older individuals
LANGUAGE	
Boston Diagnostic Aphasia Examination	Comprehensive assessment of expressive and receptive language functions
Boston Naming Test—Revised	Documents word-finding difficulty in a visual confrontation format
Verbal Fluency	Measures ability to generate words fluently within semantic categories (e.g., animals) or phonetic categories (e.g., words beginning with *S*)
Token Test	Systematically assesses comprehension of complex commands by use of standard token stimuli that vary in size, shape, and color
VISUOSPATIAL–CONSTRUCTIONAL	
Judgment of Line Orientation	Ability to judge angles of lines on a page presented in a match-to-sample format
Facial Recognition	Assesses matching and discrimination of unfamiliar faces
Clock Drawing	Useful screening technique sensitive to organization and planning as well as constructional ability
Rey-Osterreith Complex Figure Test	Ability to draw and later recall complex geometric configuration; sensitive to executive deficits in development of strategies and planning
MOTOR	
Finger Tapping	Standard measure of simple motor speed; particularly useful for documenting lateralized motor impairment
Grooved Pegboard	Ability to place notched pegs in slotted holes rapidly; measures fine finger dexterity as well as eye–hand coordination
Grip Strength	Standard measure of lateralizing differences in strength
EXECUTIVE FUNCTIONS	
Wisconsin Card Sorting Test	Measure of problem-solving efficiency is particularly sensitive to executive deficits of perseveration and impaired ability to generate alternative strategies flexibly in response to feedback
Category Test	Measure of problem-solving ability that also examines ability to benefit from feedback while flexibly generating alternative response strategies; regarded as one of the most sensitive measures of general brain dysfunction in the Halstead-Reitan battery
Trail-Making Test	Requires rapid and efficient integration of attention, visual scanning, and cognitive sequencing

in relation to vocabulary level is interpreted as reflecting an impairment in conceptual thinking.

Answers 5.30–5.34

5.30 The answer is C

5.31 The answer is D

5.32 The answer is A

5.33 The answer is B

5.34 The answer is A

The past decade has seen a virtual explosion in the growth of more sophisticated and better standardized tests and procedures for neuropsychological evaluation. Although a comprehensive listing of tests and techniques is beyond the scope of this book, excellent reviews of current techniques are found in texts by Lezak as well as Otfried Spreen and Esther Strauss. Asenath LaRue has published detailed observations about pertinent assessment issues in aging and neuropsychology. A list of examples of common neuropsychological tests and techniques is provided in Table 5.5.

Table 5.6
Selected Intelligence and Academic Achievement Tests

Intelligence tests
  Bayley Infant Scale of Development—2nd edition (1–42 months)
  McCarthy Scales of Children's Intelligence (2.5–8.5 years)
  Kaufman Assessment Battery for Children (2.5–12.5 years)
  Stanford-Binet Intelligence Test, 4th edition (2.5 years—adult)
  Wechsler Preschool and Primary Scale of Intelligence—Revised (4–6.5 years)
  Wechsler Intelligence Scale for Children—Third Edition (6–16 years)
  Test of Nonverbal Intelligence—3 (6–89 years)
  Raven's Progressive Matrices (Coloured or Standard) (5.5 years–adult)
Academic achievement tests
  Wide Range Achievement Test—3rd edition
  Woodcock Johnson Psycho-Educational Test Battery—Revised
  Peabody Individual Achievement Test—Revised
  Wechsler Individual Achievement Tests
  Bracken Basic Concept Scales (school screener)

Answers 5.35–5.37

5.35 The answer is C

5.36 The answer is A

5.37 The answer is A

The most frequently used general intelligence batteries for children are the WISC, the Stanford-Binet Test, and the Wechsler Preschool and Primary Scale of Intelligence (WPPSI). A relatively low level of general intelligence is probably the most constant behavioral result of brain damage in children.

Generally, a comprehensive evaluation screens each relevant domain to establish integrity of function. The decision to administer more detailed testing within a domain is based on the referral question, the response to screening measures, and behaviors observed during the test session. A growing number of tests is available for inclusion in an individually designed session. The choice depends on examiner experience and preference.

Table 5.6 lists commonly used intelligence and academic achievement tests. These tests vary, and the choice of instrument is based in part on the age of the child. For example, *the Stanford-Binet Intelligence Scale is appropriate for children beginning at 2½ years of age. It yields a composite IQ score and scores for four scales: verbal reasoning, abstract visual reasoning, quantitative reasoning, and short-term memory.*

Intelligence and achievement tests are not validated with respect to brain function, but they provide valuable data for a neuropsychological evaluation. *The Wechsler Intelligence Scale for Children— Third Edition is the most commonly administered general intelligence test for children at least 6 years of age.* It is a battery comprising 13 subtests (ten core tests and 32 alternates). Three summary IQs are obtained: (1) the Verbal IQ, based on five verbal subtests; (2) the Performance IQ, based on five performance subtests; and (3) the averaged index of general intellectual functioning, the Full Scale IQ. Language expression, comprehension, and application of verbal skills in problem solving are assessed within the verbal scale. Nonverbal visuoperceptual analysis, synthesis, expression, psychomotor speech, and visuomotor efficiency are assessed within the

Performance Scale. Neither scale assesses several important factors that influence successful performance, such as motivation, creativity, organizational skill, or study habits. Four additional index scores can be obtained. The Verbal Comprehension Index is based on performances on the information, similarities, vocabulary, and comprehension subtests. The perceptual Organizational Index is based on performances on the picture completion, picture arrangement, block design, and object assembly subtests. The Freedom from Distractibility Index is based on arithmetic and digit-span performances. The Processing Speed Index is based on coding and symbol search performances. The *Wechsler Preschool and Primary Scale of Intelligence (WPPSI)* is a scale for children ages 4 to 6 years, extending the range of assessment downward in age.

Answers 5.38–5.39

5.38 The answer is A

5.39 The answer is B

One of the more commonly used interview rating scales is the *Brief Psychiatric Rating Scale (BPRS). To use the BPRS, the psychologist or psychiatrist completes a mental status interview with the patient and then rates that patient on a series of 18 psychiatric symptoms such as motor retardation, blunted affect, conceptual disorganization, anxiety, and guilt.* Expanded definitions of each of these terms are provided to the examiner. The interviewer rates each domain on a seven-point scale from "not present," the lowest rating, to "extremely severe," the highest rating. An experienced interviewer can complete the ratings in 2 or 3 minutes. The BPRS has been used extensively in drug-outcome and other studies. The advantages of the BPRS are the reasonably high interrater reliability, the ease and speed of rating, and the well-defined symptom description. *The BPRS ratings are made on the basis of a mental status interview and do not require that the examiner ask any specific questions of the patient.* This approach allows flexibility but results in considerable variation due to interview style. A flexible interview results in different information being gathered by different interviewers.

The SADS *is a highly structured interview instrument.* The interviewer is required to ask each patient a series of prescribed questions to ensure that all relevant areas are addressed. For example, a patient is asked a question similar to the following: "Have you ever heard voices or other things that weren't there or that other people couldn't hear or see?" Based on the patient's response, the examiner asks other detailed, prescribed follow-up questions concerning hallucinations, or if the response was negative, the interviewer moves on to the next question in a different area. This approach ensures that all areas are covered in a comprehensive fashion. The SADS is especially helpful for establishing a reliable diagnosis. The SADS can also be used as an index of behavioral severity. Behavioral changes can be determined by repeated administration. The SADS is quite time consuming, mainly because it is comprehensive. After an initial evaluation using the complete SADS, a condensed SADS (SADS/C) can be used for follow-up.

The advantage of the test is that it is comprehensive and has reasonably good reliability. One disadvantage is its length; another is that in the structured interview the interviewer must read questions from a lengthy booklet, which makes it difficult to establish eye contact and rapport with the patient. The SADS has been used for both research and clinical purposes, probably more frequently for the former.

6 ▲

Theories of Personality and Psychopathology

All major psychological theories of personality involve the basic premise that a person's early psychosocial development shapes what comes later: that the impact of childhood events, beliefs, experiences, and fantasies, continue, consciously or unconsciously, throughout life and account for adult behavior.

The most important personality theorist of the modern era was Sigmund Freud (1856–1939). His revolutionary contributions to the understanding of the human mind and psyche continue to stimulate, provoke, and challenge students of personality and psychopathology today. His basic tenets of the unconscious mind, psychosexual development, and psychodynamics remain the bedrock of psychoanalytic theory, even though many have disagreed with, modified, or expanded on his ideas. No matter how a particular theorist may feel about

Freud's ideas, each must begin with a thorough knowledge of his contributions.

There have been many psychoanalytic personality theorists with widely varying views on development. These include Alfred Adler (1870–1937), Erik Erikson (1902–1994), Karen Horney (1885–1952), Carl Gustav Jung (1875–1961), Melanie Klein (1882–1960), Harry Stack Sullivan (1892–1949), and Heinz Kohut (1913–1981). Schools of thought, encompassing a variety of different theories, include ego psychology, object relations, self psychology, and interpersonal psychology, among others. Each approach has its own perspective on personality development and the development of psychopathology.

Students should study the questions and answers below to test their knowledge in this area.

HELPFUL HINTS

The student should know the various theorists, their schools of thought, and their theories.

- Karl Abraham
- abreaction
- acting out
- Alfred Adler
- Franz Alexander
- Gordon Allport
- analytical process
- attention cathexis
- Michael Balint
- behaviorism
- Eric Berne
- Wilfred Bion
- birth trauma
- Joseph Breuer
- cathexis
- Raymond Cattell
- character traits
- condensation
- conflict
- conscious
- day's residue
- defense mechanisms
- displacement
- dream work
- ego functions
- ego ideal

- ego psychology
- Erik Erikson
- Eros and Thanatos
- Ronald Fairbairn
- Sandor Ferenczi
- Anna Freud
- free association
- Erich Fromm
- fundamental rule
- Kurt Goldstein
- Heinz Hartmann
- Karen Horney
- hypnosis
- hysterical phenomena
- infantile sexuality
- instinctual drives
- interpretation
- Carl Gustav Jung
- Søren Kierkegaard
- Melanie Klein
- Heinz Kohut
- latent dream
- Kurt Lewin
- libido
- libido and instinct theories

- manifest dream
- Abraham Maslow
- Adolph Meyer
- multiple self-organizations
- Gardner Murphy
- Henry Murray
- narcissism
- narcissistic, immature, neurotic, and mature defenses
- nocturnal sensory stimuli
- object constancy
- object relations
- parapraxes
- Frederick S. Perls
- preconscious
- preconscious system
- pregenital
- primary and secondary gains
- primary autonomous functions
- primary process
- psychic determinism
- psychoanalytic theory
- psychodynamic thinking
- psychoneurosis
- psychosexual development
- Sandor Rado

- Otto Rank
- reality principle
- reality testing
- regression
- Wilhelm Reich
- repetition compulsion
- repression
- resistance
- secondary process
- secondary revision
- signal anxiety
- structural model
- *Studies on Hysteria*
- Harry Stack Sullivan
- symbolic representation
- symbolism
- synthetic functions of the ego
- talking cure
- *The Ego and the Id*
- *The Interpretation of Dreams*
- topographic theory
- transference
- unconscious motivation
- Donald Winnicott
- wish fulfillment
- working through

▲ QUESTIONS

DIRECTIONS: Each of the questions or incomplete statements below is followed by five suggested responses or completions. Select the *one* that is *best* in each case.

6.1 Wilhelm Reich's concept of character includes all of the following *except*

A. character is an armoring of the ego
B. punishment over sexual activity affects character formation
C. elasticity determines the difference between the healthy and the neurotic character
D. the death instinct affects character formation
E. special emphasis on repressive and inhibiting effects

6.2 Psychic determinism refers to

A. long-forgotten memories reemerging in the process of treatment
B. psychoanalysis being fundamentally a one-person (intrapsychic) psychology
C. dreams being a primary source of information about unconscious conflict
D. childhood experiences that continue to affect adult behavior
E. all of the above

6.3 The concept of birth trauma, as developed by Otto Rank, refers to which of the following constructs:

A. the mother's painful experience at the time of delivery
B. the transference
C. the Oedipus complex
D. the source of primal anxiety
E. none of the above

6.4 Transference refers to

A. removing symptoms by recovering and verbalizing repressed feelings with which they were associated
B. the displacement onto the analyst of thoughts and feelings originally associated with significant figures from the past
C. the process of saying whatever comes to mind, without censorship
D. excluding unpleasant thoughts or memories from conscious awareness
E. the compromise between a repressed impulse and the countervailing forces of repression

6.5 The concept of masculine protest

A. was introduced by Alfred Adler
B. is a universal human tendency
C. refers to a move from the female or passive role
D. is an extension of Adler's ideas about organ inferiority
E. all of the above

6.6 Ego functions include

A. reality testing
B. object relationships
C. defense mechanisms
D. control of instinctual drives
E. all of the above

6.7 The ego-ideal

A. is generally conceptualized as a set of functions contained within the structure of the superego
B. dictates what one should not do
C. is not conceptualized as an amalgam of internalized representations
D. is associated with guilt more than shame
E. none of the above

6.8 In Erik Erikson's descriptions of the stages of the life cycle

A. the stage of industry versus inferiority corresponds to Freud's phallic-oedipal stage
B. the stage of identity versus role diffusion corresponds to Freud's latency stage
C. the stage of autonomy versus shame and doubt corresponds to Freud's anal stage
D. generativity can occur only if a person has or raises a child
E. the state of integrity versus despair occurs from late adolescence through the early middle years

6.9 In the structural model of the mind

A. the superego controls the delay and the modulation of drive expression
B. the superego is the executive organ of the psyche
C. the superego's activities occur unconsciously to a large extent
D. the reality principle and the pleasure principle are aspects of the id functioning
E. the id operates under the domination of secondary process

6.10 The major defense mechanism used in paranoia is

A. projection
B. identification
C. displacement
D. undoing
E. reaction formation

6.11 Mature defenses, according to George Vaillant, include

A. altruism
B. controlling
C. intellectualization
D. rationalization
E. all of the above

6.12 Autonomous functions of the ego include all of the following *except*

A. perception
B. language
C. motor development
D. repression
E. intelligence

6.13 According to Carl Gustav Jung, archetypes are

A. instinctual patterns
B. expressed in representational images
C. expressed in mythological images
D. organizational units of the personality
E. all of the above

6.14 According to Alfred Adler, the helplessness of the infant accounts for

A. feelings of inferiority
B. a need to strive for superiority
C. fantasied organic or psychological deficits
D. compensatory strivings
E. all of the above

6.15 Donald Winnicott's contributions to the British school of object relations included hypotheses of all of the following *except*

A. a true self
B. a traditional space
C. a transitional object
D. a holding environment
E. a good-enough mother

6.16 All of the following early psychoanalysts studied with Sigmund Freud *except*

A. Carl Gustav Jung
B. Alfred Adler
C. Karl Abraham
D. Frederick S. Perls
E. Sandor Ferenczi

6.17 Which of the following statements about dreams is true as described by Freud?

A. Dreams are the conscious expression of an unconscious fantasy.
B. Dreams represent wish-fulfillment activity.
C. Latent dream content derives from the repressed part of the id.
D. Sensory impressions may play a role in initiating a dream.
E. All of the above

6.18 The superego

A. results from the resolution of the Oedipus complex
B. results from the internalization of parental moral values
C. grew out of the need for monitoring and preserving the ego-ideal
D. has primitive precursors formed early in life from the internalization of frightening perceptions of parental figures
E. all of the above

6.19 In Carl Gustav Jung's psychoanalytic school

A. the collective unconscious is a collection of impulses of the id and the ego
B. archetypes contribute to complexes
C. the male part of the self is called the persona
D. individuation is a process that is completed in childhood
E. an emphasis is placed on infantile sexuality

6.20 Self psychology

A. stresses responses from others as important to self-esteem representations
B. puts deficits at center stage rather than conflicts
C. emphasizes infantile needs
D. emphasizes building the psychic structure
E. all of the above

6.21 Lacanian theory

A. places heavy emphasis on linguistics
B. has no place for biology or drives
C. postulates that an individual is embedded in political and societal structure
D. views the analytical process as an effort to recognize alienation from one's true self
E. all of the above

6.22 All of the following statements correctly describe the theories of Erik Erikson *except*

A. Erikson described eight stages of human life cycles.
B. Erikson's stage 6, intimacy versus isolation, refers to young adulthood and later.
C. Erikson's stages do not extend beyond age 70.
D. Erikson described a corresponding zone for each of Freud's three psychosexual stages.
E. Erikson described one stage of childhood in terms similar to those of Piaget's object permanence stage.

6.23 All of the following statements correctly describe the work of Sigmund Freud *except*

A. An important innovation of Freud's was his emphasis on infant sexuality.
B. Freud considered dreams to have two levels of content: manifest and latent.
C. In Freud's tripartite model of the mind, each entity is distinguished by its function.
D. Anna O. had hysterical symptoms related to her father's illness and death, and was treated solely by Freud.
E. Freud's writings on conflicts stressed the need for "working through" to ameliorate psychic disturbances.

6.24 The fundamental rule of psychoanalysis is

A. resistance and repression
B. psychic determinism
C. abreaction
D. free association
E. the concept of the unconscious

6.25 Isolation, the defense mechanism involving the separation of an idea or memory from its attached feeling tone, is found most clearly in

A. obsessive-compulsive disorder
B. anxiety disorders
C. pain disorder
D. dissociative disorders
E. dysthymic disorder

6.26 The term "habit training" was coined by

A. Adolf Meyer
B. Carl Gustav Jung
C. Otto Rank
D. B. F. Skinner
E. Joseph Wolpe

6.27 The self-system concerns Harry Stack Sullivan's concept of the

A. unconscious
B. personality
C. libido
D. defense mechanisms
E. Oedipus complex

6.28 All of the following statements regarding the unconscious system are true *except*

A. It is characterized by secondary process thinking.
B. Its contents become conscious by passing through the preconscious.
C. Its content is limited to wishes that are seeking fulfillment.
D. It disregards logical connections and permits contradictory ideas to exist simultaneously.
E. Its memories are divorced from connections with verbal symbols.

6.29 Which of the following statements applies to the unconscious?

A. Its elements are ordinarily inaccessible to consciousness.
B. It is characterized by primary process thinking.
C. It is closely related to the pleasure principle.
D. It is closely related to the instincts.
E. All of the above

6.30 Of the following assertions about depression, Heinz Kohut would be most linked to which of the following?

A. Depression is internally directed anger.
B. Depression is the result of a harsh superego.
C. Depression is the result of aggression and greed destroying internal good objects.
D. Depression is related to a sense of despair about getting one's self-object needs met by people in the environment.
E. None of the above

DIRECTIONS: Each group of questions below consists of lettered headings followed by a list of numbered words or statements. For each numbered word or statement, select the *one* lettered heading that is most closely associated with it. Each lettered heading may be selected once, more than once, or not at all.

Questions 6.31–6.35

A. Condensation
B. Displacement
C. Symbolic representation
D. Secondary revision
E. Primary process

6.31 Several unconscious impulses are combined and attached to one manifest dream image
6.32 Primitive mode of cognitive activity characterized by illogical, bizarre, and seemingly incoherent images
6.33 Complex feelings toward a person represented by a simple, concrete, or sensory image
6.34 Unacceptable impulses or wishes toward a highly charged figure are redirected toward a neutral or less significant figure
6.35 Primitive aspects of a dream are organized into a more coherent, less bizarre form

Questions 6.36–6.40

A. Franz Alexander
B. Donald Winnicott
C. Karen Horney
D. Melanie Klein
E. Heinz Kohut

6.36 Introduced the concept of the transitional object
6.37 Believed that oedipal strivings are experienced during the first year of life, wherein gratifying experiences with the good breast reinforce basic trust
6.38 Emphasized cultural factors and disturbances in interpersonal and intrapsychic development
6.39 Introduced the concept of the corrective emotional experience
6.40 Expanded Freud's concept of narcissism; his/her theories are known as self psychology

Questions 6.41–6.45

A. Shadow
B. Anima
C. Animus
D. Persona
E. Collective unconscious

6.41 Face presented to the outside world
6.42 Another person of the same sex as the dreamer
6.43 A man's undeveloped femininity
6.44 A woman's undeveloped masculinity
6.45 Mythological ideas and primitive projections

Questions 6.46–6.50

A. Harry Stack Sullivan
B. Abraham Maslow
C. Wilhelm Reich
D. Kurt Lewin
E. Frederick S. Perls

6.46 "Group dynamics"
6.47 Peak experience
6.48 Participant observer
6.49 Character formation and character types
6.50 Gestalt therapy

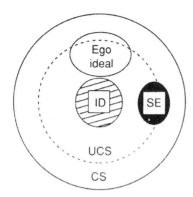

SE = Superego
CS = Conscious
UCS = Unconscious

FIGURE 6.1
Freudian topology of the psychic apparatus. (Reprinted with permission from Kaplan HI, Sadock BJ, eds. *Comprehensive Textbook of Psychiatry*. 6th ed. Baltimore: Williams & Wilkins; 1995:490.)

Questions 6.51–6.56

  A. Basic trust versus basic mistrust
  B. Integrity versus despair
  C. Initiative versus guilt
  D. Intimacy versus isolation
  E. Identity versus role diffusion

6.51 Infancy
6.52 Early childhood
6.53 Puberty and adolescence
6.54 Early adulthood
6.55 Late adulthood
6.56 Basing your response on Freud's structural model of the psychic apparatus, represented in Figure 6.1, select the lettered item (A to C) that *best* matches the function described for each of the numbered items (1 to 5) below. Each lettered item may be used once, more than once, or not at all.

  A. Ego
  B. Superego
  C. Id

1. Delays and modifies drive expression through defense mechanisms
2. Reservoir of unorganized instinctual drives
3. Provides ongoing scrutiny of a person's behavior, thoughts, and feelings
4. Functions include logical and abstract thinking and verbal expression
5. Establishes and maintains a person's moral conscience

DIRECTIONS: Each set of lettered headings below is followed by a list of numbered words or phrases: For each numbered word or phrase, select

  A. if the item is associated with *A only*
  B. if the item is associated with *B only*
  C. if the item is associated with *both A and B*
  D. if the item is associated with *neither A nor B*

Questions 6.57–6.61

  A. Primary process
  B. Secondary process
  C. Both
  D. Neither

6.57 Characteristic of very young children
6.58 The unconscious
6.59 The id
6.60 The preconscious
6.61 The ego

Questions 6.62–6.66

  A. Topographic theory
  B. Structural theory
  C. Both
  D. Neither

6.62 Set forth by Sigmund Freud in *The Interpretation of Dreams* in 1900
6.63 Presented in Freud's *The Ego and the Id* in 1923
6.64 Unconscious, preconscious, and conscious
6.65 Id, ego, and superego
6.66 First systematic and comprehensive study of the defenses used by the ego

---

ANSWERS

Theories of Personality and Psychopathology

6.1 The answer is D
Wilheim Reich viewed character as a defensive structure, an *armoring of one's ego,* both against instincts within and the world without. As a result, a defense develops that prevents flexibility, producing a loss in psychic and physical elasticity. This prevention or, rather, the degree of persisting *elasticity, determines the difference between the healthy and neurotic character.*

Reich viewed the inevitable frustrations of incestuous wishes as the core of character formation. Character formation, according to Reich, represents an attempt to end these conflicts. *Punishment over sexual activity affects character formation.*

Reich placed particular emphasis on the influence of social forces in determining character structure, especially their *repressive and inhibiting* effects.

Reich disagreed strongly with Freud's concept of *the death instinct,* and he was opposed to Freud's reference to the death instinct as the basis for masochistic phenomena.

6.2 The answer is D
Psychic determinism refers to childhood experiences that are very much alive in terms of the adult's motivations, conflicts, and wishes. As Wordsworth noted, "The child is the father of the man." It is the concept that adult actions can be understood as the end-result of a chain of psychological events beginning in child-

hood. Another central tenet of psychoanalytic theory is that behavior has meaning. Indeed, much of psychoanalytic clinical work can be described as the co-creation of meanings by patient and analyst. The meaning is partly determined by unconscious conflicts. Even when symptoms or behavior are influenced by biological factors and cultural considerations, the domain of psychoanalysis always involves meanings, and psychoanalysts are interested in how a patient uniquely interprets thoughts, feelings, and external events based on his or her past experiences.

Psychoanalytic theory is now largely a pluralistic endeavor in which several useful constructs compete as explanations for specific human behaviors. *Among the basic controversies in contemporary psychoanalysis is whether psychoanalysis is fundamentally a one-person (intrapsychic) or a two-person (interpersonal) psychology.* Is the database in psychoanalysis limited to a patient's subjective experience? Does psychopathology originate from real traumatic events or from the role of fantasy in distorting real events?

Dreams are one of the primary sources of information about unconscious conflict. Freud noted that *long-forgotten memories* reemerged in the process of the treatment, an observation that led him to conclude that the human mind has formed a censorship that deems certain memories, thoughts, and feelings unacceptable. The material is repressed or buried in the unconscious, so the person is no longer consciously aware of the phenomena that have undergone repression during conscious waking life.

6.3 The answer is D

Otto Rank hypothesized that the birth process is *the source of primal anxiety,* which is then subject to repression. Inasmuch as a subsequent desire to return to the position of original or primal pleasure gives rise to anxiety, so does any change from a pleasurable to a painful situation.

Rank maintained that the circumstances of birth are deeply imprinted on the psyche of the infant and often reappear in symbolic form in psychiatric patients. He stated that childhood was devoted to the mastery of the birth trauma, although the original or primal anxiety was displaced onto other situations and objects. Although he described the birth process as a *painful experience for the mother,* his concept of birth trauma did not relate to the mother's experience but to that of the infant.

The transference is an unconscious tendency of a person to assign to others in the person's present environment those feelings and attitudes originally linked with significant figures in the person's early life. It is a crucial process in psychoanalysis. The development of the *Oedipus complex* coincides with the phallic phase of psychosexual development as formulated by Freud.

6.4 The answer is B

Freud's concept of transference was to become a cornerstone of psychoanalytic theory and technique. *Transference refers to the displacement onto the analyst of thoughts, feelings, and behavior associated originally with significant figures from the past.*

Freud's discovery of transference contributed to his abandonment of hypnosis. In his view, hypnosis concealed aspects of the transference, so that they could not be investigated as part of the process. He also felt that hypnosis encouraged the patient to please the hypnotist, instead of learning about the origins and the meanings of symptoms. Freud also observed that many patients were simply refractory to hypnosis.

By the late 1890s Freud abandoned hypnosis. Instead, he had the patient lie on the couch and *say whatever came to mind without censorship, the method of free association* that remains a central part of psychoanalytic technique today.

In addition to Freud's discovery of transference, two other seminal psychoanalytic concepts—resistance and repression—grew out of his clinical investigations of hysterical patients in the 1890s. In the evolution of his technique from hypnosis to free association, he discerned that a stubborn refusal to cooperate was not at the root of the resistance. Many of his patients who were genuinely distressed by their symptoms were also the most resistant to the therapeutic techniques. Freud concluded that active forces in the patient's unconscious mind were *excluding unpleasant thoughts or memories from conscious awareness.* He referred to that active force as *repression.*

Freud's studies of hysterical symptoms convinced him that repression was a pivotal force in the process of symptom formation. He described the mechanism in the following manner: A traumatic experience or a series of experiences, usually of a sexual nature, that had occurred in childhood had been forgotten or repressed because of their painful or unacceptable nature, but the excitement associated with the incidents was not extinguished, and traces persist in the unconscious in the form of repressed memories. The memories may remain without pathogenic effect until a contemporary event, such as a disturbing love affair, revives them. The so-far-successful repression fails at that point, leading the patient to experience what Freud referred to as *the return of the repressed.* The original sexual excitement recurs and comes to the surface in the form of a neurotic symptom.

On the basis of his understanding of repression, *Freud postulated that symptoms arise from a compromise between a repressed impulse and the countervailing forces of repression.* In cases of hysteria Freud believed that impulses that were unacceptable and therefore repressed were diverted into somatic pathways, resulting in such symptoms as paralysis, blindness, and disturbances of sensation. He speculated that similar mechanisms are involved in the development of paranoid ideation and obsessive-compulsive symptoms. Hence, the main thrust of treatment was to assist patients in the retrieval of repressed memories so that the excitations attached to them could emerge into conscious awareness and be discharged through verbalization; removal of symptoms would be achieved by recovering and verbalizing the repressed feelings with which they were associated.

6.5 The answer is E (all)

Alfred Adler introduced the concept of masculine protest, which represents the *universal human tendency* to move from a *female or passive role* to a masculine or active role. The doctrine *is an extension of his ideas about organ inferiority.* Adler regards this concept as the main force in neurotic disease. It represents the distorted perception of sex differences caused by the striving for superiority. If it takes an active force in women, they attempt from an early age to usurp the male position. They become aggressive in manner, adopt masculine habits, and aim to dominate everyone around them. The masculine protest in a male indicates that he has never fully recovered from an infantile doubt as to whether he was really male. He strives for an ideal masculinity, invariably perceived as the self-possession of freedom and power. Adler believed that gender roles should be more similar than different in a healthy society.

6.6 The answer is E (all)

Ego psychologists have identified a set of basic ego functions that characterize the ego. The following descriptions reflect the activities that are generally regarded as fundamental to the operation of the ego.

Control and regulation of instinctual drives. The development of the capacity to delay or postpone drive discharge, like the capacity to test reality, is closely related to the progression in early childhood from the pleasure principle to the reality principle. That capacity is also an essential aspect of the ego's role as mediator between the id and the outside world. Part of the infant's socialization to the external world is the acquisition of language and secondary process or logical thinking, both of which assist in the control of instinctual drives. The capacity to think in a logical and abstract manner allows for the representation of drives in fantasy, which may circumvent the need to discharge them in action.

Relation to reality. The mediation between the internal world and external reality is a crucial function of the ego. The relationship with the outside world can be divided into three aspects: the sense of reality, reality testing, and adaptation to reality. The sense of reality develops in concert with the infant's dawning awareness of bodily sensations. The ability to distinguish what is outside the body from what is inside is an essential aspect of the sense of reality, and disturbances of body boundaries, such as depersonalization, reflect impairment in that ego function.

Reality testing is an ego function of paramount importance in that it differentiates psychotic persons from nonpsychotic persons. Reality testing refers to the capacity to distinguish internal fantasy from external reality. That function of the ego gradually develops in parallel with the increasing domination of the reality principle over the pleasure principle.

Object relationships. The significance of object relationships in normal psychological development and in psychiatric disorders was not fully appreciated until relatively late in the evolution of classical psychoanalysis. The capacity to form mutually satisfying relationships is in part linked to patterns of internalization stemming from early interactions with parents and other significant figures. That ability is also a fundamental function of the ego in that satisfying relatedness depends on the ability to integrate positive and negative aspects of others and oneself and to maintain an internal sense of others, even in their absence. Similarly, mastery of drive derivatives is crucial to the achievement of satisfying relationships.

Defensive functions of the ego. Freud acknowledged the existence of several defense mechanisms, but his writings focused predominantly on repression, which he regarded as the queen of the defenses. In many of Freud's contributions, defense and repression are used almost synonymously. Repression provides a barrier against the direct expression of impulses and wishes from the unconscious. With the ascent of the structural model, Freud shifted the function of defense to the ego.

6.7 The answer is A

The distinction between the superego and the ego-ideal has always been ambiguous. The most common usage today is to refer to the ego-ideal as an agency that *prescribes* what one should do and to refer to the superego as an agency of moral conscience that *proscribes—that is, dictates—what one should not do. Today most analysts conceptualize the ego-ideal as comprising a set of functions contained within the structure of the superego.*

The ego-ideal can be viewed as an amalgam of internalized representations. The ideal object, stemming from internal images of an admired and omnipotent parent, is one such representation. The ideal self, based on fantasies of a self-image that would result in maximal parental approval, is another representation contained within the concept. Representations of actions that should be done to attain an ideal relationship with significant figures in one's life are also involved.

The ego-ideal becomes an internal standard of what one should be. *In this regard it is intimately connected with shame (not with guilt), which is a response to an internal perception that one has not lived up to one's ego-ideal.* Although guilt is a closely related affect, it is generally regarded as a response to the transgressions of superego prohibitions, particularly sexual or aggressive wishes toward others.

6.8 The answer is C

Erik Erikson described eight stages of the life cycle, which are outlined in detail in Table 6.1. The stages are marked by one or more internal crises, which are defined as turning points—periods when the person is in a state of increased vulnerability. Ideally, the crisis is mastered successfully, and the person gains strength and is able to move on to the next stage.

Erikson's stage of autonomy versus shame and doubt occurs at about 1 to 3 years of age. Autonomy concerns children's sense of mastery over themselves and over their drives and impulses. *The stage of autonomy versus shame and doubt corresponds with Freud's anal stage* of development. For Erikson, it is the time for the child either to retain feces (holding in) or to eliminate feces (letting go); both behaviors have an effect on the mother.

The stage of initiative versus guilt occurs from 3 to 5 years and *corresponds to Freud's phallic-oedipal stage.* The stage of industry versus inferiority occurs later, from ages 6 to 11. Good teachers and good parents who encourage children to value diligence and productivity and to persevere in difficult enterprises are bulwarks against a sense of inferiority. *The stage of industry versus inferiority corresponds to Freud's latency stage, not the phallic stage, while the stage of identity role diffusion corresponds to Freud's genital stage (11 years through adolescence).* According to Erikson, developing a sense of identity is the main task of the period, which coincides with puberty and adolescence. Identity is defined as the characteristics that establish who persons are and where they are going. Healthy identity is built on success in passing through the earlier stages. Failure to negotiate the stage leaves the adolescent without a solid identity; the person suffers from role diffusion or identity confusion, characterized by not having a sense of self and by confusion about one's place in the world.

The stage of generativity versus stagnation (40 to 65 years) occurs during the decades that span the middle years of life. *Generativity can occur even if a person has not had or raised a child.* Generativity also includes a vital interest outside the home in establishing and guiding the oncoming generation or in improving society. Childless people can be generative if they develop a sense of altruism and creativity.

Table 6.1
Erik Erikson's Stages of the Life Cycle

Stage 1. Basic Trust versus Basic Mistrust (birth to about 1 year)

Corresponds to the oral psychosexual stage

Trust is shown by ease of feeding, depth of sleep, bowel relaxation

Depends on consistency and sameness of experiences provided by caretaker or outerprovider

Second 6 months: teething and biting move the infant from getting to taking

Weaning leads to nostalgia for the lost paradise

If basic trust is strong, the child maintains a hopeful attitude and develops self-confidence

Oral zone is associated with the mode of being satisfied

Stage 2. Autonomy versus Shame and Doubt (about 1 to 3 years)

Corresponds to the muscular-anal stage

Biologically includes learning to walk, feed self, talk

Need for outer control and firmness of caretaker before development of autonomy

Shame occurs when the child is overtly self-conscious through negative exposure and punishment

Self-doubt can evolve if the parents overtly shame the child (e.g., about elimination)

Anal zone is associated with the mode of holding on and letting go

Stage 3. Initiative versus Guilt (3 to 5 years)

Corresponds to the phallic psychosexual stage

Initiative arises in relation to tasks for the sake of activity, both motor and intellectual

Guilt may arise over goals contemplated (especially aggressive goals)

Desire to mimic adult world; involvement in oedipal struggle leads to resolution through social role identification

Sibling rivalry is frequent

Phallic zone is associated with the mode of competition and aggression

Stage 4. Industry versus Inferiority (6 to 11 years)

Corresponds to the latency psychosexual stage

Child is busy building, creating, accomplishing

Child receives systematic instruction and fundamentals of technology

Danger of a sense of inadequacy and inferiority if the child despairs of tools, skills, and status among peers

Socially decisive age

No dominant zone or mode

Stage 5. Identify versus Role Diffusion (11 years through the end of adolescence)

Struggle to develop ego identity (sense of inner sameness and continuity)

Preoccupation with appearance, hero worship, ideology

Group identity (with peers) develops

Danger of role confusion, doubts about sexual and vocational identity

Psychosexual moratorium, stage between morality learned by the child and the ethics developed by the adult

No dominant zone or mode

Stage 6. Intimacy versus Isolation (21 to 40 years)

Tasks are to love and to work

Intimacy is characterized by self-abandonment, mutuality of sexual orgasm, intense friendship, attachments that are life-long

Isolation is marked by separation from others and by the view that others are dangerous

General sense of productivity

No dominant zone or mode

Stage 7. Generativity versus Stagnation (40 to 65 years)

Generativity includes raising children, guiding new generation, creativity, altruism

Stagnation is not prevented by having a child; the parent must provide nurturance and love

Self-concern, isolation, and the absence of intimacy are characteristic of stagnation

No dominant zone or mode

Stage 8. Integrity versus Despair (over 65 years)

Integrity is a sense of satisfaction that life has been productive and worthwhile

Despair is a loss of hope that produces misanthropy and disgust

Persons in the state of despair are fearful of death

An acceptance of one's place in the life cycle is characteristic of integrity

---

The stage of integrity versus despair occurs in old age, not in late adolescence through the early middle years. It is Erikson's eighth stage of the life cycle. The stage (over 65 years) is described as the conflict between the sense of satisfaction that one feels in reflecting on a life productively lived versus the sense that life has had little purpose or meaning. Integrity allows for an acceptance of one's place in the life cycle and of the knowledge that one's life is one's own responsibility. There is an acceptance of one's parents, and an understanding of how they lived their lives.

6.9 The answer is C

In *The Ego and the Id,* published in 1923, Sigmund Freud developed the tripartite structural model of ego, id, and superego. This model of the psychic apparatus, which is the cornerstone of ego psychology, represented a transition for Freud from his topographical model of the mind (conscious, preconscious, and unconscious). The three provinces of id, ego, and superego are distinguished by their varying functions.

The superego's activities occur unconsciously to a large extent. The superego establishes and maintains the person's moral conscience in the complex system of ideals and values internalized from one's parents. Freud viewed the superego as the heir to the Oedipus complex. In other words, the child internalizes the parental values and standards around the age of 5 or 6 years. The superego then serves as an agency that provides ongoing scrutiny of the person's behavior, thoughts, and feelings. It makes comparisons with expected standards of behavior and offers approval or disapproval.

The superego does not control the delay and the modulation of drive expression. The delay and the modulation of drive expression are achieved by the ego. *The ego, not the superego, is the executive organ of the psyche,* through the mechanisms of defense available to it and through mobility, perception, and contact with reality. According to Freud, the ego spans all three topographical dimension of conscious, preconscious, and unconscious. Logical and abstract thinking and verbal expression are associated with its conscious and preconscious functions. Defense mechanisms reside in its unconscious domain.

Freud also believed that the ego brings influences from the external world to bear on the id, and the ego simultaneously substitutes the reality principle for the pleasure principle. Thus, in Freud's view, both *the reality principle and the pleasure principle are aspects of ego functioning, not id functioning.* The id, according to Freud, harbors the innate, biological, instinctual drives; it is the source of libido and follows the pleasure principle. *Secondary process* is the form of thinking that is logical, organized, and reality-oriented.

6.10 The answer is A

Projection is a defense mechanism in which thoughts, feelings, and impulses that are undesirable are transferred to another person and is the defense that underlies paranoia. *Identification* is a defense mechanism by which persons pattern themselves after another person. *Undoing* is an unconscious defense mechanism by which a person symbolically acts out in reverse of something unacceptable. *Reaction formation* is an unconscious defense mechanism in which a person develops a socialized attitude or interest that is the direct antithesis of some infantile wish.

Displacement transfers an emotion from the original idea to which it was attached to another idea or object. For instance a phobia is an abnormal fear reaction caused by a paralyzing conflict attached to an unconscious object. The fear is avoided by *displacement*; the conflict is displaced onto an external object or situation.

6.11 The answer is A

George Vaillant's mature defenses include *altruism,* anticipation, asceticism, humor, sublimation, and suppression. In the 1970s he published his 30-year follow-up study of people who had gone to Harvard in the 1930s. He delineated the psychological characteristics he considered essential to mental health in this group, including descriptions of defense mechanisms he thought to be healthy and those he thought to be more psychopathological. Vaillant classified four types of defenses: (1) mature defenses, which are characteristic of healthy adults; (2) narcissistic defenses, which are characteristic of young children and psychotic adults; (3) immature defenses, which are characteristic of adolescents and are also seen in psychopathological states, such as depression; (4) neurotic defenses, which are characteristic of adult functioning. At times, some of the defensive categories overlap; for instance, neurotic defenses may be seen in normally healthy, mature adults. *Controlling, intellectualization,* and *rationalization* are characterized by Vaillant as among the neurotic defenses.

Altruism is a regard for the intents and needs of others. *Controlling* is the excessive attempt to manage or regulate events or objects in the environment in the interest of minimizing anxiety and solving internal conflicts. *Intellectualization* represents the attempt to avoid unacceptable feelings by escaping from emotions into a world of abstract concepts and words. *Rationalization* is justification, making a thing appear reasonable that otherwise would be regarded as irrational. The defense mechanisms are listed and defined in Table 6.2.

6.12 The answer is D

Repression is a mechanism of defense employed by the ego to help mediate conflict within the tripartite mind's ego, superego, and id. It is not considered an autonomous ego function. Repression is defined as an unconscious defense mechanism in which unacceptable mental content is banished or kept out of consciousness.

Autonomous ego functions are based on rudimentary apparatuses that are present at birth. They develop outside the conflict with the id. Heinz Hartmann included *perception,* intuition, comprehension, thinking, *language,* some phases of *motor development,* learning, and *intelligence* among the functions of that conflict-free sphere.

6.13 The answer is E (all)

Carl Gustav Jung believed archetypes to be *instinctual patterns.* All psychic energy is transmitted in forms of experience, behavior, and emotion, which are *expressed in representational* or *mythological images.* Thus, the archetypes represent the basic motivations and drives that become *organizational units of the personality.*

6.14 The answer is E (all)

According to Alfred Adler, infants are born with certain *feelings of inferiority.* As a result, they have *a need to strive for superiority,* perfection, and totality. Adler classified those strivings under the heading of the inferiority complex, which comprises the newborns' feelings secondary to their real or *fantasied organic or psychological deficits. Compensatory strivings* are attempts to overcome feelings of inferiority.

6.15 The answer is B

A traditional space is not a term referring to one of Winnicott's concepts; the correct term is *transitional space,* the area in which a transitional object—the link to the mother—functions. This space, according to Winnicott, is a source of art, creativity, and metaphysical beliefs.

Donald Winnicott, a major figure in the British school of object relations, created several concepts of child development, including *a true self* (which emerges in a healthy environment), *a holding environment* (the context in which a true self emerges), *a good-enough mother* (one who provides adequate responses to her infant in a holding environment), and *a transitional object* (a pacifier or blanket, which substitutes for a mother as an infant matures).

6.16 The answer is D

Frederick S. Perls did not work with Sigmund Freud. Rather, he was one of the creators of Gestalt theory in Germany. According to Perls, Gestalt therapy emphasizes a patient's current life experiences and not the "there and then" of Freudian psychoanalysis.

Carl Gustav Jung, although he later broke with Freud over the latter's ideas of infantile sexuality, initially was one of Freud's disciples. After breaking with Freud, Jung created a concept of the mind that included the collective unconscious, a reservoir of humans' common, shared myths and symbols in the form of archetypes or images with universal meanings. *Alfred Adler,* another early disciple of Freud, became estranged because of Freud's stress on sexuality in neurosis. Adler emphasized the role of aggression, which he saw as more important than sexuality, and he coined the term *inferiority complex* to describe a universal, innate sense of inadequacy.

Karl Abraham, the first psychoanalyst in Germany, was an early disciple of Freud as well. Abraham elaborated Freud's stages of psychosexual development and linked each stage to a specific syndrome. He also developed a psychoanalytic view of depression, which he described as a fixation at

Table 6.2
Defense Mechanisms

Acting out. An action rather than a verbal response to an unconscious instinctual drive or impulse that brings about the temporary partial relief of inner tension. Relief is attained by reacting to a present situation as if it were the situation that originally gave rise to the drive or impulse. An immature defense.

Altruism. Regard for and dedication to the welfare of others. The term was originated by Auguste Comte (1798–1857), a French philosopher. In psychiatry the term is closely linked with ethics and morals. Sigmund Freud recognized altruism as the only basis for the development of community interest. Eugen Bleuler equated it with morality. A mature defense.

Anticipation. The act of dealing with, doing, foreseeing, or experiencing beforehand. Anticipation is characteristic of the ego and is necessary for the judgment and planning of suitable later action. Anticipation depends on reality testing—by trying in an active manner and in small doses what may happen to one passively and in unknown doses. The testing affords the possibility of judging reality and is an important factor in the development of the ability to tolerate tensions. A mature defense.

Asceticism. A mode of life characterized by rigor, self-denial, and mortification of the flesh. Asceticism is seen typically as a phase in puberty, when it indicates a fear of sexuality and a simultaneous defense against sexuality. Asceticism is also seen as an extreme type of masochistic character disorder, in which almost all activity is forbidden because it represents intolerable instinctual demands. In such cases the very act of mortifying may become a distorted expression of the blocked sexuality and may produce masochistic pleasure. Examples are eccentrics who devote their lives to the combating of some particular evil that unconsciously may represent their own instinctual demands. A mature defense.

Blocking. The involuntary cessation of thought processes or speech because of unconscious emotional factors. It is also known as thought deprivation. An immature defense.

Controlling. The excessive attempt to manage or regulate events or objects in the environment in the interest of minimizing anxiety and solving internal conflicts. A neurotic defense.

Denial. A mechanism in which the existence of unpleasant realities is disavowed. The mechanism keeps out of conscious awareness any aspects of external reality that, if acknowledged, would produce anxiety. A narcissistic defense.

Displacement. A mechanism by which the emotional component of an unacceptable idea or object is transferred to a more acceptable one. A neurotic defense.

Dissociation. A mechanism involving the segregation of any group of mental or behavioral processes from the rest of the person's psychic activity. It may entail the separation of an idea from its accompanying emotional tone, as seen in dissociative disorders. A neurotic defense.

Distortion. A misrepresentation of reality. It is based on unconsciously determined motives. A narcissistic defense.

Externalization. A general term, correlative to internalization, for the tendency to perceive in the external world and in external objects components of one's own personality, including instinctual impulses, conflicts, moods, attitudes, and styles of thinking. It is a more general term than projection, which is defined by its derivation, form, and correlation with specific introjects. A neurotic defense.

Humor. The overt expression of feelings without personal discomfort or immobilization and without unpleasant effects on others. Humor allows one to bear, yet focus on, what is too terrible to be borne, in contrast to wit, which always involves distraction or displacement away from the affective issues. A mature defense.

Hypochondriasis. An exaggerated concern about one's physical health. The concern is not based on real organic pathology. An immature defense.

Identification. A mechanism by which one patterns oneself after another person. In the process, the self may be permanently altered. An immature defense.

Identification with the aggressor. A process by which one incorporates within oneself the mental image of a person who represents a source of frustration. The classic example of the defense occurs toward the end of the oedipal stage, when a boy, whose main source of love and gratification is his mother, identifies with his father. The father represents the source of frustration, being the powerful rival for the mother; the child cannot master or run away from his father, so he is obliged to identify with his father. An immature defense.

Incorporation. A mechanism in which the psychic representation of another person or aspects of another person are assimilated into oneself through a figurative process of symbolic oral ingestion. It represents a special form of introjection and is the earliest mechanism of identification.

Inhibition. The depression or arrest of a function; suppression or diminution of outgoing influences from a reflex center. The sexual impulse, for example, may be inhibited because of psychological repression. A neurotic defense.

Intellectualization. A mechanism in which reasoning or logic is used in an attempt to avoid confrontation with an objectionable impulse and thus defends against anxiety. It is also known as brooding compulsion and thinking compulsion. A neurotic defense.

Introjection. The unconscious, symbolic internalization of a psychic representation of a hated or loved external object with the goal of establishing closeness to the object and its constant presence. In the case of a loved object, anxiety consequent to separation or tension arising out of ambivalence toward the object is diminished; in the case of a feared or hated object, internalization of its malicious or aggressive characteristics serves to avoid anxiety by symbolically putting those characteristics under one's own control. An immature defense.

Isolation. In psychoanalysis a mechanism involving the separation of an idea or memory from its attached feeling tone. Unacceptable ideational content is thereby rendered free of its disturbing or unpleasant emotional charge. A neurotic defense.

Passive-aggressive behavior. The showing of aggressive feelings in passive ways, such as through obstructionism, pouting, and stubbornness. An immature defense.

Primitive idealization. Viewing external objects as either all good or all bad and as unrealistically endowed with great power. Most commonly, the all-good object is seen as omnipotent or ideal, and the badness in the all-bad object is greatly inflated. A narcissistic defense.

Projection. An unconscious mechanism in which one attributes to another the idea, thoughts, feelings, and impulses that are unacceptable to oneself. Projection protects a person from anxiety arising from an inner conflict. By externalizing whatever is unacceptable, one deals with it as a situation apart from oneself. A narcissistic and immature defense.

Projective identification. Depositing unwanted aspects of the self into another person and feeling at one with the object of the projection. The extruded aspects are modified by and recovered from the recipient. The defense allows one to distance and make oneself understood by exerting pressure on another person to experience feelings similar to one's own. A narcissistic defense.

Rationalization. A mechanism in which irrational or unacceptable behavior, motives, or feelings are logically justified or made consciously tolerable by plausible means. A neurotic defense.

(continued)

Table 6.2 (*continued*)

Reaction formation. An unconscious defense mechanism in which a person develops a socialized attitude or interest that is the direct antithesis of some infantile wish or impulse in the unconscious. One of the earliest and most stable defense mechanisms, it is closely related to repression; both are defenses against impulses or urges that are unacceptable to the ego. A neurotic defense.

Regression. A mechanism in which a person undergoes a partial or total return to early patterns of adaptation. Regression is observed in many psychiatric conditions, particularly schizophrenia. An immature defense.

Repression. A mechanism in which unacceptable mental contents are banished or kept out of consciousness. A term introduced by Sigmund Freud, it is important in both normal psychological development and in neurotic and psychotic symptom formation. Freud recognized two kinds of repression: (1) repression proper—the repressed material was once in the conscious domain, (2) primal repression—the repressed material was never in the conscious realm. A neurotic defense.

Schizoid fantasy. The tendency to use fantasy and to indulge in autistic retreat for the purpose of conflict resolution and gratification. An immature defense.

Sexualization. The endowing of an object or function with sexual significance that it did not previously have or that it possesses to a small degree; it is used to ward off anxieties connected with prohibitive impulses. A neurotic defense.

Somatization. The defense conversion of psychic derivatives into bodily symptoms; a tendency to react with somatic rather than psychic manifestations. Infantile somatic responses are replaced by thought and affect during development (desomatization); regression to early somatic forms of response (resomatization) may result from unresolved conflicts and may play an important role in psychological reactions. An immature defense.

Splitting. Dividing external objects into all good and all bad, accompanied by the abrupt shifting of an object from one extreme category to the other. Sudden and complete reversals of feelings and conceptualizations about a person may occur. The extreme repetitive oscillation between contradictory self-concepts is another manifestation of the mechanism. A narcissistic defense.

Sublimation. A mechanism in which the energy associated with unacceptable impulses or drives is diverted into personally and socially acceptable channels. Unlike other defense mechanisms, sublimation offers some minimal gratification of the instinctual drive or impulse. A mature defense.

Substitution. A mechanism in which a person replaces an unacceptable wish, drive, emotion, or goal with one that is acceptable. A neurotic defense.

Suppression. A conscious act of controlling and inhibiting an unacceptable impulse, emotion, or idea. Suppression is differentiated from repression in that repression is an unconscious process. A mature defense.

Symbolization. A mechanism by which one idea or object comes to stand for another because of some common aspect or quality in both. Symbolization is based on similarity and association. The symbols formed protect the person from the anxiety that may be attached to the original idea or object. A mature defense.

Turning against the self. Changing an unacceptable impulse aimed at others by redirecting it against oneself. An immature defense.

Undoing. A mechanism by which a person symbolically acts out in reverse something unacceptable that has already been done or against which the ego must defend itself. A primitive defense mechanism, undoing is a form of magical action. Repetitive in nature, it is commonly observed in persons with obsessive-compulsive disorder. A neurotic defense.

Table compiled from Freud S, Freud A, Semrad E, Meissner WW, Vaillant G. Narcissistic defenses: used by children and psychotics; immature defenses: used by adolescents and in depressive disorders and obsessive-compulsive disorder; neurotic defenses: used by adults under stress and in obsessive-compulsive disorder and somatoform disorders; mature defenses: used by normal adults.

the oral stage. *Sandor Ferenczi,* who was influenced by Freud's ideas early in his career and who was psychoanalyzed by Freud, later developed his own method of analysis, in which analysts were to love their patients to compensate them for the insufficient love they had received from their parents.

6.17 The answer is E (all)

The Interpretation of Dreams, published in 1900, is generally considered to be one of Sigmund Freud's most important contributions to the field. The book includes much of the data derived from his clinical experience with patients and the insights gained from his self-analysis and free association to his own dreams. On the basis of that evidence, Freud concluded that *dreams are the conscious expression of an unconscious fantasy* or wish. Freud maintained that *dreams represent wish-fulfillment activities,* albeit activities disguised and distorted through such mechanisms as symbolism, displacement, and condensation. Dream analysis yields material that has been repressed by the ego's defensive activities. The dream, as it is consciously recalled and experienced, is termed the manifest dream, and its various elements are termed the manifest dream content; the unconscious thoughts and wishes that make up the core meaning of the dream are described as the latent dream content. *Latent dream content derives from the repressed part of the id* and includes such categories as nocturnal sensory stimuli and the day's residue. Nocturnal sensory stimuli, such as pain or thirst, are *sensory impressions that may play a role in initiating a dream.* Repressed id impulses are wishes that have their origin in oedipal and preoedipal phases of development. The day's residue comprises thoughts and ideas connected with the activities of the dreamer's waking life.

6.18 The answer E (all)

The third component of the tripartite structural model is the superego. *The superego establishes and maintains the person's moral conscience on the basis of a complex system of ideals and values internalized from one's parents.* Freud viewed the superego as the heir to the Oedipus complex; *it is, therefore, influenced by the resolution of oedipal conflict.* It conducts an ongoing scrutiny of the behavior, thoughts, and feelings of the person; makes comparisons with expected standards; and offers approval or disapproval. Criticisms and reproaches lead to a variety of painful feelings; praises and rewards raise the person's self-esteem. Those activities occur unconsciously to a large extent, reflecting the clinical observation that self-criticism operates as much outside conscious awareness as aggressive and sexual drive derivatives do.

According to Freud, the superego is a relatively mature structure resulting from the resolution of the Oedipus complex. In the case of the little boy, his love for his mother engenders murderous wishes toward his father. His observation of the genital differences between males and females leads him to fear that his oedipal wishes will be punished with castration. Under the influence of the perceived threat from his father, the little boy renounces his incestuous longings for his mother and identifies with his father. That resolution involves the installation of the parental moral values as the superego structure.

In the case of the little girl, she renounces oedipal strivings for her father because she realizes that a victory over her mother would result in the loss of her mother's love. Freud initially postulated that little girls grow up with less moral conviction and character as a result of the absence of the castration threat. That view is no longer held by contemporary psychoanalysts. Recent empirical studies suggest that moral developmental differences between boys and girls may exist but along different lines. It has been postulated that boys tend to place high moral value on achievement and fair play; girls are more likely to develop a moral code based on affiliation and relatedness to others.

Primitive superego precursors are formed early in life from the internalization of frightening and aggressive perceptions of parental figures. In some cases those perceptions are based on real behaviors of the parents; in other cases the perceptions are influenced by distortions deriving from fantasies by the child and from projections of the child's rage and sadism onto external objects. As a child matures and resolves the Oedipus complex, identifications with both parents become integrated to form an intricate and well-rounded internal object representation within the ego that interacts with the other contents of the ego as a superego. The parental identification is further reinforced by the child's struggles to repress unacceptable sexual and aggressive wishes and by the child's identification with the parents' superegos.

6.19 The answer is B
According to Carl Gustav Jung's psychoanalytic school, known as analytical psychology, *archetypes contribute to complexes.* That occurs because complexes, which are feeling-toned ideas, develop as a result of personal experiences interacting with archetypal imagery. Archetypes are representational images and confirmations that have universal meanings. Archetypal figures exist for the mother, the father, the child, and the hero, among others. Thus, a mother complex is determined not only by the mother–child interaction but also by the conflict between archetypal expectations and actual experiences with the real woman who functions in a motherly role.

Archetypes are a part of Jung's concept of the collective unconscious, which consists of all humankind's common and shared mythological and symbolic past. *The collective unconscious is not a collection of the impulses of the id and the ego.*

The persona is the mask covering the personality; it is what the person presents to the outside world. The persona may become fixed, so that the real person is hidden even from the person. *The male part of the self is called the animus, not the persona.*

The aim of Jungian treatment is to bring about an adequate adaptation to reality, which involves fulfilling one's creative potential. The ultimate goal is to achieve *individuation, a pro-* cess that continues throughout life in which persons develop unique senses of their own identities. This developmental process may lead persons down new paths that may differ from their previous directions in life.

In Jungian psychology, *an emphasis is not placed on infantile sexuality.*

6.20 The answer is E (all)
A major theoretical school in modern psychoanalysis is self psychology, derived from the work of Heinz Kohut. *The self psychology model of the mind regards the person as needing particular kinds of responses from others in the environment to develop and maintain a sense of self-esteem and well-being. It focuses on the role of actual external relationships in creating self-cohesion and self-esteem.*

Kohut's self psychology departs from classical ego psychology in a number of ways. *Deficits, rather than conflicts, take center stage in self psychology. Faulty structures are viewed as responsible for faulty functioning, and the emphasis is on infantile needs, rather than repressed wishes and drives.* Hence, the analyst's therapeutic goals involve understanding those needs and partially meeting them in the treatment, rather than frustrating infantile wishes that must ultimately be renounced. *Building the psychic structure and repairing self-defects are seen as more important than the resolution of conflict.*

6.21 The answer is E (all)
The French psychoanalyst Jacques Lacan (1901–1981) made a lasting impression on French psychoanalysis as well as on literary and film criticism in academic departments throughout the world. *Lacan's reading of Freud relies heavily on linguistics.* The notion that the human being is constituted by language is one of three basic principles endorsed by Lacan. *The unconscious is structured like a language that consists only of signifiers—biology and drives have no place in his theory.* Second, the ego does not exist as an autonomous structure. *A third principle is that an individual is inevitably embedded in political and societal structure that cannot be transcended.*

Lacan preferred to speak of "orders" rather than stages of development, and he identified three orders relevant to understanding the human condition. From 6 to 18 months there is an imaginary order involving a mirror stage, during which infants delight in identifying with their reflection. This preverbal and presymbolic order gives way to a symbolic order involving the acquisition of language and a split between the inner and the outer world. The inner world is connected with a misrecognition in the mirror stage where the "I" or the self is identified, with the father's laws and the cultural standards associated with those laws: The final order is that of the "real," *which is stark factual reality and exists somewhere outside of* language; this is viewed as unreachable and indefinable by Lacan.

Lacan thrived on being unorthodox. He denied the significance of diagnoses, rules, or established schools of thought. *He saw the analytical process as an effort to recognize the alienation from one's true self.* Analysis was also designed to bring out underlying structures and contexts in the unconscious. Historical reconstruction is downplayed whereas desire for the "Other" is examined in all its many forms.

Lacanian analysis has had little influence on the clinical practice of psychoanalysis in North America, although literary critics within American universities have made many applications of Lacan in their analyses of texts. Its antiempirical basis, its denial of the importance of preverbal human experience, and the impenetrability of much of the prose written by Lacan and Lacanian disciples have made it less popular among American clinicians than those in Europe and South America.

6.22 The answer is C

Erikson's stage integrity versus despair begins at age 65 and continues throughout life. A person in a stage of despair is fearful of death. This endpoint of the life cycle requires preparation and the feeling of having lived a productive and worthwhile life.

Erikson described eight stages of the human life cycle, ranging from 1 year to over 65 years. Each stage is marked by a crisis, which, if mastered successfully, allows a person to move on to the next stage. *Erikson's stage 6 refers to young adulthood and later,* from 21 to 40 years. This stage, called intimacy versus isolation, is characterized by successful fulfillment of the usual elements of this period: love, intimacy, and productivity.

Erikson described a corresponding zone for each of Freud's *three psychosexual stages:* oral, anal, and phallic. Each zone has a specific pattern of behavior associated with it. Erikson, however, emphasized that ego development is not only a result of intrapsychic energies but also of interactions between a child and society. *Erikson described one developmental stage of childhood in terms similar to those of Piaget's stage of object permanence.* In stage 1, basic trust versus basic mistrust, a healthy infant learns to let the mother go out of sight without experiencing fear or anger, a phenomenon related to Piaget's idea that an infant can maintain a mental image of a person or an object although the image is not always visible. Erikson considered change possible throughout the life cycle. *It did not stop at age 70.*

6.23 The answer is D

Anna O., who had many hysterical symptoms associated with her father's illness and death, was treated first by Josef Breuer and then by Sigmund Freud. Freud, a friend of Breuer, was interested in Breuer's treatment of Anna O. and investigated the reasons for symptoms appearing in patients with hysteria. His studies were a contributing factor to his developing psychoanalysis.

Freud's *emphasis on infant sexuality* was a major tenet of psychoanalytic theory, although many people found the idea difficult to accept. In Freud's concept of infantile sexuality, children from birth through puberty struggle to deal with sexual feelings and activities of different types, and with social reactions to these pleasures. *Freud considered dreams to have two levels of content.* The manifest level is recalled by dreamers; the latent content is unconscious. *Dream work* enabled latent content to be made conscious, or manifest, so that a person's conflicts could be worked through.

In Freud's tripartite model of the mind, each entity—id, ego, and superego—is distinguished by its function. The id is a reservoir of unorganized instinctual drives; the ego, which is conscious, preconscious, and unconscious, functions with logical, abstract thinking and with verbal expression; the superego functions as a conscience composed of ideals internalized from parents.

Freud's work on conflicts presumed that they occurred between instincts and external reality or between internal agencies. When conflicts have not been examined consciously and worked through, they are repressed from consciousness or otherwise defended against, and become a basis for neurotic development.

6.24 The answer is D

Free association is known as the fundamental rule of psychoanalysis. The use of free association in psychoanalysis evolved gradually from 1892 to 1895. Sigmund Freud began to encourage his patients to verbalize, without reservation or censorship, the passing thoughts in their minds. The conflicts that emerge while fulfilling the task of free association constitute *resistance,* which was first defined by Freud as the reluctance of his patients to recount significant memories. Later, Freud realized that resistance was often the result of an unconscious *repression* of conflictual material; the repression led to an active exclusion of painful or anxiety-producing feelings from consciousness. Freud thought that repression was at the core of all symptom formation.

Psychic determinism is the concept that actions as adults can be understood as the end result of a chain of psychological events that have a definable cause and effect.

Abreaction is a process in which a memory of a traumatic experience is released from repression and brought into consciousness. As the patient is able to express the affect associated with the memory, the affect is discharged, and the symptoms disappear.

The concept of the unconscious was one of Freud's most important contributions—first used to define mental material not in the field of awareness and, later, to designate a topographic area of the mind where psychic material is not readily accessible to conscious thought.

6.25 The answer is A

Obsessive-compulsive disorder comes about as a result of the separation of affects from ideas or behavior by the defense mechanisms of undoing and isolation, by regression to the anal-sadistic level, or by turning the impulses against the self. To defend against a painful idea in the unconscious, the person displaces the affect onto some other indirectly associated idea, one more tolerable that, in turn, becomes invested with an inordinate quantity of affect.

Anxiety disorders are disorders in which anxiety is the most prominent disturbance or in which patients experience anxiety if they resist giving in to their symptoms. The anxiety disorders include phobias, obsessive-compulsive disorder, posttraumatic stress disorder, and panic disorder.

Pain disorder is a disorder characterized by the complaint of pain. The pain may vary with intensity and duration and may range from a slight disturbance of the patient's social or occupational functioning to total incapacity and the need for hospitalization.

Dissociative disorders are characterized by a sudden, temporary alteration in consciousness, identity, or motor behavior. The dissociative disorders include dissociative amnesia, dissociative fugue, dissociative identity disorder, and depersonalization disorder.

Dysthymic disorder is a mood disorder characterized by depression.

6.26 The answer is A

Adolf Meyer used the term "habit training" to explain the process of therapy by which the main goal is to aid patients' adjustment by helping them to modify unhealthy adaptations. In the process of habit training, the psychiatrist always emphasized patients' current life situations by using a variety of techniques, such as guidance, suggestion, reeducation, and direction.

Carl Gustav Jung developed the school known as analytic psychology. *Otto Rank* focused on analytical aspects of what he called the birth trauma. *B. F. Skinner* and *Joseph Wolpe* are known for their work in learning theory and behavior therapy, respectively.

6.27 The answer is B

Harry Stack Sullivan's self-system concerns the concept of the *personality*. The self-system reflects maternal and paternal attitudes and any accumulated sets of experiences that begin in infancy and continue for a long time.

The *unconscious* is the topographic division of the mind in which psychic material is not readily accessible to conscious awareness by ordinary means. Its existence may be manifested in symptom formation, in dreams, in psychoanalytic treatment, or under the influence of drugs.

The *libido* is the psychic energy associated with the sexual drive or life instinct. *Defense mechanisms* are unconscious processes acting to relieve conflict and anxiety arising from one's impulses and drives.

The *Oedipus complex* is the constellation of feelings, impulses, and conflicts in the developing child that concern sexual impulses and attraction toward the opposite-sex parent and aggressive, hostile, or envious feelings toward the same-sex parent. Real or fantasied threats from the same-sex parent result in the repression of those feelings. The development of the Oedipus complex coincides with the phallic phase of psychosexual development. One of Freud's most important concepts, the term was originally applied only to boys. The female analogue of the Oedipus complex is called the Electra complex, a term attributed to Carl Jung, and is used to describe unresolved developmental conflicts influencing a woman's relationships with men.

6.28 The answer is A

The unconscious system is the dynamic one; according to Freud, its mental contents and processes are kept out of conscious awareness through the force of censorship or repression. Key features of Freud's theory of unconscious include the following:

1. The unconscious is closely related to instinctual drives, characterized by Freud as sexual and self-preservative in nature.
2. The content of the unconscious is limited to wishes that are seeking fulfillment.
3. *The unconscious system is characterized by primary process thinking,* not secondary process thinking, which is associated with the preconscious. Primary process thinking is governed by the pleasure principle and *disregards logical connections, represents wishes as fulfillments, and permits contradictory ideas to exist simultaneously.*
4. Memories in the unconscious have been divorced from their connections with verbal symbols.
5. The contents of the unconscious can become conscious only by passing through the preconscious, where censors are empowered, allowing the elements to enter into consciousness.

6.29 The answer is E (all)

Ordinarily, the repressed ideas and affects of the unconscious *are inaccessible to consciousness* because of the censorship or repression imposed by the preconscious. Those repressed elements may attain the level of consciousness when the censor is overpowered (as in neurotic symptom formation), relaxes (as in dream states), or is fooled (as by jokes).

The unconscious is associated with the form of mental activity that Freud called the primary process or *primary process thinking.* Characteristically seen in infancy and dreams, the primary process is marked by primitive, prelogical thinking and by the tendency to seek immediate discharge and gratification of instinctual demands. Consequently, the unconscious is also *closely related to the pleasure principle,* the principle by which the id seeks immediate tension reduction by direct or fantasied gratification. Similarly, the id also contains the mental representatives and derivatives of the *instinctual drives,* particularly those of the sexual instinct.

6.30 The answer is D

From the self-psychological point of view associated with Heinz Kohut, *depression is related to a sense of despair about ever getting one's self-object needs met by people in the environment.*

Freud originally understood *depression as internally directed anger.* In his view the self-reproaches and the loss of self-esteem commonly experienced by depressed patients are directed not at the self but, rather, at an ambivalently experienced introject. He noted that in some cases the only way the ego can give up an object is to introject it, so the anger directed at the ambivalently held object takes on the clinical manifestations of depression. After his development of the structural model, he expanded his understanding of depression to include *a harsh superego* that punishes the person for harboring destructive wishes toward parental figures and other loved ones.

Melanie Klein suggested that depression is linked to a reactivation of the depressive position; depressed patients are convinced that they have *destroyed their internal good objects because of their own aggression and greed.* As a result, they feel persecuted by internal bad objects while longing for the lost love objects.

From an object relations perspective, many depressed patients unconsciously experience themselves to be at the mercy of a tormenting internal object that is unrelenting in its persecution of them. In cases of psychosis, that primitive forerunner of the superego may actually be hallucinated as a voice that is unrelentingly critical.

Contemporary psychoanalytic contributors have downplayed the role of aggression in the development of depression. They are likely to view depression as a disturbance of self-esteem in the context of interpersonal relationships. A consistent observation is that depressed patients feel that they have not lived up to their internal standards of conduct. The depressed patients' awareness of the disparity between their actual performance and those internalized high expectations leads them to feel helpless and powerless. Often, their internal expectations involve eliciting a certain kind of response from important persons in the environment. Depressed persons often live their entire lives for others, rather than for themselves. Depression may begin when they feel hopeless about their life plans because they realize that their efforts have been wasted in living for someone else.

Answers 6.31–6.35

6.31 The answer is A

6.32 The answer is E

6.33 The answer is C

6.34 The answer is B

6.35 The answer is D

Condensation. In *condensation several unconscious impulses, wishes, or feelings can be combined and attached to one manifest dream image.* For example, a composite character may appear in the dream that has the name of one person in the dreamer's life, a beard like another person, and a musical instrument that reflects a third person. The feelings associated with those three persons may be disguised in the resulting amalgam and may become apparent only through analysis of the various dream elements. The converse of condensation, diffusion, can also occur in a dream when a single latent wish or impulse is distributed through multiple representations in the manifest content.

Displacement. *In displacement, the energy or intensity linked with one object is diverted to a substitute object that is related associatively but more acceptable to the dreamer's ego.* Murderous wishes toward one's mother, for example, may be redirected toward a neutral or insignificant figure in one's life. In that manner the dream censor has displaced affective energy so that the dreamer's sleep can continue undisturbed.

A special instance of displacement, projection, involves the attribution of the dreamer's own unacceptable impulses or wishes to another character in the dream. For example, a patient who finds homosexual impulses unacceptable may attribute them to his analyst in the dream. In some cases different aspects of the patient are represented in several characters in the dream.

Symbolic Representation. Freud noted that the dreamer would often represent highly charged ideas or objects by using innocent images that were in some way connected with the idea or object being represented. *An abstract concept or a complex set of feelings toward a person could be symbolized by a simple, concrete, or sensory image.* Freud noted that symbols have unconscious meanings that can be discerned through the patient's associations with the symbol. However, he also believed that certain symbols have universal meanings—for example, a flower as a symbol for female genitalia, a snake as a symbol for the penis.

Secondary Revision. The mechanisms of condensation, displacement, and symbolic representation are characteristic of a type of thinking that Freud referred to as *primary process. That primitive mode of cognitive activity is characterized by illogical, bizarre, and absurd images that seem incoherent.* Freud believed that a more mature and reasonable aspect of the ego is at work during the dream to organize some of those primitive aspects of the dream into a more coherent form. He called that process *secondary revision;* its intellectual processes of a more mature nature make the dream somewhat more rational. The process is related to the more mature activity characteristic of waking life, which Freud termed *secondary process.*

Answers 6.36–6.40

6.36 The answer is B

6.37 The answer is D

6.38 The answer is C

6.39 The answer is A

6.40 The answer is E

Donald Winnicott (1897–1971) was an influential contributor to object relations theory. He focused on the conditions that make it possible for a child to develop awareness as a separate person. One of the conditions is the provision of an environment termed "good-enough mothering." Good-enough mothering enables the child to be nurtured in a nonimpinging environment that permits the emergence of the true self. Winnicott *introduced the concept of the transitional object,* something that helps the child gradually shift from subjectivity to external reality. Such a material possession, usually blankets or a soft toy, exists in an intermediate realm as a substitute for the mother and as one of the first objects a child begins to recognize as separate from the self.

Melanie Klein (1882–1960) modified psychoanalytic theory, particularly in its application to infants and very young children. In contrast to orthodox psychoanalytic theory, which postulates the development of the superego during the fourth year of life, Klein's theory maintains that a primitive superego is formed during the first and second years. Klein further believed that aggressive, rather than sexual, drives are preeminent during the earliest stages of development. She deviated most sharply from classic psychoanalytic theory in her formulations concerning the Oedipus complex. She *believed that oedipal strivings are experienced during the first year of life,* as opposed to the classic formulation of its occurring between the ages of 3 and 5. She also believed that, *during the first year, gratifying experiences with the good breast reinforce basic trust* and that frustrating experiences can lead to a depressive position.

Karen Horney (1885–1952) was an American psychiatrist who ascribed great importance to the influence of sociocultural factors on individual development. She raised questions about the existence of immutable instinctual drives and developmental phases or sexual conflict as the root of neurosis while recognizing the importance of sexual drives. Rather than focusing on such concepts as the Oedipus complex, Horney *emphasized cultural factors and disturbances in interpersonal and intrapsychic development* as the cause of neuroses in general.

Franz Alexander (1891–1964) founded the Chicago Institute for Psychoanalysis. He *introduced the concept of the corrective emotional experience.* The therapist, who is supportive, enables the patient to master past traumas and to modify the effects of those traumas. Alexander was also a major influence in the field of psychosomatic medicine.

Heinz Kohut (1913–1981) *expanded Sigmund Freud's concept of narcissism.* In *The Analysis of the Self,* published in 1971, Kohut wrote about a large group of patients suffering from narcissistic personality disorder whom he believed to be analyzable but who did not develop typical transference neuroses in the classic sense. The conflict involves the relation between the self and archaic narcissistic objects. Those objects are the grandiose self and the idealized parent image, the reactivations of which constitute a threat to the patient's sense of integrity. Kohut's *theories are known as self psychology.*

Answers 6.41–6.45

6.41 The answer is D

6.42 The answer is A

6.43 The answer is B

6.44 The answer is C

6.45 The answer is E

With the term *persona,* Carl Gustav Jung denoted the disguised or masked attitude assumed by a person, in contrast to the deeply rooted personality components. Such persons put on a mask, corresponding to their conscious intentions, that makes up the *face presented to the outside world.* Through their identification with the persons, they deceive other people and often themselves as to their real character.

The *shadow* appears in dreams as *another person of the same sex as the dreamer.* According to Jung, one sees much in another person that does not belong to one's conscious psychology but that comes out from one's unconscious.

In Jung's terminology, anima and animus are archetypal representations of potentials that have not yet entered conscious awareness or become personalized. *Anima* is *a man's undeveloped femininity. Animus* is *a woman's undeveloped masculinity.* Those concepts are universal basic human drives from which both conscious and unconscious individual qualities develop. Usually, they appear as unconscious images of persons of the opposite sex.

The *collective unconscious* is defined as the psychic contents outside the realm of awareness that are common to humankind in general. Jung, who introduced the term, believed that the collective unconscious is inherited and derived from the collective experience of the species. It transcends cultural differences and explains the analogy between ancient *mythological ideas and primitive projections* observed in some patients who have never been exposed to those ideas.

Answers 6.46–6.50

6.46 The answer is D

6.47 The answer is B

6.48 The answer is A

6.49 The answer is C

6.50 The answer is E

Kurt Lewin (1890–1947) adapted the field approach from physics into a concept called field theory. A field is the totality of coexisting parts that are mutually interdependent. Applying field theory to groups, Lewin coined the term *"group dynamics"* and believed that a group is greater than the sum of its parts.

Abraham Maslow (1908–1970) was a developer of the self-actualization theory, which focuses on the need to understand the totality of the person. A *peak experience,* according to Maslow's school of thought, is an episodic, brief occurrence in which the person suddenly experiences a powerful transcendental state of consciousness. The powerful experience occurs most often in psychologically healthy persons.

Harry Stack Sullivan (1892–1949) made basic contributions to psychodynamic theory with his emphasis on the cultural matrix of personality development. Sullivan defined psychiatry as the study of interpersonal relationships that are manifest in the observable behavior of persons. Those relationships can be observed inside the therapeutic situation; the process is greatly enhanced when the therapist is both active and observant in the treatment. The transaction is then between the therapist, who is a *participant observer,* and a patient, whose life is disturbed or disordered.

Wilhelm Reich's (1897–1957) major contributions to psychoanalysis were in the areas of *character formation and character types.* Reich placed special emphasis on the influence of social forces in determining character structure, particularly on their repressive and inhibiting effects. Reich's basic concept was that character is a defensive structure, an armoring of the ego against instinctual forces within and the world without. It is the person's characteristic manner of dealing with threats. Reich described four major character types: hysterical, compulsive, narcissistic, and masochistic.

The evolution of *Gestalt therapy* is closely associated with the work of *Frederick S. Perls* (1893–1970), a European émigré trained in the psychoanalytic tradition. Although acknowledging its influences, Perls largely rejected the tenets of psychoanalysis and founded his own school of Gestalt therapy, borrowing the name from Gestalt theory. Gestalt theory proposes that the natural course of the biological and psychological development of the organism entails a full awareness of physical sensations and psychological needs. Perls believed that, as any form of self-control interferes with healthy functioning, modern civilization inevitably produces neurotic people; thus, the task of the therapist is to instruct the patient in discovering and experiencing the feelings and the needs repressed by society's demands.

Answers 6.51–6.55

6.51 The answer is A

6.52 The answer is C

6.53 The answer is E

6.54 The answer is D

6.55 The answer is B

The first of Erik Erikson's developmental stages, *infancy* (birth to 1 year), is characterized by the first psychosocial crisis the infant must face, that of *basic trust versus basic mistrust.* The crisis takes place in the context of the intimate relationship between the infant and its mother. The infant's primary orientation to reality is erotic and centers on the mouth. The successful resolution of the stage includes a disposition to trust others, a basic trust in oneself, a capacity to entrust oneself, and a sense of self-confidence.

During *early childhood* (ages 3 to 5 years) the crisis addressed by the child *is initiative versus guilt.* As the child struggles to resolve the oedipal struggle, guilt may grow because of aggressive thoughts or wishes. Initiative arises as the child begins to desire to mimic the adult world and as the child finds enjoyment in productive activity.

The stage of *puberty and adolescence* (age 11 years through the end of adolescence) is characterized by *identity versus role diffusion,* during which the adolescent must begin to establish a future role in adult society. During this psychosocial crisis, the adolescent is peculiarly vulnerable to social and cultural influences.

Early adulthood (21 to 40 years) is characterized by *intimacy versus isolation*. The crisis is characterized by the need to establish the capacity to relate intimately and meaningfully with others in mutually satisfying and productive interactions. The failure to achieve a successful resolution of that crisis results in a sense of personal isolation. *Late adulthood* (65 and older) is characterized by *integrity versus despair*. The crisis implies and depends on the successful resolution of all the preceding crises of psychosocial growth. It entails the acceptance of oneself and of all the aspects of life and the integration of their elements into a stable pattern of living. The failure to achieve ego integration often results in a kind of despair and an unconscious fear of death. The person who fails this crisis lives in basic self-contempt.

A further explanation of Erikson's stages appears in Table 6.3.

6.56 The answers are: 1, A; 2, C; 3, B; 4, A; and 5, B

The three provinces of Freud's structural model—id, ego, and superego—are distinguished by their different functions in the psychic apparatus. *Id* refers to a reservoir of unorganized instinctual drives. Operating under the domination of the primary process, the id lacks the capacity to delay or modify the instinctual drives with which the infant is born.

Ego is the executive organ of the psyche and functions to delay and modify drive expression through defense mechanisms. Defense mechanisms reside in the unconscious domain of the ego, whereas logical and abstract thinking and verbal expression are associated with conscious and preconscious functions of the ego. *Superego* establishes and maintains the person's moral conscience on the basis of a complex system of ideals and values internalized from one's parents. The superego provides ongoing scrutiny of the person's behavior, thoughts, and feelings. It then makes comparisons with expected standards of behavior and offers approval or disapproval. While the superego dictates what one should *not* do, the ego-ideal, often regarded as a component of the superego, prescribes what one should do according to internalized standards and values.

Answers 6.57–6.61

6.57 The answer is A

6.58 The answer is A

6.59 The answer is A

6.60 The answer is B

6.61 The answer is B

Table 6.3
Erikson's Psychosocial Stages

Psychosocial Stage	Associated Virtue	Related Forms of Psychopathology	Positive and Negative Forerunners of Identity Formation	Enduring Aspects of Identity Formation
Trust vs. mistrust (birth—)	Hope	Psychosis Addictions Depression	Mutual recognition vs. autistic isolation	Temporal perspective vs. time confusion
Autonomy vs. shame and doubt (~18 months—)	Will	Paranoia Obsessions Compulsions Impulsivity	Will to be oneself vs. self-doubt	Self-certainty vs. self-consciousness
Initiative vs. guilt (~3 years—)	Purpose	Conversion disorder Phobia Psychosomatic disorder Inhibition	Anticipation of roles vs. role inhibition	Role experimentation vs. role fixation
Industry vs. inferiority (~5 years—)	Competence	Creative inhibition Inertia	Task identification vs. sense of futility	Apprenticeship vs. work paralysis
Identity vs. role confusion (~13 years—)	Fidelity	Delinquent behavior Gender-related identity disorders Borderline psychotic episodes		Identity vs. identity confusion
Intimacy vs. isolation (~20s—)	Love	Schizoid personality disorder Distantiation		Sexual polarization vs. bisexual confusion
Generativity vs. stagnation (~40s—)	Care	Mid-life crisis Premature invalidism		Leadership and followership vs. abdication of responsibility
Integrity vs. despair (~60s—)	Wisdom	Extreme alienation Despair		Ideological commitment vs. confusion of values

Adapted from Erikson E. *Insight and Responsibility.* New York: WW Norton; 1964; Erikson E. *Identity: Youth and Crisis.* New York: WW Norton; 1968.

Primary process was Sigmund Freud's term for the laws that govern unconscious processes. It is a type of thinking *characteristic of very young children, the unconscious, the id,* and dreams. Primary process is characterized by an absence of negatives, conditionals, and other qualifying conjunctions; by a lack of any sense of time; and by the use of allusion, condensation, and symbols. It is primitive, prelogical thinking marked by the tendency to seek immediate discharge and gratification of instinctual drives.

Secondary process was Freud's term for the laws that regulate events in *the preconscious and the ego.* It is a form of thinking that uses judgment, intelligence, logic, and reality testing; it helps the ego block the tendency of the instincts toward immediate discharge.

Answers 6.62–6.66

6.62 The answer is A

6.63 The answer is B

6.64 The answer is A

6.65 The answer is B

6.66 The answer is D

The *topographic theory,* as *set forth by Sigmund Freud in* The Interpretation of Dreams *in 1900,* represented an attempt to divide the mind into three regions—*unconscious, preconscious, and conscious*—which were differentiated by their relation to consciousness. In general, all psychic material not in the immediate field of awareness—such as primitive drives, repressed desires, and memories—is in the unconscious. The preconscious includes all mental contents that are not in immediate awareness but can be consciously recalled with effort, in contrast to the unconscious, whose elements are barred from consciousness by some intrapsychic force, such as repression. The conscious is that portion of mental functioning that is within the realm of awareness at all times.

The *structural theory* of the mind was *presented in* The Ego and the Id *in 1923.* It represented a shift from the topographic model. Only when Freud discovered that not all unconscious processes can be relegated to the instincts (for example, that certain aspects of mental functioning associated with the ego and superego are unconscious) did he turn to the study of those structural components. From a structural viewpoint, the psychic apparatus is divided into three provinces—*id, ego, and superego.* Each is a particular aspect of human mental functioning and is not an empirically demonstrable phenomenon. The ego controls the apparatus of voluntary movement, perception, and contact with reality; through mechanisms of defense the ego is the inhibitor of primary instinctual drives. Freud conceived of the ego as an organized, problem-solving agent. Freud's concept of the id is as a completely unorganized, primordial reservoir of energy derived from the instincts; it is under the domination of the primary process. The id is not synonymous with the unconscious, as the structural viewpoint demonstrates that certain ego functions (for example, defenses against demands of the id) and aspects of the superego operate unconsciously. The discharge of id impulses is further regulated by the superego, which contains the internalized moral values and influence of the parental images—the conscience. The superego is the last of the structural components to develop; it results from the resolution of the Oedipus complex. Essentially, neurotic conflict can be explained structurally as a conflict between ego forces and id forces. Most often, the superego is involved in the conflict by aligning itself with the ego and imposing demands in the form of guilt. Occasionally, the superego may be allied with the id against the ego.

Sigmund Freud coined the idea of defense functions in 1894 and believed that defense mechanisms serve to keep conflictual ideation out of consciousness. However, the *first systematic and comprehensive study of the defenses used by the ego* was presented in Anna Freud's 1936 book, *The Ego and the Mechanisms of Defense,* which marked the beginning of ego psychology.

7 ▲

Clinical Examination of the Psychiatric Patient

The most comprehensive clinical examination in psychiatry involves knowing about the patient's genetic, psychological, biological, developmental, social, and cultural history. Obtaining information about these complex factors and making an accurate diagnosis involves a sophisticated interplay of listening and observational skills. To develop such skills that encourage patients to trust and confide in them, psychiatrists must convey genuine concern, empathy, and respect.

Psychiatrists often deal with patients whose thinking is chaotic or who act violently; they must be able to reach these patients as effectively as they can and interact with those who are moderately disturbed. Skilled interviewers are flexible and may change their interviewing techniques to suit different patients. They may also alter their approaches as they learn more about a patient. Nevertheless, arriving at an appropriate diagnosis and treatment requires that psychiatrists have a standard by which they organize interviews and obtain needed data. For instance, a psychiatric history must provide objective information about a patient's chief complaint, history of illnesses, family background, and so on.

The mental status examination provides a formal framework for the clinician's observations. The patient's appearance, behavior, affect, mood, speech, thought, cognitive functioning, impulse control, insight, and judgment provide valuable guideposts to diagnosis and effective treatment. The skilled psychiatrist will combine data obtained from the mental status examination and the patient's history with the use of laboratory testing.

Psychiatrists must be familiar with the array of laboratory tests available; these procedures can rule out medical disorders that may be associated with psychiatric signs and symptoms and may even help to make or confirm a diagnosis of a particular mental disorder. In ordering tests, there should be clear clinical evidence that they are warranted. For example, the use of psychotherapeutic drug serum levels should not be routine. In evidence-based medicine, a specific drug level might be indicated in a nonresponder to help clarify the situation. In the clinical setting, the best guide is to ask whether a specific test result will affect diagnosis and treatment. If the answer is affirmative, then ordering the test is probably justified.

The student should address the following questions and study the answers to gain a knowledge of the clinical examination.

HELPFUL HINTS

Students should familiarize themselves with these terms, especially the acronyms and names of laboratory tests.

- ▶ adulthood
- ▶ anamnesis
- ▶ antipsychotics
- ▶ appearance, behavior, attitude, and speech
- ▶ appropriateness
- ▶ carbamazepine
- ▶ catecholamines
- ▶ chief complaint
- ▶ clang associations
- ▶ concentration, memory, and intelligence
- ▶ confabulation
- ▶ consciousness and orientation
- ▶ countertransference

- ▶ CSF
- ▶ CT
- ▶ current social situation
- ▶ cyclic antidepressants
- ▶ data
- ▶ do's and don'ts of treating violent patients
- ▶ dreams, fantasies, and value systems
- ▶ DSM-IV-TR and Axes I–V
- ▶ early, middle, and late childhood history
- ▶ EEG
- ▶ eliciting delusional beliefs

- ▶ family history
- ▶ history of present illness; previous illnesses
- ▶ initial interview and greeting
- ▶ interviewing variations
- ▶ judgment and insight
- ▶ lithium
- ▶ marital history
- ▶ medical history
- ▶ mental status examination
- ▶ military history
- ▶ mood, feelings, and affect
- ▶ neologisms

- ▶ occupational and educational history
- ▶ paraphasia
- ▶ patient questions
- ▶ perception
- ▶ PET
- ▶ polysomnography
- ▶ prenatal history
- ▶ prognosis
- ▶ psychiatric history
- ▶ psychiatric report
- ▶ psychodynamic formulation
- ▶ psychosexual history
- ▶ punning
- ▶ rapport

▶ reliability	▶ sexuality	▶ therapeutic alliance	▶ TRH
▶ religious background	▶ social activity	▶ thought process	▶ TSH
▶ resistance	▶ stress interview	▶ time management	▶ uncovering feelings
▶ sensorium and cognition	▶ style	▶ transference	▶ VDRL
	▶ subsequent interviews	▶ treatment plan	▶ word salad

▲ QUESTIONS

DIRECTIONS: Each of the questions or incomplete statements below is followed by five suggested responses or completions. Select the *one* that is *best* in each case.

7.1 Formal thought disorders include

  A. circumstantiality
  B. clang associations
  C. neologisms
  D. flight of ideas
  E. all of the above

7.2 Tests of concentration include all of the following *except*

  A. calculations
  B. repeating a series of random numbers
  C. proverb interpretation
  D. spelling "world" backward
  E. repeating three or four unrelated objects after 5 to 10 minutes

7.3 True statements about diagnostic tests in psychiatric disorders include

  A. serum amylase may be increased in bulimia nervosa
  B. serum bicarbonate may be decreased in panic disorder
  C. decreased serum calcium has been associated with depression
  D. serum bicarbonate may be elevated in bulimia nervosa
  E. all of the above

7.4 Hypothyroidism in the elderly may commonly present with all of the following *except*

  A. lassitude
  B. fatigue
  C. cognitive impairment
  D. anorexia
  E. constipation

7.5 Laboratory tests typically used in a dementia evaluation include

  A. VDRL (serological test for syphilis)
  B. HIV
  C. CT scan of brain
  D. EEG
  E. all of the above

7.6 True statements about the lengths of time drugs of abuse can be detected in urine include

  A. morphine for 8 days
  B. benzodiazepine for 2 to 3 weeks
  C. alcohol for 7 to 12 hours
  D. marijuana for 24 to 48 hours
  E. cocaine for 1 to 2 weeks

7.7 Common pretreatment lithium tests include

  A. ECG
  B. pregnancy test
  C. serum electrolytes
  D. serum BUN
  E. all of the above

7.8 True statements about laboratory testing related to antipsychotics include

  A. There are clear pretreatment and follow-up laboratory and diagnostic evaluation strategies for most antipsychotics.
  B. Specific therapeutic blood levels have emerged for most antipsychotics.
  C. For haloperidol, gross toxic adverse effects have been associated with blood concentrations greater than 30 ng/mL.
  D. Agranulocytosis and seizures are associated only with clozapine.
  E. Serious cardiac arrhythmias have not been reported to be associated with antipsychotic use.

7.9 Polysomnography (sleep EEG) abnormalities include

  A. a decrease in the amount of REM sleep in major depressive disorder
  B. a lengthened REM latency in major depressive disorder
  C. an increase in REM sleep in dementia
  D. an increased sleep latency in schizophrenia
  E. none of the above

7.10 Each of the following statements is true *except*

  A. Sodium lactate provokes panic attacks in a majority of patients with panic disorder.
  B. Sodium lactate can trigger flashbacks in patients with posttraumatic stress disorder.
  C. Hyperventilation is as sensitive as lactate provocation in inducing panic attacks.
  D. Panic attacks triggered by sodium lactate are not inhibited by propranolol.
  E. Panic attacks triggered by sodium lactate are inhibited by alprazolam.

7.11 An abnormal finding on a dexamethasone-suppression test (DST) means that the patient may have

A. a good response to electroconvulsive therapy (ECT)
B. a good response to cyclic drugs
C. disseminated cancer
D. received high-dosage benzodiazepine treatment
E. all of the above

7.12 The first sign of beginning cerebral disease is impairment of

A. immediate memory
B. recent memory
C. long-term memory
D. remote memory
E. none of the above

7.13 The reaction of the patient to the psychiatrist may be affected by

A. the psychiatrist's attitude
B. previous experiences with physicians
C. the patient's view of authority figures in childhood
D. the patient's cultural background
E. all of the above

7.14 If a patient receiving clozapine shows a white blood count (WBC) of 2,000 per cc, the clinician should

A. increase the dosage of clozapine at once
B. terminate any antibiotic therapy
C. stop the administration of clozapine at once
D. monitor the patient's WBC every 10 days
E. institute weekly complete blood count (CBC) tests with differential

7.15 Which of the following substances has been implicated in mood disorders with a seasonal pattern?

A. luteotropic hormone (LTH)
B. gonadotropin-releasing hormone (GnRH)
C. testosterone
D. estrogen
E. melatonin

7.16 A favorable therapeutic window is associated with

A. imipramine
B. nortriptyline
C. desipramine
D. amitriptyline
E. all of the above

7.17 A good test for recent memory is to ask patients

A. their date of birth
B. what they had to eat for their last meal
C. how many siblings they have
D. to subtract 7 from 100
E. who is the President of the United States

7.18 In a psychiatric interview

A. the psychiatrist may have to medicate a violent patient before taking a history
B. a violent patient should be interviewed alone to establish a doctor–patient relationship
C. delusions should be challenged directly
D. the psychiatrist must not ask depressed patients if they have suicidal thoughts
E. the psychiatrist should have a seat higher than the patient's seat

DIRECTIONS: Each group of questions below consists of lettered headings followed by a list of numbered phrases. For each numbered phrase, select the *best* lettered heading. Each heading may be used once, more than once, or not at all.

Questions 7.19–7.23

A. Epstein-Barr virus (EBV)
B. Mean corpuscular volume (MCV)
C. Creutzfeldt-Jakob disease
D. Bulimia nervosa
E. Bromide intoxication

7.19 Elevated in alcoholism and vitamin B_{12} and folate deficiency
7.20 Causative agent for infectious mononucleosis, associated with depression, fatigue, and personality change
7.21 Decreased serum chloride
7.22 Psychosis, hallucinations, delirium
7.23 Biphasic or triphasic slow bursts on EEG

Questions: 7.24–7.28

A. Elevated level of 5-HIAA
B. Decreased level of 5-HIAA

7.24 Carcinoid tumors
7.25 Phenothiazine medications
7.26 Aggressive behavior
7.27 High banana intake
7.28 Suicidal patients

Questions: 7.29–7.33

A. Hyperthyroidism
B. Hypothyroidism
C. Porphyria
D. Hepatolenticular degeneration
E. Pancreatic carcinoma

7.29 Jaundice, sense of imminent doom
7.30 Dry skin, myxedema madness
7.31 Kayser-Fleischer rings, brain damage
7.32 Abdominal crises, mood swings
7.33 Tremor, anxiety, hyperactivity

Questions: 7.34–7.35

A. Serum ammonia
B. Cortisone
C. Copper
D. Creatinine
E. Platelet count

7.34 Increased in hepatic encephalopathy
7.35 Decreased by carbamazepine

ANSWERS

Clinical Examination of the Psychiatric Patient

7.1 The answer is E (all)

The form of thought refers to the way in which ideas are linked, not the ideas themselves. Thoughts may be logically associated and goal directed. If they are not, a disorder of thought (also called formal thought disorder or sometimes, thought disorder) may exist. A number of different formal thought disorders have been described and are listed, with examples, in Table 7.1. No thought disorder is pathognomonic for a particular disorder. However, a specific disorder of thought form is sometimes more characteristic of one diagnosis than another and may thereby convey diagnostic significance. For example, *clang associations* and *flight of ideas* are most closely associated with manic states. *Neologisms* and *circumstantiality* are associated with schizophrenia. There may be overlap, however.

7.2 The answer is C

Concentration describes the ability to sustain attention over time. Patients who forget the examiner's question, are distracted by extraneous stimuli, or lose track of what they are saying have impaired concentration. Concentration may be tested in several ways.

Table 7.1
Formal Thought Disorders

Circumstantiality. Overinclusion of trivial or irrelevant details that impede the sense of getting to the point.
> *Example:* A 79-year-old woman is describing her headaches to her doctor. "They usually start in the morning. I'll wake up at 6 or 6:30, and then by the time I have my coffee . . . well sometimes I'll have tea. I like it with lemon and just a bit of sugar . . . or honey sometimes. I always take milk with coffee. And like I was saying, after coffee I may turn on the TV for a half hour or so. Well, unless there's something really good. If I'm watching the news, I may not even notice the headaches, but by lunch they're so bad I have to lie down."

Clang association. Thoughts are associated by the sound of words rather than their meaning, for example, through rhyming or assonance.
> *Example:* A 31-year-old man in the manic phase of bipolar disorder was asked if he had any trouble sleeping. He replied, "I never have trouble sleeping. I never have trouble peeping. I never have trouble pooping."

Derailment. (Synonymous with *loose associations*) There is a breakdown in both the logical connection between ideas and the overall sense of goal-directedness. The words make sentences, but the sentences don't make sense.
> *Example:* A 19-year-old man with a first psychotic episode describes the week at home before coming into the hospital. "I . . . I watched TV, but the newspaper didn't come. I . . . David is at school, too. Sometimes it's better to be alone, you know, to save for a rainy day."

Flight of ideas. A succession of multiple associations, so that thought seems to move abruptly from idea to idea. Often (but not invariably) expressed through rapid, pressured speech.
> *Example:* A 37-year-old man who is in the middle of a manic episode is speaking with great rapidity: "I just got back from New York. Call it the Big Apple, but it's rotten to the core. Nobody can take me. I could beat up my father. He was tough, a salesman. He sold his soul for a pig in a poke."

Neologism. Invention of new words or phrases or the use of conventional words in idiosyncratic ways.
> *Example:* A 25-year-old man with a diagnosis of chronic undifferentiated schizophrenia described his activities during a pass from a psychiatric hospital: "We went to the park. It was hot, but not too hot. It was burging."

Perseveration. Repetition out of context of words, phrases, or ideas.
> *Example:* A psychiatrist is evaluating an 86-year-old woman in a nursing home.
> Psychiatrist: Do you know what day it is?
> Woman: Yes, Tuesday.
> Psychiatrist: And where are we now?
> Woman: Tuesday.

Tangentiality. In response to a question, the patient gives a reply that is appropriate to the general topic without actually answering the question.
> *Example:* A 40-year-old man with depression is being evaluated by a psychiatrist.
> Psychiatrist: Have you had trouble sleeping through the night lately?
> Patient: I usually sleep in my bed but now I'm sleeping on the sofa.

Thought blocking. A sudden disruption of thought or break in the flow of ideas.
> *Example:* A psychiatrist is interviewing a 55-year-old man.
> Psychiatrist: Have you been drinking more than usual in the last couple of months?
> Patient: Not really. I've always been a pretty big drinker . . . could hold my liquor pretty well.
> Psychiatrist: How much would you drink in a normal day?
> Patient: Maybe a pint. Two pints sometimes . . . no [pause]
> Psychiatrist: What?
> Patient: I forgot. What were we talking about? What did you ask me?

Memory, which involves concentration, must be evaluated across the spectrum of immediate to remote. One test of immediate recall is to *say* (without inflection or verbal spacing) *a series of random numbers and have the patient repeat the series.* A progressively longer sequence of numbers is presented, and both forward and backward recall are tested. Most adults can easily recall five or six numbers forward and three or four in reverse. Recent memory is for events several minutes to hours old and may be evaluated by *giving patients* the *names of three or four unrelated objects and asking them to repeat them after 5 to 10 minutes.* Remote memory describes events 2 or more years old. It is usually revealed in the course of obtaining patients' histories, although it may be necessary to confirm facts through collateral sources.

Calculations describe the ability to manipulate numbers mentally. Simple addition, subtraction, or multiplication questions may be used. Problems of money and change are often helpful with patients with limited educational background. For example, if a magazine costs $3.50 and you pay with a ten dollar bill, how much change should you be given? Other tests of concentration include counting backward by 3s, reciting the alphabet backward, *spelling "world" backward*, and naming the months of the year backward.

Abstract reasoning describes the ability to mentally shift back and forth between general concepts and specific examples. A frequently used way to test abstract reasoning is asking *proverb interpretation.* For example, a clinician might ask the patient, "What does it mean when someone says, 'People who live in glass houses shouldn't throw stones'?" A conventional response, one that is able to generalize from the specifics of the proverb to the generalization, might be, "Don't criticize others of what you are guilty yourself." A nonabstract response would address the concrete particulars without grasping the larger meaning; for example, "You would break the glass." (Some answers will be idiosyncratic and difficult to classify as either abstract or concrete: "The police would see you and would come to arrest you.")

7.3 The answer is E (all)

The patient's history and physical examination typically dictate which tests are ordered. Laboratory abnormalities are typically useful when they optimize outcomes; that is, if the test results will contribute to the detection of a previously unrecognized medical condition or otherwise influence treatment. Diagnostic testing can also serve a therapeutic function by reassuring the patient or family that other serious medical problems do not appear to be present.

Serum amylase may be increased in bulimia nervosa. Serum bicarbonate may be decreased in panic disorder and may be *elevated in patients with bulimia nervosa. Serum calcium may be decreased in depression* in addition to hyperparathyroidism and bone metastases.

7.4 The answer is D

Thyroid disease in the elderly is common and can present with an atypical picture. Nonspecific symptoms such as *lassitude, constipation,* cold intolerance, *fatigue,* and *cognitive impairment may occur.* These symptoms may be attributed to depression or degenerative dementia. Severe hypothyroidism (myxedema) is a medical emergency that occurs primarily in patients over age 50. *Anorexia* is more common in older patients with hyperthyroidism. They present with typical symptoms of heat intolerance, weight loss, tremor, palpitations, and atrial fibrillation.

7.5 The answer is E (all)

Besides a thorough medical history and physical and neurological examinations, laboratory tests typically used in a dementia evaluation include a CBC with differential, sedimentation rate, blood chemistry panel (with liver and kidney function tests), serum electrolytes (some include magnesium and zinc blood levels), thyroid function tests, B_{12} and folate levels, and a *serological test for syphilis. Human immunodeficiency virus (HIV)* testing should be considered in the laboratory evaluation of the patient with dementia because neurological involvement is a common sequela of HIV infection. Chest X-ray and ECG are usually included, and a brain imaging study such as *computed tomography (CT)* or magnetic resonance imaging (MRI) are now considered standard; *electroencephalograms (EEG)* are also obtained frequently. Some clinicians are ordering single photon emission computed tomography (SPECT) scans to further their understanding of the dementing condition. On SPECT and positron emission tomography (PET) scans, single focal perfusion defects or multiple areas of patchy hypoperfusion are suggestive of ischemic brain changes (vascular dementia), whereas dementia of the Alzheimer's type typically shows decreased perfusion in temporoparietal areas bilaterally.

7.6 The answer is C

The laboratory is useful for detecting substances of abuse and for evaluating the impact the substance use is having on the patient's body. Often the laboratory detection of abused substances and certain diagnostic test abnormalities related to the substance abuse (e.g., abnormal liver function tests in alcohol-abusing patients) are used therapeutically to confront the denial of a patient with a substance abuse disorder and to help engage the patient in treatment.

The most commonly used specimen for the detection of drugs of abuse is urine, although toxicological analyses can also be performed on blood specimens. The period of time that the clinician can detect drugs in blood specimens is typically shorter than the length of time drugs can be detected in urine specimens because drugs and their metabolites are excreted and detectable in the urine for longer periods of time than they are detectable in blood. However, the length of time that a particular drug of abuse can be detected in the urine is somewhat variable, depending on the specific drug, the duration and amounts of the substance used, and concomitant medical problems (e.g., liver or kidney disease). *Table 7.2 provides a list of some common drugs of abuse that can be detected in urine specimens, along with a typical length of time* after recent use that the substance can be detected. Other specimens that have been studied to detect substance abuse include saliva and hair samples.

7.7 The answer is E (all)

The therapeutic and toxic blood levels of lithium are very close to one another, and in certain individuals even seem to overlap. Additionally, lithium has effects on a number of organ systems of which the clinician should be aware. Lithium therapy is associated with a benign elevation of the white blood cell count (WBC), which may reach 15,000 cells per mm^3. This WBC elevation can sometimes be mistaken for signs of infection or wrongly attributed to lithium in the context of other signs of infection (e.g., fever, cough, discomfort on urination, malaise). Furthermore, lithium can have adverse effects on electrolyte balance (especially in patients on thiazide diuretics), thyroid func-

Table 7.2
Drugs of Abuse That Can Be Tested in Urine

Drug	Length of Time Detected in Urine
Alcohol	7–12 hours
Amphetamine	48 hours
Barbiturate	24 hours (short-acting)
	3 weeks (long-acting)
Benzodiazepine	3 days
Cocaine	6–8 hours (metabolites 2–4 days)
Codeine	48 hours
Heroin	36–72 hours
Marijuana	3 days to 4 weeks (depending on use)
Methadone	3 days
Methaqualone	7 days
Morphine	48–72 hours
Phencyclidine (PCP)	8 days
Propoxyphene	6–48 hours

tion, the kidney, and the heart. The common lithium pretreatment tests include *serum electrolytes, BUN,* serum creatinine, urinalysis, thyroid function tests (TFTs) (e.g., TSH, T_4, T_3RU), and an *ECG.* In patients with a history suggestive of possible kidney problems, a 24-hour urine test for creatinine and protein clearance is recommended. Some clinicians routinely order this test in patients about to begin lithium therapy. It has been argued that antithyroid antibody testing is helpful in assessing the potential of lithium-induced hypothyroidism. Because of the potential cardiac teratogenicity of lithium, *a pregnancy test* in potentially child-bearing women should be ordered. Periodic follow-up of serum electrolytes, BUN, creatinine, TFTs, ECG, and 24-hour urine for creatinine and protein clearance are recommended. The frequency and exact makeup of the follow-up testing battery should be dictated by the patient's medical condition.

7.8 The answer is C
Except for the antipsychotic clozapine (Clozaril), no clear pretreatment and follow-up laboratory and diagnostic evaluation strategies exist. Additionally, *no specific therapeutic blood levels for these agents* have emerged, although some suggested therapeutic blood concentrations for several antipsychotic agents exist in the psychiatric literature. *For haloperidol, gross toxic adverse effects,* including neuroleptic malignant syndrome, confusion, seizures, or catatonia, *have been associated with blood concentrations greater than 30 ng/mL;* blood-level reductions were associated with a reduction in these toxic adverse effects.

Clinicians need to be aware of the potential toxicities of the antipsychotic agents that they use and order laboratory and diagnostic tests accordingly. For instance, clinicians using *clozapine* need to be aware of its *potential to cause fatal agranulocytosis and seizures.* These risks exist with all antipsychotic agents, albeit to a lesser extent.

Serious cardiac arrhythmias have been reported with antipsychotic use (e.g., thioridazine [Mellaril]); hence, patients with preexisting cardiac disorder might need careful ECG follow-up when these agents are used. In patients about to start on antipsychotic agents with known cardiac effects,

obtaining a baseline ECG is prudent, especially in patients over the age of 50.

7.9 The answer is D
EEG obtained during sleep is a potentially powerful biological marker of psychiatric illness. Sleep EEG abnormalities described in major depressive disorder include *an increase in the overall amount of rapid-eye movement (REM) sleep,* not a decrease, and a *shortened (not lengthened) REM latency.* Medical conditions giving rise to pseudodepressions are typically associated with decreased REM sleep. *Patients with dementia usually have increased amounts of non-REM sleep. In schizophrenia, an increased sleep latency* has been reported, especially during relapse.

7.10 The answer is C
Even though hyperventilation can trigger panic attacks in predisposed persons, *hyperventilation is not as sensitive as lactate provocation in inducing panic attacks. Sodium lactate provokes panic attacks* in a majority (up to 72 percent) of patients with panic disorder. Therefore, lactate provocation is used to confirm a diagnosis of panic disorder. *Sodium lactate can also trigger flashbacks in patients with posttraumatic stress disorder.* Carbon dioxide (CO_2) inhalation also precipitates panic attacks in those so predisposed. *Panic attacks triggered by sodium lactate are not inhibited by* peripherally acting β-blockers, such as *propranolol* (Inderal), but are *inhibited by alprazolam* (Xanax) and tricyclic drugs.

7.11 The answer is E (all)
The dexamethasone-suppression test (DST) can help to confirm a diagnostic impression of major depressive disorder with melancholic features. In such depressions, the test result is abnormal in many cases, meaning that there is nonsuppression of endogenous cortisol production after exogenous steroid ingestion. Nonsuppression, a positive finding, indicates a hyperactive hypothalamic-pituitary-adrenal axis. The test is sometimes used to predict which patients will have *a good response to* somatic treatments, such as *electroconvulsive therapy (ECT)* and *cyclic drugs.* The clinician needs to be aware that false-positive findings can result from several factors, such as *disseminated cancer.* A false-negative finding can occur in patients who have *received high-dosage benzodiazepine treatment.*

7.12 The answer is B
Memory impairment, most notably in *recent* or short-term *memory,* is usually the first sign of beginning cerebral disease. Memory is a process by which anything that is experienced or learned is established as a record in the central nervous system, where it persists with a variable degree of permanence and can be recollected or retrieved from storage at will. *Immediate memory* is the reproduction, recognition, or recall of perceived material after a period of 10 seconds or less has elapsed after the initial presentation. *Recent memory* covers a time period from a few hours to a few weeks after the initial presentation. *Long-term memory or remote memory* is the reproduction, recognition, or recall of experiences or information from the distant past. That function is usually not disturbed early in cerebral disease.

7.13 The answer is E (all)
The reaction of patients to the psychiatrist is influenced by *the psychiatrist's attitude,* style, and orientation. If patients believe that they will lose their psychiatrist's respect as they

expose their problems, they may be unwilling to disclose such material. If, in their *previous experiences with physicians* (psychiatric or nonpsychiatric), patients felt ridiculed or that their problems were minimized, those experiences influence what they do or do not tell the psychiatrist.

Transference is a process in which patients unconsciously displace onto persons in their current life those patterns of behavior and emotional reactions that originated in childhood. *The patient's view of authority figures in childhood* influences reactions to the psychiatrist. Differences in the social, educational, and intellectual backgrounds of each patient and the psychiatrist may also interfere with the development of rapport. It is an obvious advantage for the psychiatrist to acquire as much understanding and familiarity as possible with *the patient's cultural background.*

7.14 The answer is C

A patient who shows a white blood count of 2,000 while taking clozapine (Clozaril) is at high risk for agranulocytosis. If agranulocytosis develops (that is, if the WBC is less than 1,000) and there is evidence of severe infection (for example, skin ulcerations), the patient should be placed in *protective isolation on a medical unit.* The clinician should *stop the administration of clozapine at once,* not increase the dosage of clozapine. The patient may or may not have clinical symptoms, such as fever and sore throat. *If the patient does have such symptoms, antibiotic therapy* may be necessary. Depending on the severity of the condition, the physician should *monitor the patient's WBC every 2 days, not 10 days,* or institute *daily, not weekly, CBC tests* with differential.

Table 7.3 summarizes the treatment of patients with reduced WBC.

Table 7.3
Clinical Management of Reduced White Blood Cell Count (WBC), Leukopenia, and Agranulocytosis

Problem Phase	WBC Findings	Clinical Findings	Treatment Plan
Reduced WBC count	WBC count reveals a significant drop (even if WBC count is still in normal range). "Significant drop" is (1) a drop of more than 3,000 cells from prior test or (2) three or more consecutive drops in WBC counts	No symptoms of infection	1. Monitor patient closely 2. Institute twice-weekly CBC tests with differentials if deemed appropriate by attending physician 3. Clozapine therapy may continue
Mild leukopenia	WBC = 3,000–3,500	Patient may or may not show clinical symptoms, such as lethargy, fever, sore throat, weakness	1. Monitor patient closely 2. Institute a minimum of twice-weekly CBC tests with differentials 3. Clozapine therapy may continue
Leukopenia or granulocytopenia	WBC = 2,000–3,000 or granulocytes = 1,000–1,500	Patient may or may not show clinical symptoms, such as fever, sore throat, lethargy, weakness	1. Interrupt clozapine at once 2. Institute daily CBC tests with differentials 3. Increase surveillance, consider hospitalization 4. Clozapine therapy may be reinstituted after normalization of WBC
Agranulocytosis (uncomplicated)	WBC count less than 2,000 or granulocytes less than 1,000	Patient may or may not show clinical symptoms, such as fever, sore throat, lethargy, weakness	1. Discontinue clozapine at once 2. Place patient in protective isolation in a medical unit with modern facilities 3. Consider a bone marrow specimen to determine if progenitor cells are being suppressed 4. Monitor patient every 2 days until WBC and differential counts return to normal (about 2 weeks) 5. Avoid use of concomitant medications with bone marrow–suppressing potential
Agranulocytosis (with complications)	WBC count less than 2,000 or granulocytes less than 1,000	Definite evidence of infection, such as fever, sore throat, lethargy, weakness, malaise, skin ulcerations, etc.	1. Consult with hematologist or other specialist to determine appropriate antibiotic regimen 2. Start appropriate therapy; monitor closely
Recovery	WBC count more than 4,000 and granulocytes more than 2,000	No symptoms of infection	1. Once-weekly CBC with differential counts for four consecutive normal values 2. Clozapine must not be restarted

Reprinted with permission from Sandoz Pharmaceuticals Corporation and MacKinnon RA, Yudofsky SC. *Principles of the Psychiatric Evaluation.* Philadelphia: JB Lippincott; 1991:118.

7.15 The answer is E

Melatonin is the substance that has been implicated in mood disorders with seasonal pattern. Melatonin's exact mechanism of action is unknown, but its production is stimulated in the dark, and it may affect the sleep–wake cycle. Melatonin is synthesized from serotonin, an active neurotransmitter. Decreased nocturnal secretion of melatonin has been associated with depression. A number of other substances also affect behavior, and some known endocrine diseases (for example, Cushing's disease) have associated psychiatric signs. Symptoms of anxiety or depression may be explained in some patients by changes in endocrine function or homeostasis.

Luteotropic hormone (LTH) is an anterior pituitary hormone whose action maintains the function of the corpus luteum.

Gonadotropin-releasing hormone (GnRH), produced by the hypothalamus, increases the pituitary secretion of luteotropic hormone (LTH) and the follicle-stimulating hormone (FSH). GnRH is secreted in a pulsatile manner that is critical for the control of LTH and FSH from the pituitary. GnRH also acts as a neurotransmitter whose exact function is unknown.

Testosterone is the hormone responsible for the secondary sex characteristics in men. A decreased testosterone level has been associated with erectile dysfunction and depression. Testosterone is formed in greatest quantities by the interstitial cells of the testes, but it is also formed in small amounts by the ovaries and the adrenal cortex.

Estrogen is produced by the granulosa cells in the ovaries and it is responsible for pubertal changes in girls. Exogenous estrogen replacement therapy has been associated with depression.

7.16 The answer is E (all)

A favorable therapeutic window—that is, the range within which a drug is most effective—is associated with all the drugs listed. Blood levels should be tested when using *imipramine* (Tofranil), *amitriptyline* (Elavil), *nortriptyline* (Pamelor), or *desipramine* (Norpramin) in the treatment of depressive disorders. Taking blood levels may also be of use in patients with poor responses at normal dosage ranges and in high-risk patients when there is an urgent need to know whether a therapeutic or toxic plasma level of the drug has been reached. Blood level tests should also include the measurement of active metabolites (for example, imipramine is converted to desipramine, and *amitriptyline* [Elavil] is converted to nortriptyline).

7.17 The answer is B

Recent memory is the ability to remember what has been experienced within the past few hours, days, or weeks. It is assessed by asking patients to describe how they spent the last 24 hours, such as *what they had to eat for their last meal.*

Remote memory or long-term memory is the ability to remember events in the distant past. Memory for the remote past can be evaluated by inquiring about important dates in patients' lives, such as *their date of birth, or how many siblings they have.* The answers must be verifiable. *Subtracting 7 from 100* is more a test of concentration. Asking *who the President of the United States is* tests the general fund of information.

7.18 The answer is A

Psychiatrists often encounter violent patients in a hospital setting. Frequently, the police bring a patient into the emergency room in some type of physical restraint (for example, handcuffs). The psychiatrist must establish whether effective verbal contact can be made with the patient or whether the patient's sense of reality is so impaired that productive interviewing is impossible. If impaired reality testing is an issue, *the psychiatrist may have to medicate a violent patient before taking a history.*

With or without restraints, *a violent patient should not be interviewed alone* to establish a doctor–patient relationship. At least one other person should always be present; in some situations that other person should be a security guard or a police officer. Other precautions include leaving the interview room's door open and sitting between the patient and the door, so that the interviewer has unrestricted access to an exit should it become necessary. The psychiatrist must make it clear, in a firm but nonangry manner, that the patient may say or feel anything but is not free to act in a violent way.

Delusions should never be directly challenged. Delusions are fixed false ideas that may be thought of as a patient's defensive and self-protective, albeit maladaptive, strategy against overwhelming anxiety, low self-esteem, and confusion. Challenging a delusion by insisting that it is not true or possible only increases the patient's anxiety and often leads the patient to defend the belief desperately. However, clinicians should not pretend that they believe the patient's delusion. Often, the best approach is for clinicians to indicate that they understand that the patient believes the delusion to be true but that they do not hold the same belief.

Being mindful of the possibility of suicide is imperative when interviewing any depressed patient, even if a suicidal risk is not apparent. *The psychiatrist must ask depressed patients if they have suicidal thoughts.* Doing so does not make patients feel worse. Instead, many patients are relieved to talk about their suicidal ideas. The psychiatrist should ask specifically, "Are you suicidal now?" or "Do you have plans to take your own life?" A suicide note, a family history of suicide, or previous suicidal behavior by the patient increases the risk for suicide. Evidence of impulsivity or of pervasive pessimism about the future also places patients at risk. If the psychiatrist decides that the patient is in imminent risk for suicidal behavior, the patient must be hospitalized or otherwise protected.

The way chairs are arranged in the psychiatrist's office affects the interview. *The psychiatrist should not have a seat higher than the patient's seat.* Both chairs should be about the same height, so that neither person looks down on the other.

Answers 7.19–7.23

7.19 The answer is B

7.20 The answer is A

7.21 The answer is D

7.22 The answer is E

7.23 The answer is C

There are major psychological changes that occur in psychiatric disorders, which have led many doctors to believe that all mental illness is accompanied by such changes, even though current laboratory tests do not allow all of them to be demonstrated. In some cases, as listed in Table 7.4, those changes are very much in evidence and are useful in confirming diagnoses.

Table 7.4
Some Laboratory Findings in Mental Disorder

Test	Major Psychiatric Indication	Comments
Mean corpuscular volume (average volume of a red blood cell)	Alcohol abuse	Elevated in alcoholism and vitamin B_{12} and folate deficiency
Epstein-Barr Virus (EBV); cytomegalovirus (CMV)	Cognitive/medical workup	Part of herpes virus group EBV is causative agent for infectious mononucleosis, which can present with depression, fatigue, and personality change
	Anxiety	CMV can produce anxiety, confusion, mood disorders
	Mood disorders	EBV may be associated with chronic mononucleosis-like syndrome associated with chronic depression and fatigue
Chloride (Cl), serum	Eating disorders	Decreased in patients with bulimia and psychogenic vomiting
	Panic disorder	Mild elevation in hyperventilation syndrome, panic disorder
Bromide (Br), serum	Dementia	Bromide intoxication can cause psychosis, hallucinations, delirium
	Psychosis	Part of dementia workup, especially when serum chloride is elevated
Electroencephalogram (EEG)	Cognitive/medical workup	Seizures, brain death, lesions; shortened REM latency in depression
		High-voltage activity in stupor; low-voltage fast activity in excitement, functional nonorganic cases (e.g., dissociative states), alpha activity present in the background, which responds to auditory and visual stimuli
		Biphasic or triphasic slow bursts seen in dementia of Creutzfeldt-Jakob disease

Answers 7.24–7.28

7.24 The answer is A

7.25 The answer is A

7.26 The answer is B

7.27 The answer is A

7.28 The answer is B
The serotonin metabolite 5-hydroxyindoleacetic acid (5-HIAA) is *elevated* in the urine of patients with *carcinoid tumors,* at times in patients who take *phenothiazine medications* and in persons who eat foods high in L-tryptophan, the chemical precursor of serotonin (for example, walnuts, *bananas,* and avocados). The amount of 5-HIAA in cerebrospinal fluid is *decreased* in some persons who display *aggressive behavior* and in some *suicidal patients* who have committed suicide in particularly violent ways.

Answers 7.29–7.33

7.29 The answer is E

7.30 The answer is B

7.31 The answer is D

7.32 The answer is C

7.33 The answer is A
The clinician should be aware of the many medical problems that may present as psychiatric symptoms. For example, *tremor, anxiety, and hyperactivity* are often associated with *hyperthyroidism; dry skin* and *myxedema madness* (which may mimic schizophrenia) are associated with *hypothyroidism; abdominal crises* and *mood swings* are associated with *porphyria; Kayser-Fleischer rings* and *brain damage* are associated with *hepatolenticular degeneration (Wilson's disease);* and *jaundice* and a *sense of imminent doom* are associated with *pancreatic carcinoma.*

Table 7.5 gives some examples of medical problems that may present as psychiatric symptoms.

Answers 7.34–7.35

7.34 The answer is A

7.35 The answer is E
Hepatic encephalopathy is associated with *increased serum ammonia* caused by chronic liver disease. The psychiatric signs of hepatic encephalopathy include personality changes, impaired consciousness, agitation, a musty sweet breath odor, and fetor hepaticus.

Wilson's disease is associated with an *elevated* level of *copper* caused by a disturbance in copper metabolism. The rare disease is transmitted in an autosomal recessive fashion.

Table 7.5
Medical Problems That May Present as Psychiatric Symptoms

Medical Problem	Sex and Age Prevalence	Common Medical Symptoms	Psychiatric Symptoms and Complaints	Impaired Performance and Behavior	Diagnostic Problems
Hyperthyroidism (thyrotoxicosis)	Females 3:1, 30 to 50	*Tremor,* sweating, loss of weight and strength	*Anxiety* if rapid onset; depression if slow onset	Occasional *hyperactivity* or grandiose behavior	Long lead time; a rapid onset resembles anxiety attack
Hypothyroidism (myxedema)	Females 5:1, 30 to 50	Puffy face, *dry skin,* cold intolerance	Anxiety with irritability, thought disorder, somatic delusions, hallucinations	*Myxedema madness;* delusional, paranoid belligerent behavior	Madness may mimic schizophrenia; mental status is clear, even during most disturbed behavior
Porphyria—acute intermittent type	Females, 20 to 40	*Abdominal crises,* paresthesias, weakness	Anxiety—sudden onset, severe *mood swings*	Extremes of excitement or withdrawal; emotional or angry outbursts	Patients often have truly abnormal life styles; crises resemble conversion disorder or anxiety attacks
Hepatolenticular degeneration (Wilson's disease)	Males 2:1; adolescence	Liver and extrapyramidal symptoms, *Kayser-Fleischer rings*	Mood swings—sudden and changeable; anger—explosive	Eventual *brain damage* with memory and IQ loss; combativeness	In late teens, disorder may resemble adolescent storm, incorrigibility, or schizophrenia
Pancreatic carcinoma	Males 3:1, 50 to 70	Weight loss, abdominal pain, weakness, *jaundice*	Depression, *sense of imminent doom* but without severe guilt	Loss of drive and motivation	Long lead time; exact age and symptoms of involutional depression

Carbamazepine (Tegretol) is used in psychiatry as a mood stabilizer in bipolar I disorder. The most serious potential adverse effect is agranulocytosis, including a *decrease in platelet count.*

Lithium (Eskalith) is used in the treatment of manic episodes of bipolar I disorder. A side effect is polyuria secondary to decreased resorption of fluid from the distal tubule of the kidneys. *Creatinine* clearance is a good gauge of the patient's renal function.

8 ▲

Signs and Symptoms in Psychiatry

Signs are generally defined as the objective findings observed by clinicians, symptoms as the subjective descriptions by patients of what they are experiencing. Certain clusters of signs and symptoms are associated with certain disorders, and the clinician needs to be thoroughly familiar with these. A syndrome is a group of symptoms that occur together and constitute a recognizable condition; the term "syndrome" is less specific than "disorder" or "disease." Most psychiatric conditions are more accurately defined as syndromes.

In psychiatry, the presentation of signs and symptoms is not always straightforward. A patient may insist that nothing is wrong (that there are no symptoms), when it is obvious to most observers that certain behaviors or ways of thinking are bizarre, damaging, or disruptive. These might be defined as ego-syntonic symptoms. Ego-dystonic symptoms are those of which the patient is aware and that are experienced as uncomfortable or unacceptable. Another complicating factor is that a clinician may not be able to literally observe or to hear a described symptom (such as an auditory hallucination), and may have to depend on indirect evidence (for example, a patient's preoccupation or distraction) to diagnose it.

In psychiatry there are few if any pathognomonic signs and symptoms. Human behavior is too complex for this. Complicating matters further, medical conditions can frequently present initially with psychiatric signs and symptoms, and psychiatric conditions with medical ones. Medical pathology can underlie apparent psychiatric symptomatology, and psychiatric syndromes can be expressed in physical terms. The skilled clinician must know when to have a heightened level of suspicion that a condition may not be what it first appears to be, and must know concretely how to differentiate between them.

Students should study the questions and answers below for a useful review of these topics.

HELPFUL HINTS

The student should be able to define and categorize the signs and symptoms and other terms listed below.

- ▶ affect and mood
- ▶ aggression
- ▶ agnosias
- ▶ anxiety
- ▶ aphasic disturbances
- ▶ cerea flexibilitas
- ▶ coma
- ▶ *déjà entendu*
- ▶ *déjà pensé*
- ▶ *déjà vu*
- ▶ delirium
- ▶ delusion
- ▶ dementia
- ▶ depersonalization
- ▶ disorientation
- ▶ distractibility
- ▶ disturbances in speech
- ▶ disturbances in the form and the content of thought
- ▶ disturbances of conation
- ▶ disturbances of consciousness and attention
- ▶ disturbances of intelligence
- ▶ disturbances of memory
- ▶ disturbances of perception, both those caused by brain diseases and those associated with psychological phenomena
- ▶ *folie à deux*
- ▶ hypnosis
- ▶ illusions
- ▶ insight and judgment
- ▶ *jamais vu*
- ▶ noesis
- ▶ panic
- ▶ phobias
- ▶ pseudodementia
- ▶ stereotypy
- ▶ synesthesia

▲ QUESTIONS

DIRECTIONS: Each of the incomplete statements below is followed by five suggested completions. Select the *one* that is *best* in each case.

8.1 A psychiatric patient who, although coherent, never gets to the point has a disturbance in the form of thought called

   A. word salad
   B. circumstantiality
   C. tangentiality
   D. verbigeration
   E. blocking

8.2 Loss of normal speech melody is known as

   A. stuttering
   B. stammering
   C. aphonia
   D. dysprosody
   E. dyslexia

8.3 Perceptual disturbances include all of the following *except*

   A. hallucinations
   B. hypnagogic experiences
   C. echolalia
   D. depersonalization
   E. derealization

8.4 Asking a patient to interpret a proverb is used as a way of assessing

   A. judgment
   B. impulse control
   C. abstract thinking
   D. insight
   E. intelligence

8.5 Disturbances of attention include

   A. hypervigilance
   B. twilight state
   C. somnolence
   D. sundowning
   E. all of the above

8.6 Alexithymia is

   A. an unpleasant mood
   B. a loss of interest in and withdrawal from pleasurable activities
   C. an inability to describe or to be aware of emotions or mood
   D. a normal range of mood, implying absence of depressed or elevated emotional state
   E. a state in which a person is easily annoyed and provoked to anger

8.7 Physiological disturbances associated with mood include

   A. hyperphagia
   B. anorexia
   C. hypersomnia
   D. diurnal variation
   E. all of the above

8.8 Stereotypy is

   A. temporary loss of muscle tone and weakness precipitated by a variety of emotional states
   B. pathological imitation of movements of one person by another
   C. ingrained, habitual involuntary movement
   D. repetitive fixed pattern of physical action or speech
   E. subjective feeling of muscular tension and restlessness secondary to antipsychotic or other medication

8.9 Primary process thinking is

   A. a form of magical thinking
   B. similar to that of the preoperational phase in children
   C. normally found in dreams
   D. dereistic
   E. all of the above

DIRECTIONS: Each group of questions below consists of lettered headings followed by a list of numbered phrases or statements. For each numbered phrase or statement, select the *one* lettered heading that is most associated with it. Each lettered heading may be selected once, more than once, or not at all.

Questions 8.10–8.14

   A. Loosening of associations
   B. Flight of ideas
   C. Clang association
   D. Blocking
   E. Neologism

8.10 "I was gigglifying, not just tempifying; you know what I mean."
8.11 "I was grocery training; but, when I ride the grocery, I drive the food everywhere on top of lollipops."
8.12 "Cain and Abel—they were cannibals. You see brothers kill brothers—that is laudable. If you ask me, though, never name your son Huxtibal. OK."
8.13 Patient: "I never wanted." Physician: "Go on. What were you saying?" Patient: "I don't know."
8.14 "Tired, mired, schmired, wired."

Questions 8.15–8.18

   A. Broca's (motor) aphasia
   B. Sensory aphasia
   C. Nominal aphasia
   D. Global aphasia
   E. Syntactical aphasia

8.15 Difficulty in finding the correct names for objects
8.16 Loss of the ability to comprehend the meaning of words
8.17 Loss of the ability to speak
8.18 Inability to arrange words in a proper sequence

Questions 8.19–8.22

   A. Synesthesia
   B. Paramnesia
   C. Hypermnesia
   D. Eidetic images
   E. Lethologica

8.19 Exaggerated degree of retention and recall
8.20 Temporary inability to remember a name
8.21 Confusion of facts and fantasies
8.22 Sensations that accompany sensations of another modality

Questions 8.23–8.26

   A. Dysdiadochokinesia
   B. Astereognosis
   C. Visual agnosia
   D. Autotopagnosia
   E. Simultanagnosia

8.23 Inability to recognize a body part as one's own
8.24 Inability to distinguish by touch between a quarter and a dime
8.25 Inability to perform rapid alternating movements
8.26 Inability to recognize objects or people

Questions 8.27–8.30

   A. *Déjà vu*
   B. *Déjà entendu*
   C. *Déjà pensé*
   D. *Jamais vu*
   E. Confabulation

8.27 Illusion of auditory recognition
8.28 Regarding a new thought as a repetition of a previous thought
8.29 Feeling of unfamiliarity with a familiar situation
8.30 Regarding a new situation as a repetition of a previous experience

Questions 8.31–8.34

   A. Anxiety
   B. Ambivalence
   C. Guilt
   D. Abreaction

8.31 Coexistence of two opposing impulses
8.32 Emotional discharge after recalling a painful experience
8.33 Feeling of apprehension
8.34 Emotion resulting from doing something perceived as wrong

Questions 8.35–8.37

   A. Information variance
   B. Criterion variance
   C. Observation bias
   D. Validity

8.35 Discrepancies in psychiatric evaluation caused by differences in the patient's status or in information imparted by the patient from examination to examination
8.36 Discrepancies caused by differences in perceiving and interpreting the patient's responses to questions within the interview
8.37 Discrepancies caused by differences in the observer's definition of the symptoms or signs in question

Questions 8.38–8.42

   A. Narcolepsy
   B. Cataplexy
   C. Restless legs syndrome
   D. Klein-Levin syndrome
   E. Nocturnal myoclonus

8.38 Peculiar feelings during sleep, causing an irresistible need to move around
8.39 Periods of sleepiness, alternating with confusion, hunger, and sexual activity
8.40 Sudden attacks of generalized muscle weakness, leading to physical collapse while alert
8.41 Sudden attacks of irresistible sleepiness
8.42 Repetitive jerking of the legs during sleep, waking patients as well as their partners

Questions 8.43–8.47

   A. Capgras's syndrome
   B. Frégoli's phenomenon
   C. Clérambault's syndrome
   D. Delusion of doubles
   E. Delusional jealousy

8.43 Patients believe that another person has been physically transformed into themselves
8.44 Strangers are identified as familiar persons in the patient's life
8.45 False belief that someone (usually of higher status or authority) is erotically attached to the patient
8.46 Patient believes that someone close to him or her has been replaced by an exact double
8.47 False belief about a spouse's infidelity

Questions 8.48–8.50

   A. Registration
   B. Retention
   C. Recall

8.48 Capacity to return previously stored memories to consciousness
8.49 Capacity to add new material to memory
8.50 Capacity to hold memories in storage

Questions 8.51–8.55

   A. Haptic hallucinations
   B. Olfactory hallucinations
   C. Ictal hallucinations
   D. Autoscopic hallucinations
   E. Migrainous hallucinations

8.51 Most are simple visual hallucinations of geometric patterns, but phenomena such as micropsia and macropsia may occur
8.52 Hallucinations of one's own physical self
8.53 Involve the sense of smell and are most often associated with organic brain disease or psychotic depression
8.54 Occur as part of seizure activity, and are typically brief and stereotyped
8.55 Formication

Questions 8.56–8.60

    A. Ophidiophobia
    B. Triskaidekaphobia
    C. Acrophobia
    D. Amathophobia
    E. Gatophobia

8.56 Fear of heights
8.57 Fear of cats
8.58 Fear of the number 13
8.59 Fear of snakes
8.60 Fear of dust

Questions 8.61–8.64

    A. Cluster A
    B. Cluster B
    C. Cluster C

8.61 Borderline personality disorder
8.62 Paranoid personality disorder
8.63 Obsessive-compulsive personality disorder
8.64 Schizoid personality disorder

ANSWERS

Signs and Symptoms in Psychiatry

8.1 The answer is C

Tangentiality is the inability to have a goal-directed association of thoughts. The patient never gets from the desired point to the desired goal. *Word salad* is an incoherent mixture of words and phrases. *Circumstantiality* is indirect speech that is delayed in reaching the point but eventually gets there. Circumstantiality is characterized by an overinclusion of details and parenthetical remarks. *Verbigeration* is a meaningless repetition of specific words or phrases. *Blocking* is an abrupt interruption in the train of thinking before a thought or idea is finished. After a brief pause, the person indicates no recall of what was being said or what was going to be said. It is also known as thought deprivation.

8.2 The answer is D

Loss of normal speech melody is known as *dysprosody*. A disturbance in speech inflection and rhythm results in a monotonous and halting speech pattern, which occasionally suggests a foreign accent. It can be the result of a brain disease, such as Parkinson's disease, or it can be a psychological defensive mechanism (seen in some people with schizophrenia). As a psychological device, it can serve the function of maintaining a safe distance in social encounters.

Stuttering is a speech disorder characterized by repetitions or prolongations of sound syllables and words and by hesitations or pauses that disrupt the flow of speech. It is also known as *stammering*. *Aphonia* is a loss of one's voice. *Dyslexia* is a specific learning disability involving a reading impairment that is unrelated to the person's intelligence.

8.3 The answer is C

A disturbance in perception is a disturbance in the mental process by which data—intellectual, sensory, and emotional—are organized. Through perception, people are capable of making sense out of the many stimuli that bombard them. Perceptual disturbances do not include *echolalia,* which is the repetition of another's words or phrases. Echolalia is a disturbance of thought form and communication. Examples of perceptual disturbances are *hallucinations,* which are false sensory perceptions without concrete external stimuli. Common hallucinations involve sights or sounds, although any of the senses may be involved, and *hypnagogic experiences,* which are hallucinations that occur just before falling asleep. Other disturbances of perception include *depersonalization,* which is the sensation of unreality concerning oneself or one's environment,

and *derealization,* which is the feeling of changed reality or the feeling that one's surroundings have changed.

8.4 The answer is C

Asking a patient to interpret a proverb is generally used as a way of assessing whether the person has the capacity for abstract thought. *Abstract thinking*, as opposed to concrete thinking, is characterized primarily by the ability to shift voluntarily from one aspect of a situation to another, to keep in mind simultaneously various aspects of a situation, and to think symbolically. Concrete thinking is characterized by an inability to conceptualize beyond immediate experience or beyond actual things and events. Psychopathologically, it is most characteristic of persons with schizophrenia or organic brain disorders.

Judgment, the patient's ability to comprehend the meaning of events and to appreciate the consequences of actions, is often tested by asking how the patient would act in certain standard circumstances; for example, if the patient smelled smoke in a crowded movie theater. *Impulse control* is the ability to control acting on a wish to discharge energy in a manner that is, at the moment, felt to be dangerous, inappropriate, or otherwise ill-advised. *Insight* is a conscious understanding of forces that have led to a particular feeling, action, or situation. *Intelligence* is the capacity for learning, recalling, integrating, and applying knowledge and experience.

8.5 The answer is A

Attention is the amount of effort exerted in focusing on certain portions of an experience; ability to sustain a focus on one activity; and ability to concentrate. Examples of disturbances of attention include:

Hypervigilance: excessive attention and focus on all internal and external stimuli, usually secondary to delusional or paranoid states.
Selective inattention: blocking out only those things that generate anxiety.
Distractibility: inability to concentrate attention; state in which attention is drawn to unimportant or irrelevant external stimuli.
Trance: focused attention and altered consciousness, usually seen in hypnosis, dissociative disorders, and ecstatic religious experiences.

Apperception is perception modified by a person's own emotions and thoughts; sensorium is the state of cognitive functioning of the special senses (sometimes used as a synonym for consciousness); disturbances of consciousness are most often associated with brain pathology. Examples include:

Twilight state: disturbed consciousness with hallucinations.
Somnolence: abnormal drowsiness.
Sundowning: syndrome in older people that usually occurs at night and is characterized by drowsiness, confusion, ataxia, and falling as the result of being overly sedated with medications; also called sundowner's syndrome.

8.6 The answer is C

Mood is a pervasive and sustained emotion, subjectively experienced and reported by a patient and observed by others; examples include depression, elation, and anger. *Euthymic mood* is a normal range of mood, implying absence of depressed or elevated mood.

Irritable mood is a state in which a person is easily annoyed and provoked to anger.
Anhedonia is a loss of interest in and withdrawal from all regular and pleasurable activities, often associated with depression.
Alexithymia is a person's inability to describe, or difficulty in describing or being aware of, emotions or mood.

8.7 The answer is E (all)

Physiological disturbances associated with mood are signs of somatic (usually autonomic) dysfunction, most often associated with depression (also called vegetative signs). They include:

Anorexia: loss of or decrease in appetite.
Hyperphagia: increase in appetite and intake of food.
Insomnia: lack of or diminished ability to sleep.

   a. Initial: difficulty in falling asleep.
   b. Middle: difficulty in sleeping through the night without waking up and difficulty in going back to sleep.
   c. Terminal: early morning awakening.

Hypersomnia: excessive sleeping.
Diurnal variation: mood is regularly worse in the morning, immediately after awakening, and improves as the day progresses.
Diminished libido: decreased sexual interest, drive, and performance (increased libido is often associated with manic states).
Constipation: inability to defecate or difficulty in defecating.
Fatigue: a feeling of weariness, sleepiness, or irritability following a period of mental or bodily activity.
Pica: craving and eating of nonfood substances, such as paint and clay.
Pseudocyesis: rare condition in which a nonpregnant patient has the signs and symptoms of pregnancy.
Bulimia: insatiable hunger and voracious eating; seen in bulimia nervosa and atypical depression.

8.8 The answer is D

Motor behavior is that aspect of the psyche that includes impulses, motivations, wishes, drives, instincts, and cravings, as expressed by a person's behavior or motor activity.

Stereotypy is a *repetitive fixed pattern* of physical action or speech.
Echopraxia is a *pathological imitation* of movements of one person by another.

Cataplexy is *a temporary loss* of muscle tone and weakness precipitated by a variety of emotional states.
Mannerism is an *ingrained, habitual* involuntary movement.
Akathisia is *a subjective feeling of muscular tension* secondary to antipsychotic or other medication, which can cause *restlessness*, pacing, and repeated sitting and standing; can be mistaken for psychotic agitation.

8.9 The answer is E (all)

Thinking is the goal-directed flow of ideas, symbols, and associations initiated by a problem or task and leading toward a reality-oriented conclusion; when a logical sequence occurs, thinking is normal; parapraxis (an unconsciously motivated lapse from logic also called a freudian slip) is considered part of normal thinking. Disturbances in the form of process of thinking include dereism, a form of mental activity not concordant with logic or experience; *magical thinking*, a form of *dereistic thought*; thinking similar to that of the *preoperational phase in children* (Jean Piaget), in which thoughts, words, or actions assume power (for example, to cause or prevent events); and primary process thinking, which is a general term for thinking that is dereistic, illogical, magical and is normally found in *dreams*, abnormally in psychosis.

Answers 8.10–814

8.10 The answer is E

8.11 The answer is A

8.12 The answer is B

8.13 The answer is D

8.14 The answer is C

All the lettered responses are examples of specific disturbances in form of thought. *Neologisms* are new words created by the patient, often by combining syllables of other words, for idiosyncratic psychological reasons. *Loosening of associations* is a flow of thoughts in which ideas shift from one subject to another in completely unrelated ways. When the condition is severe, the patient's speech may be incoherent. *Flight of ideas* is a rapid, continuous verbalization or play on words that produces a constant shifting from one idea to another; the ideas tend to be connected, and when the condition is not severe, a listener may be able to follow them; the thought disorder is most characteristic of someone in a manic state. *Blocking* is an abrupt interruption in a train of thinking before a thought or idea is finished; after a brief pause, the person indicates no recall of what was being said or what was going to be said. The condition is also known as thought deprivation. A person who is using *clang association* uses an association of words similar in sound but not in meaning; the words used have no logical connections and may include examples of rhyming and punning.

Answers 8.15–8.18

8.15 The answer is C

8.16 The answer is B

8.17 The answer is A

8.18 The answer is E

Nominal aphasia, also known as anomia, is *difficulty in finding the correct names for objects.* A person who experiences an organic *loss of the ability to comprehend the meaning of words* suffers from *sensory aphasia;* speech is fluid and spontaneous but incoherent and nonsensical. A person who retains language comprehension but who suffers the *loss of the ability to speak* has *Broca's (motor) aphasia;* speech is halting, laborious, and inaccurate. *Syntactical aphasia* is the *inability to arrange words in a proper sequence. Global aphasia* is a combination of a grossly nonfluent aphasia and a severe fluent aphasia; the person has difficulty in both the comprehension and the production of language.

Answers 8.19–8.22

8.19 The answer is C

8.20 The answer is E

8.21 The answer is B

8.22 The answer is A

In *synesthesia* the patient experiences *sensations that accompany sensations of another modality;* for example, an auditory sensation is accompanied by or triggers a visual sensation, or a sound is experienced as being seen or accompanied by a visual experience. *Paramnesia* is a *confusion of facts and fantasies;* it leads to a falsification of memory with the distortion of real events by fantasies. *Hypermnesia* is an *exaggerated degree of retention and recall* or an ability to remember material that ordinarily is not retrievable. *Eidetic images,* also known as primary memory images, are *visual memories* of almost hallucinatory vividness. *Lethologica* is the *temporary inability to remember a name* or a proper noun.

Answers 8.23–8.26

8.23 The answer is D

8.24 The answer is B

8.25 The answer is A

8.26 The answer is C

The lettered responses are examples of cognitive disorders. *Autotopagnosia* is the *inability to recognize a body part as one's own;* it is also known as somatopagnosia. *Astereognosis* is the *inability to distinguish objects by touch,* such as a quarter and a dime. *Dysdiadochokinesia* is the *inability to perform rapid alternating movements;* it is usually a cerebellar dysfunction. *Visual agnosia* is the *inability to recognize objects or persons. Simultanagnosia* is the *inability to comprehend* more than one element of a *visual scene* at a time or to integrate the parts into a whole.

Answers 8.27–8.30

8.27 The answer is B

8.28 The answer is C

8.29 The answer is D

8.30 The answer is A

Déjà vu is *regarding a new situation as a repetition of a previous experience. Déjà entendu* is an *illusion of auditory recogni-* tion. *Déjà pensé* is *regarding a new thought as a repetition of a previous thought. Jamais vu* is a *feeling of unfamiliarity with a familiar situation. Confabulation* is the *unconscious filling in of memory* by imagining experiences that have no basis in fact.

Answers 8.31–8.34

8.31 The answer is B

8.32 The answer is D

8.33 The answer is A

8.34 The answer is C

Anxiety is a *feeling of apprehension* caused by anticipation of danger, which may be internal or external. *Ambivalence* is the *coexistence of two opposing impulses* toward the same thing in the same person at the same time. *Guilt* is an *emotion resulting from doing something perceived as wrong. Abreaction* is an *emotional discharge after recalling a painful experience.*

Answers 8.35–8.37

8.35 The answer is A

8.36 The answer is C

8.37 The answer is B

Among the core difficulties in psychiatric evaluation has been that multiple observers may note different symptoms or interpret signs differently when interviewing the same patient. *These discrepancies may be caused by differences in the patient's status or in* information imparted by the patient from examination to examination, in the *observers' definitions of the symptoms or signs* in question, and *differences in perceiving and interpreting the patient's responses* to general presentation or *questions within* the interview. These three types of reliability problems are called *information variance, criterion variance,* and *observation bias.*

Although good interrater reliability can be achieved for most symptoms of Axis I disorders, this may not hold true for personality disorders or for some specific symptoms. Furthermore, good interrater reliability may occur consistently only under optimal circumstances and may not be as common in clinical practice.

Even when simply responding to direct questions about symptoms, patients may answer differently depending on the interviewer's manner, how the questions are asked, their personal sense of trust or safety, whether they have answered these questions before, the amount of cuing that may signal the desired response, fatigue, or a host of other variables.

Most clinicians still rely heavily on their own clinical intuition and subjective responses to patients as part of a diagnostic assessment. Unfortunately, whether accurate or not, these clinical judgments are often based on unconscious assumptions, comparisons with other patients not well remembered, or distortions based on the clinician's own personal experiences. When the basis for these intuitions can be identified and described clearly, they may prove to be reliable and valid. However, intuitions are often wrong—simple trust in intuition alone is not sufficient. Thus, a clinician's sense that a patient is angry and potentially violent may result from the patient's subtle (but verifiable) body language and tone of voice—or it may represent a countertransference distortion that is not prompted by any observable patient behavior.

Often, clinicians too quickly label behaviors as inappropriate when they fail to appreciate and understand contextual or cultural considerations. Appropriateness depends heavily on context, and definitions of what is proper in a given context may also be highly subjective. Appropriate behavior or clothing in some parts of California may be inappropriate in Boston. A low intensity of emotional expression leading to a clinical description of "constricted affect" may reflect cultural norms or a psychopathological state.

Validity reflects that a designated disorder is actually what is described.

Answers 8.38–8.42

8.38 The answer is C

8.39 The answer is D

8.40 The answer is B

8.41 The answer is A

8.42 The answer is E
In *narcolepsy*, the patient has *sudden attacks of irresistible sleepiness,* a symptom that may be part of a broader syndrome that includes *cataplexy* (*sudden attacks of generalized muscle weakness leading to physical collapse* in the presence of alert consciousness).

Periodic hypersomnia occurs in the *Klein-Levin syndrome,* a condition that typically affects young men, in which *periods of sleepiness alternate with confusional states, ravenous hunger, and protracted sexual activity.*

Sensory symptoms during sleep, typically described by patients as peculiar feelings in their *legs, causing an irresistible need to move* around, are characteristic of *restless legs syndrome.* The motor abnormality of *repetitive myoclonic jerking of the legs, awakening both patients and their partners,* is known as *nocturnal myoclonus.*

Answers 8.43–8.47

8.43 The answer is D

8.44 The answer is B

8.45 The answer is C

8.46 The answer is A

8.47 The answer is E
Delusions are fixed, false beliefs, strongly held and immutable in the face of refuting evidence, that are not consonant with the person's education, social, and cultural background.

Delusions of misidentification are prominently reported because of their inherently intriguing nature. In *Capgras's syndrome,* the patient believes that someone close to him has been replaced by an exact double. In *Frégoli's phenomenon, strangers are identified as familiar persons in the patient's life.* In the *delusion of doubles, patients believe that another person has been physically transformed into themselves.* In *Clérambault's syndrome,* patients believe that a person is erotically attached to them, when in fact they are not. *Delusional jealousy* is a false belief about a spouse's infidelity.

Answers 8.48–8.50

8.48 The answer is C

8.49 The answer is A

8.50 The answer is B
Memory functions have been divided into three stages: registration, retention, and recall. *Registration or acquisition refers to the capacity to add new material to memory.* The material may be sensory, perceptual, or conceptual and may come from the environment or from within the person. In order for new material to be acquired, the person must attend to the information presented; it must then be processed or cortically organized. *Retention* is the *ability to hold memories in storage.* Large numbers of neurons are thought to be involved in the storage of a specific memory, and it is believed that reverberating circuits are formed in which memory traces are held by means of changes in proteins or synaptic connectivity, or both. *Recall is the capacity to return previously stored memories to consciousness.*

Registration and short-term memory retention are usually impaired in disorders that affect vigilance and attention, such as head trauma, delirium, intoxication, psychosis, spontaneous or induced seizures, anxiety, depression, and fatigue. A variety of other metabolic and structural brain disturbances can affect short-term memory as well, particularly lesions affecting the mammillary bodies, hippocampus, fornix, and closely associated areas. Patients with impaired attention and concentration who are able to demonstrate immediate recall may not be able to retain or recollect these items from short-term memory. Benzodiazepine use has been associated with working memory difficulties, especially in the elderly. Some short-acting high-potency benzodiazepines used as sleeping pills may be particularly troublesome in this regard.

The retention of memories is impaired in posttraumatic amnesia as well as in a number of cognitive disorders, such as dementia of the Alzheimer's type and the Wernicke-Korsakoff syndrome. The latter, which ordinarily results from the chronic thiamine deficiency seen with alcoholism, is associated with pathological alterations in the mammillary bodies and thalamus.

Disturbances in recall can occur even when memories have been registered and are in storage. Research has shown that memories are not passively retrieved but are actively reconstructed. Each act of recollection requires an act of putting the memory together, not simply lifting it ready made from a file. Because memories are often retrieved for specific purposes to meet the individual's particular needs and agendas, this act of reconstruction is often subject to the introduction of distortions and falsification. As a result, memories may fail to truly represent past events. At times, failure to recall may signify that the memory traces themselves have disappeared and are no longer retrievable. However, difficulties in recall can occur separately, as in the everyday event of forgetting the name of a person or object, only to spontaneously remember it hours or days later.

Answers 8.51–8.55

8.51 The answer is E

8.52 The answer is D

8.53 The answer is B

8.54 The answer is C

8.55 The answer is A

Hallucinations are perceptions that occur in the absence of corresponding sensory stimuli. Phenomenologically, hallucinations are ordinarily subjectively indistinguishable from normal perceptions. Hallucinations are often experienced as being private, so that others are not able to see or hear the same perceptions. The patient's explanation for this is typically delusional. Hallucinations can affect any sensory system and sometimes occur in several concurrently.

Autoscopic hallucinations are *hallucinations of one's own physical self.* Such hallucinations may stimulate the delusion that one has a double (*Doppelgänger*). Reports of near-death out-of-body experiences in which individuals see themselves rising to the ceiling and looking down at themselves in a hospital bed may be autoscopic hallucinations. In *Lilliputian hallucinations,* the individual sees figures in very reduced size, like midgets or dwarfs. They may be related to the perceptual distortions of *macropsia* and *micropsia,* respectively, the perceptions of objects as much bigger or smaller than they actually are.

Haptic hallucinations involve touch. Simple haptic hallucinations, such as the feeling that *bugs are crawling over one's skin (formication)* are common in alcohol withdrawal syndromes and in cocaine intoxication. When unkempt and physically neglectful patients complain of these sensations, they may be caused by the presence of real physical stimuli such as lice. Some tactile hallucinations, having sexual intercourse with God, for example, are highly suggestive of schizophrenia, but may also occur in tertiary syphilis and other conditions, and may in fact be stimulated by local genital irritation. *Olfactory* and gustatory *hallucinations, involving smell and taste* respectively, have most often been associated with organic brain disease, particularly with the uncinate fits of complex partial seizures. Olfactory hallucinations may also be seen in psychotic depression, typically as odors of decay, rotting, or death.

Ictal hallucinations, occurring as *part of seizure activity,* are typically brief, lasting only seconds to minutes, and stereotyped. They may be simple images—such as flashes of light—or elaborate ones, such as visual recollections of past experiences. During the hallucinations the patient ordinarily experiences altered consciousness or a twilight sleep.

Migrainous hallucinations are reported by about 50 percent of patients with migraines. Most are simple *visual hallucinations of geometric patterns, but fully formed visual hallucinations, sometimes with micropsia and macropsia,* may also occur. This complex has been called the *Alice in Wonderland syndrome* after Lewis Carroll's descriptions of the world in *Through the Looking Glass,* which mirrored some of his own migrainous experiences. In turn, these phenomena closely resemble visual hallucinations induced by psychedelic drugs such as mescaline.

Answers 8.56–8.60

8.56 The answer is C

8.57 The answer is E

8.58 The answer is B

8.59 The answer is A

8.60 The answer is D

Phobias are irrational fears. In an effort to reduce the intense anxiety attached to phobic objects and situations, patients do their best to avoid the feared stimuli. Thus, phobias consist both of the fears and the avoidance components. The fear itself may include all the symptoms of extreme anxiety, up to and including panic. In *specific phobias,* persistent, irrational fears are provoked by specific stimuli. Table 8.1 lists some illustrative phobias. Common specific phobias include *fear of dust,* excreta, *snakes,* spiders, *heights,* and blood.

Answers 8.61–8.64

8.61 The answer is B

8.62 The answer is A

8.63 The answer is C

8.64 The answer is A

DSM-IV-TR uses a categorical approach to personality. The large overlap among the DSM personality disorders and the clustering of these personality disorders into three broad groups

Table 8.1
Specific Phobias

Acrophobia	Fear of heights
Agoraphobia	Fear of open spaces
Amathophobia	Fear of dust
Apiphobia	Fear of bees
Astrapophobia	Fear of lightning
Blennophobia	Fear of slime
Claustrophobia	Fear of enclosed spaces
Cynophobia	Fear of dogs
Decidophobia	Fear of making decisions
Electrophobia	Fear of electricity
Eremophobia	Fear of being alone
Gamophobia	Fear of marriage
Gatophobia	Fear of cats
Gephyrophobia	Fear of crossing bridges
Gynophobia	Fear of women
Hydrophobia	Fear of water
Kakorrhaphiophobia	Fear of failure
Katagelophobia	Fear of ridicule
Keraunophobia	Fear of thunder
Musophobia	Fear of mice
Nyctophobia	Fear of night
Ochlophobia	Fear of crowds
Odynophobia	Fear of pain
Ophidiophobia	Fear of snakes
Pnigerophobia	Fear of smothering
Pyrophobia	Fear of fire
Scholionophobia	Fear of school
Sciophobia	Fear of shadows
Spheksophobia	Fear of wasps
Technophobia	Fear of technology
Thalassophobia	Fear of the ocean
Triskaidekaphobia	Fear of number 13
Tropophobia	Fear of moving or making changes

imply a lack of clear boundaries to the currently defined categories. The three DSM-IV-TR clusters describe odd or eccentric types (*Cluster A*); dramatic, emotional, and erratic types (*Cluster B*); and anxious and fearful types (*Cluster C*).

The odd or eccentric group includes *paranoid, schizoid,* and schizotypal personality disorders. Patients with these personality disorders have the core traits of being interpersonally distant and emotionally constricted. People with paranoid personality disorder are quick to feel slighted and jealous, carry grudges, and expect to be exploited and harmed by others. People with schizoid personality disorder lack friendships or close relationships with others and are indifferent to praise or criticism by others. People with schizotypal personality disorder display odd beliefs, engage in odd and eccentric gestures and practices, and exhibit odd speech.

The dramatic, emotional, and erratic group includes *borderline,* histrionic, narcissistic, and antisocial personality disorders. Patients with these personality disorders characteristically have chaotic lives, emotions, and relationships. People with borderline personality disorder are impulsive, unpredictable, angry, temperamental, unstable in relationships, compulsively interpersonal, and self-damaging with regard to sex, money, and substance use. People with histrionic personality disorder are attention-seeking, exhibitionistic, seductive, and self-indulgent; exhibit exaggerated expressions of emotions; and are overconcerned with physical appearance. People with narcissistic personality disorder tend to be hypersensitive to criticism,

exploitative of others, egocentric with an inflated sense of self-importance, feel entitled to special treatment, and demand constant attention. People with antisocial personality disorder are described almost exclusively in behavioral rather than affective or relational terms. They commit truancy, lie, steal, start fights, break rules, are unable to sustain work or school, and shirk day-to-day responsibilities.

The anxious and fearful group includes patients with avoidant, dependent, and *obsessive-compulsive* personality disorders. Patients with these disorders are characterized by constricting behaviors that serve to limit risks. People with avoidant personality disorder avoid relationships, people with dependent personality disorder avoid being responsible for decisions, and people with obsessive-compulsive personality disorder use rigid rules that preclude new behaviors. People with avoidant personality disorders are hypersensitive to rejection and are reluctant to enter close relationships in spite of strong desires for affection. Those with dependent personality disorders show excessive reliance on others to make major life decisions, stay trapped in abusive relationships for fear of being alone, have difficulty initiating projects on their own, and constantly seek reassurance and praise. Individuals with obsessive-compulsive personality disorders exhibit restricted expressions of warmth, tenderness, and generosity, and also exhibit stubbornness with a need to be right and to control decisions; indecisive at times, they often apply rules and morals too rigidly, to the point of being inflexible.

9

Classification in Psychiatry and Psychiatric Rating Scales

The revised fourth edition of *Diagnostic and Statistical Manual of Mental Disorders, Text Revision* (DSM-IV-TR) and the tenth revision of *International Statistical Classification of Diseases and Related Health Problems* (ICD-10), are the two official classification systems used in psychiatry. ICD-10 was published by the World Health Organization in 1992 and is used in Europe. Although similar, the two systems are not identical. DSM was first published in 1952 by the American Psychiatric Association. The most recent edition (DSM-IV-TR) was published in 2000. Both systems aim to increase the use of a standard language in describing diagnoses and defining data specific to different disorders.

While this common vocabulary has greatly improved the ability of clinicians to speak the same language with each other (to know that when they use, for instance, the term schizophrenia they are speaking of the same entity), it can be badly misused in incompetent hands. DSM-IV-TR is not a cookbook, and human behavior and thought cannot be reduced to simplistic prescriptions. A meaningful classification system is meant to be used as a rigorous guideline, a framework in which to begin to define often baffling and complicated syndromes, but it is also meant to be understood as an approximation. No one person is simply the compilation of a particular set of signs and symptoms.

The student should study the questions and answers below for a useful review of these topics.

HELPFUL HINTS

The student should be able to define the terms below, especially the diagnostic categories.

- age of onset
- agoraphobia
- alcohol delirium
- amnestic disorders
- associated and essential features
- atheoretical
- bipolar I disorder
- body dysmorphic disorder
- classification
- clinical syndromes
- cognitive disorders
- competence
- complications
- conversion disorder
- course
- delusional disorder
- dementia precox
- depersonalization disorder

- depressive disorders
- descriptive approach
- diagnostic criteria
- differential diagnosis
- disability determination
- dissociative disorders
- dissociative fugue
- dissociative identity disorder
- DSM-IV-TR
- dysthymic disorder
- ego-dystonic and ego-syntonic
- familial pattern
- general medical conditions
- generalized anxiety disorder
- Global Assessment of Functioning Scale

- gross social norms
- highest level of functioning
- hypochondriasis
- ICD-10
- impairment
- Emil Kraepelin
- mood disorders
- multiaxial system
- obsessive-compulsive disorder
- panic disorder
- paraphilias
- partial and full remission
- personality disorders
- pervasive developmental disorders
- phobias
- posttraumatic stress disorder

- predictive validity
- predisposing factors
- premenstrual dysphoric disorder
- prevalence
- psychological factors affecting medical condition
- psychosis
- psychosocial and environmental stressors
- reality testing
- residual type
- schizophrenia
- severity-of-stress rating
- sex ratio
- sexual dysfunctions
- somatization disorder
- somatoform disorders
- validity and reliability

▲ QUESTIONS

DIRECTIONS: Each of the incomplete statements below is followed by five suggested completions. Select the *one* that is *best* in each case.

9.1 The term neurosis

    A. is not found in DSM-IV-TR, but it is still found in ICD-10

    B. encompasses a narrow range of disorders with very specific and easily definable signs and symptoms

    C. signifies that gross reality testing may not be intact

    D. is now defined as disorders characterized mainly by depression

    E. refers to a disturbance limited to a transitory reaction to stressors

9.2 DSM-IV-TR

    A. uses the term disorders because most of the entities lack the features necessary to warrant the term disease

    B. never specifies cause

    C. officially employs the term psychopathy as a disorder

    D. is not compatible with ICD-10

    E. none of the above

9.3 DSM-IV-TR

    A. strives to be neutral or atheoretical with regard to etiology

    B. provides specific diagnostic criteria that tend to increase the reliability of clinicians

    C. makes no mention of management or treatment

    D. provides explicit rules to be used in making a diagnosis when the clinical information is insufficient

    E. all of the above

9.4 The Global Assessment of Functioning scale (GAF)

    A. is recorded on Axis IV

    B. is a 50-point scale, with 50 representing the highest level of functioning

    C. evaluates impairment in functioning due to physical or environmental limitation

    D. conceptualizes functioning as a composite of two major areas: social and occupational functioning

    E. none of the above

9.5 The Social and Occupational Functioning Assessment Scale (SOFAS)

    A. is scored independently of the person's psychological symptoms

    B. does not include impairment in functioning that is caused by a general medical condition

    C. may not be used to rate functioning at the time of the evaluation

    D. may not be used to rate functioning of a past period

    E. is included on Axis III

9.6 True statements about DSM-IV-TR include

    A. Axis I and Axis II comprise the entire classification of mental disorders.

    B. Many patients have one or more disorders on both Axis I and Axis II.

    C. The habitual use of a particular defense mechanism can be indicated on Axis II.

    D. On Axis III, the identified physical condition may be causative, interactive, and effect, or unrelated to the mental state.

    E. All of the above

9.7 Dementia in Alzheimer's disease may be characterized by each of the following terms *except*

    A. mixed type

    B. atypical type

    C. of acute onset

    D. with late onset

    E. with early onset

DIRECTIONS: Each set of lettered headings below is followed by a list of numbered phrases or statements. For each numbered phrase or statement select the *one* lettered heading that is most closely associated with it. Each lettered heading may be selected once, more than once, or not at all.

Questions 9.8–9.13

    A. Axis I

    B. Axis II

    C. Axis III

    D. Axis IV

    E. Axis V

9.8 Alcohol abuse

9.9 Threat of job loss

9.10 Frequent use of denial

9.11 Mood disorder due to hypothyroidism, with depressive features

9.12 GAF = 45 (on admission), GAF = 65 (at discharge)

9.13 Mental retardation

Questions 9.14–9.17

    A. Brief Psychiatric Rating Scale

    B. Hamilton Rating Scale

    C. Yale-Brown Scale

    D. Social and Occupational Functioning Assessment Scale

    E. None of the above

9.14 Obsessive-compulsive symptoms

9.15 Psychotic disorders

9.16 Depression and anxiety

9.17 Abnormal involuntary movements

ANSWERS

Classification in Psychiatry and Psychiatric Rating Scales

9.1 The answer is A

The term *neurosis* is now defined as a chronic or recurrent non-psychotic disorder, characterized mainly by anxiety that is experienced or expressed directly, or is altered through defense mechanisms. It appears as a symptom, such as an obsession, a compulsion, a phobia, or a sexual dysfunction. *Although not used in DSM-IV-TR, the term is still found in ICD-10.*

DSM-III redefined *neurotic disorder* as a mental disorder in which the predominant disturbance is a symptom or group of symptoms that is distressing to the individual and is recognized by him or her as unacceptable and alien (ego-dystonic); reality testing is grossly intact. Behavior does not actively violate gross social norms although it may be quite disabling. The disturbance is relatively enduring or recurrent without treatment, and it is *not limited to a transitory reaction to stressors.*

In ICD-10, a class called "neurotic, stress-related, and somatoform disorders" encompasses the following: phobic anxiety disorders, other anxiety disorders (including panic disorder, generalized anxiety disorder, and mixed anxiety and *depressive disorder*), obsessive-compulsive disorder, adjustment disorders, dissociative (conversion) disorders, and somatoform disorders. ICD-10 also includes neurasthenia as a neurotic disorder characterized by mental and physical fatigability, a sense of general instability, irritability, anhedonia, and sleep disturbances. Many cases diagnosed as neuroses outside the United States fit the descriptions of anxiety disorders as defined by American psychiatrists.

There are no diagnoses called "neuroses" in DSM-IV-TR. For those who still adhere to the term, *neurosis encompasses a broad range of disorders* with various signs and symptoms. Beyond *signifying that gross reality testing is intact*, neurosis has lost the precision currently necessary for a diagnostic category. In terms of an individual's functioning, it can reflect an intermediate level of impairment in a number of areas.

9.2 The answer is A

As with DSM-I and -II, the development of DSM-III was coordinated with the development of the ninth revision of *International Statistical Classification of Diseases and Related Health Problems* (ICD-9) and published in 1980 by the APA. It represented a return to a descriptive system of diagnosis based on explicit operational diagnostic criteria, theoretically neutral, and multiaxial in format. The revised third edition of DSM (DSM-III-R) (1987) and DSM-IV-TR (1994) along with DSM-IV-TR (2000) refined the diagnostic categories based on available empirical data, and proceeded to make the current diagnostic system compatible with that of the latest revision of *International Statistical Classification of Diseases and Related Health Problems (ICD-10)* system.

As late as the end of the 19th century, the adjective *psychopathic* meant psychopathological and applied to any form of mental disorder. However, Koch, Gross, Morel, and others were narrowing the concept to apply to less severe forms of pathology that would eventually evolve into the contemporary concepts of personality disorders.

Psychopathic personality became a subclass of the larger group of abnormal personalities. In the conceptualization of discordant adaptation, Eugen Khan used the term psychopathic to designate these conditions as complex states that lay intermediately between mental health and illness. Although Sigmund Freud was less interested in the issue, other psychodynamic and psychoanalytic writers like Daniel Stern and Wilhelm Reich contributed significantly to the understanding of character pathology. Carl Gustav Jung reinvigorated views of personality by shifting the focus away from archaic views of stereotyped behavioral forms to the contemporary perspective of combinations of dimensions and typologies. Erne Kretschmer proposed typology based on biological speculation that followed Kraepelin's approach to the psychoses. These perspectives led incrementally to the current concepts of personality disorder that, like the current nosological paradigm, are primarily descriptive and directed towards neurobiological explanatory hypotheses. Although *psychopathy* does not appear in the current official nosology, a residue of the concept is retained in DSM-IV-TR's antisocial personality disorder and ICD-10's dissocial personality disorder.

The official diagnostic nomenclature in *DSM-IV-TR uses the term disorder because most of the entities lack the features necessary to warrant the term disease. Cause is not specified* except for cases of posttraumatic stress disorder, mental disorders due to a general medical condition, and substance-induced mental disorders. Other than some of the dementias, even these disorders lack a specified mechanism; most psychiatric illnesses and many medical illnesses are not diseases in the strict sense of the word.

9.3 The answer is E (all)

DSM-IV-TR is the current classification of mental disorders; it is used by mental health professionals of all disciplines and is cited in insurance reimbursement, disability deliberations, statistical determinations, and forensic matters. Although there has been substantial criticism of each consecutive version of the DSM, DSM-IV-TR is the official nomenclature and is used throughout this textbook.

Specified diagnostic criteria are provided for each mental disorder. Those criteria include a list of features and, in most cases, how many must be present for the diagnosis to be made. The use of specific criteria *tends to increase the reliability of the diagnostic process among clinicians.*

DSM-IV-TR also systematically describes each disorder in terms of its associated features: specific age-, culture-, and gender-related aspects; prevalence, incidence, and predisposing factors; course; complications; familial pattern; and differential diagnosis. In cases where many of the specific disorders share common features, that information is included in the introduction to the entire section. Laboratory findings and associated physical examination signs and symptoms are described when relevant. DSM-IV-TR explicitly states that it is not a textbook. *No mention is made of causal theories, management, or treatment*; nor are the controversial issues surrounding particular diagnostic categories discussed.

DSM-IV-TR provides explicit rules to be used when the information is insufficient (diagnosis to be deferred or provisional), or the patient's clinical presentation and history do not meet the required criteria of a prototypical category (atypical type, residual, or not otherwise specified).

9.4 The answer is E (none of the above)

Axis V is the *Global Assessment of Functioning (GAF) scale* with which the clinician judges the patient's overall level of functioning during a particular time period (e.g., the patient's level of functioning at evaluation or the patient's highest level of functioning for at least a few months during the past year). Functioning is conceptualized as a composite of three major areas: social functioning, occupational functioning, and psychological functioning. The GAF scale, based on a continuum of severity, is a 100-point scale with 100 representing the highest level of functioning in all areas.

The GAF does not include functional impairment due to physical or environmental limitations.

9.5 The answer is A

The *Social and Occupational Functioning Assessment Scale (SOFAS)* (Table 9.1) is a new scale included in a DSM-IV-TR appendix. The scale differs from the Global Assessment of Functioning (GAF) Scale in that it focuses only on the per-

son's level of social and occupational functioning. It is scored independent of the severity of the person's psychological symptoms. And, unlike the GAF scale, the SOFAS may include *impairment in functioning* that is caused by a general *medical condition.* The SOFAS may be used to rate functioning at the time of the evaluation, or *it may be used to rate functioning of a past period.* The SOFAS is included on Axis V, not Axis III.

9.6 The answer is E (all)

DSM-IV-TR is a multiaxial system that comprises five axes and evaluates the patient along each. *Axis I and Axis II comprise the entire classification of mental disorders:* 17 major groupings, more than 300 specific disorders, and almost 400 categories. In many instances the patient has *one or more disorders on both Axes I and II.* For example, a patient may have major depressive disorder noted on Axis I and borderline and narcissistic personality disorders on Axis II. In general, multiple diagnoses on each axis are encouraged.

Axis II consists of personality disorders and mental retardation. The *habitual use of a particular defense mechanism can be indicated on Axis II.*

Axis III lists any physical disorder or general medical condition that is present in addition to the mental disorder. The *identified physical condition may be causative* (e.g., hepatic failure causing

Table 9.1
Social and Occupational Functioning Assessment Scale (SOFAS)

Consider social and occupational functioning on a continuum from excellent functioning to grossly impaired functioning. Include impairments in functioning due to physical limitations, as well as those due to mental impairments. To be counted, impairment must be a direct consequence of mental and physical health problems; the effects of lack of opportunity and other environmental limitations are not to be considered.

Code (**Note:** Use intermediate codes when appropriate, e.g., 45, 68, 72.)

Code		Code	
100	Superior functioning in a wide range of activities.	50	Serious impairment in social, occupational, or school functioning (e.g., no friends, unable to keep a job).
91		41	
90	Good functioning in all areas, occupationally and socially effective.	40	Major impairment in several areas, such as work or school, family relations (e.g., depressed man avoids friends, neglects family, and is unable to work; child frequently beats up younger children, is defiant at home, and is failing at school).
81		31	
80	No more than a slight impairment in social, occupational, or school functioning (e.g., infrequent interpersonal conflict, temporarily falling behind in schoolwork).	30	Inability to function in almost all areas (e.g., stays in bed all day; no job, home, or friends).
71			
70	Some difficulty in social, occupational, or school functioning, but generally functioning well, has some meaningful interpersonal relationships.	21	
61		20	Occasionally fails to maintain minimal personal hygiene; unable to function independently.
60	Moderate difficulty in social, occupational, or school functioning (e.g., few friends, conflicts with peers or coworkers).	11	
51		10	Persistent inability to maintain minimal personal hygiene. Unable to function without harming self or others or without considerable external support (e.g., nursing care and supervision).
		1	
		0	Inadequate information.

Note: The rating of overall psychological functioning on a scale of 0–100 was operationalized by Luborsky in the Health-Sickness Rating Scale. Luborsky L. Clinicians' judgments of mental health. *Arch Gen Psychiatry.* 1962;7:407. Spitzer and colleagues developed a revision of the Health-Sickness Rating Scale called the Global Assessment Scale (GAS) (Endicott J, Spitzer RL, Fleiss JL, et al. The Global Assessment Scale: a procedure for measuring overall severity of psychiatric disturbance. *Arch Gen Psychiatry.* 1976;33:766). The SOFAS is derived from the GAS and its development is described in Goldman HH, Skodol AE, Lave TR. Revising Axis V for DSM-IV: a review of measures of social functioning. *Am J Psychiatry.* 1992;149:1148. Reprinted with permission from American Psychiatric Association. *Diagnostic and Statistical Manual of Mental Disorders.* 4th ed. Text rev. Washington, DC: American Psychiatric Association; copyright 2000.

delirium), interactive (e.g., gastritis secondary to alcohol dependence), and effect (e.g., dementia and human immunodeficiency virus [HIV]–related pneumonia), or unrelated to the mental disorder. When a medical condition is causally related to a mental disorder, a mental disorder due to a general condition is listed on Axis I and the general medical condition is listed on both Axes I and III.

9.7 The answer is C

Acute onset refers to vascular dementia, not to dementia in Alzheimer's disease, which has a slow onset. The other four types—*mixed, atypical, with late onset,* and *with early onset*— all refer to dementia in Alzheimer's disease.

Answers 9.8–9.13

9.8   The answer is A

9.9   The answer is D

9.10 The answer is B

9.11 The answer is C

9.12 The answer is E

9.13 The answer is B

DSM-IV-TR uses a multiaxial scheme of classification consisting of five axes, each of which covers a different aspect of functioning. Each axis should be covered for each diagnosis. *Axis I* consists of all clinical syndromes as well as other conditions that may be a focus of clinical syndromes and other conditions that may be a focus of clinical attention. Examples include schizophrenia, mood disorders, and *alcohol abuse. Axis II* consists of personality disorders, *mental retardation,* and *frequent use of a defense mechanism such as denial. Axis III* consists of general medical conditions. The condition may be causative (for example, hypothyroidism causing depression), secondary (e.g., acquired immune deficiency syndrome [AIDS] as a result of a substance-related disorder), or unrelated. *Axis IV* consists of psychosocial and environmental problems that are related to the current mental disorder. Examples include divorce, *threat of job loss,* and inadequate health insurance. *Axis V* is a global assessment in which the clinician evaluates the highest level of functioning by the patient in the past year. The *Global Assessment of Functioning (GAF) Scale* is a 100-point scale, with 100 representing the highest level of functioning in all areas.

Answers 9.14–9.17

9.14 The answer is C

9.15 The answer is A

9.16 The answer is B

9.17 The answer is E

Psychiatric rating scales, also called rating instruments, provide a way to quantify aspects of a patient's psyche, behavior, and relationships with individuals and society. The measurement of

pathology in these areas of a person's life may initially seem to be less straightforward than is the measurement of pathology—hypertension, for example—by other medical specialists. Nevertheless, many psychiatric rating scales are able to measure carefully chosen features of well-formulated concepts. Moreover, psychiatrists who do not use these rating scales are left with only their clinical impressions, which are difficult to record in a manner that allows for reliable future comparison and communication. Without psychiatric rating scales, quantitative data in psychiatry are crude (for example, length of hospitalization or other treatment, discharge and readmission to hospital, length of relationships or employment, and presence of legal troubles).

Rating scales can be specific or comprehensive, and they can measure both internally experienced variables (e.g., mood) and externally observable variables (e.g., behavior). Specific scales measure discrete thoughts, moods, or behaviors, such as *obsessive thoughts* and temper tantrums; comprehensive scales measure broad abstractions, such as *depression* and anxiety. Well-known rating scales include the Hamilton Rating Scale for depression and anxiety and the Yale-Brown Scale for obsessive-compulsive symptoms.

Classic items from the mental status examination are the most frequently assessed items on rating scales. These items include *thought disorders, mood disturbances,* and gross behaviors (i.e., the Brief Psychiatric Rating Scale). Another type of information covered by rating scales is the assessment of adverse effects from psychotherapeutic drugs. *Social adjustments* (e.g., *occupational success* and quality of relationships with the SOFAS) and psychoanalytic concepts (e.g., ego strength and defense mechanisms) are also measured by some rating scales, although the reliability and the validity of such scales are lowered by the absence of agreed-on norms, the high level of inference required on some items, and the lack of independence between measures.

Other characteristics of rating scales include the time covered, the level of judgment required, and the method of recording answers. The time covered by a rating scale must be specified, and the rate must adhere to this period. For example, a particular rating scale may rate a 5-minute observation period, a week-long period, or a patient's entire life.

The most reliable rating scales require a limited amount of judgment or inference on the part of the rater. Whatever the level of judgment required, clear definitions of the answer scale, preferably with clinical examples, should be provided by the developer of the scale and should be read by the rater.

The actual answer given may be recorded as either a dichotomous variable (for example, true or false, present or absent) or a continuous variable. Continuous items may ask the rater to choose a term to describe severity (absent, slight, mild, moderate, severe, or extreme) or frequency (never, rarely, occasionally, often, very often, or always). Although many psychiatric symptoms are thought of as existing in dichotomous states—for example, the presence or absence of *delusions*—most experienced clinicians know that the world is not so simple.

10

Delirium, Dementia, and Amnestic and Other Cognitive Disorders and Mental Disorders Due to a General Medical Condition

Severe disturbance in cognitive function is the hallmark of delirium, dementia, and amnestic and other cognitive disorders. The fourth edition of the *Diagnostic and Statistical Manual of Mental Disorders* (DSM-IV-TR) classifies these three groups of disorders into a broad category that encompasses the primary common symptoms of these disorders. These symptoms are impairments in memory, judgment, attention, and orientation.

Dementia is also characterized by marked cognitive deficits, but unlike delirium, these deficits occur in the context of a clear sensorium. The deficits include impairments in intelligence, learning and memory, language, problem solving, orientation, perception, attention and concentration, judgment, and social skills. The clinical work-up of etiology is crucial. Clinicians need

to be especially familiar with dementias of the Alzheimer's type as well as vascular dementias. Knowledge of the course and prognosis of both these dementia types is essential. Principles of treatment, and perhaps most importantly, long-term management of people with these disorders, must be learned in order to most effectively assist patients and their families.

Amnestic disorders are characterized by memory impairments that are associated with significant deficits in social or occupational functioning. The amnestic disorders are causally related to general medical conditions, such as head trauma. This characteristic distinguishes them from the dissociative disorders involving memory impairments.

The questions and answers below can test knowledge of the subject.

HELPFUL HINTS

The student should be able to define the signs, symptoms, and syndromes listed below.

- abstract attitude
- Addison's disease
- AIP
- ALS
- amnestic disorders
- anxiety disorder due to a general medical condition
- auditory, olfactory, and visual hallucinations
- beclouded dementia
- beriberi
- black-patch
- catastrophic reaction
- cognitive disorders
- confabulation
- cretinism
- Creutzfeldt-Jakob disease

- Cushing's syndrome
- delirium
- delusional disorder
- dementia
- dementia of the Alzheimer's type
- diabetic ketoacidosis
- dissociative amnesia
- Down's syndrome
- dysarthria
- epilepsy
- general paresis
- granulovacuolar degeneration
- Huntington's disease
- hypnagogic and hypnopompic hallucinations

- hypoglycemic, hepatic, and uremic encephalopathy
- intellectual functions
- interictal
- intoxication and withdrawal
- intracranial neoplasms
- Korsakoff's syndrome
- kuru
- Lilliputian hallucinations
- manifestations
- memory
- mood disorder due to a general medical condition
- multiple sclerosis

- myxedema
- neurofibrillary tangles
- normal aging
- normal pressure hydrocephalus
- orientation
- parkinsonism
- partial versus generalized seizures
- pellagra
- pernicious anemia
- personality change due to a general medical condition
- Pick's disease
- postoperative
- prion disease
- pseudobulbar palsy

► pseudodementia
► retrograde versus anterograde amnesia
► senile plaques
► short-term versus long-term memory loss
► SLE
► sundowner syndrome
► tactile or haptic hallucinations
► TIA
► transient global amnesia
► vascular dementia
► vertebrobasilar disease

▲ QUESTIONS

DIRECTIONS: Each of the questions or incomplete statements below is followed by five suggested responses or completions. Select the *one* that is *best* in each case.

10.1 The most common cause of delirium within 3 days postoperatively in a 40-year-old man with a history of alcohol dependence is

A. stress of surgery
B. postoperative pain
C. pain medication
D. infection
E. delirium tremens

10.2 Delirium

A. has an insidious onset
B. rarely has associated neurological symptoms
C. generally has an underlying cause residing in the central nervous system
D. may be successfully treated with lithium
E. generally causes a diffuse slowing of brain activity

10.3 Which of the following drugs is best used to treat acute delirium?

A. chlorpromazine (Thorazine)
B. diazepam (Valium)
C. haloperidol (Haldol)
D. amobarbital (Amytal)
E. physostigmine salicylate (Antilirium)

10.4 The electroencephalogram (EEG) shown in Figure 10.1 is an example of

A. partial seizure
B. grand mal epilepsy
C. petit mal epilepsy or absence seizure
D. psychomotor epilepsy
E. none of the above

10.5 A person with a complex partial seizure disorder

A. has no alteration in consciousness during the seizure
B. may exhibit a personality disturbance, such as religiosity
C. usually does not experience preictal events (auras)
D. usually displays a characteristic electroencephalogram (EEG) pattern
E. may have acute intermittent porphyria as the underlying cause

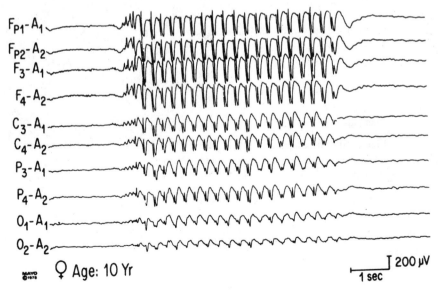

FIGURE 10.1
Electroencephalogram (EEG).

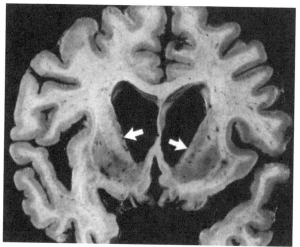

FIGURE 10.2

Reprinted with permission from Golden A, Powell DE, Jennings CD, eds. *Pathology: Understanding Human Disease.* 2nd ed. Baltimore: Williams & Wilkins; 1985:278.

10.6 The gross neuropathology in Figure 10.2, demonstrating marked atrophy of the caudate nuclei (*arrows*), corresponds with a disorder characterized by which of the following manifestations?

    A. urinary incontinence, gait disturbance, progressive dementia

    B. confusion, ataxia, ophthalmoplegia

    C. psychomotor slowing, difficulty with complex tasks, choreiform movements

    D. memory impairment, aphasia, personality changes

    E. bradykinesia, rigidity, resting tremor

10.7 The SPECT image on the right in Figure 10.3 demonstrates an area of hypoperfusion (compared to normal on the left) in a patient showing behavioral disinhibition and features of Klüver-Bucy syndrome, with subsequent onset of dementia. The most likely diagnosis is

    A. normal pressure hydrocephalus

    B. pseudodementia

    C. neurosyphilis

    D. Pick's disease

    E. progressive supranuclear palsy

10.8 The SPECT image in Figure 10.4, demonstrating a 50 percent reduction in blood flow in the posterior temporal-parietal cortex, is most consistent with the pathological changes found in which of the following?

    A. Pick's disease

    B. Huntington's disease

    C. normal pressure hydrocephalus

    D. Alzheimer's disease

    E. Parkinson's disease

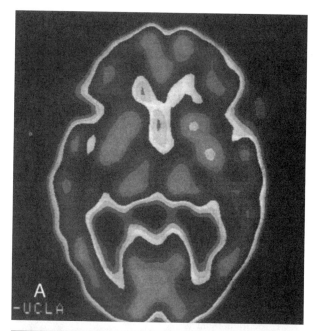

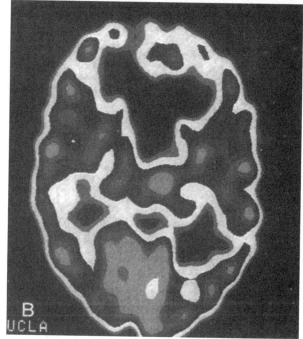

FIGURE 10.3

Reprinted with permission from Kaplan HI, Sadock BJ, eds. *Comprehensive Textbook of Psychiatry.* 6th ed. Baltimore: Williams & Wilkins; 1995:260, 263.

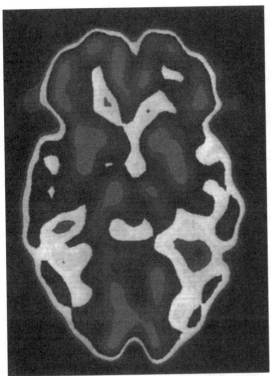

FIGURE 10.4
Reprinted with permission from Kaplan HI, Sadock BJ, eds. *Comprehensive Textbook of Psychiatry.* 6th ed. Baltimore: Williams & Wilkins; 1995:262.

10.9 Microscopic examination of the gross pathological specimen shown in Figure 10.5 revealed, among other abnormalities, plaques composed of β/A_4 protein, a breakdown product of amyloid precursor protein. In life, the patient would have had

A. fluctuation of cognitive impairment during the course of the day
B. progressive memory impairment and aphasia
C. sudden onset of dementia with discrete, stepwise deterioration
D. marked variability in performance of tasks of similar difficulty
E. early and prominent loss of social skills

10.10 All of the following statements regarding the neuropathological specimen shown in Figure 10.6 are false *except*

A. A cholinergic deficit is implicated in the pathophysiology of the patient's disease.
B. The course of the patient's disease (from onset until death) was likely to have been under 6 months.
C. The patient's symptoms would have improved with L-dopa administration.
D. Motor dysfunction was the initial and predominant manifestation of this patient's disease.
E. The patient suffered from a treatable condition.

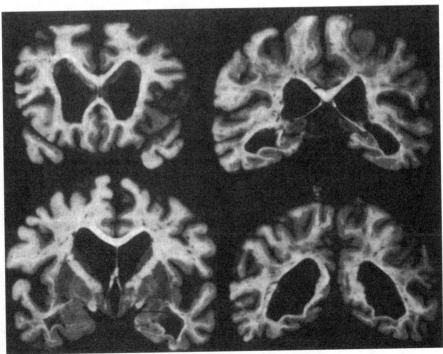

FIGURE 10.5
Reprinted with permission from Kaplan HI, Sadock BJ, eds. *Comprehensive Textbook of Psychiatry.* 4th ed. Baltimore: Williams & Wilkins; 1985:863.

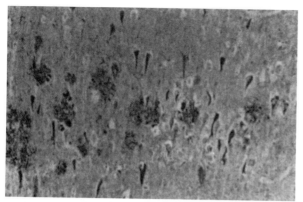

FIGURE 10.6
Reprinted with permission from Kaplan HI, Sadock BJ, eds. *Synopsis of Psychiatry.* 8th ed. Baltimore: Williams & Wilkins; 1998:1294.

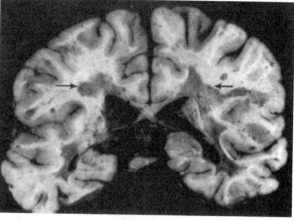

FIGURE 10.7
Reprinted with permission from Golden A, Powell DE, Jennings CD, eds. *Pathology: Understanding Human Disease.* 2nd ed. Baltimore: Williams & Wilkins; 1985:281.

10.11 The coronal section depicted in Figure 10.7 reveals, adjacent to the lateral ventricles (*arrows*), large, sharply demarcated plaques as part of a chronic disease characterized pathologically by multiple areas of white matter inflammation, demyelination, and glial scarring. In addition to manifestations such as motor weakness, paresthesias, ataxia, and diplopia, common neuropsychiatric symptoms of this disorder include all of the following *except*

A. depression
B. psychosis
C. memory impairment
D. euphoric mood
E. personality changes

10.12 The gross neuropathology shown in Figure 10.8 shows depigmentation of the substantia nigra and locus ceruleus in a patient's diseased tissue on the left (*arrows*), with normal tissue shown on the right. Physical examination of this patient might have revealed all of the following *except*

A. sucking reflexes
B. positive Babinski signs
C. impairment of fine movements
D. intention tremor
E. cogwheel rigidity

10.13 Of the following cognitive functions, the one most likely to be difficult to evaluate and interpret on formal testing is

A. memory
B. visuospatial and constructional ability
C. reading and writing
D. abstraction
E. calculations

10.14 Creutzfeldt-Jakob disease is characterized by

A. rapid deterioration
B. myoclonus
C. diffuse, symmetric, rhythmic slow waves in EEG
D. postmortem definitive diagnosis
E. all of the above

10.15 True statements about Alzheimer's disease include all of the following *except*

A. Age at onset is earlier in patients with a family history of the disease.
B. There is clear phenomenological separation between early-onset and late-onset cases.
C. The early-onset type may have a more rapidly progressive course.
D. No features of the physical examination or laboratory evaluation are pathognomonic.
E. Brain-imaging studies are used to exclude other identifiable causes.

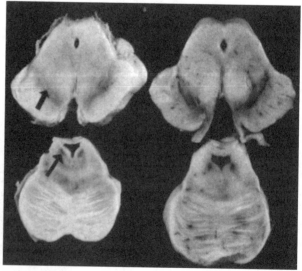

FIGURE 10.8
Reprinted with permission from Golden A, Powell DE, Jennings CD, eds. *Pathology: Understanding Human Disease.* 2nd ed. Baltimore: Williams & Wilkins; 1985:277.

10.16 True statements about Parkinson's disease include

    A. It is a prototype of a cortical degenerative disease.

    B. It cannot be distinguished from parkinsonian syndromes that arise from a variety of causes.

    C. It is the result of the degeneration of the substantia nigra, globus pallidus, putamen, and caudate.

    D. The only cells affected are those containing dopamine.

    E. Dementia is more common in early-onset disease.

10.17 Features supportive of the diagnosis of dementia with Lewy bodies include

    A. recurrent visual hallucinations that are typically well formed and detailed

    B. fluctuating cognition with profound variations in attention and alertness

    C. spontaneous motor features of parkinsonism

    D. neuroleptic sensitivity

    E. all of the above

10.18 Risk factors for the development of delirium include

    A. increased severity of physical illness

    B. older age

    C. preexisting dementia

    D. the use of anticholinergics

    E. all of the above

10.19 True statements about the epidemiology of dementia include all of the following *except*

    A. The estimated prevalence in a population over 65 years is consistently reported to be about 5 percent.

    B. Dementia of Alzheimer's type is the most common dementing disorder in North America, Scandinavia, and Europe.

    C. The risk for vascular dementia is six times greater than that for Alzheimer's among people older than 75 years.

    D. There appears to be a higher rate of vascular dementia in men, and a higher rate of Alzheimer's in women.

    E. In geriatric psychiatric populations, Alzheimer's is much more common than vascular dementia.

10.20 Frontal lobe degeneration is associated with

    A. disinhibition

    B. social misconduct

    C. lack of insight

    D. apathy

    E. all of the above

10.21 True statements about vascular etiologies of dementia include

    A. Together they comprise the second most common cause of dementia.

    B. It is believed that tissue damage in infarction underlies vascular dementia.

    C. The most common cause of cerebral infarction is thromboembolism from a large vessel plaque.

    D. Approximately 15 percent of cerebrovascular disease is due to cerebral hemorrhage related to hypertension.

    E. All of the above

10.22 Clinical characteristics of vascular dementia

    A. are the same regardless of the area of infarction

    B. are the same regardless of the number of infarctions

    C. are the same regardless of the type of vasculature involved

    D. are the same regardless of whether or not deficits accumulate or resolve quickly after small strokes

    E. none of the above

10.23 Amnestic disorders

    A. may be diagnosed in the context of delirium

    B. may be diagnosed in the context of dementia

    C. are secondary syndromes caused by primary etiologies

    D. are most often due to nutritional deficiencies related to chronic alcohol dependence

    E. none of the above

10.24 Amnestic disorders

    A. are invariably persistent, lasting at least a month

    B. are defined by a better memory for remote events than recent ones

    C. do not typically impair the ability to immediately repeat a sequential string of information (e.g., digit span)

    D. typically have a gradual onset

    E. none of the above

DIRECTIONS: Each group of questions below consists of lettered headings followed by a list of numbered phrases or statements. For each numbered phrase or statement, select the *one* lettered heading that is most closely associated with it. Each lettered heading may be used once, more than once, or not at all.

Questions 10.25–10.28

    A. Lead poisoning

    B. Manganese madness

    C. Mercury poisoning

    D. Thallium intoxication

    E. None of the above

10.25 Alopecia

10.26 Succimer (Chemet)

10.27 Mad Hatter syndrome

10.28 Masked facies

Questions 10.29–10.33

    A. Creutzfeldt-Jakob disease

    B. Normal-pressure hydrocephalus

    C. Neurosyphilis

    D. Huntington's disease

    E. Multiple sclerosis

10.29 Death occurring 15 to 20 years after the onset of the disease, with suicide being common

10.30 Slow virus, with death occurring within 2 years of the diagnosis

10.31 Manic syndrome with neurological signs in up to 20 percent of cases

10.32 Treatment of choice being a shunt

10.33 More prevalent in cold and temperate climates than in the tropics and subtropics

Questions 10.34–10.39

A. Delirium
B. Dementia
C. Both
D. Neither

10.34 Hallucinations
10.35 Sundowning
10.36 Catastrophic reaction
10.37 High mortality rate
10.38 Decreased acetylcholine activity
10.39 Insight present

Questions 10.40–10.43

A. CT scan
B. MRI
C. Both
D. Neither

10.40 Acute cerebral hemorrhage or hematomas
10.41 Better discriminates the interface between gray and white matter
10.42 Its greatest utility in the evaluation of dementia arises from what it may exclude (tumors, vascular disease) rather than what it can demonstrate specifically
10.43 Use is prohibited in patients with pacemakers or metal implants

Questions 10.44–10.50

A. Cortical dementia
B. Subcortical dementia
C. Both
D. Neither

10.44 Huntington's chorea
10.45 Alzheimer's disease
10.46 Early decline in calculation, naming, and copying skills
10.47 Fine and gross motor movements are generally preserved until later in the disease process
10.48 Language is relatively spared
10.49 Presenting symptoms more likely to be a personality change or mood disturbance
10.50 Presenting symptoms more often reflect cognitive impairment

Questions 10.51–10.54

A. dominant temporal lobe
B. subcortical or limbic
C. bilateral occipital lobe, optic tract
D. nondominant parietal lobe
E. none of the above

10.51 Complex delusions
10.52 Anton's syndrome
10.53 Auditory hallucinations
10.54 Anosognosia

ANSWERS

Delirium, Dementia, and Amnestic and Other Cognitive Disorders and Mental Disorders Due to a General Medical Condition

10.1 The answer is E

The most common cause of delirium in this case is *delirium tremens* (called alcohol withdrawal delirium in DSM-IV-TR). It is a medical emergency that results in mortality in about 20 percent of cases if left untreated. It occurs within 1 week after the person stops drinking. It usually develops on the third hospital day in a patient admitted for an unrelated condition (such as surgery) who has no access to alcohol and stops drinking suddenly. Another less common cause of postoperative delirium is *stress*, especially in major procedures such as cardiac or transplantation surgery. *Pain, pain medication*, and *infection* must also be considered in the postoperative period.

10.2 The answer is E

Delirium *generally causes a diffuse slowing of brain activity* on the electroencephalogram (EEG), which may be useful in differentiating delirium from depression and psychosis. The EEG of a delirious patient sometimes shows focal areas of hyperactivity. In rare cases, differentiating delirium related to epilepsy from delirium related to other causes may be difficult. In general, *delirium has a sudden, not insidious, onset*. Patients with delirium *commonly (not rarely) have associated neurological* symptoms, including dysphasia, tremor, asterixis, incoordination, and urinary incontinence. Delirium does not generally have an underlying cause residing in the central nervous system. Delirium has many causes, all of which result in a similar pattern of symptoms relating to the patient's level of consciousness and cognitive impairment. *Most of the causes of delirium lie outside the central nervous system*—for example, renal and hepatic failures. Delirium *cannot be successfully treated with lithium (Eskalith)*. Patients with variable lithium serum concentrations may be at risk for delirium.

10.3 The answer is C

Of the drugs listed, the best choice is *haloperidol (Haldol)*, a butyrophenone. Depending on the patient's age, weight, and physical condition, the initial dose may range from 0.5 to 10 mg intramuscularly, repeated in an hour if the patient remains agitated. As soon as the patient is calm, oral medication in liquid concentrate or tablet form should begin. Two daily oral doses should suffice, with two-thirds of the dose being given at bedtime. To achieve the same therapeutic effect, the clinician should give an oral dose about 1.5 times higher than a parenteral dose. The effective total daily dosage of haloperidol may range from 5 to 50 mg for the majority of delirious patients. The patient's response should always be closely monitored for possible side effects.

Phenothiazines, such as *chlorpromazine (Thorazine)*, should be avoided in delirious patients because those drugs are associated with significant anticholinergic activity. *Benzodiazepines* with long half-lives, such as *diazepam (Valium)*, and barbiturates, such as *amobarbital (Amytal)*, should be avoided unless they are being used as part of the treatment for the underlying disorder (for example, alcohol withdrawal). Sedatives can increase cognitive disorganization in delirious patients. When the delirium is due to anticholinergic toxicity, the use of *physostigmine salicylate (Antilirium)* may be indicated; but it is not the first drug to be used in an acute delirium in which the cause has not been determined.

10.4 The answer is C

Petit mal epilepsy or absence seizure is associated with a characteristic generalized, bilaterally synchronous, 3-hertz spike-and-wave pattern in the electroencephalogram (EEG) and is often easily induced by hyperventilation. Petit mal epilepsy occurs predominantly in children. It usually consists of simple absence attacks lasting 5 to 10 seconds, during which the patient has an abrupt alteration in awareness and responsiveness and an interruption in motor activity. The child often has a blank stare associated with an upward deviation of the eyes and some mild twitching movements of the eyes, eyelids, face, or extremities. Petit mal epilepsy is usually a fairly benign seizure disorder, often resolving after adolescence.

A *partial seizure* (also known as jacksonian epilepsy) is a type of epilepsy characterized by recurrent episodes of focal motor seizures. It begins with localized tonic or clonic contraction, increases in severity, spreads progressively through the entire body, and terminates in a generalized convulsion with loss of consciousness. *Grand mal epilepsy* is the major form of epilepsy. Gross tonic-clonic convulsive seizures are accompanied by loss of consciousness and, often, incontinence of stool or urine. *Psychomotor epilepsy* is a type of epilepsy characterized by recurrent behavior disturbances. Complex hallucinations or illusions, frequently gustatory or olfactory, often herald the onset of the seizure, which typically involves a state of impaired consciousness resembling a dream, during which paramnestic phenomena, such as *déjà vu* and *jamais vu,* are experienced, and the patient exhibits repetitive, automatic, or semipurposeful behaviors. In rare instances, violent behavior may be prominent. The EEG reveals a localized seizure focus in the temporal lobe.

10.5 The answer is B

A person with a complex partial seizure disorder *may exhibit a personality disturbance, such as religiosity.* The most frequent psychiatric abnormalities reported in epileptic patients (especially patients with partial complex seizures of temporal lobe origin) are *personality disturbances.* In a person displaying *religiosity,* the religiosity may be striking and may be manifested not only by increased participation in overtly religious activities but also by unusual concern for moral and ethical issues, preoccupation with right and wrong, and heightened interest in global and philosophical concerns. The hyperreligious features can sometimes seem like the prodromal symptoms of schizophrenia and can result in a diagnostic problem in an adolescent or a young adult.

Partial seizures are classified as complex if they are associated with alterations in consciousness during the seizure episode. Thus, a person with a complex partial seizure disorder always has *an alteration in consciousness* during the seizure.

The person also *experiences preictal events (auras).* Preictal events in complex partial seizures include autonomic sensations (for example, fear, panic, depression, and elation) and, classically, automatisms (for example, lip smacking, rubbing, and chewing).

A person with a complex partial seizure disorder *does not display a characteristic electroencephalogram (EEG) pattern.* On the contrary, multiple normal EEGs are often obtained from a patient with complex partial seizures; therefore, normal EEGs

cannot be used to exclude a diagnosis of complex partial seizures. The use of long-term EEG recordings (usually 24 to 72 hours) can help the clinician detect a seizure focus in some patients. Only in petit mal epilepsy does one see a characteristic EEG pattern of three-per-second spike-and-wave activity.

Acute intermittent porphyria is not the underlying cause of complex partial seizures. The porphyrias are disorders of heme biosynthesis, resulting in the excessive accumulation of porphyrins. However, a disease that may lead to the development of complex partial seizures is herpes simplex encephalitis.

10.6 The answer is C

The neuropathology is consistent with that found in Huntington's disease, which involves atrophy of the caudate nuclei and putamen. Huntington's disease is an autosomal dominant disorder characterized by *choreiform movements* and by subcortical dementia, which may present with *psychomotor slowing and difficulty with complex tasks.*

Urinary incontinence, gait disturbance, and progressive dementia are characteristic of normal-pressure hydrocephalus. *Confusion, ataxia, and ophthalmoplegia* are characteristic of Wernicke's encephalopathy, a disorder caused by deficiency of thiamine (vitamin B_1) as seen in chronic alcoholism. *Memory impairment, aphasia, and personality changes* are characteristic of dementia, such as dementia of the Alzheimer's type and vascular dementia. *Bradykinesia, resting tremor, and rigidity* are characteristic of Parkinson's disease.

10.7 The answer is D

Pick's disease is characterized by a preponderance of atrophy in the frontal and anterior temporal lobes, *seen as frontal,* sparing the temporal-parietal regions (in contrast to Alzheimer's disease, which mainly affects the temporal-parietal regions). Initial symptoms of Pick's disease often involve behavior and personality changes, with dementia symptoms occurring later. Common early symptoms include apathy and behavioral disinhibition, with some patients showing features of the Klüver-Bucy syndromes (hypersexuality, placidity, hyperorality).

Normal-pressure hydrocephalus often appears as global cerebral hypoperfusion on SPECT and is characterized by urinary incontinence, gait disturbance, and progressive dementia. *Neurosyphilis* appears 10 to 15 years after the primary *Treponema* infection and generally affects the frontal lobe, resulting in personality changes, impaired judgment, irritability, and decreased care for self with later development of dementia and tremor. *Pseudodementia* refers to clinical features resembling a dementia not caused by an organic condition, most often caused by depression. *Progressive supranuclear palsy* is a heterogeneous deterioration involving the brainstem, basal ganglia, and cerebellum with nuchal dystonia and dementia.

10.8 The answer is D

Parietal-temporal hypoperfusion on SPECT imaging is consistent with the distribution of pathology found in *Alzheimer's disease.*

In contrast, *Pick's disease* appears on SPECT imaging as frontal hypoperfusion. *Huntington's disease* is visualized on SPECT as hypoperfusion of the caudate regions. Patients with *normal-pressure hydrocephalus* do not show the Alzheimer's pattern of selective parietal-temporal changes. The neuropathology of *Parkinson's disease* involves degeneration of subcortical structures, primarily the substantia nigra but also the globus pallidus, caudate, and putamen.

10.9 The answer is B

The patient suffered from Alzheimer's disease. Pathological examination of the brain tissue is the only means by which this diagnosis can be established with certainty. As shown in the photograph, the classic gross neuroanatomical observation of the brain from a patient with Alzheimer's disease is diffuse cerebral atrophy with dilation of ventricles and widening of the cortical sulci. Senile plaques composed of β/A$_4$ protein (a breakdown product of amyloid precursor protein) is a classic microscopic finding. Other neuropathologic changes in Alzheimer's disease include neurofibrillary tangles, synaptic loss, and granulovacuolar degeneration of neurons.

The DSM-IV-TR diagnostic criteria for dementia of the Alzheimer's type (DAT) emphasize the *presence of memory impairment* and the associated presence of at least one other symptom of cognitive decline (*aphasia*, apraxia, agnosia, or abnormal executive functioning). *The sudden onset of dementia with discrete, stepwise deterioration* is characteristic of vascular dementia rather than DAT, which is characterized by insidious onset and slow progression of symptoms over 8 to 10 years. *Fluctuation of cognitive impairment during the course of the day* is characteristic of delirium rather than dementia. Although both delirium and dementia involve cognitive impairment, the changes in dementia are more stable over time and tend not to fluctuate over the course of a day. The differential diagnosis of dementia includes depression-related cognitive dysfunction, referred to as pseudodementia. *Early and prominent loss of social skills* and *marked variability in performance of tasks of similar difficulty* are characteristic of pseudodementia rather than dementia. Patients with dementia often retain social skills and show consistently poor performance of tasks of similar difficulty.

10.10 The answer is A

Figure 10.6 shows the microscopic appearance of the hippocampus from a patient with Alzheimer's disease, showing large numbers of neurofibrillary tangles and senile plaques. Although neurofibrillary tangles are not unique to Alzheimer's disease, senile plaques (also referred to as amyloid plaques) are much more indicative of Alzheimer's. The neurotransmitters acetylcholine and norepinephrine are among the factors *implicated in the pathophysiology of Alzheimer's disease*, both of which are hypothesized to be hypoactive.

The course of Alzheimer's is characteristically one of gradual decline over 8 to 10 years; *disease progression of less than 6 months would not be expected*. The mean survival of patients with Alzheimer's disease is approximately 8 years, with a range of 1 to 20 years. Cognitive dysfunction, rather than *motor dysfunction*, is the initial and predominant manifestation of Alzheimer's disease. Memory impairment is accompanied by such deficits as aphasia, apraxia, agnosia, and disturbances in executive functioning. The general sequence of deficits is memory, language, and visuospatial functions. *Dementia of Alzheimer's type has no known prevention or cure. Treatment is palliative*, and medication may be helpful in managing agitation and behavior disturbances. *L-Dopa* is a medication used in the treatment of Parkinson's disease.

10.11 The answer is B

The neuropathology is consistent with multiple sclerosis (MS), the most common demyelinating disorder. Pathologically, MS consists of multifocal demyelination, producing irregularly shaped areas (plaques) of demyelination with sharp borders. In addition to multiple exacerbations and remissions of neurological deficits, MS often features behavioral symptoms including *depression, personality changes, and euphoric mood*, as well as cognitive impairment. *Memory is the most commonly affected cognitive function. Psychosis* is a rare complication of MS.

10.12 The answer is D

The neuropathology is consistent with Parkinson's disease, which results from a loss of cells in the substantia nigra, a decrease in the concentration of dopamine, and a degeneration of dopaminergic tracts. The major finding on observation of gross neuropathology is depigmentation of the substantia nigra and locus ceruleus.

Parkinson's disease is a progressive disease, usually of late adult life, with characteristic symptoms of *bradykinesia, rigidity*, and tremor at rest (*not intention tremor*, which is characteristic of cerebellar dysfunction). Physical examination of a patient with Parkinson's disease reveals an *impairment of fine movements, cogwheel rigidity, sucking reflexes, positive Babinski signs*, and other evidence of pyramidal tract involvement.

Apathy, intellectual impairment, depression, and dementia are commonly seen in Parkinson's disease. The prevalence of *depression* in Parkinson's disease has been reported to be between 40 and 60 percent, whereas *dementia* is present in 30 to 60 percent.

10.13 The answer is D

When testing cognitive functions the clinician should evaluate *memory*; *visuospatial and constructional abilities*; *reading and writing*, and *mathematical abilities*. *Abstraction ability* is also valuable to assess, although a patient's performance on tasks, such as proverb interpretation, may be difficult to evaluate when abnormal. Proverb interpretation may be a useful bedside projective test in some patients, but the specific interpretation may result from a variety of factors, such as poor education, low intelligence, and failure to understand the concept of proverbs, as well as a broad array of primary and secondary psychopathological disturbances. Although testing similarities are also education-sensitive, similarities may be more easily understood by patients.

10.14 The answer is E (all)

Creutzfeldt-Jakob disease is an infection that causes a rapidly progressive cortical-pattern dementia. The infectious agent, a *prion,* is a subviral replicative protein that is now known to cause a variety of so-called spongiform diseases in animals and humans. The 1998 Nobel Prize for Medicine was awarded to Stanley Prusiner for his work describing this novel biological entity. The age at onset of Creutzfeldt-Jakob disease is usually in the sixth or seventh decade, although onset can occur at any age. The incidence is 1 in 1,000,000. The clinical symptoms vary with progression of the illness and depend on the regions of the brain that become involved. Patients may present initially with nonspecific symptoms, including lethargy, depression, and fatigue. Within weeks, however, more fulminant symptoms develop, including progressive cortical-pattern dementia, myoclonus, and pyramidal and extrapyramidal signs. Although blood, CSF, and imaging studies are unremarkable, the *EEG can demonstrate a characteristic pattern of diffuse, symmetric, rhythmic slow waves. A presentation with rapid deterioration, myoclonus, and the characteristic EEG pattern* should raise suspicion of

Creutzfeldt-Jakob disease. The *definitive diagnosis is made by postmortem microscopic examination,* which demonstrates spongiform neural degeneration and gliosis throughout the cortical and subcortical gray matter; white matter tracts are usually spared. Prion disease can incubate for decades before the emergence of clinical symptoms and subsequent rapid progression. Reported routes of transmission include invasive body contacts, such as direct tissue transplantation (e.g., corneal transplants) or hormonal extracts (e.g., human growth hormone, before synthetic supplies were developed). Familial patterns have also been reported, which suggests that there may be genetic susceptibility to infection or vertical transmission of the disease agent. No antiviral agents have been shown to be effective in retarding or slowing disease progress, although amantadine (Symmetrel) has been reported occasionally to have had some success. Death usually ensues within 6 months to 2 years of onset. During the past several years, a pathologically similar condition, bovine spongiform encephalopathy, has been described. Diagnosed primarily in the United Kingdom, this disease underscores the effects of modern animal husbandry methods on the amplification of rare diseases and the continuing threat of xenobiotic transmission of these to humans.

10.15 The answer is B

Alzheimer's disease is the prototype of a cortical degenerative disease. Alzheimer's original description in 1906 detailed most of the familiar clinical and neuropathological features. Of note, his patient suffered from paranoia in addition to cognitive decline. Currently, the diagnosis of Alzheimer's disease requires neuropathological confirmation, but the diagnosis is used clinically for cases identified antemortem. *Age at onset is earlier in patients with a family history of the disease.* Despite some data to suggest distinctive age-related clinical patterns, *no phenomenological separation between early-onset and late-onset cases has been found consistently* enough for age to substitute for detailed clinical description; however, *early-onset dementia of the Alzheimer's type may have a more rapidly progressive course.* A major component of the presenting symptoms is usually subjective complaints of memory difficulty, language impairment ("I can't find the word"), and dyspraxia (e.g., difficulty driving). Diagnosis at this juncture is primarily based on exclusion of other possible etiologies for dementia. *No features of the physical examination or laboratory evaluation are pathognomonic for dementia of the Alzheimer's type.* Some studies have apparently discriminated patients with dementia of the Alzheimer's type from patients with dementia of other etiologies and from normal controls by using techniques such as EEG, MRI, and SPECT. These studies have been difficult to replicate consistently, and at present, *brain-imaging studies are best used to exclude other identifiable causes.* Indeed, available technological diagnostic methods have not proved more sensitive and specific than astute clinical evaluation in comparisons of patients with dementia of the Alzheimer's type and healthy control subjects. PET holds promise but currently is too expensive for routine clinical diagnostic use.

10.16 The answer is C

Described by James Parkinson in 1817, Parkinson's disease is *a prototype of a subcortical, not cortical, degenerative disease.* It is idiopathic *and must be distinguished from parkinsonian syndromes that arise from a variety of causes.*

Parkinson's disease is the result of the degeneration of subcortical structures, *primarily the substantia nigra but also the globus pallidus, putamen, and caudate. Cells containing dopamine are predominantly affected, although serotonergic and other systems are disrupted as well.* Just as the appellation "cortical pattern" is pseudoanatomical, so in subcortical Parkinson's disease there can be significant degeneration of cortical structures. The parkinsonian syndrome manifests with structural damage that reflects the underlying process or insult. Medication-induced parkinsonism presumably involves only a dysfunction of the basal ganglia structures, without any obvious pathoanatomical abnormality. The typical age at onset of Parkinson's disease is between 50 and 60 years but may vary widely, with onset sometimes occurring 1 to 2 decades earlier. The clinical course is chronic and progressive, with severe disability attained after approximately 10 years. A smaller proportion of patients have a more rapidly progressive disease, and a yet smaller group has a slowly progressive disorder in which deterioration plateaus or remains minimal for two to three decades.

In general, subcortical diseases are thought to impinge on the three Ms—movement, mentation, and mood. In Parkinson's disease all three of these areas are affected, although not always uniformly. The movement abnormalities are characterized by the triad of tremor, rigidity, and bradykinesia. The tremor and rigidity can be unilateral or bilateral. Bradykinesia is manifested by slowness in the initiation and execution of movement. The typical presentation, with a mask-like facies, minimal blink, and monotonic speech, is a concomitant of the rigidity and slowness of movement. Other prominent characteristics include postural changes such as chin-to-chest flexion and gait abnormalities. The gait is characteristically slow and shuffling, and the patient has difficulty turning (en bloc turning) and trouble initiating and stopping walking. Seborrhea, sialorrhea, excessive fatigue, and constipation are also common.

Mentation or cognition in Parkinson's disease is an area of controversy. Most patients complain of slowed thinking, sometimes called bradyphrenia. In general, approximately 20 to 30 percent of patients with Parkinson's disease are found to have *dementia, with the likelihood greater in those with late-onset disease (after 70 years).* Approximately 40 percent of nondemented patients with Parkinson's disease, however, demonstrate some neuropsychological impairment in most studies. The impairments are primarily in visuospatial capacities, as measured by copying, tracing, and tracking tasks, and in the shifting of cognitive sets, as measured by the Wisconsin Card Sorting Test or the Stroop Test. Such deficits have been noted in the absence of cognitive-based functional decline or other evidence of cognitive impairment. Controversy has emerged over whether these two patterns represent a single continuum of dementia integral to the process of Parkinson's disease or are two separate processes indicative of two distinct diseases. Neuropathologically, cases intermediate between Parkinson's disease and Alzheimer's disease exist, with the characteristic microscopic features of the latter and Lewy bodies in the substantia nigra suggesting the former. There is no clear line of division as yet between a process resembling dementia of the Alzheimer's type on which abnormal parkinsonian movements are superimposed and a clinical presentation of Parkinson's disease in which the patient slowly develops a global progressive dementia.

10.17 The answer is E (all)

Since the late 1980s research has revealed that, beyond dementia of the Alzheimer's type and vascular dementia, a common cause of progressive dementia may be related to the presence of Lewy bodies in the brainstem and cerebral cortex. Lewy bodies—intracytoplasmic, spherical, eosinophilic neuronal inclusion bodies—are scattered through the brainstem, subcortical nuclei, limbic cortex (cingulate, entorhinal, amygdala), and neocortex (temporal, frontal, parietal). Parkinson's disease, in contrast, manifests Lewy bodies in subcortical nuclei, in addition to degeneration of dopamine cell bodies in substantia nigra. Table 10.1 lists the pathological features of dementia with Lewy bodies; Table 10.2 includes recently developed consensus guidelines for clinical diagnosis. Neuropsychiatric features, including *visual hallucinations*, delusions, fluctuating attention, and executive or managerial *cognitive deficits*, are prominent; although not specific, mood disturbances are common.

10.18 The answer is E (all)

There have been relatively few studies of the incidence and prevalence of delirium. Little is known about the epidemiology of delirium in community or other nonpatient, noninstitutionalized populations. An estimated 10 to 15 percent of general medical inpatients are delirious at any given time, and studies indicate that as many as 30 to 50 percent of acutely ill geriatric patients become delirious at some point during their hospital stay. Rates of delirium in psychiatric and nursing home populations are not well established but are clearly substantial. Risk factors for the development of delirium include *increased severity of physical illness, older age, baseline cognitive impairment (e.g., due to dementia),* and *use of anticholinergics.*

Delirium is frequently unrecognized by treating physicians. Because of its wide array of associated symptoms, it may be detected but misdiagnosed as depression, schizophrenia, or another psychiatric disorder. Delirium is a frequent cause for psychiatric consultation in the general hospital but often is not recognized as such by the referring physician.

10.19 The answer is C

The prevalence of dementia rises exponentially with age. *The estimated prevalence* of moderate to severe dementia in a population aged 65 years or older is consistently reported at *approximately 5 percent.* Within that age group the exponential curve is pronounced

Table 10.1
Pathological Features Associated with Dementia with Lewy Bodies

Essential for diagnosis
  Lewy bodies
Associated but not essential
  Lewy-related neurites
  Plaques (all morphological types)
  Neurofibrillary tangles
  Regional neuronal loss—especially brainstem (substantia nigra and locus ceruleus) and nucleus basalis of Meynert
  Microvacuolation (spongiform change) and synapse loss
  Neurochemical abnormalities and neurotransmitter deficits

Reprinted with permission from McKeith IG, Galasko D, Kosaka K, et al. For the Consortium on Dementia with Lewy Bodies. *Neurology.* 1996;47:1113.

Table 10.2
Consensus Criteria for the Clinical Diagnosis of Probable and Possible Dementia with Lewy Bodies

1. The central feature required for a diagnosis of dementia with Lewy bodies is progressive cognitive decline of sufficient magnitude to interfere with normal social or occupational function. Prominent or persistent memory impairment may not necessarily occur in the early stages but is usually evident with progression. Deficits on tests of attention and of frontal-subcortical skills and visuospatial ability may be especially prominent.
2. Two of the following core features are essential for a diagnosis of probable dementia with Lewy bodies, and one is essential for possible dementia with Lewy bodies:
   a. Fluctuating cognition with profound variations in attention and alertness
   b. Recurrent visual hallucinations that are typically well formed and detailed
   c. Spontaneous motor features of parkinsonism
3. Features supportive of the diagnosis are:
   a. Repeated falls
   b. Syncope
   c. Transient loss of consciousness
   d. Neuroleptic sensitivity
   e. Systematized delusions
   f. Hallucinations in other modalities
4. A diagnosis of dementia with Lewy bodies is less likely in the presence of
   a. Stroke disease, evident as focal neurologic signs or on brain imaging
   b. Evidence on physical examination and investigation of any physical illness or other brain disorder sufficient to account for the clinical picture

Reprinted with permission from McKeith IG, Galasko D, Kosaka K, et al. For the Consortium on Dementia with Lewy Bodies. *Neurology.* 1996;47:1113.

so that the prevalence in the subgroup aged 65 to 69 years is 1.5 to 2 percent; in the subgroup aged 75 to 79 years it is 5.5 to 6.5 percent; and in the subgroup aged 85 to 89 years it is 20 to 22 percent. *Dementia of the Alzheimer's type is the most common dementing* disorder in clinical and neuropathological prevalence studies reported from North America, Scandinavia, and Europe. Prevalence studies from Russia and Japan show vascular dementia to be more common in those countries. It remains unclear whether those apparent clinical differences reflect true etiological distinctions or inconsistent uses of diagnostic criteria. Dementia of the Alzheimer's type becomes more common with increasing age; among persons older than 75 years, the risk is six times greater than *the risk for vascular dementia.* There is a suggestion of *higher rates of dementia of the Alzheimer's type in females and higher rates of vascular dementia in males. In geriatric psychiatric patient samples, dementia of the Alzheimer's type is a much more common etiology (50 to 70 percent) than vascular dementia (15 to 25 percent).*

Studies of the incidence of dementia have been plagued by widely differing methodology and results. Again, there is an exponential increase in incidence with age, although some reports have noted a leveling off starting around age 75 years.

10.20 The answer is E (all)

In recent years several authors have sought to distinguish dementias of the frontal lobe from other disorders. The uncertain status of dementias of the frontal lobe as distinct clinical and neuropathological entities has not yet warranted their formal inclusion in DSM-IV-TR or ICD-10. They are described as cortical dementias that are found in as many as 10 to 20 percent of cases in some neuropathological series. Age at onset is apparently between 50 and 60 years for the majority, but the reported range is broad—20 to 80 years. The early clinical features of frontal lobe dementias are typified by damage to the frontal lobes and include prominent changes in personality and behavior. *The personality changes include disinhibition, social misconduct, and lack of insight; these changes progress to apathy, mutism, and repetitive behaviors.*

Neuropsychological testing in patients suspected of having dementia of frontal lobe origin may demonstrate disproportionate impairment in tasks related to frontal lobe function, such as deficiency in abstract thinking, attentional shifting, or set formation. Structural neuroimaging, such as CT or MRI, may reveal prominent atrophy of the frontal lobe, especially early in the disease process. Functional neuroimaging may prove more reliable for distinguishing dementia of frontal lobe origin from dementia of the Alzheimer's type. Regional cerebral blood flow studies using radioactively labeled xenon and SPECT studies have demonstrated disproportionate decreases in blood flow, radio tracer uptake, and glucose metabolism in the frontal lobes in patients with suspected or autopsy-confirmed frontal lobe dementia.

At present, the definitive diagnosis of any degenerative dementia rests on postmortem neuropathological examination. Only one type of frontal lobe dementia, Pick's disease, is associated with distinctive histopathological abnormalities that allow for certain diagnosis. Swollen neurons known as Pick bodies define the disorder neuropathologically. Demyelination and gliosis of the frontal lobe white matter may also be found. Other frontal lobe dementias have been referred to as dementia of the frontal lobe type or frontal lobe degeneration of non-Alzheimer's type. They have been distinguished from Alzheimer's disease by their marked gross morphological involvement of frontal and anterior temporal lobes, with relative sparing of the postcentral and temporoparietal areas mostly affected in Alzheimer's disease, and by the absence of amyloid plaques and neurofibrillary tangles microscopically. The lack of positive neuropathological inclusion criteria leaves many of these clinical conditions as disease entities of uncertain status, defined histopathologically by the absence of specific features. Whenever the hallmark findings of Alzheimer's disease are present, that diagnosis has been applied, irrespective of prior clinical findings. Thus, there are no data available to determine how many clinically diagnosed cases of frontal lobe dementia have been recast as Alzheimer's disease after death.

Of the potentially multiple forms of dementia associated with progressive frontal lobe dysfunction, only one type can be distinguished from Alzheimer's disease neuropathologically; the others show no defining postmortem signs. They may also be difficult to distinguish clinically in life. In the early stages of disease, the predominance of behavioral and personality disturbance, the presence of primitive reflexes, and neuropsychological and neuroimaging evidence of disproportionate frontal lobe involvement can help with a more confident premortem diagnosis of frontal lobe dementia. Some authors have assumed that there are many variants of dementia of frontal lobe origin that cannot be distinguished from each other clinically; at present, only Pick's disease has definitive neuropathological features.

10.21 The answer is E (all)

Cerebrovascular diseases together comprise the second most common cause of dementia. This category of dementia was referred to in the past as arteriosclerotic dementia, reflecting the belief that vascular insufficiency was responsible for the cognitive degeneration. That has now been supplanted by the belief that *tissue damage or infarction underlies the vascular dementias.* Cerebral infarction can be the result of a number of processes, of which *thromboembolism* from a large vessel plaque or cardiothrombus is the most common. Anoxia due to cardiac arrest, hypotension, anemia, or sleep apnea can also produce ischemia and infarction. *Cerebral hemorrhage* related to hypertension or an arteriovenous malformation accounts for approximately *15 percent of cerebrovascular disease.*

10.22 The answer is E (none)

The clinical characteristics of a vascular dementia depend on the area of infarction. As such, there is a wide variability in the possible presenting features of a vascular dementia. *Single infarctions may result in the discrete loss of one particular function* (e.g., language) without dementia per se. *However, some strategically located infarctions can affect more than one domain of cognitive function* and mimic the clinical picture of a global dementia. An example is the angular gyrus syndrome that can occur with large posterior lesions in the dominant hemisphere. It has been characterized as manifesting with alexia with agraphia, aphasia, constructional disturbances, and Gerstmann syndrome (acalculia, agraphia, right-left disorientation, and finger agnosia). Although the findings are similar to those of dementia of the Alzheimer's type, angular gyrus syndrome can be distinguished by its abrupt onset; the presence of focal neurological, EEG, and imaging abnormalities; and preservation of memory and ideomotor praxis.

Vascular dementia is more commonly associated with multiple infarctions. The infarctions may take the form of numerous large infarctions accompanied by widespread cognitive and motor deficits. Tiny, deep infarctions, *lacunae,* result from disease of the small arteries that usually involves subcortical structures, such as the basal ganglia, thalamus, and internal capsule. The neurological and cognitive *deficits may resolve quickly after each of the small strokes; however, the deficits may accumulate,* leading to a persisting functional and intellectual decline. In the past a stepwise pattern of deterioration was described for that type of vascular dementia, but it was dropped from the DSM-IV-TR criteria, as no specific pattern of deterioration has been reliably demonstrated for vascular dementias. Similarly, the description of patchy deficits has been deleted, in light of the *marked variability in presentation of vascular dementia, depending on the type of vasculature and the site and extent of infarction.*

10.23 The answer is C

The essential feature of amnestic disorders is the acquired impaired ability to learn and recall new information, coupled variably with the inability to recall previously learned knowledge or past events. The impairment must be sufficiently severe to compromise personal, social, or occupational functioning. The diagnosis is not made if the memory impairment exists in the context of reduced ability to maintain and shift attention, as encountered in *delirium,* or in association with significant functional problems due to the compromise of multiple intellectual abilities, as seen in *dementia. Amnestic disorders are secondary syndromes* caused by systemic medical or primary cerebral diseases, substance-use disorders, or medication adverse effects, as evidenced by findings from clinical history, physical examination, or laboratory examination.

The number of individuals given amnestic diagnoses due to nutritional deficiency, often related to *chronic alcohol dependence,* has declined. In contrast, traumatic causes have increased dramatically during recent decades.

10.24 The answer is C

For some forms of amnestic disorder, events from the *remote past may be better remembered than more recent events.* However, such a gradient of recall is not present uniformly among individuals with amnestic disorders. *Typically, the ability to immediately repeat a sequential string of information (e.g., a digit span) is not impaired* in amnestic disorder; when such impairment is evident, it suggests the presence of attentional dysfunction that may be indicative of delirium. Amnestic disorders *may be transient, lasting for several hours to a few days, as in transient global amnesia, or persistent, lasting at least 1 month.* In the context of a newly developed but unresolved memory impairment, the term *provisional* should be added to a diagnosis of transient amnesia.

Transient global amnesia is a form of transient amnestic disorder associated with episodes that are characterized by a dense, transitory inability to learn new information (i.e., to form sustained memories), with a variable (ultimately shrinking on recovery) inability to recall events that occurred during the duration of the disturbance. The episode is followed by restoration to a completely intact cognitive state. There are no data to suggest that the memory impairment is associated with disturbed or abnormal behavior beyond the mild confusion or perplexity that may be manifest during the episode.

Depending on the cause of the disorder, the *onset of amnesia may be sudden or gradual.* Head trauma, vascular events, or specific types of neurotoxic exposure (e.g., carbon monoxide poisoning) may lead to acute mental status changes. Prolonged substance abuse, chronic neurotoxic exposure, or sustained nutritional deficiency exemplify conditions that may lead to an insidious memory decline, eventually causing a clinically definable cognitive impairment.

Amnestic disorder may develop as a result of alcohol dependence associated with dietary and vitamin deficiency. Alternatively, it may be the primary clinical deficit arising from traumatic head injury and may present as the major feature of a postconcussional state. When memory dysfunction exceeds other features of a postconcussional syndrome, it is preferable to diagnose the condition as amnestic disorder due to head trauma.

Answers 10.25–10.28

10.25 The answer is D

10.26 The answer is A

10.27 The answer is C

10.28 The answer is B

In acute *mercury poisoning,* the central nervous system symptoms of lethargy and restlessness may occur, but the primary symptoms are secondary to severe gastrointestinal irritation, with bloody stools, diarrhea, and vomiting leading to circulatory collapse because of dehydration. *Mad Hatter syndrome,* named for the *Mad Hatter* in *Alice's Adventures in Wonderland,* is a parody of the madness resulting from the inhalation of mercury nitrate vapors; mercury nitrate was used in the past in the processing of felt hats.

Early intoxication with manganese produces *manganese madness,* with symptoms of headache, irritability, joint pains, and somnolence. Lesions involving the basal ganglia and pyramidal system result in gait impairment, rigidity, monotonous or whispering speech, tremors of the extremities and tongue, *masked facies (manganese mask),* micrographia, dystonia, dysarthria, and loss of equilibrium.

Thallium intoxication initially causes severe pains in the legs, as well as diarrhea and vomiting. Within a week, delirium, convulsions, cranial nerve palsies, blindness, choreiform movements, and coma may occur. Behavioral changes include paranoid thinking and depression, with suicidal tendencies. *Alopecia* is a common and important diagnostic clue.

Chronic *lead poisoning* occurs when the amount of lead ingested exceeds the ability to eliminate it. Toxic symptoms appear after several months. Treatment should be instituted as rapidly as possible, even without laboratory confirmation, because of the high mortality. The treatment of choice to facilitate lead excretion is the oral administration of *succimer (Chemet).*

Answers 10.29–10.33

10.29 The answer is D

10.30 The answer is A

10.31 The answer is C

10.32 The answer is B

10.33 The answer is E

Huntington's disease, inherited in an autosomal dominant pattern, leads to major atrophy of the brain with extensive degeneration of the caudate nucleus. The onset is usually insidious and most commonly begins in late middle life. The course is one of gradual progression; *death occurs 15 to 20 years after the onset* of the disease, and *suicide* is common.

Creutzfeldt-Jakob disease is a rare degenerative brain disease caused by a *slow virus,* with death occurring within 2 years of the diagnosis. A computed tomography (CT) scan shows cerebellar and cortical atrophy.

Neurosyphilis (also known as general paresis) is a chronic dementia and psychosis caused by the tertiary form of syphilis that affects the brain. The presenting symptoms include a *manic syndrome* with neurological signs in up to 20 percent of cases.

Normal pressure hydrocephalus is associated with enlarged ventricles and normal cerebrospinal fluid (CSF) pressure. The characteristic signs include dementia, a gait disturbance, and urinary incontinence. *The treatment of choice is a shunt* of the CSF from the ventricular space to either the atrium or the peritoneal space. Reversal of the dementia and associated signs is sometimes dramatic after treatment.

Multiple sclerosis is characterized by diffuse multifocal lesions in the white matter of the central nervous system (CNS). Its clinical course is characterized by exacerbations and remissions. It has no known specific cause, although research has focused on slow viral infections and autoimmune disturbances. Multiple sclerosis is much *more prevalent in cold and temperate climates* than in the tropics and subtropics, is *more* common in women than in men, and is predominantly a disease of young adults.

Answers 10.34–10.39

10.34 The answer is C

10.35 The answer is C

10.36 The answer is B

10.37 The answer is A

10.38 The answer is C

10.39 The answer is D

The differentiation between delirium and dementia can be difficult. Several clinical features help in the differentiation. In contrast to the sudden onset of delirium, dementia usually has an insidious onset. Although both conditions include cognitive impairment, the changes in dementia are relatively stable over time and do not fluctuate over the course of a day, for example. A patient with dementia is usually alert; a patient with delirium has episodes of clouding of consciousness. Both delirium and dementia are reversible, although delirium has a better chance of reversing if treatment is timely. *Insight*, defined as the awareness that one is mentally ill, is absent in both conditions. *Hallucinations* can occur in both conditions and must be differentiated from those that occur in schizophrenia. In general, the hallucinations of schizophrenic patients are more constant and better formed than are the hallucinations of delirious patients. *Sundowning* is observed in both demented and delirious patients. Sundowning is characterized by drowsiness, confusion, ataxia, and accidental falls just about bedtime. Kurt Goldstein described a *catastrophic reaction* in demented patients; it is marked by agitation secondary to the subjective awareness of one's intellectual deficits under stressful circumstances. The presence of delirium is a bad prognostic sign. Patients with delirium have a *high mortality rate*. The 3-month mortality rate of patients who have an episode of delirium is estimated to be 23 to 33 percent; the 1-year mortality rate may be as high as 50 percent. The major neurotransmitter hypothesized to be involved in delirium and dementia is acetylcholine. Several types of studies of delirium and dementia have shown a correlation between *decreased acetylcholine activity* in the brain and both delirium and dementia.

Answers 10.40–10.43

10.40 The answer is A

10.41 The answer is B

10.42 The answer is C

10.43 The answer is B

CT scanning and *MRI* have proved to be powerful neuropsychiatric research tools. Recent developments in MRI allow the direct measurement of structures such as the thalamus, basal ganglia, hippocampus, and amygdala, as well as temporal and apical areas of the brain and the structures of the posterior fossa. MRI has largely replaced CT as the most utilitarian and cost-effective method of imaging in neuropsychiatry. *Patients with acute cerebral hemorrhages or hematomas must continue to be assessed using CT,* but these patients present infrequently in psychiatric settings. *MRI better discriminates the interface between gray and white matter* and is useful in detecting a variety of white matter lesions in the periventricular and subcortical regions. The pathophysiological significance of such findings, designated by such terms as rims, caps, unidentified bright objects, and leukoariosis, remains to be defined. Such abnormalities are detected in younger patients with multiple sclerosis or HIV infection and in older patients with hypertension, vascular dementia, or dementia of the Alzheimer's type. However, their prevalence is also increased in healthy, aging individuals who have no defined disease processes. At present, those types of findings should be viewed in the same light as one would consider atrophic changes; namely, they are detected in a highly sensitive fashion but are usually nonspecific or nondiagnostic in meaning. White matter hyperintensities are more extensive and more frequent in individuals with disease, particularly those with disorders involving cognitive dysfunction, but they are too variable to contribute to the diagnosis or prognosis in an individual case. Like CT, *the greatest utility of MRI when used in the evaluation of patients with dementia* arises from what it may exclude (tumors, vascular disease) rather than what it can demonstrate specifically.

Because of MRI's ability to delineate brain anatomy and its sensitivity to white matter changes, these guidelines remain utilitarian when modified appropriately. Indications for ordering MRI in psychiatric patients include (1) delirium or dementia of unknown etiology; (2) a first episode of psychosis of unknown etiology; (3) a movement disorder of unknown etiology; (4) the initial evaluation of anorexia nervosa; (5) prolonged catatonia; (6) the initial onset of a major mood disorder or personality change after age 50 years; (7) the presence of unanticipated behavioral, intellectual, or functional decline in an already-diagnosed psychiatric patient in whom the clinician would normally expect long-term stability or, at worst, a relapsing-remitting course with a return to baseline between episodes; and (8) the presence of any new behavioral or intellectual disorder in a patient infected with HIV.

Imaging studies have been overused in the periodic monitoring or reassessment of patients with suspected dementia of the Alzheimer's type in whom earlier examinations showed characteristic cerebral changes. Unless one suspects a missed diagnosis such as of normal pressure hydrocephalus, or perhaps failure to detect microinfarctions on CT when such a finding on MRI might have ruled out Alzheimer's type, repeated scans are not warranted.

Occasional patients may become agitated in the MRI tube; premedication with a benzodiazepine can minimize the problem. The magnetic field *prohibits use of MRI in patients with pacemakers or metal implants*, including metallic surgical clips, although many patients now receive MRI-compatible clips at surgery.

Answers 10.44–10.50

10.44 The answer is B

10.45 The answer is A

10.46 The answer is A

10.47 The answer is A

10.48 The answer is B

10.49 The answer is B

10.50 The answer is A

Degenerative CNS diseases can be distinguished clinically from one another by the relative impairment and sparing of various cognitive and behavioral functions. *Two basic clinical patterns of dementia have been characterized clinically: cortical and subcortical.* The cortical pattern of dementia is characterized by impairments in memory (primarily a storage and recall deficit) and gnostic-practice abilities (primarily involving language, visuospatial abilities, calculation, and motor praxis). Executive or managerial functions such as organization, judgment, abstraction, emotional control or modulation, and insight and social judgment are similarly affected. *Fine and gross motor movements* are generally preserved until later in the disease course. Personality often remains intact or displays subtle variations, with patients becoming more passive or less spontaneous, or becoming coarse and crude in their interactions. With disease progression the changes in personality become more common and pronounced. Affective expression is generally preserved, although again a coarsening may be noted in the form of emotional lability. Early in the disease, patients frequently discern and express dismay about their intellectual decline.

The subcortical pattern is characterized by a generalized slowing of mental processing. Specific cognitive skills, such as *calculation, naming, or copying are less* affected initially, in contrast to their early decline in the cortical degenerative processes. Verbal and visual memory impairment may be present early in the course, although such impairment more often takes the form of forgetfulness or a failure of retrieval that is initially amenable to prompting, in contrast to the more severe recall deficits of cortical dementia. Patients also show deficits in learning new motor movements or complex psychomotor procedures. Planning and organizational skills are disrupted. Abnormal movements are common and manifest as a slowing and awkwardness in normal movement or as the intrusion of such extraneous movements as chorea or tremor. *In contrast to the early impairment of language function in cortical disease, language is relatively spared,* although the motor production of speech may be abnormal. The personality change is often marked, with striking patterns of apathy, inertia, and diminished spontaneity. Mood disorders, including major depression and mania, occur frequently. The presenting symptoms in subcortical degenerative processes may be those of a *personality change or a mood disorder* at a time when cognitive impairment or motor dysfunction is not yet obvious. In the cortical processes, by contrast, the presenting symptoms more often reflect *cognitive impairment,* particularly memory and language dysfunction. As the dementia and the degenerative process progress, the clinical presentations of cortical and subcortical diseases become nearly indistinguishable from one another.

The term subcortical dementia was first used to describe the cognitive and behavioral deficits seen in patients with *Huntington's disease.* A similar clinical pattern was soon described for other subcortical diseases, such as progressive supranuclear palsy and Parkinson's disease. Although the term was initially used in reference to a clinical picture that could be localized to the subcortex, *subcortical dementia is*

now considered a pseudoanatomical designation. It is clear from imaging and neuropathological studies that cortical dementia (e.g., *dementia of the Alzheimer's* type) is not restricted pathologically to the cortex; major affected cholinergic fiber pathways are subcortical in origin. Subcortical diseases similarly affect regions outside the subcortex, especially the frontal lobes, because of the brain's robust frontal-subcortical connections. Moreover, failure of subcortical nuclei that directly receive cortical efferent pathways can lead to clinical symptoms whose cerebral level of origin cannot be differentiated. Nonetheless, the cortical-subcortical distinction has been of clinical utility in defining patterns of cognitive, behavioral, mood, personality, and motor impairment, especially in the early stages of the degenerative disease process.

Answers 10.51–10.54

10.51 The answer is B

10.52 The answer is C

10.53 The answer is A

10.54 The answer is D

Secondary psychotic syndromes were categorized in DSM-II as psychoses associated with organic brain syndromes. The syndromes included in that category were the dementias, deliria, and psychoses associated with other cerebral and systemic conditions. Entry into the category depended on cognitive symptoms, such as disturbances of orientation, memory, judgment, and lability of affect. The term "psychosis" continued to be used for the sake of historic continuity, with the acknowledgment that "many patients for whom these diagnoses are clinically justified are not in fact psychotic." DSM-III improved on the nosology by establishing the general rubric of organic brain syndromes, with six specific syndromes, including organic hallucinosis and organic delusional syndrome. In DSM-IV-TR, psychotic disorder due to a general medical condition (with its available subtypes) has been moved out of the organic group to the phenomenological cluster to which it is related. This shift underscores the need for differential diagnosis, the clinical importance of defining etiology whenever possible, and the idea that primary psychopathology is idiopathic—that is, without known cause.

The differential diagnosis involves first establishing that the symptoms and signs encountered are in fact psychotic, according to the more specific modern definition. Confabulation may be mistaken for delusions. Confabulation is the spontaneous or prompted production of inconsistent and fabricated statements, often in response to questions or environmental stimuli. Although memory impairment is present in those who confabulate, the more salient cognitive deficit involves an inability to suppress or self-analyze the automatic fabrications and responses. Confabulation differs from delusions in that the fabricated beliefs are quite transient and varying. A behavioral response to the confabulated belief is usually absent. The presence of confabulation is also suggestive of brain disease, often involving the anterior temporal lobe (memory impairment) and the frontal lobes (loss of self-analysis). Perceptual disturbances that result in illusions or other misinterpretations of environ-

Table 10.3
Psychotic Symptoms Associated with Abnormality of Specific Brain Regions

Symptoms	Site	Laterality

First-rank symptoms
  Thoughts spoken aloud
  Voices commenting
  Third-person voices arguing
  Made actions
  Made feelings
  Thought withdrawal
  Thought diffusion
  Delusional perception
	Temporal lobe	Dominant hemisphere

Complex delusions	Subcortical or limbic	
Anton's syndrome	Occipital lobe, optic tract	Bilateral
Anosognosia	Parietal lobe	Nondominant hemisphere

Misidentification syndromes
  Capgras syndrome
  Reduplicative paramnesia
  Fregoli syndrome
  Intermetamorphosis syndrome
	Parietal, temporal, frontal lobes	Nondominant hemisphere, bilateral

mental stimuli must be distinguished from hallucination, which are experienced as true perceptual experiences, but without an actual stimulus.

Agnosias, or deficit syndromes, such as *prosopagnosia, topographic agnosia,* or *phonagnosia* (inability to recognize familiar faces, places, or sounds, respectively), can occur in the context of intact peripheral perception and can be mistaken

for delusional beliefs as well as *hallucinations.* It is important to distinguish these deficit syndromes and to recognize that *they point to parietal lobe dysfunctions* that are not associated with other psychotic symptoms. The phenomenology or type of psychotic symptom does not help distinguish idiopathic from secondary etiologies. However, once the suspicion of a secondary etiology has arisen, the specific psychotic presentation may suggest a particular brain region or direction for further investigation. Table 10.3 lists a number of specific psychotic symptoms that have been consistently associated with disease in particular brain regions. First-rank symptoms such as *auditory hallucinations,* originally described by Kurt Schneider as pathognomonic symptoms of schizophrenia, are now accepted as nonspecific psychotic symptoms occurring in all psychotic disorders. Although nonspecific for diagnosis, they have been associated with abnormalities in the left temporal lobe. *Complex delusions* have been associated with lesions in subcortical regions. Simple persecutory ideas are more common than complex or systematized delusions in patients with significant cognitive deficits. Patients apparently require a variety of intact intellectual abilities (and presumably underlying brain substrate) in order to produce psychotic symptoms of greater complexity. *Anton's syndrome* refers to denial of blindness, classically described in patients with acquired cortical blindness arising from bilateral occipital cortex damage. More recently, it has been described in patients with peripheral optic neuropathy, suggesting that the syndrome may be a variation of the other denial-of-deficit syndromes, such as anosognosia. *Misidentification syndromes,* such as anosognosia, have been described primarily in idiopathic psychotic disorders, although recent studies have pointed to nondominant parietal and frontal lesions as the basis for many. One recent neuropsychological theory proposes that the right hemisphere plays a role in the appreciation of the individuality or uniqueness of people, places, and objects, and that lesions in the right hemisphere can result in delusions of misidentification.

11 ▲

Neuropsychiatric Aspects of Human Immunodeficiency Virus (HIV) Infection and Acquired Immune Deficiency Syndrome (AIDS)

Psychiatrists play an important role in the diagnosis, treatment, and management of HIV-positive people and people with AIDS. Not infrequently, psychiatrists are the first physicians to make the diagnosis, and are then often fundamentally involved in treating and managing the psychological, emotional, and neuropsychiatric sequelae of the conditions.

With the advent of revolutionary new treatments, many HIV-positive people and people with AIDS are now able to live longer and more symptom-free lives. For these patients, the conditions have taken on the qualities of living with a chronic but manageable illness. However, as effective as many of these new treatments seem to be, there are still many complicated and difficult issues. Many treatments have uncomfortable and even disabling side effects. Many people do not have access to the treatments due to prohibitive cost, ignorance, or lifestyle issues that make compliance with the rigorous and complicated regimens untenable. There has been much commentary on the concern that younger at-risk people are once again engaging in high-risk behaviors out of ignorance and the misperception that the conditions have been cured. While much progress has been made, much work obviously still needs to be done. AIDS is still an illness that kills people.

Psychiatrists must be part of the multidisciplinary team that works with people with HIV-related disorders. This team will include infectious disease specialists, social workers, nurses, and others. Public education campaigns have been helpful and have resulted in significant reductions in high-risk behaviors, and thus in new infections. These campaigns must continue to reach new generations of people at risk.

All clinicians must be knowledgeable about and comfortable with discussing the issues of AIDS and HIV infection with their patients and patients' significant others and families.

The student should study the questions and answers below for a useful review of all of these topics.

HELPFUL HINTS

The following terms should be known by the student.

- ▶ AIDS dementia complex
- ▶ AIDS in children
- ▶ astrocytes
- ▶ AZT
- ▶ *Candida albicans*
- ▶ CNS infections
- ▶ confidentiality
- ▶ ddI
- ▶ ELISA
- ▶ false-positives
- ▶ high-risk groups
- ▶ HIV encephalopathy
- ▶ HIV-1 and HIV-2
- ▶ institutional care
- ▶ Kaposi's sarcoma
- ▶ neuropsychiatric syndromes

- ▶ *Pneumocystis carinii* pneumonia
- ▶ pretest and posttest counseling
- ▶ protease inhibitors
- ▶ psychopharmacology
- ▶ psychotherapy
- ▶ retrovirus
- ▶ safe sex guidelines
- ▶ seropositive
- ▶ T4 lymphocytes
- ▶ *Toxoplasma gondii* and *Cryptococcus neoformans*
- ▶ transmission
- ▶ tuberculosis
- ▶ wasting syndrome
- ▶ Western blot analysis
- ▶ worried well

▲ QUESTIONS

DIRECTIONS: Each of the questions or incomplete statements below is followed by five suggested responses or completions. Select the *one* that is *best* in each case.

11.1 In persons infected by HIV

   A. seroconversion usually occurs 2 weeks after infection

   B. the estimated length of time from infection to the development of AIDS is 5 years

   C. 10 percent have neuropsychiatric complications

   D. the T4-lymphocyte count usually falls to abnormal levels during the asymptomatic period

   E. the majority are infected by HIV type 2 (HIV-2)

11.2 In the treatment of HIV and HIV-related disorder

   A. Azidothymidine (AZT) acts by inhibiting the adherence of glycoprotein-120 (GP-120) to the CD4 receptor on T4 lymphocytes.

   B. AZT has caused increased neuropsychiatric symptoms.

   C. Patients taking haloperidol (Haldol) have decreased sensitivity to the drug's extrapyramidal effects.

   D. The entire range of psychotherapeutic approaches may by appropriate.

   E. Pentamidine is used prophylactically to guard against the development of *Cryptosporidium* infection.

11.3 In a test for HIV

   A. Assays usually detect the presence of viral proteins.

   B. The enzyme-linked immunosorbent assay (ELISA) is used to confirm positive test results of the Western blot analysis.

   C. The results cannot be shared with other members of a medical treatment team.

   D. Pretest counseling should not inquire why a person desires HIV testing.

   E. A person may have a true-negative result, even if the person is infected by HIV.

11.4 Diseases affecting the central nervous system (CNS) in patients with AIDS include

   A. atypical aseptic meningitis

   B. *Candida albicans* abscess

   C. primary CNS lymphoma

   D. cerebrovascular infarction

   E. all of the above

11.5 The multinucleated giant cells shown in Figure 11.1 are part of a neuropathological picture that includes diffuse astrocytosis, microglial nodules, and white matter vacuolation and demyelination in this HIV-positive patient. This neuropathology is consistent with a diagnosis of

   A. *Toxoplasma gondii* infection

   B. primary central nervous system (CNS) lymphoma

   C. HIV encephalopathy

   D. metastatic Kaposi's sarcoma

   E. cryptococcal meningitis

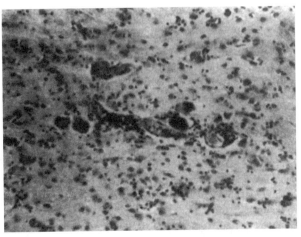

FIGURE 11.1

Reprinted with permission from Pajeau AK, Roman GC. HIV encephalopathy and dementia. *Psychiatr Clin North Am.* 1992; 15:461.

11.6 Clinical symptoms associated with this patient's diagnosis include all of the following *except*

   A. early-onset aphasia

   B. mood and personality changes

   C. hyperreflexia and paraparesis

   D. psychomotor slowing

   E. problems with memory and concentration

11.7 Mild neurocognitive deficits associated with HIV infection

   A. include attentional problems, slowing of information processing, and deficiencies in learning

   B. do not suggest selective involvement of subcortical structures

   C. are often characterized by confabulatory responses on formal memory testing

   D. do not occur independently of depression or anxiety

   E. are rarely associated with difficulties in abstract reasoning

11.8 Mania in people with AIDS

   A. may have a rate of up to ten times the general population rates

   B. may be precipitated by steroids, zidovudine, and ganciclovir

   C. is associated with personal or family history of bipolar I disorder, if the onset is early in HIV illness

   D. is associated with a higher prevalence of comorbid dementia if the onset is late in the course of HIV illness, and there is no personal or family history of mood disorders

   E. all of the above

11.9 Psychotic symptoms associated with HIV infection

   A. are usually early-stage complications

   B. are rare

   C. most often take the form of persecutory, grandiose, or somatic delusions

   D. rarely are associated with bizarre behavior

   E. are also associated with frequent and specific neurological findings

11.10 Protease inhibitors can increase plasma levels of all of the following *except*

  A. bupropion
  B. fluoxetine
  C. alprazolam and zolpidem
  D. nefazodone
  E. depakote

11.11 True statements associated with the treatment of delirium in HIV illness include

  A. There is no increased incidence of extrapyramidal symptoms associated with high-potency typical agents in advanced HIV illness.
  B. Patients with underlying HIV-associated dementia do not appear to be at higher risk for medication-induced movement disorders.
  C. The use of benzodiazepines alone appears to be effective in delirious states.
  D. Symptoms of delirium in HIV illness can be managed effectively with low-potency antipsychotics such as chlorpromazine.
  E. None of the above

11.12 Potential complications in the treatment of mania in patients with AIDS include

  A. Lithium and antipsychotic medications may be poorly tolerated by individuals with HIV-related neurocognitive disorders.
  B. Valproate is usually poorly tolerated by individuals with evidence of brain atrophy on MRI.
  C. The gastrointestinal disturbances associated with AIDS (e.g., vomiting and diarrhea) rarely affect lithium absorption or excretion.
  D. Carbamazepine may increase serum concentrations of protease inhibitors.
  E. Protease inhibitors increase valproate concentrations.

11.13 True statements about the association of suicide and HIV disease include

  A. Studies suggest that patients with advanced HIV disease have a 30-fold risk of committing suicide compared to matched seronegative persons.
  B. Some reports indicate that high-risk seronegative persons have an elevated lifetime prevalence of suicidal ideation and attempt compared to community controls.
  C. Psychiatric disorder is strongly implicated in suicidal ideation and attempted suicide.
  D. HIV-infected adolescents are at a particularly high risk for suicide.
  E. All of the above

11.14 Neuropathic pain related to HIV

  A. is generally more effectively treated with SSRIs than with tricyclic antidepressants
  B. is rarely effectively treated with opioid analgesics
  C. is not effectively managed with anticonvulsants such as phenytoin (Dilantin) or carbamazepine (Tegretol)
  D. should not be treated with acetaminophen (Tylenol), because it may diminish the metabolism of zidovudine
  E. all of the above

ANSWERS

Neuropsychiatric Aspects of HIV Infection and AIDS

11.1 The answer is D

The T4-lymphocyte count usually falls to abnormal levels during the asymptomatic period of HIV infection. The normal values are greater than 1,000/mm³ and grossly abnormal values can be fewer than 200/mm³.

Seroconversion is the change after infection with HIV from a negative HIV antibody test result to a positive HIV antibody test result. *Seroconversion usually occurs 6 to 12 weeks after infection.* In rare cases, seroconversion can take 6 to 12 months. The estimated length of *time from infection to the development of AIDS is 8 to 11 years*, although that time is gradually increasing because of the early implementation of treatment. *At least 50 percent* of HIV-infected patients *have neuropsychiatric complications,* which may be the first signs of the disease in about 10 percent of patients. At least two types of HIV have been identi-

fied, HIV type 1 (HIV-1) and HIV type 2 (HIV-2). *The majority of HIV-positive patients are infected by HIV-1.* However, HIV-2 infection seems to be increasing in Africa.

11.2 The answer is D

The entire range of psychotherapeutic approaches may be appropriate in the treatment of HIV and HIV-related disorders. Treatment with *AZT does not cause increased neuropsychiatric symptoms,* rather, it prevents or reverses the neuropsychiatric symptoms associated with HIV encephalopathy. Although dopamine receptor antagonists such as haloperidol (Haldol) may be required for control of agitation, they should be used in as low dosage as possible because *patients taking haloperidol have increased sensitivity to the drug's extrapyramidal effects.* Also, the prophylactic use of aerosolized *pentamidine (NebuPent)* and of trimethoprim (Bactrim) and sulfamethoxazole (Gantanol) against the development of *Pneumocystis carinii* is now in common practice. Aerosolized *pentamidine is not used prophylacti-*

Table 11.1
Pretest HIV Counseling

1. Discuss the meaning of a positive result and clarify distortions (e.g., the test detects exposure to the AIDS virus; it is not a test for AIDS).
2. Discuss the meaning of a negative result (e.g., seroconversion requires time, recent high-risk behavior may require follow-up testing).
3. Be available to discuss the patient's fears and concerns (unrealistic fears may require appropriate psychological intervention).
4. Discuss why the test is necessary (not all patients will admit to high-risk behaviors).
5. Explore the patient's potential reactions to a positive result (e.g. "I'll kill myself if I'm positive"). Take appropriate necessary steps to intervene in a potentially catastrophic reaction.
6. Explore past reactions to severe stresses.
7. Discuss the confidentiality issues relevant to the testing situation (e.g., is it an anonymous or nonanonymous setting?). Inform the patient of other possible testing options where the counseling and testing can be done completely anonymously (e.g., where the result is not made a permanent part of a hospital chart). Discuss who has access to the test results.
8. Discuss with the patient how being seropositive can potentially affect social status (e.g., health and life insurance coverage, employment, housing).
9. Explore high-risk behaviors and recommend risk-reducing interventions.
10. Document discussions in chart.
11. Allow the patient time to ask questions.

Reprinted with permission from Rosse RB, Giese AA, Deutsch SI, Morihisa JM. *Laboratory and Diagnostic Testing in Psychiatry.* Washington, DC: American Psychiatric Press; 1989:55.

cally to guard against the development of Cryptosporidium, which causes intermittent or severe watery diarrhea, primarily in HIV-positive homosexual men.

11.3 The answer is E

A person may have a true negative result, even if the person is infected by HIV, if the test takes place after infection but before seroconversion. *Assays do not usually detect the presence of viral proteins. The enzyme-linked immunosorbent assay (ELISA) is not used to confirm positive test results of the Western blot analysis.* Rather, the ELISA is used as an initial screening test because it is less expensive than the Western blot analysis and more easily used to screen a large number of samples. The ELISA is sensitive and reasonably specific; although it is unlikely to report a false-negative result, it may indicate a false-positive result. For that reason, positive results from an ELISA are confirmed by using the more expensive and cumbersome Western blot analysis, which is sensitive and specific.

Confidentiality is a key issue in serum testing. No persons should be given HIV tests without their prior knowledge and consent, although various jurisdictions and organizations (for example, the military) now require HIV testing for all their inhabitants or members. *The results can be shared with other members of a medical treatment team* but should be provided to no one else.

Any person who wants to be screened should probably be tested, although *pretest counseling should inquire why a person desires HIV testing* to detect unspoken concerns and motivations that may merit psychotherapeutic intervention. Table 11.1 lists general guidelines for HIV testing and counseling.

Table 11.2
Diseases Affecting the CNS in Patients with AIDS

Primary viral diseases
  HIV encephalopathy
  Atypical aseptic meningitis
  Vacuolar myelopathy
Secondary viruses (encephalitis, myelitis, retinitis, vasculitis)
  Cytomegalovirus
  Herpes simplex virus types 1 and 2
  Herpes varicella-zoster virus
  Papovavirus (PML)
Nonviral infections (encephalitis, meningitis, abscess)
  Toxoplasma gondii
  Cryptococcus neoformans
  Candida albicans
  Histoplasma capsulatum
  Aspergillus fumigatus
  Coccidioides immitis
  Acremonium albamensis
  Rhizopus species
  Mycobacterium avium-intracellulare
  Mycobacterium tuberculosis hominis
  Mycobacterium kansasii
  Listeria monocytogenes
  Nocardia asteroides
Neoplasms
  Primary CNS lymphoma
  Metastatic systemic lymphoma
  Metastatic Kaposi's sarcoma
Cerebrovascular diseases
  Infarction
  Hemorrhage
  Vasculitis
Complications of systemic therapy

Reprinted with permission from Beckett A. The neurobiology of human immunodeficiency virus infection. In: Tasman A, Goldfinger SM, Kaufman CA, eds. *American Psychiatric Press Review of Psychiatry.* Vol 9. Washington: American Psychiatric Press; 1990:595.

11.4 The answer is E (all)

Most of the infections secondary to HIV involvement of the central nervous system (CNS) are viral or fungal. *Atypical aseptic meningitis,* Candida albicans *abscess, primary CNS lymphoma,* and *cerebrovascular infarction* can all affect a patient with AIDS. Table 11.2 lists the most common diseases affecting the CNS in patients with AIDS.

11.5 The answer is C

The neuropathology described for this patient is consistent with a diagnosis of *HIV encephalopathy.* HIV enters the CNS, where it infects primarily glial cells, particularly astrocytes. The virus is also harbored within immune cells in the CNS. The neuropathology of HIV encephalopathy is characterized by multinucleated giant cells, microglial nodules, diffuse astrocytosis, perivascular lymphocyte cuffing, cortical atrophy, and white matter vacuolation and demyelination. The severely disabled cellular immune system of HIV-infected patients permits the development of a staggering array of infections and neoplasms. The most common infections are from protozoa such as *Toxoplasma gondii,* fungi such as *Cryptococcus neoformans* and *Candida albicans*, bacteria such as *Mycobacterium avium-cellulare*, and viruses such as cytomegatovirus and herpes simplex. *Kaposi's sarcoma* is a skin cancer related to HIV infection, which can metastasize. CNS neoplasms, such as *lymphomas*, are not uncommon.

11.6 The answer is A

HIV encephalopathy is a subacute encephalitis that results in a progressive subcortical dementia without focal neurological signs. The major differentiating feature between subcortical dementia and cortical dementia is the absence of classical cortical symptoms (for example, *aphasia*) until late in the illness. Patients with HIV encephalitis or their friends usually notice *subtle mood and personality changes, problems with memory and concentration*, and some *psychomotor slowing*. The presence of motor symptoms may also suggest a diagnosis of HIV encephalopathy. Motor symptoms associated with subcortical dementia include *hyperreflexia*, spastic or ataxic gait, *paraparesis*, and increased muscle tone.

11.7 The answer is A

A person experiencing mild neurocognitve disorder associated with HIV infection will typically have some difficulty concentrating, may experience unusual fatigability when engaged in demanding mental tasks, may feel subjectively slowed down, and may notice *difficulty in remembering*. Such persons may say that they are not as sharp or as quick as they once were.

Such a set of presenting complaints, especially in younger individuals who may be struggling to accept their seropositive status, may lead the clinician to conclude *that anxiety, depression*, or hypochondriasis is responsible. Although affective features are occasionally the best explanation for such complaints, that is not generally the case. Rather, comprehensive neuropsychological testing may reveal that the individual does indeed have difficulties with speeded information processing, divided attention, and sustained effortful processing as well as deficiencies in learning and recalling new information.

Some individuals with mild neurocognitive disorder also have difficulties with tasks involving problem solving and *abstract reasoning*, and there may also be slowing of simple motor performance (e.g., speed of finger tapping). Verbal skills are less affected, although there may be some decrement in fluency (e.g., quickly reciting as many animals as possible or as many words beginning with a particular letter as possible).

These neuropsychological findings, which emphasize *attentional problems, slowing of information processing*, and *deficiencies in learning*, are reminiscent of neuropsychological patterns seen in patients with so-called subcortical dementias (e.g., Huntington's disease and Parkinson's disease). Fine-grained analysis of memory breakdown in HIV-infected persons also confirms a subcortical pattern. For example, persons with HIV-associated cognitive disorders have difficulty recalling words from a list, but do not make intrusion errors (i.e., *confabulatory responses*) the way patients with cortical dementias (e.g., dementia of the Alzheimer's type) tend to do. Neuropsychological features that suggest *selective involvement of subcortical structures* are consistent with neuropathological findings. It is important to stress that these mild neurocognitive deficits occur independently of depression, anxiety, and other non-HIV sources of cognitive deficit.

11.8 The answer is E (all)

Mood disorders with manic features, with or without hallucinations, delusions, or a disorder of thought process can complicate any stage of HIV infection, but most commonly occur in late-stage disease complicated by neurocognitive impairment.

Precise estimates of prevalence or incidence of mania are not available but may approach 1 percent. *Some evidence suggests the rate in AIDS is up to ten times the general population rates.*

In non–HIV-infected patients, mood disorders with manic features are noted to occur at therapeutic dosages of many medications and in a wide variety of neurological conditions, such as cerebrovascular disorder, meningitis, and tumor, and these sources can also be causative in HIV illness. *Steroids, zidovudine, and ganciclovir are the most frequently reported iatrogenic causes.* There are two typical onsets of mania in HIV. *Manic states with onset early in HIV are associated with personal or family history of bipolar I disorder.* Manic syndromes in persons without previous personal or family history of mood disorder usually have their onset late in the course of HIV illness and have a higher prevalence of comorbid dementia; in these cases the etiology is presumed to be related to the pathophysiology of HIV infection of the CNS.

11.9 The answer is C

Psychotic symptoms are usually later-stage complications of HIV infection. They require immediate medical and neurological evaluation and often require management with antipsychotic medications. Whereas psychotic symptoms can obviously occur in deliria or can reflect neurological or primary psychiatric disorders or iatrogenic origins, there is also considerable interest in new-onset psychosis, wherein these etiologies do not seem to be present (e.g., psychotic disorder due to HIV disease).

Prevalence estimates vary widely depending on methodology: large-scale surveys find a prevalence of new-onset psychosis at less than 0.5 percent whereas chart review methods find frequencies ranging from 3 to 15 percent in persons for whom obvious causes (e.g., delirium) have been excluded. Thus, *psychotic symptoms may be uncommon, but not rare* in HIV-infected populations.

The clinical presentation in new-onset psychosis is extremely variable. The most prevalent symptom seems to be *delusions* (occurring in almost 90 percent of cases in some series) with *persecutory, grandiose*, or *somatic* components. Persecutory themes can be quite elaborate, with patients proclaiming messianic themes or believing that they have been accorded superhuman powers by God. Somatic delusions may include being shot through with electricity or lasers. Delusions of thought insertion, thought broadcasting, and of passivity and control are also described. Most patients experience auditory hallucinations, with perhaps one-half of those also experiencing visual hallucinations. A majority of series also report disorders of thought process, including looseness of associations or frankly disorganized thinking. Disturbances of mood commonly coexist, with anxiety being the most prevalent symptom, followed by depressed mood, euphoria, or irritability, and mixed depressed and euphoric states. Lability, flatness, and inappropriate laughter or anger are also described; *bizarre behavior is commonplace*. There are reports of persons eating dirt to conquer their fear of germs, and one patient painted himself and his entire apartment, including furniture and appliances, with green paint in an effort to "celebrate life."

Table 11.3
Antiretroviral Agents

Generic Name	Trade Name	Usual Abbreviation
Nucleoside reverse transcriptase inhibitors		
Zidovudine	Retrovir	AZT or ZDV
Didanosine	Videx	ddI
Zalcitabine	Hivid	ddC
Stavudine	Zerit	d4T
Lamivudine	Epivir	3TC
Abacavir	Ziagen	
Nonnucleoside reverse transcriptase inhibitors		
Nevirapine	Viramune	
Delavirdine	Rescriptor	
Efavirenz	Sustiva	
Protease inhibitors		
Saquinavir	Invirase	
Ritonavir	Norvir	
Indinavir	Crixivan	
Nelfinavir	Viracept	

Bedside examination reveals impairment in memory or other cognitive functions in perhaps one-third of patients; more comprehensive and formal neuropsychological assessment would be likely to detect neurocognitive difficulties in a larger proportion of cases, but many psychotic individuals are unable to complete such examinations.

Neurological findings are infrequent and nonspecific, usually consisting of ataxia, mild increases in motor tone, hyperreflexia, and tremor, but bizarre grimacing and posturing can also be present. Cerebrospinal fluid is generally unremarkable except for the mild pleocytosis common to HIV infection. Diffuse cortical slowing has been reported in about one-half of patients on whom an EEG was performed. CT and MR scans reveal nonspecific cerebral atrophy in about one-half of cases; rarely, focal abnormalities are evident, suggesting tumor, opportunistic infection, or vascular etiology.

11.10 The answer is E
A growing list of agents that act at different points of viral replication has raised for the first time the hope that HIV can be permanently suppressed or actually eradicated from the body. At the time of this writing, the active agents were in two general classes: the reverse transcriptase inhibitors and the protease inhibitors. The reverse transcriptase inhibitors are further subdivided into the nucleoside reverse transcriptase inhibitor group and the nonnucleoside reverse transcriptase inhibitors. Table 11.3 lists the currently available agents in each of these three categories.

The antiretroviral agents have many adverse effects, too numerous to describe. Of importance to psychiatrists is that protease inhibitors are metabolized by the hepatic cytochrome P-450 oxidase system, and can therefore increase levels of certain psychotropic drugs that are similarly metabolized. These include *bupropion* (Wellbutrin), meperidine (Demerol), various benzodiazepines, and selective serotonin reuptake inhibitors (SSRIs). Therefore, prescribing psychotropic drugs to persons taking protease inhibitors must be done with caution.

All protease inhibitors will increase psychotropic drug concentrations if the major route of metabolism of the psychotropic agent is the 3 cytochrome P450 (CYP) CYP 3A system. If the CYP 2D6 system is the primary route of metabolism (e.g., tricyclic medica-

tions, SSRIs), ritonavir (Norvir) will specifically inhibit their metabolism. Thus the protease inhibitors may inhibit the metabolism of many antidepressants and antipsychotic agents as well as benzodiazepines. For example, plasma concentrations of *alprazolam* (Xanax), midazolam (Versed), triazolam (Ilalcion), and *zolpidem* (Ambien), may be increased and dosage reduction and careful monitoring may be required to prevent oversedation or other toxic effects. Protease inhibitors have been reported to increase concentrations of bupropion, *nefazodone* (Serzone), and *fluoxetine* (Prozac) to toxic levels, and to increase desipramine plasma concentrations by 100 to 150 percent. Drug interactions with antipsychotic agents are less well studied, but here ritonavir particularly may increase concentrations. Concentrations of methadone and meperidine are also reported to be elevated. Additionally, concentrations of some drugs of abuse such as methylenedioxymethamphetamine (MDMA) may be increased. In turn, protease inhibitors may induce the metabolism of valproate (*Depakene*) and of lorazepam (Ativan) and lead to *lower plasma concentrations*.

Some psychotropic medications may induce metabolism of protease inhibitors. Carbamazepine and phenobarbital may reduce serum concentrations of protease inhibitors. The clinical relevance of this potential interaction is not clear, but use of an alternate mood stabilizer may be indicated. Interactions with lithium (Eskalith) and gabapentin (Neurontin) have not been reported.

Finally, psychotropic drugs may reduce the metabolism of some protease inhibitors, with an increase of protease inhibitor adverse effects; this has been reported with *nefazodone* and fluoxetine.

11.11 The answer is D
Symptoms of delirium in HIV illness can be managed effectively with modest dosages of either low-potency antipsychotic agents, such as chlorpromazine at 10 to 25 mg once to three times daily, or with high-potency agents, such as haloperidol (Haldol) at 0.25 mg to 5 mg once to three times daily, or with atypical serotonin-dopamine agonists, including risperidone (Risperdal) at 0.5 mg to 2 mg daily, or olanzapine (Zyprexa) at 10 mg daily. There may well be *an increased incidence of extrapyramidal symptoms* associated with high-potency typical agents in advanced HIV illness, and *patients with underlying HIV-associated dementia appear to be at higher risk for medication-induced movement disorders*. For patients who do not respond to low-dosage oral therapy, excellent results have been reported with intravenous haloperidol given in individual boluses ranging from up to 2 to 10 mg every hour. Some clinicians have also had good results with a combination of intravenous haloperidol and lorazepam, with an average daily intravenous dose of less than 50 mg of haloperidol and 10 mg of lorazepam. In general, no serious adverse effects have been noted with those more aggressive intravenous regimens, although nearly one-half of the patients treated may have extrapyramidal symptoms and extreme care must be utilized.

Benzodiazepines alone (e.g., lorazepam) do not appear to be effective in delirious states and they may accentuate confusion.

11.12 The answer is A
For immediate control of manic excitement up to 10 mg of clonazepam (Klonopin) daily is effective in many instances although the risk for disinhibition or delirium must always be monitored. If psychotic features are present, low doses of antipsychotic agents, such as risperidone at 0.5 to 2 mg daily, olanzapine up to 10 mg daily, chlorpromazine at 25 to 150 mg daily, or haloperidol at

0.5 to 5 mg daily, may be employed. For longer-term management lithium is effective but may not be as well tolerated as is carbamazepine and valproate (depakene). For example, *in some studies lithium and antipsychotic medications are poorly tolerated* by individuals with HIV-associated neurocognitive disorders, especially if brain MRI abnormalities are present (e.g., atrophy), whereas *valproate* (dosage range, 750 to 1,750 mg daily; plasma concentration >50 μg per mL) is more successful. Good control is usually possible within 7 days, and treatment gains have been maintained for up to 4-year follow-up. Lithium has been used to treat patients who develop manic syndromes as an adverse effect of zidovudine, with good control of symptoms, which allows a patient to continue antiretroviral therapy. It may be that valproic acid and carbamazepine would be effective in these iatrogenic manias.

In HIV-infected patients treated with lithium for the control of bipolar I disorder care must be taken to monitor lithium concentrations closely, especially if the patient has significant *gastrointestinal disturbances* (e.g., vomiting and diarrhea) that may affect lithium absorption and excretion. *Carbamazepine may reduce serum concentrations of protease inhibitors, and these agents themselves may lower valproate concentrations.*

11.13 The answer is E (all)

Studies based on coroners' reports suggest that *patients with advanced HIV disease have a 30-fold risk of committing suicide* compared to seronegative persons matched for age and social position. Some survey reports indicate that seronegative persons who are in a high-risk group for HIV infection, as well as seropositive persons at all stages of HIV infection, have *an elevated lifetime prevalence of suicidal ideation and suicide attempt* compared with community controls. It is important to note that both sources of data suggest that *psychiatric disorder is strongly implicated in suicide, attempted suicide, and suicidal ideation.* Psychological autopsies from coroners' cases have identified psychiatric histories in almost 50 percent of cases. Suicide attempt and suicidal ideation are correlated with histories of major depressive disorder or substance-related disorders, and in over half of cases these suicidal behaviors commenced before the likely date of seroconversion. Conflicts about sexual orientation may be associated with suicide attempts by adolescents. This, together with the increase in HIV infection in adolescents, may place *HIV-infected youths at particularly high risk.* Suicide rates in women are not noted to be elevated, but the epidemic is now just starting to affect large numbers of women, and their greater vulnerability to major depressive disorder may mean that women are at increased risk. Advances in therapy may heighten hope and reduce the risk of suicide. However, those whose hopes are first raised but who then do not respond to or cannot tolerate these agents may require psychotherapeutic intervention. Thus, while debate over the distinction between suicide and the right to choose death or to refuse unwanted treatment are important issues, it is imperative that persons expressing suicidal behaviors or ideas be examined for a major psychiatric disorder and be offered appropriate treatment.

11.14 The answer is D

Pain probably remains the most underrecognized and undertreated symptom in HIV disease, as it is in other life-threatening illnesses, such as cancer. Undertreatment of pain is especially prevalent in injection drug users. The etiology and pathogenesis of pain in HIV-related disorders is just beginning to be understood. Psychiatric disorders may complicate persisting pain, and, because no one specialty addresses pain syndromes, patient care is often fragmented between anesthesiologists, neurologists, internists, and psychiatrists.

Neuropathic pain related to HIV usually presents as a persisting, painful sensorimotor neuropathy with dysesthesia, stocking-glove sensory loss, diminished distal reflexes, and distal weakness. Similarly, postherpetic neuralgia (herpes zoster radiculitis) may involve pain of the face or trunk. Treatment of neuropathic pain syndromes is usually with low-dosage tricyclic antidepressant agents, such as desipramine or nortriptyline at 10 to 25 mg a day. The typical steady-state dosage is 50 mg a day, although some patients require higher amounts (75 to 100 mg daily). A response will often ensue within 1 to 2 weeks, but 4 to 6 weeks of treatment may be necessary before response occurs or another tricyclic agent is chosen. In general, *tricyclic antidepressants are more effective than SSRIs* for chronic neuropathic pain. *Opioid analgesics* are also useful. *Anticonvulsants* such as phenytoin (Dilantin) or carbamazepine, at usual therapeutic concentrations required for seizure management, may also be effective. Postherpetic neuralgia may likewise be treated with topical capsaicin (Dolorac) and may respond to clonazepam at 1 to 5 mg daily.

Chronic headache may appear as a residual symptom from acute aseptic meningitis in seroconversion illness or as an effect of zidovudine (which may persist after drug discontinuation). It is known that imipramine, desipramine, amitriptyline, and nortriptyline can be effective in treating migraine and mixed migraine–tension headache syndromes in non-HIV populations, and there is speculation that persisting headache following aseptic meningitis may also respond to low-dosage regimens of these agents (e.g., nortriptyline or desipramine at 10 to 25 mg daily with increases up to 75 mg).

Among the rheumatological disorders are arthralgias, myalgias, and arthritides involving large joints of the leg. HIV-related arthralgias may respond to nonsteroidal antiinflammatory agents, although *acetaminophen (Tylenol) should be avoided* because it may diminish the metabolism of zidovudine. HIV may also be associated with a polymyositis, which involves pain, weakness, and elevated CPK, along with changes on electromyography indicating a myopathic process. Long-term administration of zidovudine may also produce a myositis that persists when the medication is discontinued. Psychopharmacological interventions are not of demonstrated efficacy in these states.

Multidisciplinary pain-treatment approaches, which employ coordinated efforts of experts in various disciplines, may be as useful in chronic HIV-related pain as they are in chronic, non-HIV pain syndromes. Such approaches employ education about the nature of persisting pain, activity scheduling, self-monitoring and relaxation training, and cognitive therapies to reduce disability related to pain.

Finally, studies of acute postoperative pain and chronic cancer pain generally indicate that for those conditions in which opiate analgesia is indicated, those medications are often underprescribed, or irrationally prescribed, in subtherapeutic doses at too extended an interval. The clinician should always be alert to that possibility in advanced HIV disease.

12 ▲

Substance-Related Disorders

Comorbidity between psychiatric disorders and substance-related disorders is very common, each complicating the presentation of the other. People with substance-related disorders frequently exhibit psychiatric signs and symptoms, and those with psychiatric disorders often abuse substances. It may be difficult to determine if a person is self-medicating psychiatric symptoms (such as depression, anxiety, or auditory hallucinations), or if the substance use has led to the symptoms. The opportunity for a vicious cycle to be set up is obvious. Also obvious is that substances can cause neuropsychiatric symptoms that are indistinguishable from those of common psychiatric disorders with no known causes. This observation can then be taken to suggest that psychiatric disorders and disorders involving the use of brain-altering substances are related. The study of brain-altering chemicals can provide important clues regarding how the brain functions in both normal and abnormal states.

Diagnosing a psychiatric disorder in the context of substance abuse can be complicated. Was the person depressed and anxious before the alcohol or drug abuse started, or did the mood disorder develop as the result of ongoing use? Is the person who experiences paranoia and hallucinations suffering from a primary psychotic disorder, or are the symptoms the result of chronic methamphetamine or other drug abuse? A careful and detailed chronological history of symptom development and its relationship to substance use is critical to clarifying diagnosis. However, even with this, questions about primary diagnosis can remain.

What does seem clear is that substance abuse worsens the course, prognosis, and presentation of any preexisting psychiat-

ric disorder. The schizophrenic patient abusing crack, or the depressed patient abusing cocaine or benzodiazepines, will undoubtedly be more impaired than the patient who is not. In fact, most experienced clinicians would agree that effectively treating any psychiatric disorder in the context of ongoing substance abuse is not possible.

Clinicians need to be clear about the definitions of addiction, dependence, abuse, tolerance, cross-tolerance, intoxication, and withdrawal. Dependence is currently the preferred term to addiction, but both imply a psychological and physical reliance on a drug or alcohol that leads to substance-seeking behavior, an inability to stop using, an increasing tolerance to its effects, and a deterioration in physical and mental health as a result of continued use.

Tolerance is the need for increased amounts of the substance to achieve the desired effect. Cross-tolerance is when tolerance to one substance develops as the result of tolerance to another. The cross-tolerance of alcohol and benzodiazepines is the reason benzodiazepines are often used in the clinically controlled withdrawal from alcohol. Tolerance may differ in people of different ethnic backgrounds. Substance abuse is a pattern of abuse that is problematic but may or may not lead to dependence. Intoxication and withdrawal syndromes are unique to the specific substance involved.

Each substance-related disorder has its own definition, epidemiology, and clinical features, and skilled clinicians must be knowledgeable about each one.

The student should study the questions and answers below for a useful review of these disorders.

HELPFUL HINTS

The student should know each of the terms below and the revised fourth edition *Diagnostic and Statistical Manual of Mental Disorders* (DSM-IV-TR) diagnostic criteria.

- AA
- abuse
- addiction
- AIDS
- Al-Anon
- alcohol delirium
- alcohol psychotic disorder
- alcohol withdrawal

- amotivational syndrome
- anabolic
- anabolic steroids
- anticholinergic side effects
- arylcyclohexylamine
- belladonna alkaloids
- binge drinking

- blackouts
- caffeine
- cocaine delirium
- cocaine intoxication and withdrawal
- cocaine psychotic disorder
- codependence
- comorbidity

- cross-tolerance
- DEA
- delta alcohol dependence
- dementia
- dispositional tolerance
- disulfiram
- DMT
- DOM

- ► DPT
- ► drug-seeking behavior
- ► DSM-IV-TR course modifiers
- ► DTS
- ► dual diagnosis
- ► fetal alcohol syndrome
- ► flashback
- ► freebase
- ► gamma alcohol dependence
- ► hallucinogen
- ► hallucinogen persisting perception disorder
- ► idiosyncratic alcohol intoxication

- ► illicit drug use
- ► inhalant intoxication
- ► ketamine
- ► Korsakoff's and Wernicke's syndromes
- ► LAMM
- ► LSD
- ► MDMA
- ► methadone withdrawal
- ► miosis
- ► misuse
- ► MPTP-induced parkinsonism
- ► mydriasis
- ► nicotine receptor
- ► NIDA
- ► nitrous oxide

- ► opiate
- ► opioid
- ► opioid antagonists
- ► opioid intoxication
- ► opioid withdrawal
- ► pathological alcohol use
- ► patterns of pathological use
- ► PCP
- ► persisting amnestic disorder
- ► persisting dementia
- ► physical dependence
- ► psychedelics
- ► psychoactive
- ► psychological dependence

- ► RFLP
- ► "roid" rage
- ► sedative-hypnotic-anxiolytic
- ► STP alcohol intoxication; blood levels
- ► substance abuse
- ► substance dependence
- ► sympathomimetic signs
- ► THC
- ► tolerance
- ► type I alcoholism
- ► type II alcoholism
- ► volatile hydrocarbons
- ► WHO
- ► WHO definitions
- ► withdrawal

▲ QUESTIONS

DIRECTIONS: Each of the questions or incomplete statements below is followed by five suggested responses or completions. Select the *one* that is *best* in each case.

12.1 Match the lettered blood alcohol level with the appropriate numbered item.

- A. 0.05 percent
- B. 0.10 percent
- C. 0.15 percent
- D. 0.30 percent
- E. 0.50 percent

1. legal intoxication in most states
2. judgment impaired
3. clumsy voluntary motor action
4. coma
5. confusion or stupor

12.2 Match the lettered headings with the appropriate numbered phrases.

- A. Alcohol dehydrogenase
- B. Aldehyde dehydrogenase
- C. Both
- D. Neither

1. involved in alcohol metabolism
2. converts alcohol into acetaldehyde
3. inhibited by disulfiram (Antabuse)
4. converts acetaldehyde into acetic acid
5. decreased in Asian people

12.3 The effects of alcohol on the cardiovascular system include all of the following *except*

- A. increased risk of myocardial infarction
- B. decreased cardiac output
- C. increased heart rate
- D. increased incidence of esophageal cancer
- E. increased level of estradiol in women

12.4 All of the following statements about seizures associated with alcohol withdrawal are true *except*

- A. They are tonic-clonic in character.
- B. They usually recur 3 to 6 hours after the first seizure.
- C. They often progress to status epilepticus.
- D. They do not respond to anticonvulsants.
- E. They may be associated with hypomagnesemia.

12.5 All of the following statements about dehydroepiandrosterone (DHEA) are false *except*

- A. DHEA is a Food and Drug Administration (FDA)–regulated drug.
- B. DHEA is a precursor of serotonin.
- C. DHEA can decrease low-density lipoproteins.
- D. DHEA produces reversible gynecomastia in men.
- E. DHEA has addictive potential.

12.6 Cocaine

- A. competitively blocks dopamine reuptake by the dopamine transporter
- B. does not lead to physiological dependence
- C. -induced psychotic disorders are most common in those who snort cocaine
- D. has been used by 40 percent of the United States population since 1991
- E. is no longer used as a local anesthetic

12.7 The lifetime use of inhalants is highest in

- A. young adults aged 18 to 25 years
- B. adults aged 26 to 34 years
- C. youths aged 12 to 17 years
- D. adults 40 to 65 years old
- E. adults over the age of 65

12.8 Adverse effects on the brain that have been associated with long-term inhalant use include all the following *except*

A rhabdomyolysis
B. brain atrophy
C. decreased intelligence quotient (IQ)
D. electroencephalographic (EEG) changes
E. decreased cerebral blood flow

12.9 Acute phencyclidine (PCP) intoxication is *not* treated with

A. diazepam (Valium)
B. cranberry juice
C. phentolamine (Regitine)
D. phenothiazines
E. all of the above

12.10 Which of the following drugs is an opioid antagonist?

A. naloxone
B. naltrexone
C. nalorphine
D. apomorphine
E. all of the above

12.11 The symptoms of benzodiazepine withdrawal include

A. dysphoria
B. intolerance for bright lights
C. nausea
D. muscle twitching
E. all of the above

12.12 The SPECT image (Fig. 12.1) shows multifocal areas of hypoperfusion in a patient with chronic substance abuse. The patient's ischemic cerebrovascular disorder is most likely precipitated by which of the following substances?

A. PCP
B. cocaine
C. heroin
D. cannabis
E. barbiturates

Questions 12.13–12.14

An 18-year-old high school senior was brought to the emergency room by police after being picked up wandering in traffic on the Triborough Bridge. He was angry, agitated, and aggressive, and he talked of various people who were deliberately trying to confuse him by giving him misleading directions. His story was rambling and disjointed, but he admitted to the police that he had been using speed. In the emergency room he had difficulty focusing his attention and had to ask that questions be repeated. He was disoriented as to time and place and was unable to repeat the names of three objects after 5 minutes. His family gave a history of the patient's regular use of pep pills over the previous 2 years, during which time he was frequently high and did poorly in school.

12.13 Which of the following would *not* be a clinical effect of amphetamine intoxication in this patient?

A. increased libido
B. formication
C. delirium
D. catatonia
E. all of the above

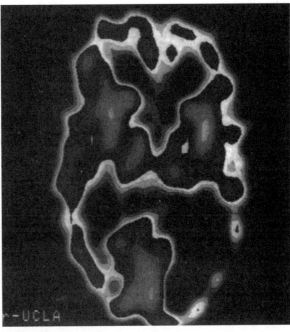

FIGURE 12.1
Reprinted with permission from Kaplan HI, Sadock BJ, eds. *Comprehensive Textbook of Psychiatry.* 6th ed. Baltimore: Williams & Wilkins; 1995:268.

12.14 The abrupt discontinuation of amphetamine in this patient would produce

A. fatigue
B. dysphoria
C. nightmares
D. agitation
E. all of the above

12.15 The patient is a 20-year-old man who was brought to the hospital, trussed in ropes, by his four brothers. It was his seventh hospitalization in the past 2 years, each for similar behavior. One of his brothers reported that he "came home crazy" late one night, threw a chair through a window, tore a gas heater off the wall, and ran into the street. The family called the police, who apprehended him shortly thereafter as he stood, naked, directing traffic at a busy intersection. He assaulted the arresting officers, escaped, and ran home screaming threats at his family. There his brothers were able to subdue him.

On admission, the patient was observed to be agitated, his mood fluctuating between anger and fear. He had slurred speech and he staggered when he walked. He remained extremely violent and disorganized for the first several days of his hospitalization; then he began having longer and longer lucid intervals, still interspersed with sudden, unpredictable periods during which his speech was slurred, he displayed great suspiciousness, and he assumed a fierce expression and clenched his fists.

After calming down, the patient denied ever having been violent or acting in an unusual way ("I'm a peaceable man") and said that he could not remember how he got to the hospital. He admitted to using alcohol and marijuana socially but denied phencyclidine (PCP) use except once, experimentally, 3 years previously. Nevertheless, blood and urine tests were positive for PCP, and a brother said that "he gets dusted every day."

After 3 weeks of hospitalization, the patient was released, still sullen, watchful, and quick to remark sarcastically on the smallest infringement of the respect due him. He was mostly quiet and isolated from others but was easily provoked to fury. His family reported that "this is as good as he gets now." He lived and ate most of his meals at home and kept himself physically clean, but mostly he lay around the house, did no housework, and had not held a job for nearly 2 years. The family did not know how he got his spending money or how he spent his time outside the hospital.

Which of the following diagnoses does not apply in this case?

A. substance intoxication
B. phencyclidine-induced psychotic disorder with hallucinations
C. substance dependence
D. hallucinogen persisting perception disorder
E. all of the above

12.16 DSM-IV-TR states specifically that the diagnosis of dependence can be applied to every class of substances *except*

A. nicotine
B. caffeine
C. anabolic steroids
D. nitrous oxide
E. none of the above

12.17 Substance withdrawal

A. is invariably associated with substance dependence
B. is seen only when the substance is completely stopped
C. varies with the specific class of drug
D. generally does not vary in severity based on amount used or duration and patterns of use
E. none of the above

12.18 True statements about the biological substrates of substance-use disorders include

A. Critical reinforcing pathways for a number of dependence-producing drugs have their origins in the ventral tegmental area, with projections to the nucleus accumbens.
B. The medial part of the nucleus accumbens is a particularly important site in the reinforcing affects of cocaine and amphetamines.
C. Some research indicates that all positive reinforcement critically depends on the mesolimbic dopaminergic circuit.
D. Cocaine acts primarily at the nerve endings of the serotonergic, dopaminergic, and noradrenergic neurons.
E. All of the above

12.19 With regard to the epidemiology of alcohol use, all of the following statements are true *except*

A. At some time during their lives, 90 percent of the population in the United States drinks.
B. At any time two out of three men are current drinkers.
C. The age of highest prevalence of drinking and of greatest alcohol intake is from the mid to early 30s.
D. Higher levels of education and socioeconomic status are associated with the greatest proportion of current drinkers.
E. Conservative Protestants and Catholics use alcohol less than liberal Protestants and Catholics.

12.20 True statements concerning alcohol abuse or dependence include

A. The lifetime risk for alcohol dependence is approximately 10 percent for men and 3 to 5 percent for women.
B. The rate of abuse and dependence combined may be as high as 20 percent for men and 10 percent for women.
C. The leading causes of death among alcoholic men and women are accidents, suicide, cancer, and heart disease.
D. Alcoholics make up one-quarter to one-third of the usual patient load in psychiatric settings.
E. All of the above

12.21 Laboratory tests useful in making the diagnosis of alcohol abuse or dependence include

A. GGT
B. MCV
C. triglycerides
D. all of the above
E. none of the above

12.22 Which of the following three diagnoses are most likely to predate alcohol abuse or dependence and to be considered true comorbid conditions?

A. antisocial personality disorder, schizophrenia, and bipolar I disorder
B. antisocial PD, panic disorder, and bipolar I disorder
C. bipolar I disorder, major depression, and schizophrenia
D. major depressive disorder, agoraphobia, and obsessive-compulsive disorder
E. none of the above

12.23 Amphetamines and cocaine are similar in

A. their mechanisms of action at the cellular level
B. their duration of action
C. their metabolic pathways
D. the induction of paranoia and production of major cardiovascular toxicities
E. all of the above

12.24 In distinguishing schizophrenia from amphetamine-induced toxic psychosis, the presence of which of the following is most helpful?

    A. paranoid delusions
    B. auditory hallucinations
    C. clear consciousness
    D. tactile or visual hallucinations
    E. intact orientation

12.25 MDMA ("Ecstasy")

    A. produces selective, long-lasting damage to serotonergic nerve terminals in animals
    B. produces sympathomimetic effects of tachycardia, palpitations, increased blood pressure, sweating, and bruxism
    C. can cause psychotic reactions
    D. produces feelings of increased self-confidence, sensory sensitivity, peacefulness, and decreased appetite
    E. all of the above

12.26 Pharmacologic agents that have been confirmed to reduce cocaine use include

    A. dopaminergic agonists
    B. bupropion
    C. SSRIs
    D. desipramine
    E. none of the above

12.27 Opioid intoxication is generally characterized by

    A. pupillary dilation
    B. piloerection
    C. increased blood pressure
    D. depressed respiration
    E. increased body temperature

12.28 True statements about methadone treatment program outcomes include

    A. The methadone dose itself appears not to be critical.
    B. Confrontational techniques appear to be more effective than supportive ones.
    C. Positive behavioral change generally occurs immediately upon entry into treatment, then tapers off.
    D. Treatments lasting less than 90 days usually have the greatest impact.
    E. None of the above

12.29 Signs and symptoms of the benzodiazepine discontinuation syndrome commonly include

    A. grand mal seizures
    B. psychosis
    C. nightmares
    D. hyperpyrexia
    E. death

12.30 The amotivational syndrome associated with chronic cannabis use

    A. appears to be generally irreversible
    B. has been definitely demonstrated and confirmed to exist
    C. may correlate with the reversible decrement in cerebral blood flow that has been documented as an effect of marijuana
    D. is proven not to be related to persistent functional and structural changes in hippocampal neurons (seen in animals subjected to long-term THC administration)
    E. none of the above

12.31 Anabolic steroids

    A. have no legitimate medical applications
    B. are associated with hypomanic and manic symptoms
    C. have a low rate of use among American adolescents
    D. routinely cause psychotic symptoms
    E. appear to cause depressive symptoms in withdrawal that are invariably brief and self-limited

DIRECTIONS: Each set of lettered headings below is followed by a list of numbered words or phrases. For each numbered word or phrase, select

    A. if the item is associated with *A only*
    B. if the item is associated with *B only*
    C. if the item is associated with *both A and B*
    D. if the item is associated with *neither A nor B*

Questions 12.32–12.36

    A. Benzodiazepines
    B. Barbiturates
    C. Both
    D. Neither

12.32 Cause rapid eye movement (REM)–sleep suppression
12.33 Have symptoms of withdrawal that usually appear within 3 days
12.34 Are associated with high suicide potential when used alone
12.35 Are clinically used as muscle relaxants
12.36 Are antipsychotics

Questions 12.37–12.45

    A. Intoxication
    B. Withdrawal
    C. Both
    D. Neither

12.37 Alcohol-induced psychotic disorders
12.38 Alcohol-induced mood disorders
12.39 Cannabis-induced psychotic disorders
12.40 Cannabis-induced anxiety disorders
12.41 Anabolic-steroid–induced mood disorders
12.42 Amphetamine-induced psychotic disorders
12.43 Alcohol-induced sleep disorders
12.44 Cocaine-induced mood disorders
12.45 Cocaine-induced psychotic disorders

DIRECTIONS: The questions below consist of lettered headings followed by a list of numbered words or phrases. For each numbered word or phrase, select the *one* lettered heading that is most closely associated with it. Each lettered heading may be selected once, more than once, or not at all.

Questions 12.46–12.52

  A. γ-Aminobutyric acid (GABA) receptor system
  B. Opioid receptor system
  C. Glutamate receptor system
  D. Adenosine receptor system
  E. Acetylcholine receptor system

12.46 Ethanol
12.47 Phenobarbital
12.48 Diazepam
12.49 Heroin
12.50 Phencyclidine (PCP)
12.51 Caffeine
12.52 Nicotine

ANSWERS

Substance-Related Disorders

12.1 The answers are: 1, C; 2, A; 3, B; 4, E; and 5, D
At a level of *0.05 percent* alcohol in the blood, thought, *judgment*, and restraint are loosened and sometimes disrupted. At a concentration of *0.1 percent,* voluntary motor actions usually become perceptibly clumsy. In most states, legal intoxication ranges from *0.1 to 0.15 percent* blood alcohol level. At *0.2 percent* the function of the entire motor area of the brain is measurably depressed; the parts of the brain that control emotional behavior are also affected. At *0.3 percent* a person is commonly confused or may become *stuporous*; at *0.4 to 0.5 percent* the person falls into a *coma*. At higher levels, the primitive centers of the brain that control breathing and heart rate are affected, and death ensues. People with long-term histories of alcohol abuse, however, can tolerate much higher concentrations of alcohol than can alcohol-naive people. Their alcohol tolerance may cause them to appear less intoxicated than they really are.

12.2 The answers are: 1, C; 2, A; 3, B; 4, B; and 5, C
Alcohol is metabolized by two enzymes: *alcohol dehydrogenase* (ADH) and *aldehyde dehydrogenase*. ADH catalyzes the conversion of alcohol into acetaldehyde, which is a toxic compound, and aldehyde dehydrogenase catalyzes the conversion of acetaldehyde into acetic acid. Aldehyde dehydrogenase is *inhibited by disulfiram (Antabuse),* often used in the treatment of alcohol-related disorders. Some studies have shown that women have a lower ADH blood content than do men; this fact may account for women's tendency to become more intoxicated than do men after drinking the same amount of alcohol. The decreased function of *alcohol-metabolizing enzymes in some Asian people* can also lead to easy intoxication and toxic symptoms.

   About 90 percent of absorbed alcohol is metabolized through oxidation in the liver; the remaining 10 percent is excreted unchanged by the kidney and the lungs. The rate of oxidation by the liver is constant and independent of the body's energy requirements. The body is capable of metabolizing at 15 mg/dL an hour, the range of 10 to 34 mg/dL an hour. Stated another way, the average person oxidizes three-fourths of an ounce of 40 percent (80 proof) alcohol in an hour. In people with a history of alcohol consumption, an up-regulation of the necessary enzymes results in fast metabolism of alcohol.

12.3 The answer is B
Alcohol *increases, not decreases, the cardiac output* among alcoholics and among people who do not drink on a regular basis. A significant intake of alcohol has been associated with increased blood pressure, dysregulation of lipoproteins and triglycerides, and *increased risk of myocardial infarctions* and cerebrovascular diseases. Alcohol has been shown to affect the hearts of people who do not usually drink: it *increases the heart rate* and the myocardial oxygen consumption. Evidence indicates that alcohol intake can adversely affect the hematopoietic system and can increase the incidence of cancer, particularly head, neck, *esophageal*, stomach, hepatic, colonic, and lung *cancer*. Acute intoxication may also be associated with hypoglycemia, which, when unrecognized, may be responsible for some of the sudden deaths of people who are intoxicated. Muscle weakness is another side effect of alcoholism. Recent evidence shows that alcohol intake *raises the blood concentration of estradiol* in women. The increase in estradiol correlates with the blood alcohol level.

12.4 The answer is C
Status epilepticus is relatively rare (not common), occurring in fewer than 3 percent of all patients. Seizures associated with alcohol withdrawal are stereotyped, generalized, and *tonic-clonic* in character. Patients often have *more than one seizure 3 to 6 hours after the first seizure.* Although anticonvulsant medications are not required routinely for the management of alcohol-withdrawal seizures, the cause of the seizures is difficult to establish when a patient is first assessed in the emergency room; thus, many *patients with withdrawal seizures receive anticonvulsant medications,* which are discontinued once the cause of the seizures is recognized. Seizure activity in patients with known alcohol-abuse histories should still prompt clinicians to consider other causative factors, such as head injuries, CNS infections, CNS neoplasms, and other cerebrovascular diseases; long-term severe alcohol abuse can result in hypoglycemia, hyponatremia, and *hypomagnesemia*, all of which can also be associated with seizures.

12.5 The answer is E
DHEA is an adrenal androgen marketed as a food supplement and *sold over the counter* in health food stores. It is *not approved* by the FDA or regulated by it.

   DHEA is *a steroid precursor of both androgens and estrogens (not of serotonin),* and persons taking the substance report an increase in physical and psychological well-being. The adverse effects of the drug are hirsutism and *nonreversible gynecomastia in men.* Because DHEA is available in health food stores and *may have addictive potential,* increased reports of misuse and adverse effects should be expected.

12.6 The answer is A
Cocaine *competitively blocks dopamine reuptake by the dopamine transporter.* This primary pharmacodynamic effect is believed to be related to cocaine's behavioral effects, including elation, euphoria, heightened self-esteem, and perceived improvement on mental and physical tasks. Cocaine *does lead to physiological dependence,* although cocaine withdrawal is mild compared with the effects of withdrawal from opiates and opioids. A psychological dependence on cocaine can develop after a single use because of its potency as a positive reinforcer of behavior. *Cocaine-induced psychotic disorders are most common in intravenous (IV) users and crack users, not in those who snort cocaine.* The National Institute of Drug Abuse (NIDA) reported that cocaine *has been used by 12 percent, not 40 percent, of the United States population since 1991.* The highest use was in the 18- to 25-year-old age group; 18 percent of them had used cocaine at least once, and 2 percent were current users. In that age group, 3.8 percent had used crack at least once. Although cocaine use is highest among the unemployed, cocaine is also used by highly educated persons in high socioeconomic groups. Cocaine use among males is twice as frequent as cocaine use among females.

Despite its reputation as the most addictive commonly abused substance and one of the most dangerous, cocaine does have some important medical applications. Cocaine *is still used as a local anesthetic,* especially for eye, nose, and throat surgery, for which its vasoconstrictive effects are helpful.

12.7 The answer is A
According to the National Institute of Drug Abuse (NIDA), *young adults aged 18 to 25 years make up the largest group* to have used inhalants in their lifetimes; 10.9 percent of that age group have used inhalants. Among the *adults aged 26 to 34 years,* 9.2 percent have used inhalants; 7 percent of *youths aged 12 to 17 years* have used inhalants, and only 2.5 percent of adults over 35, including *adults 40 to 65 years old,* have used inhalants. Inhalant use is minimal in *adults over the age of 65.*

12.8 The answer is A
Rhabdomyolysis does not affect the brain. It is a potentially fatal disease that entails destruction of skeletal muscles. It is a reported adverse effect of inhalant use that if not fatal results in permanent muscle damage.

The combination of organic solvents and high concentrations of copper, zinc, and heavy metals has been associated with the development of *brain atrophy,* temporal lobe epilepsy, *decreased intelligence quotient (IQ)*, and a variety of *electroencephalographic (EEG) changes.* Several studies of house painters and factory workers who have been exposed to solvents for long periods have found evidence of brain atrophy on computed tomography (CT) scans and *decreased cerebral blood flow.*

12.9 The answer is D
Phenothiazines are not used in the treatment of acute phencyclidine (PCP) intoxication because they have anticholinergic effects that may potentiate the adverse effects of PCP, such as seizures. *Diazepam (Valium)* is useful in reducing agitation. If agitation is severe, however, the antipsychotic haloperidol (Haldol) may have

to be used. *Cranberry juice* is used to acidify the urine and to promote the elimination of the drug. Ammonium chloride or ascorbic acid also serves the same purpose. *Phentolamine (Regitine)* is a hypotensive agent that may be needed to deal with severe hypertensive crises produced by PCP.

12.10 The answer is E (all)
Opioid antagonists block or antagonize the effects of opiates and opioids. Unlike methadone, they do not in themselves exert narcotic effects and do not cause dependence. The antagonists include the following drugs: *naloxone,* which is used in the treatment of opiate and opioid overdose because it reverses the effects of narcotics; *naltrexone,* which is the longest-acting (72 hours) antagonist; *nalorphine,* levallorphan, and *apomorphine.*

12.11 The answer is E (all)
The severity of the withdrawal syndrome associated with the benzodiazepines varies significantly according to the average dose and the duration of use. However, a mild withdrawal syndrome can follow even the short-term use of relatively low doses of benzodiazepines. A significant withdrawal syndrome is likely to occur at the cessation of dosages in the 40 mg a day range for diazepam, for example, although 10 to 20 mg a day taken for a month, can also result in a withdrawal syndrome when the drug is stopped. The onset of withdrawal symptoms usually occurs 2 to 3 days after the cessation of use, but with long-acting drugs, such as diazepam, the latency before onset may be 5 or 6 days.

The symptoms of benzodiazepine withdrawal include anxiety, *dysphoria, intolerance for bright lights* and loud noises, *nausea,* sweating, *muscle twitching,* and sometimes seizures (generally at dosages of 50 mg a day or more of diazepam).

12.12 The answer is B
The development of an ischemic cerebrovascular disorder is *an adverse effect of cocaine abuse.* The most common cerebrovascular diseases associated with cocaine use are nonhemorrhagic cerebral infarctions. When hemorrhagic infarctions do occur, they can include subarachnoid hemorrhages. Other adverse effects of cocaine use include seizures, myocardial infarction, and arrhythmias.

12.13 The answer is D
Catatonia is not a clinical effect of amphetamine intoxication. When amphetamine is taken intravenously, the user experiences a characteristic rush of well-being and euphoria. Intoxication with high doses can lead to transient ideas of reference, paranoid ideation, *increased libido,* tinnitus, hearing one's name being called, and *formication* (tactile sensation of bugs crawling on the skin). Stereotyped movements may occur. *Delirium* with episodes of violence and substance-induced psychotic disorder may also be seen.

12.14 The answer is E (all)
Abrupt discontinuation of an amphetamine results in a letdown or crash characterized by the onset of *fatigue, dysphoria, nightmares,* and *agitation.* According to DSM-IV-TR, the syndrome may develop within a few hours to several days after the cessation of heavy amphetamine use. The withdrawal dysphoria may be treated with antidepressant medication. The agitation of the immediate letdown syndrome responds to diazepam (Valium).

12.15 The answer is D
Hallucinogen persisting perception disorder does not apply in this case. This disorder is characterized by the reexperiencing

of the signs and symptoms of hallucinogen intoxication after having stopped the drug. The patient is mostly quiet and isolated and shows no loss of contact with reality or perceptual distortions unrelated to hallucinogen ingestion.

On the basis of information given in the case of the 20-year-old man, the patient showed agitation, fluctuating mood, suspiciousness, and disorientation after the ingestion of a substance. Therefore, a general diagnosis of *substance intoxication* can apply. The substance, identified as phencyclidine (PCP), is an arylcyclohexylamine, a class of drugs (similar to hallucinogens) that produce hallucinations, loss of contact with reality, and other changes in thinking and feeling. PCP is a potent drug that may be taken orally, intravenously, or by sniffing. The disorder is diagnosed specifically as PCP intoxication. A patient who is found naked, directing traffic, screaming threats, and displaying great suspiciousness can be presumed to be suffering from delusions, hallucinations, or both, and a diagnosis of *phencyclidine-induced psychotic disorder, with hallucinations, can be made.* A history of the regular use of PCP with resultant impairment of functioning allows for a diagnosis of *substance dependence.*

12.16 The answer is B

The DSM-IV-TR section dealing with substance dependence and substance abuse presents descriptions of the clinical phenomena associated with the use of 11 designated classes of pharmacological agents: alcohol, amphetamines or similarly acting agents; *caffeine*; cannabis; cocaine; hallucinogens; inhalants; *nicotine*; opioids; phencyclidine (PCP) or similar agents; and sedatives, hypnotics, and anxiolytics. A residual twelfth category includes a variety of agents, such as *anabolic steroids* and *nitrous oxide*, that are not in the 11 designated classes.

The revised third edition of DSM (DSM-III-R), DSM-IV-TR, and ICD-10 formulations for substance abuse and dependence closely follow the concepts and terminology developed in 1980 by an International Working Group sponsored by the World Health Organization (WHO) and the Alcohol, Drug Abuse, and Mental Health Administration (ADAMHA) of the United States, which defined substance dependence as follows:

> A syndrome manifested by a behavioral pattern in which the use of a given psychoactive drug, or class of drugs, is given a much higher priority than other behaviors that once had higher value. The term "syndrome" is taken to mean no more than a clustering of phenomena so that not all the components need always be present or not always present with the same intensity. . . . The dependence syndrome is not absolute, but is a quantitative phenomenon that exists in different degrees. The intensity of the syndrome is measured by the behaviors that are elicited in relation to using the drug and by the other behaviors that are secondary to drug use. . . . No sharp cut-off point can be identified for distinguishing drug dependence from non-dependent but recurrent drug use. At the extreme, the dependence syndrome is associated with "compulsive drug-using behavior."

That central notion is continued in DSM-IV-TR, which states

> The essential feature of dependence is a cluster of cognitive, behavioral, and physiological symptoms indicating that

the individual continues substance use despite significant substance-related problems.

In addition to requiring the clustering of three criteria in a 12-month period, DSM-IV-TR includes a few other qualifications. *It states specifically that the diagnosis of dependence can be applied to every class of substances except caffeine.* That point is admittedly controversial, and some researchers believe, on the basis of the same DSM-IV-TR generic criteria, that caffeine produces a distinct form of dependence, although it is relatively benign for most persons.

12.17 The answer is C

Substance withdrawal, as used in DSM-IV-TR, is a diagnostic term rather than a technical term. Thus, minor symptoms that technically are due to *cessation of substance use* (e.g., the coffee drinker's early morning pre-coffee lethargy or minor headache) would not by themselves fulfill the criteria for substance withdrawal, unless they are accompanied by a maladaptive behavior change and cause some clinically significant distress or impairment in social, occupational, or other important area of functioning. DSM-IV-TR does not recognize withdrawal from caffeine, cannabis, or PCP, although some observers believe that specific signs and symptoms can be observed when those agents are abruptly discontinued after a period of heavy use. ICD-10 does describe a cannabinoid withdrawal state.

Withdrawal is commonly, but not invariably, associated with substance dependence. The signs and symptoms of withdrawal *vary with the specific class of drug.* In general, the *severity of withdrawal is related to the amount of substance used and the duration and patterns of use.* Withdrawal is seen not only when substance use is stopped but also when reduced use of a substance or a change in metabolism results in lower tissue levels.

12.18 The answer is E (all)

Knowledge about the neurobiology of drug reinforcement and the mechanisms underlying tolerance and dependence has increased substantially. For opioids (and probably for other drugs as well) the neural systems involved in drug reinforcement and self-administration are distinct from those responsible for some of the other actions (e.g., opioid-induced analgesia) as well as from those that mediate the more visible signs of the withdrawal syndrome characteristic for that drug class. The *pathways critical for the reinforcing actions of a number of dependence-producing drugs,* such as opioids, amphetamines, cocaine, and to some degree nicotine and alcohol, have their origins in dopaminergic neurons with cell bodies in the ventral tegmental area and projections to the nucleus accumbens and the related structures that make up the "extended amygdala." This comprises several neural structures receiving input from the limbic cortex, hippocampus, lateral amygdala and midbrain, and projecting axons to the ventral pallidum, the medial ventral tegmental area, and the lateral hypothalamus. *The medial part of the nucleus accumbens is a particularly important site*; dopamine release here is critical for the reinforcing effects of cocaine and amphetamines. It is also important for the reinforcing effects of opioids, but there are opioid receptors on neurons in the nucleus accumbens, and opioids can exert reinforcing effects at that site even when the dopaminergic terminals are destroyed. Evidence suggests that such drugs as nicotine, cannabinoids, and alcohol also activate dopaminergic pathways linked to the nucleus accumbens. Some researchers have proposed that all *positive reinforcement*, including the reinforcement associated with food reward and sex, critically *depends on this dopaminergic circuit.*

Dopamine release from mesolimbic dopaminergic neurons may play more than one role in the genesis of drug seeking and drug dependence. Dopamine release has been postulated to facilitate learning which events and behaviors lead to important consequences for the organism and to alert the organism to pay greater attention to such events. In this way, drug-induced dopamine release leads to a greater salience of drug-using opportunities and is linked to wanting and craving.

As a reinforcing drug, *cocaine acts* primarily *at the nerve endings of the serotonergic, dopaminergic, and noradrenergic neurons.* When transmitters are released from these neurons into the synapse, they are transported back into the nerve endings by transporter proteins. By occupying these transporter sites, cocaine prevents the reuptake of the transmitters, thus increasing their concentration in the synapse. Cocaine's binding to the dopamine transporter is primarily responsible for its reinforcing effects, but the actions on other neurotransmitters also influence its subjective effects. Amphetamine, too, increases dopamine levels at the synapse and binds to the dopamine transporter to some degree. But amphetamine actions at the transporter are not as important as its major action, which is to displace dopamine and norepinephrine from their storage sites in the neuron and thereby lead to their release.

12.19 The answer is C

At some time during their lives, *90 percent of the population in the Unites States drinks,* with most persons beginning their alcohol intake in the early-to mid-teens years (Table 12.1). At any time *two out of three men are current drinkers,* with a ratio of persisting alcohol intake of approximately 1.3 men to 1 woman. A *current drinker* is defined most commonly as anyone who has used alcohol during the preceding 1 to 3 months, and is differentiated from persons with alcohol problems. *The age of highest prevalence of drinking* and of greatest alcohol intake is from the mid-or late-teens years to the mid 20s.

Different groups in the United States have different proportions of drinkers. *Generally, those who have high education and high socioeconomic status have the greatest proportion who are current drinkers.* Among religious groups, Jews have the highest proportion who consume alcohol, but the lowest

number of persons with alcohol problems. *Conservative Protestants and Catholics use alcohol less frequently than liberal Protestants and Catholics.* Other groups, such as the Irish, have higher rates of severe alcohol problems, but they also have significantly higher rates of abstention. High rates of alcohol problems are also found among Native Americans and Eskimos.

In the United States in the early 1990s the average person over the age of 14 years consumed 2.3 gallons of absolute alcohol a year. This amount sounds substantial, but it is considerably less than the over 5 gallons of absolute ethanol consumed each year at the time of the American Revolution. The current figure also represents a significant decrease from the amounts consumed during the mid 1970s, and the 2.7 gallons per capita in 1981.

12.20 The answer is E (all)

The lifetime risk for alcohol dependence is approximately 10 percent for men and 3 to 5 percent for women. *The rate of alcohol abuse and dependence combined* may be as high as 20 percent for men and 10 percent for women. Those figures translate to perhaps a total of 25,000 deaths a year in the United States from *accidents* (some 25,000 persons a year alone), suicide, cancer, and heart disease—*the leading causes of death among alcoholic men and women.* Cirrhosis is also found at increased rates; 15 percent of alcoholic persons meet the criteria for cirrhosis. Because alcoholism is associated with numerous medical and psychiatric problems, *alcoholic persons are overrepresented in psychiatric settings, where they make up one-quarter to one-third of the usual patient load,* even in facilities that serve the affluent.

The age of peak onset of alcohol problems severe enough to lead to a diagnosis of alcohol dependence is probably in the middle 20s to approximately age 40. Despite multiple difficulties in social relationships, families, and jobs, high functioning in some areas is likely to remain. Thus, the stereotypical alcoholic person who is a homeless bum is very much the exception rather than the rule, representing only 5 percent of all persons with severe, recurring alcohol-related difficulties.

Age-related differences are found in the pattern of alcohol-related problems. As is true with almost all psychiatric and many medical disorders, the earlier the onset of alcoholism, the greater the chance that the disorder is severe and that another psychiatric disorder preexisted. Therefore, when alcohol dependence is noted in a teenager, the person probably has another problem, usually conduct disorder (i.e., early antisocial personality disorder). In that instance, the alcohol-related problems are likely to be associated with severe drug difficulties and antisocial problems in school and with family or peers that occurred before the onset of alcohol dependence. At the other extreme, although most alcoholic persons have their problems early in life, perhaps 10 percent or so have an onset of recurring difficulties after the age of 55. The late onset of the disorder tends to be associated with less severe social difficulties and more subtle signs and symptoms, but a greater likelihood of associated medical problems than among younger alcoholic persons.

12.21 The answer is D (all)

Establishing the diagnosis for alcohol abuse or dependence centers on obtaining from the patient and a resource person a history of the patient's life problems and the possible role played by alcohol. Up to one-third of all psychiatric patients are

Table 12.1
Alcohol Epidemiology

Condition	Population (%)
Ever had a drink	90
Current drinker	60–70
Temporary problems	40+
Abuse*	Male: 10+
	Female: 5+
Dependence*	Male: 10
	Female: 3–5

*20–30 percent of psychiatric patients.

Table 12.2
State Markers of Heavy Drinking Useful in Screening for Alcoholism

Test	Relevant Range of Results
γ-Glutamyltransferase (GGT)	>30 U/L
Carbohydrate-deficient transferrin (CDT)	>20 mg/L
Mean corpuscular volume (MCV)	>91 μm³
Uric acid	>6.4 mg/dL for men
	>5.0 mg/dL for women
Serum glutamic-oxaloacetic transaminase (aspartate aminotransferase) (SGOT [AST])	>45 IU/L
Serum glutamic-pyruvic transaminase (alanine aminotransferase) (SGPT [ALT])	>45 IU/L
Triglycerides	>160 mg/dL

likely to have an alcohol problem that either caused or exacerbated the presenting clinical condition.

The process of identification can also be facilitated by a series of blood tests, outlined in Table 12.2. Those state markers of heavy drinking reflect physiological alterations likely to be observed if the patient regularly ingests four or more drinks a day over many days or weeks. One of the most sensitive and specific of the markers (perhaps 60 to 80 percent sensitivity and specificity) is a level of 30 or more units per liter of γ-*glutamyltransferase (GGT)*, an enzyme that aids in the transport of amino acids and that is found in most areas of the body. Because this enzyme is likely to return to normal levels after 2 to 4 weeks of abstinence, even 20 percent increases in enzyme levels above those observed after 4 weeks of abstinence can be useful in identifying patients who have returned to drinking after treatment. Equally impressive results have been reported for the measure of a deglycosylated form of the protein transferrin, known as carbohydrate-deficient transferrin (CDT). Using a commercially available assay, CDTect, and employing a cutoff of 20 mg/L, this test has both a sensitivity and a specificity of 65 to 80 percent for the identification of the heavy consumption of alcohol (e.g., five to eight drinks per day for a week); these figures might be slightly lower for women. With a biological half-life of about 16 days, this test can also be useful in monitoring abstinence in alcoholics. It appears that patients not identified by higher GGT values might still have elevations in CDT so that both tests should be used for identification and abstinence-monitoring functions in alcoholics.

The *MCV blood test*, with perhaps 70 percent sensitivity and specificity, is a state marker when the size of the red blood cell is 91 or more cubic micrometers. The 120-day life span of the red cell does not allow the test to be used as an indicator of a return to drinking after about 1 month of abstinence. Other tests that can be helpful in identifying patients who are regularly consuming heavy doses of alcohol include those for high-normal concentrations of uric acid (greater than 6.4 mg/dL, with a range that depends on the sex of the person); mild elevations in the usual liver function tests, including asparatate aminotransferase and alanine aminotransferase; and elevated levels of *triglycerides* or LDL cholesterol.

12.22 The answer is A
When the emphasis on the chronological development of symptoms is used, at least three diagnoses—*antisocial personality*

disorder, schizophrenia, and *bipolar I disorder*—are likely to predate alcohol abuse or dependence and to be true comorbid conditions. Antisocial personality disorder, listed on Axis II, begins early in life and has major effects on many aspects of life functioning. The diagnosis is based on evidence of severe antisocial behaviors in many areas beginning before the age of 15 years and continuing into adulthood. Persons with antisocial personality disorder are described as impulsive, frequently violent, highly likely to take risks, and unable to learn from their mistakes or to benefit from punishment. A person who carries these characteristics into adolescence, the typical time for experimentation with alcohol and drugs, can be expected to have difficulty controlling substance use. Thus, perhaps 80 percent or more of persons with antisocial personality disorder are likely to have severe secondary alcohol problems in the course of their lives. A diagnosis of preexisting antisocial personality disorder with subsequent alcohol abuse or dependence indicates someone who is more likely than the average alcoholic person to have severe coexisting drug problems, to be violent, to discontinue treatment prematurely, and to have a much less than optimistic prognosis.

Debate continues on the optimal manner of viewing the co-occurrence of antisocial personality disorder and alcoholism, but most researchers agree that the personality disorder is a separate entity worthy of diagnosis. The genetic factors that increase the risk for antisocial personality disorder may be separate from those that affect the development of alcoholism. In most treatment programs, perhaps 5 percent of alcoholic women and between 10 and 20 percent of alcoholic men have preexisting antisocial personality disorder. Other Axis II-type symptoms are often observed during intoxication and as part of the acute and protracted abstinence syndromes, but they have not been documented to predate the alcohol-related disorders.

A second disorder in which secondary alcohol problems are more common than in the general population is *schizophrenia*. Characterized by what is usually a slow onset of paranoid delusions and auditory hallucinations in a clear sensorium and typically beginning in the mid-teens to the 20s, schizophrenia is likely to be severe and debilitating. Possibly because of a lack of long-term treatment facilities, persons with schizophrenia are likely to live in inner-city areas and to spend a great deal of time on the streets. Perhaps because they use alcohol to decrease feelings of isolation or to self-medicate their symptoms, persons with schizophrenia are more likely than those in the general population to go on to have severe alcohol-related life problems. Their alcohol intake is likely to undercut the effectiveness of appropriate antipsychotic medications, to increase mood swings and signs of psychoses, and to contribute to a downward course of schizophrenia that entails repeatedly revolving into and out of inpatient care. Because most alcohol treatment programs exclude actively psychotic patients, schizophrenic persons rarely appear in inpatient alcohol treatment programs. However, severe alcohol-related disorders are observed in 30 percent or so of schizophrenic persons being treated in public mental-health facilities.

Finally, there are data from recent studies that support a small but statistically significant association between independent (i.e., not alcohol-induced) *panic disorder* and perhaps independent social phobia and alcohol dependence. One large investigation involved over 3,000 personal interviews carried out across six centers in different parts of the United States. While about 90 percent of alcohol-dependent men and women did not have a major anxiety disorder and there was no evidence for a significant increased risk for most major anxiety disorders, the rates of independent panic disorder and independent social phobia were significantly higher than in controls.

Debate in the literature continues about whether *major depressive disorder*, *agoraphobia*, *obsessive-compulsive disorder*, and other major psychiatric diagnoses are overrepresented in the histories of alcoholic persons. Several studies indicate that, when the time-line method is used and a history is obtained from many informants, little evidence is found for very high rates of most independent psychiatric disorders among alcoholic persons, other than the three disorders noted above. Therefore, although the majority of alcoholic persons have temporary psychiatric symptoms, they are not more likely than are persons in the general population to carry an independent psychiatric syndrome other than the three exceptions discussed above.

12.23 The answer is D

The reinforcing and toxic effects of amphetamines and amphetamine-like drugs play an important role in the genesis of amphetamine dependence and other amphetamine-related disorders. Amphetamines produce subjective effects very similar, if not identical, to those produced by cocaine. Both categories of drugs can produce a sense of alertness, euphoria, and well-being. Performance impaired by fatigue is usually improved. There may be decreased hunger and decreased need for sleep. Patterns of toxicity are also similar, although not identical. Both the amphetamines and cocaine *can induce paranoia*, suspiciousness, and overt psychosis that can be difficult to distinguish from paranoid-type schizophrenia; both *can produce major cardiovascular toxicities*. However, the *amphetamines and cocaine differ distinctly in their mechanisms of action at the cellular level*, their *duration of action*, and their *metabolic pathways*.

Although amphetamines inhibit reuptake of monoamines to a small degree, their major action is the release of monoamines from storage sites in axon terminals, which in turn increases monoamine concentrations in the synaptic cleft. The release of dopamine in the nucleus accumbens and related structures is thought to account for their reinforcing and mood-elevating effects; the release of norepinephrine is probably responsible for the cardiovascular effects. In contrast to cocaine, which binds to neurotransporters and inhibits reuptake of the neurotransmitters released into the synapse, amphetamine-like drugs are taken into the neurons where they are transported into the neurotransmitter storage vesicles. By changing the internal environment of the vesicles, the drugs cause the neurotransmitters to leak out into the cytoplasm and into the synaptic cleft. The dopamine released into the cytoplasm may undergo oxidation, which results in the production of several highly toxic and reactive chemicals (oxygen radicals, peroxides, and hydroxyl-quinones). Some of the neuronal toxicity of methamphetamine is due, therefore, not to the drug per se, but to the intracellular accumulation of dopamine.

Amphetamine and methamphetamine are extensively metabolized in the liver, but much of what is ingested is excreted unchanged in the urine. The half-lives of amphetamine and methamphetamine (weak bases) are considerably shortened when the urine is acidic. The half-life of amphetamine after therapeutic doses ranges from 7 to 19 hours and that of methamphetamine appears slightly longer. Thus, after toxic dosage, resolution of symptoms may take far longer (up to several days) with amphetamines than with cocaine, depending on the pH of the urine.

12.24 The answer is D

Amphetamine-induced toxic psychosis can be exceedingly difficult to differentiate from schizophrenia and other psychotic disorders characterized by hallucinations or delusions. *Paranoid delusions* occur in about 80 percent of patients, and *hallucinations* in 60 to 70 percent. *Consciousness is clear* and *disorientation is uncommon. The presence of vivid visual or tactile hallucinations should raise suspicion of a drug-induced disorder.* In areas and populations where amphetamine use is common it may be necessary to provide only a provisional diagnosis until the patient can be observed and drug test results are obtained. Even then, there may be difficulties because in some urban areas a high percentage of persons with established diagnoses of schizophrenia also use amphetamines or cocaine. Typically, symptoms of amphetamine psychosis remit within a week, but in a small proportion of patients, psychosis may last for more than a month.

12.25 The answer is E (all)

MDMA ("Ecstasy," "Adam") is one of a series of substituted amphetamines that also includes N-ethyl-3,4-methylenedioxy-ethylamphetamine (MDEA, "Eve"), 3,4-methylenedioxyamphetamine (MDA), 2,5-dimethoxy-4-bromoamphetamine (DOB), paramethoxyamphetamine (PMA), and others. These drugs produce subjective effects resembling those of amphetamine and lysergic acid diethylamide (LSD), and in that sense, MDMA and similar analogues may represent a distinct category of drugs ("entactogens").

A methamphetamine derivative that came into use in the 1980s, MDMA was not technically subject to legal regulation at the time. Although it has been labeled a designer drug in the belief that it was deliberately synthesized to evade legal regulation, it was actually synthesized and patented in 1914. Several psychiatrists used it as an adjunct to psychotherapy and concluded that it was of value. At one time it was advertised as legal and was used in psychotherapy for its subjective effects. However, it was never approved by the FDA. Its use raised questions of both safety and legality, since the related amphetamine derivatives MDA, DOB, and PMA had caused a number of overdose deaths, and MDA was known to cause extensive destruction of serotonergic nerve terminals in the CNS. Using emergency scheduling authority, the Drug Enforcement Agency made MDMA a Schedule I drug under the CSA, along with LSD, heroin, and marijuana. Despite its illegal status, MDMA continues to be manufactured, distributed, and used in the United States, Europe, and Australia.

The unusual properties of the drugs may be a consequence of the different actions of the optical isomers: the R(−) isomers produce LSD-like effects and the amphetamine-like properties are linked to S(+) isomers. The LSD-like actions, in turn, may be linked to the capacity to release serotonin. The various derivatives may exhibit significant differences in subjective effects and toxicity. Animals in laboratory experiments will self-administer the drugs, suggesting prominent amphetamine-like effects.

After taking usual doses (100 to 150 mg), MDMA users experience elevated mood and, according to various reports, *increased self-confidence and sensory sensitivity; peaceful feelings* coupled with insight, empathy, and closeness to people; and *decreased appetite.* Difficulty in concentrating and an increased capacity to focus have both been reported. Dysphoric reactions, psychotomimetic effects, and *psychosis* have *also* been *reported.* Higher doses seem more likely to produce psychotomimetic effects. *Sympathomimetic effects of tachycardia, palpitations, increased blood pressure, sweating, and bruxism are common.* The subjective effects are reported to be prominent for about 4 to 8 hours, but they may not last as long or may last longer, depending on the dose and route of administration. The drug is usually taken orally, but it has been snorted and injected. Both tachyphylaxis and some tolerance are reported by users.

The acute adverse effects reported include precipitation of episodes of panic and anxiety. More severe brief psychiatric disturbances can also occur, and preexisting pathology does not appear to be a requisite for severe reactions. A healthy drug-free subject, known to be without personal and family psychiatric illness, was given a 40-mg IV dose of the drug and developed a psychosis lasting 2 1/2 hours that included vivid auditory and visual hallucinations and a belief that people were making noise to annoy him intentionally.

Although it is not as toxic as MDA, various somatic toxicities attributable to MDMA use have been reported, as well as fatal overdoses. It does not appear to be neurotoxic when injected into the brain of animals, but it is metabolized to MDA in both animals and humans. *In animals MDMA produces selective, long-lasting damage to serotonergic nerve terminals.* It is not certain if the levels of the MDA metabolite reached in humans after the usual doses of MDMA suffice to produce lasting damage. Nonhuman primates are more sensitive than are rodents to MDMA's toxic effects and show more prolonged or permanent neurotoxicity at doses not much higher than those used by humans (Fig. 12.1). Users of MDMA show differences in neuroendocrine responses to serotonergic probes, and studies of former MDMA users show global and regional decreases in serotonin transporter binding, as measured by positron emission tomography. Although psychological assessment of a small sample of users did not reveal evidence of current anxiety or a mood disorder, eight of nine subjects had at least some impairment on at least one test of neuropsychological function.

Other reported toxicities include arrhythmias, cardiovascular collapse, hyperthermia, rhabdomyolysis, disseminated intravascular coagulation, acute renal failure, and hepatotoxicity. The role that contaminants in illicit MDMA played in the toxic reactions is uncertain, but significant elevations of blood pressure and temperature have been observed after administration of pure MDMA.

Following the acute effects of MDMA there may be a combination of some diminishing residual effects gradually superseded by feelings of drowsiness, fatigue, depression, and difficulty concentrating, somewhat comparable to the crash after cessation of amphetamine use. When young adults who were Saturday-night MDMA users were compared with alcohol-only users who frequented the same club, the MDMA users reported elevated mood on the following day but feelings of depression (Beck Depression Inventory scores of about 12) by the fifth day. In contrast, alcohol-only users showed relatively little mood change over the 5-day period; their highest Beck depression scores (about 8) occurred on the second day. In a double-blind placebo-controlled study of normal volunteers given 1.7 mg per kg of body weight of MDMA, some subjects continued to report symptoms typical of MDMA actions (suppressed appetite, jaw clenching, restlessness, heaviness in the legs, difficulty concentrating) 24 hours later. More persistent neuropsychiatric adverse effects associated with MDMA use include anxiety, depression, flashbacks, irritability, panic disorder, psychosis, and memory disturbance.

12.26 The answer is E (none)

Presently no pharmacological treatments produce decreases in cocaine use that compare with the decreases in opioid use seen when heroin users are treated with methadone, levomethadyl acetate (ORLAAM) (commonly called L-α-acetylmethadol [LAAM]), or buprenorphine. However, a variety of pharmacological agents, most of which are approved for other uses, have been and are being tested clinically for the treatment of cocaine dependence and relapse. Some of these agents are being used routinely by clinicians although little solid evidence exists for their efficacy. The most common premises on which pharmacological interventions are based are as follows: (1) chronic cocaine use alters dopaminergic systems, so that giving up the drug is associated with a hypodopaminergic state characterized by dysphoria or anhedonia; (2) some cocaine users are taking the drug to ameliorate a preexisting psychiatric disorder, such as major depressive disorder, dysthymic disorder, attention-deficit disorder, or cyclothymic disorder; (3) cocaine produces a sensitization, or kindling, effect that somehow predisposes to continued use; and (4) relapse is related to memories of the reinforcing and euphoric effects of cocaine, craving for which can be elicited by stress, other drugs, or environmental stimuli.

Cocaine users presumed to have preexisting attention-deficit/hyperactivity disorder or mood disorders have been treated with methylphenidate (Ritalin) and lithium (Eskalith), respectively. Those drugs are of little or no benefit in patients without the disorders, and clinicians should adhere strictly to maximal diagnostic criteria before using either of them in the treatment of cocaine dependence. In patients with attention-deficit/hyperactivity disorder, slow-release forms of methylphenidate may be less likely to trigger cocaine craving, but the impact of such pharmacotherapy on cocaine use remains to be demonstrated.

Many pharmacological agents have been explored on the premise that chronic cocaine use alters the function of multiple neurotransmitter systems, especially the dopaminergic and serotonergic transmitters regulating hedonic tone, and that cocaine induces a state of relative dopaminergic deficiency. Although the evidence for such alterations in dopaminergic function has been growing, it has been difficult to demonstrate that agents theoretically capable of modifying dopamine function can alter the course of treatment. This has been so even when studies in animal models and open-label studies suggested that they would be successful. In well-designed, controlled trials that obtained objective evidence of drug use, the following agents are among those that have not been found to reduce cocaine use: neurotransmitter precursors (e.g., dopa, tyrosine); *dopaminergic agonists (bromocriptine [Parlodel]*, lisuride, pergolide [Permax]); and antiparkinson drugs that may also affect the dopaminergic system (amantadine [Symmetrel]).

Tricyclic antidepressant drugs such as desipramine and imipramine (Tofranil) have been tried as well. Although some double-blind studies that relied heavily on self-reports of drug use yielded positive results, other studies have not found them significantly beneficial in inducing abstinence or preventing relapse. *There is no consensus that the effects of desipramine are robust or reliable enough to justify routine use, but used early in treatment, it may have some transient benefit for patients who are less severely dependent.*

Also tried in pilot or open-label studies, but not confirmed effective in controlled studies, are other antidepressants, such as *bupropion (Wellbutrin)*; monoamine oxidase (MAO) inhibitors (selegiline [Eldepryl]); *selective serotonin reuptake inhibitors (SSRIs)* (e.g., fluoxetine [Prozac]); mazindol (Sanorex); pemoline (Cylert); antipsychotics (e.g., flupenthixol); lithium; several different calcium channel inhibitors; and anticonvulsants (e.g., carbamazepine [Tegretol] and valproic acid [Depakene]). One double-blind study not yet replicated found that 300 mg a day of phenytoin (Dilantin) reduced cocaine use.

12.27 The answer is D

Opioid Intoxication. Intoxication can vary in severity. In extreme cases of opioid overdose there is usually coma, *severely depressed respiration*, and pinpoint pupils. There may be *gross pulmonary edema* with frothing at the mouth, but X-ray evidence of pulmonary changes is seen even in less extreme cases. Pulmonary edema is an opioid effect and is sometimes seen with overdoses of oral opioids that have been medically prescribed. Depending on when the patient is seen, there may also be cyanosis, cold clammy skin, and *decreased body temperature. Blood pressure is decreased,* but only falls dramatically with severe anoxia, at which point the *pupils may dilate.* Cardiac arrhythmias have been reported and may be related either to anoxia or to the presence of quinine as an adulterant in the opioid.

Opioid Withdrawal. The opioid withdrawal syndrome can vary greatly in intensity, depending primarily on the dose of the opioid used, the degree to which the opioid effects on the CNS were continuously exerted, the duration of use, and the rate at which the opioid is removed from the receptors. These generalizations appear to apply as well to other categories of drugs, such as barbiturates and benzodiazepines.

The clinical syndrome observed consists of purposive behavior, which is dependent on the observer and environment (e.g., complaints, pleas, and manipulations directed at getting more drugs), and nonpurposive behavior (e.g., *piloerection* and dilated pupils*), which is not goal oriented and is relatively independent of the observer and environment. The opioid withdrawal syndrome, while often exquisitely uncomfortable and distressing, is not, in contrast to withdrawal from alcohol or

barbiturates, life-threatening in healthy adults. Deaths have occurred during abrupt opioid withdrawal in debilitated patients with other medical disorders.

12.28 The answer is E (none)

The majority of patients treated in methadone programs show significantly decreased opioid and nonopioid drug use, criminal behavior, and symptoms of depression and increased gainful employment. Differences in effectiveness across programs are due in some measure to the characteristics of the patients treated, but certain program features tend to make some programs more effective than others. In 1980 the average retention rate for a group of methadone clinics participating in a national prospective study was 81 percent at 1 month, 67 percent at 3 months, and 52 percent at 6 months. *Higher retention rates are associated with* the provision of high-quality social services (especially within the first months), *higher doses of methadone (60 mg or more)* and allowing patients to know their dosage, the ease of accessibility, no fees or very low fees, *and the use of supportive rather than confrontational techniques.*

It bears repeating that the effectiveness of opioid maintenance treatment is powerfully influenced by the quality of the additional services provided. Effective individual drug counseling (e.g., one session per week) can result in significantly better outcome in terms of illicit opioid and cocaine use, needle-sharing, crime, employment, and psychological well-being. Treatment outcome can be further improved by the provision of psychiatric services, employment counseling, and family therapy. However, such additional services increase the overall cost of treatment, and in terms of improved outcomes it is more cost effective to ensure that all patients have competent standard drug counseling. Providing additional group therapy to patients in maintenance programs does not appear to produce better outcomes.

It has been confirmed repeatedly that *positive behavioral change, including* decreases in illicit drug use and other criminal behavior, *does not typically occur immediately upon entry into treatment but takes place over a period of many months. Treatments lasting less than 90 days usually have little or no impact;* consequently, retention in treatment is critical. Several studies have shown a direct relation between methadone dose and the probability of treatment retention.

In Australia patients on doses of 80 mg or higher were twice as likely to remain in treatment as those receiving 60 to 79 mg, who were twice as likely to remain as those receiving less than 60 mg. *Dosage has also been shown to have a profound effect on whether or not patients will continue to use illicit heroin.* In a study of six clinics in the United States there was an inverse relationship between methadone dosage (over the range from 20 to ≤80 mg daily) and the percentage of patients using heroin. Although some programs persist in using low doses that have been shown to correlate with both high dropout rates and continued heroin use, their number has decreased as the data on the importance of adequate dosage has become more generally accepted.

Other program factors that influence outcome and retention are the perceived range and quality of the social services provided to the patient early in the course of treatment, whether the program is flexible or confrontational and punitive about occasional illicit drug use, and the competence and quality of the program leadership and the counselors. Outcome correlates with services actually delivered and the degree to which patients perceive that the services are those they believe are important to them. Some of the better-funded programs with better staff-patient ratios did not deliver as many services as did less well-endowed programs. The retention of drug users in treatment programs and the successful reduction of injecting drug use are particularly important in an era when such drug use often results in transmitting or acquiring HIV infection. Older, black, married, and employed patients tend to remain in methadone programs longer; patients with extensive criminal backgrounds tend to drop out sooner and to perform more poorly while in treatment. The severity or duration of opioid use does not correlate with retention or performance in treatment, and patients who enter treatment under what they perceive as legal coercion show improvement comparable to that of patients who report no such external pressure.

12.29 The answer is C
Studies in the early 1960s by Leo Hollister established that abrupt discontinuation of high doses of chlordiazepoxide or diazepam could lead to a withdrawal syndrome.

The American Psychiatric Association's *Task Force Report on Benzodiazepine Dependence, Toxicity, and Abuse* defined withdrawal as a true abstinence syndrome consisting of "new signs and symptoms and worsening of preexisting symptoms following drug discontinuance that were not part of the disorder for which the drugs were originally prescribed." Many authorities have taken issue with that definition of withdrawal and prefer to distinguish withdrawal only from recurrence, not from rebound symptoms, viewing the true abstinence syndrome as consisting of rebound symptoms plus new signs and symptoms.

The signs and symptoms of the benzodiazepine discontinuation syndrome (Table 12.3) have been classified as major or minor, like those of the alcohol withdrawal syndrome. According to that classification, minor symptoms include anxiety, insomnia, and *nightmares*. Major symptoms (which are extremely rare) include *grand mal seizures, psychosis, hyperpyrexia*, and death.

Table 12.3
Signs and Symptoms of the Benzodiazepine Discontinuation Syndrome

The following signs and symptoms may be seen when benzodiazepine therapy is discontinued; they reflect the return of the original anxiety symptoms (recurrence), worsening of the original anxiety symptoms (rebound), or emergence of new symptoms (true withdrawal)

Disturbances of mood and cognition:
  Anxiety, apprehension, dysphoria, pessimism, irritability, obsessive rumination, paranoid ideation
Disturbances of sleep:
  Insomnia, altered sleep–wake cycle, daytime drowsiness
Physical signs and symptoms:
  Tachycardia, elevated blood pressure, hyperreflexia, muscle tension, agitation—motor restlessness, tremor, myoclonus, muscle and joint pain, nausea, coryza, diaphoresis, ataxia, tinnitus, grand mal seizures
Perceptual disturbances:
  Hyperacusis, depersonalization, blurred vision, illusions, hallucinations

The discontinuance syndrome may also be divided into symptoms of rebound, recurrence, and withdrawal. *Rebound symptoms* are symptoms for which the benzodiazepine was originally prescribed that return in a more severe form than they had before treatment. They have a rapid onset following termination of therapy and a brief duration. *Recurrence* refers to return of the original symptoms at or below their original intensity. The pattern and course of these symptoms will reflect the anxiety disorder for which treatment was originally instituted.

Withdrawal symptoms (Table 12.3) are categorized loosely into four types: (1) disturbance of mood and cognition, (2) disturbances of sleep, (3) physical signs and symptoms, and (4) perceptual disturbances. Mood and cognitive symptoms are anxiety, apprehension, dysphoria, irritability, obsessive ruminations, and paranoia. Sleep disturbances include insomnia, altered sleep–wake cycle, and daytime drowsiness. Somatic symptoms are agitation, tachycardia, palpitations, motor restlessness, muscle tension, tremor myoclonus, nausea, coryza, diaphoresis, lethargy, muscle and joint pain, hyperreflexia, ataxia, tinnitus, and seizures. Perceptual disturbances include hyperacusis, depersonalization, blurred vision, illusions, and hallucinations.

The temporal sequence of symptom development is not well established, but upon the abrupt cessation of benzodiazepines with short elimination half-lives, symptoms may appear within 24 hours and peak at 48 hours. Symptoms arising from abrupt discontinuation of benzodiazepines with long half-lives may not peak until 2 weeks later. Although some investigators suggest that a subgroup of patients had withdrawal syndromes that lasted for many months, no medical or scientific evidence validates the existence of such a syndrome. Prolonged symptoms are almost certainly attributable to recurrence of the original anxiety or progression of the anxiety disorder itself.

12.30 The answer is C
An amotivational syndrome associated with chronic cannabis use was described in the older clinical literature from the Middle East, Asia, and the United States. The syndrome is marked by apathy, poor concentration, social withdrawal, and loss of interest in achievement. Those features *may correlate with the reversible decrement in cerebral blood flow that has been documented as an effect of marijuana*. However, most of the reports are not rigorously scientific and lack controls that distinguish between the effects of cannabis and preexisting psychological and social conditions. Subsequent reports using different populations and better scientific methods *have failed to demonstrate the syndrome*. Several authors have noted that it is difficult to determine which came first, the drug or the amotivation. Most plausible perhaps is the suggestion that in certain persons the pharmacological effects of the drug interact with psychological and social factors to retard motivation and productivity.

Thus, the direct causal role of marijuana in the amotivational syndrome has been seriously questioned. Symptoms may indicate ongoing intoxication or represent normal psychosocial variants that predispose to the use of cannabis and other substances. However, *because persistent functional and structural changes in hippocampal neurons in animals subjected to long-term THC administration have been observed, the concept that a developing personality can be altered by chronic intoxication should not be entirely dismissed*. In any event, cessation may lead to gradual improvement. Despite those potential adverse effects, many regard cannabis as a relatively safe drug because lethal doses are unknown in humans.

12.31 The answer is B

The anabolic steroids are a family of drugs comprising the natural male hormone testosterone and a group of many synthetic analogues of testosterone synthesized since the 1940s. All these drugs possess various degrees of *anabolic* (muscle-building) and *androgenic* (masculinizing) effects. Thus, they should more correctly be called anabolic-androgenic steroids; however, the terms anabolic steroids and, simply, steroids are used for brevity. *Steroids have a number of legitimate medical applications,* such as in the treatment of hypogonadal men, and in the treatment of certain diseases, such as muscular dystrophy, various anemias, and the wasting syndrome associated with acquired immune deficiency syndrome (AIDS). However, steroids are widely used illicitly by individuals seeking to gain increased muscle mass and strength, either for athletic purposes or simply to improve personal appearance.

Various studies of high school students in the United States have produced high (not low) *estimates of the prevalence of anabolic steroid use among adolescents.* For example, one study of 3,403 twelfth-grade boys in 46 public and private hospitals in the United States found that 6 percent of students reported current or past use of anabolic steroids, with two-thirds of the users reporting that they had first tried these drugs when they were 16 years of age or less. Similarly, high estimates have emerged from other studies of high school and college students in the United States; the prevalence of steroid use among male students has generally been many times greater than that among female students in these studies. One possible criticism of these results, however, is that some students may have misunderstood the survey questions and claimed that they had used anabolic steroids when in fact they had used only corticosteroids, prescribed to them for conditions such as asthma or dermatological problems. *Even allowing for this possible source of error,* it is evident that *rates of anabolic steroid use among American adolescents are high.*

Irritability, aggressiveness, hypomania, and frank mania associated with anabolic steroid use probably represent one of the most important public health issues associated with these drugs. Although athletes using these drugs have long recognized that syndromes of anger and irritability (sometimes called "roid rage") could be associated with steroid use, these syndromes were little recognized in the scientific literature until the late 1980s and 1990s. Since than a series of observational field studies of athletes has suggested that *some steroid users develop prominent hypomanic or even manic symptoms* during steroid use. Of the 12 such studies that have appeared to date, 11 have found at least some such effects in association with anabolic steroid use, with an apparent association between the dosage of steroids used and the frequency of psychiatric effects. Specifically, in individuals using the equivalent of 300 mg of testosterone a week or less, psychiatric effects appear rare; in individuals taking intermediate dosages, between 300 and 1,000 mg of testosterone equivalent per week, mood syndromes appear more common; and in individuals taking the equivalent of more than 1,000 mg of testosterone equivalent per week, mood syndromes appear more common; and in individuals tak-

ing the equivalent of more than 1,000 mg a week, mood syndromes become quite common and are occasionally severe.

Anabolic steroid-induced depressive syndromes have generally not been reported in laboratory studies, but have been documented in field studies. Case reports of completed suicides associated with steroid withdrawal have also appeared. *In some instances it appears that a brief and self-limited syndrome of depression occurs upon steroid withdrawal,* probably as a result of the depression of the hypothalamic-pituitary-gonadal axis following exogenous steroid administration. Such syndromes might be expected to occur more often in the field than in laboratory settings because athletes typically take steroids for longer intervals than would occur in the laboratory, resulting in more pronounced neuroendocrine depression and shrinkage of the testes.

Not all depressive syndromes of this nature, however, are self-limited. Some reports have described episodes of depression that continued for months after discontinuing steroids, and which required treatment with fluoxetine (Prozac), tricyclic antidepressant agents, or electroconvulsive therapy (ECT). Again, however, given the uncontrolled and retrospective quality of these observations, it is difficult to judge the true frequency of such syndromes in the field.

Psychotic symptoms are rare in association with anabolic steroid use but have been described in a few cases, primarily in individuals who were using the equivalent of more than 1,000 mg of testosterone a week. Usually these symptoms have consisted of grandiose or paranoid delusions, generally occurring in the context of a manic episode, although occasionally occurring in the absence of a frank manic syndrome. In most cases reported, psychotic symptoms have disappeared promptly (within a few weeks) after the discontinuation of the offending agent, although temporary treatment with antipsychotic agents was sometimes required. As with manic reactions to steroids, the mechanism for these seemingly idiosyncratic psychotic reactions is unknown. It is interesting to note, however, that the chemically related family of hormones, corticosteroids, also produce idiosyncratic manic and psychotic symptoms in occasional individuals while creating few psychiatric effects in the great majority of patients. The mechanism of action of these idiosyncratic effects with corticosteroids is also unknown.

12.32 The answer is B

12.33 The answer is C

12.34 The answer is B

12.35 The answer is A

12.36 The answer is D

Barbiturates *cause rapid eye movement (REM) sleep suppression.* An abrupt withdrawal of a barbiturate will cause a marked increase or rebound in REM sleep. *Symptoms of withdrawal* from both benzodiazepines and barbiturates *usually appear within 3 days.* Barbiturates have a *high suicide potential.* Virtually no cases of successful suicide have occurred in patients taking benzodiazepines by themselves. In addition to treating anxiety, benzodiazepines are used in alcohol detoxification, for anesthetic induction, *as muscle relaxants,* and as anticonvulsants. *Neither* benzodiazepines nor barbiturates *are antipsychotics.*

12.37 The answer is C

12.38 The answer is C

12.39 The answer is A

12.40 The answer is A

12.41 The answer is C

12.42 The answer is A

12.43 The answer is C

12.44 The answer is C

12.45 The answer is A

In addition to dependence, abuse, intoxication, and withdrawal, the use of certain psychoactive drugs can induce syndromes that used to be called organic mental disorders. To avoid implying that other psychiatric disorders do not have an organic basis, DSM-IV-TR designates these syndromes as substance-induced disorders and recognizes the following categories: substance intoxication, substance withdrawal, substance-induced withdrawal delirium, substance-induced intoxication delirium, substance-induced persisting dementia, substance-induced persisting amnestic disorder, *substance-induced mood disorder*, *substance-induced anxiety disorder*, *substance-induced psychotic disorder*, substance-induced sexual dysfunction, and *substance-induced sleep disorder*.

In recording a diagnosis of a substance-related disorder, the clinician should indicate the specific agent causing the disorder, if known, rather than the broad drug category, that is, substance-induced intoxication, pentobarbital (Nembutal) rather than substance-induced intoxication, sedative-hypnotics. However, the diagnostic code should be selected from the list of classes of substances provided in sets of criteria for the substance-induced disorder being recorded. For each of the substance-induced disorders (other than intoxication and withdrawal), the clinician is asked to specify whether the onset was during intoxication or during withdrawal. Thus, a specific substance-induced disorder would have a three-part name delineating (1) the specific substance, (2) the context (whether the disorder occurred during intoxication or during withdrawal or occurs or persists beyond those stages), and (3) the phenomenological presentation (e.g., diazepam [Valium]-induced anxiety disorder with onset during withdrawal).

12.46 The answer is A

12.47 The answer is A

12.48 The answer is A

12.49 The answer is B

12.50 The answer is C

12.51 The answer is D

12.52 The answer is E

Ethanol acts on the γ-aminobutyric acid (GABA) receptor system and has effects on noradrenergic neurons in the locus ceruleus and on the dopaminergic neurons of the ventral tegmental area. Barbiturates, such as *phenobarbital*, also act primarily on the GABA system, specifically on the GABA receptor complex, which includes a binding site for the inhibitory amino acid GABA, a regulatory site that binds benzodiazepines, and a chloride ion channel. The binding of the barbiturate results in the facilitation of chloride ion influx into the neuron, making the neuron more negatively charged and less likely to be stimulated.

Diazepam (Valium), a benzodiazepine, affects the GABA receptor complex by binding to the site for benzodiazepines. When diazepam or another benzodiazepine binds to that site, the chloride ions flow through the channel, resulting in inhibition of the neuron. The benzodiazepine antagonist flumazenil (Mazicon) reverses the effects of benzodiazepines.

Opiates such as *heroin* bind to specific sites in the brain labeled opioid receptors. Changes in the number or the sensitivity of the opiate receptors may occur as the result of continuous exposure to an opiate, producing dependence on the substance. The activity of adrenergic neurons in the locus ceruleus also decreases with long-term use.

Phencyclidine (PCP) binds to specific receptor sites located in the ion channel associated with the receptor for glutamate, an excitatory amino acid. Tolerance to PCP does not occur.

The leading theory regarding a mechanism of action for *caffeine* involves antagonism of the adenosine receptors. Adenosine appears to function as a neuromodulator, possibly as a neurotransmitter in the brain. Caffeine may also affect dopaminergic systems and adrenergic systems.

Nicotine is believed to exert its effects on the central nervous system through the nicotinic receptors, one subclass of *acetylcholine receptors*. Nicotine affects the nicotinic receptors in the receptor-gated ion channels of the receptor system.

13 ▲

Schizophrenia

Schizophrenia is one of the most fascinating and disturbing disorders in psychiatry. It is no longer thought of as one illness, but rather as a spectrum of disorders, with a range of presentations and prognoses. Although once thought of as having an unrelentingly downhill course, this is not necessarily the case for many people with the diagnosis. As psychiatry becomes ever more sophisticated in its understanding of the brain's functioning, advances are continually being made in the effective psychopharmacological and psychosocial interventions utilized in the treatment of schizophrenia.

The DSM-IV-TR diagnostic criteria for schizophrenia owe a debt to the early observations of clinicians such as Emil Kraepelin, Eugen Bleuler, Karl Jaspers, and Kurt Schneider. The history of the description and diagnosis of schizophrenia is important in better understanding how the current ideas about the diagnosis have evolved.

However, with all the advances in our understanding of this spectrum of disorders, and of the brain, there is still no known or agreed-upon etiology of schizophrenia. Many researchers and clinicians believe that the various presentations of the disorder represent "final common pathways" of multiple initial etiologic injuries to the brain. These injuries may be infectious, genetic, neurochemical, or traumatic, affecting the frontal lobes, limbic system, and basal ganglia. All of the various etiologies produce similar signs and symptoms, but the range of severity of presentation and prognosis may depend in part on which areas of the brain are most affected.

A useful paradigm for understanding the development of symptoms in schizophrenia is what has been termed the stress–diathesis model of the disorder. This model postulates that a particular diathesis, or underlying vulnerability, must be present for the disease to develop, and that this vulnerability interacts in some way with particular stresses to lead to symptoms. The severity of the diathesis and stress, be they biological, psychological, and/or environmental, determines the presentation of the illness. An individual with a very strong underlying diathesis may develop the illness with very little stress, while an individual with no diathesis will theoretically never develop the illness no matter how much stress is present. Minimal stress in people with a very strong schizophrenic diathesis can provoke both the initial presentation of the disorder, and subsequent episodes of the illness. It is this concept that has led to the understanding that the effective management of stress in the lives of schizophrenic people can very positively affect prognosis and course. Optimal psychosocial treatments have been shown to reduce the number of relapses, the frequency and length of hospitalizations, and the amounts of needed medications. Education of family members has been shown to be critically important in many cases.

Biological theories of schizophrenia strongly emphasize neurochemical dysfunctions. Students must be familiar with the strengths and weaknesses of the dopamine hypothesis, as well as more recent advances in understanding the role of other neurotransmitters, such as serotonin, in the development of schizophrenia. Knowledge of how crucial neurotransmitters are involved in the presentation of the illness and in psychopharmacologic treatment and side effects is essential. The neural pathways and affected areas of the brain must be familiar to the student.

The student should study the questions and answers below for a useful review of this topic.

HELPFUL HINTS

The following names and terms, including the schizophrenic signs and symptoms listed, should be studied and the definitions learned.

- antipsychotics
- autistic disorder
- Gregory Bateson
- Eugen Bleuler
- *bouffée délirante*
- brain imaging— CCT, PET, MRI
- catatonic type
- deinstitutionalization
- delusions
- dementia precox
- disorganized type
- dopamine hypothesis
- double bind
- downward-drift hypothesis
- ECT
- ego boundaries
- electrophysiology— EEG
- expressed emotion
- first-rank symptoms
- flat affect and blunted affect
- forme fruste
- fundamental and accessory symptoms
- genetic hypothesis
- hallucinations
- impulse control, suicide, and homicide
- Karl Jaspers
- Karl Kahlbaum

▶ Emil Kraepelin	▶ paranoia	▶ psychosocial	▶ soft signs
▶ Gabriel Langfeldt	▶ paranoid type	treatments	▶ stress–diathesis
▶ mesocortical and	▶ paraphrenia	▶ residual type	model
mesolimbic tracts	▶ positive and negative	▶ RFLPs	▶ Harry Stack Sullivan
▶ Adolf Meyer	symptoms	▶ schizoaffective disorder	▶ tardive dyskinesia
▶ Benedict Morel	▶ projective testing	▶ Kurt Schneider	▶ the four As
▶ neurotransmitters and	▶ psychoanalytic and	▶ seasonality of birth	▶ thought disorders
neurodegeneration	learning theories	▶ serotonin hypothesis	▶ undifferentiated type
▶ orientation, memory,	▶ psychoimmunology and	▶ social causation	
judgment, and insight	psychoendocrinology	hypothesis	

▲ QUESTIONS

DIRECTIONS: Each of the questions or incomplete statements below is followed by five suggested responses or completions. Select the *one* that is *best* in each case.

13.1 Which of the following lettered choices best describes a characteristic of the epidemiology of schizophrenia?

A. Schizophrenia patients occupy about 50 percent of all hospital beds.

B. Some regions of the world have an unusually high prevalence of schizophrenia.

C. Female patients with schizophrenia are more likely to commit suicide than are male patients.

D. In the northern hemisphere, schizophrenia occurs more often among people born from July to September than in those born in the other months.

E. Reproduction rates among people with schizophrenia are typically higher than those among the general population.

13.2 Investigations into the cause of schizophrenia have revealed that

A. no significant abnormalities appear in the evoked potentials in schizophrenic patients

B. a monozygotic twin reared by adoptive parents has schizophrenia at the same rate as his/her twin raised by biological parents

C. a specific family pattern plays a causative role in the development of schizophrenia

D. the efficacy and potency of most antipsychotics correlate with their ability to act primarily as antagonists of the dopamine type 1 (D_1) receptor

E. a particular defective chromosomal site has been found in all schizophrenic patients

13.3 Epidemiological studies of schizophrenia have found all of the following *except*

A. Hospital records suggest that the incidence of schizophrenia in the U.S. has remained unchanged for the past 100 years.

B. The peak age of onset for schizophrenia is the same for men and women.

C. Schizophrenia is equally prevalent among men and women.

D. Approximately 50 percent of schizophrenic patients attempt suicide at least once in their lifetimes.

E. The lifetime prevalence is usually between 1 and 1.5 percent of the population.

13.4 The mortality rate among schizophrenic patients

A. is higher than the rate for normal persons

B. is lower than the rate for normal persons

C. is the same as the rate for normal persons

D. has never been studied

E. is the same as the rate for patients with phobias

13.5 All of the following statements are factors with an increased risk of schizophrenia *except*

A. having a schizophrenic family member

B. having a history of temporal lobe epilepsy

C. having low levels of monoamine oxidase, type B, in blood platelets

D. having previously attempted suicide

E. having a deviant course of personality maturation and development

13.6 A schizophrenic patient who states that he feels his brain burning is most likely experiencing a

A. delusional feeling

B. gustatory hallucination

C. cenesthetic hallucination

D. haptic hallucination

E. hypnopompic hallucination

13.7 The majority of computed tomographic (CT) studies of patients with schizophrenia have reported

A. enlarged lateral and third ventricles in 10 to 50 percent of patients

B. cortical atrophy in 10 to 35 percent of patients

C. atrophy of the cerebellar vermis

D. findings that are not artifacts of treatment

E. all of the above

13.8 In general, pooled studies show concordance rates for schizophrenia in monozygotic twins of

A. 0.1 percent
B. 5 percent
C. 25 percent
D. 40 percent
E. 50 percent

13.9 Features weighing toward a good prognosis in schizophrenia include all of the following *except*

A. depression
B. a family history of mood disorders
C. paranoid features
D. undifferentiated or disorganized features
E. an undulating course

13.10 Thought disorders in schizophrenia are characterized by

A. delusions
B. loss of ego boundaries
C. sexual confusion
D. looseness of associations
E. all of the above

13.11 Clozapine (Clozaril)

A. is an appropriate first-line drug for the treatment of schizophrenia
B. is associated with a 10 to 20 percent incidence of agranulocytosis
C. requires monthly monitoring of blood chemistry
D. has been associated with few, if any, extrapyramidal side effects
E. is believed to exert its therapeutic effect mainly by blocking dopamine receptors

13.12 Electrophysiological studies of persons with schizophrenia show

A. decreased alpha activity
B. spikes in the limbic area that correlate with psychotic behavior
C. increased frontal lobe slow-wave activity
D. increased parietal lobe fast-wave activity
E. all of the above

Questions 13.13–13.14

A 40-year-old man is brought to the hospital, his 12th admission, by his mother, because she is afraid of him. He is dressed in a ragged overcoat, bedroom slippers, and a baseball cap, and wears several medals around his neck. His affect ranges from anger at his mother ("She feeds me shit . . . what comes out of other people's rectums") to a giggling, obsequious seductiveness toward his interviewer. His speech and manner have a child-like quality, and he walks with a mincing step and exaggerated hip movements. His mother reports that he stopped taking his medication about a month ago and has since begun to hear voices and to look and act more bizarrely. His spontaneous speech is often incoherent and marked by frequent rhyming and clang associations. His first hospitalization occurred after he dropped out of school at age 16, and since that time he has never been able to attend school or hold a job.

13.13 As described, the patient's condition is best diagnosed as

A. schizophrenia, paranoid type
B. schizophrenia, disorganized type
C. schizophrenia, catatonic type
D. schizophrenia, undifferentiated type
E. schizophrenia, residual type

13.14 Which of the following neuroleptics is a serotonin-dopamine antagonist (SDA) that would lessen the need for antiparkinsonian medication in this patient?

A. haloperidol
B. fluphenazine
C. trifluoperazine
D. risperidone
E. pimozide

13.15 A 23-year-old schizophrenic patient is under your care. Two months after you have placed him on medication, haloperidol (Haldol), the patient's family begins to complain that he has recently begun to drool and that when he walks he has a shuffling gait. They also state that the patient seems to have a tremor around his mouth and appears to be indifferent to his surroundings. All of the following treatments could improve the patient's condition *except*

A. starting the patient on an anticholinergic agent
B. decreasing the dosage of haloperidol
C. giving the patient diphenhydramine
D. switching the patient to risperidone
E. adding an antidepressant

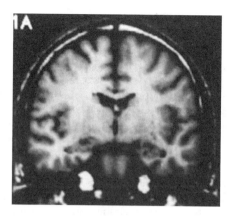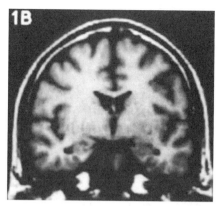

FIGURE 13.1

Reprinted with permission from Suddath RL, Christison GW, Torrey EF, Casanova MF, Weinberger DR. Anatomical abnormalities in the brains of monozygotic twins discordant for schizophrenia. *N Engl J Med.* 1990;322:789.

13.16 The magnetic resonance images shown in Figure 13.1 demonstrate a difference in lateral ventricular size in monozygotic twins discordant for schizophrenia. Panel 1A shows normal lateral ventricles; Panel 1B shows abnormal lateral ventricles. With regard to the ventricular size in schizophrenia, which of the following statements is true?

A. Ventricular enlargement is a pathognomonic finding in schizophrenia.

B. Ventricular changes in schizophrenia are likely to be specific for the pathophysiological processes underlying this disorder.

C. Patients with schizophrenia invariably demonstrate significant enlargement of the lateral ventricles.

D. All of the above

E. None of the above

13.17 MRI studies of schizophrenics have found evidence for

A. increased cortical gray matter

B. increased volume of the amygdala

C. increased volume of basal ganglia nuclei

D. increased temporal cortex gray matter

E. increased volume of the hippocampus

13.18 Prefrontal cortex and limbic system hypotheses are the predominant neuroanatomical theories of schizophrenia because of the demonstration of

A. decreased volume of prefrontal gray or white matter

B. prefrontal cortical interneuron abnormalities

C. disturbed prefrontal metabolism and blood flow

D. disarray or abnormal migration of hippocampal neurons

E. all of the above

13.19 The rationale for the role of excess dopamine in schizophrenia is based on observations that

A. Dopaminergic drugs can induce paranoid psychosis.

B. Drugs that block postsynaptic dopamine receptors reduce symptoms of schizophrenia.

C. Metabolic alterations in limbic anatomy are consistent with a disturbance in dopamine metabolism.

D. Increased concentrations of dopamine have been found in the amygdalas in postmortem brains of schizophrenic patients.

E. All of the above

13.20 True statements about the premorbid adjustment of patients with schizophrenia include

A. Seventy-five percent of patients with schizophrenia have abnormal premorbid adjustment.

B. Signs and symptoms include diminished social drive and delayed developmental milestones.

C. Disturbances in social behavior have not been observed as early as infancy.

D. Evidence of a positive formal thought disorder developing before the occurrence of hallucinations and delusions has not been found.

E. None of the above

13.21 Possible risk factors for the development of schizophrenia include

A. birth during winter months

B. increased number of birth complications

C. social class

D. recent immigration status

E. all of the above

13.22 True statements about structural brain abnormalities in patients with schizophrenia include

A. abnormalities are present from birth

B. cortical involvement is multifocal rather than diffuse

C. abnormalities are present in a minority of patients

D. abnormalities have not been correlated with cognitive deficits

E. none of the above

13.23 True statements about hypothesized neurobiological models of schizophrenia include

A. Genes function in part by increasing vulnerability to environmental factors.
B. Environmental factors increase risk by producing subtle brain damage.
C. The apparent lack of gliosis in postmortem studies implicates in utero factors.
D. As the prefrontal cortex matures, behavioral and cognitive sequelae of subtle structural deficits become manifest.
E. All of the above

13.24 Pathognomonic symptoms of schizophrenia include

A. loosening of association
B. bizarre behavior
C. blunting of emotional response
D. deterioration of social habits
E. none of the above

13.25 Paranoid schizophrenia is prominently characterized by

A. disorganized speech
B. disorganized behavior
C. flat or inappropriate affect
D. persecutory delusions
E. all of the above

13.26 In simple deteriorative disorder

A. Hallucinations are common.
B. Delusions are common.
C. Homelessness is common.
D. Early diagnosis is common.
E. All of the above

13.27 Childhood schizophrenia

A. is not diagnosed using the same symptoms as are used for adult schizophrenia
B. tends to have an abrupt onset
C. tends to have a chronic course
D. tends to have a better prognosis that adult schizophrenia
E. all of the above

13.28 Disturbances of thinking in schizophrenia include

A. archaic modes of mystical or magical thought
B. concretization
C. overinclusion
D. believing two things are identical because they have identical properties
E. all of the above

13.29 True statements about violence and schizophrenia include all of the following *except*

A. Patients with schizophrenia are more violent as a group than the general population.
B. Patients with disorganized schizophrenia are at much greater risk to commit violence than those with paranoid schizophrenia.
C. Command hallucinations do not appear to play a particularly important role in violence.
D. Violence in a hospital setting can result from undiagnosed neuroleptic-induced acute akathisia.
E. It is easier to prevent most schizophrenic homicides compared to the general population, because there are usually clear warning signs.

13.30 Factors associated with relapse in schizophrenia include

A. noncompliance with maintenance medication
B. history of sudden social or psychological traumas
C. exposure to critical emotions
D. previous relapse
E. all of the above

13.31 In selecting an antipsychotic medication for a patient with schizophrenia

A. Haloperidol (Haldol) should not be given to pregnant women.
B. Sensitivity to extrapyramidal adverse effects weighs against the use of serotonin-dopamine.
C. A dysphoric subjective response to a particular drug is not predictive of compliance.
D. It is possible that the use of an SDA in patients with prominent cognitive symptoms is more effective than using a dopamine receptor antagonist.
E. All of the above

DIRECTIONS: Each group of questions consists of lettered headings followed by a list of numbered words or statements. For each numbered word or statement, select the *one* lettered heading that is most closely associated with it. Each lettered heading may be selected once, more than once, or not at all.

Questions 13.32–13.35

A. Eugen Bleuler
B. Emil Kraepelin

13.32 Latinized the term *démence précoce*
13.33 Classified patients as being afflicted with manic-depressive psychoses, dementia precox, or paranoia
13.34 Coined the term schizophrenia
13.35 Described the four As of schizophrenia—associations, autism, affect, and ambivalence

Questions 13.36–13.41

  A. Schneiderian first-rank symptom
  B. Schneiderian second-rank symptom

13.36 Sudden delusional ideas
13.37 Perplexity
13.38 Audible thoughts
13.39 Voices commenting
13.40 Thought withdrawal
13.41 The experience of having one's thoughts controlled

Questions 13.42–13.46

  A. Neologism
  B. Echolalia
  C. Verbigeration
  D. Clang association
  E. Loosening of associations

13.42 Loss of logical relations between thoughts
13.43 Creation of a new expression or word
13.44 Repetition of interviewer's words when answering a question
13.45 Words associated by sound rather than meaning
13.46 Use of words in stereotypically repetitive fashion

Questions 13.47–13.51

  A. Echopraxia
  B. Negativism
  C. Anhedonia
  D. Stereotypies
  E. Mutism

13.47 Functional inhibition of speech
13.48 Imitation of movements
13.49 Repetitive, often bizarre, speech or behavior
13.50 Unwillingness to cooperate without apparent reason
13.51 Diminution in ability to experience pleasure

ANSWERS

Schizophrenia

13.1 The answer is B

An important epidemiological factor in schizophrenia is that *some regions of the world have an unusually high prevalence* of the disorder. Certain researchers have interpreted this geographic inequity as supporting an infectious cause for schizophrenia, whereas others emphasize genetic or social factors.

Schizophrenic patients occupy 50 percent of mental hospital beds, not of all hospital beds.

Female patients with schizophrenia are no more likely to commit suicide than are male patients; the risk factors are equal.

There is a difference in prevalence of schizophrenia according to season, but *in the northern hemisphere, schizophrenia occurs more often among people* born from January to April, not from July to September. The latter time range refers to seasonal preference for the disorder in the southern hemisphere. *Reproduction rates among people with schizophrenia* have been rising in recent years because of newly introduced medications and changes in laws and policies about hospitalization and community-based care. The fertility rate among people with schizophrenia, however, is only approaching the rate for the general population and does not exceed it.

13.2 The answer is B

The cause of schizophrenia is not known. However, a wide range of genetic studies strongly suggest a genetic component to the inheritance of schizophrenia. *Monozygotic twins have the highest concordance rate for schizophrenia.* The studies of adopted monozygotic twins show that twins who are reared by adoptive parents have schizophrenia at the same rate as their twin siblings raised by their biological parents. That finding suggests that the genetic influence outweighs the environmental influence. In further support of the genetic basis is the observation that the more severe the schizophrenia, the more likely the twins are to be concordant for the disorder.

Nevertheless, *a particular genetic defect has not been found in all schizophrenic patients.* Many associations between particular chromosomal sites and schizophrenia have been reported in the literature since the widespread application of the techniques of molecular biology. More than half of the chromosomes have been associated with schizophrenia in those various reports, but the long arms of chromosomes 5, 11, 18, and 22; the short arms of chromosomes 6, 8, and 19; and the X chromosome have been the most commonly reported. At this time, the literature is best summarized as indicating a potentially heterogeneous genetic basis for schizophrenia.

The research literature also reports that *a large number of abnormalities appear in the evoked potentials in schizophrenic patients.* The P300, so far the most studied, is defined as a large positive evoked-potential wave that occurs about 300 milliseconds after a sensory stimulus is detected. The major source of the P300 wave may be in the limbic system structures of the medial temporal lobes. In schizophrenic patients the P300 has been reported to be statistically smaller and later than in comparison groups.

Except for the serotonin-dopamine antagonists, *the efficacy and the potency of most antipsychotics correlate* with their ability to act as antagonists of the dopamine type 2 (D_2) (not type 1) receptor.

No well-controlled evidence indicates that any specific family pattern plays a causative role in the development of schizophrenia. Some schizophrenic patients do come from dysfunctional families, just as many persons who are not psychiatrically ill come from dysfunctional families.

13.3 The answer is B

Men have an earlier onset of schizophrenia than do women. The peak ages of onset for men are 25 to 35. However, *schizophrenia is equally prevalent in men and women.*

Hospital records suggest that the *incidence of schizophrenia in the United States has probably remained unchanged* for the past 100 years and possibly throughout the entire history of the country, despite tremendous socioeconomic and population changes.

Suicide is a common cause of death among schizophrenic patients. *About 50 percent of patients with schizophrenia attempt suicide* at least once in their lifetimes, and 10 to 15 percent of schizophrenic patients die by suicide during a 20-year follow-up period.

The lifetime prevalence of schizophrenia is usually between 1 and 1.5 percent of the population. Consistent with that range, the National Institute of Mental Health (NIMH)-sponsored Epidemiologic Catchment Area (ECA) study reported a lifetime prevalence of 1.3 percent.

13.4 The answer is A

The mortality rate among schizophrenic patients *is higher than the rate for normal persons and higher than in patients with phobias.* The *reasons for the high rate* are *not readily explainable.* Poor nutrition, not attending to personal hygiene, and possible immunological issues, may contribute to premature death rates.

13.5 The answer is D

Having previously attempted suicide does not increase the risk for developing schizophrenia, although at least 50 percent of schizophrenic patients attempt suicide once in their lifetimes. *Having a schizophrenic family member*, especially having one or two schizophrenic parents or a monozygotic twin who is schizophrenic, *increases the risk for schizophrenia.* Other risk factors include the following: (1) having lived through a difficult obstetrical delivery, presumably with trauma to the brain; (2) having, for unknown reasons, *a deviant course of personality maturation and development* that has produced an excessively shy, daydreaming, withdrawn, friendless child; an excessively compliant, good, or dependent child; a child with idiosyncratic thought processes; a child who is particularly sensitive to separation; a child who is destructive, violent, incorrigible, and prone to truancy; or an anhedonic child; (3) having a parent who has paranoid attitudes and formal disturbances of thinking; (4) *having low levels of monoamine oxidase, type B, in the blood platelets;* (5) having abnormal pursuit eye movements; (6) having taken a variety of drugs—particularly lysergic acid diethylamide (LSD), amphetamines, cannabis, cocaine, and phencyclidine; and (7) *having a history of temporal lobe epilepsy,* Huntington's disease, homocystinuria, folic acid deficiency, and the adult form of metachromatic leukodystrophy.

None of those risk factors invariably occurs in schizophrenic patients; they may occur in various combinations. The vast majority of people who ingest psychotomimetic drugs do not become schizophrenic. Not every schizophrenic patient has abnormal pursuit eye movements, and some well relatives of schizophrenic patients may also have abnormal pursuit eye movements.

13.6 The answer is C

A person with schizophrenia often experiences a *cenesthetic hallucination,* a sensation of an altered state in body organs without any special receptor apparatus to explain the sensation—for example, *a burning sensation in the brain*, a pushing sensation in the abdominal blood vessels, or a cutting sensation in the bone marrow.

A *delusional feeling* is a feeling of false belief, based on an incorrect inference about external reality. A *gustatory hallucination* involves primarily taste. A tactile or *haptic hallucination* involves the sense of touch (for example, formication—the feeling of bugs crawling under the skin). A *hypnopompic hallucination* is a hallucination that occurs as one awakes. Neither hallucinations nor delusions are pathognomonic of schizophrenia; they may occur in other disorders.

13.7 The answer is E (all)

The majority of computed tomographic (CT) studies of patients with schizophrenia have reported *enlarged lateral and third ventricles in* 10 to 50 percent of patients and *cortical atrophy* in 10 to 35 percent of patients. Controlled studies have also revealed *atrophy of the cerebellar vermis,* decreased radiodensity of brain parenchyma, and reversals of the normal brain asymmetries. Those *findings are not artifacts of treatment* and are not progressive or reversible. The enlargement of the ventricles seems to be present at the time of diagnosis, before the use of medication. Some studies have correlated the presence of CT scan findings with the presence of negative or deficit symptoms (for example, social isolation), neuropsychological impairment, frequent motor side effects from antipsychotics, and a poor premorbid adjustment.

13.8 The answer is E

In general, pooled studies show *concordance rates of about 50 percent* in monozygotic twins. This is the most robust finding pointing to a genetic etiologic component to the disorder.

13.9 The answer is D

Poor prognostic features in schizophrenia include a family history of schizophrenia; poor premorbid social, sexual, and work histories; and *undifferentiated or disorganized features.* Features weighting toward a good prognosis in schizophrenia include mood symptoms (especially *depression*), *a family history of mood disorders, paranoid features,* and *an undulating course.* Table 13.1 presents a summary of the factors used to assess prognosis in schizophrenia.

13.10 The answer is E (all)

Disordered thought is characteristic of schizophrenia. Thought disorders may be divided into disorders of content, form, and process. Disorders of content reflect ideas, beliefs, and interpretations of stimuli. *Delusions* are the most obvious examples of disorder of thought content. The delusions may be persecutory, grandiose, religious, or somatic. *Loss of ego boundaries* is the patient's lack of a clear sense of where the patient's own body, mind, and influence end and where those of other animate and inanimate objects begin. For example, the content of thought may include ideas of reference that other people, persons on television, or newspaper items are making reference to the patient. Other symptoms include a sense of fusion with outside objects (for example, a tree or

Table 13.1
Features Weighting toward Good to Poor Prognosis in Schizophrenia

Good Prognosis	Poor Prognosis
Late onset	Young onset
Obvious precipitating factors	No precipitating factors
Acute onset	Insidious onset
Good premorbid social, sexual, and work histories	Poor premorbid social, sexual, and work histories
Mood disorder symptoms (especially depressive disorders)	Withdrawn, autistic behavior
Married	Single, divorced, or widowed
Family history of mood disorders	Family history of schizophrenia
Good support systems	Poor support systems
Positive symptoms	Negative symptoms
	Neurological signs and symptoms
	History of perinatal trauma
	No remissions in 3 years
	Many relapses
	History of assaultiveness

another person) or a sense of disintegration. Given that state of mind, patients with schizophrenia may have *sexual confusion* and doubts as to what sex they are or what their sexual orientation is. Disorders in thought form or process reflect how thoughts are conveyed. *Looseness of associations*, a disorder of thought form, was once thought to be pathognomonic for schizophrenia; however, that form of thought may be seen in other psychotic states as well. It is characterized by thoughts that are connected to each other by meanings known only to the patient and conveyed in a manner that is diffuse, unfocused, illogical, and even incoherent.

13.11 The answer is D

Clozapine (Clozaril) *has been associated with few, if any, extrapyramidal side effects* or tardive dyskinesia. It is an antipsychotic medication that is appropriate in the treatment of schizophrenic patients who have not responded to first-line dopamine receptor antagonists or who have tardive dyskinesia. It *is not an appropriate first-line drug for the treatment of schizophrenia*. Clozapine *has been associated with a 1 to 2 percent (not 10 to 20 percent) incidence of agranulocytosis* and thus *requires weekly, not monthly, monitoring of blood chemistries*. Clozapine *is believed to exert its therapeutic effect by* blocking serotonin type 2 (5-HT$_2$) and, secondarily, dopamine receptors.

13.12 The answer is E (all)

Electrophysiological studies of schizophrenia patients include electroencephalogram (EEG) studies. Those studies indicate a higher than usual number of patients with abnormal recordings, increased sensitivity (for example, frequent spike activity) to activation procedures (for example, sleep deprivation), *decreased alpha activity*, increased theta and delta activity, possibly more epileptiform activity, and possibly more left-sided abnormalities. Evoked potential studies have generally shown increased ampli-

tude of early components and decreased amplitude of late components. That difference may indicate that although schizophrenia patients are more sensitive to sensory stimulation than other persons, they compensate for that increased sensitivity by blunting their processing of the information at higher cortical levels.

Other central nervous system (CNS) electrophysiological investigations include depth electrodes and quantitative EEG (QEEG). One study reported that schizophrenic patients showed *spikes in the limbic area that correlate with psychotic behavior*; however, no control subjects were examined. QEEG studies of schizophrenia show *increased frontal lobe slow-wave activity* and *increased parietal lobe fast-wave activity*.

13.13 The answer is B

The patient's condition is best diagnosed as *schizophrenia, disorganized type*, characterized by a marked regression to primitive, disinhibited, and unorganized behavior and by the absence of symptoms that meet the criteria for the catatonic type. The onset is usually early, before age 25. Disorganized patients are usually active but in an aimless, nonconstructive manner. Their thought disorder is pronounced, with symptoms such as marked loosening of associations, and their contact with reality is poor. Their personal appearance is disheveled, and their social behavior is strange. Their emotional responses are inappropriate, and they often burst out laughing without any apparent reason. Incongruous grinning and grimacing are common in disorganized patients whose behavior is best described as silly or fatuous.

Schizophrenia, paranoid type is marked by preoccupation with delusions or auditory hallucinations. However, for that diagnosis to be made, there must be no (or little) disorganized speech or behavior, both of which are present in this case.

Schizophrenia, catatonic type, although common several decades ago, is now rare in Europe and North America. The classic feature of the catatonic type is a marked disturbance in motor function, which may involve stupor, negativism, rigidity, excitement, or posturing. Sometimes the patient shows a rapid alteration between extremes of excitement and stupor. Associated features include stereotypies, mannerisms, and waxy flexibility. Mutism is particularly common.

Frequently, patients who are clearly schizophrenic cannot be easily fitted into one of the other types. The fourth revised edition of *Diagnostic and Statistical Manual of Mental Disorders* (DSM-IV-TR) diagnoses their condition as *schizophrenia, undifferentiated type*.

Schizophrenia, residual type is characterized by the presence of continuing evidence of the schizophrenic disturbance and the absence of a complete set of active symptoms. Emotional blunting, social withdrawal, eccentric behavior, illogical thinking, and mild loosening of associations are common in the residual type. If delusions or hallucinations are present, they are not prominent and are not accompanied by strong affect.

13.14 The answer is D

Risperidone is chemically distinct from *all other antipsychotics*. In addition to its significant affinity for the dopamine (D$_2$) receptors, risperidone is a potent antagonist of serotonin type 2 (5-HT$_2$) receptors. Drugs of this class are referred to as serotonin-dopamine antagonists (SDAs). In addition to risperidone, this group includes clozapine, olanzapine, sertindole, quetiapine, and ziprasidone.

13.15 The answer is E

Adding an antidepressant may increase the levels of the antipsychotics within the patient, leading to a worsening of neuroleptic-induced parkinsonism. For this reason, drug interactions have to be carefully monitored. All of the other options involve standard acceptable interventions for the treatment of neuroleptic-induced parkinsonism.

13.16 The answer is E (none)

Magnetic resonance imaging (MRI) studies have consistently shown that the brains of many schizophrenic patients have *lateral* and *third ventricular enlargement* and some degree of reduction in cortical volume, as shown in *Panel 1B*. Those findings can be interpreted as consistent with the presence of less than usual brain tissue in affected patients; whether that decrease is due to abnormal development or to degeneration remains undetermined.

However, the abnormalities reported in MRI studies of schizophrenic patients have also been reported in other neuropsychiatric conditions, including mood disorders, alcohol-related disorders, and dementias. Thus, those *changes are not likely to be pathognomonic for the pathological processes underlying schizophrenia.* Although the *enlarged ventricles* in schizophrenic patients can be shown when groups of patients and controls are used, the difference between affected and unaffected persons is variable and usually small.

One of the most important MRI studies examined monozygotic twins who were discordant with schizophrenia. The study found that virtually all of the affected twins had larger cerebral ventricles than did the nonaffected twins, although most of the affected twins had cerebral ventricles within a normal range.

13.17 The answer is C

Studies employing MRI have found evidence in schizophrenic patients for *decreased (not increased) cortical gray matter, especially in the temporal cortex,* decreased volume of limbic system structures (e.g., *the amygdala, hippocampus,* and parahippocampus), and *increased volume of basal ganglia nuclei.* These findings are consistent with the findings of neuropathological examinations of postmortem tissue, including ultrastructural examination, which in some cases indicates cell loss, misalignment of cells, altered intracellular structure, and protein expression, or gliosis.

13.18 The answer is E (all)

Prefrontal cortex and limbic system hypotheses are the predominant neuroanatomical theories of schizophrenia. The demonstration of *decreased volumes of prefrontal gray or white matter, prefrontal cortical interneuron abnormalities, disturbed prefrontal metabolism and blood flow,* decreased volumes of hippocampal and entorhinal cortex, and *disarray or abnormal migration of hippocampal* and entorhinal *neurons* provide strong support for the involvement of these brain regions in the pathophysiology of schizophrenia. In the context of neural circuit hypotheses linking the prefrontal cortex and limbic system, studies demonstrating a relation between hippocampal morphological abnormalities and disturbances in prefrontal cortex metabolism or function are particularly interesting.

13.19 The answer is E (all)

The hyperdopaminergic hypothesis of schizophrenia arose from two sets of observations of drug action relating to the dopaminergic system. *Drugs that increase dopamine system activity,* such as D-amphetamine, cocaine, levodopa (Larodopa), and methylphenidate (Ritalin), *can induce a paranoid psychosis* that is similar to some aspects of schizophrenia. Substantial evidence supports the *role of postsynaptic dopamine blockade* as an initiating factor in a cascade of events responsible for the mode of therapeutic action of antipsychotic drugs.

However, despite the compelling evidence for the role of dopamine in schizophrenia, testing the hypothesis has proven problematic. Clinical studies across a broad range of indices of dopamine metabolism have been characterized by marked variability in results. The most decisive clinical testing of the hypothesis has been at the level of observed drug action and symptom manipulation. Studies aimed at measuring abnormal concentrations of dopamine or its metabolites in blood, urine, and spinal fluid are confronted by problems that are almost insurmountable. In large fluid compartments, alterations in dopamine metabolism associated with schizophrenia will represent only a minor contribution to the particular index of dopamine metabolism; spinal fluid necessarily provides a summation of total brain activity, most of which is not considered germane to schizophrenia, and blood and urine provide even more indirect indices.

Functional imaging studies provide indirect evidence of dopamine involvement through the examination of metabolic rates in brain regions where dopamine is an important neurotransmitter. For example, data confirming *metabolic alterations in limbic anatomy are consistent with a disturbance in dopamine metabolism,* but it is not possible to determine the extent to which this reflects an alteration of dopamine biochemistry versus an alteration of any one of a number of interacting neurotransmitter and neuromodulatory systems. A more informative approach for assessing abnormal dopamine metabolism in patients with schizophrenia is to infuse subjects with an indirect dopamine agonist and then to determine the extent to which radioligand occupancy of postsynaptic dopamine receptors is reduced by competition with the increased endogenous dopamine. The comparison of preinfusion and postinfusion radioligand occupancy provides an index of dopamine release and reuptake rates. PET studies of dopamine receptor distribution and the density of receptor expression may offer an alternative approach for documenting the dopamine hypothesis. The observation of an increased quantity of dopamine type 2 (D_2) receptors in the caudate nucleus of drug-free schizophrenic patients is an example of this approach, but replication has been difficult. The extension of this approach to other dopamine receptor types is an important new direction of research.

Finally, there is the potential for the relatively precise biochemical study of dopamine in postmortem tissue, but here, as with the use of body fluids, sources of artifact and imprecision have been difficult to manage.

Despite these methodological limitations, postmortem studies have reported differences between schizophrenic and control brains. For example, *increased concentration of dopamine has been found in the left amygdala* (a limbic system structure) in the postmortem brains of patients with schizophrenia. This finding has been replicated and, since it is lateralized, is not likely to be an artifact. There has also been a report of an increase in D_2 postsynaptic receptors in postmortem tissue of schizophrenic patients whose medical records provided a diagnosis of schizophrenia but did not reveal neuroleptic drug use.

These results suggest that the increase in binding (receptor) number is not secondary to neuroleptic drugs. The investigation of receptor abnormalities has been extended to other dopamine receptor types, and an increase of D_4 receptors in the entorhinal cortex, independent of antipsychotic use, has been reported.

13.20 The answer is B
Premorbid adjustment refers to symptoms that appear prior to the onset of positive symptoms. *Twenty-five to 50 percent* (not 75 percent) of patients with schizophrenia *have abnormal premorbid adjustment*, which may be manifested as poor social and scholastic adjustment or *diminished social drive;* decreased emotional responsivity; withdrawn, introverted, suspicious, or impulsive behavior; idiosyncratic responses to ordinary events or circumstances; short attention span; and *delayed developmental milestones* or poor motor and sensorimotor coordination. Childhood asociality, a trait that has been referred to in the past as a poor prognostic indicator, is probably more appropriately conceptualized as the early morbid manifestation of deficit symptomatology. *Disturbances in social behavior have been picked up as early as infancy* by workers who have noticed a lack of responsiveness and emotional expression in infants who later developed schizophrenia. It is also evident, however, that deficit symptoms may have their onset following psychosis and become part of the progression of the illness during the initial years of psychosis. *Subtle forms of positive formal thought disorder may also be manifest* before overt hallucinations and delusions occur. Studies that have evaluated the development of the offspring of mothers with schizophrenia have observed cognitive difficulties during the pre-teen and teenage years in these high-risk children.

13.21 The answer is E (all)
Studies have shown *that a disproportionate number of persons with schizophrenia are born during winter months* (seasonal excess of approximately 10 percent); which, together with a birth pattern in their nonschizophrenic siblings that is similar to that seen in the general population, suggests the presence of a seasonal factor. Proposed explanations for this seasonal effect include deleterious environmental factors in the winter (such as temperature, nutritional deficiencies, infectious agents); a genetic factor in those with a propensity for schizophrenia that protects against infection and other insults and thus increases the likelihood of survival; and more frequent conception in the spring and summer by the parents of persons with schizophrenia.

Although no experimental testing has been conducted, studies appear to favor the harmful-effects hypothesis that schizophrenia involves infectious agents, but the other hypotheses have not been ruled out conclusively. Although some studies in the southern hemisphere confirm a higher birth rate for schizophrenic persons in winter than in other seasons, further study of that hypothesis is needed. There are a number of methodological problems with previous studies. If there are statistically significant increases of schizophrenic births during the southern hemisphere winter, environmental factors should be favored over sociocultural ones. Whether winter- and summer-born persons with schizophrenia differ is not clear, but that would not necessarily be expected if the causative agent is active all year but more active in the colder months.

When compared with controls, persons with schizophrenia as a group, and especially male infants, experience a greater number of birth complications. Some studies have also reported

a relationship between perinatal complications and early onset of disease, negative symptoms, and poorer prognosis. The crucial factor appears to be transient perinatal hypoxia, although not all infants so affected later develop a psychiatric disorder. There is, however, a general trend toward psychopathology in persons who have suffered obstetrical complications; such events appear to increase the vulnerability to development of schizophrenia and probably are not a specific cause. Some have proposed that complications at birth may be the result of preexisting fetal neurodevelopmental abnormalities or a vulnerability to such abnormalities. No prospective studies have been done, and retrospective case control studies may be biased if informants interviewed about a relative with schizophrenia try harder to remember birth complications than do informants reporting on healthy controls. Obstetrical records often refer only to severe complications.

Social class can be specified in various ways using some combinations of income, occupation, education, and place of residence. In previous studies *the prevalence and number of newly identified cases of schizophrenia have been reported to be higher among members of the lower than the upper social classes.* Two different explanations have been proposed. One explanation is that socioenvironmental factors found at lower socioeconomic levels are a cause of schizophrenia (social causation theory). Those factors include more life event stressors, increased exposure to environmental and occupational hazards and infectious agents, poorer prenatal care, and fewer support resources if stress does occur.

The other explanation is that lower socioeconomic status is a consequence of the disorder (social selection or drift theory). The insidious onset of inherited schizophrenia is believed to preclude elevating one's status or to cause a downward drift in status. Prospective studies have shown that persons with schizophrenia have less upward mobility from generation to generation than do the general population and that there is downward drift after the onset of symptoms. Many continue to argue this unsettled question, but a recent study strongly suggests that social drift processes are more important than social causation.

A higher risk for schizophrenia among recent immigrants than in native populations has been reported, but no study to date has confirmed that immigration stress leads to schizophrenia. Indeed, the ECA study found a low prevalence of schizophrenia among Mexican-Americans followed in Los Angeles, most of whom were immigrants. The generally reported increased prevalence of schizophrenia among immigrants could result from selection (i.e., persons with schizophrenia may be more likely to leave their families); from the failure to control for such other factors as social class, age, and sex; or from the failure to compare immigrant patients to nonimmigrant controls from the same homeland. These methodological issues limit any conclusions that can be drawn from existing reports.

13.22 The answer is E (none)
Structural abnormalities in schizophrenia, such as enlarged ventricles and reduced cortical volume, are a prominent feature. *It is unclear whether cortical involvement is multifocal or diffuse.* Temporal and frontal lobe regions are certainly involved. These abnormalities are present very early in the illness. *It is too early to say, however, whether they are present from birth or develop at a later stage. Structural abnormalities may be*

present in a majority of patients, although the exact percentage is unknown. The prevalence is most apparent when compared to ideally matched genetic controls. Structural abnormalities are *correlated to some degree with clinical aspects of the illness, such as cognitive deficits.* A key issue remains unresolved: what neurobiological processes account for these enigmatic changes?

13.23 The answer is E (all)

The essential neurobiological features of schizophrenia may place some constraints on plausible pathophysiological processes. First, there is a major genetic contribution. *Many genes are likely to be involved and these may function in part by increasing vulnerability to the deleterious effects of environmental factors. Several environmental factors have been hypothesized to increase the risk of schizophrenia, perhaps by producing subtle brain damage.* Structural abnormalities have played an important role in placing theoretical constraints on mechanisms. Since they are present from early in the illness and do not appear to progress, they may predate the onset of illness. Neuropathological data and studies of obstetric and perinatal complications support the idea that an early lesion may account for structural changes. *The apparent lack of gliosis in postmortem studies is particularly critical and implicates in utero factors.* Structural and functional neuroimaging, as well as neuropsychological data and animal studies present converging evidence for the importance of frontal and temporal regions. Finally, altered dopamine and glutamate neurotransmission is likely to play a part in the expression of psychotic symptoms.

The neurodevelopmental model can account for many of these findings. In short, some process (genetic or environmental) produces damage to selected brain areas early in life. Temporal lobe regions such as the hippocampus may be particularly vulnerable. Secondary functional abnormalities develop later. *As the prefrontal cortex matures in late adolescence, the behavioral and cognitive sequelae of subtle structural deficits become manifest.* One result is hypofrontality and cognitive impairment. Alterations in limbic and prefrontal function then produce downstream, secondary alterations in subcortical dopamine, glutamate, and other neurotransmitter systems. Dopamine dysfunction, in particular, may lead to positive psychotic symptoms. The feasibility of this model has received substantial validation from animal studies showing the delayed behavioral and neurobiological effects of minor damage to the hippocampus in neonatal rats. Observations that children at risk for schizophrenia have a number of subtle neuropsychiatric abnormalities, such as deficits in attention, motor control, and social interactions, also support the neurodevelopmental model.

13.24 The answer is E (none)

The presence of some key symptoms for schizophrenia (e.g., blunting of emotional response or a strikingly inappropriate emotional response) weighs heavily in favor of a diagnosis of schizophrenia *but none are strictly pathognomonic for the disease.* For instance, what is *emotional blunting*, and what is an inappropriate emotional reaction? For example, is the embarrassed adolescent's sheepish or defying smile an inappropriate emotional reaction? Considerable clinical experience is required to be certain about the presence of such symptoms.

The *loosening of association*—the specific thought disorder of the schizophrenic—is perhaps one of the most valuable diagnostic criteria, but a good knowledge of psychopathology is required to be sure of its presence and to avoid confusing it with other forms of disturbed thinking, such as manic flight of ideas, disintegration of thought processes due to clouding of consciousness, and impaired reasoning due to fatigue or distraction. It is not sufficient to ask a patient the meaning of a proverb and then, on the basis of one's personal impression, declare that the patient has a pronounced schizophrenic thinking disturbance. It is sometimes impossible to distinguish, on the basis of a proverb test, between the disordered thinking of a schizophrenic and a manic patient, except for the greater verbosity of the manic.

The *patient's behavior* may furnish significant clues for the diagnosis of schizophrenia. *Bizarre* postures and grimacing are certainly characteristic of schizophrenic conditions, but identifying a bizarre posture is not always easy. For instance, religious rituals and special positions for meditation or dancing with which the observer is not familiar may be called bizarre. But in a recent case of a withdrawn, suicidal young girl, a possible diagnosis of depression was ruled out in favor of schizophrenia when the girl began eating raw chicken, pouring hot tea over herself, and openly trying to get into bed with her brother-in-law during a weekend home visit.

True catalepsy may be almost pathognomonic of schizophrenia, but it is not a common symptom. A stupor strongly suggests catatonic schizophrenia, but hysteria or a depressive stupor must be carefully ruled out in the differential diagnosis.

The *deterioration of social habits,* even involving the smearing of feces, does not suffice for the diagnosis of schizophrenia. Such deterioration can occur in various toxic and organic psychoses, temporarily in hysterical twilight states, and even at the peak of a manic episode in bipolar I disorder.

Pronounced social withdrawal also occurs under many conditions, ranging from simple sulking to anxiety and depression. Sustained passivity and lack of spontaneity should suggest the diagnosis of schizophrenia only if organic and depressive conditions can be definitely ruled out.

Stereotypies and verbigeration strongly suggest schizophrenia, but they occur almost exclusively in chronic, institutionalized patients and are rarely seen today. Frequent and lengthy staring into a mirror and other odd mannerisms also strongly suggest a diagnosis of schizophrenia.

13.25 The answer is D

The paranoid type of schizophrenia is characterized mainly by the presence of delusions of persecution or grandeur. Patients with paranoid schizophrenia are usually older than patients with other subtypes of schizophrenia when they break down (i.e., they are usually in their late 20s or their 30s). Patients who have been well up to that age have usually established a place and an identity for themselves in the community. Their ego resources are greater than those of catatonic and disorganized patients. *Paranoid schizophrenics show less regression of mental faculties, emotional response, and behavior* than those with the other subtypes of schizophrenia.

Typical patients with paranoid schizophrenia are tense, suspicious, guarded, and reserved. They are often hostile and aggressive. They usually conduct themselves relatively well socially, and their intelligence in areas not invaded by delusions may remain high. Paul Murphy, an American chess champion in the first half of the 19th century and one of the greatest chess masters in history, developed paranoid schizophrenia in his middle 20s and was hospitalized for years. But even many years after he had become ill, he played an original and masterly game of chess when he could be persuaded to accept the challenge.

13.26 The answer is C

The DSM-IV-TR diagnosis of simple deteriorative disorder (simple schizophrenia) is characterized by a gradual, insidious loss of drive, interest, ambition, and initiative. *Hallucinations and delusions are uncommon, and if those symptoms do occur, they do not persist.* Patients with simple deteriorative disorder withdraw from contact with other people, tend to stay in their rooms, avoid meeting or eating with other members of the family, stop working, and stop seeing friends. If they are still in school, their marks drop to a low level, even if they were consistently high in the past.

These patients avoid going out into the street during the day but may go for long walks alone at 2:00 or 3:00 A.M. They tend to sleep until noon or later, after staying up alone most of the night. During the early stages of the illness they may have many somatic complaints, variously described as fatigue, nervousness, neurosis, psychosomatic disease, and laziness. *Patients are often treated for a year or more before the correct diagnosis is made. In many cases patients with simple deteriorative disorder later become homeless.* They become increasingly shallow in their emotional responses and are quite content to drift aimlessly through life as long as they are left alone.

Although patients appear to be indifferent to their environment, they may react with sudden rage to persistent nagging by family members. The immediate reason for admission of patients with simple schizophrenia to a hospital is often an outburst of violence directed against their mothers or fathers for a trivial reason.

Patients with simple deteriorative disorder may resemble personalities of the schizoid type. The distinguishing feature is the disorder makes its appearance at some time during or after puberty and from then on goes on to definite deterioration; personality deviations usually start earlier and remain the same over the years.

To meet the ICD-10 diagnostic criteria for simple schizophrenia, the individual must show over a period of at least 1 year all of the following manifestations: (1) a significant and consistent change in the overall quality of some aspect of personal behavior such as loss of drive and interest; (2) gradual appearance and deepening of negative symptoms such as marked apathy; and (3) a marked decline in social, scholastic, or occupational performance.

13.27 The answer is C

Recent studies have established that *the diagnosis of childhood schizophrenia may be based on the same symptoms used for adult schizophrenia.* What characterizes childhood schizophrenia is not the nature but the dramatic intensity of its symptoms. *Its onset is usually insidious, its course tends to be chronic, and the prognosis is mostly unfavorable.* Briefly, it resembles the typical Kraepelinian case of dementia precox. What gives childhood schizophrenia unique importance for research is the observation that anatomical features of the brain that are often associated with adult-onset schizophrenia (e.g., enlarged ventricles) are also present in this early-onset form of the disease. Neurobiological studies of children with schizophrenia may therefore provide significant clues to the developmental pathogenesis of adult-onset schizophrenia.

13.28 The answer is E (all)

Disturbance of thinking and conceptualization is one of the most characteristic features of schizophrenia. Thought disorder is characterized by patients thinking and reasoning in autistic terms according to their own intricate private rules of logic. Schizophrenic patients may be highly intelligent, not confused, and they may be painstaking in their abstractions and deductions. But their thought processes are strange and do not lead to conclusions based on reality or universal logic.

One study emphasized the fact that the patient with schizophrenia may *consider two things identical merely because they have identical predicates or properties.* By contrast, in normal logical thought, identity is based on identical subjects and not on identical predicates. The patient with schizophrenia may reason (to quote Silvano Arieti), "The Virgin Mary was a virgin; I'm a virgin; therefore, I'm the Virgin Mary." However, this particular fallacy is not specific for schizophrenia and may be commonly committed, for instance, by college students who are distracted or fatigued. Arieti believed that schizophrenic cognition uses isolated segments and parts, rather than the whole of the concept.

Patients with schizophrenia may reason: "John is Peter's father; therefore, Peter is John's father." Such symmetrical reasoning is sometimes justified (e.g., John is Peter's brother, therefore, Peter is John's brother), but at other times such conclusions are not justified, and patients do not seem to know when they may apply them and when they may not.

Patients with schizophrenia use archaic modes of mystical or magical thinking. Such primitive modes of thinking are closely related to the psychoanalytic concept of primary thought processes that are at work in normal dreaming and allow condensation, reversal, substitution, displacement, and other distortions of conceptual relations impossible in rationally controlled thought. Jung, in fact, compared the psychotic processes of schizophrenic patients who are awake to those of normal persons who are dreaming with their eyes open.

Kurt Goldstein described *a concretization of thought and a loss of the abstract attitude as typical of schizophrenic* thinking. Patients lose their ability to generalize correctly and exhibit in the ordering of their concepts a defect similar to a loss of the figure-ground relation in perceptual performance. That defect is often brought out by the simple clinical test of asking a patient to interpret a well-known proverb. One patient interpreted the saying "A stitch in time saves nine" as "I should sew nine buttons on my coat," an overly personalized and concrete explanation.

Norman Cameron *identified overinclusion as a typical feature of schizophrenic thought disorder.* In contrast to patients whose mental functions are impaired by an organic brain lesion and who tend to omit important items in thought and speech, patients with schizophrenia tend to include many irrelevant items in their ideational and verbal behavior. That tendency seems to result from a loosening of associations in the schizophrenia patient. Studies have shown that overinclusive thinking is not a learning defect but an impairment of a central filtering process that normally inhibits external sensations and internal thoughts that are irrelevant to a given focus of attention. Only a well-functioning, filtering-inhibiting process makes rational thinking possible. Overinclusive thinking usually develops within the setting of a delusional mood, when things look different, sensations are more intense, and everything seems to have some strange special significance.

13.29 The answer is B

Patients with schizophrenia are more violent as a group than the general population. This is particularly a problem for patients with the paranoid type who may act quite suddenly and impulsively on a delusional idea. Patients with paranoia tend to be intelligent and capable of forming plans; therefore, they represent a much greater risk than individuals who are disorganized and cannot plan an effective attack. *Despite earlier beliefs, command hallucinations do not appear to play a particularly important role in violence.* Violence between patients in hospitals frequently results from the attacking patient's mistaken belief that another patient is behaving in a threatening way or getting physically too close. *Studies have revealed that violence in a hospital setting can result from undiagnosed neuroleptic-induced acute akathisia.* Persistently violent inpatients often do well in special treatment units that provide a more structured program and a less crowded environment. The patients who fail to respond to this kind of care usually show neurological signs in addition to their diagnosis.

Unfortunately, it is exceedingly difficult to prevent most schizophrenic homicides, since there is usually no clear warning. Most of the homicides come as a horrifying surprise. Patients who are known to be paranoid with homicidal tendencies should not, as a rule, be allowed to move about freely as long as they retain their delusions and their aggressive tension.

13.30 The answer is E (all)

Several important observations have been made about the factors that determine whether a patient in remission will suffer a relapse. *The most important protective factor is undoubtedly maintenance therapy with antipsychotic drugs.* One study noted a *history of sudden social or psychological traumas* (e.g., the death of a parent, moving from one apartment to another) during the 3 weeks preceding schizophrenic relapses in about 60 percent of cases.

The type of home in which the patient in remission resides plays a vital role. In one American study patients with schizophrenia fared better in conjugal homes than in parental homes, but some British investigators made the opposite observation in their sample. Most importantly, *clear correlations exist between exposure to expressed negative critical emotions (called EE, expressed emotion) in the household of a patient with schizophrenia* in remission and the likelihood of relapse. The critical time limit seemed to be about 35 hours of such exposure a week. When that time limit was exceeded, even maintenance drug therapy was often inadequate in preventing relapse.

The risk of personality deterioration increases with each schizophrenic relapse. Schizophrenia recoveries are often called remissions because many of the patients later relapse.

Although patients may remit again, each schizophrenic attack carries a greater probability of some permanent personality damage. Risk of personality deterioration increases rapidly after the second relapse. However, chronic schizophrenia does not inevitably lead to intellectual deterioration. In fact, in one sample, patients with chronic schizophrenia retained or improved their mean intelligence scores in spite of old age and prolonged institutionalization over a period of 14 years. In a group of schizophrenia patients who were followed over a 10-year period, schizophrenic symptoms decreased by 15 percent.

13.31 The answer is D

The introduction of new antipsychotic agents has made the selection of an antipsychotic much more complicated. Prior to the development of the new antipsychotics, all the drugs were equally effective for schizophrenia. Many clinicians believed that different subtypes of schizophrenia responded differently to different antipsychotics. For example, it was proposed that more agitated patients responded better to more sedating drugs whereas more withdrawn patients responded better to less sedating agents; however, controlled trials failed to support this. The differences among antipsychotics were confined to their side effects, the available formulations, and, to some extent, their cost. The newer antipsychotics challenged this view, suggesting that certain populations of individuals with schizophrenia were likely to do better on a newer antipsychotic.

Antipsychotic drugs can be categorized into two main groups: the older conventional ones, which have also been called *dopamine receptor antagonists*, and the newer second-generation drugs, which have been called *serotonin-dopamine antagonists (SDAs)*, or more broadly, atypical antipsychotics. *Dopamine receptor antagonist* refers to the theory that the antipsychotic effects of this group of drugs result from the blockade of dopamine type 2 (D_2) receptors. The SDAs differ in having effects related to their ratios of D_2 and serotonin (5-hydroxytryptamine [5-HT]) type 2A (5-HT_{2A}) antagonism. The dopamine receptor antagonists are further categorized as being low, mid, or high potency with the higher-potency drugs having a greater affinity for D_2 receptors and a greater tendency to cause extrapyramidal side effects. Low-potency drugs are less likely to cause extrapyramidal side effects, but more likely to cause postural hypotension, sedation, and anticholinergic effects.

A number of factors should be considered in selecting an antipsychotic medication. Perhaps the most important consideration should be the patient's prior experience with drug treatment. This includes both the patient's clinical and subjective response. Regarding the subjective response, studies by Theodore Van Putten and others found that a patient's early response to a query such as "How does this medication agree with you?" was a powerful predictor of whether that patient would comply with taking that particular medication. In other words, *if the patient has uncomfortable side effects on a medication, compliance is likely to be poor if that medication is prescribed.*

Prior to the introduction of the SDAs, few options were available for patients who developed extrapyramidal effects. At times, dosage reduction or changing the patient to a lower-potency dopamine receptor antagonist may be helpful. Unfortunately, many patients experience extrapyramidal or other

Table 13.2
Factors Influencing Antipsychotic Drug Selection

Factors	Considerations
Subjective response	A dysphoric subjective response to a particular drug predicts poor compliance with that drug
Sensitivity to extrapyramidal adverse effects	A serotonin-dopamine antagonist (SDA)
Tardive dyskinesia	Clozapine or (possibly another SDA)
Poor medication compliance or high risk of relapse	Injectable form of a long-acting antagonist (haloperidol or fluphenazine)
Pregnancy	Probably haloperidol (most data supporting its safety)
Cognitive symptoms	Possibly an SDA
Negative symptoms	Possibly an SDA

adverse effects at the lowest effective dosage that is clinically effective. *The introduction of the SDAs provides an opportunity for treating these individuals with agents that seldom cause extrapyramidal side effects at their effective dosage.*

With these factors in mind, clinicians should consider the factors included in Table 13.2. In some cases these recommendations are based on incomplete data. *For example, it remains unproven that patients with prominent negative or cognitive symptoms will respond better to an SDA than to a dopamine receptor antagonist. Haloperidol (Haldol) is recommended for pregnant patients* because more data support its safety and not because it had proved safer than other drugs.

An important nonclinical factor is the cost of the drug; the SDAs are much more expensive. However, evidence indicates that the higher drug costs of these agents may be offset by other factors. Studies found that patients treated with clozapine required fewer hospital days than patients treated with a conventional dopamine receptor antagonist. Clozapine use was associated with a reduced suicide rate in schizophrenic suicidal patients and was approved for use in 2002.

In selecting a drug for first-episode patients, clinicians should give a high priority to minimizing adverse effects. Many of these individuals are ambivalent about drug treatment and may discontinue antipsychotics when they experience relatively mild adverse effects. Unpleasant experiences with medications during this initial episode may be frightening to these individuals and may influence their future attitudes toward pharmacotherapy. These considerations may lead to the selection of an SDA or a relatively low dosage of a high-potency dopamine receptor antagonist. A number of studies indicate that both olanzapine and risperidone are effective for first-episode patients.

Answers 13.32–13.35

13.32 The answer is B

13.33 The answer is B

13.34 The answer is A

13.35 The answer is A

Emil Kraepelin (1856–1926) *latinized the term* démence précoce *to dementia precox*, a term that emphasized a distinct cognitive process (dementia) and the early onset (precox) that is characteristic of the disorder. Kraepelin *classified patients as being afflicted with manic-depressive psychoses, dementia precox, or paranoia.*

Eugen Bleuler (1857–1939) *coined the term "schizophrenia"* and *described the four As of schizophrenia: Associations* are loose; ideas have *autistic* qualities with meanings only the patient can understand; *affect* is restricted or flat; and the patient has conscious *ambivalent* feelings about almost everything.

Answers 13.36–13.41

13.36 The answer is B

13.37 The answer is B

13.38 The answer is A

13.39 The answer is A

13.40 The answer is A

13.41 The answer is A

Kurt Schneider (1887–1967) described a number of *first-rank symptoms* of schizophrenia that are considered of pragmatic value in making the diagnosis of schizophrenia, although they are not specific to the disease. The symptoms include *audible thoughts* (hearing one's thoughts aloud); *voices* or auditory hallucinations *commenting* on the patient's behavior; *thought withdrawal* (the removal of the patient's thoughts by others); and *the experience of having one's thoughts controlled.* Schneider pointed out that schizophrenia can be diagnosed by second-rank symptoms when accompanied by a typical clinical presentation. *Second-rank symptoms* include *sudden delusional ideas, perplexity,* and feelings of emotional impoverishment. Schneider's diagnostic criteria for schizophrenia are listed in Table 13.3.

Table 13.3
Kurt Schneider's Diagnostic Criteria for Schizophrenia

1. First-rank symptoms
   a. Audible thoughts
   b. Voices arguing or discussing or both
   c. Voices commenting
   d. Somatic passivity experiences
   e. Thought withdrawal and other experiences of influenced thought
   f. Thought broadcasting
   g. Delusional perceptions
   h. All other experiences involving volition, made affects, and made impulses
2. Second-rank symptoms
   a. Other disorders of perception
   b. Sudden delusional ideas
   c. Perplexity
   d. Depressive and euphoric mood changes
   e. Feelings of emotional impoverishment
   f. " . . . and several others as well"

Answers 13.42–13.46

13.42 The answer is E

13.43 The answer is A

13.44 The answer is B

13.45 The answer is D

13.46 The answer is C
Occasionally, patients with schizophrenia *create a completely new expression, a neologism*, when they need to express a concept for which no ordinary word exists.

A woman with schizophrenia who had been hospitalized for several years kept repeating (in an otherwise quite rational conversation) the word "polamolalittersjitterstittersleelitla." Her psychiatrist asked her to spell it out, and she proceeded to explain the meaning of the various components, which she insisted were to be used as one word. "Polamolalitters" was intended to recall the disease poliomyelitis, because the patient wanted to indicate that she felt she was suffering from a serious disease affecting her nervous system; the component "litters" stood for untidiness or messiness, the way she felt inside; "jitterstitters" reflected her inner nervousness and lack of ease; "leelita" was a reference to the French *le lit là* (that bed there), meaning that she both depended on and felt handicapped by her illness. That single neologistic production thus enabled the patient to express—in a condensed, autistic manner—information about her preoccupations and apprehensions that otherwise would have taken a whole paragraph to explain in common language.

It is assumed that the disorders of language reflect an underlying disorder of thinking. A variety of features have been reported by clinicians for the last 100 years as characteristic of this syndrome. These include the loss of the logical relations between antecedent and subsequent associations that is termed *loosening of associations*. Words can be combined on the basis of sound rather than on meaning called *clang association*. New words may be generated, which are called *neologisms*. *Verbigeration* involves the use of words in a stereotypically repetitive fashion. This rare symptom is found almost exclusively in chronic and very regressed patients with schizophrenia. It consists of the senseless repetition of the same words or phrases, and it may go on for days. Like neologisms and echolalia, verbigeration is a rare symptom today and is almost restricted to long-term institutionalized schizophrenia patients. Many psychiatrists working with schizophrenia patients in the community may never encounter these manifestations of deterioration.

Echolalia involves the repetition of the examiner's words.

Examiner: How did you sleep last night?
Patient: I slept well last night.
Examiner: Can you tell me the name of your head nurse?
Patient: The name of my head nurse is Miss Brown.

Echolalia seems to signal two facts, patients are aware of some shortcomings in their ideation and they are striving to maintain active rapport with the interviewer. They act much like someone learning a new language who answers the teacher's questions with as many of the teacher's words in the strange language as they can possibly manage.

Thought blocking involves the sudden and inexplicable blocking of thoughts manifested by the patient's inability to speak.

Loosening of associations is based on the late 19th century association theory. According to association theory language is determined by purpose. This purposefulness is often lost in schizophrenic speech. A sentence completion test illustrates the point. The sentence to be completed was "The man fell on the street . . . ." The patient's response was "because of World War I." Although the thought of falling might be associated with falling in combat, it was an inappropriate association for the stimulus.

It can be helpful to look at disorders of association as disorders of the word and disorders of the sentence. Disorders of the word range from loss of symbolic meaning of the word, as in clang associations, to inability to maintain the correct semantic context for a word, to approximate use of words, to the creation of new words. Disorders of the sentence include associative failures and failures of system placement. Most words have multiple meanings. Even a simple question such as "Where is your husband?" must be answered in terms of the frame of reference. In one context, the question might ask for the physical location of the husband, and in another context it might ask for his identification in his graduating class picture. An example of system shifting was reported by Silvano Arieti. Commenting on the Japanese attack on Pearl Harbor, a patient said, "The next time they may attack Diamond Harbor or Emerald Harbor." The patient had lost the contextual system of Pearl Harbor as a geographical military base and had substituted a contextual system in which pearls are precious stones.

Answers 13.47–13.51

13.47 The answer is E

13.48 The answer is A

13.49 The answer is D

13.50 The answer is B

13.51 The answer is C
The motor symptom *echopraxia* is analogous to echolalia in the verbal sphere. It is the *imitation of movements* and gestures of the person the patient is observing.

Negativism refers to a patient's *unwillingness to cooperate without any apparent reason* for that lack of cooperation. It does not appear to be related to fatigue, depression, suspicion, or anger. Negativism may even take the form of unwillingness to follow a request for a physical movement. It can become so severe that the patient will do the opposite of what is asked. For example, when asked to raise an arm, he or she may lower it.

Anhedonia is a particularly distressing symptom. Sandor Rado considered anhedonia to be a cardinal feature of schizophrenia. There is frequently a *diminution in the patient's ability to experience pleasure* and, in some severe cases, even to imagine a pleasant feeling. Patients may not meet the criteria for the diagnosis of clinical depression but will describe an emotional emptiness or barrenness. Anhedonia can become unbearable enough to contribute to a suicide attempt.

Stereotyped behavior is primarily seen in patients with chronic schizophrenia, including those in the community. *At times it may take a motoric form and be expressed in a repetitive pattern of walking or pacing.* It may also be demonstrated in repetitive strange gestures, which may or may not have a magical meaning to the patient. Finally, *in language one can have the repetition of phrases or comments for long periods.* This is separate from perseveration and distinct from verbigeration. Interestingly, when schizophrenia patients are engaged psychosocially, this symptom tends to diminish. It appears to be a consequence of psychosocial isolation.

Functional inhibition of speech and vocalization may last for hours or days, but before the use of modern treatment methods, it often lasted for years in patients with catatonic schizophrenia. Many of these patients tend to be monosyllabic and answer questions as briefly as possible. They attempt to restrict contact with the interviewer without being altogether uncooperative.

14

Other Psychotic Disorders

The fourth revised edition of the *Diagnostic and Statistical Manual of Mental Disorders* (DSM-IV-TR) includes a classification of psychotic disorders that do not meet the diagnostic criteria for schizophrenia or for mood disorders with psychotic features. These include schizophreniform disorder, schizoaffective disorder, delusional disorder, brief psychotic disorder, postpartum psychosis, and shared psychotic disorder (or *folie à deux*). The obvious common factor among these diverse disorders is the presence of psychotic symptoms. The causes are varied and many.

Schizophreniform disorder is similar in all ways to schizophrenia except for the shorter duration of symptoms required to make the diagnosis: from 1 to 6 months. Brief psychotic disor-

der also has symptoms similar to schizophrenia but has a duration of less than a month. Schizoaffective disorder is characterized by symptoms typical of both schizophrenia and mood disorders. Delusional disorder is characterized by a generally intact personality, a relatively later age of onset, nonbizarre delusions, and nonprominent hallucinations. Postpartum psychosis must be considered a potential psychiatric emergency, as it can involve hallucinations and delusions that may lead to the mother harming her children or herself. Shared psychotic disorder occurs when two people closely attached to each other develop the same delusion.

The student should study the questions and answers below for a useful review of these disorders.

HELPFUL HINTS

Students should know the psychotic syndromes and other terms listed here.

- age of onset
- amok
- antipsychotic drugs:
    clozapine
    dopamine receptor antagonists
- Arctic hysteria
- atypical psychoses
- autoscopic psychosis
- *bouffée délirante*
- brief psychotic disorder
- Norman Cameron
- Capgras's syndrome
- Clérambault's syndrome
- conjugal paranoia
- Cotard's syndrome
- course
- culture-bound syndromes
- Cushing's syndrome
- delusional disorder
- delusions
- denial
- differential diagnosis
- double insanity
- EEG and CT scan
- erotomania
- family studies
- *folie à deux*

- Fregoli's syndrome
- Ganser's syndrome
- good-prognosis schizophrenia
- heutoscopy
- homicide
- ICD-10
- incidence
- inclusion and exclusion criteria
- *koro*
- Gabriel Langfeldt
- lifetime prevalence
- limbic system and basal ganglia
- lithium
- lycanthropy
- marital status
- mental status examination
- mood-congruent and -incongruent psychotic features
- neuroendocrine function
- neurological conditions
- neuropsychological testing
- nihilistic delusion
- paranoia
- paranoid pseudocommunity
- paranoid states
- paraphrenia
- passive person and dominant person

- *piblokto*
- postpartum blues
- postpartum psychosis
- postpsychotic depressive diorder of schizophrenia
- prognostic variables
- projection
- pseudocommunity
- psychodynamic formulation
- psychosis of association
- psychotherapy
- psychotic disorder not otherwise specified
- reaction formation
- reduplicative paramnesia
- schizoaffective disorder
- schizophreniform disorder
- Daniel Paul Schreber
- SES
- shared psychotic disorder
- significant stressor
- simple schizophrenia
- suicidal incidence
- *suk-yeong*
- TRH stimulation test
- wihtigo psychosis

▲ QUESTIONS

DIRECTIONS: Each of the questions or incomplete statements below is followed by five suggested responses or completions. Select the *one* that is *best* in each case.

14.1 Erotomania, the delusional disorder in which the person makes repeated efforts to contact the object of the delusion, through letter, phone call, and stalking, is also referred to as

A. Cotard's syndrome
B. Clérambault's syndrome
C. Fregoli's syndrome
D. Ganser's syndrome
E. Capgras's syndrome

14.2 A successful, 34-year-old interior designer was brought to a clinic by her 37-year-old husband and attorney. The husband lamented that for the past 3 years his wife had made increasingly shrill accusations that he was unfaithful to her. He declared that he had done everything in his power to convince her of his innocence, but there was no shaking her conviction. An examination of the facts revealed no evidence that the man had been unfaithful. When his wife was asked what her evidence was, she became vague and mysterious, declaring that she could tell such things by a faraway look in his eyes.

The patient experienced no hallucinations; her speech was well-organized; she interpreted proverbs with no difficulty; she seemed to have a good command of current events and generally displayed no difficulty in thinking, aside from her conviction of her husband's infidelity. She described herself as having a generally full life, with a few close friends and no problems except those centering on her experiences of unhappiness in the marriage. The husband reported that his wife was respected for her skills but that she had had difficulties for most of her life in close relationships with friends. She had lost a number of friends because of her apparent intolerance of differences in opinion. The patient reported that she did not want to leave the marriage, nor did she want her husband to leave her; instead, she was furious about his "injustice" and demanded that it be confessed and redeemed.

The patient's condition is best diagnosed as

A. schizophrenia, paranoid type
B. delusional disorder, jealous type
C. schizophreniform disorder
D. schizoaffective disorder, depressive type
E. delusional disorder, persecutory type

14.3 Delusional disorder

A. involves bizarre delusions
B. has a prevalence in the United States of 5 percent
C. may lead to the development of a pseudocommunity
D. has a mean age of onset in the early 20s
E. of the somatic type is the most common

14.4 Schizoaffective disorder patients

A. tend to have a deteriorating course
B. do not usually respond to lithium
C. may exhibit symptoms of schizophrenia and a mood disorder in an alternating fashion
D. have a suicide rate of at least 50 percent
E. have a poorer prognosis than patients with schizophrenia

14.5 A 45-year-old, single woman was taken to the hospital by her parents. Over the preceding year, the patient had begun to believe that her parents and state government officials were involved in a plan to get her to give away a piece of land she owned in the country. She began accusing the officials of putting substances in her food that damaged her hair and caused her to have receding gums. She wrote numerous letters to federal officials complaining of those events, yet all the while she worked efficiently at her job of examining income tax forms. She had had no previous contact with mental health professionals. The mental status examination revealed no hallucinations, incoherence, or loosening of associations.

The most likely diagnosis is

A. schizophrenia, paranoid type
B. schizophreniform disorder
C. delusional disorder
D. a mood disorder with psychotic features
E. paranoid personality disorder

14.6 True statements concerning brief psychotic disorder include all the following *except*

A. The stressor must be of sufficient severity to cause significant stress to any person in the same socioeconomic and cultural class.
B. Many patients also have preexisting personality disorders.
C. Prodromal symptoms appear before the onset of the precipitating stressor.
D. Mood disorders may be common in the relatives of affected probands.
E. Good prognostic features include a severe precipitating stressor, acute onset, and confusion or perplexity during psychosis.

14.7 Most studies of normal pregnant women indicate that the percentage who report the "blues" in the early postpartum period is about

A. 10 percent
B. 25 percent
C. 50 percent
D. 75 percent
E. 100 percent

14.8 All of the following are true statements about postpartum psychosis *except*

A. The risk is increased if the patient had a recent mood disorder.
B. Hallucinations involve voices telling the patient to kill her baby.
C. It is found in 1 to 2 per 1,000 deliveries.
D. Generally, it is not considered a psychiatric emergency.
E. Delusional material may involve the idea that the baby is dead.

14.9 In schizoaffective disorder, all of the following variables indicate a poor prognosis *except*

A. depressive type
B. no precipitating factor
C. a predominance of psychotic symptoms
D. bipolar type
E. early onset

14.10 True statements concerning the treatment of shared psychotic disorder include all of the following *except*

A. Recovery rates have been reported to be as low as 10 percent.
B. The submissive person commonly requires treatment with antipsychotic drugs.
C. Psychotherapy for nondelusional members of the patient's family should be undertaken.
D. Separation of the submissive person from the dominant person is the primary intervention.
E. The submissive person and the dominant person usually move back together after treatment.

14.11 Which of the following statements is correct?

A. The delusions of schizophrenia, paranoid type, tend to be bizarre and fragmented, in contrast to the better-organized delusions of delusional disorder.
B. In the few patients who have hallucinations in conjunction with delusional disorder, the hallucinations are not primary and are associated with the delusions, whereas hallucinations in schizophrenia are not necessarily connected with the delusion.
C. In paranoid patients with a depressed affect, the affect is secondary to the delusional system, whereas in depressed patients the delusions are secondary to the depression.
D. Delusions seen in cognitive disorders are characterized by concomitant forgetfulness and disorientation, whereas delusional disorder is characterized by intact orientation and memory.
E. All of the above

14.12 A 17-year-old high school junior was brought to the emergency room by her distraught mother, who was at a loss to understand her daughter's behavior. Two days earlier, the patient's father had been buried: he had died of a sudden myocardial infarction earlier in the week. The patient had become wildly agitated at the cemetery, screaming uncontrollably and needing to be restrained by relatives. She was inconsolable at home, sat rocking

in a corner, and talked about a devil that had come to claim her soul. Before her father's death, her mother reported, she was a "typical teenager, popular, a very good student, but sometimes prone to overreacting." The girl had no previous psychiatric history.

The most likely diagnosis is

A. grief
B. brief psychotic disorder
C. schizophrenia
D. substance intoxication
E. delusional disorder

14.13 Delusional disorder

A. is less common than schizophrenia
B. is caused by frontal lobe lesions
C. is an early stage of schizophrenia
D. usually begins by age 20
E. is more common in men than in women

14.14 Which of the following combinations best characterizes the occurrence of mental disorders among the relatives of patients with schizoaffective disorder?

A. a frequency of schizophrenia comparable to that seen among the relatives of schizophrenic patients and a frequency of mood disorders greater than that expected for the general population
B. a frequency of schizophrenia less than that seen in the general population and a frequency of mood disorders greater than that expected for the relatives of patients with mood disorders
C. a frequency of schizoaffective disorder greater than that seen in the general population and a frequency of mood disorders less than that seen among the relatives of patients with mood disorders
D. a frequency of schizophrenia less than that seen in the relatives of schizophrenic patients and a frequency of mood disorders comparable to that seen in the relatives of patients with mood disorders
E. a frequency of schizoaffective disorder comparable with that of the general population and a frequency of schizophrenia greater than that of the general population

14.15 Shared diagnostic criteria between schizophrenia and schizophreniform disorder include all of the following *except*

A. social and occupational dysfunction
B. delusions
C. hallucinations
D. disorganized speech
E. disorganized behavior

14.16 The typical presentation of schizophreniform disorder is

A. insidious-onset psychosis
B. poor premorbid functioning
C. blunted affect
D. hallucinations and delusions present
E. none of the above

14.17 The differential diagnosis of brief psychotic disorder includes

   A. substance-induced psychotic disorder
   B. psychotic disorder due to a general medical condition
   C. severe personality disorders
   D. malingering
   E. all of the above

14.18 False statements about brief psychotic disorder include all of the following *except*

   A. Approximately 50 percent of patients diagnosed retain the diagnosis and 50 percent evolve either to schizophrenia or major mood disorder.
   B. There are clear distinguishing features between brief psychotic disorder and acute-onset schizophrenia on initial presentation.
   C. There are clear distinguishing features between brief psychotic disorder and mood disorders with psychosis on initial presentation.
   D. Poor prognosis is associated with emotional turmoil at the height of the episode.
   E. None of the above

14.19 Major features of delusional disorder include

   A. presence of bizarre delusions
   B. presence of other significant psychopathology
   C. patients with the disorder are more often seen by lawyers, police, or medical specialists
   D. patients with the disorder generally do not appear eccentric or odd
   E. none of the above

14.20 Delusional disorder may include

   A. tactile hallucinations
   B. olfactory hallucinations
   C. auditory hallucinations
   D. visual hallucinations
   E. all of the above

14.21 The best-documented risk factor for delusional disorder is

   A. sensory impairment
   B. recent immigration
   C. advanced age
   D. family history
   E. social isolation

14.22 Evidence that suggests delusional disorder is a separate entity from schizophrenia or mood disorders includes

   A. epidemiological data
   B. family or genetic studies
   C. natural history of the disorder
   D. premorbid personality data
   E. all of the above

14.23 Pimozide (ORAP) is reported to be especially effective in treating delusional disorder of the

   A. erotomanic type
   B. grandiose type
   C. somatic type
   D. persecutory type
   E. jealous type

14.24 True statements about patients with delusional disorder, erotomanic type, include

   A. they exhibit what has been called "paradoxical conduct"
   B. the course of the disorder is invariably chronic
   C. separation from the love object is usually not an effective treatment
   D. women predominate in forensic populations
   E. all of the above

14.25 Of the following somatic treatments for delusional disorder, which is considered the least likely to be successful?

   A. dopamine receptor antagonists
   B. serotonin-dopamine antagonists
   C. selective serotonin reuptake inhibitors
   D. electroconvulsive treatment
   E. all of the above are considered equally effective

14.26 *Nervios* is a culture-bound syndrome that commonly includes symptoms of

   A. headaches and brain aches
   B. easy tearfulness
   C. tingling sensations
   D. dizziness
   E. all of the above

14.27 *Bouffée délirante* refers to

   A. a syndrome observed in West Africa and Haiti
   B. a sudden outburst of agitated and aggressive behavior
   C. episodes that may be accompanied by visual and auditory hallucinations
   D. episodes that resemble brief psychotic disorder
   E. all of the above

14.28 Treatment of culture-bound syndromes

   A. does not include use of antipsychotic drugs
   B. should not include collaboration with indigenous healers
   C. can involve psychotherapy
   D. is generally the same as that of other syndromes
   E. none of the above

14.29 Puerperal psychosis

   A. has a prevalence of 10 to 15 percent
   B. usually does not occur until 2 to 3 months postpartum
   C. usually has insidious onset
   D. is most likely to occur in patients with a previous history of the disorder
   E. all of the above

DIRECTIONS: Each group of questions below consists of lettered headings followed by a list of numbered words or statements. For each numbered word or statement, select the *one* lettered heading that is most closely associated with it. Each lettered heading may be selected once, more than once, or not at all.

Questions 14.30–14.34

    A. Delusions of guilt
    B. Delusions secondary to perceptual disturbances
    C. Grandiose delusions
    D. Bizarre delusions of being controlled
    E. Delusions of jealousy

14.30 Delusional disorder
14.31 Schizophrenia
14.32 Mania
14.33 Depressive disorders
14.34 Cognitive disorders

Questions 14.35–14.39

    A. Paranoid personality disorder
    B. Delusional disorder
    C. Schizophrenia
    D. Manic episode
    E. Major depressive episode

14.35 Psychomotor retardation
14.36 Thought broadcasting
14.37 Easy distractibility with an elevated, expansive, or irritable mood
14.38 Nonbizarre persecutory or grandiose delusions
14.39 Suspiciousness and mistrust of people, without psychotic symptoms

Questions 14.40–14.44

    A. Cortical impairment
    B. Subcortical impairment

14.40 Simple, transient delusions
14.41 Persecutory delusions
14.42 Elaborate and systematic delusions
14.43 Delusions with strong affective components
14.44 Delusions associated with Alzheimer's disease

Questions 14.45–14.49

    A. *Dhat*
    B. *Zar*
    C. *Hwa-byung*
    D. *Latah*
    E. *Taijin kyofu sho*

14.45 Hypersensitivity to sudden fright, often with echopraxia, echolalia, and dissociative behavior
14.46 Severe anxiety and hypochondriacal concerns associated with discharge of semen
14.47 Term applied to the experience of spirits possessing a person
14.48 Intense social phobia in which there is intense fear that one's body is offensive to other people
14.49 Known as "anger syndrome" and attributed to the suppression of anger

ANSWERS

Other Psychotic Disorders

14.1 The answer is B
Erotomania, the delusional disorder in which the person makes repeated efforts to contact the object of the delusion, through letters, phone calls, gifts, visits, surveillance, and even stalking, is also called *Clérambault's syndrome*. Most patients with erotomania are women. In forensic samples in which harm is done to another person, most are men. In *Cotard's syndrome*, patients may believe that they have lost everything: possessions, strength, and even bodily organs. *Fregoli's syndrome* is the delusion that a persecutor is taking on a variety of faces, like an actor. *Ganser's syndrome* is the voluntary production of severe psychiatric symptoms, sometimes described as the giving of approximate answers. *Capgras's syndrome* is the delusion that familiar people have been replaced by identical impostors.

14.2 The answer is B
The patient's condition is best diagnosed as *delusional disorder, jealous type*. Not all complaints of infidelity are unfounded, but in this case the evidence supported the idea that the wife's jealousy was delusional. Delusional jealousy may be seen in schizophrenia, but in the absence of the characteristic psychotic symptoms of schizophrenia, such as bizarre delusions, halluci-

nations, and disorganized speech, it is a symptom of delusional disorder. As is commonly the case in delusional disorder, the woman's impairment because of her delusion did not affect her daily functioning apart from her relationship with her husband.

The patient's condition cannot be diagnosed as *schizophrenia, paranoid type,* because of the absence of the characteristic psychotic symptoms of schizophrenia, such as bizarre delusions and hallucinations. Furthermore, the woman showed no evidence since the onset of the disturbance of a deterioration of functioning in the areas of work, self-care, and other interpersonal relationships not involved in the delusion. A person with *schizophreniform disorder* has symptoms identical to those of schizophrenia except that the symptoms last at least 1 month but less than 6 months; in schizophrenia, the symptoms must be present for at least 6 months. The patient's condition cannot be diagnosed as *schizoaffective disorder, depressive type* because she showed no evidence of schizophrenia or a major depressive episode. In *delusional disorder, persecutory type*, the delusion usually involves a single theme or a series of connected themes, such as being conspired against, cheated, spied on, followed, poisoned or drugged, maliciously maligned, harassed, or obstructed in the pursuit of long-term goals. The patient in this question did not have such a delusion.

14.3 The answer is C

Delusional disorder *may lead to the development of a pseudocommunity*. Elaboration of the delusion to include imagined persons and the attribution of malevolent motivations to both real and imagined people results in the organization of the pseudocommunity—that is, a perceived community of plotters. That delusional entity hypothetically binds together projected fears and wishes to justify the patient's aggression and to provide a tangible target for the patient's hostilities.

Delusional disorder, unlike schizophrenia, *does not involve bizarre delusions that are impossible*. For example, patients with delusional disorder may feel that they are being followed by the Federal Bureau of Investigation, which is possible; schizophrenia patients may feel that they are being controlled by Martians, which is impossible.

Delusional disorder *has a prevalence in the United States of 0.025 to 0.03 percent*. Thus, delusional disorder is much rarer than schizophrenia, which has a prevalence of about 1 percent, and the mood disorders, which have a prevalence of about 5 percent. Many persons with delusional beliefs do not talk about them, so the prevalence may be higher.

Delusional disorder *has a mean age of onset of about 40 years*, but the range for the age of onset runs from 18 to the 90s. Delusional disorder *of the somatic type is not the most common*. The persecutory type is the most common.

14.4 The answer is C

Schizoaffective disorder patients *may exhibit symptoms of schizophrenia and a mood disorder in an alternating fashion*. As a group, schizoaffective disorder patients *tend to have a nondeteriorating course and usually respond to lithium*. Also as a group, schizoaffective disorder patients tend to *have a better prognosis than do patients with schizophrenia* and a worse prognosis than do patients with mood disorders. Schizoaffective disorder patients *have a suicide rate of 10 percent, not 50 percent*.

14.5 The answer is C

On the basis of the information given, the most likely diagnosis in the case described is *delusional disorder*. The central features are the nonbizarre delusions involving situations that occur in real life—such as being followed, poisoned, and deceived—of at least 1 month's duration. The age of onset for delusional disorder is usually between 40 and 55. Intellectual and occupational functioning is usually satisfactory, whereas social and marital functioning is often impaired. The diagnosis is made only when no organic factor can be found that has initiated or maintained the disorder.

By definition, delusional disorder patients do not have prominent or sustained hallucinations, and the relatively nonbizarre quality of the delusion cited rule out *schizophrenia, paranoid type, and schizophreniform disorder*. In addition, as compared with schizophrenia, delusional disorder usually produces less impairment in daily functioning. Another consideration in the diagnostic criteria of schizophreniform disorder is the specification that the episode lasts 6 months (the patient described had symptoms over 1 year). The differential diagnosis with *mood disorders with psychotic features* can be difficult, as the psychotic features associated with mood disorders often involve nonbizarre delusions, and prominent hallucinations are unusual. The differential diagnosis depends on the relationship of the mood disturbance and the delusions. In a major depression with psychotic features, the onset of the depressed mood usually antedates the appearance of psychosis and is present after the psychosis remits. Also, the depressive symptoms are usually prominent and severe. If depressive symptoms occur in delusional disorder, they occur after the onset of the delusions, are usually mild, and often remit while the delusional symptoms persist. In *paranoid personality disorder*, there are no delusions, although there is suspiciousness and mistrust.

14.6 The answer is C

Prodromal symptoms do not appear before the onset of the precipitating stressor in brief psychotic disorder. A significant stressor may be a causative factor for brief psychotic disorder, and the *stressor must be of sufficient severity to cause significant stress to any person in the same socioeconomic and cultural class*. However, *many patients also have preexisting personality disorders*. Although schizophrenia has not been found to be common in the relatives of persons with brief psychotic disorder, *mood disorders may be common in the relatives of affected probands*. Good prognostic features include a *severe precipitating stressor, acute onset, and confusion or perplexity during the psychosis*.

14.7 The answer is C

Postpartum psychosis should not be confused with postpartum "blues," a normal condition that *occurs in about 50 percent of women after childbirth*. The "blues" are self-limited, last only a few days, and are characterized by tearfulness, fatigue, anxiety, and irritability that begin shortly after childbirth and lessen in severity each day postpartum. Postpartum psychosis is characterized by agitation, severe depression, and thoughts of infanticide.

14.8 The answer is D

Postpartum psychosis is found in 1 to 2 per 1,000 deliveries. The risk is increased if the patient or the patient's mother had a previous postpartum illness or mood disorder. The symptoms are usually experienced within days of delivery and almost always within the first 8 weeks after giving birth. The patient begins to complain of insomnia, restlessness, and fatigue, and she shows lability of mood with tearfulness. Later symptoms include suspiciousness, confusion, incoherence, irrational statements, and obsessive concerns about the baby's health. *Delusional material may involve the idea that the baby is dead* or defective. The birth may be denied, or ideas of persecution, influence, or perversity may be expressed. *Hallucinations may involve voices telling the patient to kill her baby. Postpartum psychosis is a psychiatric emergency.* In one study, 5 percent of patients killed themselves, and 4 percent killed the baby. Postpartum psychosis is not to be confused with postpartum "blues."

14.9 The answer is D

The course and the prognosis of schizoaffective disorder are variable. As a group, patients with this disorder have a prognosis intermediate between patients with schizophrenia and patients with mood disorders. Schizoaffective disorder, *bipolar type*, typically has a better prognosis. A poor prognosis is associated with the *depressive type* of schizoaffective disorder. A poor prognosis is also associated with the following variables: *no precipitating factor, a predominance of psychotic symptoms, early* or insidious *onset*, a poor premorbid history, and a positive family history of schizophrenia.

14.10 The answer is C

Psychotherapy for nondelusional *members of the patient's family is usually not necessary*. Clinical reports vary, but the prognosis is guarded—recovery rates have been reported to be *as low as 10 percent.* The *submissive person often requires treatment with antipsychotic drugs,* as does the dominant person. *Separation* of the submissive person from the dominant person is the primary intervention. The submissive person and the dominant person usually *move back together after treatment.*

14.11 The answer is E (all)
The delusions of schizophrenia, paranoid type, tend to be bizarre and fragmented, in contrast to the *better-organized delusions of delusional disorder.* In the few patients who have hallucinations in conjunction with delusional disorder, *the hallucinations are associated with the delusions,* whereas hallucinations in schizophrenia are not necessarily connected with the delusions. *In paranoid patients* with a depressed affect *the affect is secondary to the delusional system, whereas in depressed patients the delusions are secondary* to the depression. *Delusions seen in cognitive disorders are characterized by forgetfulness and disorientation,* whereas *delusional disorder is characterized by intact orientation and memory.*

14.12 The answer is B
The sudden onset of a florid psychotic episode immediately after a marked psychosocial stressor, such as the death of a loved one, in the absence of increasing psychopathology before the stressor indicates the diagnosis of *brief psychotic disorder. Grief* is an expected and normal reaction to the loss of a loved one. The girl's reaction, however, was not only more severe than would be expected (wildly agitated, screaming) but also involved psychotic symptoms (the devil). Typically, the psychotic symptoms in brief psychotic disorder last for more than a day but no more than a month. In *schizophrenia* the symptoms last for at least 6 months. *Substance intoxication* can mimic brief psychotic disorder, but the case presented shows no evidence of substance use. *Delusional disorder* presents with nonbizarre delusions of at least 1 month's duration, with otherwise relatively normal behavior.

14.13 The answer is A
Delusional disorder *is less common than schizophrenia.* Its prevalence in the United States is estimated to be 0.03 percent—in contrast with schizophrenia, 1 percent, and mood disorders, 5 percent.

The neuropsychiatric approach to delusional disorder derives from the observation that delusions are a common symptom in many neurological conditions, particularly those involving the limbic system and the basal ganglia. *No evidence indicates that the* disorder *is caused by frontal lobe lesions.* Long-term follow-up of patients with delusional disorder has found that their diagnoses are rarely revised as schizophrenia or mood disorders; hence, delusional disorder *is not an early stage of schizophrenia* or mood disorders. Moreover, delusional disorder has a later onset than does schizophrenia or mood disorders. The mean age of onset is 40 years; the disorder *does not usually begin by age 20.* The disorder *is slightly more common in women than in men.*

14.14 The answer is D
The occurrence of mental disorders among the relatives of patients with schizoaffective disorder includes an increased risk of schizoaffective disorder, *a frequency of schizophrenia less (not more) than that seen in the relatives of schizophrenic* patients, and a frequency of mood disorders comparable to (not greater than) that seen in the relatives of patients with mood disorders but greater than that expected for the general population. In fact, most of the ill relatives of patients with schizoaffective disorders suffer from uncomplicated mood disorders.

14.15 The answer is A
Schizophreniform disorder shares an overlap with schizophrenia with two exceptions: the duration of illness is from 1 to 6 months and *social or occupational dysfunction is not required to meet the diagnosis,* although it may occur at some point in the illness. Given the requirement of 1 month of psychotic symptoms, however, it seems quite unlikely that a person's social and occupational functioning would not be disrupted. DSM-IV-TR describes two possible conditions for this diagnosis: (1) when a person has recovered within the 6-month period (the "pure" form of schizophreniform disorder) and (2) when a person has not had the illness long enough (6 months) to meet the diagnosis of schizophrenia. For this latter condition the term "provisional" is used. A guide for clinicians is given as a part of the diagnosis, which should be qualified by the presence or absence of good prognostic signs. The following are listed, and two are required for the qualifier of good prognosis: (1) rapid onset of psychotic symptoms, (2) confusion at the peak of psychotic symptomatology, (3) good premorbid social and occupational functioning, and (4) maintenance of a range of affect.

As with most psychiatric diagnoses, schizophreniform disorder should not be used if substance abuse or a secondary medical condition causes the symptoms.

14.16 The answer is D
Schizophreniform disorder *in its typical presentation is a rapid-onset psychotic disorder without a significant prodrome. Hallucinations, delusions, or both will be present;* negative symptoms of alogia and avolition may be present. *Affect may be flattened, which is seen as a poor prognostic sign.* Speech may be grossly disorganized and confused, and behavior may be disorganized or catatonic. The symptoms of psychosis, the negative symptoms, and those affecting speech and behavior will last at least 1 month but may last longer. The patient's degree of perplexity about what is happening should be assessed, as this is a differentiating prognostic sign.

Although the above is the typical presentation, a picture exactly resembling that of schizophrenia may also occur. In that case, the onset may be insidious, premorbid functioning may have been poor, and affect is quite blunted. The only differentiation from schizophrenia for this type of presentation will be duration of the total episode of illness. When it has lasted 6 months, the diagnosis becomes schizophrenia. In making the diagnosis in the case with insidious onset, the "attenuated symptoms" of the acute episode may have lasted for some time. If they have been present for at least 5 months and then the acute episode lasts 1 month, the diagnosis of schizophrenia is appropriate, without a prior diagnosis of schizophreniform disorder.

In the typical form of the disorder, the patient returns to baseline functioning by the end of 6 months. Theoretically, repeated episodes of schizophreniform illness are possible, each lasting less than 6 months, but rarely is functioning not lost with repeated episodes of this severe illness, and schizophrenia is a more likely consideration.

14.17 The answer is E (all)

Sharing rapid onset of symptoms, brief psychotic disorder must be differentiated from *substance-induced psychotic disorders* and *psychotic disorders due to a general medical condition.* A thorough medical evaluation, including a physical examination, laboratory studies, and brain imaging, will help rule out many of those conditions. With only cross-sectional information, brief psychotic disorder is difficult to differentiate from other types of functional psychosis.

The relationship between brief psychotic disorder and both schizophrenia and affective disorders remains uncertain. DSM-IV-TR has made the distinction between brief psychotic disorder and schizophreniform disorder clearer by now requiring a full month of psychotic symptoms for the latter. If psychotic symptoms are present longer than 1 month, the diagnoses of schizophreniform disorder, schizoaffective disorder, schizophrenia, mood disorders with psychotic features, delusional disorder, and psychotic disorder not otherwise specified need to be entertained. If psychotic symptoms of sudden onset are present for less than a month in response to an obvious stressor, the diagnosis of brief psychotic disorder is strongly suggested. Other diagnoses to differentiate include factitious disorder, *malingering, and severe personality disorders,* with consequent transient psychosis possible.

14.18 The answer is A

The course of brief psychotic disorder is found in the diagnostic criteria of DSM-IV-TR. It is a psychotic episode that lasts more than 1 day but less than 1 month, with eventual return to premorbid level of functioning. *Approximately 50 percent patients diagnosed with brief psychotic disorder retain this diagnosis; the other 50 percent will evolve into either schizophrenia or a major affective disorder.* There are *no apparent distinguishing features* between brief psychotic disorder, acute-onset schizophrenia, and mood disorders with psychotic features on initial presentation. Several prognostic features have been proposed to characterize the illness, but they are inconsistent across studies. The *good prognostic features* are similar to those found in schizophreniform disorder: acute onset of psychotic symptoms, *confusion or emotional turmoil at the height of the psychotic episode,* good premorbid functioning, the presence of affective symptoms, and short duration of symptoms. There is a relative dearth of information on the recurrence of brief psychotic episodes, however, so the course and prognosis of this disorder have not been well characterized.

14.19 The answer is C

Once viewed as too rare to warrant a separate classification, delusional disorder has emerged in recent years as a focus of clinical research and treatment innovation. Better definition and a growing literature have revitalized the efforts to characterize, understand, and treat these conditions. Limited but growing evidence supports not only its occurrence, but its distinctiveness from schizophrenia and mood disorder as well as its treatability. Delusional disorder refers to a group of disorders, the chief feature of which is the *presence of a nonbizarre delusion.* It is the delusion and the *relative absence of other psychopathology* that unify these disorders in terms of natural history and impact on functioning.

Despite such advances, clinicians are relatively ill-informed about delusional disorders and many have only seen an occasional example. There are several possible reasons why this is

so. Persons with this condition do not regard themselves as mentally ill and actively oppose psychiatric referral. Because they may experience little impairment, they generally remain outside hospital settings, *appearing reclusive, eccentric, or odd, rather than ill.* If they do have contact with professionals, it is more likely to be with *lawyers* regarding litigious concerns; with *medical specialists* regarding health concerns; or with the *police* regarding complaints of trespass, persecution, or threat, rather than with psychiatric clinicians regarding complaints of emotional disorder. A hallmark of these disorders is that the patient does not believe that he or she is deluded or in need of psychiatric assistance. In the infrequent psychiatric encounter, clinicians tend to diagnose these disorders as other conditions, often as schizophrenia or mood disorders.

14.20 The answer is E (all)

Generally in delusional disorders, the patient's delusions are well systematized and have been developed logically. The person *may experience auditory or visual hallucinations,* but these are not prominent features. *Tactile or olfactory hallucinations* may be present and prominent if they are related to the delusional content or theme; examples are the sensation of being infested by bugs or parasites, associated with delusions of infestation; and the belief that one's body odor is foul, associated with somatic delusions. The person's behavioral and emotional responses to the delusion appear to be appropriate. Impairment of functioning is not marked and personality deterioration is minimal, if it occurs at all. General behavior is neither obviously odd nor bizarre.

14.21 The answer is D

The cause of delusional disorder is unknown. The epidemiological and clinical literature suggests that certain risk factors may be relevant to etiology and deserve further research elaboration. These risk factors are found in Table 14.1. Whether they are risk predictors or simply characteristics or markers of the disorder, is unknown. *Familial psychiatric disorder,* including delusional disorder, is the *best-documented risk factor at present.*

14.22 The answer is E (all)

An issue that is central to attributing causation is whether delusional disorder represents a separate group of conditions or is an atypical form of schizophrenic and mood disorders. The relevant data come from a limited number of studies and are inconclusive. *Epidemiology data suggest that delusional disorder is a separate condition;* it is far less prevalent than schizophrenic or mood disorders; age of onset is later than in schizophrenia, although men tend to experience the illness at earlier ages than women; and the sex ratio is different from that of mood disorder, which occurs disproportionately among

Table 14.1
Risk Factors Associated with Delusional Disorder

Advanced age
Sensory impairment/isolation
Family history
Social isolation
Personality features (e.g., unusual interpersonal sensitivity)
Recent immigration

women. Findings *from family or genetic studies* also support the theory that delusional disorder is a distinct entity. If delusional disorder is simply an unusual form of schizophrenic or mood disorders, the incidence of these latter conditions in family studies of delusional disorder patient probands should be higher than that of the general population. However, this has not been a consistent finding. A recent study concluded that patients with delusional disorder are more likely to have family members who show suspiciousness, jealousy, secretiveness, even paranoid illness, than families of controls. Other investigative efforts have found paranoid personality disorder and avoidant personality disorder to be more common in the relatives of patients with delusional disorder than in the relatives of controls or of schizophrenic patients. A recent study documented modest evidence for an increased risk of alcoholism among the relatives of patients with delusional disorder as compared to probands with schizophrenia, probands with psychotic disorder not otherwise specified, and probands with schizophreniform disorder.

Investigations into *patient's natural history* also lend support to the suggestion that delusional disorder is a distinct category: age of onset appears to be later than in schizophrenia and outcome generally is better for delusional disorder patients than for schizophrenia patients. Although fraught with methodological shortcomings, *premorbid personality data* indicate that schizophrenia patients and patients with delusional disorder differ early in life. The former are more likely to be introverted, schizoid, and submissive; the latter extroverted, dominant, and hypersensitive. Delusional disorder patients may have below-average intelligence. Precipitating factors, especially related to social isolation, conflicts of conscience, and immigration, are more closely associated to delusional disorder than schizophrenia. These characteristics support the view that environmental factors may play an important etiological role. Clinical characteristics such as greater intensity of delusions, uncommon occurrence of negative symptoms, and possible association with cerebrovascular disorder in late-onset cases also suggest differences from late-onset schizophrenia. Recent observations of successful treatment with pimozide (Orap) in several subtypes of delusional disorders suggest the possibility of a common pathogenetic mechanism in these disorders. Follow-up studies indicate that the diagnosis of delusional disorder remains fairly stable: only a small proportion of cases (3 to 22 percent) are diagnosed as having schizophrenia, and even fewer (6 percent) are diagnosed as having a mood disorder. Outcome in terms of hospitalization and occupational adjustment is markedly more favorable for delusional disorder than for schizophrenia. When social or occupational functioning is poor in delusional disorder, it generally occurs as the result of the delusional beliefs themselves, not because of cognitive impairment or negative symptoms.

The evidence argues in favor of the distinctiveness of delusional disorder, but it is likely that at least some patients diagnosed as having delusional disorder will develop schizophrenia or mood disorders. Hence, current clinical criteria have limitations and need improvement, which may be possible with the use of laboratory techniques or more specified clinical definitions. Furthermore, the data suggest that delusional disorder is relatively chronic and is probably biologically distinct from other psychotic disorders.

14.23 The answer is C

Data from treatment reports on delusional disorder suggest that pimozide (Orap), a highly specific dopamine-blocking agent, has greater effectiveness than typical antipsychotic drugs in this condition; some data even suggest that it has a unique role. Several pharmacological effects of pimozide, in addition to dopamine receptor blockade, may help explain its effectiveness: (1) relative lack of noradrenergic-blocking action, (2) calcium channel antagonism, and (3) opioid receptor blockade. The effect of opiate receptor blockade has been proposed as relevant to reported specific effectiveness in delusional infestation partly based on observations of opiate receptor–blocking interventions in delusional disorder, somatic type, with delusions of infestation. Intravenous administration of the opioid agonist fentanyl (Sublimaze) led to intensified cutaneous sensations. That *pimozide is especially effective in delusional disorder, somatic type,* supports the notion that its opiate receptor antagonism blocks central recognition of abnormal peripheral sensation.

14.24 The answer is A

Patients with erotomania have delusions of secret lovers. Most frequently the patient is a woman, but men are also susceptible to the delusion. The patient believes that a suitor, usually more socially prominent than herself, is in love with her. The delusion becomes the central focus of the patient's existence and the onset can be sudden.

Erotomania, the *psychose passionelle,* is also referred to as Clérambault's syndrome to emphasize its occurrence in different disorders. Besides being the key symptom in some cases of delusional disorder, it is known to occur in schizophrenia, mood disorder, and other organic disorders. There is no mention of erotomania in DSM-III: the condition was termed *atypical psychosis.* DSM-III-R reinstated the condition, and it remains in DSM-IV-TR.

Patients with erotomania frequently show certain characteristics: they are generally but not exclusively women, may be considered unattractive in appearance, are in low-level jobs, and lead withdrawn, lonely lives, being single and having few sexual contacts. They select secret lovers who are substantially different from themselves. *They exhibit what has been called "paradoxical conduct,"* the delusional phenomenon of interpreting all denials of love, no matter how clear, as secret affirmations of love. The *course may be chronic, recurrent, or brief. Separation from the love object may be the only satisfactory means of intervention.* Although men are less commonly afflicted by this condition than women, they may be more aggressive and possibly violent in their pursuit of love. Hence, *in forensic populations men with this condition predominate.* The object of aggression may not be the loved individual but companions or protectors of the love object who are viewed as trying to come between the lovers. The tendency toward violence among men with erotomania may lead initially to police rather than psychiatric contact. In certain cases resentment and rage in response to an absence of reaction from all forms of love communication may escalate to a point that the love object is in danger.

14.25 The answer is D

Delusional disorder is a psychotic disorder by definition, and the natural presumption has been that the condition would respond to antipsychotic medication. Because controlled studies are limited and the disorder is uncommon, the results required to support this practice empirically have been only partially obtained.

The disparate findings in the recent literature on delusional disorder treatment have been summarized recently, with several qualifications. Of approximately 1,000 articles published since 1961, the majority since 1980, 257 cases of delusional disorder (consistent with DSM-IV-TR criteria), of which 209 provided sufficient treatment detail to make comparison, were assessed. Overall treatment results indicated that 80.8 percent of cases either recovered fully or partially. Pimozide (the most frequently reported treatment) produced full recovery in 68.5 percent and partial recovery in 22.4 percent of cases treated, whereas there was full recovery in 22.6 percent and partial recovery in 45.3 percent of cases treated with *dopamine-receptor antagonists* that are typical neuroleptic agents (e.g., thioridazine [Mellaril], haloperidol [Haldol], chlorpromazine [Thorazine], loxapine, perphenazine [Trilafon], and others). The remaining cases were noncompliant with any treatment. There were no specific conclusions drawn regarding treatment with *selective serotonin reuptake inhibitors (SSRIs)*, although a number of such reports have been published.

The results of treatment with the *serotonin-dopamine antagonists* (i.e., clozapine [Clozaril], risperidone [Risperdal], olanzapine [Zyprexa], and others) is preliminary. Unfortunately, systematic case series will develop slowly, but these early results suggest that the atypical neuroleptic agents may add to the available treatment options.

The impression is growing that antipsychotic drugs are effective, and a trial, especially with pimozide or a serotonin-dopamine antagonist, is warranted. Certainly, trials of antipsychotic medication make sense when the agitation, apprehension, and anxiety that accompany delusions are prominent.

Delusional disorders *respond less well generally to electroconvulsive treatment* than do major mood disorders with psychotic features. Some cases may respond to SSRIs, especially cases of body dysmorphic disorder with delusional concerns. Table 14.2 summarizes the somatic agents with reports of successful use in delusional disorder.

14.26 The answer is E (all)

Nervios is a common idiom of distress among Latinos in the United States and Latin America. A number of other ethnic groups have related, though often somewhat distinctive, ideas of nerves (such as *nerva* among Greeks in North America). *Nervios* refers both to a general state of vulnerability to stressful life experiences and to a syndrome brought on by difficult life circumstances. The term *nervios* includes a wide range of symptoms of emotional distress, somatic disturbance, and inability to function. *Common symptoms include headaches*

Table 14.2
Pharmacological Agents with Reports of Successful Use in Delusional Disorder

Dopamine-receptor antagonists (particularly pimozide)
Serotonin-dopamine antagonists
Selective serotonin reuptake inhibitors

and brain aches, irritability, stomach disturbances, sleep difficulties, nervousness, *easy tearfulness,* inability to concentrate, trembling, *tingling sensations,* and mareos (*dizziness* with occasional vertigo-like exacerbations). Nervios tends to be an ongoing problem, although variable in the degree of disability that is manifest. *Nervios* is a very broad syndrome that spans the range from patients free of a mental disorder to presentations resembling adjustment, anxiety, depressive, dissociative, somatoform, or psychotic disorders. Differential diagnosis depends on the constellation of symptoms experienced, the kind of social events that are associated with the onset and progress of *nervios,* and the level of disability experienced.

14.27 The answer is E (all)

Bouffée délirante is a syndrome observed in *West Africa and Haiti.* The French term refers to a *sudden outburst of agitated and aggressive behavior* marked by confusion and psychomotor excitement. It may sometimes be accompanied by *visual and auditory hallucinations* or paranoid ideation. The episodes may resemble an episode of *brief psychotic disorder.*

14.28 The answer is C

Because cross-culture syndromes may share the presence of psychosis, pharmacotherapy *frequently involves the use of antipsychotic drugs.* Some evidence indicates that the dosage of antipsychotic drugs necessary for acute transient psychotic disorders is significantly lower than that required for other psychotic conditions, especially schizophrenia. It is thus prudent to use the lowest dose that can control the patient's symptoms. Since acute and transient psychotic disorders are often episodic, intermittent use of antipsychotic drugs, guided by the emergence of psychotic symptoms, is worth considering.

The importance of cultural issues in the evaluation and treatment of atypical psychoses can hardly be exaggerated, especially when dealing with patients from non-Western and ethnic minority populations. *Cultural information* is not only crucial for accurate diagnosis, but also *indispensable in the formulation of treatment plans.* Treatment approaches that do not take the patient's sociocultural background into account are likely to fail, no matter how well intentioned the therapists may be. For example, while *psychotherapy can be very effective* in cultures in which family and group harmony and unity are valued over individual independence, the rigid application of Western-based psychotherapeutic techniques may exacerbate, rather than ameliorate, the patient's psychopathological condition. Consideration of the intercultural elements in the clinician-patient relationship is also fundamental for establishment of rapport and effective engagement of the patient and the family in the treatment process.

One *promising avenue is collaboration with indigenous healers.* Several researchers have reported on their success in the use of indigenous and traditional healers in the treatment of psychiatric patients, especially those whose psychotic conditions are substantially connected to culture-specific beliefs (e.g., fear of voodoo death). Others have mentioned the potential pitfalls and problems in such collaboration. Decisions about involving indigenous healers should be individualized and planned thoughtfully, taking into consideration the setting, the conscientiousness and flexibility of the available healers, the type of psychopathology, and the patient's characteristics.

Determining the meaning and particularly their belief about what has caused the distress is an important entry point in facilitating therapeutic management and enhancing adherence to the treatment plan. As part of taking the history, ask these patients what they think could have caused the problem, requesting the "patient's explanatory model": (1) What do you think has caused your problem? (2) Why do you think it started when it did? (3) What do you think your sickness does to you? How does it work? (4) How severe is your sickness? Will it have a short or long course? (5) What kind of treatment do you think you should receive?

Such insight into the dynamics of the patient's world facilitates the clinician's efforts to adapt his or her techniques (e.g., general activity level, mode of verbal intervention, content of remarks, tone of voice) to the cultural background of clients; communicate acceptance of and respect for the patients in terms that make sense within their cultural frame of reference; and be open to the possibility of more direct intervention in the life of the patient than conventional approaches might suggest.

In conclusion, the *treatment* of patients experiencing acute transient psychotic disorders and culture-bound syndromes, even more than that of patients with other psychiatric disorders, *should be personalized and comprehensive*, using judiciously all biological, psychological, and social therapies pertinent to the problem at hand and keeping in mind the cultural framework of the patients and their families.

14.29 The answer is D

Puerperal psychosis is the most severe form of postpartum psychiatric illness. In contrast to postpartum blues and depression, puerperal psychosis is a *rare event that occurs in approximately 1 to 2 per 1,000 women after childbirth. Its presentation is often dramatic, with onset of psychosis as early as the first 48 to 72 hours postpartum. Most women with puerperal psychosis develop symptoms within the first 2 to 4 weeks after delivery.*

In women with this disorder, psychotic symptoms and disorganized behavior are prominent and cause significant dysfunction. Puerperal psychosis *resembles a rapidly evolving affective psychosis* with restlessness, irritability, and insomnia. Women with this disorder may exhibit a rapidly shifting depressed or elated mood, disorientation or depersonalization, and disorganized behavior. Delusional beliefs often center on the infant and include delusions that the child may be defective or dying, that the infant has special powers, or that the child is either Satan or God. Auditory hallucinations that instruct the mother to harm or kill herself or her infant are sometimes reported. Although most believe that this illness is indistinguishable from an affective (or manic) psychosis, some have argued that puerperal psychosis may be clinically distinct in that it is more commonly associated with confusion and delirium than nonpuerperal psychotic mood disorder.

Although it has been difficult to identify specific demographic and psychosocial variables that consistently predict risk for postpartum illness, there is a well-defined association between all types of postpartum psychiatric illness and a personal history of mood disorder (Table 14.3). At highest risk are women with a history of postpartum psychosis; *up to 70 percent of women who have had one episode of puerperal psychosis will experience another episode following a subsequent pregnancy.* Similarly, women with histories of postpartum

Table 14.3
History of Psychiatric Illness and Risk for Puerperal Relapse

Disorders	Risk of Relapse at Future Pregnancy (%)
Postpartum psychosis	70
Postpartum depression	50
Bipolar I disorder	20–50
Major depressive disorder	30

depression are at significant risk, with rates of postpartum depression recurrence as high as 50 percent. Women with bipolar disorders also appear to be particularly vulnerable during the postpartum period, with rates of bipolar relapse ranging from 20 to 50 percent.

Answers 14.30–14.34

14.30 The answer is E

14.31 The answer is D

14.32 The answer is C

14.33 The answer is A

14.34 The answer is B

In *delusional disorder, delusions of jealousy* are most commonly found. In *schizophrenia, bizarre delusions* may occur, for instance of being controlled by outside persons or forces and delusions of persecution. *Grandiose delusions* are most often seen in *mania* but can be observed in other psychotic disorder as well. In *depressive disorders, delusions of guilt* are especially characteristic. In *cognitive disorders,* such as dementia, *delusions secondary to perceptual disturbances* are most often evident.

Answers 14.35–14.39

14.35 The answer is E

14.36 The answer is C

14.37 The answer is D

14.38 The answer is B

14.39 The answer is A

Psychomotor retardation is a general slowing of mental and physical activity. It is often a sign of a *major depressive episode,* which is characterized by feelings of sadness, loneliness, despair, low self-esteem, and self-reproach. *Thought broadcasting* is the feeling that one's thoughts are being broadcast or projected into the environment. Such feelings are encountered in *schizophrenia.*

A patient in a *manic episode* is *easily distracted, with an elevated, expansive, or irritable mood* with pressured speech and hyperactivity.

Delusional disorder is characterized by nonbizarre *persecutory or grandiose delusions* and related disturbances in mood, thought, and behavior.

The essential feature of *paranoid personality disorder* is a long-standing *suspiciousness and mistrust of people without the presence of psychotic symptoms*. Patients with this disorder are hypersensitive and continually alert for environmental clues that will validate their original prejudicial ideas.

Answers 14.40–14.44

14.40 The answer is A

14.41 The answer is A

14.42 The answer is B

14.43 The answer is B

14.44 The answer is A

As in most psychiatric conditions, there is no evidence of localized brain pathology to correlate with clinical psychopathology in patients with delusional disorder. These patients seldom die early and show no consistent abnormalities on neurological examination. Delusions can complicate many disorders and virtually all brain disorders. Certain disorders produce delusions at rates greater than that expected in the general population: for example, epilepsy (especially of the temporal lobe), degenerative dementias (dementia of the Alzheimer's type and vascular dementia), cerebrovascular disease, extrapyramidal disorders, and traumatic brain injury.

Although many types of delusions have been reported in patients with brain disorders, there appear to be particular connections between delusion phenomenology and certain kinds of brain dysfunction. For example, patients with *more severe cortical impairment tend to experience simpler, transient, persecutory delusions*. This type of delusional experience is characteristic of conditions such as *Alzheimer's disease,* dementia, and metabolic encephalopathy that are also associated with significant cognitive disturbance. *More complex (i.e., elaborate and systematic) delusional experiences* tend to be more chronic, intensely held, resistant to treatment, and associated with neurological conditions producing less intellectual impairment and *strong affective components*. Those features occur in patients with neurological lesions involving the limbic system or *subcortical* nuclei rather than cortical areas. That, coupled with the observation of response of some patients to drug treatment, such as pimozide and other medications, provides a rational basis on which to hypothesize the presence of subcortical pathology, possibly involving systems subserving temporolimbic areas. Available evidence suggests that if there is a lesion, it will be subtle.

Answers 14.45–14.49

14.45 The answer is D

14.46 The answer is A

14.47 The answer is B

14.48 The answer is E

14.49 The answer is C

Latah. *Hypersensitivity to sudden fright*, often with echopraxia, echolalia, command obedience, and dissociative or trance-like behavior. The term *latah* is of Malaysian or Indonesian origin, but the syndrome has been found in many parts of the world. Other terms for the condition are *amurakh, irkunil, ikota, olan, myriachit,* and *menkeiti* (Siberian groups); *bah tschi, bah-tsi, baah-ji* (Thailand); *imu* (Ainu, Sakhalin, Japan); and *mali-mali* and *silok* (Philippines). In Malaysia it is more frequent in middle-aged women.

Dhat. A folk diagnostic term used in India to refer to *severe anxiety and hypochondriacal concerns associated with the discharge of semen*, whitish discoloration of the urine, and feelings of weakness and exhaustion. Similar to *jiryan* (India), *sukra prameha* (Sri Lanka), and *shen-k'uei* (China).

Zar. A general term applied in Ethiopia, Somalia, Egypt, Sudan, Iran, and other North African and Middle Eastern societies to the *experience of spirits possessing a person*. Persons possessed by a spirit may experience dissociative episodes that may include shouting, laughing, hitting the head against a wall, singing, or weeping. They may show apathy and withdrawal, refusing to eat or carry out daily tasks, or may develop a long-term relationship with the possessing spirit. Such behavior is not considered pathological locally.

Taijin kyofu sho. A culturally distinctive phobia in Japan, in some ways *resembling social phobia* in DSM-IV-TR. The syndrome refers to an *intense fear that one's body*, its parts, or its functions, displease, embarrass, or are *offensive* to other people in appearance, odor, facial expressions, or movements. The syndrome is included in the official Japanese diagnostic system for mental disorders.

Hwa-byung. (also known as *wool-hwa-byung*) A Korean folk syndrome literally translated into English as *"anger syndrome"* and *attributed to the suppression of anger*. The symptoms include insomnia, fatigue, panic, fear of impending death, dysphoric affect, indigestion, anorexia, dyspnea, palpitations, generalized aches and pains, and a feeling of a mass in the epigastrium.

15

Mood Disorders

Mood disorders have been studied and described for as many years as has schizophrenia. In fact, Emil Kraepelin, who was one of the first clinicians to explain schizophrenia, was also one of the first to explicate the major mood disorders. He called these the manic-depressive insanities and distinguished their presentation, course, and prognosis from those of schizophrenia. In the fourth revised edition of the *Diagnostic and Statistical Manual of Mental Disorders* (DSM-IV-TR), mood disorders are classified as depressive, bipolar, and other mood disorders. Specifiers are employed to describe the most recent mood episode as mild, moderate, or severe, and with or without psychotic features. The depressive disorders include major depressive, dysthymic, and not otherwise specified. The bipolar disorders include bipolar I, bipolar II, cyclothymic, and not otherwise specified. Other mood disorders include those due to a general medical condition, substance-induced, and not otherwise specified.

The two major mood disorders, and the ones that most closely resemble those described by Kraepelin, are major depressive disorder and bipolar I disorder. The former is characterized by one or more major depressive episodes, and the latter by one or more manic or mixed episodes, usually associated with a history of major depressive episodes as well. Mood disorders are common. The lifetime prevalence of major depressive disorder is particularly so, with 10 percent of women and 6 percent of men being affected. The lifetime prevalence of bipolar I disorder is about 1 percent, similar to that of schizophrenia.

Mood disorders can sometimes be difficult to diagnose, given the subjective nature of the symptoms. All people have normal periods of feeling either blue or elated, and most of these obviously are not diagnosable as disorders. A mood disorder is characterized by the intensity, duration, and severity of the symptoms. People with mood disorders cannot control their symptoms, the most severe of which are psychotic. Symptoms interfere with normal thought process and content, and cognitive, speech, and social functioning. Many people with depressive disorders unfortunately go untreated, as their symptoms are minimized or misinterpreted. People with bipolar disorders are more often treated, as their symptoms more frequently are bizarre or disruptive enough to bring them to medical and psychiatric attention.

Mood disorders are caused by a complex interplay of biological and psychological factors. Biologic theories involve the role of the biogenic amines, in particular dysfunction in the norepinephrine, serotonin, dopamine, and GABA neurotransmitter systems. Most antidepressant medications involve complex manipulations of these systems. There appears to be dysregulation as well in the adrenal, thyroid, and growth hormone axes, all of which have been implicated in the etiology of mood disorders. Abnormalities in the sleep cycle and in regulation of circadian rhythms have also been studied.

Genetics always play an important role in the etiology of mental disorders, but genetic input is especially relevant in mood disorders. Bipolar I disorder is one of the most genetically determined disorders in psychiatry. However, as with any mental disorder, psychosocial factors play a crucial role in the development, presentation, course, and prognosis of mood disorders. Issues of real and symbolic loss, family relationships and dynamics, environmental stress, and unconscious conflicts all strongly contribute to and determine mood symptoms. Some clinicians believe that these factors are particularly important in the first episodes of mood disorders, but in one form or another they play a role in all episodes.

Skilled clinicians will be knowledgeable about all available treatment modalities, their indications, side effects, limitations, and advantages. They will know how best to combine different treatments, and which treatments are most effective for which disorders, from psychopharmacologic interventions, to the different psychotherapies, to ECT.

The student should study the questions and answers below for a useful review of these disorders.

HELPFUL HINTS

The student should know the following terms that relate to mood disorders.

- ▶ adrenal axis
- ▶ affect
- ▶ age-dependent symptoms
- ▶ amphetamine
- ▶ antipsychotics
- ▶ anxiety-blissfulness psychosis
- ▶ atypical features
- ▶ biogenic amines
- ▶ bipolar I disorder
- ▶ bipolar II disorder
- ▶ carbamazepine
- ▶ catatonic features
- ▶ clinical management

- ▶ cognitive, behavioral, family, and psychoanalytic therapies
- ▶ cognitive theories
- ▶ cyclothymic disorder
- ▶ depression rating scales
- ▶ depressive equivalent
- ▶ differential diagnosis
- ▶ double depression
- ▶ dysthymic (early and late onset) disorder
- ▶ ECT
- ▶ euthymic
- ▶ *folie à double forme*
- ▶ *folie circulaire*
- ▶ *forme fruste*
- ▶ GABA

- ▶ genetic studies
- ▶ GH
- ▶ 5-HT
- ▶ hypomania
- ▶ hypothalamus
- ▶ incidence and prevalence
- ▶ Karl Kahlbaum
- ▶ kindling
- ▶ Heinz Kohut
- ▶ Emil Kraepelin
- ▶ learned helplessness
- ▶ LH, FSH
- ▶ life events and stress
- ▶ lithium
- ▶ major depressive disorder

- ▶ mania
- ▶ MAOIs
- ▶ melancholic features
- ▶ melatonin
- ▶ mild depressive disorder
- ▶ mixed episode
- ▶ mood
- ▶ mood-congruent and mood-incongruent psychotic fear
- ▶ neurological, medical, and pharmacological causes of mood disorders
- ▶ norepinephrine
- ▶ phototherapy
- ▶ postpartum onset

- ▶ premenstrual dysphoric disorder
- ▶ premorbid factors
- ▶ pseudodementia
- ▶ rapid cycling
- ▶ REM latency, density
- ▶ RFLP
- ▶ seasonal pattern
- ▶ sex ratios of disorders
- ▶ SSRI
- ▶ suicide
- ▶ T3
- ▶ thymoleptics
- ▶ TSH, TRH
- ▶ vegetative functions
- ▶ *Zeitgebers*

▲ QUESTIONS

DIRECTIONS: From the following list of lettered lifetime prevalence criteria, select the best estimated percentage for each disorder in questions 15.1 to 15.3.

- A. Lifetime prevalence is about 6 percent.
- B. Lifetime prevalence is about 0.5 percent.
- C. Lifetime prevalence is about 0.4 to 1.6 percent.
- D. Lifetime prevalence is about 3 to 5 percent.
- E. Lifetime prevalence is about 0.4 to 1 percent.

15.1 Bipolar I disorder
15.2 Bipolar II disorder
15.3 Cyclothymic disorder

DIRECTIONS: Each of the questions or incomplete statements below is followed by five suggested responses or completions. Select the *one* that is *best* in each case.

15.4 All of the following statements about patients with bipolar I disorder are true *except*

- A. They have a poorer prognosis than do patients with major depressive disorder.
- B. They may have bizarre and mood-incongruent delusions and hallucinations when manic.
- C. About 75 percent of female patients have had a manic episode before exhibiting their first depressive disorder.
- D. Only 50 to 60 percent of these patients achieve significant control of their symptoms with lithium.
- E. When manic, they may be emotionally labile and not easily interrupted while they are speaking.

15.5 Which of the following is helpful in the differential diagnosis and the formulation of a treatment plan for a patient with a mood disorder?

- A. family history of psychiatric illness
- B. knowledge of the type of psychiatric medication used in the past
- C. medical problems
- D. past or present substance abuse
- E. all of the above

15.6 The defense mechanism most commonly used in depression is

- A. projection
- B. introjection
- C. sublimation
- D. undoing
- E. altruism

15.7 The percentage of depressed patients who eventually commit suicide is estimated to be

- A. 0.5 percent
- B. 5 percent
- C. 15 percent
- D. 25 percent
- E. 35 percent

15.8 All of the following statements about bipolar I disorder are true *except*

- A. Bipolar I disorder most often starts with depression.
- B. About 10 to 20 percent of patients experience only manic episodes.
- C. An untreated manic episode lasts about 3 months.
- D. As the illness progresses, the amount of time between episodes often increases.
- E. Rapid cycling is much more common in women than in men.

15.9 Of the following neurological diseases, which is most often associated with depression?

    A. epilepsy

    B. brain tumor

    C. Parkinson's disease

    D. dementia of the Alzheimer's type

    E. huntington's disease

Questions 15.10–15.11

A 25-year-old junior executive was referred to a health service because he had been drinking excessively over the previous 2 weeks. The patient reported that he had been "down" for about a month, cried frequently, and had no interest in sex or work. His history revealed that he had suffered those down periods for several years; but he also described himself as having experienced periods of elation during which he was gregarious, productive, and optimistic. During those times, he said, he did not drink at all. The young man also stated that the behavior had been present on and off since he was about 15 years old.

15.10 The best diagnosis for this patient is most likely

    A. major depressive disorder

    B. bipolar I disorder

    C. cyclothymic disorder

    D. dysthymic disorder

    E. bipolar II disorder

15.11 If the patient was treated with a tricyclic antidepressant (TCA), which of the following is *least likely* to result?

    A. tachycardia, flattened T waves, and prolonged QT intervals

    B. suicidal ideation

    C. excessive involvement in pleasurable activities with a high potential for painful consequences

    D. myoclonic twitches and tremors of the tongue

    E. a hypomanic state

15.12 A 40-year-old man was taken to the psychiatric emergency room after becoming involved in a fist fight at a bar. He was speaking rapidly, jumping from one thought to another in response to simple, specific questions (for example, "When did you come to New York?" "I came to New York, the Big Apple, it's rotten to the core, no matter how you slice it, I sliced a bagel this morning for breakfast."). The patient described experiencing his thoughts as racing. He was unable to explain how he got into the fight other than to say that the other person was jealous of the patient's obvious sexual prowess, the patient having declared that he had slept with at least 100 women. He made allusions to his father as being God and he stated that he had not slept in 3 days. "I don't need it," he said. The patient's speech was full of amusing puns, jokes, and plays on words.

    Typical associated findings consistent with the patient's probable diagnosis include all of the following *except*

    A. emotional lability

    B. hallucinations

    C. flight of ideas

    D. nocturnal electroencephalographic (EEG) changes

    E. mood-incongruent delusions

15.13 The lifetime prevalence of dysthymic disorder is

    A. 1 percent

    B. 3 percent

    C. 6 percent

    D. 9 percent

    E. 11 percent

15.14 The course of major depressive disorder usually includes all of the following *except*

    A. an untreated episode of depression lasting 6 to 13 months

    B. a treated episode of depression lasting about 3 months

    C. the return of symptoms after the withdrawal of antidepressants before 3 months have elapsed

    D. an average of five to six episodes over a 20-year period

    E. progression to bipolar II disorder

15.15 Which of the following medications may produce depressive symptoms?

    A. Analgesics

    B. Antibacterials

    C. Antipsychotics

    D. Antihypertensives

    E. All of the above

15.16 L-Tryptophan

    A. is the amino acid precursor to dopamine

    B. has been used as an adjuvant to both antidepressants and lithium

    C. has been used as a stimulant

    D. has not been associated with any serious side effects

    E. all of the above

15.17 Drugs that may precipitate mania include all of the following *except*

    A. bromocriptine

    B. isoniazid

    C. propranolol

    D. disulfiram

    E. all of the above

15.18 Figure 15.1 depicts the distribution, according to age and sex, of which of the following?

    A. incidence of anorexia nervosa

    B. prevalence of mood disorders

    C. incidence of obsessive-compulsive disorder

    D. prevalence of schizophrenia

    E. incidence of somatization disorder

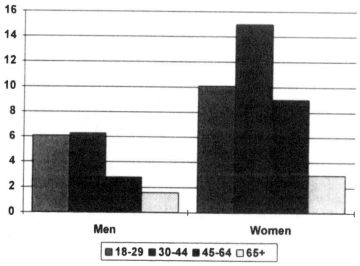

FIGURE 15.1
Data derived from the Epidemiologic Catchment Area study.

15.19 A 37-year-old white man comes to your office at the urging of his wife. A few years earlier he had an asymptomatic thyroid mass removed, which was followed by dramatic mood changes a month later. The patient would experience 25 days of remarkable energy, hyperactivity, and euphoria, followed by 5 days of depression during which he slept a lot and felt he could hardly move. That rapid pattern of alternating periods of elation and depression, apparently with few "normal" days, repeated itself continuously to the present time. The patient denies any drug use and states that his last batch of hospital tests revealed some evidence of thyroid hypofunctioning but that he was without clinical signs of thyroid disease. The patient also states that he has been minimally cooperative and noncompliant with several medications that were prescribed for him, including lithium, neuroleptics, and antidepressants.

The correct first-line treatment for this patient's disorder is

A. lithium
B. electroconvulsive therapy (ECT)
C. valproate or carbamazepine
D. tricyclic antidepressants
E. clozapine (Clozaril)

15.20 The most common mood disorder is reported to be

A. major depressive disorder
B. bipolar disorder
C. dysthymia
D. cyclothymia
E. none of the above

15.21 Recent clinical experience suggests comorbidity patterns between bipolar II disorder and

A. panic symptoms
B. obsessive-compulsive symptoms
C. social phobia symptoms
D. all of the above
E. none of the above

15.22 Most studies in developed countries estimate the distribution of major depressive disorder to be greater

A. in middle and old age than in young adulthood
B. in rural residents than in urban residents
C. in women than in men
D. among married persons than among single or divorced persons
E. in blacks than in whites

15.23 True statements about changing prevalence rates related to mood disorders include all the following *except*

A. The risk of first-onset depression is higher for younger birth cohorts than older in Sweden.
B. There is a progressively lower age of onset of depression disorder in community studies.
C. Suicide rates are not much higher in young people today than they were 30 years ago.
D. Suicide rates in older adults have increased by 25 percent since 1980.
E. There is an increase in childhood mood disorders seen by pediatricians and mental health workers.

15.24 True statements about the association of early childhood experience with onset of mood disorder later in life include all of the following *except*

A. Parental loss before adolescence has not been well documented as a risk factor for adult-onset depression.
B. A deprived and disrupted home constitutes a risk.
C. Objective study of childhood trauma and deprivation is difficult.
D. Divorce and separation of parents are events that can be documented reliably.
E. Reports of parental neglect tend to be subjective and vary depending on state at time of interview.

15.25 True statements about the natural history of mood disorders include

A. Relapse rates are lower for major depressive disorder immediately following recovery.

B. Bipolar I disorder patients with only manic episodes had worse outcome than those with major depressive disorder.

C. Bipolar I patients with a mixed episode or rapid cycling had worse outcomes than those with major depressive disorder.

D. Following diagnosis with either bipolar I disorder or major depressive disorder, about 70 percent of subjects recovered during the first year, and more than 50 percent of the others resolved during subsequent years.

E. None of the above

15.26 True statements about the genetics of mood disorders include

A. The morbid risk of bipolar disorder in first-degree relatives of bipolar disorder probands is between 3 and 8 percent, compared to 1 percent in the general population.

B. Depressive disorders are typically the most common mood disorder in families of probands with bipolar disorder.

C. The concordance rate for mood disorder in general in monozygotic twins is two to four times that in dizygotic twins.

D. There is greater genetic involvement in bipolar disorders than in unipolar depressive disorders.

E. All of the above

15.27 Serotonin

A. is an important regulator of sleep, appetite, and libido

B. helps to regulate circadian rhythms

C. permits or facilitates goal-directed motor and consummatory behavior in conjunction with norepinephrine and dopamine

D. stores are increased by transient stress and depleted by chronic stress

E. all of the above

15.28 True statements concerning the role of the thyroid in mood disorders include

A. About 0.5 to 1 percent of people evaluated for depression have primarily undetected or subclinical thyroid dysfunction.

B. Depressed patients receiving a TRH challenge test usually show a blunted TSH response.

C. A blunted TSH response has not been associated with heightened relapse risk.

D. Elevated antithyroid antibody levels rarely compromise response to treatment in women with rapid-cycling bipolar disorder.

E. None of the above

15.29 The most consistent CT and MRI abnormality observed in depressive disorders is

A. ventricular enlargement

B. increased frequency of hyperintensities in subcortical regions

C. cortical atrophy

D. sulcal widening

E. none of the above

15.30 Mirroring, twinship, and idealization are terms associated with

A. Sigmund Freud

B. Melanie Klein

C. Edith Jacobson

D. Heinz Kohut

E. Charles Brenner

15.31 Of the following personality disorders, which is the *least* likely to decompensate into depression?

A. Paranoid

B. Borderline

C. Histrionic

D. Obsessive-compulsive

E. Dependent

15.32 DSM-IV-TR criteria for melancholic features of depression include

A. mood reactivity to pleasurable stimuli

B. long-standing patterns of interpersonal rejection sensitivity

C. depression is regularly worse in the morning

D. hypersomnia

E. significant weight gain

15.33 All of the following are DSM-IV-TR criteria for manic episode or bipolar disorder *except*

A. hyposomnia

B. denial and lack of insight

C. distractibility

D. irritability

E. impulsive behavior

15.34 Common features of normal bereavement include

A. the presence of marked psychomotor retardation

B. lack of reactivity to the environment

C. suicidal ideation

D. delusions of worthlessness and guilt

E. none of the above

15.35 True statements about ECT as a treatment in mood disorders include all of the following *except*

A. ECT is effective in the treatment of both psychotic and nonpsychotic depressions.

B. Usually 15 to 20 treatments are needed.

C. Bilateral ECT is more effective than unilateral ECT.

D. Unilateral ECT is associated with fewer cognitive adverse effects.

E. ECT is effective even in patients who have failed to respond to one or more medications or combined treatment.

15.36 Nefazodone (Serzone) and mirtazapine (Remeron) are considered to be

A. norepinephrine reuptake inhibitors

B. 5-HT reuptake inhibitors

C. 5-HT norepinephrine reuptake inhibitors

D. presynaptic and postsynaptic active agents

E. dopamine-reuptake inhibitors

15.37 Augmentation strategies in the treatment of a bipolar patient include the use of

A. p.r.n. high-potency benzodiazepine
B. a second or third mood stabilizer
C. p.r.n. antipsychotic
D. clonidine
E. all of the above

DIRECTIONS: Each set of lettered headings below is followed by a list of phrases or statements. For each numbered phrase or statement, select

A. if the item is associated with *A only*
B. if the item is associated with *B only*
C. if the item is associated with *both A and B*
D. if the item is associated with *neither A nor B*

Questions 15.38–15.40

A. Minor depressive disorder
B. Recurrent brief depressive disorder
C. Both
D. Neither

15.38 Symptoms meet most of the diagnostic criteria for major depressive disorder
15.39 Symptoms are equal in duration, but fewer in number than those in major depressive disorder
15.40 Treatment may include the use of antidepressants

Questions 15.41–15.44

A. Major depressive disorder, recurrent
B. Dysthymic disorder
C. Both
D. Neither

15.41 Episodic periods of depression
15.42 Family history of mood disorders, decreased rapid eye movement latency, and therapeutic response to antidepressants
15.43 DSM-IV-TR–defined subtypes based on onset before and after age 21
15.44 Possible psychotic symptoms

Questions 15.45–15.46

A. Cyclothymic disorder
B. Bipolar II disorder
C. Both
D. Neither

15.45 Characterized by episodes of hypomanic-like symptoms and periods of mild depression
15.46 Characterized by major depressive episodes and hypomanic episodes

DIRECTIONS: Each group of questions below consists of lettered headings followed by a list of numbered words or statements. For each numbered word or statement, select the *one* lettered heading that is most closely associated with it. Each lettered heading may be selected once, more than once, or not at all.

Questions 15.47–15.51

A. Sigmund Freud
B. Adolph Meyer
C. Aaron Beck
D. Emil Kraepelin
E. Martin Seligman

15.47 Depression is a result of aggressive impulses directed against an ambivalently loved internalized object
15.48 Negative cognitive schemata lead to depressive symptoms
15.49 Learned helplessness as a model for depression
15.50 Established manic-depressive illness as a nosological and disease entity
15.51 Coined the term "psychobiology" to emphasize that both psychological and biological facts could cause depression

Questions 15.52–15.55

A. Period effects
B. Age effects
C. Cohort effects
D. All of the above
E. None of the above

15.52 The genetic predisposition to develop major depressive disorder is probably greater during the 30s, and the predisposition to develop bipolar disorder is greatest during the 20s
15.53 The uncertainty of employment among college graduates and the trend to delay marriage during the 1990s
15.54 The association between age and suicide in white males
15.55 People born between 1915 and 1925 exhibit lower suicide rates at all ages than either those born in 1900 or 1940

ANSWERS

Mood Disorders

15.1 The answer is C

Bipolar I disorder is characterized by one or more manic or mixed episodes and sometimes by one or more major depressive episodes. People with this disorder have a rate of suicide that may be as high as 10 to 15 percent. Child or spouse abuse or other violent behavior can occur during severe manic episodes or in patients whose disorders show psychotic features. Other problems include antisocial behavior, occupational failure, and divorce. The *lifetime prevalence* of bipolar I disorder *is about 0.4 to 1.6 percent.*

15.2 The answer is B

Bipolar II disorder is characterized by one or more major depressive episodes accompanied by at least one hypomanic episode. The presence of a manic or mixed disorder precludes the diagnosis of bipolar II disorder. People with bipolar II disorder are at significant risk for suicide, which occurs in 10 to 15 percent of those with this disorder. Associated features similar to those of bipolar I disorder include occupational failure and divorce. This disorder may be more common in women than in men. *Lifetime prevalence* of bipolar II disorder *is about 0.5 percent.*

15.3 The answer is E

Cyclothymic disorder is a chronic fluctuating mood disturbance with many periods of hypomanic and depressive symptoms. The hypomanic symptoms are too few and not severe, pervasive, or long-lasting enough to satisfy the criteria for a manic episode, and the depressive symptoms are too few and not severe, pervasive, or long-lasting enough to satisfy the criteria for a major depressive episode. Although some people function well during some periods of hypomania, there is usually a significant level of impairment or distress in social, occupational, or other important areas of functioning. The disorder apparently occurs at the same rate in both women and men, on the basis of community sampling, but women seek treatment more than do men. *The lifetime prevalence rate of* cyclothymic disorder *is about 0.4 to 1 percent.*

15.4 The answer is C

Patients with bipolar I disorder *usually have had a depressive episode before exhibiting their first manic episode.* That has been found true 75 percent of the time in women and 67 percent of the time in men. Most patients experience both depressive and manic episodes, although 10 to 20 percent experience only manic episodes.

Patients with bipolar I disorder *have a poorer prognosis than do patients with major depressive disorder.* About 40 to 50 percent of bipolar I disorder patients may have a second manic episode within 2 years of the first episode. Although lithium (Eskalith) prophylaxis improves the course and the prognosis of bipolar I disorder, probably *only 50 to 60 percent of patients achieve significant control of their symptoms with lithium.*

Patients may be emotionally labile when manic, switching from laughter to irritability to depression in minutes or hours. Patients *are not easily interrupted while they are speaking when manic,* and they are often intrusive nuisances to those around them. Patients *may have bizarre and mood-incongruent (as well as mood-congruent) delusions and hallucinations when manic.*

15.5 The answer is E (all)

A patient's history and *family history of psychiatric illness* can provide valuable information about the patient's clinical picture. Suicide in a parent, for example, increases the risk of suicide in the patient. If a patient has been depressed before, *knowledge of the type of medication used in the past* can provide the physician with a head start. Knowing whether the patient has ever had a period of mania or has had a recent severe emotional trauma is essential in making the correct diagnosis and formulating an effective treatment plan. For example, a history of a manic episode is indicative of bipolar I disorder. *Medical problems of many types,* such as cancer of the pancreas, multiple sclerosis, and a space-occupying lesion of the brain, can produce depression. *Past or present substance abuse* is also important, since certain substances, such as alcohol and amphetamines, can mimic the clinical picture of depression.

15.6 The answer is B

In Sigmund Freud's structural theory, the *introjection* of the lost object into the ego leads to the typical depressive symptoms of a lack of energy available to the ego. The superego, unable to retaliate against the lost object externally, flails out at the psychic representation of the lost object, now internalized in the ego as an introject. When the ego overcomes or merges with the superego, energy previously bound in the depressive symptoms is released, and a mania supervenes with the typical symptoms of excess.

Projection is the unconscious defense mechanism in which a person attributes to another person those generally unconscious ideas, thoughts, feelings, and impulses that are personally undesirable or unacceptable. *Sublimation* is an unconscious defense mechanism in which the energy associated with unacceptable impulses or drives is diverted into personally and socially acceptable channels. *Undoing* is an unconscious defense mechanism by which a person symbolically acts out to reverse something unacceptable that has already been done or against which the ego must defend itself. *Altruism* is regard for and dedication to the welfare of others.

15.7 The answer is C

Approximately two-thirds of depressed patients have suicidal ideation, and about *15 percent* do eventually commit suicide.

15.8 The answer is D

As the illness progresses, the amount of time between episodes often decreases, not increases. After approximately five episodes, however, the interepisode interval often stabilizes at about 6 to 9 months. *Bipolar I disorder most often starts with depression* (75 percent of the time in females, 67 percent in males). Most patients experience both depression and mania, although *about 10 to 20 percent of patients experience only manic episodes. An untreated manic episode lasts about 3 months;* therefore, it is unwise to discontinue drugs before that time. Some patients develop rapidly cycling bipolar I disorder episodes. *Rapid cycling is much more common in women than in men,* although it is not related temporally to the menstrual cycle. Rapid cycling may be associated with treatment with tricyclic drugs, and patients often respond to treatment with Depakote or valproic acid.

15.9 The answer is C

Parkinson's disease is most often associated with depression. Up to 90 percent of Parkinson's disease patients may have marked depressive symptoms that are not correlated with their degree of physical disability or age or duration of their illness. The symptoms of depression may be masked by the almost identical motor symptoms of Parkinson's disease. The depressive symptoms of Parkinson's disease often respond to antidepressant drugs or electroconvulsive therapy.

Other neurological diseases less often associated with depression are *epilepsy, brain tumors, dementia of the Alzheimer's type,* and *Huntington's disease.* Table 15.1 lists physical diseases associated with onset of depression.

15.10 The answer is C

The patient was suffering from *cyclothymic disorder;* he had symptoms of both depression and hypomania. His down or depressed periods were marked by crying and loss of interest in sex and work, and his excessive use of alcohol during those times was a defense against depression and not the primary illness from which he suffered. When elated, the patient was gregarious, optimistic, and productive.

Table 15.1
Physical Diseases Associated
with Onset of Depression

Pharmacological	Steroidal contraceptives
	Reserpine; α-methyldopa
	Anticholinesterase insecticides
	Amphetamine or cocaine withdrawal
	Alcohol or sedative-hypnotic withdrawal
	Cimetidine; indomethacin
	Phenothiazine antipsychotic drugs
	Thallium; mercury
	Cycloserine
	Vincristine; vinblastine
Endocrine	Hypothyroidism and hyperthyroidism
	Hyperparathyroidism
	Hypopituitarism
	Addison's disease
	Cushing's disease
	Diabetes mellitus
Infectious	General paresis (tertiary syphilis)
	Toxoplasmosis
	Influenza; viral pneumonia
	Viral hepatitis
	Infectious mononucleosis
	AIDS
Collagen	Rheumatoid arthritis
	Lupus erythematosus
Nutritional	Pellagra
	Pernicious anemia
Neurological	Multiple sclerosis
	Parkinson's disease
	Head trauma
	Complex partial seizures
	Sleep apnea
	Cerebral tumors
	Cerebrovascular disorder
Neoplastic	Abdominal malignancies
	Disseminated carcinomatosis

The essential feature of *major depressive disorder* is a severe dysphoric mood and persistent loss of interest or pleasure in all usual activities. Because of the patient's hypomanic episodes and mild depressive symptoms, major depressive disorder is ruled out.

Bipolar I disorder is characterized by severe alterations in mood that are usually episodic and recurrent. The patient in this case had mood changes similar to those seen in bipolar I disorder, but the mildness of his symptoms precluded the full diagnosis of bipolar I disorder.

A diagnosis of *dysthymic disorder* is excluded because the patient showed episodes of elated moods. In dysthymic disorder, the patient's mood is chronic depression; in adult patients, a 2-year history of such depression is required before the diagnosis can be made.

Bipolar II disorder is characterized by one or more major depressive episodes, at least one hypomanic episode, and no manic episodes. This patient had no major depressive episodes.

15.11 The answer is B
Tricyclic drugs have cardiac, neurological, and physiological adverse effects. Cardiac effects include *tachycardia, flattened T waves, and prolonged QT intervals.* Neurological effects include *myoclonic twitches and tremors of the tongue.* Some patients may become *hypomanic* or develop delusions and hallucinations, but this is rare. A manic episode, characterized by *involvement in pleasurable activities with a high potential for painful consequences, may occur.* The least likely effect would be *suicidal ideation.*

15.12 The answer is E
Mood-incongruent delusions are usually not part of bipolar disorder, which typically includes mood-congruent delusions and hallucinations. Mood-incongruent delusions may point to a diagnosis of schizophrenia. The patient was experiencing a manic episode, characterized by a predominantly elevated, expansive, or irritable mood. The mood may be characterized by *emotional lability,* with rapid shifts to brief depression from mania. The essential feature of a manic episode is a distinct period of intense psychophysiological activation with a number of accompanying symptoms, such as lack of judgment of the consequences of actions, pressure of speech, *flight of ideas,* inflated self-esteem, and at times hypersexuality. Delusions of grandiosity, *hallucinations,* and ideas of reference may also be present. *Nocturnal electroencephalographic* (EEG) *changes* in mania include a decreased total sleep time, a decreased percentage of dream time, and an increased dream latency. Those findings have been interpreted as indicating that circadian rhythm activities are delayed in mania because the activity of the intrinsic pacemaker is increased. In DSM-IV-TR the diagnosis of a manic episode requires not a specific duration, such as 3 days, but rather only a distinct period of abnormally and persistently disordered mood.

15.13 The answer is C
The lifetime prevalence of dysthymic disorder has been reported by a number of studies to be *approximately 6 percent.*

15.14 The answer is E
The course of major depressive disorder by definition does not include *bipolar II disorder,* but it usually includes *an untreated episode of depression lasting 6 to 13 months, a treated episode of depression lasting about 3 months, the return of symptoms after the withdrawal of antidepressants before 3 months have elapsed,* and *an average of five to six episodes over a 20-year period.*

15.15 The answer is E (all)
Many substances used to treat somatic illnesses may trigger depressive symptoms. Commonly prescribed medications associated with depressive symptoms include *analgesics* (for example, ibuprofen), *antipsychotics* (for example, phenothiazines), *antihypertensives* (for example, propranolol [Inderal]), and *antibacterials* (for example, ampicillin). Certain substances used to treat medical disorders may also trigger a manic response. The most commonly encountered manic response is to steroids. In some cases spontaneous manic and depressive episodes originated some years later in patients whose first illness episode seemed to be triggered by the medical use of steroids. Other drugs are also known to have the

Table 15.2
Pharmacological Causes of Depressive Symptoms

Analgesics and antiinflammatory drugs
    Ibuprofen
    Indomethacin
    Opiates
    Phenacetin
Antibacterials and antifungals
    Ampicillin
    Cycloserine
    Ethionamide
    Griseofulvin
    Metronidazole
    Nalidixic acid
    Nitrofurantoin
    Streptomycin
    Sulfamethoxazole
    Sulfonamides
    Tetracycline
Antihypertensives and cardiac
  drugs
    Bethanidine
    β-Blockers (propranolol)
    Clonidine
    Digitalis
    Guanabenz acetate
    Guanethidine
    Hydralazine
    Lidocaine
    α-Methyldopa
    Prazosin
    Procainamide
    Rescinnamine
    Reserpine
    Veratrum
Antineoplastics
    C-Asparaginase
    Azathioprine (AZT)

  6-Azauridine
  Bleomycin
  Trimethoprim
  Vincristine
Neurological and psychiat-
  ric drugs
    Amantadine
    Antipsychotics (buty-
      rophenones, phe-
      nothiazines,
      oxyindoles)
    Baclofen
    Bromocriptine
    Carbamazepine
    Levodopa
    Phenytoin
    Sedatives and hypnotics
      (barbiturates, benzodi-
      azepines, chloral
      hydrate)
Steroids and hormones
    Corticosteroids (includ-
      ing ACTH)
    Danazol
    Oral contraceptives
    Prednisone
    Triamcinolone
Miscellaneous
    Acetazolamide
    Choline
    Cimetidine
    Cyproheptadine
    Diphenoxylate
    Disulfiram
    Methysergide
    Stimulants (amphet-
      amines, fenfluramine)

ACTH, adrenocorticotropic hormone.

Table 15.3
Drugs Associated with Manic Symptoms

Amphetamines
Baclofen
Bromide
Bromocriptine
Captopril
Cimetidine
Cocaine
Corticosteroids (including ACTH)
Cyclosporine
Disulfiram
Hallucinogens (intoxication and flashbacks)
Hydralazine
Isoniazid
Levodopa
Methylphenidate
Metrizamide (following myelography)
Opiates and opioids
Procarbazine
Procyclidine

ACTH, adrenocorticotropic hormone.

potential for initiating a manic syndrome, including amphetamines and tricyclic drugs (for example, imipramine [Tofranil] and amitriptyline [Elavil, Endep]). Table 15.2 lists drugs that can cause depression.

15.16 The answer is B

L-Tryptophan, the amino acid precursor to serotonin, *has been used as an adjuvant to both antidepressants and lithium* in the treatment of bipolar I disorder. Tyrosine *is the amino acid precursor to dopamine.* L-Tryptophan has also been used alone as a hypnotic and an antidepressant. L-Tryptophan and L-tryptophan-containing products have been recalled in the United States because L-tryptophan *has been associated with eosinophilia-myalgia syndrome.* The symptoms include fatigue, myalgia, shortness of breath, rashes, and swelling of the extremities. Congestive heart failure and death can also occur. Although several studies have shown that L-tryptophan is an efficacious adjuvant in the treatment of mood disorders, it should not be used for any purpose until the problem with eosinophilia-myalgia syndrome is resolved. Current evidence points to a contaminant in the manufacturing process.

15.17 The answer is C

Propranolol (a β-blocker) is an antihypertensive and may actually cause depressive symptoms. Many pharmacological agents,

such as *bromocriptine* (Parlodel), *isoniazid* (Nydrazid), cimetidine (Tagamet), and *disulfiram* (Antabuse), may precipitate mania, as can antidepressant treatment or withdrawal. Table 15.3 lists pharmacological causes of depressive symptoms associated with manic symptoms.

15.18 The answer is B

The graph depicts the lifetime *prevalence of mood disorder.* Anorexia nervosa occurs 10 to 20 times more often in females than in males, and the most common age of onset of anorexia nervosa is the mid-teenage years.

Regarding *obsessive-compulsive disorder,* men and women are equally likely to be affected (however, adolescent boys are more commonly affected than adolescent girls). The mean age of onset is about 20 years and about two-thirds of patients have the onset of symptoms before age 25. *Schizophrenia* is equally prevalent among men and women, with the peak ages of onset for men 15 to 25 and women 25 to 35. Women with *somatization disorder* outnumber men 5 to 20 times. Somatization disorder is defined as beginning before age 30; it most often begins during a person's teens.

15.19 The answer is C

This patient may be experiencing rapid-cycling or mixed episodes of bipolar I disorder. The treatment of bipolar I disorder has been changed by the many studies that have demonstrated the efficacy of two anticonvulsants—*carbamazepine* and *valproate* (Depakene)—in the treatment of manic episodes and in the prophylaxis of manic and depressive episodes in bipolar I disorder. Although the data in support of the efficacy of *lithium* are numerous (though presence of thyroid impairment might mitigate against its use), sufficient data have accumulated to warrant the use of the two anticonvulsants as first-line treatments of bipolar I disorder. Such a decision should be based primarily on the compatibility between the patient and the relevant side effects of the drugs. The long-term treatment of bipolar I disorder is an indication for those anticonvulsants, but the initial stages of manic episodes often require the addition of drugs with potent sedative effects. Drugs commonly used at the initiation of therapy for bipolar I disorder include clonazepam (Klonopin) (1 mg every 4 to 6 hours), lorazepam (Ativan) (2 mg every 4 to 6 hours), and haloperidol (Haldol) (5 mg every 2 to 4 hours). The physician should taper those medications and discontinue them as soon as the initial phase of the manic episode has subsided and the effects of lithium, carbamazepine, or valproate are beginning to be seen clinically.

The patient in this case was *noncompliant* with lithium, neuroleptics, and antidepressants; that is a further indication to try valproate or carbamazepine. In addition, obtaining a history of why the patient was noncompliant is helpful. Some patients cannot tolerate anticholinergic symptoms, which are most likely with *tricyclic antidepressants*. *Clozapine* is rarely considered a first-line treatment for bipolar I disorder, given its serious side-effect profile. *ECT* may be indicated in extremely severe or drug-resistant cases.

15.20 The answer is A
Major depressive disorder (unipolar depression) is reported to be the most common mood disorder. The lifetime prevalence is 10 to 25 percent for women and 5 to 12 percent for men. It may manifest as a single episode or as recurrent episodes. The course may be somewhat protracted—up to 2 years or longer—in those with the single-episode form. Whereas the prognosis for recovery from an acute episode is good for most patients with major depressive disorder, three out of four patients experience recurrences throughout life, with varying degrees of residual symptoms between episodes. Bipolar disorders (previously called *manic-depressive psychosis)* consist of at least one hypomanic, manic, or mixed episode. The lifetime prevalence of *bipolar disorder* is 0.4 to 1.6 percent. Mixed episodes represent a simultaneous mixture of depressive and manic or hypomanic manifestations, although a minority of patients experience only manic polarity. Manias predominate in men, depression and mixed states in women. The bipolar disorders were classically described as psychotic mood disorders with both manic and major depressive episodes (now termed bipolar I disorder), but recent clinical studies have shown the existence of a spectrum of ambulatory depressive states that alternate with milder, short-lived periods of hypomania rather than full-blown mania (bipolar II disorder). Bipolar II disorder, which is not always easily discriminable from recurrent major depressive disorder, illustrates the need for more research to elucidate the relationship between bipolar disorder and major depressive disorder. The prevalence of *dysthymic disorder* is 6 percent and of *cyclothymic disorder* is 0.4 to 1.0 percent.

15.21 The answer is D (all)
Mood disorders overlap considerably with anxiety disorders. As summarized in an NIMH monograph, anxiety disorders can occur during an episode of depression, may be a precursor to the depressive episode, and, less commonly, may occur during the future course of a mood disorder. Those findings suggest that at least some depressive disorders share a common diathesis with certain anxiety disorders. *More recent clinical experience suggests intriguing comorbidity patterns between bipolar II disorder on one hand and panic, obsessive-compulsive, and social phobic states on the other.* Furthermore, bipolar II disor-

ders are particularly likely to be complicated by use of alcohol, stimulants, or both. In many cases the alcohol or substance abuse represents an attempt at self-treatment of the mood disorder. Finally, physical illness—both systemic and cerebral—occurs in association with depressive disorders with a greater frequency than expected by chance alone. Unless properly treated, such depression negatively affects the prognosis of the physical disorder. More provocatively, there is current reawakening to the contribution of cerebral and cardiovascular factors in the origin of late-onset psychotic depressions (previously classified as involutional melancholia).

15.22 The answer is C
Most studies in developed countries estimate the distribution of major depressive disorder to be greater in women than in men, in young adulthood than in midlife and old age, in urban residents than in rural residents, and among single or divorced persons than among married persons. Few studies document a racial difference when social class and education are controlled. In a recent comparison of population-based epidemiologic studies in ten countries—the United States, Canada, Puerto Rico, France, West Germany, Italy, Lebanon, Taiwan, Korea, and New Zealand—the lifetime prevalence for major depressive disorder ranged from 1.5 percent in Taiwan to 19 percent in Beirut. Current prevalence ranged from 0.8 percent in Taiwan to 5.8 percent in New Zealand. The difference in prevalence estimates across countries suggests that cultural differences or differences in risk factors may influence the expression of major depression.

15.23 The answer is C
The higher prevalence of depression in younger age groups than in older ones has led to the hypothesis that *cohorts born after World War II are at appreciably greater risk for major depressive disorder than older birth cohorts in advanced Western society.* The trend has been observed not only in the United States but also in Sweden, Germany, Canada, and New Zealand.

A number of observations made prior to the ECA study suggest that prevalence rates of depressive disorders are changing. Relevant factors include a *progressively lower age of onset* of depressive disorders reported in community studies, an *increase in childhood mood disorders* seen by pediatricians and mental health workers, a decrease in deaths from suicide among the elderly (until about 1980), and a lower average age of onset for depressive disorders in clinical samples since World War II. For example, the *risk of first-onset depression* was higher for younger birth cohorts than for older birth cohorts in Sweden. The trends in suicide data parallel the trends in mood disorders (*i.e., suicide rates are much higher in younger persons today than they were in younger persons 30 years ago*). Suicide rates *in older adults have increased by 25 percent* since 1980.

15.24 The answer is A
Much attention has been directed to the association of early childhood experience with onset of mood disorders later in life. Although the complexities of a psychodynamic investigation of childhood traumas cannot be applied in community-based epidemiological studies, even cursory investigation of childhood experiences has revealed correlates. *Parental loss before adolescence is a well-documented risk factor for adult-onset depression. A deprived and disrupted home environment also*

constitutes a risk. Methodological problems make *objective study of childhood trauma and deprivation difficult. Some events (e.g., divorce or separation of parents) can be documented reliably,* but others (e.g., parental neglect) are quite subjective. *The report of parental neglect by a depressed adult may vary depending on the respondent's emotional state at the time of the interview.*

15.25 The answer is C
A number of *natural history* studies of mood disorders have been performed on clinical samples. The most extensively studied cohort derives from the Psychobiology of Depression Study and consists of over 500 young adult and middle-aged subjects diagnosed with either bipolar I disorder or major depressive disorder. *Following diagnosis about 50 percent of subjects recovered during the first year, but fewer than 30 percent of the others recovered during subsequent years.* Comorbid dysthymic disorder with a slow onset accompanying psychotic symptoms was associated with less likelihood of recovery. *Relapse rates are high for major depressive disorder immediately following recovery.* Superimposed dysthymic disorder and a history of three or more major depressive episodes were associated with relapse. *Bipolar I disorder patients with only manic episodes had better outcomes than those with major depressive disorder.* However, *Bipolar I patients with a mixed episode (depression and mania) or with rapid cycling had worse outcomes than those with major depressive disorder.*

15.26 The answer is E (all)
Family studies address the question of whether a disorder is familial. More specifically, is the rate of illness in the family members of someone with the disorder greater than that of the general population? Typically, all subjects with the disorder in a given environment or population are identified and questioned about illness in their first-degree relatives of control subjects. Rates of illness are typically adjusted for age to indicate the morbid risk (i.e., the risk that an individual will develop an illness at some point in his or her life).

Table 15.4 illustrates several such studies of bipolar disorders. They indicate *a morbid risk of bipolar disorder in first-degree relatives of bipolar disorder probands that ranges between 3 and 8 percent. Compared with a 1 percent rate in the general population,* this reflects a substantial familial increase. Similarly, studies of families of probands with depressive disorder (unipolar) reveal morbid risks for depressive disorders among first-degree relatives that are two to three times those of

the general population. These data argue strongly for the familial nature of mood disorders. Furthermore, depressive disorders generally occur at a higher rate in the families of probands with bipolar disorders, and the rate of bipolar disorder is elevated in the families of probands with depressive disorders. In fact, *depressive disorders are typically the most common mood disorder in families of probands with bipolar disorders.* This familial overlap suggests some common genetic underpinnings between these two forms of mood disorders.

The family study data clearly indicate that mood disorders are familial. However, such studies cannot distinguish whether genetic or environmental factors mediate the familial transmission. Families might share a variety of different environmental factors that could transmit the illness. Such factors might be behavioral but could also be shared exposure to infectious agents, toxins, or other brain insults. Twin studies provide the most powerful approach to separating genetic from environmental factors, or "nature" from "nurture." Many strategies for twin studies have been used, but most commonly both monozygotic (MZ) and same-sex dizygotic (DZ) twin pairs are identified in which one twin has a mood disorder. The other twins are then examined to determine the proportion of twin pairs in which both twins are affected, termed the *concordance rate.* Typically, twin pairs are selected who have been raised together so that environmental factors are shared equally. A difference in concordance rate between the MZ and DZ pairs, therefore, reflects the role of heritable genetic factors. An alternative powerful strategy is to study twin pairs raised apart; however, such samples are much more difficult to obtain.

Considering depressive and bipolar disorders together, studies find that the concordance rate for mood disorder in the MZ twins is two to four times that in the DZ twins. These are the most compelling data for the role of genetic factors in mood disorders. Further, the concordance rate for MZ twins is not 100 percent. Thus, nonheritable environmental factors also play a significant role in mood disorders. In studies that distinguish bipolar from unipolar disorders, the MZ to DZ concordance ratio for bipolar–bipolar pairs is higher than that for unipolar–unipolar pairs, which indicates *greater genetic involvement in bipolar disorders than in unipolar depressive disorders.* Furthermore, the rate of depressive disorders is elevated in monozygotic co-twins of probands with bipolar disorders, and to a lesser extent, the rate of bipolar disorders is elevated in the co-twins of probands with depressive disorders. This is consistent with the family data, and it argues for a genetic overlap between bipolar and depressive disorders.

15.27 The answer is E (all)
Serotoninergic neurons project from the brainstem dorsal raphe nuclei to the cerebral cortex, hypothalamus, thalamus, basal ganglia, septum, and hippocampus (Fig. 15.2). Serotonin pathways have both inhibitory and facilitatory functions in the brain. For example, much evidence suggests that 5-HT is *an important regulator of sleep, appetite, and libido.* Serotonergic neurons projecting to the suprachiasmatic nucleus of the hypothalamus *help to regulate circadian rhythms* (e.g., sleep–wake cycles, body temperature, and hypothalamic-pituitary-adrenocortical axis function). *Serotonin also permits or facilitates goal-directed motor and consummatory behaviors in conjunction with norepinephrine and dopamine.* Moreover, serotonin inhibits aggressive behavior across mammalian and reptilian species.

Table 15.4
Selected Family Studies of Bipolar Disorders

Study	Relatives at Risk (N)	Morbid Risk (%)	
		Bipolar	Depressive (Unipolar)
Dunner et al., 1980	1,199	4.2	8.2
Gershon et al., 1982	598	8.0	14.9
Rice et al., 1987	557	5.7	23.0*
Sadovnick et al., 1994	1,102	3.5	5.7

*Observed rates rather than morbid risk.

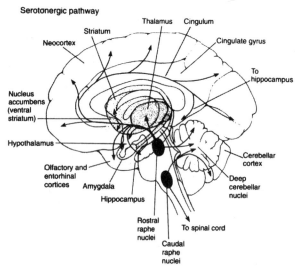

FIGURE 15.2

A lateral view of the brain demonstrates the course of the major serotonergic pathways. Although the raphe nuclei form a fairly continuous collection of cell groups throughout the brain stem, they are graphically illustrated here as two groups, one rostral and one caudal. (Reprinted with permission from Kandel ER, Schwartz JH, Jessell TM, eds. *Principles of Neural Science.* 3rd ed. Stanford, CT: Appleton & Lange; 1991.)

There is some evidence that serotonin neurotransmission is partly under genetic control. *Nevertheless, acute stress increases serotonin release transiently, whereas chronic stress eventually will deplete serotonin stores.* Chronic stress may also increase synthesis of 5-HT$_{1A}$ autoreceptors in the dorsal raphe nucleus, which further decrease serotonin transmission. Elevated glucocorticoid levels tend to enhance serotonergic functioning and thus may have significant compensatory effects on chronic stress.

15.28 The answer is B

About 5 to 10 percent of people (not 0.5 to 1 percent) evaluated for depression have previously undetected or subclinical thyroid dysfunction, as reflected by an elevated basal thyroid-stimulating hormone (TSH) concentration or an increased TSH response to a 500-μg infusion of the hypothalamic neuropeptide thyrotropin-releasing hormone (TRH). Such abnormalities are often associated *with elevated antithyroid antibody levels and, unless corrected with thyroid hormone replacement therapy, may compromise response to treatment. These findings are especially relevant to women with rapid cycling bipolar disorder.*

More commonly, *depressed patients receiving a TRH challenge test show a blunted TSH response. This abnormality, which may be state-independent, has been associated with a heightened relapse risk following pharmacotherapy or ECT.* The TSH response may represent pituitary downregulation consequent to a prolonged elevation of TRH secretion. In turn, increased TRH secretion could result from a homeostatic response intended to enhance noradrenergic neurotransmission. Some researchers further speculate that the therapeutic benefit of liothyronine (Cytomel) augmentation therapy is the result of correction of this failed homeostatic response.

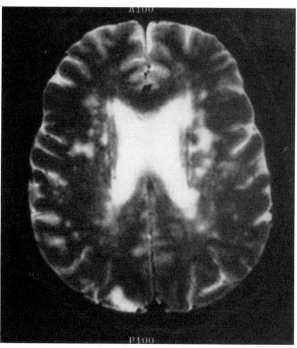

FIGURE 15.3

This magnetic resonance imaging (MRI) scan of a patient with late-onset major depressive disorder illustrates extensive periventricular hyperintensities associated with diffuse cerebrovascular disease.

15.29 The answer is B

Computed axial tomography and magnetic resonance imaging scans provide sensitive, noninvasive methods to assess the brain, including cortical and subcortical tracts, as well as white matter lesions. *The most consistent abnormality observed in the depressive disorders is increased frequency of abnormal hyperintensities in subcortical regions, especially the periventricular area, basal ganglia, and thalamus* (Fig. 15.3). More common in bipolar I disorder and among the elderly, these hyperintensities appear to reflect the deleterious neurodegenerative effects of recurrent mood episodes. Ventricular enlargement, cortical atrophy, and sulcal widening also have been reported in patients with mood disorders as compared to normal controls. In addition to age and illness duration, structural abnormalities are associated with increased illness severity, bipolar status, and increased cortisol levels. Some depressed patients also may have reduced caudate nucleus volumes, suggesting a defect in the mesocorticolimbic system. Cerebrovascular factors often involve subcortical frontal and basal ganglia structures, and appear particularly relevant to late-life depression.

15.30 The answer is D

Heinz Kohut's theory, known as self psychology, rests on the assumption that the developing self has specific needs that must be met by parents to give the child a positive sense of self-esteem and self-cohesion and that similar responses are required from others throughout the course of the life cycle. He *referred to those needs as mirroring, twinship, and idealization.* The *mirroring* responses required by the self are equated with the gleam in the mother's eye when the child exhibitionistically shows off for her. Admiration, validation, and affirmation are responses that are included in the category of mirroring. *Twinship* responses refer to the child's need to be like or identify with significant others. A small boy who is outside playing with his toy lawn mower while his father is mowing the lawn is meeting important psychological needs in asserting his commonality with his father. Finally, the need for *idealization* is an important aspect of the development of the self. Children who grow up with parents they can respect and idealize develop healthy standards of conduct and morality.

Kohut referred to those needs collectively as self-object needs. In other words, the responses demanded from others are required by the self, and the needs of the object as a separate person are not taken into account. The other person serves as an object who meets the needs of the self. Self-object needs essentially refer to certain functions that persons in the environment provide rather than to those persons themselves. Kohut felt that self-object responses continue to be needed throughout life and are as necessary for emotional health as oxygen is for physical health. Within that conceptual framework, depression involves the failure of self-objects in the environment to provide the self of the depressed person with mirroring, twinship, or idealizing responses necessary for the self to feel whole and sustained. The massive loss of self-esteem seen in depression is regarded by Kohut and the self psychologists as a serious disruption of the self–self-object connection or bond.

A common finding in depressed patients is profound self-depreciation. *Sigmund Freud,* in his classic 1917 paper "Mourning and Melancholia," attributed that self-reproach to anger turned inward, which he related to object loss, which may or may not be real. A fantasied loss may suffice to trigger a severe depression. Moreover, the patient may actually be unaware of any specific feelings of loss, since the fantasied loss may be entirely unconscious.

Although *Melanie Klein* understood depression as involving the internalized expression of aggression toward loved ones, much as Freud did, the developmental theory on which her view was based is quite different from freudian theory. During the first year of life, Klein believed, the infant progresses from the paranoid-schizoid position to the depressive position. In the first few months of life, according to Klein, the infant projects highly destructive fantasies onto its mother and then becomes terrified of the mother as a sadistic persecutor. That terrifying "bad" mother is kept separate from the loving, nurturing "good" mother through the defense mechanism of splitting. In that manner the infant's blissful feeding experience remains uncontaminated and undisturbed by persecutory fears of attack by the "bad" mother. In the course of normal development, according to Klein, the positive and negative images of the mother are integrated into a more ambivalent view. In other words, the infant recognizes that the "bad" mother it fears and hates is the same mother as the "good" mother it loves and adores. The recognition that one can hurt loved ones is the essence of the depressive position.

Edith Jacobson compared the state of depression to a situation in which the ego is a powerless, helpless child, victimized by the superego, which becomes the equivalent of a sadistic and powerful mother who takes delight in torturing the child. Like Freud, Jacobson assumed that depressed persons have identified with ambivalently regarded lost love objects. The self is experienced as identified with the negative aspects of the object, and ultimately the sadistic qualities of the lost love object are transformed into the cruel superego. Hence, depressed persons feel that they are at the mercy of a sadistic internal tormentor that is unrelenting in its victimization. Jacobson also noted that the boundary between self and object may disappear, resulting in a fusion of the bad self with the bad object.

Some contemporary ego psychologists believe that depression is not truly a psychiatric disorder or illness. Instead, depression is regarded as an affect reflecting conflict and compromise formation. *Charles Brenner,* the principal architect of that view, suggested that concern about such childhood calamities as object loss, loss of love, castration, and punishment are associated with two kinds of unpleasure. One form of unpleasure is anxiety, which involves an anticipated calamity or danger. The other form of unpleasure, depressive affect, involves a calamity that has already happened. That theory of depressive affect differs sharply from the classical views of Freud and Abraham. Brenner pointed out that depression is not always related to object loss or to oral wishes. He also asserted that identification with a lost object is found in some depressed persons but not in all and that anger turned inward is a result of depression, rather than a cause. Depressive affect, in Brenner's view, can be linked to any of the childhood calamities, rather than uniquely to object loss. People can experience depressive affect because they feel unloved, because they feel powerless, or because they feel punished in a variety of ways. In this view, depressive affect is a normal and universal part of the human condition.

15.31 The answer is A
A comprehensive psychodynamic understanding of depression must include premorbid personality factors in the equation. All persons may become depressed, given sufficient environmental stress, but certain personality types or traits appear to dispose one to depression. For example, the harsh, perfectionistic superego characteristic of persons with *obsessive-compulsive personality* disorder may lead them to feel that they are always falling short of their own excessive expectations of themselves. That intrapsychic constellation may be critical in the development of a major depressive episode. Similarly, Axis II personality disorders involving dependent yearnings for care—such as *dependent, histrionic,* and *borderline* personality disorders—may also be more vulnerable to depression. *Personality disorders that use projection and other externalizing defense mechanisms, such as* antisocial and *paranoid personality disorders, are less likely to decompensate into depression.* No particular premorbid personality type has been associated with the development of bipolar disorder, although narcissistic personality disorder should be considered.

Evidence is accumulating that an Axis II diagnosis of a personality disorder may complicate the course and treatment of depression. Depressed patients with personality disorders generally have poorer outcomes in the area of social functioning than those without personality disorders. Furthermore, residual depressive symptoms are more likely to present in recovering depressed patients with an Axis II diagnosis. Psychoanalytic clinicians have observed that personality factors frequently serve to maintain a depressed state once it has occurred.

15.32 The answer is C
The Greeks considered depression a somatic illness and ascribed it to black bile; hence the term "melancholia." The mood change in depressive disorder is accompanied by measur-

able alterations of biorhythms that implicate midbrain dysfunction. Once the changes occur, they tend to be independent of the environment throughout much of the episode, and as a consequence, they *do not respond to interpersonal feedback of a pleasant and upbeat nature.* The biological concomitants of melancholia include profound reductions in appetite, sleep, and sexual functioning as well as alterations in other circadian rhythms, especially *morning worsening of mood* and psychomotor performances. These disturbances are central to the DSM-IV-TR concept of melancholia, a form of depression in which such biological concomitants predominate. A smaller subgroup of depressed persons exhibits a reversal of the vegetative and circadian functions, with *increases in appetite and sleep*—and sometimes in sexual functioning—and an evening worsening of mood; in this atypical pattern, patients characteristically exhibit mood reactivity and *sensitivity to rejection.*

15.33 The answer is B

The bipolar or manic patient exhibits inflated self-esteem and a grandiose sense of confidence and achievements. Behind that facade, however, may be a vague and painful recognition that the positive self-concepts do not represent reality. However, such insight (if present at all) is transient, and manic patients are notoriously refractory to self-examination and insight. *Denial and lack of insight, cardinal psychological derangements of mania, are not listed in the DSM-IV-TR criteria for manic episode or bipolar disorders.* This is a serious omission because this lack of insight leads manic patients to engage in activities that harm themselves and their loved ones. It also explains, in part, their noncompliance with medication regimens during the manic phase. Finally, because of their lack of insight, mania nearly always reaches delusional proportions, including delusions of exceptional mental and physical fitness and exceptional talent; delusions of wealth, aristocratic ancestry, or other grandiose identity; delusions of assistance (i.e., well-placed persons or supernatural powers are assisting their endeavors); or delusions of reference and persecution, based on the belief that enemies are observing or following them out of envy of their special abilities.

The cardinal sign of mania is *decreased need for sleep*—the patient sleeps only a few hours but feels energetic on awakening. Some patients may actually go sleepless for several days or even longer. This practice could lead to dangerous escalation of manic activity, which might continue despite signs of physical exhaustion.

The prevailing positive mood in mania is not stable, and momentary crying or bursting into tears is common. Also, the high is so excessive that many patients experience it as intense nervousness. When crossed, patients can become extremely irritable and hostile. Thus, lability and *irritable hostility* are as much features of the manic mood as is elation.

Manic patients are typically *impulsive,* disinhibited, and meddlesome. They are intrusive in their increased involvement with others, leading to friction with family members, friends, and colleagues. They *are distractible* and move quickly, not only from one thought to another, but also from one person to another, showing heightened interest in every new activity that strikes their fancy. They are indefatigable and engage in various activities in which they usually display poor social judgment. Examples include preaching or dancing in the street; abuse of

long-distance calling; buying new cars, hundreds of records, expensive jewelry, or other unnecessary items; paying the bills of total strangers in bars; giving away furniture; impulsive marriages; engaging in risky business ventures; gambling; and sudden trips. Such pursuits can lead to personal and financial ruin.

15.34 The answer is E (none)

Bereaved persons exhibit many depressive symptoms during the first 1 to 2 years after their loss, so how can the 5 percent of bereaved persons who have progressed to a depressive disorder be identified?

Grieving persons and their relatives perceive bereavement as a normal reaction, while those with depressive disorder often view themselves as sick and may actually believe they are losing their minds.

Unlike the melancholic person, the *grieving person reacts to the environment and may show a range of positive affects.*

Marked psychomotor retardation is *not usually observed in normal grief.*

Although bereaved persons often feel guilty about not having done certain things that might have saved the life of the deceased loved one (guilt of omission), they typically do not experience guilt of commission (i.e., believing they caused the person's death).

Delusions of worthlessness or sin and psychotic experiences in general point toward mood disorder.

Active suicidal ideation is rare in grief but common in major depressive disorder.

Mummification (i.e., keeping the belongings of the deceased person exactly as they were before his or her death for extended periods of time) indicates serious psychopathology.

Severe anniversary reactions should alert the clinician to the possibility of psychopathology.

In another form of bereavement depression, the sufferer simply pines away, unable to live without the departed person, usually a spouse. Although not necessarily pathological by the foregoing criteria, such persons do have a serious medical condition. Their immune function is often depressed, and their cardiovascular status is precarious. Death can ensue within a few months of that of a spouse, especially among elderly men. Such considerations (highlighted in the work of Sidney Zisook and his San Diego colleagues at the University of California) suggest that it would be clinically unwise to withhold antidepressants from many persons experiencing an intensely mournful form of grief.

15.35 The answer is B

ECT (electroconvulsive therapy) is effective, even in patients who have *failed to respond* to one or more medications or combined treatment. It is *effective in both psychotic and nonpsychotic* forms of depression. *Usually 8 to 12 (not 15 to 20)* treatments are needed. *Bilateral ECT* is somewhat more effective than unilateral ECT, but it appears to have *more (not fewer)* cognitive adverse effects.

15.36 The answer is D

Table 15.5 lists commonly used antidepressant agents presently available in the United States and groups them on the basis of their presumed mechanisms of action (e.g., *presynaptic activity*). However, as basic neuroscientific knowledge expands, further actions will likely be discovered. For example, the number of

Table 15.5
Antidepressant Medications*

Generic (Brand) Name	Usual Daily Dosage (mg)	Common Side Effects	Clinical Caveats
Norepinephrine reuptake inhibitors			
Desipramine (Norpramin, Pertofrane)	75–300	Drowsiness, insomnia, agitation, OSH, CA, weight ↑, anticholinergic[†]	Overdose may be fatal; dose titration needed
Protriptyline (Vivactil)	20–60	Drowsiness, insomnia, agitation, OSH, CA, anticholinergic[†]	Overdose may be fatal; dose titration needed
Nortriptyline (Aventyl, Pamelor)	40–200	Drowsiness, OSH, CA, weight ↑, anticholinergic[†]	Overdose may be fatal; dose titration needed
Maprotiline (Ludiomil)	100–225	Drowsiness, CA, weight ↑, anticholinergic[†]	Overdose may be fatal; dose titration needed
5-HT reuptake inhibitors		All SSRIs may cause insomnia, agitation, sedation, GI distress, sexual dysfunction	All SSRIs have various effects on cytochrome P450 enzyme systems, are better tolerated than tricyclic drugs, and have high safety in overdose
Citalopram (Celexa)	20–40		
Escitalopram (Lexapro)	20–40		
Fluoxetine (Prozac)	10–40		
Fluvoxamine (Luvox)	100–300		
Paroxetine (Paxil)	20–50		
Sertraline (Zoloft)	50–150		
5-HT-norepinephrine reuptake inhibitors			
Amitriptyline (Elavil, Endep)	75–300	Drowsiness, OSH, CA, weight ↑, anticholinergic[†]	Overdose may be fatal; dose titration needed
Doxepin (Adapin, Sinequan)	75–300	Drowsiness, OSH, CA, weight ↑, anticholinergic[†]	Overdose may be fatal
Imipramine (Janimine, Tofranil)	75–300	Drowsiness, insomnia/agitation, OSH, CA, GI distress, weight ↑, anticholinergic[†]	Overdose may be fatal; dose titration needed
Trimipramine (Surmontil)	75–300	Drowsiness, OSH, CA, weight ↑, anticholinergic[†]	
Venlafaxine (Effexor)	150–375	Sleep changes, GI distress	Higher dosages may cause hypertension; dose titration needed
Presynaptic and postsynaptic active agents			
Nefazodone (Serzone)	300–600	Sedation	Dose titration needed; no sexual dysfunction
Mirtazapine (Remeron)	15–30	Sedation, weight ≤	No sexual dysfunction
Dopamine reuptake inhibitor			
Bupropion (Wellbutrin)	200–400	Insomnia, agitation, CA, GI distress	b.i.d. dosing with sustained release; no sexual dysfunction
Mixed-action agents			
Amoxapine (Asendin)	100–600	Drowsiness, insomnia/agitation, CA, weight ↑, OSH, anticholinergic[†]	Movement disorders may occur; dose titration needed
Clomipramine (Anafranil)	75–300	Drowsiness, weight ↑	Dose titration needed
Trazodone (Desyrel)	150–600	Drowsiness, OSH, CA, GI distress, weight ↑	Priapism possible

5-HT, serotonin; CA, cardiac arrhythmia; GI, gastrointestinal; OSH, orthostatic hypotension.
*Dosage ranges are for adults in good general medical health, taking no other medications, aged 18 to 60. Doses vary depending on the agent, concomitant medications, the presence of general medical or surgical conditions, age, genetic constitution, and other factors. Brand names are those used in the United States.
[†]Dry mouth, blurred vision, urinary hesitancy, constipation.

serotonin receptor types has increased faster than our understanding of their physiological roles. Moreover, the actions of some (e.g., venlafaxine [Effexor]) are affected by the dosages used or levels attained in the central nervous system (CNS). Venlafaxine exerts proportionally more serotonin than *norepinephrine reuptake* blockade at lower dosages than at higher dosages.

15.37 The answer is E (all)
The new range of psychopharmacological agents raises a series of important issues for the clinician, particularly when these agents must be chosen on the basis of an inadequate literature on relative efficacy or clinical and biological markers of responsiveness. There is a consensus that, with the exception of ECT, no antidepressant modality is more effective or more rapid in onset than another. Thus, the choice of agents is typically based on their adverse-effect profile and clinical lore regarding syndromal selectivity of response.

Fortunately, as the limitations of lithium as a mood stabilizer have been increasingly recognized, a variety of other treatment modalities have become available, particularly the anticonvulsants carbamazepine (Tegretol), valproate (Depakene), and divalproex (Depakote), as well as the calcium channel inhibitors. Other promising anticonvulsants are being explored as possible third-generation mood stabilizers, including lamotrigine (Lamictal) and possibly gabapentin (Neurontin) and topiramate (Topamax). However, as with targeting therapeutic modalities to specific patients in the depressive disorders, the data are not yet adequate to choose among the accepted mood stabilizers or to establish how to use them in combination, which has been increasingly necessary in recurrent bipolar disorders.

Thus, the clinician often has to resort to educated guesses and systematic and sequential clinical trials in individual patients to delineate optimal responsivity (Table 15.6). Even with the availability of many new treatments, episodes of illness can often emerge through otherwise partially successful pharmacoprophylaxis and necessitate adjunctive measures. The role of complex combination therapies is well recognized in many branches of medicine and is indispensable in the approach to tuberculosis, acquired immune deficiency syndrome (AIDS), congestive heart failure, or cancer chemotherapy. Systematic research of combination therapies has lagged markedly behind clinical practice, and clinicians are often left to their own devices, without the aid of controlled studies in the literature to guide the optimal algorithm for approaching the patient who is refractory to standard treatment interventions. Thus, *augmentation strategies in the treatment of bipolar disorder include benzodiazepines, a second or third mood stabilizer, antipsychotics, and clonidine.*

Answers 15.38–15.40

15.38 The answer is B

15.39 The answer is A

15.40 The answer is C

Recurrent brief depressive disorder is characterized by multiple, relatively brief (less than 2 weeks) episodes of depressive *symptoms* that *meet most of the diagnostic criteria for major depressive disorder.* The clinical features of recurrent brief depressive disorder are almost identical to those of major depressive disorder. One subtle difference is that the lives of patients with recurrent brief depressive disorder may seem more disrupted or chaotic because of the frequent changes in their moods when compared with the lives of patients with major depressive disorder, whose depressive episodes occur at a measured pace.

The treatment of patients with recurrent brief depressive disorder should be similar to the treatment of patients with major depressive disorder. The main treatment should be psychotherapy (insight-oriented psychotherapy, cognitive therapy, interpersonal therapy, or behavior therapy). *Treatment may include the use of antidepressants.*

In *minor depressive disorder, the symptoms are equal in duration, but fewer in number than those in major depressive disorder.* The treatment of minor depressive disorder can include psychotherapy or pharmacotherapy or both. *Treatment may include the use of antidepressants.*

Answers 15.41–15.44

15.41 The answer is A

Table 15.6
Steps in the Treatment Algorithm of the Bipolar Patient

A. *Diagnostic clarification*
  1. Retrospective course (bipolar I disorder, bipolar II disorder, bipolar disorder not otherwise specified, recurrent brief mania, or cycling)
  2. Medication history (antidepressant-induced, tolerance, or seasonal pattern)
  3. Family history of bipolar disorder and medication response
  4. Principle: treat first, determine blood concentrations and chemistries later
B. *Maximize current regimen*
  1. Increase dosage if adverse effects allow
  2. Change timing of dose (especially at night—for sleep adverse effects, compliance)
  3. Treat dose-limiting adverse effects:
    a. Use another antimanic agent if possible (i.e., one with two-for-one return)
      1. Propranolol (for lithium tremor)
      2. Calcium channel inhibitor (for lithium diarrhea)
      3. Lithium (for carbamazepine → ↓ WBC)
      4. Thyroid (for lithium → ↓ thyroid)
    b. Decrease dosage (if response allows)
    c. Discontinuation (for intolerable adverse effects)
C. *Augment;* especially with partial efficacy; occasionally with little or no efficacy (i.e., do not discontinue ineffective lithium without careful reconsideration of risk to benefit ratio, including its antisuicidal effects)
  1. p.r.n. high-potency benzodiazepine (clonazepam or lorazepam)
  2. With second mood stabilizer (especially acute efficacy)
  3. Use third mood stabilizer if needed
  4. p.r.n. antipsychotic (low dose)
      Typical: haloperidol, primozide, chlorpromazine
      Atypical: olanzapine, clozapine, risperidone
  5. Use drug with new mechanism of action (i.e., with profile of effects in different cycle frequencies or illness patterns)
    a. Calcium channel inhibitor (for ultradian cycling)
    b. Clonidine (for panic and opiate withdrawal)
    c. Valproate (for migraine)
    d. Carbamazepine (as atypical antidepressant-mood stabilizer) active at peripheral-type benzodiazepine receptor
    e. Consider trimipramine as atypical antidepressant with D_2 blocking and antipsychotic effects
D. *Discontinuation of potential mania-inducing or cycle-inducing agents such as*
  1. Antidepressants and alprazolam
  2. Cocaine and related stimulants
  3. Steroids (if possible)
E. *Substitution* (if adverse effects occur and drug is ineffective)
  1. Drug with different adverse-effects profile
  2. Use drugs with different mechanisms of action
F. *Refocus on early warning system (EWS) and prophylaxis*
  1. Mood chart and contract of medication changes and contact doctor for given degrees of symptom emergence
  2. Education and compliance
  3. Principle: maintain effective prophylaxis
    a. Be conservative when good medication responses are achieved
    b. Be more radical and make changes in face of previous inefficacy

15.42 The answer is C

15.43 The answer is B

15.44 The answer is A
Dysthymic disorder does not include patients who have *episodic periods of depression.* By definition, dysthymic disorder symptoms do not occur exclusively during the course of a chronic psychotic disorder; dysthymic disorder *does not have psychotic symptoms.* Dysthymic disorder has nonpsychotic signs and symptoms of depression that meet specific diagnostic criteria but do not meet the diagnostic criteria for major depressive disorder. About 5 to 10 percent of patients with *major depressive disorder have psychotic symptoms,* including both delusions and hallucinations. *Major depressive disorder, recurrent,* is characterized by *episodic periods of depression. Many patients* with major depressive disorder and some patients with dysthymic disorder *have a positive family history of mood disorders, decreased rapid eye movement latency, and a positive therapeutic response to antidepressants. DSM-IV-TR defines subtypes of dysthymic disorder based on onset before and after age 21.*

Answers 15.45–15.46

15.45 The answer is A

15.46 The answer is B
Cyclothymic disorder is *characterized by episodes of hypomanic-like symptoms and periods of mild depression.* In DSM-IV-TR, cyclothymic disorder is differentiated from *bipolar II disorder,* which is *characterized by major depressive episodes and hypomanic episodes.*

Answers 15.47–15.51

15.47 The answer is A

15.48 The answer is C

15.49 The answer is E

15.50 The answer is D

15.51 The answer is B
Sigmund Freud was initially interested in a psychoneural project for all mental phenomena. Limitations of the brain sciences of the day led him to adopt instead a model that relied on a concept of mental function borrowed from physics. The notion that *depressed affect is derived from retroflexion of aggressive impulses* directed against an ambivalently loved internalized object was actually formulated by his Berlin disciple Karl Abraham and later elaborated by Freud. Abraham and Freud hypothesized that turned-in anger was intended as punishment for the love object that had thwarted the depressed patient's need for dependency and love. Because, in an attempt to prevent the traumatic loss, the object had already been internalized, the patient now became the target of his or her own thanatotic impulses. A central element in those psychic operations was the depressed patient's ambivalence toward the object, which was perceived as a frustrating parent. Aggression directed at a loved object (parent) was therefore attended by considerable guilt. In the extreme, such ambivalence, guilt, and retroflexed anger could lead to suicidal behavior.

Bridging the divide between psyche and soma was the ambition of Swiss-born *Adolf Meyer* (1866–1950), who dominated

psychiatry from his chair at Johns Hopkins University during the first half of the 20th century. Meyer *coined the term psychobiology* to emphasize that both psychological and biological factors could enter into the causation of depressive and other mental disorders. Because of the nascent state of brain science during Meyer's time, he was more adept at biography than biology and therefore paid greater attention to psychosocial causation. He preferred the term *depression* (pressed down) to *melancholia* because of its lack of biological connotation. He conceived of depressive states in terms of unspecified constitutional or biological factors interacting with a series of life situations beginning at birth or even at conception. From that viewpoint arose the unique importance accorded personal history in depressive reactions to life events.

The cognitive model, developed by *Aaron Beck* at the University of Pennsylvania, *hypothesizes that thinking along negative lines* (e.g., thinking that one is helpless, unworthy, or useless) *is the hallmark of clinical depression.* In effect, depression is redefined in terms of a cognitive triad, according to which patients think of themselves as helpless, interpret most events unfavorably vis-à-vis the self, and believe the future to be hopeless. In more recent formulations in academic psychology, these cognitions are said to be characterized by a negative attributional style that is global, internal, and stable and to exist in the form of latent mental schemata that generate biased interpretations of life events.

Emil Kraepelin's (1856–1926) unique contribution was not so much grouping together all the forms of melancholia and mania, but his methodology and painstaking longitudinal observations, *which established manic-depressive illness as a nosological entity and* (he hoped) *a disease entity.* His rationale was that (1) the various forms had a common heredity measured as a function of familial aggregation of homotypic and heterotypic cases; (2) frequent transitions from one form to the other occurred during longitudinal follow-up; (3) a recurrent course with illness-free intervals characterized most cases; (4) the superimposed episodes were commonly opposite to the patient's habitual temperament; that is, mania was superimposed on a depressive temperament and depression was superimposed on a hypomanic temperament; and (5) both depressive and manic features could occur during the same episode (mixed states).

The learned helplessness model is in some ways an experimental analogue of the cognitive model. The model proposes that the depressive posture is learned from past situations in which the person was unable to terminate undesirable contingencies. The model is based on experiments in dogs that were prevented from taking adaptive action to avoid unpleasant electrical shock and subsequently showed no motivation to escape such aversive stimuli, even when escape avenues were readily available. Armed with evidence from many such experiments, a University of Pennsylvania psychologist, *Martin Seligman,* postulated a trait of learned helplessness (a belief that it is futile to initiate personal action to reverse aversive circumstances) formed from the accumulation of past episodes of uncontrollable helplessness.

Answers 15.52–15.55

15.52 The answer is B

15.53 The answer is A

15.54 The answer is B

15.55 The answer is C

Three factors influenced historical trends in the relative prevalence of mood disorders by age: period effects, age effects, and cohort effects.

Period effects are changes in the prevalence of an illness secondary to environmental stressors on the population or particular age groups within the population at a specific period in history. For example, *the uncertainty of employment among college graduates and the trend among younger persons to delay marriage during the 1990s may place young adults at greater risk for depression and suicide* because of economic impairment and lack of affiliative relations.

Age effects are the biological and psychosocial factors that predispose an individual to develop a particular disorder during a specific part of the life cycle. For example, *the genetic predisposition to develop major depressive disorder is probably greatest during the 30s, whereas the predisposition to develop a bipolar disorder is greatest during the 20s.* Age-related changes in the brain, such as increased subcortical hyperintensities on brain magnetic resonance imaging, may also be associated with mood disorders. Perhaps *the most consistently observed age effect relevant to mood disorders that has been observed during the 20th century is the positive association between age and suicide among white males in the United States.*

Cohort effects are the relative differences in rates of illness across different generations. A cohort is usually defined by the year or decade of birth. Persons born in a given year may be at greater risk for an illness, such as major depressive disorder, throughout their lives. Suicide data reveal marked cohort trends throughout the 20th century. *For example, persons currently 75 to 85 years of age (approximately the birth cohorts of 1915–1925) have exhibited lower suicide rates at all ages than either the 1900 or the 1940 birth cohorts.*

Considerable statistical and methodological problems confound sorting out the relative contribution of period, age, and cohort effects upon the prevalence and incidence of mood disorders by age. First, these effects undoubtedly interact. Stressors during a particular period interact with age-related vulnerability. For example, the current high rate of substance abuse among adolescents may reflect both the vulnerability of adolescents to substance abuse, which is an age effect, and the greater availability of drugs to adolescents, a period effect. Second, older persons may not recognize major depressive episodes as such, and so do not report them, thus setting the higher threshold for identifying depression among community-dwelling elders. Yet age does not appear to affect the rate of hospitalization for mood disorders. The more severe cases of major depressive disorder are hospitalized, regardless of age, and the relative cohort differences persist in hospitalization rates.

Most investigators have explained the current data as reflecting a period effect. They argue that the risk for depressive disorders increased dramatically for all ages from about 1965 to 1975 but has since stabilized at a higher incidence. Young persons are more vulnerable to that period effect, however, and therefore carry the greater burden of depressive disorders. A young person who experiences a major depressive episode is likely to exhibit ongoing and severe depressive episodes for many years. Therefore, clinicians can expect to see the current cohort of younger persons endure major depressive disorders for a long time. Despite being the healthiest and most affluent generation of the 20th century, younger persons may be placed at greater risk for major depressive disorders by a variety of environmental risk factors, including increased urbanization, more social isolation and anomie, changes in occupational roles and career trajectories for both men and women, heightened secularization, and expanding geographic mobility.

16 ▲

Anxiety Disorders

Anxiety is a ubiquitous human emotion. In fact, the complete absence of a sense of anxiety is felt by most clinicians to be pathologic. In some circumstances, anxiety is not only normal, it is adaptive. Defining anxiety disorders, then, can be problematic, and diagnostic criteria need to be well described and as precise as possible. The revised fourth edition of the *Diagnostic and Statistical Manual of Mental Disorders* (DSM-IV-TR) attempts to do this by delineating a number of specific anxiety disorders with clear diagnostic criteria. These include panic attack, agoraphobia, panic disorder with and without agoraphobia, specific phobia, social phobia, obsessive-compulsive disorder, posttraumatic stress disorder, acute stress disorder, generalized anxiety disorder, anxiety disorder due to a general medical condition, substance-induced anxiety disorder due to a general medical condition, substance-induced anxiety disorder, and anxiety disorder not otherwise specified.

Anxiety symptoms can be produced by purely biological means, or they can be the direct result of solely psychological factors. However, anxiety disorders, like most psychiatric disorders, are usually the result of a complex interplay of biological, psychological, and psychosocial elements. The role of temperament has been investigated. Treatment of these disorders can be correspondingly complex, with an array of approaches from psychoanalytic, to cognitive, to behavioral, to psychopharmacologic. Many times, a combination of these treatments is utilized to best address the multiplicity of etiologic forces.

Students need to be aware of the role of specific neurotransmitters in the development of anxiety and anxiety disorders, and the mechanisms of anxiolytic medications. They need to study the neuroanatomical areas of the brain, such as the locus ceruleus and the raphe nucleus, and their projections to the limbic system, which have been implicated in the etiology and treatment of anxiety disorders.

The student should study the questions and answers below for a useful review of these disorders.

HELPFUL HINTS

The student should know the following names, cases, terms, and acronyms related to anxiety disorders.

- acute stress disorder
- adrenergic
- aggression
- ambivalence
- anticipatory anxiety
- anxiety
- *Aplysia*
- aversive conditioning
- benzodiazepines
- cerebral cortex
- cleanliness
- clomipramine (Anafranil)
- conflict
- counterphobic attitude
- Jacob M. DaCosta
- Charles Darwin
- disorders associated with anxiety
- dopamine

- ego-dystonic
- fear
- Otto Fenichel
- flooding
- Sigmund Freud
- GABA
- generalized anxiety disorder
- hypnosis
- imipramine (Tofranil)
- implosion
- intrapsychic conflict
- isolation
- lactate infusion
- limbic system
- Little Albert
- Little Hans
- locus ceruleus and raphe nuclei
- magical thinking

- MHPG
- mitral valve prolapse
- MMPI, Rorschach
- norepinephrine
- numbing
- obsessive-compulsive disorder
- panic attack
- panic disorder
- panicogens
- peripheral manifestations
- PET
- phobias:
  agoraphobia
  social
  specific
- posttraumatic stress disorder

- propranolol (Inderal)
- reaction formation
- repression
- secondary gain
- serotonin
- shell shock
- sleep EEG studies
- soldier's heart
- stress
- systematic desensitization
- thought stopping
- time-limited psychotherapy
- trauma
- undoing
- John B. Watson
- Joseph Wolpe

▲ QUESTIONS

DIRECTIONS: Each of the questions or incomplete statements below is followed by five suggested responses or completions. Select the *one* that is *best* in each case.

16.1 A patient with obsessive-compulsive disorder might exhibit all of the following brain-imaging findings *except*

A. abnormalities in frontal lobes, cingulum, and basal ganglia
B. decreased caudate volumes bilaterally compared with normal controls
C. lower metabolic rates in basal ganglia and white matter than in normal controls
D. longer mean T1 relaxation times in the frontal cortex than normal controls
E. significantly more gray matter and less white matter than normal controls

16.2 Which of the following choices most accurately describes the role of serotonin in obsessive-compulsive disorder?

A. Serotonergic drugs are an ineffective treatment.
B. Dysregulation of serotonin is involved in the symptom formation.
C. Measures of platelet binding sites of titrated imipramine are abnormally low.
D. Measures of serotonin metabolites in cerebrospinal fluid are abnormally high.
E. None of the above

16.3 The most common form of phobia is

A. photophobia
B. thanatophobia
C. acrophobia
D. agoraphobia
E. nyctophobia

16.4 Sigmund Freud postulated that the defense mechanisms necessary in phobias are

A. repression, displacement, and avoidance
B. regression, condensation, and projection
C. regression, repression, and isolation
D. repression, projection, and displacement
E. regression, condensation, and dissociation

16.5 All of the following may be used effectively in the treatment of phobias *except*

A. diazepam
B. chlordiazepoxide
C. imipramine
D. hypnosis
E. chlorpromazine

16.6 Therapy for phobias may include all of the following *except*

A. propranolol (Inderal)
B. systematic desensitization
C. phenelzine (Nardil)
D. flooding
E. counterphobic attitudes

16.7 Medications used to treat posttraumatic stress disorder include

A. amitriptyline
B. imipramine
C. phenelzine
D. clonidine
E. all of the above

16.8 In acute stress disorder, the symptoms

A. must last for a minimum of 2 days
B. can last for a maximum of 8 weeks
C. must occur within 1 year of the trauma
D. must occur within 6 months of the trauma
E. must occur within 2 months of the trauma

16.9 Unexpected panic attacks are required for the diagnosis of

A. panic disorder
B. social phobia
C. specific phobia
D. generalized anxiety disorder
E. all of the above

16.10 Isolated panic attacks without functional disturbances

A. are uncommon
B. occur in less than 2 percent of the population
C. are part of the criteria for diagnostic panic disorder
D. usually involve anticipatory anxiety or phobic avoidance
E. none of the above

16.11 In posttraumatic stress disorder

A. ordinary traumatic events can produce it, although they must involve a threat of death or physical injury
B. anyone exposed to particular traumatic events would be expected to develop it
C. the number of previous traumatic events has little influence
D. previous psychiatric history of the exposed person does not seem to play a major role in its development
E. none of the above

16.12 Induction of panic attacks in patients with panic disorder can occur with

A. yohimbine
B. carbon dioxide
C. doxapram
D. cholecystokinin
E. all of the above

16.13 First-line medication treatments of anxiety disorders may generally include all of the following *except*

A. fluoxetine (Prozac)
B. fluvoxamine (Luvox)
C. venlafaxine (Effexor)
D. diazepam (Valium)
E. nefazodone (Serzone)

16.14 Cognitive-behavioral therapy

A. is not as effective in treating panic disorder as tricyclic drugs or benzodiazepines
B. usually does not result in long-term positive response after completion of therapy in panic disorder patients
C. is effective for social phobia and obsessive-compulsive disorder
D. is not effective for generalized anxiety disorder
E. none of the above

16.15 In panic disorder, panic attacks

A. can be precipitated only by exposure to a feared situation
B. can be due to a physical disorder
C. must be recurrent
D. tend not to occur before the development of agoraphobia
E. none of the above

16.16 Tourette's disorder has been shown to possibly have a familial and genetic relationship with

A. panic disorder
B. social phobia
C. generalized anxiety disorder
D. obsessive-compulsive disorder
E. none of the above

16.17 In generalized anxiety disorder

A. as many as 30 percent of patients do not respond to benzodiazepines
B. worrying serves a defensive function to avoid thinking about more disturbing issues
C. there is a link to an insecure or complicated attachment in childhood
D. there is an increased prevalence of past traumas
E. all of the above

16.18 In treating a patient with uncomplicated panic disorder

A. the physician should start with low doses of an SSRI
B. there is often an initial supersensitivity syndrome in the first week or two, which involves an increase in frequency of panic attacks
C. for full panic blockade, most patients require dosages equivalent to those used in depression
D. nonrespondents to initial SSRI treatment can be offered a second SSRI or Venlafaxine
E. all of the above

DIRECTIONS: Each group of questions below consists of lettered headings followed by a list of numbered statements. For each numbered phrase or statement, select the *one* lettered heading that is most closely associated with it. Each lettered heading may be used once, more than once, or not at all.

Questions 16.19–16.22

A. Classic psychoanalytic theories of anxiety
B. Behavioral theories of anxiety
C. Existential theories of anxiety

16.19 Anxiety is a conditioned response to specific environmental stimuli

16.20 Persons become aware of a profound nothingness in their lives

16.21 Anxiety is a signal to the ego that an unacceptable drive is pressing for conscious representation

16.22 Treatment is usually with some form of desensitization to the anxiogenic stimulus

Questions 16.23–16.25

A. Norepinephrine
B. Serotonin
C. γ-Aminobutyric acid (GABA)

16.23 The cell bodies of the neurotransmitter's neurons are confined primarily to the locus ceruleus

16.24 Benzodiazepines enhance the neurotransmitter's effects at its receptors

16.25 The cell bodies of the neurotransmitter's neurons are localized primarily within the raphe nuclei

Questions 16.26–16.31

A. Generalized anxiety disorder
B. Obsessive-compulsive disorder
C. Specific phobia
D. Social phobia
E. Posttraumatic stress disorder

16.26 Fear of flying
16.27 Fear of public speaking
16.28 Isolation, undoing, and reaction formation
16.29 Shell shock
16.30 Buspirone is a drug of choice
16.31 Possibility of associated Tourette's disorder

DIRECTIONS: Each set of lettered headings below is followed by a list of numbered words or phrases. For each numbered word or phrase, select

    A. if the item is associated with *A only*
    B. if the item is associated with *B only*
    C. if the item is associated with *both A and B*
    D. if the item is associated with *neither A nor B*

Questions 16.32–16.35

    A. Little Hans
    B. Little Albert
    C. Both
    D. Neither

16.32 Fear of horses
16.33 Castration anxiety
16.34 Conditioned response
16.35 Fear of rabbits

Questions 16.36–16.39

    A. Panic disorder
    B. Agoraphobia
    C. Both
    D. Neither

16.36 Higher rates for women than for men
16.37 Lifetime prevalance of 3 to 5.6 percent
16.38 Lifetime prevalance of 0.6 to 6 percent
16.39 Relatives have higher rates of both panic disorder and agoraphobia than relatives of controls

Questions 16.40–16.44

    A. Generalized anxiety disorder
    B. Panic disorder
    C. Both
    D. Neither

16.40 Response rates between 60 and 80 percent have been reported to buspirone
16.41 Patients with the disorder may still be responsive to buspirone after being exposed to benzodiazepine
16.42 Buspirone's use is limited to potentiating the effects of other antidepressants and counteracting the adverse sexual effects of SSRIs
16.43 Relapse rates are generally high after discontinuation of medication
16.44 Tricyclic drugs have been reported to worsen anxiety symptoms in patients where first symptoms were precipitated by cocaine use

Questions 16.45–16.48

    A. Cognitive-behavioral therapy
    B. Psychodynamic therapy
    C. Both
    D. Neither

16.45 Produces 80 to 90 percent panic-free status in panic disorder within at least 6 months of treatment
16.46 May be nearly twice as effective in the treatment of social phobia as a more educational-supportive approach
16.47 Goals are more ambitious and require more time to achieve
16.48 Combining treatment with medication may be superior to either treatment alone

Questions 16.49–16.50

    A. Acute stress disorder
    B. Posttraumatic stress disorder
    C. Both
    D. Neither

16.49 Characterized by the onset of psychiatric symptoms following exposure to a traumatic event
16.50 Characterized by reexperiencing trauma, avoidance, and increased arousal

ANSWERS

Anxiety Disorders

16.1 The answer is C

Brain-imaging studies of obsessive-compulsive disorder (OCD) patients using positron emission testing (PET) have found *abnormalities in frontal lobes, cingulum, and basal ganglia.* PET scans have shown *higher levels of metabolism* and blood flows to those areas in OCD patients than in controls. Volumetric computed tomography (CT) scans have shown *decreased caudate volumes bilaterally in OCD patients* compared with normal controls. Morphometric magnetic resonance imaging (MMRI) has revealed that *OCD patients have significantly more gray matter and less white matter* than normal controls. MRI has also shown *longer mean T1 relaxation times in the frontal cortex in OCD patients* than is seen in normal controls.

16.2 The answer is B

Clinical trials of drugs have supported the hypothesis that *dysregulation of serotonin is involved in the symptom formation* of obsessions and compulsions. Data show that *serotonergic drugs are* an effective, not *an ineffective treatment*, but it is unclear whether serotonin is involved in the cause of obsessive-compulsive disorder.

Clinical studies have shown that *measures of platelet binding sites of imipramine* and of *serotonin metabolites in cerebrospinal fluid are* variable, neither consistently *abnormally low* nor *abnormally high*.

16.3 The answer is D

Agoraphobia, a dread of open spaces, seems to be one of the most common forms of phobia, constituting some 60 percent of all phobias. *Photophobia* usually means an organically determined hypersensitivity to light (as in many acute infectious diseases with conjunctivitis) that results in severe pain and marked tearing when the patient is exposed to very strong light. Photophobia can also be defined as a neurotic fear or avoidance of light. *Thanatophobia* is the fear of death. *Acrophobia* is the fear of high places. *Nyctophobia* is the fear of night or darkness.

16.4 The answer is A

Sigmund Freud viewed phobias as resulting from conflicts centered on an unresolved childhood oedipal situation. In the adult, because the sexual drive continues to have a strong incestuous coloring, its arousal tends to create anxiety that is characteristically a fear of castration. The anxiety then alerts the ego to exert *repression* to keep the drive away from conscious representation and discharge. Because repression is not entirely successful in its function, the ego must call on auxiliary defenses. In phobic patients, the defenses, arising genetically from an earlier phobic response during the initial childhood period of the oedipal conflict, involves primarily the use of *displacement*—that is, the sexual conflict is transposed or displaced from the person who evoked the conflict to a seemingly unimportant, irrelevant object or situation, which has the power to elicit the entire constellation of affects, including anxiety. The phobic object or situation selected has a direct associative connection with the primary source of the conflict and has thus come naturally to symbolize it. Furthermore, the situation or object is usually such that the patient is able to keep out of its way and by the additional defense mechanism of *avoidance,* to escape suffering from serious anxiety.

Regression is an unconscious defense mechanism in which a person undergoes a partial or total return to early patterns of adaptation. *Condensation* is a mental process in which one symbol stands for a number of components. *Projection* is an unconscious defense mechanism in which persons attribute to another person generally unconscious ideas, thoughts, feelings, and impulses that are undesirable or unacceptable in themselves. Projection protects persons from anxiety arising from an inner conflict. By externalizing whatever is unacceptable, persons deal with it as a situation apart from themselves. In psychoanalysis, *isolation* is a defense mechanism involving the separation of an idea or memory from its attached feeling tone. Unacceptable ideational content is thereby rendered free of its disturbing or unpleasant emotional charge. *Dissociation* is an unconscious defense mechanism involving the segregation of any group of mental or behavioral processes from the rest of the person's psychic activity. Table 16.1 describes a more current view of seven of the psychodynamic themes in phobias.

16.5 The answer is E

Chlorpromazine (Thorazine) is a phenothiazine derivative used primarily as an antipsychotic agent and in the treatment of nausea and vomiting. It is not used in phobias.

Table 16.1
Psychodynamic Themes in Phobias

▶ Principal defense mechanisms include: displacement, projection, and avoidance.

▶ Environmental stressors, including humiliation and criticism from an older sibling, parental fights, or loss and separation from parents, interact with a genetic-constitutional diathesis.

▶ A characteristic pattern of internal object relations is externalized in social situations in the case of social phobia.

▶ Anticipation of humiliation, criticism, and ridicule is projected onto individuals in the environment.

▶ Shame and embarrassment are the principal affect states.

▶ Family members may encourage phobic behavior and serve as obstacles to any treatment plan.

▶ Self-exposure to the feared situation is a basic principle of all treatment.

Diazepam (Valium) and *chlordiazepoxide* (Librium) may be useful in decreasing symptoms of anxiety. They should be prescribed with caution for patients who have a history suggesting a tendency for psychological or physical dependence on substances. *Imipramine* (Tofranil) may be useful in decreasing phobic or depressive symptoms. All of these drugs should be used with caution in patients suffering from serious physical illness. Imipramine in particular may precipitate symptoms of delirium in patients suffering from serious medical illness.

Hypnosis is useful not only in enhancing the suggestion that is a part of the therapist's generally supportive approach, but indirectly combating the anxiety arising from the phobic situation. The psychiatrist can teach patients the techniques of autohypnosis, through which they can achieve a degree of relaxation that will enable them to tolerate the phobic situation when they must face it. Patients who cannot be hypnotized may be taught techniques of muscle relaxation. Some clinicians find that selective serotonin reuptake inhibitors (SSRIs), such as paroxetine (Paxil) and fluoxetine (Prozac), are also useful in treating phobias.

16.6 The answer is E

A *counterphobic attitude* is not a therapy for phobias, although it may lead to counterphobic behavior. Many activities may mask phobic anxiety, which can be hidden behind attitudes and behavior patterns that represent a denial, either that the dreaded object or situation is dangerous or that one is afraid of it. Basic to this phenomenon is a reversal of the situation in which one is the passive victim of external circumstances to a position of attempting actively to confront and master what one fears. The counterphobic person seeks out situations of danger and rushes enthusiastically toward them. The devotee of dangerous sports, such as parachute jumping, rock climbing, bungee jumping, and parasailing, may be exhibiting counterphobic behavior. Such patterns may be secondary to phobic anxieties or may be used as a normal means of dealing with a realistically dangerous situation.

Both behavioral and pharmacological techniques have been used in treating phobias. The most common behavioral technique is *systematic desensitization*, in which the patient is exposed serially to a predetermined list of anxiety-provoking stimuli graded in a hierarchy from the least frightening to the most frightening. Patients are taught to self-induce a state of relaxation in the face of each anxiety-provoking stimulus.

In *flooding,* patients are exposed to the phobic stimulus (actually [in vivo] or through imagery) for as long as they can tolerate the fear until they reach a point at which they can no longer feel it. The social phobia of stage fright in performers has been effectively treated with such β-adrenergic antagonists as *propranolol (Inderal),* which blocks the physiological signs of anxiety (for example, tachycardia). *Phenelzine (Nardil),* a monoamine oxidase inhibitor, is also useful in treating social phobia.

16.7 The answer is E (all)

Tricyclic drugs, especially *amitriptyline* (Elavil) and *imipramine* (Tofranil), and the monoamine oxidase inhibitor *phenelzine* (Nardil) are drugs used to treat posttraumatic stress disorder. They are indicated particularly when depression or panic symptoms are present. Increasing numbers of clinicians report therapeutic success with *clonidine* (Catapres), and a few reports suggest that propranolol (Inderal) may be an effective treatment. Other medications have been effectively used, including SSRIs and some mood stabilizers. Antipsychotic medications may be necessary for brief periods during treatment if behavior is particularly agitated.

16.8 The answer is A

In acute stress disorder, the symptoms *must last for a minimum of 2 days,* can last for a maximum of 4 weeks (not 8 weeks), and *must occur within 4 weeks (not 1 year, 6 months, or 2 months) of the trauma.*

16.9 The answer is A

Unexpected panic attacks are required for the diagnosis of *panic disorder,* but panic attacks can occur in several anxiety disorders. The clinician must consider the context of the panic attack when making a diagnosis. Panic attacks can be divided into two types: (1) unexpected panic attacks, which are not associated with a situational trigger, and (2) situationally bound panic attacks, which occur immediately after exposure in a situational trigger or in anticipation of the situational trigger. Situationally bound panic attacks are most characteristic of *social phobia* and *specific phobia.* In *generalized anxiety disorder* the anxiety cannot be about having a panic attack.

16.10 The answer is E (none)

Some differences between DSM-IV-TR and earlier versions in the diagnostic criteria of panic disorder are interesting. For example, no longer is a specific number of panic attacks necessary in a specific period of time to meet *criteria for panic disorder. Rather, the attacks must be recurrent and at least one attack must be followed by at least 1 month of anticipatory anxiety or phobic avoidance.* This recognizes for the first time that although the panic attack is obviously the seminal event for diagnosing panic disorder, the syndrome involves a number of disturbances that go beyond the attack itself. Isolated panic attacks without functional disturbances are not diagnosed as panic disorder. Furthermore, *isolated panic attacks without functional disturbance are not uncommon, occurring in approximately 15 percent of the population.*

16.11 The answer is A

There has been significant alteration in criteria for posttraumatic stress disorder between DSM-III and DSM-IV-TR. The criteria for the earlier version suggest that anyone exposed to particular traumatic events would be expected to develop posttraumatic stress disorder. Furthermore, the qualifying traumas were considered "outside of the range of ordinary human experience." Two things changed this view. First, *fairly ordinary traumatic events can produce posttraumatic stress disorder* and there is no adequate definition of "outside the range of ordinary human experience." Second, *only a subset of people exposed to the same traumatic event actually develop posttraumatic stress disorder. The number of previous traumatic events,* the severity of the events, and certain precipitating factors such as *previous psychiatric illness all seem to increase the likelihood that an individual exposed to severe traumatic stress will in fact develop posttraumatic stress disorder.* Hence, the DSM-IV-TR criteria make no statement about the commonality of the required traumatic events but stipulate that they *must involve a threat of death or physical injury*—and that the person's response must involve intense fear, helplessness, or horror.

16.12 The answer is E (all)

Since the original finding that sodium lactate infusion can induce panic attacks in patients with panic disorder, many substances have shown similar panicogenic properties including the noradrenergic stimulant *yohimbine* (Yocon), *carbon dioxide, the respiratory stimulant doxapram* (Dopram), *and cholecystokinin.* Disordered serotonergic, noradrenergic, and respiratory systems are doubtless implicated in panic disorder, and the condition appears to be caused both by a genetic predisposition and some type of traumatic distress. More recently, neuroimaging studies revealed that patients with panic disorder have abnormally brisk cerebral vascular responses to stress, showing greater vasoconstriction during hypocapnic respiration than normal controls.

16.13 The answer is D

Antidepressant medication is increasingly seen as the medication treatment of choice for the anxiety disorders. More specifically, drugs with primary effects on the serotonin neurotransmission system have become first-line recommendations for panic disorder, social phobia, obsessive-compulsive disorder, and posttraumatic stress disorder. Evidence now exists that such medications are also effective for generalized anxiety disorder. Although they typically take longer to work than benzodiazepines, the selective serotonin reuptake inhibitors such as *fluoxetine (Prozac),* sertraline (Zoloft), paroxetine (Paxil), *fluvoxamine (Luvox),* and citalopram (Celexa), as well as *venlafaxine (Effexor) and nefazodone (Serzone) are probably more effective than benzodiazepines and easier to discontinue.* Increasingly, benzodiazepines such as *diazepam (Valium)* are used only for the temporary relief of extreme anxiety as clinician and patient wait for the effects of antidepressants to take hold. Longer-term administration of benzodiazepines is reserved for patients who do not respond to, or cannot tolerate, antidepressants.

Placebo-controlled trials leave little doubt that newer antidepressants are effective for anxiety disorders. Because they work fairly quickly and have fewer adverse effects than tricyclic drugs and monoamine oxidase inhibitors, a low threshold for prescribing them to anxious patients should be maintained. However, most clinicians believe that the best result for anxiety disorder patients comes with the combination of medication with one or more types of psychotherapy.

16.14 The answer is C

A large number of studies have now shown that cognitive-behavior therapy of various types is effective for panic disorder. *The response rate after acute treatment is comparable to that achieved with tricyclic drugs or benzodiazepines. Furthermore, some, but not all, studies indicate that once a patient with panic disorder has completed this therapy, the response may be long-lived.* Many different techniques are incorporated into standard cognitive-behavioral packages for panic disorder, including breathing retraining, deconditioning, cognitive restructuring, relaxation, exposure, and psychoeducation. It is not clear which among these is critical for favorable outcome. Studies are also needed to determine if some kind of maintenance, or booster, therapy would help prevent symptomatic relapse.

At least one group has shown that *cognitive-behavioral therapy is effective for social phobia, and many studies have documented its benefits for obsessive-compulsive disorder. Studies also report favorable outcome with patients suffering from generalized anxiety disorder or posttraumatic stress disorder.* These treatments may be given as first-line approaches to patients who refuse or cannot tolerate medication or in combination with medication. The latter approach may be particularly effective, but empirical justification for it is lacking.

Not only has cognitive-behavioral research provided another effective way to treat anxiety disorders, it has also heartened psychotherapists in general because it proves that one can demonstrate scientifically that psychotherapy works. This should be considered just as exciting a development as anything generated by the neuroscience community. One intriguing challenge for research will be understanding how the psychosocial treatments affect central nervous system processes. Indeed, some imaging studies already suggest that psychotherapy may alter abnormal patterns of brain activation, but much more work is required in this area.

16.15 The answer is C

The key feature of panic disorder in DSM-III is the occurrence of three or more panic attacks within a 3-week period. These *attacks cannot be precipitated only by exposure to a feared situation, cannot be due to a physical disorder,* and must be accompanied by at least four of the following symptoms: dyspnea, palpitations, chest pain, smothering or choking, dizziness, feelings of unreality, paresthesias, hot and cold flashes, sweating, faintness, trembling, or shaking. In DSM-III-R, the definition was revised to require four attacks in 4 weeks or one or more attacks followed by a persistent fear of having another attack, and the list of potential symptoms was revised to include nausea or abdominal distress and to exclude depersonalization or derealization.

More importantly, DSM-III-R changed the diagnostic hierarchy so that panic disorder could be diagnosed as a primary disorder with or without agoraphobia and dropped the category of agoraphobia with panic attacks. This change placed the emphasis on identifying panic disorder as a discrete entity and reflected *the clinical experience that panic attacks tended to occur before development of agoraphobia,* which was increasingly viewed as a phobic avoidance response to the frightening experience of spontaneous panic attacks, near-panic experiences, or limited symptom attacks.

DSM-IV-TR expands the criteria to *require recurrent unexpected panic attacks* and persistent concern about having further attacks, worry about the implications of the attacks, or a significant change in behavior because of the attacks. No epidemiological data using these criteria are available.

16.16 The answer is D

An interesting set of findings concerns the possible relationship between a subset of cases of obsessive-compulsive disorder and certain types of motor tic syndromes (i.e., Tourette's disorder and chronic motor tics). *Increased rates of obsessive-compulsive disorder, Tourette's disorder, and chronic motor tics were found in the relatives of Tourette's disorder patients as compared to relatives of controls* whether or not the patient had obsessive-compulsive disorder. However, most family studies of probands with obsessive-compulsive disorder have found elevated rates of Tourette's disorder and chronic motor tics only among the relatives of probands with obsessive-compulsive disorder who also have some form of tic disorder. Taken together these data suggest that *there is a familial and perhaps genetic relationship between Tourette's disorder and chronic motor tics and some cases of obsessive-compulsive disorder.* Cases of the latter in which the individual also manifests tics are the most likely to be related to Tourette's disorder and chronic motor tics. As there is considerable evidence of a genetic contribution to Tourette's disorder, this finding also supports a genetic role in a subset of cases of obsessive-compulsive disorders.

16.17 The answer is E (all)

Most of the systematic studies on generalized anxiety disorder have involved behavioral or cognitive treatments, which have been shown to be helpful, or pharmacotherapy, which also is efficacious in reducing anxiety. However, there is a variety of limitations inherent in using benzodiazepines, including the fact that *as many as 30 percent of patients do not respond to them.* Other problems include the fact that benzodiazepines often do not affect the core symptom of worry; cause a variety of adverse effects; have a potential for abuse, physical dependence, and withdrawal; and result in fairly high relapse rates when the medication is withdrawn. Whereas generalized anxiety disorder was formerly thought to be something of a "wastebasket" category into which all other forms of anxiety were placed, more recent research has begun to identify specific interpersonal issues and traumatic events connected with the diagnosis. In a survey study of over 1,000 subjects, *the individuals meeting criteria for generalized anxiety disorder had more frequent traumatic events in their history than those who did not meet the criteria.* Subjects with this disorder reported trauma involving injury, illness, or death at a rate that was one and a half times greater than the reports from normal controls. Also, traumas related to assault, emotional events, and miscellaneous other occurrences were four to six times more prevalent in subjects with generalized anxiety disorder than in those without this condition. *Affected patients also tend to avoid thinking about the past events they consider traumatic; worrying appears to distract these patients with superficial matters that prevent them from worrying about more disturbing underlying concerns. In addition to this characteristic defensive pattern of avoidance, generalized anxiety disorder has also been linked to an insecure or conflicted attachment in childhood.*

Because the object of the worry is often misleading, the psychodynamic clinician must embark on a collaborative

Table 16.2
Psychodynamic Themes in Generalized
Anxiety Disorder

▶ Worrying serves a defensive function to avoid thinking about more disturbing issues.

▶ Increased prevalence of past trauma is highly characteristic.

▶ Link with an insecure/conflicted attachment in childhood.

▶ The underlying conflict that creates the anxiety can be related to any number of developmental themes.

▶ The unconscious conflict continues to be "alive" in self-defeating patterns in relationships.

▶ Resistance is common in moving below the level of symptoms to underlying sources of conflict.

Table 16.3
Recommended Dosages for Antipanic Drugs
(Daily Unless Indicated Otherwise)

Drug	Starting (mg)	Maintenance (mg)
SSRIs		
Paroxetine	5–10	20–60
Fluoxetine	2–5	20–60
Sertraline	12.5–25	50–200
Fluvoxamine	12.5	100–150
Citalopram	10	20–40
Tricyclic antidepressants		
Clomipramine	5–12.5	50–125
Imipramine	10–25	150–500
Desipramine	10–25	150–200
Benzodiazepines		
Alprazolam	0.25–0.5 t.i.d	0.5–2 t.i.d
Clonazepam	0.25–0.5 b.i.d	0.5–2 b.i.d
Diazepam	2–5 b.i.d	5–30 b.i.d
Lorazepam	0.25–0.5 b.i.d	0.5–2 b.i.d
MAOIs		
Phenelzine	15 b.i.d	15–45 b.i.d
Tranylcypromine	10 b.i.d	10–30 b.i.d
RIMAs		
Moclobemide	50	300–600
Brofaromine	50	150–200
Atypical antidepressants		
Venlafaxine	6.25–25	50–150
Nefazodone	50 b.i.d	100–300 b.i.d
Other agents		
Valproic acid	125 b.i.d	500–750 b.i.d
Inositol	6,000 b.i.d	6,000 b.i.d

Courtesy of Laszlo Papp, M.D.

search with the patient to discover the underlying conflicts and the true source of anxiety. As noted previously, the developmental hierarchy may help guide such a search, but the clinician must remain open to surprises rather than forcing the data to fit within a favorite theoretical formulation. Often the deeper conflicts surface in maladaptive and repetitive relationship patterns that are ultimately self-defeating. Table 16.2 illustrates the common psychodynamic themes in generalized anxiety disorder.

16.18 The answer is E (all)

Current consensus is to start treating a patient with uncomplicated panic disorder with low dosages of an SSRI (Table 16.3). Even at these low starting dosages, many panic patients may experience initial agitation and more frequent panic attacks. This so-called supersensitivity syndrome is usually limited to the first week or two of treatment. Further dosage reduction, switching to a different compound in the same family, or addition of a high-potency benzodiazepine, such as clonazepam (Klonopin) or alprazolam (Xanax), usually gets the patient through this relatively short period. Dosages can subsequently be increased over several weeks until they reach therapeutic range. *For full panic blockade, most patients require dosages equivalent to those used in depression.* A therapeutic trial with these agents should last for at least 5 weeks. Panic blockade often leads to improvement in both anticipatory anxiety and phobic avoidance. Preliminary evidence suggests that improvement in phobic avoidance may require higher dosages than panic blockade.

Approximately 60 percent of patients respond to this approach. Partial responders can benefit from the addition of a short-term, high-potency benzodiazepine or buspirone. Partial responders with tachycardia may try a combination of an SSRI and β-adrenergic receptor antagonists. β-adrenergic receptor antagonists may also alleviate cardiac discomfort associated with mitral valve prolapse. Contraindications to using β-adrenergic receptor antagonists include bradycardia, heart block, and asthma. Drug–drug interactions between some SSRIs and some β-adrenergic receptor antagonists should be kept in mind.

Nonresponders may be tapered off the SSRI and offered several different options, including a second SSRI, venlafaxine (Effexor), a high-potency benzodiazepine, a tricyclic or tetracyclic, or an MAOI. Persistent adverse effects, such as weight gain, hypomania, or sexual dysfunction, may also necessitate a switch from an SSRI in otherwise fully responding panic patients, although first an attempt should be made to address these negative effects.

Originally, one of the most important advantages of SSRI treatment was considered the absence of withdrawal reaction upon discontinuation. However, withdrawal reactions ranging from mild, transient anxiety and insomnia to severe headache, nausea, dizziness, and "electric jolts" lasting for several months have since been reported in a high percentage of patients who abruptly discontinue taking SSRIs. Therefore, gradual tapering over several weeks is strongly recommended. Anecdotal reports suggest that the addition of benzodiazepines, or trazodone for sleep, may alleviate untoward effects of SSRI withdrawal.

Answers 16.19–16.22

16.19 The answer is B

16.20 The answer is C

16.21 The answer is A

16.22 The answer is B

Psychoanalytic, behavioral, and existential schools of psychological theory, among others, have contributed theories regarding the causes of anxiety. Within the classic *psychoanalytic* school of thought, Sigmund Freud proposed that *anxiety is a signal to the ego that an unacceptable drive is pressing for conscious representation and discharge. Behavioral* theories state that *anxiety is a conditioned response to specific environmental stimuli.* In a model of classic conditioning, a person who does not have any food allergies may become sick after eating contaminated shellfish in a restaurant. Subsequent exposures to shellfish may cause that person to feel sick. Through generalization, such a person may come to distrust all food prepared by others. *Treatment is usually with some form of desensitization to the anxiogenic stimulus,* coupled with cognitive psychotherapeutic approaches. In *existential* theories of anxiety, *persons become aware of a profound nothingness in their lives,* feelings that may be even more profoundly discomforting than an acceptance of their inevitable death. Anxiety is the person's response to that vast void.

Answers 16.23–16.25

16.23 The answer is A

16.24 The answer is C

16.25 The answer is B

The three major neurotransmitters associated with anxiety are norepinephrine, serotonin, and γ-aminobutyric acid (GABA). The general theory regarding the role of *norepinephrine* in anxiety disorders is that affected patients may have a poorly regulated noradrenergic system that has occasional bursts of activity. In that system *the cell bodies of the neurotransmitter's neurons are localized primarily to the locus ceruleus* in the rostral pons, and they project their axons to the cerebral cortex, the limbic system, the brainstem, and the spinal cord. Experiments in primates have shown that stimulation of the locus ceruleus produces a fear response.

The interest in *serotonin* was initially motivated by the observation that serotonergic antidepressants have therapeutic effects in some anxiety disorders—for example, clomipramine (Anafranil) in obsessive-compulsive disorder. The effectiveness of buspirone (BuSpar), a serotonergic type 1A ($5\text{-}HT_{1A}$) receptor agonist, in the treatment of anxiety disorders also suggests the possibility of an association between serotonin and anxiety. *The cell bodies of most of the serotonergic neurons are in the raphe nuclei* in the rostral brainstem, especially the amygdala in the hippocampus, and the hypothalamus.

The role of *GABA* in anxiety disorders is most strongly supported by the undisputed efficacy of *benzodiazepines, which enhance the activity of GABA at the $GABA_A$ receptor in the treatment of some types of anxiety disorders.*

Answers 16.26–16.31

16.26 The answer is C

16.27 The answer is D

16.28 The answer is B

16.29 The answer is E

16.30 The answer is A

16.31 The answer is B

Excessive *fear of flying* is an example of a *specific phobia. Fear of public speaking* is an example of a *social phobia.*

Sigmund Freud described three major psychological defense mechanisms that determine the form and the quality of *obsessive-compulsive disorder: isolation, undoing, and reaction formation.* Isolation is a defense mechanism wherein the affect and the impulse of which it is a derivative are separated from the ideational component and are pushed out of consciousness. Undoing is a compulsive act that is performed in an attempt to prevent or undo the consequences that the patient irrationally anticipates from a frightening obsessional thought or impulse. Reaction formation involves manifest patterns of behavior and consciously experienced attitudes that are exactly the opposite of the underlying impulses.

In World War I, *posttraumatic stress disorder* was called *shell shock* and was hypothesized to result from brain trauma caused by the explosion of shells. The psychiatric morbidity associated with Vietnam War veterans brought the concept of posttraumatic stress disorder into full fruition as it is known today.

Buspirone is a drug of choice in *generalized anxiety disorder.* The drug has been reported to be effective in 60 to 80 percent of patients with the disorder. Data indicate that buspirone is more effective in reducing the cognitive symptoms of generalized anxiety disorder than in reducing the somatic symptoms.

Patients with *obsessive-compulsive disorder may have associated Tourette's disorder.* The characteristic symptoms of Tourette's disorder are motor and vocal tics that occur frequently and virtually every day. About 90 percent of Tourette's disorder patients have compulsive symptoms, and as many as two-thirds meet the diagnostic criteria for obsessive-compulsive disorder.

Answers 16.32–16.35

16.32 The answer is A

16.33 The answer is A

16.34 The answer is B

16.35 The answer is B

In Sigmund Freud's case history of *Little Hans*, a 5-year-old boy who had a *fear of horses,* Hans' fear represented *castration anxiety,* a displaced fear that his penis would be cut off by his father.

In 1920 John B. Watson recounted his experiences with Little Albert, an infant with a phobia of rabbits. Unlike Freud's Little Hans, who showed his symptoms in the natural course of his maturation, Little Albert's difficulties were the direct result of the scientific experiments of two psychologists, who used techniques that had successfully induced *conditioned responses* in laboratory animals. They produced a loud noise paired with the rabbit, so that a *fear of rabbits* was elicited in Little Albert.

Answers 16.36–16.39

16.36 The answer is C

16.37 The answer is D

16.38 The answer is B

16.39 The answer is B

Analyses of relative risks show *higher rates of agoraphobia for women than for men, just as with panic disorder.*

Some individuals with panic disorder also develop agoraphobia while some do not and the reasons for this variation are not known. It is possible that panic disorder with agoraphobia is a more severe form of panic disorder. Alternatively, the development of agoraphobia may be related to separate inherited or environmental factors, or some mixture of these. Two studies have addressed these questions. Rates of panic disorder with and without agoraphobia in relatives of three groups of individuals: patients with panic disorder and no agoraphobia, patients with panic disorder and agoraphobia, and nonanxious controls were compared; results indicated *that relatives of the agoraphobia patients had higher rates of both panic disorder (7.0 versus 3.5) and agoraphobia (14.9 versus 3.5) than the relatives of the controls, although the difference reached the .05 level of significance only in the latter group.* In contrast, the relatives of the panic disorder patients had significantly higher rates of panic disorder (14.9 versus 3.5, P<.005) but no agoraphobia (1.7 versus 3.5, not significant) as compared to relatives of controls. These data may be interpreted as indicating that with respect to intergenerational transmission, agoraphobia (with panic attacks) is either a more severe form of panic disorder or possibly a different but partially overlapping illness. The lifetime prevalence of panic attacks (not panic disorder) is 3 to 5.6 percent. Panic disorder is 1.5 to 5 percent. Lifetime prevalence of agoraphobia has been reported to range from as low as 0.6 percent to as high as 6 percent.

Answers 16.40–16.44

16.40 The answer is A

16.41 The answer is A

16.42 The answer is B

16.43 The answer is C

16.44 The answer is B

Buspirone was promoted as a less sedating alternative to benzodiazepines in the treatment of panic disorder. Buspirone has lower potential for abuse and dependence than benzodiazepines and produces relatively few adverse effects and no withdrawal syndrome. Buspirone does not alter cognitive or psychomotor function, does not interact with alcohol, and is not a muscle relaxant or an anticonvulsant. However, the efficacy of buspirone in panic disorder is disappointing, and with its further handicap of delayed onset of action and the need for multiple dosings, its *use is limited to potentiating the efficacy of other antidepressants and counteracting the adverse sexual effects of SSRIs.* Also, *buspirone seems even less effective in patients previously exposed to benzodiazepines.*

Bupropion, maprotiline (Ludiomil), and trazodone have not been found efficacious for panic disorder in controlled studies, while the anticonvulsants divalproex (Depakote) and gabapentin (Neurontin), the polyol second-messenger precursor inositol, nefazodone, and the calcium-channel inhibitor verapamil (Calan, Isoptin) have shown promise as antipanic agents.

While the short-term efficacy of antipanic medications has been established, the question of how long to treat a panic patient who responds to treatment remains open. The results of follow-up studies are mixed. *Several reports indicate that most panic patients relapse within 2 months to 2 years after the medication is discontinued.* A recent review concludes that following medication discontinuation, only about 30 to 45 percent of the patients remain well, and even remitted patients rarely revert back to significant phobic avoidance or serious vocational or social disability. Improvement may continue for years following a single course of medication treatment. This favorable outcome may be explained by the heterogeneity of panic disorder, spontaneous learning experience of patients in clinical trials, and concomitant self-monitoring. Given the uncertainty about the optimal duration of treatment, the current recommendation is to continue full-dosage medication for panic-free patients for at least 1 year. Medication taper should be slow, with careful monitoring of symptoms. Distinction should be made among return symptoms, withdrawal, and rebound anxiety.

Since longer duration of illness at baseline predicts poor long-term outcome, all efforts should be made to identify and treat panic patients as early as possible. More severe phobic avoidance and comorbid depression and social phobia at baseline also predict poor long-term outcome. Higher depression scores coincide with greater severity of avoidance and disability. The poorer overall outcome in panic disorder patients with comorbid recurrent depression is more likely due to the simultaneous presence of the two conditions. Comorbid depression usually improves in parallel with panic symptoms.

Atypical responses to medications have been reported in panic patients whose first panic attacks were precipitated by cocaine use. These patients respond preferentially to benzodiazepines and anticonvulsants, *while tricyclic drugs seem to worsen their anxiety symptoms.* This pattern of medication response suggests that cocaine-induced panic attacks may be related to a kindling-like phenomenon.

Patients with generalized anxiety disorder suffer from excessive and uncontrollable anxiety and worry for at least 6 months and experience a series of somatic symptoms such as restlessness, irritability, insomnia, and muscle tension. The illness is chronic, with periodic exacerbations and relative quiescence. The relative sparsity of biological data and pharmacotherapy research is due to a number of factors. First, because of their multiple somatic complaints, patients with generalized anxiety disorder are usually seen by generalists and medical specialists other than psychiatrists; generalized anxiety disorder is more likely to be diagnosed as a comorbid condition in psychiatric practices. Second, pharmacotherapy is considered less effective in generalized anxiety disorder than in some other anxiety disorders. Third, the diagnostic features are not clear-cut, and comorbid conditions make the diagnosis difficult.

The efficacy of benzodiazepines in the pharmacological treatment of generalized anxiety disorder gave rise to theories implicating the benzodiazepine γ-aminobutyric acid (GABA) receptor system in the pathophysiology of generalized anxiety disorder, but evidence exists for the involvement of the serotonergic and noradrenergic systems as well. Data do not support the advantage of any one benzodiazepine over others, and no correlation has been established between clinical response and dosage or plasma concentration. A daily equivalent of 15 to 25 mg of diazepam usually suffices to relieve most symptoms in up to 70 percent of generalized anxiety disorder patients. Both somatic and psychic anxiety symptoms respond within the first week of treatment. Tolerance to the sedative effects of benzodiazepines develops quickly, but the antianxiety effect of a given dosage is well maintained over time in generalized anxiety disorder. *However, the relapse rate upon discontinuation of benzodiazepines is high, as is the risk for dependency.*

Buspirone, the only currently available azaperone, is a potential alternative to benzodiazepine treatment in generalized anxiety disorder. *Response rates between 60 and 80 percent have been reported at levels ranging from 30 to 60 mg a day in three divided doses.* While response rates seem comparable, more patients drop out of buspirone trials than benzodiazepine trials. The relative merits of buspirone and benzodiazepines are further detailed under panic disorder. One notable exception is that *generalized anxiety disorder patients exposed to benzodiazepines may still be responsive to buspirone, unlike panic patients.*

Answers 16.45–16.48

16.45 The answer is A

16.46 The answer is A

16.47 The answer is B

16.48 The answer is C

Some studies have shown that cognitive-behavioral treatment of panic disorder, or panic control therapy, produces 80 to 90 percent panic-free status within at least 6 months of treatment. Two-year follow-up indicates that more than 50 percent of those patients who originally responded to panic control therapy have occasional panic attacks and more than a quarter will seek additional treatment. Nonetheless, these treatment responders do tend to have a significant decline in panic-related symptoms and most maintain many of their treatment gains.

As with panic disorder, considerable progress in the psychological treatment of social anxiety or social phobia is linked to the application of cognitive-behavioral methods. Unlike more traditional psychotherapies, cognitive-behavioral approaches do not focus on the origins of social anxiety, but instead focus on the use of coping strategies that can be implemented in current fearful situations. The most thoroughly studied form of cognitive-behavioral therapy for social phobia is a group therapy consisting of several discrete entities including (1) presentation of a three-system (cognitive-behavioral-physiological) model of social anxiety; (2) training in identification and restructuring of irrational beliefs regarding social performance; (3) in-session exposure to feared social situations via group role-playing scenarios; and (4) homework assignments directing patients to utilize cognitive and exposure techniques in vivo. Groups are particularly amenable to the treatment of social phobia in that they provide natural opportunities for patients to practice feared behaviors in a supportive and informative context.

Outcome research is somewhat limited but one study showed that cognitive-behavioral group therapy was nearly twice as effective as standard educational-supportive group psychotherapy. Responders to cognitive-behavioral group therapy were also shown to maintain treatment gains to a considerable extent at 5-year follow-up. Questions remain as to the effective treatment component in these therapies that blend cognitive and exposure-based methods. For example, it is unclear whether exposure to feared situations alone, without cognitive therapy, would be just as effective as the combined treatment. Also, it is not known whether group therapies other than educational or supportive group therapy, such as interpersonal group therapy, may be effective in treating social phobia.

Psychodynamic psychotherapy is based on the concept that symptoms result from mental processes that may be outside of the patient's conscious awareness and that elucidating these processes can lead to remission of symptoms. Moreover, in order to lessen the patient's vulnerability to panic, the psychodynamic therapist considers it necessary to identify and alter core conflicts. *The goals of psychodynamic psychotherapy are more ambitious and require more time to achieve than those of a more symptom-focused treatment approach.* Thus, these therapies are inherently more difficult to study than more concrete, focused, manual-based therapies. There are some case reports of brief dynamic psychotherapies that took no longer than cognitive-behavioral therapy to achieve reasonable treatment goals for patients with panic disorder.

In psychodynamic psychotherapy, the successful emotional and cognitive understanding of the various elements of psychic conflict (impulses, conscience, internal standards that are often excessively harsh, psychological defense patterns, and realistic concerns) and reintegration of these elements in a more adaptive way may result in symptom resolution and fewer relapses. To achieve this insight and acceptance, the therapist places the symptoms in the context of the patient's life history and current realities and extensively uses the therapeutic relationship to focus on unconscious symptom determinants.

Investigators have examined use of the combination of medication and cognitive behavior therapy for patients with panic disorder and agoraphobia. *Several short-term treatment studies have shown that the combination* of the tricyclic medication imipramine (Tofranil) with one component of cognitive behavior therapy, behavioral exposure, *may be superior to either treatment alone.* Another study showed that selective serotonin reuptake inhibitors, such as paroxetine (Paxil), plus cognitive therapy worked significantly better for patients with panic disorder than cognitive therapy plus placebo. There has been one study of the combination of psychodynamic psychotherapy with medication. *This study suggested that psychodynamic psychotherapy may improve the long-term outcome of medication-treated patients.*

Answers 16.49–16.50

16.49 The answer is C

16.50 The answer is C

Both PTSD and acute stress disorder are characterized by the onset of psychiatric symptoms immediately following exposure to a traumatic event. DSM-IV-TR specifies that the traumatic event involves either witnessing or experiencing threatened death or injury or witnessing or experiencing threat to physical integrity. Further, the response to the traumatic event must involve intense fear or horror. Such traumatic experiences might include being involved in or witnessing an accident or crime, military combat, assault, being kidnapped, being involved in natural disasters, being diagnosed with a life-threatening illness, or experiencing systematic physical or sexual abuse. Both PTSD and acute stress disorder also require characteristic symptoms following such trauma. There is evidence of a relationship between the degree of trauma and the likelihood of symptoms. The proximity to, and intensity of, the trauma bear on the probability of developing symptomatology.

In PTSD, the individual develops symptoms in three domains: *reexperiencing the trauma, avoiding stimuli* associated with the trauma, and experiencing symptoms of *increased autonomic arousal*, such as an enhanced startle response. Flashbacks represent the classic form of reexperiencing; the individual may act and feel as if the trauma were recurring. Other forms of reexperiencing include distressing recollections or dreams and either physiological or psychological stress reactions upon exposure to stimuli linked to the trauma. An individual must exhibit at least one symptom of reexperiencing to meet criteria for PTSD. Symptoms of avoidance associated with PTSD include efforts to avoid thoughts or activities related to the trauma, anhedonia, reduced capacity to remember events related to the trauma, blunted affect, feelings of detachment or derealization, and a sense of a foreshortened future. An individual must exhibit at least three such symptoms. Symptoms of increased arousal include insomnia, irritability, hypervigilance, and exaggerated startle. An individual must exhibit at least two such symptoms. Finally, the diagnosis of PTSD is only made when these symptoms persist for at least 1 month; the diagnosis of acute stress disorder is made in the interim. DSM-IV-TR acknowledges three subtypes of PTSD that differentiate syndromes with varying time courses. *Acute* PTSD refers to an episode that lasts less than 3 months. *Chronic* PTSD refers to an episode lasting 3 months or longer. PTSD *with delayed onset* refers to an episode that develops 6 months or more after exposure to the traumatic event.

The diagnosis of acute stress disorder is applied to syndromes that resemble PTSD but last less than 1 month after a trauma. *Acute stress disorder is characterized by reexperiencing, avoidance, and increased arousal, much like PTSD.*

17

Somatoform Disorders

Medical symptoms without evidence of organic pathology may represent malingering and are often greeted with hostility and suspicion by clinicians. Somatoform disorders may be mistaken for malingering, but this is not an accurate assessment, and the unfortunate consequence is that these patients may be frequently misdiagnosed. While there is no definable medical condition to explain the presented symptoms, the patients experience the symptoms as real, distressing, and often frightening. The diagnosis of somatoform disorders under the best of circumstances is difficult, as they are characterized by physical symptoms that suggest a general medical condition but are not explained by a general medical condition, by the effects of a substance, or by another mental disorder.

The fourth revised edition of the *Diagnostic and Statistical Manual of Mental Disorders* (DSM-IV-TR) classifies them as somatization disorder, conversion disorder, hypochondriasis, body dysmorphic disorder, and pain disorder, as well as undifferentiated somatoform disorder not otherwise specified.

Before a somatoform disorder is diagnosed, the clinician must initiate a thorough medical evaluation to rule out the presence of actual medical pathology. A certain percentage of these patients will turn out to have real underlying medical pathology, but it does not usually account for the symptoms described by the patient. The disorders may be chronic or episodic, they may be associated with other mental disorders, and the symptoms described are always worsened by psychological stress.

Treatment is often very difficult, as the symptoms tend to have deeply rooted and unconscious psychological meanings for most patients, and these are patients who do not or cannot express their feelings verbally. Unconscious conflicts are expressed somatically and seem to have a particular tenaciousness and resistance to psychological treatment.

Treatment involves both biological and psychological strategies, including cognitive-behavioral treatments, psychodynamic therapies, and psychopharmacologic approaches. If other psychiatric disorders, such as depression or anxiety disorders, are also present, they must be treated concomitantly. Different medications are effective with the range of disorders and the student should be knowledgeable about this.

The student should study the questions and answers below for a useful review of these disorders.

HELPFUL HINTS

The student should be able to define the terms listed below.

- amobarbital (Amytal) interview
- anorexia nervosa
- antidepressants
- antisocial personality disorder
- astasia-abasia
- autonomic arousal disorder
- biofeedback
- body dysmorphic disorder
- Briquet's syndrome
- conversion disorder
- cytokines
- depression
- differential diagnosis
- dysmorphophobia
- endorphins
- generalized anxiety disorder
- hemianesthesia
- hypochondriasis
- hysteria
- identification
- instinctual impulse
- *la belle indifférence*
- major depressive disorder
- malingering
- pain disorder
- pimozide (Orap)
- primary gain and secondary gain
- pseudocyesis
- pseudoseizures
- secondary symptoms
- somatization disorder
- somatoform disorder not otherwise specified
- somatosensory input
- stocking-and-glove anesthesia
- symbolization and projection
- undifferentiated somatoform disorder
- undoing

▲ QUESTIONS

DIRECTIONS: Each of the questions or incomplete statements below is followed by five suggested responses or completions. Select the *one* that is *best* in each case.

17.1 True statements about somatoform disorders include all of the following *except*

A. Patients present with somatic complaints that suggest major medical illness but have no associated serious and demonstrable peripheral organ disorder.
B. Psychological factors and conflict are important in initiating and maintaining the disorders.
C. Patients with these disorders are not malingerers.
D. Symptoms or magnified health concerns are under the patient's conscious control.
E. None of the above

17.2 Conversion reactions

A. are always transient
B. are invariably sensorimotor as opposed to autonomic
C. conform to usual dermatomal distribution of underlying peripheral nerves
D. seem to change the psychic energy of acute conflict into a personally meaningful metaphor of bodily dysfunction
E. all of the above

17.3 Historically, conversion disorders have been associated with

A. Pierre Briquet
B. Jean-Martin Charcot
C. Sigmund Freud
D. Pierre Janet
E. all of the above

17.4 The most frequently occurring of the somatoform disorders is

A. conversion disorder
B. somatization disorder
C. hypochondriasis
D. pain disorder
E. body dysmorphic disorder

17.5 Evidence used to support a theory of brain localization in conversion disorders includes

A. preponderance of left-sided, unilateral symptoms
B. strong association with depressive disorders
C. the left hemisphere is phylogenetically associated with inhibitory influences
D. the increased occurrence of the disorder in women
E. all of the above

17.6 Many patients with pseudoseizures have

A. interictal EEG abnormalities
B. neuropsychological impairment
C. abnormalities on MRI and CT scan
D. true convulsions or other true neurological conditions
E. all of the above

17.7 True statements about hypochondriasis include all of the following *except*

A. Depression accounts for a major part of the total picture in hypochondriasis.
B. Hypochondriasis symptoms can be part of dysthymic disorders, generalized anxiety disorder, or adjustment disorder.
C. Hypochondriasis is a chronic and somewhat disabling disorder.
D. Recent estimates are that 4 to 6 percent of the general medical population meet the specific criteria for the disorder.
E. Significant numbers of patients with hypochondriasis report traumatic sexual contacts, physical violence, and major parental upheaval before the age of 17.

17.8 The MADISON scale

A. is helpful in determining the extent of the emotional component of chronic pain
B. has not been validated rigorously
C. defines authenticity as the patient's being more interested in the clinician's acceptance of pain as genuine than in a cure
D. describes seven markers of considerable emotional overlay in chronic pain presentation
E. all of the above

17.9 Body dysmorphic disorder is associated with

A. major depressive disorder
B. obsessive-compulsive disorder
C. social phobia
D. family history of substance abuse
E. all of the above

17.10 According to DSM-IV-TR, a patient with conversion disorder would most typically have

A. feigned symptoms
B. sexual dysfunction
C. *la belle indifférence*
D. an urban background
E. symptom onset after age 50

17.11 A 29-year-old mother of two requested medical clearance for impending surgery for cysts in her breasts. She described the cysts as rapidly enlarging and unbearably painful. While drawing attention to her breasts, she noted, "They are so large and so tender to the touch. And I just can't have relations—forget that."

She also had disabling back pain that spread up and down her spine and made her legs give out on her suddenly, causing her to fall. When discussing this symptom, she winced visibly, and added, "Oh, there it goes; my back keeps clicking. The pain is so severe it affects me with my kids. Pain like that will make anyone into a beast." (She had previously been suspected of child abuse.) She also complained of dyspnea and a dry cough that prevented her from walking uphill.

Her medical history began at menarche with dysmenorrhea and menorrhagia. At 18 she had exploratory surgery for a possible ovarian cyst and subsequently underwent another operation for suspected abdominal adhesions. She also had a history of recurrent urinary tract symptoms, although no organisms were ever clearly documented, and she had a normal workup for "an enlarged thyroid." At various times, she had received the diagnoses of spastic colon, migraine, and endometriosis.

Two marriages, both to alcoholic and abusive men who refused to pay child support, had ended in divorce. She had lost several clerical jobs because of excessive absences. During the periods when she felt worst, she spent most of the day at home in a bathrobe while her relatives cared for her children. She had a history of narcotic dependence and claimed that she began using analgesics for her back pain and then "overdid it."

The physical examination at the time of her visit revealed inconsistencies in the breast tissue but no frank masses, and mammography findings were normal. (Courtesy of Arthur J. Barsky, M.D.)

The patient is probably suffering from

A. hypochondriasis
B. conversion disorder
C. pain disorder
D. somatization disorder
E. body dysmorphic disorder

17.12 A 38-year-old married woman had complained of nervousness since childhood. She also said she was sickly since her youth, with a succession of physical problems that doctors often indicated were caused by her nerves or depression. She, however, believed that she had a physical problem that had not yet been uncovered by the doctors. Besides nervousness, she had chest pain and had been told by a variety of medical consultants that she had a nervous heart. She also consulted doctors for abdominal pain and had been told she had a spastic colon. She had seen chiropractors and osteopaths for backaches, for pains in her extremities, and for anesthesia of her fingertips. Three months previously, she was vomiting and had chest pain and abdominal pain, and she was admitted to a hospital for a hysterectomy. Since the hysterectomy, she had had repeated anxiety attacks, fainting spells that she

claimed were associated with unconsciousness, vomiting, food intolerance, weakness, and fatigue. She had been hospitalized several times for medical workups for vomiting, colitis, vomiting of blood, and chest pain. She had had a surgical procedure for an abscess of the throat. She said she felt depressed but thought that it was all because her "hormones were not straightened out." She was still looking for a medical explanation for her physical and psychological problems.

The most likely diagnosis is

A. somatization disorder
B. conversion disorder
C. hypochondriasis
D. dysthymic disorder
E. none of the above

17.13 The most accurate statement regarding hypochondriasis is

A. Patients with hypochondriasis usually believe that they have multiple diseases.
B. Hypochondriasis may be the result of an unconscious desire to assume the sick role.
C. The patient's belief that a particular disease is present can have delusional intensity.
D. More men than women are affected by hypochondriasis.
E. The incidence of hypochondriasis is affected by educational level and marital status.

17.14 Characteristic signs of conversion disorder include all of the following *except*

A. astasia-abasia
B. stocking-and-glove anesthesia
C. hemianesthesia of the body beginning precisely at the midline
D. normal reflexes
E. cogwheel rigidity

17.15 In body dysmorphic disorder

A. plastic surgery is usually beneficial.
B. a comorbid diagnosis is unusual.
C. anorexia nervosa may also be diagnosed.
D. some 50 percent of patients may attempt suicide.
E. serotonin-specific drugs are effective in reducing the symptoms.

17.16 The most accurate statement regarding pain disorder is

A. Peak ages of onset are in the second and third decades.
B. First-degree relatives of patients have an increased likelihood of having the same disorder.
C. It is least common in persons with blue-collar occupations.
D. It is diagnosed equally among men and women.
E. Depressive disorders are no more common in patients with pain disorder than in the general public.

17.17 A patient with somatization disorder

    A. presents the initial physical complaints after age 30

    B. has had physical symptoms for 3 months

    C. has complained of symptoms not explained by a known medical condition

    D. usually experiences minimal impairment in social or occupational functioning

    E. may have a false belief of being pregnant with objective signs of pregnancy, such as decreased menstrual flow or amenorrhea

17.18 Medical disorders to be considered in a differential diagnosis of somatization disorder include

    A. multiple sclerosis

    B. systemic lupus erythematosus

    C. acute intermittent porphyria

    D. hyperparathyroidism

    E. all of the above

DIRECTIONS: Each set of lettered headings below is followed by a list of numbered phrases. For each numbered phrase, select

    A. if the item is associated with *A only*

    B. if the item is associated with *B only*

    C. if the item is associated with *both A and B*

    D. if the item is associated with *neither A nor B*

Questions 17.19–17.23

    A. Somatization disorder

    B. Pain disorder

    C. Both

    D. Neither

17.19 Affects women more than men

17.20 Most often begins during a person's teens

17.21 Responds to antidepressants

17.22 May involve serotonin in its pathophysiology

17.23 Is commonly associated with anorexia nervosa

Questions 17.24–17.29

    A. Hypochondriasis

    B. Somatization disorder

    C. Both

    D. Neither

17.24 Is found approximately equally in men and women

17.25 Has peak incidence during the 40s or 50s

17.26 Is likely to have a hysterical cognitive and interpersonal style

17.27 Includes disease conviction or disease fear

17.28 Is associated with anhedonia

17.29 May include hallucinations

Questions 17.30–17.35

    A. Somatization disorder

    B. Conversion disorder

    C. Both

    D. Neither

17.30 Prevalence is highest in rural areas and among the poorly educated.

17.31 Is associated with Pierre Briquet.

17.32 Comorbidity with an Axis II disorder is common.

17.33 Only one or two complaints.

17.34 Is chronic and relapsing, by definition.

17.35 Most symptoms remit spontaneously.

Questions 17.36–17.37

    A. Undifferentiated somatoform disorder

    B. Somatization disorder

    C. Both

    D. Neither

17.36 Estimated lifetime prevalence of between 4 and 11 percent

17.37 Course is generally chronic and relapsing

ANSWERS

Somatoform Disorders

17.1 The answer is D

Characteristic of somatoform disorders are three enduring clinical features: (1) *somatic complaints that suggest major medical maladies yet have no associated serious and demonstrable peripheral organ disorder;* (2) *psychological factors and conflicts that seem important in initiating, exacerbating, and maintaining the disturbance;* and (3) *symptoms or magnified health concerns that are not under the patient's conscious control.*

Because of their intense bodily perceptions, restricted level of physical functioning, and morbid beliefs, these patients have become convinced they harbor serious physical problems. Moreover, their symptoms are not willfully controlled. Whatever their faults and problems, *these patients are not malingerers.* Yet their physicians' physical and laboratory examinations persistently fail to evince significant substantiating data about physical infirmity other than the patients' vigorous and sincere complaints. Patients with somatoform disorders are convinced that their suffering comes from some type of presumably undetected and untreated bodily derangement.

17.2 The answer is D

Many conversion disorders simulate acute neurological pathology (e.g., strokes and disturbances of speech, hearing, or vision). However, conversion disorders are not associated with the usual pathological neurodiagnostic signs or the underlying somatic pathology. *Conversion symptoms* (e.g., anesthesias and paresthesias produced by a conversion disorder) *do not conform to usual dermatomal distribution of the underlying peripheral nerves;* rather, the signs and symptoms of a conversion disorder typically conform to the patient's concept of the medical condition.

Conversion disorders seem to change or convert the psychic energy of the turmoil of acute conflict into a personally mean-

ingful metaphor of bodily dysfunction. Turbulence of the mind is transformed into a somatic statement, condensing and focusing concepts, role models, and communicative meanings into one or several physical signs or symptoms of dysfunction. These somatic representations often simulate an acute medical calamity; initiate urgent, sometimes expensive medical investigation; and produce disability. In primitive settings, however, certain conversion symptoms have been taken as tokens of religious faith and even as expressions of witchcraft.

Although most conversion reactions are transient (hours to days), some can persist. Chronic conversion disorders can actually produce permanent conversion complications, such as disuse contractures of a "paralyzed" limb that remains long after the psychic strife that prompted the conversion has been resolved. In many cases a chronic conversion disorder serves to help stabilize an otherwise dysfunctional family. *In addition to sensorimotor symptoms, marked autonomic disturbances such as protracted (psychogenic) vomiting, hyperemesis gravidarum, urinary retention, and pseudocyesis are also seen, although less commonly.* Conversion disorders challenge the diagnostic competence of internists, neurologists, otolaryngologists, ophthalmologists, and psychiatrists.

Like the other somatoform disorders, conversion disorders are not volitional. Rather, ego defense mechanisms of repression and dissociation act outside of the patient's awareness. Many patients with conversion disorders experience *la belle indifférence,* an emotional unconcern or even flatness in a setting of catastrophic illness; but some patients do experience considerable anguish over their new symptoms. Table 17.1 lists some common symptoms of conversion disorder. Table 17.2 lists neurological conditions in the differential diagnosis of conversion disorder. Table 17.3 lists psychiatric conditions in the differential diagnosis of conversion disorder.

17.3 The answer is E (all)

Until the middle of the 19th century, somatization disorder and conversion disorder (which often travel together) were considered to be one condition called *hysteria.* The term hysteria was derived from the Greek word *hystera,* meaning uterus. Descriptions of conversion disorders appeared as far back as 1900 B.C.

Table 17.1
Common Symptoms of Conversion Disorder

Motor symptoms	Sensory deficits
Involuntary movements	Anesthesia, especially of extremities
Tics	Midline anesthesia
Blepharospasm	Blindness
Torticollis	Tunnel vision
Opisthotonos	Deafness
Seizures	**Visceral symptoms**
Abnormal gait	Psychogenic vomiting
Falling	Pseudocyesis
Astasia-abasia	*Globus hystericus*
Paralysis	Swooning or syncope
Weakness	Urinary retention
Aphonia	Diarrhea

Courtesy of Frederick G. Guggenheim, M.D.

Table 17.2
Neurological Conditions in the Differential Diagnosis of Conversion Disorder

Myasthenia gravis
Periodic paralysis
Brain tumor
Multiple sclerosis
Optic neuritis
Partial vocal cord paralysis
Guillain-Barré syndrome
On-off syndrome of Parkinson's disease
Degenerative diseases of basal ganglia and peripheral nerves
Acquired myopathies, including polymyositis
Subdural hematoma
Acquired and hereditary dystonias
Drug-induced dystonia
Creutzfeldt-Jakob disease
Early manifestations of acquired immune deficiency syndrome (AIDS)

when multiple symptoms were attributed by Egyptian physicians to a wandering of the uterus within the body.

In the middle of the century, *Pierre Briquet originated the modern concept of conversion disorder.* He considered the disorder to result from a dysfunction of the central nervous system (CNS). He proposed that conversion symptoms occurred in those with a constitutional predisposition when a receptive part of the brain was affected by extreme stress. Later, Russell Reynolds described clinical cases in which the loss of function or the persistence of severe pain could be attributed to an idea that the patient had about the body.

Jean-Martin Charcot then expanded on the biological concepts of Briquet and the psychological constructs of Reynolds, adding heredity to factors that influence predisposition. Moreover, Charcot suggested that a traumatic event gave rise to the idea, which then led to the brain's dynamic dysfunction; Charcot also suggested that the idea could be produced in the brain by hypnosis.

The term conversion was first used by Sigmund Freud and his associate Josef Breuer. It was used to describe the clinical case of Anna O., whose undischarged psychic energy was bound in a somatic symptom. This symptom represented the unconscious

Table 17.3
Psychiatric Conditions in the Differential Diagnosis of Conversion Disorder

Major depressive episodes
Catatonic schizophrenia
Pain disorder
Somatization disorder
Histrionic personality disorder
Adjustment disorder
Posttraumatic stress disorder
Malingering

conflict. That is, a repressed thought was converted to a somatic symptom. Freud then worked out his concept of talking therapy as a catharsis through which unconsciously repressed material might become conscious. With catharsis in psychotherapy and with hypnotic suggestion, somatic conversion symptoms were shown to diminish and even disappear.

In 1929, following from Charcot, *Pierre Janet observed that conversion disorders were preceded by a lowering of consciousness threshold and were associated with dissociation.* He recognized that a constitutional weakness in an individual might be accentuated by shock or fatigue, resulting in aspects of consciousness being split off. His concept of what is now considered to be conversion disorder did not, however, include the concept of repression; thus, he was not concerned with the significance of the dynamic unconscious as Freud was.

17.4 The answer is A

Conversion disorders may be the most frequently occurring of the somatoform disorders. DSM-IV-TR gives a range from a low of 11 to a high of 500 cases per 100,000 population. Affected persons can range in age from early childhood into old age. The annual incidence of conversion disorders seen by psychiatrists in a New York county has been estimated to be 22 cases per 100,000 population. In a general hospital setting 5 to 16 percent of all psychiatric consultation patients manifest some conversion symptoms. In a study of a rural Veterans Administration general hospital, 25 to 30 percent of all male patients had a conversion symptom at some time during their admission. By contrast, in a psychiatric emergency room or psychiatric clinic, the incidence of conversion disorder is far lower (1 percent of all psychiatric admissions), as different selection factors supervene. Lifetime figures for ever having any conversion symptoms, even if only on a transient basis, are far higher, with some studies reporting a 33 percent prevalence rate. Conversion disorder occurs mainly in women, with a ratio of 2 to 1 up to 5 to 1 in some studies. However, there does not seem to be an overrepresentation of conversion disorder in female children.

17.5 The answer is E (all)

Taken together, clinical and research findings could suggest that patients with conversion disorder under extraordinary circumstances experience impaired intercortical communication and blockade of ordinary channels of verbal associations. *The preponderance of left-sided, unilateral symptoms seen in conversion disorder plus the strong association of conversion disorders with depressive disorders could be used as evidence of a nondominant right-hemispheric vulnerability.* Additional complementary evidence for localization comes from the fact that the left hemisphere is phylogenetically associated with inhibitory influences. Thus, the motor and sensory symptoms of conversion suggest defects in processing and in analysis of sensorimotor signals, which leads to a failure in the integration of endogenous somatic signals. The proposed defect in understanding the signals in a conversion disorder is in some ways analogous to the failure of comprehension in a stroke (i.e., with receptive and expressive aphasia when acoustic-motor coordination of auditory signals involving language fails to occur).

The fact that conversion disorders occur mainly in women is another piece of evidence used to support a theory of brain localization. Studies from a variety of sources indicate that women have greater instability of right-hemispheric organization. Thus, it has been proposed that a primary defect in the left

hemisphere interferes with the normal transcallosal inhibitory stabilizing functions of the unstable contralateral right hemisphere. These circumstances could account for the symptoms of conversion disorder and for its almost exclusive restriction to the described pattern of cerebral organization.

Much more clinical and experimental work remains to be done if these heuristic hypotheses are to have widespread clinical relevance. The phenomena of conversion disorder and hypnosis have both been considered to result from blockade of corticofugal impulses induced by emotional rapport or intense emotional experience. Both conditions can lead to selective diminution of awareness of a bodily function. Interestingly, hypnosis can bring about temporary remission of conversion symptoms and can also produce a mimicry of conversion symptoms in those not afflicted with the condition.

These biomedical theories attempt to account for the *how*, but not the *what* or the *why* of conversion disorder. Obviously a multifactorial explanation is needed to render an understanding of the patient's plight and to serve as a framework for testing the most effective and efficient methods of treatment. Conversion symptoms represent a common pathway for the expression of a complex biopsychosocial event. A patient with conversion disorder, having a specific diathesis, experiences and creates (outside of his or her level of awareness) an illness in a setting of stress that is shaped to some extent on his or her model of disease.

17.6 The answer is E (all)

Pseudoseizures are paroxysmal episodes of altered behavior resembling epileptic attacks but devoid of the characteristic clinical epileptic and electrographic features. Convulsive behaviors identified as a conversion disorder often take place when the clinician walks into the patient's room or when the family visits. Variously termed *psychogenic* or *hysterical seizures* in the past, these clinical episodes terminate without the patient having a period of sluggishness, sleepiness, or confusion (as might be seen following a true convulsion). Pseudoseizures, but not complex partial seizures, tend not to manifest extreme stereotypy in the overt motor sequence and lack a neurological indicator. These patients do not show evidence of an elevated serum prolactin level immediately following the clinical episode. The EEG of the pseudoseizure patient during the clinical episode does not show any of the correlates of an epileptic seizure, such as increasing frequency of spike discharges, sudden onset of focal or diffuse rhythmic activity, or postictal slow waves.

The induction of a seizure by suggestion, formerly considered a hallmark of hysterical seizures, is also seen in complex partial seizures when there is elevated electrical lability. Semi-purposeful movements, thrashing, and pelvic thrusting, often considered to be the hallmarks of pseudoseizures, can be seen with direct stimulation of the cingulate region and are common correlates of complete partial seizures with frontotemporal foci. *Moreover, more than 70 percent of patients with pseudoseizures without documented bona fide seizures show interictal EEG abnormalities, neuropsychological impairment, or abnormalities on magnetic resonance imaging (MRI) and computed tomography (CT) scans.*

Although tongue-biting, urinary incontinence, injury during falls, and seeming loss of consciousness do not usually occur with a pseudoseizure, all of these can occur. However, the preservation of corneal, pupillary, and gag reflexes, plus the absence of extensor plantar responses and the preservation of normal color during the attack, all suggest a pseudoseizure.

The proportion of pseudoseizures in a given study typically reflects the nature of the referral source and their relationship with the evaluation. From a clinician's perspective, about *one-third of patients evaluated for a pseudoseizure do not have a convulsive disorder or pseudoseizures but rather have some other neurological condition; another third of patients have true convulsions as well as pseudoseizures; and another third have just pseudoseizures.*

17.7 The answer is A

Hypochondriacal symptoms can be a part of another disorder such as major depressive disorder, dysthymic disorders, generalized anxiety disorder, or adjustment disorder. However, primary hypochondriasis or hypochondriacal disorder is a chronic and somewhat disabling disorder with hypochondriacal symptoms, not merely a part of another psychiatric condition.

Hypochondriasis was included as a diagnostic entity in DSM-I. The diagnostic criteria continued to be revised in DSM-II, DSM-III, and DSM-III-R; however, the changes have been primarily linguistic, not substantive. The only change between DSM-III-R and DSM-IV-TR is the addition of a specifier to note that the patient has poor insight during the current episode. The ICD-10 criteria for hypochondriasis are essentially the same as those of DSM-IV-TR.

Hypochondriasis is rather common in primary care settings. In various locales, the prevalence has varied from 3 to 14 percent. Recent work indicates that in a 6-month period of observation, *4 to 6 percent of the general medical population meet the specific criteria for this disorder.* The prevalence in either sex is comparable to that within the general medical population. There are no specific tendencies for overrepresentation based on social position, education, marital status, or other sociodemographic descriptors. There is a wide range of ages at onset. Although the disorder can begin at any age, onset is thought to be most common between 20 and 30 years of age. A preliminary family study of 19 cases and their 72 first-degree relatives demonstrated no increase in the rate of hypochondriasis among their relatives compared with a control group.

Comorbidity with other psychiatric disorders is common with hypochondriasis and must be treated accordingly. As an example, when case-matched controls and 42 hypochondriasis patients from a medical clinic were evaluated psychiatrically, the hypochondriasis patients had twice as many lifetime Axis I disorders and three times the number of personality disorders. Of the hypochondriasis patients in the study, 88 percent had one or more additional Axis I disorders, the overlap being greatest with depressive and anxiety disorders. *Depression only accounts for a minor part of the total picture in hypochondriasis, however, so it is a mistake to think that all hypochondriasis is the result of some other Axis I disorder.*

The developmental background of hypochondriacal patients is of interest in that significantly more of these patients than matched controls report traumatic sexual contacts, physical violence, and major parental upheaval before the age of 17.

17.8 The answer is E (all)

Determining the extent of the emotional component of chronic pain is helpful, and care plans might then be effected, along with appropriate expectations and appropriate treatment. The well-known MADISON scale (Table 17.4) has not been rigorously validated but has been of considerable help to those working in the field. Another instrument that has proven to be clinically valuable in assessing whether a patient has an organic lesion that is amenable to a corrective surgical approach is the Mensana Pain Test, a 10-minute structured medical interview.

Table 17.4
MADISON Scale for Markers of Considerable Emotional Overlay

M = Multiplicity: Pain is either in more than one place or of more than one variety; when treated, may recur elsewhere.

A = Authenticity: More interested in clinician's acceptance of pain as genuine than in a cure.

D = Denial: Especially exaggerated marital or family harmony; when admitting depression or anxiety, no impact on pain is admitted.

I = Interpersonal relationship: Although the connection to the presence of any particular person's company as worsening the pain may be denied, observation of the patient's nonverbal and interactive behavior indicates otherwise.

S = Singularity: When the pain is described as unlike that of anyone else, ever.

O = "Only you": When the patient immediately idealizes the physician as savior, despite numerous failures by other competent experts.

N = Nothing helps, or no change: When there is no relief whatsoever from any type of intervention, although all are tried (including narcotics), and there is no hour-to-hour or day-to-day fluctuation under a variety of circumstances.

Table adapted from Hackett TP, Cassem NH. *Massachusetts General Handbook of General Hospital Psychiatry.* St. Louis: 1978.

17.9 The answer is E

Body dysmorphic disorder is not uncommon as a comorbid condition in patients with major depressive disorder, obsessive-compulsive disorder, and social phobia. Indeed in one study of 30 patients, all met DSM-III-R criteria for at least one other psychiatric diagnosis at some point in their lives, and usually concurrently.

The cause of body dysmorphic disorder is unknown. The high comorbidity with depressive disorders, a higher-than-expected family history of mood disorders and obsessive-compulsive disorder, and the reported responsiveness to SSRIs indicates that, in at least some patients, the pathophysiology of the disorder may involve serotonin and may be related to other disorders. There may be significant cultural or social effects on patients with body dysmorphic disorder because of the emphasis on stereotyped concepts of beauty that may be emphasized in certain families and within the culture at large. In psychodynamic models, body dysmorphic disorder is seen as reflecting the displacement of a sexual or an emotional conflict onto a nonrelated body part; such a putative association occurs through the defense mechanisms of repression, dissociation, distortion, symbolization, and projection.

Family histories of substance abuse and mood disorder are common in documented cases. Also predisposing to the disorder may be certain types of personality characteristics, especially a mixture of obsessional and avoidant traits, but no single personality pattern predominates. Reportedly, the patients are shy, self-absorbed, and overly sensitive to their imagined defect as a focus of notice or criticism.

17.10 The answer is C

In conversion disorder, a patient has symptoms or deficits that affect voluntary motor or sensory functions and that suggest a neurological or other general medical condition. Psychological factors are thought to be connected with the symptom or deficit, which is usually preceded by conflict or other stress. The disorder is ruled out if the symptoms or deficits can be explained by a medical condition, by the effects of a substance, or by cultural standards. It is ruled out if the symptoms are limited to pain or sexual dysfunction, occur only during somatization disorder, or are better accounted for by another mental disorder.

La belle indifférence, an apparent lack of concern about symptoms, can occur with conversion disorder, although other patients may exhibit their symptoms dramatically or histrionically. In conversion disorder, there is no question of *feigned symptoms;* patients do not intentionally produce symptoms to obtain certain benefits.

Sexual dysfunction may appear in conversion disorder, but it cannot be the only symptom. *An urban background* is less likely than a rural one; it occurs more commonly among rural populations, people of lower socioeconomic status, and those less familiar with medical and psychological ideas.

Symptom onset after age 50 is unlikely. Although it has been reported in the ninth decade, onset generally occurs from late childhood to early adulthood, rarely before the age of 10 years or after the age of 35 years. When conversion disorder seems to appear in a patient of middle or old age, there is probably an occult neurological or other general medical condition. The onset is usually acute, and the symptoms typically do not last long. Recurrence, however, is common; it occurs within 1 year in one-fifth to one-quarter of people; a single recurrence predicts future episodes.

17.11 The answer is D

The patient is probably suffering from *somatization disorder,* since she fits the diagnostic criteria. The patient complained of at least four pain symptoms (breast, back, urinary, and migraine), two gastrointestinal symptoms (spastic colon and adhesions), one sexual symptom ("I can't have relations"), and one pseudoneurological symptom (falling)—none of which is completely explained by physical or laboratory examinations. In addition, her symptoms had their onset before age 30.

Hypochondriasis is characterized by the false belief that one has a specific disease; in contrast, somatization disorder is characterized by concern with many symptoms. The symptoms of *conversion disorder* are limited to one or two neurological symptoms, rather than the wide-ranging symptoms of somatization disorder. *Pain disorder* is limited to one or two complaints of pain symptoms.

Body dysmorphic disorder is not distinguished by any type of symptoms. Instead, body dysmorphic disorder entails the preoccupation with an imagined defect in appearance. No such preoccupation was found in the patient described.

17.12 The answer is A

Nearly all of the physical symptoms that the patient described were apparently without an organic basis. That suggested a somatoform disorder, and the large number of symptoms involving multiple organ systems suggested *somatization disorder.* She had symptoms relating to the gastrointestinal, cardiovascular, pulmonary, neurological, and gynecological systems, which meet the criteria for that diagnosis. *Conversion disorder* was ruled out because the patient's symptoms were not limited to the sensorimotor areas alone; they covered a far broader range. *Hypochondriasis* is distinguished from somatization disorder in that it includes the fear of disease and bodily preoccupation. In *dysthymic disorder,* patients show cognitive (slow thinking), behavioral (early morning awakening, lethargy), and mood (depression or suicidal ideation) symptoms.

17.13 The answer is B

A number of theories attempt to explain the cause of hypochondriasis. One theory is that *hypochondriasis is the result of an unconscious desire to assume the sick role* by a person facing seemingly insurmountable and insolvable problems. The sick role offers a way out, because the sick patient is allowed to avoid unpleasant obligations and to postpone unwelcome challenges and is excused from usually expected duties. The diagnostic criteria for hypochondriasis require that patients be preoccupied with the false belief that they have a serious disease and that the false belief be based on a misinterpretation of physical signs or sensations. *Patients with hypochondriasis usually believe that they have a specific disease, not multiple diseases. The patient's belief that a particular disease is present is not of delusional intensity.* If it were of such intensity, a delusional disorder, somatic type, would be diagnosed. Hypochondriacs are usually reassured by a normal physical examination; delusional persons are not. *Men are not affected by hypochondriasis more than women;* in fact, men and women are equally affected. *The incidence of hypochondriasis is not affected by educational level or marital status.*

17.14 The answer is E

Cogwheel rigidity is an organic sign secondary to disorders of the basal ganglia and not a sign of conversion disorder. In conversion disorder, anesthesia and paresthesia, especially of the extremities, are common. All sensory modalities are involved, and the distribution of the disturbance is inconsistent with that of either central or peripheral neurological disease. Thus, one sees the characteristic *stocking-and-glove anesthesia* of the hands or feet or *hemianesthesia of the body beginning precisely at the midline.* Motor symptoms include abnormal movements and gait disturbance, which is often a wildly ataxic, staggering gait accompanied by gross, irregular, jerky truncal movements and thrashing and waving arms (also known as *astasia-abasia*). *Normal reflexes* are seen. The patient shows no fasciculations or muscle atrophy, and electromyography findings are normal.

17.15 The answer is E

Serotonin-specific drugs such as clomipramine (Anafranil) and fluoxetine (Prozac) *are effective in reducing the symptoms* in at least 50 percent of patients with body dysmorphic disorder. In any patient with a coexisting mental disorder or an anxiety disorder, the coexisting disorder should be treated with the appropriate pharmacotherapy and psychotherapy. How long treatment should be continued when the symptoms of body dysmorphic disorder have remitted is unknown. *Plastic surgery is not usually beneficial* in the treatment of patients with body dysmorphic disorder. In fact, surgical, dermatological, dental, and other medical procedures to address the alleged defects rarely satisfy the patient.

A comorbid diagnosis is not unusual. Body dysmorphic disorder commonly coexists with other mental disorders. One study found that more than 90 percent of body dysmorphic disorder patients had experienced a major depressive episode in their lifetimes, about 70 percent had had an anxiety disorder, and about 30 percent had a psychotic disorder. However, *anorexia nervosa should not be diagnosed* along with body dysmorphic disorder, since distortions of body image occur in anorexia nervosa, gender identity disorders, and some specific types of brain damage (for example, neglect syndromes).

The effects of body dysmorphic disorder on a person's life can be significant. Almost all affected patients avoid social and occupational exposure. As many as a third of the patients may be housebound by their concern about being ridiculed for their alleged deformities, and as many as *20 percent, not 50 percent, of patients attempt suicide.*

17.16 The answer is B

The most accurate statement about pain disorder is that *first-degree relatives of pain disorder patients have an increased likelihood of having the same disorder*, thus indicating the possibility of genetic inheritance or behavioral mechanisms in the transmission of the disorder. Pain disorder is in fact *diagnosed twice as frequently in women as in men.* The *peak ages of onset are in the fourth and fifth decades*, when the tolerance for pain declines. Pain disorder is *most common in persons with blue-collar occupations*, perhaps because of increased job-related injuries. *Depressive disorders, anxiety disorders, and substance abuse are also more common in families of pain disorder patients* than in the general population.

17.17 The answer is C

During the course of somatization disorder, the patient *has complained of* pain, gastrointestinal, sexual, and pseudoneurological symptoms that are *not explained by a known medical condition.* In addition, the patient *presents the initial physical complaints before, not after, age 30.* The patient *has had physical symptoms for at least several years, not just 3 months.* The patient has had interpersonal problems and tremendous psychological distress and *usually experiences significant, not minimal, impairment in social or occupational functioning.* A patient who has *a false belief of being pregnant* and objective signs of pregnancy, such as decreased menstrual flow or amenorrhea, does not have somatization disorder. Instead, the patient has pseudocyesis, a somatoform disorder not otherwise specified.

17.18 The answer is E (all)

The clinician must always rule out organic causes for the patient's symptoms. Medical disorders that present with non-specific, transient abnormalities pose the greatest diagnostic difficulty in the differential diagnosis of somatization disorder. The disorders to be considered include *multiple sclerosis, systemic lupus erythematosus, acute intermittent porphyria*, and *hyperparathyroidism*. In addition, the onset of many somatic symptoms late in life must be presumed to be caused by a medical illness until testing rules it out. Table 17.5 lists a few of the disorders commonly confused with somatoform disorders, especially early in their courses.

Answers 17.19–17.23

17.19 The answer is C

17.20 The answer is A

17.21 The answer is C

17.22 The answer is C

17.23 The answer is D

Both somatization disorder and pain disorder affect *women more than men.* Somatization disorder has a 5 to 1 female-to-male ratio. The lifetime prevalence of somatization disorder

Table 17.5
Conditions Commonly Confused with Somatoform Disorder

Multiple sclerosis
Central nervous system syphilis
Brain tumor
Hyperparathyroidism
Acute intermittent porphyria
Lupus erythematosus
Hyperthyroidism
Myasthenia gravis

among women in the general population may be 1 to 2 percent. Pain disorder is diagnosed twice as commonly in women as in men. Somatization disorder is defined as beginning before age 30, and it *most often begins during a person's teens.* As for pain disorder, the peak of onset is in the fourth and fifth decades, perhaps because the tolerance for pain decreases with age.

Antidepressants, such as fluoxetine (Prozac), sertraline (Zoloft), and clomipramine (Anafranil), *are effective* in the treatment of pain disorder and somatization disorder. *Serotonin may be involved in the pathophysiology of both disorders.* It is probably the main neurotransmitter in the descending inhibitory pathways. Endorphins also play a role in the central nervous system modulation of pain. *Anorexia nervosa is not commonly associated with either pain disorder or somatization disorder.* Anorexia nervosa is an eating disorder that presents a dramatic picture of self-starvation, peculiar attitudes toward food, weight loss (leading to the maintenance of the patient's body weight at least 15 percent below that expected), and an intense fear of weight gain.

Answers 17.24–17.29

17.24 The answer is A

17.25 The answer is A

17.26 The answer is B

17.27 The answer is A

17.28 The answer is C

17.29 The answer is D

Hypochondriasis, which is an excessive concern about disease and a preoccupation with one's health, *is found approximately equally in men and women.* Somatization disorder, which is a chronic syndrome of multiple somatic symptoms that cannot be explained medically, is much more common in women than in men. The *peak incidence* of hypochondriasis is thought to occur *during the 40s or 50s*, whereas somatization disorder begins before age 30. *Somatization disorder patients are likely to have a hysterical cognitive and interpersonal style*, as opposed to obsessional hypochondriac patients. *Anhedonia* (the inability to experience pleasure) is a sign of depression but may be present in both hypochondriasis and somatization disorders. *Hallucinations are not present* in either disorder.

Answers 17.30–17.35

17.30 The answer is C

17.31 The answer is C

17.32 The answer is C

17.33 The answer is B

17.34 The answer is A

17.35 The answer is B

The prevalence of conversion *is highest in rural areas and among the undereducated* and the lower socioeconomic classes. It is more prevalent in military populations, especially in those exposed to combat. It is also more common in underprivileged persons, in those of subnormal intelligence, and in industrial settings where compensation neurosis may become an issue. There may be a tendency for familial aggregation and for the patient to be the youngest sibling in the family. The incidence of the disorder may be on the decline.

Persons that meet the full criteria for somatization disorder are typically unmarried, nonwhite, *poorly educated, and from rural areas.*

In 1859 Pierre Briquet emphasized the multisymptomatic aspects of somatization and its protracted course. His report of the 430 cases observed at the Hospital de la Charité in Paris focused on polysymptomatic facets of the disorder. Briquet also recognized hysteria in men and attributed the disorder to emotional causes.

In the early 1960s two studies confirmed the original findings of a definable clinical syndrome, demonstrating diagnostic stability of the multisymptomatic concept of hysteria. In 1970 the eponym *Briquet's syndrome* was proposed to denote multi-symptomatic hysteria. The disorder, characterized by at least 25 symptoms from ten symptom groups, was known as *Briquet's syndrome* until the publication of the DSM-III. Ironically, after the decision was made to incorporate Briquet's syndrome as part of the new diagnostic nomenclature, an unrelated decision was made to drop all eponyms. Hence a new name—*somatization disorder*—had to be created. *Pierre Briquet also originated the modern concept of conversion disorder.*

Axis II personality disorders frequently accompany a conversion disorder, especially the histrionic type (in 5 to 21 percent of cases), the passive-dependent type (9 to 40 percent of cases), and the passive-aggressive type of personality disorder. However, conversion disorders can occur in persons with no predisposing medical, neurological, or psychiatric disorder. Several recent studies using structured diagnostic interviews in patients from primary care settings found that 61 to 72 percent of *patients with somatization disorder also have co-occurring personality disorders.* This rate would seem to be 2.5 to 11.6 times more common in somatization disorder patients than in general medical patients. *Conversion disorder is characterized by focus on any one or two symptoms*, whereas somatization patients focus on complaints about multisystem symptoms that lead them to have an inordinately high number of surgical procedures and consume an excessive amount of health care.

By definition, somatization disorder is a chronic relapsing condition with no known cure. It usually begins in middle to late adolescence, but may start as late as the third decade of life. Most patients diagnosed with conversion disorder experience a quick symptomatic recovery. Rapid improvement is especially seen in cases where symptoms are of recent onset.

Most conversion symptoms remit spontaneously or after behavioral treatment, suggestion, and a supportive environment. Thus,

for symptoms of very recent onset a variety of other therapies have also been utilized successfully. In practice, clinicians tend to choose therapies that reflect their training. Irrespective of the technique used, most approaches seem to work when symptoms are not reinforced and when the patient's psychosocial plight is the focus of attention.

A favorable prognosis of conversion disorder is associated with sudden onset; readily identifiable stressful events; good premorbid health with no comorbid psychiatric, medical, or neurological disease; and no ongoing compensation litigation.

Because the cause of somatization disorder is unknown and no curative or amelioriative treatment has been found, the clinician needs to focus on management rather than treatment, on coping rather than curing (care rather than cure).

Answers 17.36–17.37

17.36 The answer is A

17.37 The answer is C

Many who work in the general medical setting find the diagnosis of undifferentiated somatoform disorder helpful. Research indicates the validity of distinguishing undifferentiated somatoform disorder from somatization disorder. There appears to be a dimensional or quantitative difference between undifferentiated somatoform disorder and somatization disorder rather than a qualitative difference between the two. However, the natural history of both disorders seems to be similar. The disorder was not included in DSM-I, DSM-II, and DSM-III; it was first introduced in DSM-III-R because somatization disorder was considered to be too restrictive by primary care providers to provide adequate coverage for many patients with significant somatoform complaints. Thus the subsyndromal grouping was formalized to facilitate learning about the natural course of a large cluster of patients. The criteria for undifferentiated somatoform disorder in ICD-10 are similar to the diagnostic criteria in DSM-IV-TR.

Undifferentiated somatoform disorder is characterized by one or more unexplained physical complaints of at least 6 months' duration. These symptoms impair the patient in some domain and are temporally associated with a stressor. Psychological factors are assumed to be associated with the symptoms or complaints because of a contemporaneous relationship between the initiation or exacerbation of the symptoms and stressors, conflicts, or needs. The complaint must be unattributable to any other known psychiatric condition or pathophysiological mechanism or, when it is related to a nonpsychiatric condition, the physical complaints or resulting social and occupational impairments must be grossly in excess of what would ordinarily be expected from the findings.

The importance of undifferentiated somatoform disorder comes from the fact that it may be 30 to 100 times more prevalent than full-blown somatization disorder. *Undifferentiated somatoform disorder has an estimated lifetime prevalence in the general population of between 4 and 11 percent.* The estimated lifetime prevalence of somatization disorder is 0.2 to 2 percent in women and less in men.

The course of undifferentiated somatoform disorder is generally chronic and relapsing just as with somatization disorder; however, little systematic research on the disorder has been accomplished to date. It is likely that some cases of the disorder can resolve after a single episode.

18 ▲

Chronic Fatigue Syndrome and Neurasthenia

Neither neurasthenia nor chronic fatigue syndrome is classified in the revised fourth edition of the *Diagnostic and Statistical Manual for Mental Disorders* (DSM-IV-TR). Neurasthenia is included in the tenth revision of the *International Statistical Classification of Diseases and Related Health Problems* (ICD-10) as a neurotic disorder. Chronic fatigue syndrome was identified by the U.S. Centers for Disease Control and Prevention (CDC) in 1988, and is classified in ICD-10 as Malaise and Fatigue, a poorly defined condition of unknown etiology. The CDC in 1994 provided guidelines for chronic fatigue syndrome that serve as a good source for its clinical features.

Neurasthenia is most commonly diagnosed in China and other areas of Asia, as well as in Europe. In the U.S., it is categorized as an undifferentiated somatoform disorder in DSM-IV-TR. The major symptoms of neurasthenia have been defined as fatigue and a heightened concern over bodily symptoms. Neurasthenia as a syndrome is historically interesting in that it was described in the 1800s by such observers as Sigmund Freud, who felt it was the result of disturbed sexual functioning. The American neuropsychiatrist, George Miller Beard, coined the term in the 1860s, and postulated that it was the result of a "nervous diathesis," or of a particular vulnerability to stress. Current biological theorists postulate that prolonged stress lowers and ultimately depletes the level of neurotransmitters, causing symptoms of anxiety and depression. More psychodynamically oriented theorists might see the disorder as the result of unfulfilled dependency or other psychologically determined needs.

Chronic fatigue syndrome is a controversial diagnosis that has been observed to occur primarily in younger adults and is said to be twice as common in women as in men. Described treatments have been both pharmacologic as well and psychotherapeutic.

The student should study the questions and answers below for a useful review of this syndrome.

▲ QUESTIONS

DIRECTIONS: Each of the questions or incomplete statements below is followed by five lettered responses or completions. Select the *one* that is most appropriate in each case.

18.1 Neurasthenia

A. is included as a diagnosis in DSM-IV-TR
B. is rarely diagnosed in Asia or Russia
C. was first described by George M. Beard at the end of the 19th century
D. has a reported prevalence of 20 percent in people who meet diagnostic criteria for more than a month during the past 10 years
E. none of the above

18.2 Chronic fatigue syndrome

A. is proved to be a viral or postviral syndrome
B. has not been linked with fibromyalgia
C. has been viewed as a vehicle for negotiation of change in interpersonal worlds
D. patients in MRI studies displayed a specific pattern of white matter abnormality
E. prevalence reports show that fewer than 10 percent of cases have antecedent psychiatric disorders

18.3 True statements about chronic fatigue syndrome include

A. Studies indicate that many chronic fatigue syndrome patients have somatization disorder.
B. The syndrome is most likely to be a heterogeneous condition with fatigue as a final common pathway.
C. Treatment is invariably physiologic.
D. Cognitive-behavioral therapy (CBT) has been shown to have little or no impact on the disability and symptoms of patients.
E. None of the above

18.4 George M. Beard's concept of nerve exhaustion might include all of the following *except*

A. low serotonin levels
B. increased testosterone levels
C. low neuronal dopamine activity
D. decreased basal levels of luteinizing hormone
E. decreased basal levels of follicle-stimulating hormone

18.5 The symptoms of neurasthenia include

A. paresthesia
B. tachycardia
C. headaches
D. physical aches and pains
E. all of the above

18.6 All of the following statements correctly describe current approaches in treating neurasthenia *except*

A. Psychiatric intervention is helpful.
B. Clinicians must recognize objective symptoms.
C. Patients must recognize environmental stresses.
D. Somatic symptoms must be treated when possible.
E. Benzodiazepines are useful drugs for long-term treatment.

ANSWERS

Chronic Fatigue Syndrome and Neurasthenia

18.1 The answer is C

Neurasthenia, literally a lack of nerve energy, was described by George M. Beard at the end of the 19th century to account for the physical and mental exhaustion arising from the depletion of nervous resources. This finding has given rise to numerous theories but little controlled research. *The diagnosis is not included in DSM-IV-TR,* nor was it included in DSM-III or DSM-III-R. In DSM-I the condition was called psychologic nervous system reaction and in DSM-II it was called neurasthenic neurosis.

Neurasthenia is still diagnosed with some frequency in Asia and Russia but not in the United States. Particularly in Asia, researchers have found neurasthenia to be a culturally sanctioned idiom of distress. In ICD-10, two main types of neurasthenia occur, with considerable overlap. One type has a predominance of increased fatigue after mental effort, thus associated with a decrease in job performance or coping with activities of daily living. Difficulty in concentration, unpleasant distracting associations or recollections, and generally inefficient thinking have all been

reported. The other type has physical weakness and exhaustion after only a minimal physical effort, accompanied by muscular aches and pains and an inability to relax. Both types also have a variety of unpleasant physical feelings, including dizziness, tension headaches, and feelings of general instability. Patients also worry about decreased mental or physical well-being and have irritability and anhedonia. Varying degrees of minor anxiety and depression are also common. Sleep may be disturbed with initial- or middle-phase insomnia or hypersomnia.

According to ICD-10, the condition must be present for more than 3 months and have either (1) persistent and distressing complaints of feelings of exhaustion after minor mental effort or (2) persistent and distressing complaints of feelings of fatigue and bodily weakness after minor physical effort. Moreover, the patient is unable to recover from the symptoms of exhaustion or fatigue by rest, relaxation, or entertainment.

Prevalence studies indicate that, using ICD-10 criteria, about 1 percent of the population have had this condition for more than 3 months and *10 percent (not 20 percent) have it for more than a month during the past 10 years.* An epidemiological study of

Chinese-Americans reported that 6.4 percent of the subjects had neurasthenia, and only 3.6 percent of those had no other current or lifetime psychiatric diagnoses.

The cause of neurasthenia seems to be pleomorphic, with proponents implicating mood disorders, anxiety disorders, or conversion disorders. Others propose viral sequelae while still other investigators search for trace mineral deficiencies. Obscure neuromuscular conditions, immune dysfunction, and chronic fatigue syndrome have also been linked to the cause of neurasthenia. Despite the broad range of unproven theories, individuals can be considerably incapacitated with symptoms of fatigue and fatigability, with or without accompanying anxiety. Diagnostic workup of the fatigue syndrome by definition is unrewarding because a medical condition causing fatigue would necessarily exclude the diagnosis of neurasthenia.

18.2 The answer is C

In the absence of a clear cause, chronic fatigue syndrome has been disparagingly called "the yuppie flu," neurasthenia, and masked depression. Viral or postviral etiologies have also been considered, with diagnoses such as myalgic encephalomyelitis and chronic Epstein-Barr virus disorder being in vogue for a while. *Studies of these viral etiologies have not seemed to be relevant to a large segment of those with chronic fatigue syndrome,* but recent research notes a persistent enterovirus or herpesvirus 6 in some cases. *An overlap with fibrositis or fibromyalgia has also been considered,* but this is not particularly illuminating because it only links a poorly understood rheumatic condition with another even less clearly defined, fatigue-centered condition of uncertain etiology.

Medical anthropologists have seen chronic fatigue syndrome as a vehicle for negotiation of change in interpersonal worlds. A physiologist recently suggested that there might be a nasal fatigue reflex, akin to the diving reflex (bradycardia in cold water). According to this hypothesis, the nasal fatigue reflex could produce the debilitating fatigue that would in turn give the afflicted individual the time to heal before having to face a hostile environment. Brain magnetic resonance imaging (MRI) studies of 43 patients with chronic fatigue syndrome, compared to controls, demonstrated that *no MRI pattern of white matter abnormalities is specific.*

Psychiatric factors have been strongly associated with the etiology of chronic fatigue syndrome. For example, certain clinical samples have reported that *almost half of their cases have had antecedent psychiatric disorders such as depression, phobias, or other anxiety disorders.* In a recent matched study of 214 subjects with chronic fatigue syndrome from a nonspecialist, nonreferral setting, most of the index subjects were at considerably greater risk of current psychiatric disorder than were control subjects. The likelihood of psychiatric disorder was six times greater in these chronic fatigue syndrome patients than in the matched controls when evaluated either by interview or by questionnaire. Other studies of subjects who have undergone neuropsychological testing indicate that at least a subset of patients with chronic fatigue syndrome experience significant impairments in learning and memory. However, a primary psychiatric etiology for chronic fatigue syndrome is, typically, stoutly denied by patients with this syndrome, especially by those who are members of the chronic fatigue syndrome national peer support groups.

18.3 The answer is B

Fatigue is one of the most common symptoms in all of medical practice. The nature of chronic fatigue syndrome, however,

Table 18.1
CDC Criteria for Chronic Fatigue Syndrome

A. Severe unexplained fatigue for over 6 months that is:
  (1) of a new or definite onset
  (2) not due to continuing exertion
  (3) not resolved by rest
  (4) functionally impairing
B. The presence of four or more of the following new symptoms:
  (1) impaired memory or concentration
  (2) sore throat
  (3) tender lymph nodes
  (4) muscle pain
  (5) pain in several joints
  (6) new pattern of headaches
  (7) unrefreshing sleep
  (8) postexertional malaise lasting more than 24 hours

remains very controversial. This syndrome was defined by the Centers for Disease Control (CDC) in 1988 as a disabling disorder with a combination of a certain number of nonspecific symptoms such as fluctuating levels of fatigue, various combinations of neuromuscular and neuropsychological symptoms, chronic pain, malaise, mild fevers, and anxiety. According to the latest CDC criteria, it is a condition that has been clinically evaluated and still remains an unexplained, persistent, or relapsing chronic fatigue that is of new or definite onset in a previously healthy person; is not the result of exertion; is not substantially alleviated by rest; and leads to substantial reduction in previous levels of occupational, educational, social, or personal activities (Table 18.1).

Chronic fatigue syndrome is most likely to be a heterogenous condition, with fatigue being only a final common pathway. At this phase of research on the condition, it is not possible to speak with certainty about its etiology.

Whether chronic fatigue syndrome should be considered as a special class of mood disorder with somatic symptoms (specifically fatigue), or a somatoform disorder not otherwise specified, or a combination of a psychiatric disorder with an unidentified infectious agent, or even some composite of these conditions, remains to be clarified. Using strict DSM-IV-TR criteria, one study demonstrates that *very few chronic fatigue syndrome patients have somatization disorder.*

Treatments for a presumably heterogenous condition with an unknown cause typically should involve a multidisciplinary approach involving psychological, physiological, and social factors. Possible concomitant psychiatric disorders could most likely benefit from a psychopharmacological trial. Many other types of treatments are being used for this debilitating illness, with even electric plum blossom needle therapy having its adherents in the literature. Two randomized controlled trials of cognitive-behavioral therapy (compared with relaxation therapy or routine practitioner care) indicate that *cognitive-behavioral therapy has substantial impact on the disability and symptoms of patients with this disorder.*

18.4 The answer is B

The present-day depletion hypothesis, which holds that prolonged stress lowers the levels of neurotransmitters in neurons, bears a striking resemblance to George M. Beard's concept of nerve exhaustion. Brain amines, when depleted, cause symp-

Table 18.2
Signs and Symptoms Reported by Patients with Neurasthenia

General fatigue	Sexual dysfunction, e.g., erectile disorder, anorgasmia
Exhaustion	
General anxiety	Dysmenorrhea
Difficulty concentrating	Paresthesia
Physical aches and pains	Insomnia
Dizziness	Poor memory
Headache	Pessimism
Intolerance of noise (hyperacusis) or bright lights	Chronic worry
	Fear of disease
Chills	Irritability
Indigestion	Feelings of hopelessness
Constipation or diarrhea	Dry mouth or hypersalivation
Flatulence	Arthralgias
Palpitations	Heat insensitivity
Extrasystole	Dysphagia
Tachycardia	Pruritus
Excess sweating	Tremors
Flushing of skin	Back pain

Table 18.3
Signs and Symptoms Reported by Patients with Chronic Fatigue Syndrome

Fatigue or exhaustion
Headache
Malaise
Short-term memory loss
Muscle pain
Difficulty concentrating
Joint pain
Depression
Abdominal pain
Lymph node pain
Sore throat
Lack of restful sleep
Muscle weakness
Bitter or metallic taste
Balance disturbance
Diarrhea
Constipation
Bloating
Panic attacks
Eye pain
Scratchiness in eyes
Blurring of vision
Double vision
Sensitivity to bright lights
Numbness and/or tingling in extremities
Fainting spells
Light-headedness
Dizziness
Clumsiness
Insomnia
Fever or sensation of fever
Chills
Night sweats
Weight gain
Allergies
Chemical sensitivities
Palpitations
Shortness of breath
Flushing rash of the face and cheeks
Swelling of the extremities or eyelids
Burning on urination
Sexual dysfunction
Hair loss

Adapted from Bell DS. *The Doctor's Guide to Chronic Fatigue Syndrome: Understanding, Treating, and Living with CFIDS.* Reading: Addison-Wesley; 1995:10.

toms of anxiety or depression. *Low neuronal dopamine activity* occurs in depression; the noradrenergic and adrenergic systems are affected in anxiety and depression; and *serotonin levels are low* in depression. Neuroendocrine dysregulations in people with mood and anxiety disorders do not include *increased testosterone levels.* On the contrary, testosterone levels are decreased, and testosterone replacement is sometimes attempted. Long-term treatment with testosterone, however, can have serious adverse affects such as prostate cancer. *Decreased basal levels of luteinizing hormone* and *of follicle-stimulating hormone* are additional neuroendocrine abnormalities. These hormones are also altered during prolonged stress states and presumably in neurasthenia as well.

18.5 The answer is E (all)
All the listed choices—*paresthesia, tachycardia, headaches, and physical aches and pains*—are symptoms of neurasthenia. There are many more symptoms, such as difficulty in concentrating, dizziness, indigestion, constipation and diarrhea, palpitations, excess sweating, chills, noise or light intolerance, flushing, insomnia, and tremors. The similarity between the signs and symptoms reported by patients with neurasthenia and those with chronic fatigue syndrome are apparent when comparing Table 18.2 and Table 18.3.

18.6 The answer is E
Benzodiazepines are not useful drugs for long-term treatment of neurasthenia. Physicians should be careful when prescribing drugs for this disorder; patients may misuse them and become dependent. As benzodiazepines have the potential for abuse, they must be used only briefly and with careful supervision, for anxiety, phobias, or insomnia. *Psychotherapeutic intervention* is helpful during treatment for neurasthenia. Along with medications, *patients must recognize environmental stresses* that help to produce the disorder, the coping mechanisms with which they deal with the stresses, and the interaction between mind and body. Without insight-oriented psychotherapy, neurasthenia may well continue without

improvement. *Clinicians must recognize objective symptoms* and *somatic symptoms must be treated.* Symptoms can be produced by emotions that influence the autonomic nervous system, which in turn affects bodily functions. Stress can produce structural change in organ systems; in some cases the results can be life threatening.

19

Factitious Disorders

Just as with somatoform disorders, factitious disorders are often mistakenly diagnosed as malingering. However, unlike patients who malinger, patients with factitious disorders have no external incentive, such as collecting disability, to explain their presentation of symptoms. In fact, the goal of people with factitious disorders appears to be solely to take on the sick role, to be a patient. The motivations for this behavior are unclear, but interestingly the disorders occur most frequently in people with some type of medical background, as well as in people with some type of serious history of illness or hospitalization in childhood. In factitious disorder by proxy, one person (often a mother with a child) intentionally produces physical signs or symptoms in another person who is under the first person's care. In this case, a mother might go as far as inducing injury, or even, on occasion, death in the child.

The best known factitious disorder is perhaps factitious disorder with predominately physical signs and symptoms, popularly known as Munchausen syndrome. This presentation involves persons who travel from hospital to hospital, gaining admission, receiving multiple diagnoses and treatments, until they are found out by staff, and then quickly move on to the next hospital to repeat the same rituals again. Common complaints or presenting symptoms include hematomas, abdominal pain, fever, and seizures. Patients have been known to do such bizarre things as inject themselves with feces to induce infections or to willingly undergo repeated unnecessary surgeries.

The revised fourth edition of the *Diagnostic and Statistical Manual of Mental Disorders* (DSM-IV-TR) characterizes factitious disorders as intentionally produced physical or psychological signs and symptoms to assume a sick role. The DSM-IV-TR categories for the disorder include predominant physical signs and symptoms, predominantly psychological signs and symptoms, both physical and psychological signs and symptoms, and factitious disorder not otherwise specified.

The student should study the questions and answers below for a useful review of these disorders.

HELPFUL HINTS

The student should be able to define each of these terms.

- ▶ approximate answers
- ▶ as-if personality
- ▶ borderline personality disorder
- ▶ Briquet's syndrome
- ▶ depressive-masochistic personality
- ▶ dissociative disorder not otherwise specified
- ▶ factitious disorder:
  by proxy
  not otherwise specified
  with predominantly physical signs and symptoms
  with predominantly psychological signs and symptoms
- ▶ Ganser's syndrome
- ▶ gridiron abdomen
- ▶ identification with the aggressor
- ▶ impostorship
- ▶ malingering
- ▶ Munchausen syndrome
- ▶ pseudologia fantastica
- ▶ pseudomalingering
- ▶ regression
- ▶ schizophrenia
- ▶ sick role
- ▶ somatoform disorders
- ▶ substance abuse
- ▶ symbolization
- ▶ unmasking ceremony

▲ QUESTIONS

DIRECTIONS: Each of the questions incomplete statements below is followed by five suggested responses completions. Select the *one* that is *best* in each case.

19.1 A 22-year-old male ambulance driver who complained of severe abdominal pain and tenderness was admitted to the hospital through the emergency room. The patient demanded an appendectomy. When test after test returned with a negative result, the patient grew abusive and threatening. A likely diagnosis is

A. malingering
B. hypochondriasis
C. Ganser's syndrome
D. Briquet's syndrome
E. Munchausen syndrome

19.2 The differential diagnosis of a factitious disorder includes

A. somatization disorder
B. hypochondriasis
C. antisocial personality disorder
D. malingering
E. all of the above

19.3 Factitious disorders

A. usually begin in childhood
B. are best treated with psychoactive drugs
C. usually have a good prognosis
D. are synonymous with Ganser's syndrome
E. may occur by proxy

19.4 A leading predisposing factor in the development of factitious disorder with predominantly physical signs and symptoms is employment as a

A. teacher
B. healthcare worker
C. police officer
D. banker
E. waitress

19.5 Factitious disorder with predominantly physical signs and symptoms is synonymous with all of the following *except*

A. hospital addiction
B. Munchausen syndrome
C. professional patient syndrome
D. Briquet's syndrome
E. polysurgical addiction

19.6 Persons displaying a factitious disorder are often characterized by

A. a history of being exposed to genuine illness in a family member
B. employment in a health-related field
C. a history of early parental rejection
D. a tendency to view the physician as a loving parent
E. all of the above

19.7 You are asked by the court to evaluate a 21-year-old man arrested in a robbery because his lawyer raised the issue of his competence to stand trial. He has no known psychiatric history, and no psychotic symptoms have been previously reported. During the interview the man appears calm and in control, sits slouched in the chair, and has good eye contact. His affect shows a good range. His thought processes are logical, sequential, and spontaneous even when he describes many difficulties with his thinking. He seems guarded in his answers, particularly to questions about his psychological symptoms.

He claims to have precognition on occasion, knowing, for instance, what is going to be served for lunch in the jail, and that he does not like narcotics because Jean Dixon doesn't like narcotics either, and she is in control of his thoughts. He states that he has seen a vision of General Lee in his cell as well as "little green men from Mars," and that his current incarceration is a mission in which he is attempting to be an undercover agent for the police, although none of the local police realize this. Despite the overtly psychotic nature of these thoughts as described, the patient does not seem to be really engaged in the ideas; he seems to be simply reciting a list of what appears to be crazy rather than recounting actual experiences and beliefs. When the interviewer expresses some skepticism about his described beliefs, he responds by saying that he has "many other crazy ideas" that he can share.

Which of the following is the most likely diagnosis?

A. malingering
B. schizophrenia, paranoid type
C. factitious disorder with predominantly psychological symptoms
D. delusional disorder
E. Capgras's syndrome

19.8 Factitious disorder patients with Munchausen syndrome are typically

A. middle-aged men
B. unmarried
C. unemployed
D. estranged from their families
E. all of the above

19.9 True statements about factitious disorder by proxy include all of the following *except*

A. The average length of time to establish a diagnosis after the initial presentation is about 2 months.
B. Often a sibling has died of undiagnosed causes before the disorder is recognized.
C. The disorder currently accounts for fewer than 1,000 of the almost 3,000,000 cases of child abuse reported each year in the United States.
D. Prevalence of the disorder has been estimated to be approximately 5 percent in children presenting with allergies.
E. The prevalence of the disorder in life-threatening episodes treated with cardiopulmonary resuscitation has been estimated to be as high as 9 percent.

19.10 Psychodynamic factors proposed in the etiology of factitious disorders include

A. dependency needs
B. identity needs
C. mastery needs
D. masochistic needs
E. all of the above

19.11 Patients with factitious disorders, either physical or psychological, most often demonstrate

    A. a below-average IQ
    B. a formal thought disorder
    C. poor sexual adjustment
    D. generally adequate frustration tolerance
    E. all of the above

19.12 True statements about patients with factitious disorder with predominantly psychological signs and symptoms include

    A. Virtually all patients with this type of factitious disorder have a personality disorder.
    B. The rate of suicide is generally reported to be low in this population.
    C. Prognosis is slightly better than for most other Axis I disorders.
    D. Factitious psychosis, in particular, almost never represents the prodrome to an authentic psychosis.
    E. None of the above

19.13 Clinical indicators of poor treatment responsiveness in patients with factitious disorders include

    A. the coexistence of other Axis I disorders, such as mood, anxiety, or substance-related disorders
    B. borderline or antisocial elements
    C. religious affiliations
    D. capacity to accept confrontation in therapy
    E. all of the above

19.14 The presentation of factitious physical symptoms may take the form of

    A. total fabrications
    B. simulations
    C. illness inductions
    D. illness aggravations
    E. all of the above

19.15 The perpetrators in factitious disorder by proxy

    A. often suffer from psychotic or dissociative disorders
    B. rarely have personal histories of factitious or somatoform disorders
    C. most often suffered direct abuse in childhood themselves
    D. are commonly unresponsive to their infants when their behavior is unwitnessed
    E. all of the above

ANSWERS

Factitious Disorders

19.1 The answer is E

Munchausen syndrome is another name for factitious disorder with predominantly physical signs and symptoms. Munchausen syndrome was named after Baron von Munchausen, an 18th century German traveler and raconteur. He wrote many fantastic travel and adventure stories and wandered from tavern to tavern, telling tall tales. Patients who suffer from Munchausen syndrome wander from hospital to hospital, where they manage to be admitted because of the dramatic stories they relay about being dangerously ill. Sometimes the patients are called "hospital hobos."

Other names for Munchausen syndrome are hospital addiction, polysurgical addiction, and professional patient syndrome. A primary feature of this disorder is a patient's ability to present physical symptoms so well that he or she gains admission to a hospital. A patient may feign symptoms of a severe disorder with which he or she is familiar and may also give a history good enough to deceive a skilled clinician. The patient usually demands surgery or other treatment and can become abusive when negative test results threaten to reveal the factitious behavior. As these features are similar to our ambulance driver's behavior, a diagnosis of Munchausen syndrome is justified.

Malingering, by contrast, is a voluntary production of false or exaggerated physical or psychological symptoms, which arises from an external motivation to avoid difficult situations, to receive some sort of compensation, or to retaliate when one feels guilty or has suffered a loss. Malingering is differentiated from factitious disorders primarily because of its clearly identifiable secondary gain or goal.

Hypochondriasis, a person's concern or preoccupation with disease, is a genuine feeling and is not produced voluntarily. *Ganser's syndrome* is a controversial condition that may occur most often among prison inmates. Those with Ganser's syndrome respond to simple questions with amazingly incorrect answers. In DSM-IV-TR, Ganser's syndrome is classified as a dissociative disorder not otherwise specified. In *Briquet's syndrome*, or somatization disorder, the symptoms are not produced voluntarily, hospitalization is not frequent, and patients do not seek to undergo numerous mutilating procedures.

19.2 The answer is E (all)

A factitious disorder is differentiated from *somatization disorder* (Briquet's syndrome) by the voluntary production of factitious symptoms, the extreme course of multiple hospitalizations, and the patient's seeming willingness to undergo an extraordinary number of painful, even mutilating, procedures.

Hypochondriasis differs from factitious disorder in that the hypochondriacal patient does not voluntarily initiate the production of symptoms, and hypochondriasis typically has a later age of onset. As is the case with somatization disorder, patients with hypochondriasis do not usually submit to potentially mutilating procedures.

Because of their pathological lying, lack of close relationships with others, hostile and manipulative manner, and associated substance and criminal history, factitious disorder patients are often classified as having *antisocial personality disorder.* However, persons with antisocial personality disorder do not usually volunteer for invasive procedures or resort to a way of life marked by repeated or long-term hospitalizations.

Factitious disorder must be distinguished from *malingering.* Malingerers have an obvious, recognizable environmental goal in producing signs and symptoms of illness. They may seek hospitalization to secure financial compensation, evade the police, avoid work, or merely obtain free bed and board for the night; yet they always have some apparent end for their behavior.

19.3 The answer is E

Factitious disorders *may occur by proxy*; such disorders are dually classified as factitious disorder by proxy and factitious disorder not otherwise specified.

Factitious disorders *usually begin in early adult life*, although they may appear during childhood or adolescence. The onset of the disorder or of discrete episodes of treatment-seeking may follow a real illness, loss, rejection, or abandonment. Usually, the patient or a close relative had a hospitalization in childhood or early adolescence for a genuine physical illness. Thereafter, a long pattern of successive hospitalizations unfolds, beginning insidiously.

Factitious disorders *are not best treated with psychoactive drugs.* Pharmacotherapy is of limited use. No specific psychiatric therapy has been effective in treating factitious disorders. Although no adequate data are available about the ultimate outcome for patients, a number of them probably die as a result of needless medication, instrumentation, or surgery. They *usually have a poor prognosis.*

Factitious disorders *are not synonymous with Ganser's syndrome,* a controversial condition that is characterized by the use of approximate answers. Ganser's syndrome may be a variant of malingering, in that patients avoid punishment or responsibility for their actions. Ganser's syndrome is classified as a dissociative disorder not otherwise specified.

19.4 The answer is B

Employment as a *healthcare worker* is considered a leading predisposing factor in the development of factitious disorder with predominantly physical signs and symptoms; nurses make up one of the largest risk groups.

Employment as a *teacher, police officer, banker, or waitress* is not a predisposing factor in the development of factitious disorders.

19.5 The answer is D

Briquet's syndrome (somatization disorder) *is not synonymous with factitious disorder with predominantly physical signs and symptoms.* A factitious disorder is differentiated from Briquet's syndrome by the voluntary production of factitious symptoms, the extreme course of multiple hospitalizations, and the patient's seeming willingness to undergo an extraordinary number of arduous, if not actually mutilating procedures. Factitious disorder with predominantly physical signs and symptoms has been designated by a variety of labels, the best known of which is *Munchausen syndrome.*

19.6 The answer is E (all)

A frequent occurrence in the histories of factitious disorder patients is a personal history of serious illness or disability *or a*

history of being exposed to genuine illness in a family member or significant extrafamilial figure. Prior or current *employment in a health-related field* as a nurse, laboratory technician, ambulance driver, or physician is so common that it suggests inclusion as a clinical feature and a causal factor. Consistent with the concept of poor identity formation is the observation that patients vacillate between two separate roles—health professional and patient—with momentary confusion as to which role is being played at the time.

Psychological models of factitious disorders generally emphasize the causal significance of *a history of parental rejection.* The usual history reveals that one or both parents are experienced as rejecting figures who are unable to form close relationships.

Patients have *a tendency to view the physician as a loving parent*, a potential source of sought-for love, and a person who will fulfill their unmet dependence needs.

19.7 The answer is A

Malingering is the most likely diagnosis based on the clinical presentation. Until his arrest, there was no previous psychiatric history or previously reported psychiatric symptoms. The man's mental status examination is apparently normal; there are no disorganized thoughts or loosening of associations. The patient claims a variety of unrelated bizarre beliefs, presenting responses in a manner that is inconsistent with the disorganization of psychological functioning that would be expected if the symptoms were genuine. In this case the "psychotic" symptoms are under voluntary control, and since there is external incentive (avoiding prosecution) and no evidence of an intrapsychic need to maintain a sick role, the diagnosis of *factitious disorder with predominantly psychotic features* is ruled out. The patient expresses no paranoid feelings, as would be seen in *schizophrenia, paranoid type.* His delusions lack conviction and are therefore not indicative of the unshakable beliefs in a *delusional disorder. Capgras's syndrome,* the delusion that familiar people have been replaced by identical impostors, is not seen here.

19.8 The answer is E (all)

Overall, demographic analyses of factitious disorders in the literature have distinguished two general patterns. Factitious disorder patients with Munchausen syndrome are *typically middle-aged men who are unmarried, unemployed, and estranged from their families*; the remaining patients are generally women aged 20 to 40 years. A number of reports suggest that those in the second group are commonly employed in or intimately familiar with healthcare occupations such as nursing and physical therapy. In a 10-year retrospective study of hospitalized patients, 28 of 41 patients with factitious disorder identified worked in medically related fields, 15 as nurses.

19.9 The answer is A

Factitious disorder by proxy currently accounts for *fewer than 1,000 of the almost 3 million cases of child abuse reported each year in the United States,* but this number may rise as mass media and professional attention increase recognition of these cases. Authors have attempted to elucidate the prevalence of factitious disorder by proxy within particular populations, such as children presenting with apnea (0.27 percent), *allergy (5 percent)*, asthma (1 percent), apparent life-threatening episodes (1.5

percent), and *life-threatening episodes treated with cardiopulmonary resuscitation (over 9 percent* among children in whom final diagnoses were established). *The average length of time to establish a diagnosis of factitious disorder by proxy after the initial presentation is 15 months,* and *often a sibling has died of undiagnosed causes before the disorder is recognized.* summarizes the most common presentations of the disorder.

19.10 The answer is E (all)

A number of psychodynamic causes for Munchausen syndrome have been proposed, and they appear applicable to persons with non-Munchausen factitious disorders as well. For many patients, the production of illness simultaneously meets multiple needs ranging from conscious to fully unconscious. *Dependency needs* are typically among the salient ones. These patients often have had emotionally deprived backgrounds with parents who were rejecting, and illness becomes a way of inducing others to gratify these needs and to satisfy the longing for nurturance. For other patients, particularly those prone to a decline in reality testing, factitious behavior organizes them, establishing a role to be played. Through this role, a helpless individual becomes a clever manipulator able to control healthcare providers, who may also represent surrogates of the parents. Similarly, factitious behavior meets the *need for identity.* Patients with factitious disorders frequently have a poor sense of self and have failed to define their value systems and goals. By simulating or inducing disease, they assume the well-defined role of sick persons; through the pseudologia fantastica in Munchausen syndrome, they even become important and interesting people with exotic backgrounds.

Pseudologia fantastica is typified by stories that are not entirely improbable and that often contain a matrix of truth and falsehood. The stories have a self-aggrandizing component. As a result, the medical history presented by these patients has been described as being fraught with harrowing episodes of dubious veracity.

19.11 The answer is C

Patients with factitious disorders, whether physical or psychological, most often demonstrate *an average or above-* average intelligence quotient (IQ), absence of a formal thought disorder, a poor sense of identity, poor sexual adjustment, poor frustration tolerance, strong dependency needs, and narcissism.

19.12 The answer is A

The literature on factitious disorder with predominantly psychological signs and symptoms is notable for the magnitude of the psychological dysfunction present in patients. *Almost all have serious personality disorders,* often associated with substance abuse. Several authors have reported that *there is a high rate of suicide in this population* and that factitious psychological disorders *have a worse prognosis than most other Axis I disorders.*

The patient's simulation of a mental disorder *may actually represent the prodrome to an authentic mental disorder* with a serious outcome. In particular, clinicians *should be cautious in diagnosing factitious psychosis because in two small studies a majority of these patients eventually manifested clear-cut psychotic disorders such as schizophrenia.* In other cases, an ostensibly feigned condition such as depression has responded to psychotropic medications, validating at least some element of the presentation. Since virtually all patients with this type of factitious disorder have a personality disorder (usually borderline, histrionic, or antisocial), caregivers must also recognize that the simulated mental disorder coexists with an authentic one. Comorbidity with substance-related disorders and somatoform disorders has been reported as well, and dissociative disorders may result in alterations of memory and the patient's providing inconsistent factual information.

19.13 The answer is B

Overall, several clinical indicators of *enhanced* treatment responsiveness in patients with factitious disorders have been elucidated. They include: (1) *underlying psychiatric syndromes, such as mood, anxiety, substance-related,* or conversion disorders; (2) *personality traits without borderline or antisocial elements;* (3) psychosocial supports, such as ongoing relationships with significant others, employment or employability, or *religious affiliations;* and (4) ability to establish a therapeutic alliance as characterized by the capacity to establish and maintain rapport, *accept confrontation,* and comply with treatment recommendations.

19.14 The answer is E (all)

The presentation of factitious physical symptoms spans a considerable range. Individuals may engage in: (1) *total fabrications* (e.g., asserting falsely that one is infected with the human immunodeficiency virus [HIV]), (2) *simulations* (e.g., mimicking a grand mal seizure), (3) *illness aggravations* (e.g., manually manipulating a preexisting wound so it will not heal), or (4) *illness inductions* (e.g., injecting oneself with fecal bacteria to cause sepsis). The specific examples in the literature are as varied and intricate as the human imagination, and are constrained only by the limitation of the particular individual's creativity and motivation. The maladies may be relatively common (e.g., urinary tract infections) or so esoteric that most physicians would have only a passing familiarity with them (e.g., intermittent Mediterranean fever; necrotizing fasciitis).

Table 19.1
Ranking of the Most Common Bibliographic References to Signs and Symptoms of Factitious Disorder by Proxy

Poisoning (includes Munchausen syndrome by proxy and intentional poisonings)

Seizures or vomiting

Apnea

Diarrhea

Unconsciousness

Fevers

Lethargy

Dehydration or hematemesis

Ataxia or hematuria

Adapted from Schreier HA, Libow JA. *Hunting for Love: Munchausen by Proxy Syndrome.* New York: Guilford Press; 1993; and Rosenberg DA. Web of deceit: a literature review of Munchausen syndrome by proxy. *Child Abuse Negl.* 1987;11:533.

Table 19.2
Clinical Indicators That May Suggest
Factitious Disorder by Proxy

The symptoms and pattern of illness are extremely unusual, or inexplicable physiologically.

Repeated hospitalizations and workups by numerous caregivers fail to reveal a conclusive diagnosis or cause.

Physiological parameters are consistent with induced illness; e.g., apnea monitor tracings disclose massive muscle artifact prior to respiratory arrest, suggesting that the child has been struggling against an obstruction to the airways.

The patient fails to respond to appropriate treatments.

The vitality of the patient is inconsistent with the laboratory findings.

The signs and symptoms abate when the mother has not had access to the child.

The mother is the only witness to the onset of signs and symptoms.

Unexplained illnesses have occurred in the mother or her other children.

The mother has had medical or nursing education, or exposure to models of the illnesses afflicting the child (e.g., a parent with sleep apnea).

The mother welcomes even invasive and painful tests.

The mother grows anxious if the child improves.

Maternal lying is proved.

Medical observations yield information that is inconsistent with parental reports.

Adapted from Feldman MD, Eisendrath SJ. *The Spectrum of Factitious Disorders.* Washington, DC: American Psychiatric Press; 1996.

19.15 The answer is D

By definition, factitious disorder by proxy requires that any external gains for the victim's fabricated or induced illnesses, such as disability payments or respite from child-rearing responsibilities during hospitalization, are incidental to the pursuit of the vicarious sick role. Several analyses have referred to a disorder of empathy among perpetrating mothers fueled by depression and isolation. With their spouses typically unavailable or uninvolved, they vitiate these painful feelings by mobilizing attention and nurturance through this disorder. A related hypothesis involves projective identification. Through this defense mechanism, the mother projects onto her child her own unconscious longings for nurturance, then ensures—through her own indefatigable attention as well as that of healthcare providers and others—that the child receives the attention she herself so desperately craves. Others have referred to factitious disorder by proxy as an epiphenomenon of the parent's narcissism and sociopathy, with glee arising from the capacity to dupe highly educated professionals. The perpetrator may also be displacing onto the child sadistic impulses toward herself or others. A recent theory suggests that an unsatisfactory relationship with a desired but unavailable father contributes to a perverse relationship with physicians and hospital staff members, surrogate parents whom the abusing mother simultaneously pursues and punishes. In this context the mother perceives her child as an object to be used to manipulate an intensely ambivalent relationship with the medical establishment. Concrete evidence for this last observation has been provided through covert videotapes. In contrast to the devoted, even symbiotic, parenting style they reveal in public, these mothers *are commonly unresponsive to their infants* when their behavior is unwitnessed. Despite the perversity of their behavior, they *rarely suffer from psychotic or dissociative disorders,* although they *often have personal histories of factitious or somatoform disorders.* Although they may have been neglected or undervalued, most perpetrators *did not suffer direct abuse in childhood.*   lists the clinical indicators that may suggest factitious disorder by proxy.

20

Dissociative Disorders

Dissociative disorders have been characterized as representing defensive reactions to traumatic experiences. The revised fourth edition of the *Diagnostic and Statistical Manual of Mental Disorders* (DSM-IV-TR) classifies dissociative disorders as dissociative amnesia, dissociative fugue, dissociative identity disorder (or more popularly, multiple personality disorder), depersonalization disorder, and dissociative disorder not otherwise specified.

Feelings of dissociation or depersonalization can occur in normal people under a variety of circumstances, such as fatigue, isolation, or hypnosis. These feelings tend to be fleeting and temporary, and, while perhaps briefly uncomfortable, are not experienced as overly distressful. In dissociative disorders, the dissociation and depersonalization are much more severe and disabling. Pathological dissociative states are associated with histories of childhood physical, emotional, and sexual abuse, or may be seen in people who have undergone traumatic wartime or disaster experiences. People with dissociative disorders often describe themselves as lacking a sense of a coherent self, and as a result experience their thoughts, emotions, and behavior as easily disintegrated and fragmentary. Patients with borderline personality disorders frequently experience dissociative symptoms and disorders.

A careful and thorough medical evaluation is necessary to rule out any possible organic cause for the dissociative symptoms.

The student should study the questions and answers below for a useful review of these disorders.

HELPFUL HINTS

The terms below relate to dissociative disorders and should be defined.

- anterograde amnesia
- approximate answers
- automatic writing
- brainwashing
- coercive persuasion
- continuous amnesia
- crystal gazing
- denial
- depersonalization
- derealization disorder
- dissociation
- dissociative amnesia
- Dissociative Experience Scale
- dissociative fugue
- dissociative identity disorder
- dissociative trance
- dominant personality
- double orientation
- doubling
- epidemiology of dissociative disorders
- false memory syndrome
- Ganser's syndrome
- hemidepersonalization
- highway hypnosis
- hypnotizability
- Korsakoff's syndrome
- localized amnesia
- malingering
- multiple personality disorder
- paramnesia
- possession state
- reduplicative paramnesia
- repression
- retrograde amnesia
- secondary gain
- selective amnesia
- sleepwalking disorder
- temporal lobe functions
- transient global amnesia
- unitary sense of self
- wandering

▲ QUESTIONS

DIRECTIONS: Each of the questions or incomplete statements below is followed by five suggested responses or completions. Select the *one* that is *best* in each case.

20.1 A patient normally without cognitive deficits, who seems out of touch with the environment and in a dream-like state for a brief period of time, and who has amnesia for the experience when it is ended is likely to have

A. dementia
B. dissociative fugue
C. localized amnesia
D. generalized amnesia
E. sleepwalking disorder

20.2 DSM-IV-TR includes dissociative symptoms in the criteria for all but which of the following mental disorders?

A. acute stress disorder
B. somatization disorder
C. posttraumatic stress disorder
D. obsessive-compulsive disorder
E. none of the above

20.3 Transient global amnesia is differentiated from dissociative amnesia by

A. the presence of anterograde amnesia in dissociative amnesia
B. the greater upset in patients with transient global amnesia
C. the loss of personal identity in patients with transient global amnesia
D. the older age of the dissociative amnesia patient
E. the absence of a psychological stressor in dissociative amnesia

20.4 Each of the following statements about dissociative identity disorder is true *except*

A. The transition from one personality to another is often sudden and dramatic.
B. The patient generally has amnesia for the existence of the other personalities.
C. Each personality rarely seeks treatment.
D. The host personality rarely seeks treatment.
E. The personalities may be of both sexes.

20.5 Depersonalization disorder is characterized by

A. impaired reality testing
B. ego-dystonic symptoms
C. occurrence in the late decades of life
D. gradual onset
E. a brief course and a good prognosis

20.6 All of the following are true statements about dissociative fugue *except*

A. It is a rare type of dissociative disorder.
B. It is not characterized by behavior that appears extraordinary to others.
C. It is characterized by a lack of awareness of the loss of memory.
D. It is usually a long-lasting state.
E. Recovery is spontaneous and rapid.

20.7 Patients predisposed to dissociative fugue include those with all of the following *except*

A. mood disorders
B. schizophrenia
C. histrionic personality disorders
D. heavy alcohol abuse
E. borderline personality disorders

20.8 Dissociative disorders as classified in DSM-IV-TR include all of the following *except*

A. amnestic disorders
B. dissociative identity disorder
C. depersonalization disorder
D. Ganser's syndrome
E. dissociative trance disorder

20.9 Which of these statements regarding the prognosis of dissociative identity disorder is *incorrect*?

A. Recovery is generally complete.
B. The earlier the onset of dissociative identity disorder, the poorer the prognosis is.
C. The level of impairment is determined by the number and types of various personalities.
D. Individual personalities may have their own separate mental disorders.
E. One or more of the personalities may function relatively well.

20.10 Dissociative symptoms

A. increase with age
B. are always considered pathological
C. are more common in women than men
D. psychologically represent a self-defense against trauma
E. all of the above

20.11 Patients with dissociative amnesia

A. do not retain the capacity to learn new information
B. commonly retain awareness of personal identity, but have amnesia for general information
C. present very similarly to patients with dementia
D. typically behave in a confused and disorganized way
E. none of the above

20.12 Dissociative amnesia is thought to be

A. the least common of the dissociative disorders
B. more common in women than men
C. more common in older adults than younger
D. decreased in times of war and natural disaster
E. none of the above

20.13 Organic amnesias are distinguished from dissociative amnesias by which of the following?

A. They do not normally involve recurrent identity alteration.
B. The amnesia is not selectively limited to personal information.
C. The memories do not focus on an emotionally traumatic event.
D. The amnesia is more often anterograde than retrograde.
E. All of the above

20.14 The most common cause of organic fugue is probably

A. head trauma
B. hypoglycemia
C. epilepsy
D. brain tumors
E. migraines

20.15 Culture-bound syndromes in which dissociative fugue is a prominent feature include

A. *latah*
B. amok
C. *grisi siknis*
D. *piblokto*
E. all of the above

20.16 The mainstay of treatment of dissociative fugue is

   A. psychodynamic psychotherapy
   B. hypnosis
   C. sodium amobarbital interviewing
   D. antidepressant medication
   E. none of the above

20.17 Pathological depersonalization can be distinguished from common, mild depersonalization by the

   A. context of the symptom
   B. frequency of the symptom
   C. duration of the symptom
   D. all of the above
   E. none of the above

20.18 Dissociative identity disorder

   A. has been linked only weakly to severe experiences of early childhood trauma
   B. has been observed only in Western cultures
   C. is not related to early disturbances in the attachment relationship with the primary caregiver
   D. has been associated with high levels of dissociation in the mothers of the patients
   E. is more common in boys in early childhood

DIRECTIONS: The lettered headings below are followed by a list of numbered statements. For each numbered statement, select the *one* lettered heading that is most closely associated with it. Each lettered heading may be selected once, more than once, or not at all.

Questions 20.19–20.22

   A. Dissociative amnesia
   B. Dissociative fugue
   C. Dissociative identity disorder
   D. Depersonalization disorder

20.19 a 25-year-old man comes to the emergency room and cannot remember his name

20.20 a 35-year-old man states that his body feels unreal, not attached to him

20.21 a 16-year-old girl is found in another city far from her home and does not recall how she got there

20.22 a 30-year-old woman suddenly has a new child-like voice in the interview

DIRECTIONS: These lettered headings are followed by a list of numbered phrases. For each numbered phrase, select

   A. if the item is associated with *A only*
   B. if the item is associated with *B only*
   C. if the item is associated with *both A and B*
   D. if the item is associated with *neither A nor B*

Questions 20.23–20.26

   A. Dissociative amnesia
   B. Amnesia secondary to organic etiology
   C. Both
   D. Neither

20.23 more likely to involve interruption of the episodic-autobiographical memory

20.24 more likely to involve interruption of general cognitive functioning

20.25 more likely to involve interruption of language capacity

20.26 more likely to be localized

ANSWERS

Dissociative Disorders

20.1 The answer is E
Patients with *sleepwalking disorder*, classified in DSM-IV-TR as a type of sleep disorder, often behave like someone in a dissociative state. They appear out of touch with their environment and preoccupied with a private world; they may act emotionally upset and speak excitedly and incomprehensibly. When the episode has ended, patients have amnesia for it. By contrast, patients with *localized* or *generalized amnesia* do not seem out of touch with the environment and do not appear to be dreaming; to observers, they seem to act normally and are alert both before and after amnesia appears.

   Dissociative fugue is similar to dissociative amnesia, but in dissociative fugue patients' behavior seems more integrated with their amnesia than it is for patients with dissociative amnesia.

   Patients with dissociative fugue travel away from home or work and forget their name, occupation, and other aspects of their identity. Patients often take on a new identity and profession.

When patients with *dementia* have symptoms of amnesia, the dementia is often advanced, and the amnesia does not give way to a clear memory. Social awareness and ability to perform complex activities are also diminished, and personality is affected.

20.2 The answer is D
DSM-IV-TR does not include dissociative symptoms in the criteria for *obsessive-compulsive disorder*. *Acute stress disorder, somatization disorder,* and *posttraumatic stress disorder* all include dissociative symptoms in their criteria as given in DSM-IV-TR. A diagnosis of dissociative disorder is not given if the symptoms occur exclusively during the course of one of these disorders. DSM-IV-TR notes that neurological or other medical conditions should be considered before diagnosing conversion disorder.

20.3 The answer is B
Transient global amnesia can be differentiated from dissociative amnesia in several ways, for example, the *greater upset* in patients with transient global amnesia than in those with dissociative amnesia; the *presence of anterograde amnesia* in transient global amne-

sia but not in dissociative amnesia; the *loss of personal identity* in patients with dissociative amnesia but not in transient global amnesia; *the older age* of the transient global amnesia patient than the dissociative disorder patient; and the *presence of a psychological stressor* in dissociative amnesia but not in transient global amnesia.

20.4 The answer is D

In dissociative identity disorder, *the host personality (not each personality)* is usually the one who *seeks treatment*. The *transition from one personality to another* is often sudden and dramatic. The patient generally has *amnesia for the existence of the other personalities* and for the events that took place when another personality was dominant. Each personality has a characteristic behavioral pattern. The *personalities may be of both sexes,* of various races and ages, and from families different from the patient's family of origin. The most common subordinate personality is child-like. Often, the personalities are disparate and may even be opposites.

20.5 The answer is B

Depersonalization disorder is characterized by *ego-dystonic symptoms*—that is, symptoms distressing to the patient. However, the person maintains *intact (not impaired) reality testing;* he or she is aware of the disturbances. Depersonalization *rarely occurs in the late decades of life;* it most often starts between the ages of 15 and 30 years. In the large majority of patients, the symptoms first appear suddenly; only a few patients report a *gradual onset.* A few follow-up studies indicate that in more than half the cases, depersonalization disorder tends to have *a long-term (not brief) course and a poor (not good) prognosis.*

20.6 The answer is D

A dissociative fugue is *usually brief (not long-lasting)* (i.e., hours to days). Generally, *recovery is spontaneous and rapid,* and recurrences are rare. Dissociative fugue is considered *rare,* and like dissociative amnesia, it occurs most often during wartime, after natural disasters, and as a result of personal crises with intense conflict. Dissociative fugue is characterized by a *lack of awareness of the loss of memory* but *not by behavior that appears extraordinary* to others.

20.7 The answer is B

Schizophrenia does not predispose patients to dissociative fugue state. *Heavy alcohol abuse* may predispose a person to dissociative fugue, but the cause is thought to be basically psychological. The essential motivating factor appears to be a desire to withdraw from emotionally painful experiences. Patients with *mood disorders* and certain personality disorders (for example, *borderline,* schizoid, and *histrionic personality disorders*) are predisposed to dissociative fugue.

20.8 The answer is A

The *amnestic disorders* are classified with the cognitive disorders (for example, dementias), not the dissociative disorders. The dissociative disorders are dissociative amnesia, dissociative fugue, *dissociative identity disorder, depersonalization disorder,* and dissociative disorder not otherwise specified. *Ganser's syndrome* is listed in the fourth revised edition of *Diagnostic and Statistical Manual of Mental Disorders* (DSM-IV-TR) as an example of dissociative disorder not otherwise specified. In Ganser's syndrome, patients give approximate answers to questions (for example, 2 + 2 = 5). Another example of dissociative disorder not otherwise specified is *dissociative trance disorder.*

20.9 The answer is A

In dissociative identity disorder, while *recovery is possible*, it is *generally incomplete.* This is considered the most severe and chronic of the dissociative disorders. The earlier the onset of dissociative identity disorder, *the poorer the prognosis is.* The *level of impairment* ranges from moderate to severe and is determined by variables such as the number, the type, and the chronicity of the various personalities. The *individual personalities* may have their own separate mental disorders; mood disorders, personality disorders, and other distinctive disorders are most common. One or more of the *personalities may function relatively well,* while others function marginally.

20.10 The answer is D

Patients with these disorders exhibit a range of dissociative experiences *from normal to pathological.* The *normal* range of dissociative phenomena can be studied from several perspectives. Many researchers and clinicians consider hypnotizability to be related to these disorders. Normal people vary in their hypnotizability. Patients with dissociative disorders are not necessarily more hypnotizable than are people without the disorder, but hypnosis is an example of a dissociative state in normal people.

Researchers have developed several scales to measure dissociative experiences, one of which is the Dissociative Experience Scale. Using this scale, therapists question interviewees about mild and common dissociative phenomena (such as periods of inattention during conversations) and about pathological dissociative phenomena. Studies using such scales have shown that the scores of about 5 percent of the general population are greater than three times the mean score. Other studies of dissociative phenomena have reported that dissociative symptoms *decrease (not increase) with age* and that they are about *equally common in women and men.* Many types of studies have indicated an association between traumatic events, especially childhood physical and sexual abuse, and the development of dissociative symptoms and disorders.

Dissociation arises as a *self-defense against trauma.* Dissociative defenses perform the dual function of helping people remove themselves from trauma at the time that it occurs and also of delaying the working through needed to place the trauma in perspective within their lives.

20.11 The answer is E (none)

The symptom of amnesia is common to dissociative amnesia, dissociative fugue, and dissociative identity disorder. Dissociative amnesia is the appropriate diagnosis when the dissociative phenomena are limited to amnesia. Its key symptom is the inability to recall information, usually about stressful or traumatic events in people's lives. This inability cannot be explained by ordinary forgetfulness, and there is no evidence of an underlying brain disorder. People retain the *capacity to learn new information.*

A common form of dissociative amnesia involves *amnesia for personal identity,* but *unimpaired memory of general information.* This *clinical picture is exactly the reverse of the one seen in dementia,* in which patients may remember their names but forget general information, such as what they had for lunch. Except for their amnesia, patients with dissociative amnesia appear completely intact and *function coherently.* By contrast, in most amnesias due to a general medical condition (such as postictal and toxic amnesias), patients may be confused and behave in a disorganized manner. Other types of amnesias (for example, transient global amnesia and post-concussion amnesia) are associated with an ongoing anterograde amnesia, which does not occur in patients with dissociative amnesia.

20.12 The answer is B
Amnesia is the most common dissociative symptom and occurs in almost all the dissociative disorders. Dissociative amnesia is thought to be the *most common of the dissociative disorders,* although epidemiological data for all the dissociative disorders are limited and uncertain. Dissociative amnesia is thought to occur *more often in women than in men* and *more often in young adults than in older adults.* Inasmuch as the disorder is usually associated with stressful and traumatic events, its incidence probably *increases during times of wars and natural disasters.* Cases of dissociative amnesia related to domestic settings—for example, spouse abuse and child abuse—are probably constant in number.

20.13 The answer is E (all)
Amnestic disorders are caused by a variety of organic conditions. Examples of organic causes of amnesia are epileptic seizure, head trauma, alcoholic blackouts, Korsakoff's syndrome, stroke, postoperative amnesia, postinfectious amnesia, post-ECT, surgery, infection, electroconvulsive therapy (ECT), and transient global amnesia. Less common causes are cerebrovascular disease, metabolic abnormalities, and toxic states.

Organic amnesias have several distinguishing features: they *do not normally involve recurrent identity alteration,* the amnesia is *not selectively limited to personal information,* the memories *do not focus on or result from an emotionally traumatic event,* and the amnesia is *more often anterograde* than retrograde. In cases of amnesia of organic etiology (excluding substance abuse, transient global amnesia, or metabolic abnormalities), the amnesia is usually permanent and does not lend itself to therapeutic technique. Whereas dissociative amnesia represents a displacement of the memory from awareness, organic amnesias represent the erasure or destruction of that memory through disturbance of the neuropsychological process.

20.14 The answer is C
The differential diagnosis of fugue states is vast. Genuine dissociative fugue must be excluded as a diagnosis if dissociative identity disorder is present or if the fugue is caused by the direct physiological effects of drugs, medications, or alcohol; it cannot be diagnosed if it is due to a general medical condition such as epilepsy.

Probably the most common organic fugue is secondary to *epilepsy,* especially complex partial seizure disorder. During such seizures or postictally the individual may exhibit wandering behaviors. The clinical differentiation is usually fairly easily accomplished by a good clinical history regarding epileptic symptoms and electroencephalographic studies.

Several medical conditions besides epilepsy can cause organic fugue. These conditions include *brain tumor, head trauma, migraine,* cerebrovascular accidents, hypertensive neuropathy, limbic system dysfunction, *hypoglycemia,* uremia, dementia, and malaria.

Organic fugue states may be caused by a wide variety of medications including hallucinogenic drugs, steroids, barbiturates, phenothiazines, triazolam (Halcion), and L-asparaginase. The alcohol blackout can be easily confused with dissociative fugue, but this can be differentiated through a good clinical history and alcohol concentrations, if drawn during acute intoxication. The clinician should remember, however, that dissociative fugue and alcohol blackouts may coexist in the same individual.

20.15 The answer is E (all)
There are a number of culture-bound psychiatric syndromes in which fugue is a prominent feature. These syndromes include the "running" syndromes, which include *latah* and amok, that occur in several nations along the western Pacific rim; *grisi siknis,* occurring among the Miskito of Nicaragua and Honduras; and *piblokto* (Arctic hysteria), occurring among the Eskimos of northern Greenland. These syndromes are characterized by a high level of agitation, running about, trance-like states, and amnesia for the episode.

20.16 The answer is A
The mainstay of treatment of dissociative fugue is *psychodynamic psychotherapy.* A gently exploratory and expressive form is preferred in most cases, although a largely supportive form will usually suffice for those of low ego strength. The clinician should begin with a thorough clinical history and pay close attention to possible precipitating events. In many cases, encouraging persons with dissociative fugue to talk about what they already remember will bring the return of other memories; in some cases free association has proven helpful.

In situations where acute traumatic events have precipitated the dissociative fugue, a gentle abreaction of the trauma is indicated. However, the clinician should be very careful to not proceed with abreactive work until a stable therapeutic alliance has been established. In addition, abreactive work should be suspended, at least temporarily, if the patient's condition worsens (e.g., if the patient becomes depressed or suicidal).

If the individual with dissociative fugue continues to be densely amnesic for identity and autobiographical memory, the use of *hypnosis* or *sodium amobarbital interviewing* may be tried cautiously, keeping in mind that the dissociative fugue serves a defensive purpose, and that if the amnesia is suddenly lifted the individual may become depressed or even suicidal. Also, after the hypnotic session is completed, the amnesia may recur. Informed consent should be obtained whenever hypnosis or sodium amobarbital is used.

After the amnesia has been lifted, continued psychotherapy is indicated to help the individual cope with the underlying psychological conflicts that initially caused the dissociative fugue. Ideally, the patient should be helped to integrate the memories of the dissociative fugue state into a cohesive self and memory. *Antidepressant medication* may be helpful in the treatment of depressive symptoms that may accompany the fugue state.

20.17 The answer is D (all)
As an occasional isolated experience in the lives of many people, depersonalization is common and not necessarily pathological. Pathological depersonalization is *persistent* or *recurrent* episodes of depersonalization that lead to significant distress or impairment in such *contexts* as social, occupational, and other important areas of functioning. In general, the diagnosis of depersonalization disorder is reserved for those conditions in which depersonalization constitutes the predominating symptom.

The differential diagnosis of patients who experience depersonalization should take into account both psychological and organic causes of depersonalization. Patients who present with recurrent depersonalization should receive a comprehensive psychiatric evaluation, including a specialized diagnostic interview in order to rule out the presence of a dissociative disorder.

20.18 The answer is D

Clinicians have long noted gender differences in the frequency of dissociative identity disorder. Clinical studies report between 5 to 1 to 9 to 1 female to male ratios for diagnosed cases. Research with dissociation measures, however, finds no evidence of gender differences in the propensity or capacity to dissociate. Developmental studies indicate that the *ratio of female to male dissociative identity disorder cases* steadily increases from 1:1 in early childhood to about 8 to 1 by late adolescence. Reasons proposed for the increased numbers of female patients relative to males include sex-related differences in the types, age of onset, and duration of maltreatment experienced by males and females; differences in clinical presentations such that male cases are more likely to be missed; and the possibility that more male cases end up in the criminal justice system or alcohol and other substance treatment programs rather than the general mental health system.

Pathological levels of dissociation are *strongly associated with histories of antecedent trauma.* This has proven true across many types of trauma (e.g., rape, combat, natural disasters, and child maltreatment) in clinical and nonclinical samples. In some, but not all, studies indices of the severity of the trauma (e.g., age of onset and number of perpetrators for child abuse or intensity and duration combat) are related significantly to the degree of dissociation. Studies of peritraumatic dissociation, dissociation manifest in the immediate context of trauma, consistently find that it is the best predictor of subsequent posttraumatic stress disorder 6 or more months later. Multiple lines of research strongly associate increased levels of dissociation with antecedent trauma for many different kinds of trauma.

Dissociative identity disorder is *linked strongly to severe experiences of early childhood trauma,* usually maltreatment, in studies *in both Western and non-Western cultures* that have systematically examined this question. The rates of reported severe childhood trauma for both child and adult patients range from 85 to 97 percent of cases. Physical and sexual abuse, usually in combination, are the most frequently reported sources of childhood trauma in clinical research studies. Critics have raised questions about the validity of patients' self-reports of childhood trauma. Recent studies that now include rigorous independent corroboration of the patients' reports of maltreatment continue to strongly support a developmental linkage between childhood trauma and dissociative identity disorder.

Early life experiences resulting in *disturbances in attachment relationship* with the primary caregiver and other abnormal family processes *have been implicated* in the genesis of pathological levels of dissociation and the development of dissociative identity disorder. Recent research indicates that *high levels of dissociation in mothers* are associated with disturbed, often dissociative-like, attachment behavior in their children. In another study, early presence of these attachment disturbances prospectively predicted higher levels of dissociation in late adolescence. The contribution of genetic factors is only now being assessed systematically, but preliminary studies have not found evidence of a significant genetic contribution.

Answers 20.19–20.22

20.19 The answer is A

20.20 The answer is D

20.21 The answer is B

20.22 The answer is C

Dissociative amnesia, as in the case of the man who *cannot remember his name,* is characterized by inability to remember information, usually related to a stressful or traumatic event, that cannot be explained by ordinary forgetfulness, the ingestion of substances, or a general medical condition. *Dissociative fugue,* as in the case of the girl who is *found in another city* far from her home, is characterized by sudden and unexpected travel away from home or work, associated with an inability to recall one's past, confusion about one's past, and confusion about one's personal identity or the adoption of a new identity. *Dissociative identity disorder,* as in the case of the woman who suddenly has *a new child-like voice* in the interview, is characterized by the presence of two or more distinct personalities within a single person; dissociative identity disorder is generally considered the most severe and chronic of the dissociative disorders. *Depersonalization disorder,* as in the case of the man who states that *his body feels unreal,* is characterized by recurrent or persistent feelings of detachment from one's body or mind.

Answers 20.23–20.26

20.23 The answer is A

20.24 The answer is B

20.25 The answer is B

20.26 The answer is A

Dissociative amnesia is more likely to involve *interruption of the episodic-autobiographical memory* than the implicit-semantic memory. The memories unavailable for recall tend toward historical factual information (i.e., where was I; who was I with; and what did I do, think, and feel during the unaccountable period of time?) rather than *interruption of general cognitive functioning* or *language capacity.* This period of amnesia usually centers around a traumatic event or series of events and is *usually localized,* occurring during a specific period of time lasting anywhere from a few hours to several years. Occasionally the amnesia may be selective or systematized, whereby it is restricted to certain memories such as those involving a particular individual. Other forms of amnesia also occur (generalized amnesia, when the amnesia extends over the patient's entire life, and continuous amnesia, when the amnesia extends from a specific time up to the present), but are much more rare and are often associated with more severe dissociative disorders.

Dissociative amnesia is one of the most difficult disorders to assess because it cannot be observed directly except in cases of global amnesia; patients rarely complain about amnesia itself. Clinically, the patient may present symptoms of anxiety, depression, confusion, difficulty concentrating, and a history of blank spells or gaps in memory. Even once amnesia is confirmed, clinicians typically find it difficult to obtain from patients reliable estimates of the frequency and extent of their amnestic episodes.

21

Human Sexuality

The field of psychiatry has always had a large responsibility in describing and defining behaviors that could be classified as abnormal sexuality. The range of normal sexual expression is vast, diverse, and creative. What constitutes abnormal sexuality for one group can be considered basic to sexual expression for another. Increasing cultural sophistication expands the realm of what is generally considered normal and healthy, and psychiatry has been influenced positively by these cultural forces.

Abnormal sexuality is defined as that which is destructive, compulsive, associated with overwhelming guilt and anxiety, unable to be directed toward a partner, and is generally pervasive, recurrent, and habitual. The revised fourth edition of the *Diagnostic and Statistical Manual of Mental Disorders (DSM-IV-TR)* broadly classifies sexual disorders as sexual dysfunctions, paraphilias, and sexual disorder not otherwise specified. There is also a classification for gender identity disorders, and this will be discussed in Chapter 22.

Sexual dysfunctions describe disturbed sexual desire and psychophysiologic changes in the sexual response cycle. Paraphilias are characterized by recurrent sexual urges or fantasies involving unusual objects, activities, or situations. Sexual disorder not otherwise specified describes sexual dysfunction not classifiable in any other category.

There are several terms related to human sexuality that are often misunderstood and misused. Sexual identity is a person's biological sexual characteristics, including genes, external and internal sexual organs, hormonal makeup, and secondary sex characteristics. Gender identity is a person's sense of being female or male. Sexual orientation describes the object of a person's sexual impulses: heterosexual, homosexual, or bisexual. Sexual behavior is the physiological experience triggered by psychological and physical stimuli.

Clinicians should be familiar with the sexual disorders as well as with the variety of treatments available to address these disorders. Students should study the following questions and answers related to the topic for a helpful review.

HELPFUL HINTS

The student should know the following terms and their definitions.

- anorgasmia
- autoerotic asphyxiation
- biogenic versus psychogenic
- bisexuality
- castration
- chronic pelvic pain
- clitoral versus vaginal orgasm
- coming out
- coprophilia
- cystometric examination
- desensitization therapy
- Don Juanism
- dual-sex therapy
- dyspareunia
- erection and ejaculation
- excitement
- exhibitionism
- female orgasmic disorder
- female sexual arousal disorder
- fetishism
- frotteurism
- FSH
- gender role
- heterosexuality
- HIV, AIDS
- homophobia
- homosexuality
- hymenectomy
- hypoactive sexual desire disorder
- hypoxyphilia
- incest
- infertility
- intersexual disorders
- intimacy
- Alfred Kinsey
- libido
- male erectile disorder
- male orgasmic disorder
- William Masters and Virginia Johnson
- masturbation
- moral masochism
- necrophilia
- nocturnal penile tumescence
- orgasm
- orgasm disorders
- orgasmic anhedonia
- paraphilias
- penile arteriography
- Peyronie's disease
- phases of sexual response
- postcoital dysphoria
- postcoital headache
- premature ejaculation
- prenatal androgens
- prosthetic devices
- psychosexual stages
- rape (male and female)
- refractory period
- resolution
- retarded ejaculation
- retrograde ejaculation
- satyriasis
- scatologia
- sensate focus
- sex addiction
- sexual arousal disorders
- sexual aversion disorder
- sexual desire disorders
- sexual dysfunction not otherwise specified
- sexual identity and gender identity
- sexual masochism and sexual sadism
- sexual orientation distress

▶ sexual pain disorders
▶ spectatoring
▶ spouse abuse
▶ squeeze technique
▶ statutory rape

▶ steal phenomenon
▶ sterilization
▶ stop–start technique
▶ sympathetic and parasympathetic nervous systems

▶ telephone scatologia
▶ transvestic fetishism
▶ tumescence and detumescence
▶ unconsummated marriage

▶ urophilia
▶ vagina dentata
▶ vaginismus
▶ vaginoplasty
▶ voyeurism
▶ zoophilia

▲ QUESTIONS

DIRECTIONS: Each of the questions or incomplete statements below is followed by five suggested responses or completions. Select the *one* that is *best* in each case.

21.1 Which of the following is *not* an intersexual disorder?

A. hypoxyphilia
B. Turner's syndrome
C. Klinefelter's syndrome
D. 5α-reductase deficiency
E. 17-hydroxysteroid dehydrogenase deficiency

21.2 Paraphilias

A. are usually not distressing to the person with the disorder
B. are found equally among men and women
C. according to the classic psychoanalytic model, are due to a failure to complete the process of genital adjustment
D. with an early age of onset are associated with a good prognosis
E. such as pedophilia usually involve vaginal or anal penetration of the victim

21.3 Figure 21.1 shows a man with gynecomastia and small testes. He has positive Barr bodies and an XXY karyotype. The most likely diagnosis is

A. androgen insensitivity
B. Klinefelter's syndrome
C. Turner's syndrome
D. hermaphroditism
E. Cushing's syndrome

21.4 Which of the following statements about fetishism is *false*?

A. A fetish is an inanimate object that is used as the preferred or necessary adjunct to sexual arousal.
B. A fetish may be integrated into sexual activity with a human partner.
C. A fetish is a device that may function as a hedge against separation anxiety.
D. A fetish is a device with magical phallic qualities that is used to ward off castration anxiety.
E. Fetishism is a disorder found equally in males and females.

21.5 A man with a chief complaint of premature ejaculation is best treated with

A. antianxiety agents
B. psychoanalysis
C. squeeze technique
D. cognitive therapy
E. none of the above

21.6 Measures used to help differentiate organically caused impotence from functional impotence include

A. monitoring of nocturnal penile tumescence
B. glucose tolerance tests
C. follicle-stimulating hormone (FSH) determinations
D. testosterone level tests
E. all of the above

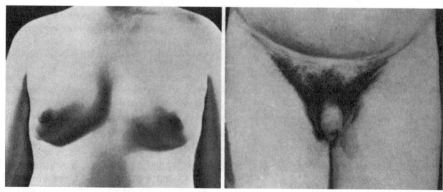

FIGURE 21.1
Courtesy of Robert B. Greenblatt, M.D., and Virginia P. McNamara, M.D.

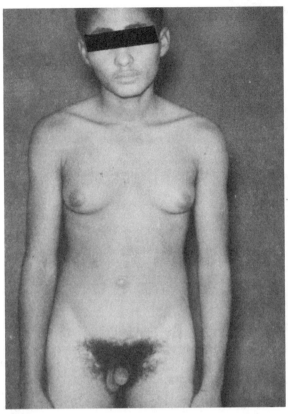

FIGURE 21.2
Courtesy of Robert B. Greenblatt, M.D., and Virginia P. McNamara, M.D.

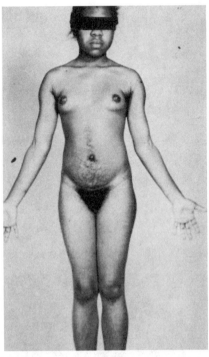

FIGURE 21.3
Courtesy of Robert B. Greenblatt, M.D., and Virginia P. McNamara, M.D.

21.7 Which of the following medications is *least likely* to impair ejaculation?

A. amitriptyline
B. spironolactone
C. haloperidol
D. phentolamine
E. fluoxetine

21.8 On the biopsy of gonadal structures in the patient shown in Figure 21.2, an abdominal ovary and scrotal testis were found. The most likely diagnosis is

A. androgen insensitivity syndrome
B. pseudohermaphroditism
C. Klinefelter's syndrome
D. true hermaphroditism
E. adrenogenital syndrome

21.9 The patient in Figure 21.3 has an XX genotype and a diagnosis of congenital adrenal hyperplasia. All of the following statements regarding her condition are true *except*

A. It is the most common female intersex disorder.
B. Patients have no uterus.
C. The condition results from excess fetal androgens.
D. Clitoral enlargement and adolescent hirsutism are characteristic.
E. Patients have a vagina.

21.10a Figure 21.4 shows a phenotypic woman with an XY karyotype. The most likely diagnosis is

A. pseudohermaphroditism
B. testicular feminization syndrome
C. Turner's syndrome
D. adrenogenital syndrome
E. true hermaphroditism

21.10b This patient's condition results from

A. insufficient androgen production
B. testicular agenesis
C. inability of target tissues to respond to androgens
D. excess estrogen production
E. pituitary dysfunction

21.10c Which of the following statements regarding the patient's condition is *false*?

A. Secondary sex characteristics at puberty are female.
B. Internal sexual organs are minimal or absent at birth.
C. The condition is an X-linked recessive trait.
D. External genitalia appear ambiguous at birth.
E. Patients are born with cryptorchid testes.

21.11 Which of the following substances has *not* been associated with sexual dysfunction?

A. cocaine
B. trazodone
C. amoxapine
D. antihistamines
E. all of the above

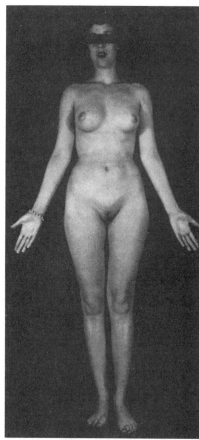

FIGURE 21.4
A phenotypic female with abdominal testes and an XY chromosomal karyotype.

21.12 Which of the following conditions is classified as a psychological or behavioral disorder associated with sexual development or orientation?

    A. fetishism
    B. voyeurism
    C. frotteurism
    D. necrophilia
    E. transsexualism

21.13 Which of the following conditions is classified as a disorder of sexual development or orientation?

    A. transvestism
    B. exhibitionism
    C. gender identity disorder
    D. sexual relationship disorder
    E. all of the above

21.14 With regard to innervation of sex organs, all of the following are true *except*

    A. Penile tumescence occurs through the synergistic activity of parasympathetic and sympathetic pathways.
    B. Clitoral engorgement results from parasympathetic stimulation.
    C. Vaginal lubrication results from sympathetic stimulation.
    D. Sympathetic innervation is responsible for ejaculation.
    E. Sympathetic innervation facilitates the smooth muscle contraction of the vagina, urethra, and uterus during orgasm.

21.15 Among the following, the sexual dysfunction *not* correlated with phases of the sexual response cycle is

    A. sexual aversion disorder
    B. vaginismus
    C. premature ejaculation
    D. post-coital dysphoria
    E. male erectile disorder

21.16 True statements about erectile dysfunction include

    A. From 35 to 40 percent of all men treated for sexual disorders have erectile dysfunction as the chief complaint.
    B. Some studies indicate that depending on age, a relatively high percentage of men with erectile dysfunction may have a medical basis for their problem.
    C. The incidence of erectile dysfunction in young men is about 8 percent.
    D. The most common medical etiologies of erectile dysfunction are probably diabetes and vascular disease.
    E. All of the above

21.17 Premature ejaculation

    A. is less common among college-educated men than among men with less education
    B. is mediated via the parasympathetic nervous system
    C. is strongly influenced by the sex partner in an ongoing relationship
    D. is not defined within a specific time frame
    E. all of the above

21.18 Female orgasmic dysfunction has been associated with

    A. tricyclic drugs
    B. monoamine oxidase inhibitors (MAOIs)
    C. serotonin reuptake inhibitors
    D. CNS stimulants
    E. all of the above

21.19 Of the following antipsychotic drugs, which causes retrograde ejaculation?

    A. trifluoperazine (Stelazine)
    B. haloperidol (Haldol)
    C. thioridazine (Mellaril)
    D. all of the above
    E. none of the above

21.20 Pharmacologic agents used to enhance libido and improve sexual functioning include

A. bromocriptine
B. bupropion
C. selegiline
D. sildenafil
E. all of the above

21.21 True statements about what research has shown about gay men and lesbians include

A. A majority of lesbians and gay men report being in a committed romantic relationship.
B. Lesbian couples tend more frequently to be sexually exclusive than male couples.
C. Gay men and lesbians, in comparison with heterosexual couples, generally have more equality in their relationships.
D. Gay men and lesbians report the same degree of global satisfaction in their relationships as heterosexual men and women.
E. All of the above

21.22 When compared to children of heterosexual parents, children of gay and lesbian parents

A. have significantly different outcomes in gender identity
B. have significantly different outcomes in gender role
C. have significantly different outcomes in sexual orientation
D. may have to struggle with their difference from heterosexual families
E. all of the above

21.23 In the most severe forms of paraphilia

A. persons never experience any sexual behavior with partners
B. the specific paraphilia imagery or activity is absolutely necessary for any sexual function
C. the need for sexual behavior consumes so much money, time, concentration, and energy that the person describes self as out of control
D. orgasm does not produce satiety in same way it typically does for age mates
E. all of the above

21.24 Child molesters

A. are always pedophiles
B. are somewhat more frequently male than female
C. when women, are often deteriorated by substance abuse, major mental illness, major organic illness, or have been coerced by a dominant man
D. are almost always indiscriminate in their choice of victim
E. none of the above

21.25 Psychiatric interventions used to assist the paraphilia patient include

A. dynamic psychotherapy
B. external control
C. cognitive-behavioral therapy
D. treatment of comorbid conditions
E. all of the above

21.26 Research has indicated that

A. a majority of married people are unfaithful to their spouses
B. the median number of sexual partners over a lifetime for men is six and for women two
C. vaginal intercourse is considered the most appealing type of sexual experience by a large majority of men and women
D. masturbation is more common among those 18 to 24 than among those 24 to 34 years old
E. the percentage of single women reporting "usually or always" having an orgasm during intercourse is greater than the percentage of married women reporting this

DIRECTIONS: Each group of questions below consists of lettered headings followed by a list of numbered words or phrases. For each numbered word or phrase, select the *one* lettered heading that is most closely associated with it. Each lettered heading may be used once, more than once, or not at all.

Questions 21.27–21.31

A. Desire phase
B. Excitement phase
C. Orgasm phase
D. Resolution phase

21.27 Vaginal lubrication
21.28 Orgasmic platform
21.29 Testes increase in size by 50 percent
21.30 Slight clouding of consciousness
21.31 Detumescence

Questions 21.32–21.34

A. Fetishism
B. Voyeurism
C. Frotteurism
D. Exhibitionism
E. Sexual masochism
F. Sexual sadism
G. Transvestic fetishism
H. Hypoactive sexual desire disorder
I. Sexual aversion disorder
J. Dyspareunia
K. Vaginismus

21.32 Rubbing up against a fully clothed woman to achieve orgasm
21.33 Involuntary muscle constriction
21.34 Persistent genital pain occurring before, during, or after intercourse

Questions 21.35–21.39

A. Sexual identity
B. Gender identity
C. Sexual orientation
D. Sexual behavior

21.35 Sense of maleness or femaleness
21.36 The object of a person's sexual impulses
21.37 Chromosomes
21.38 Gonads and secondary sex characteristics
21.39 Desire and fantasies

Questions 21.40–21.42

    A. Sensate focus exercises

    B. Squeeze technique

21.40 Intercourse is interdicted initially

21.41 Raises the threshold of penile excitability

21.42 Attempts to decrease "spectatoring"

ANSWERS

Human Sexuality

21.1 The answer is A

Intersexual disorders include several syndromes that produce gross anatomical or physiological aspects of the opposite sex. *Hypoxyphilia* is not an intersexual disorder but rather a desire to experience an altered state of consciousness during orgasm by producing hypoxia with drugs or mechanical pressure.

    Turner's syndrome (see Figure 21.5) results from the absence of a second female sex chromosome (XO). The infants are usually assigned as females because of their female-looking genitals. In *Klinefelter's syndrome,* the genotype is XXY; infants have a male habitus with a small penis and rudimentary testes caused by low androgen production. They are usually assigned as males. *5α-Reductase deficiency* and *17-hydroxysteroid dehydrogenase deficiency* are types of enzymatic defects in the XY genotype resulting in congenital interruption of dihydrotestosterone and testosterone production, respec-

tively. As a result, infants have a female habitus and ambiguous genitals. They are usually assigned as females because of their female-looking genitalia.

21.2 The answer is C

Paraphilias, *according to the classic psychoanalytic model,* are due to a failure to complete the process of genital adjustment. However bizarre its manifestation, the paraphilia provides an outlet for the sexual and aggressive drives that would otherwise have been channeled into proper sexual behavior. Paraphilias are *usually distressing* to the person with the disorder. Paraphilias are *not found equally among men and women.* As usually defined, paraphilias seem to be largely male conditions. Paraphilias with an *early age of onset* are associated with a poor prognosis, as are paraphilias with a high frequency of the acts (Table 21.1), no guilt or shame about the acts, and substance abuse. Paraphilias such as *pedophilia* usually do not involve vaginal or anal penetration of the victim. The majority of child molestations involve genital fondling or oral sex.

21.3 The answer is B

Klinefelter's syndrome is a chromosomal abnormality in which an extra sex chromosome exists; instead of the normal 46, the affected child is born with 47 chromosomes. For example, there is an XXY pattern, instead of the usual XX or XY pairs. The persons affected are male in development, with small, firm testes, eunuchoid habitus, variable gynecomastia and other signs of androgen deficiency, and elevated gonadotropin levels.

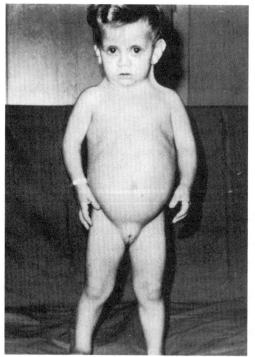

FIGURE 21.5
Photograph of patient with Turner's syndrome. The main characteristics are webbed neck, short stature, broad chest, and absence of sexual maturation. (Reprinted with permission from Sadler T. *Langman's Medical Embryology.* 5th ed. Baltimore: Williams & Wilkins; 1985:121, with permission.)

TABLE 21.1

Frequency of Paraphiliac Acts Committed by Paraphilia Patients Seeking Outpatient Treatment

Diagnostic Category	Paraphilia Patients Seeking Outpatient Treatment (%)	Paraphiliac Acts per Paraphilia Patient[a]
Pedophilia	45	5
Exhibitionism	25	50
Voyeurism	12	17
Frotteurism	6	30
Sexual masochism	3	36
Transvestic fetishism	3	25
Sexual sadism	3	3
Fetishism	2	3
Zoophilia	1	2

[a]Median number.
Courtesy of Gene G. Abel, M.D.

Androgen insensitivity is a congenital disorder resulting from an inability of target tissues to respond to androgen. *Turner's syndrome* is a chromosome disorder affecting girls. Instead of an XX sex chromosome, an XO sex chromosome exists, and the girl has a total of 45 chromosomes, rather than the usual 46. *Hermaphroditism* is a state in which a person has both female and male gonads, usually with one sex dominating. *Cushing's syndrome,* or hyperadrenocorticism, is named for an American neurosurgeon, Harvey W. Cushing (1869–1939). It is characterized by muscle wasting, obesity, osteoporosis, atrophy of the skin, and hypertension. Emotional lability is common, and frank psychoses are occasionally observed.

21.4 The answer is E

Fetishism is a disorder *found almost exclusively in males.* The essential feature of a fetish is a nonliving object that is used as the preferred or necessary *adjunct to sexual arousal.* Sexual activity may involve the fetish alone, or the fetish may be *integrated into sexual activities with a human partner.* In the absence of the fetish, the male may be impotent. According to psychoanalytic theory, the fetish may function as *a hedge against separation anxiety* from the love object and may be *used to ward off castration anxiety.*

21.5 The answer is C

A man with a chief complaint of premature ejaculation is best treated with the *squeeze technique.* In this method the woman squeezes the coronal ridge of the erect penis just before ejaculation or the time of ejaculatory inevitability. That moment is signaled to the woman by the man in a manner previously agreed to, at which time the woman forcefully applies the squeeze technique. The erection subsides slightly, and ejaculation is postponed. Eventually, the threshold of ejaculatory inevitability is raised, and the condition thereby improves.

Even though premature ejaculation is accompanied by anxiety, drug therapy with *antianxiety agents* is not indicated. Positive results have been obtained using the side effects of fluoxetine (Prozac), which delays orgasm in some men. *Psychoanalysis* may reveal unconscious fears of women that contribute to premature ejaculation, but it is not the most effective therapy. Psychoanalysis can be used if the patient does not respond to the squeeze technique because of deep-seated psychological conflicts. *Cognitive therapy* is used as a treatment of depression and is of limited use as a primary treatment approach to any of the sexual disorders. If the patient has a depression secondary to the sexual disorder, however, cognitive therapy may be useful.

21.6 The answer is E (all)

A variety of measures is used to differentiate organically caused impotence from psychologically caused impotence. The *monitoring of nocturnal penile tumescence* is a noninvasive procedure; normally, erections occur during sleep and are associated with rapid eye movement (REM) sleep periods. Tumescence may be determined with a simple strain gauge. In most cases in which organic factors account for the impotence, the man has minimal or no nocturnal erections. Conversely, in most cases of psychologically caused or psychogenic impotence, erections do occur during REM sleep.

Other diagnostic tests that delineate organic bases of impotence include *glucose tolerance tests, follicle-stimulating hor-*

mone (FSH) determinations, and *testosterone level tests.* The glucose tolerance curve measures the metabolism of glucose over a specific period and is useful in diagnosing diabetes, of which impotence may be a symptom. FSH is a hormone produced by the anterior pituitary that stimulates the secretion of estrogen from the ovarian follicle in the female; it is also responsible for the production of sperm from the testes in men. An abnormal finding suggests an organic cause for impotence. Testosterone is the male hormone produced by the interstitial cells of the testes. In the male, a low testosterone level produces a lack of desire as the chief complaint, which may be associated with impotence. If the measure of nocturnal penile tumescence is abnormal, indicating the possibility of organic impotence, a measure of plasma testosterone is indicated.

21.7 The answer is B

Spironolactone (Aldactone), an antihypertensive drug, is the medication least likely to impair ejaculation. *Amitriptyline* (Elavil) is a tricyclic antidepressant that occasionally causes impaired ejaculation. *Haloperidol* (Haldol), *phentolamine* (Regitine), and *fluoxetine* (Prozac) have all been shown to be implicated in impaired or delayed ejaculation.

21.8 The answer is D

True hermaphroditism is the presence of both ovarian and testicular tissue in one individual; it is a rare condition. *Pseudohermaphroditism,* or false hermaphroditism, is a state in which the individual has unambiguous gonadal sex (for example, possessing either ovaries or testes) but has ambiguous external genitalia. *Androgen insensitivity syndrome* is a congenital X-linked recessive trait disorder that results in an inability of target tissues to respond to androgens. The syndrome is characterized by female genitalia and cryptorchid testes. Patients are assigned as females even though they have an XY genotype. *Klinefelter's syndrome* is a chromosomal anomaly with XXY sex chromosome constitution, characterized by a male habitus presenting with a small penis and rudimentary testis because of low androgen production. *Adrenogenital syndrome,* also known as congenital virilizing adrenal hyperplasia, results from excess androgens in a fetus with an XX genotype, causing androgenization of the external genitals. Table 21.2 lists a classification of intersexual disorders.

21.9 The answer is B

Congenital virilizing adrenal hyperplasia, also known as adrenogenital syndrome, *the most common female intersex disorder,* results from *excess androgens* in a fetus with XX genotype. The syndrome is characterized by androgenization of the external genitals, ranging from mild *clitoral enlargement* to external genitals that look like a normal scrotal sac, testes, and a penis, but *hidden behind those external genitals are a vagina and uterus.* The patients are otherwise normally female.

21.10a The answer is B

21.10b The answer is C

21.10c The answer is D

The phenotypic female with XY karyotype has *androgen insensitivity syndrome,* also known as *testicular feminization syndrome,* a congenital *X-linked recessive trait* disorder that results in an inability of target tissues to respond to a mutant allele on

TABLE 21.2

Classification of Intersexual Disorders[a]

Syndrome	Description
Virilizing adrenal hyperplasia (adreno-genital syndrome)	Results from excess androgens in fetus with XX genotype; most common female intersex disorder; associated with enlarged clitoris, fused labia, hirsutism in adolescence
Turner's syndrome	Results from absence of second female sex chromosome (XO); associated with web neck, dwarfism, cubitus valgus; no sex hormones produced; infertile; usually assigned as females because of female-looking genitals
Klinefelter's syndrome	Genotype is XXY; male habitus present with small penis and rudimentary testes because of low androgen production; weak libido; usually assigned as male
Androgen insensitivity syndrome (testicu-lar-feminizing syn-drome)	Congenital X-linked recessive disorder that results in inability of tissues to respond to androgens; external genitals look female and cryptorchid testes present; assigned as females, even though they have XY genotype; in extreme form patient has breasts, normal external genitals, short blind vagina, and absence of pubic and axillary hair
Enzymatic defects in XY genotype (e.g., 5α-reductase deficiency, 17-hydroxy-steroid deficiency)	Congenital interruption in production of testosterone that produces ambiguous genitals and female habitus; usually assigned as female because of female-looking genitalia
Hermaphroditism	True hermaphrodite is rare and characterized by both testes and ovaries in same person (may be 46 XX or 46 XY)
Pseudohermaphroditism	Usually the result of endocrine or enzymatic defect (e.g., adrenal hyperplasia) in persons with normal chromosomes; female pseudohermaphrodites have masculine-looking genitals but are XX; male pseudohermaphrodites have rudimentary testes and external genitals and are XY; assigned as males or females, depending on morphology of genitals

[a]Intersexual disorders include a variety of syndromes that produce persons with gross anatomical or physiological aspects of the opposite sex.

androgens. Because it is X-linked recessive, the person needs only one X chromosome. In an XX genotype, the person would carry the gene but not express it phenotypically. The infant *at birth appears to be an unremarkable girl*, although she is later found to have *cryptorchid testes*, which produce the testosterone to which the tissues do not respond, and *minimal or absent internal sexual organs*. Secondary *sex characteristics at puberty* are female because of the small but *sufficient amounts of estrogens* typically produced by the testes. The patients invariably sense themselves as female and are feminine.

True hermaphroditism is the presence in one individual of both ovarian and testicular tissue. *Pseudohermaphroditism* is

a state in which the individual has an unambiguous gonadal sex (for example, possessing either ovaries or testes) but has ambiguous external genitalia. *Turner's syndrome* is a chromosomal anomaly with only a single X chromosome (XO genotype), resulting in *absence (agenesis)* or minimal development (dysgenesis) of the gonads and no significant production of sex hormones. *Adrenogenital syndrome* results from excess androgens in a fetus with an XX genotype, causing androgenization of the external genitals.

21.11 The answer is E

Intoxication with *cocaine* and alcohol, among other substances, produces sexual dysfunction. Medications such as *antihistamines,* antidepressants, and antiepileptics, among others, can cause arousal and orgasmic disorders as well as decreased sexual interest. *Trazodone* is one of the substances associated with priapism, and *amoxapine* is associated with painful orgasm. Still other substances implicated in sexual dysfunction include antihypertensives, antiparkinsonian agents, anxiolytics, hypnotics, sedatives, amphetamines, and anabolic steroids.

21.12 The answer is E

Transsexualism is described as a gender identity disorder that is characterized by a desire to live and be accepted as a member of the opposite sex, rather than a disorder of sexual preference. In transsexualism, a person feels uncomfortable about his or her own anatomic sex and often wishes to undergo treatments to change the body to the preferred sex.

The other choices refer to disorders of sexual preferences. *Fetishism* is a reliance on a nonliving object as a stimulus for sexual arousal and gratification. Many fetishes are extensions of the human body, such as shoes or articles of clothing; others have a particular texture, such as leather or plastic. When fetishes are used, they need not always be primary but may simply enhance sexual excitement.

In *voyeurism*, a person feels impelled to look at people engaging in sexual activity or other intimate behavior, such as undressing. *Frotteurism* is a desire to seek sexual stimulation by rubbing against people in crowded places, such as on a subway. *Necrophilia* refers to a desire to be near dead bodies or to have an impulse to have sex with a dead body.

21.13 The answer is E (all)

Sexual relationship disorder is defined in ICD-10 as a gender identity abnormality that produces difficulties in relationships with sexual partners. Other disorders in this ICD-10 category include sexual maturation disorder, in which people are uncertain about their gender identity or sexual orientation, and ego-dystonic sexual orientation, in which people wish for a different gender identity or sexual preference because of associated psychological and behavioral disorders.

Transvestism, transsexualism, and gender identity disorder of childhood are classified as *gender identity disorders*, a category rather than a specific disorder. *Exhibitionism*, voyeurism, pedophilia, and fetishism are classified as sexual preference disorders, also a category rather than a specific disorder. Transvestism is a desire to wear clothes of the opposite sex and to enjoy temporary membership in the opposite sex, without any wish for permanent sex change. Exhibitionism is a tendency to expose the genitalia to people in public places, without any desire for closer contact. Some people experience this tendency only during periods of stress.

21.14 The answer is C

Innervation of the sexual organs is mediated primarily through the autonomic nervous system (ANS). *Penile tumescence* occurs through the synergistic activity of two neurophysiologic pathways. A parasympathetic (cholinergic) component mediates reflexogenic erections via impulses that pass through the pelvic splanchnic nerves (S2, S3, and S4). A thoracolumbar, mainly sympathetic, pathway transmits psychologically induced impulses. Both parasympathetic and sympathetic mechanisms are thought to play a part in relaxing the smooth muscles of the penile corpora cavernosa, which allow the penile arteries to dilate and cause the inflow of blood that results in penile erection. Relaxation of cavernosal smooth muscles is aided by the release of nitric oxide, an endothelium-derived relaxing factor. *Clitoral engorgement* and *vaginal lubrication* also result from parasympathetic stimulation that increases blood flow to genital tissue. Adrian Zorgniotti has compared the erection phenomenon that results from increased penile blood inflow and decreased blood outflow with the inflation of an automobile tire, which requires an inflow of air and an intact casing.

Evidence indicates that the sympathetic (adrenergic) system is responsible for *ejaculation*. Through its hypogastric plexus the adrenergic impulses enervate the urethral crest, the muscles of the epididymis, and the muscles of the vas deferens, seminal vesicles, and prostate. Stimulation of the plexus causes emission. In women, the sympathetic system facilitates the *smooth muscle contraction* of the vagina, urethra, and uterus that occurs during orgasm.

The ANS functions outside of voluntary control and is influenced by external events (e.g., stress, drugs) and internal events (hypothalamic, limbic, and cortical stimuli). It is not surprising, therefore, that erection and orgasm are so vulnerable to dysfunction.

21.15 The answer is B

Seven major categories of sexual dysfunction are listed in DSM-IV-TR: (1) sexual desire disorders, (2) sexual arousal disorders, (3) orgasm disorders, (4) sexual pain disorders, (5) sexual dysfunction due to a general medical condition, (6) substance-induced sexual dysfunction, and (7) sexual dysfunction not otherwise specified.

In DSM-IV-TR sexual dysfunctions are categorized as Axis I disorders. All of the syndromes listed except *vaginismus*, including *sexual aversion disorder, premature ejaculation, post-coital dysphoria,* and *male erectile disorder,* are correlated with the sexual physiological response cycle, which is divided into four phases: desire, excitement, orgasm, and resolution. The essential feature of the sexual dysfunctions is inhibition in one or more of the phases, including disturbance in the subjective sense of pleasure or desire, or disturbance in the objective performance. Either type of disturbance can occur alone or in combination. Sexual dysfunctions are diagnosed only when they are a major part of the clinical picture. They can be lifelong or acquired, generalized or situational, and can be due to psychological factors, physiological factors, or combined factors. If they are attributable entirely to a general medical condi-

tion, substance use, or adverse effects of medication, then sexual dysfunction due to a general medical condition or substance-induced sexual dysfunction is diagnosed.

Vaginismus is an involuntary muscle constriction of the outer third of the vagina that interferes with penile insertion and intercourse. It can also occur during a gynecological exam. It is not correlated with phases of the sexual response cycle.

21.16 The answer is E (all)

Male erectile disorder is also called erectile dysfunction and impotence. A man with lifelong male erectile disorder has never obtained an erection sufficient for vaginal insertion. In acquired male erectile disorder, the man successfully achieved vaginal penetration at some time in his sexual life but later cannot do so. In situational male erectile disorder, the man can have coitus in certain circumstances but not in others; for example, a man may function effectively with a prostitute but not with his wife. Kinsey estimated that a few men (2 to 4 percent) are dysfunctional at age 35, but 77 percent are at age 80. Ten percent of the men in the University of Chicago study reported an experience with erectile dysfunction in the past year, and between 15 and 20 percent experienced anxiety about performing. More recently it was estimated that the incidence of *erectile dysfunction in young men* is about 8 percent. Masters and Johnson reported a fear of impotence in all men over 40, which the researchers believed reflects the masculine fear of loss of virility with advancing age. (As it happens, however, erectile dysfunction is not a regularly occurring phenomenon in aged men; good health and an available sexual partner are more closely related to continuing potency than is age per se.) From 35 to 40 percent of all men treated for sexual disorders have *erectile dysfunction as the chief complaint.*

Many recent studies have focused on the relative incidences of psychological and organic erectile dysfunction. Physiologically, erectile dysfunction *may be due to a variety of medical causes* (Table 21.3). In the United States it is estimated that two million men cannot gain erections because they suffer from *diabetes mellitus*; an additional 300,000 are dysfunctional because of other endocrine diseases; 1.5 million are dysfunctional as a result of *vascular disease*; 180,000 because of multiple sclerosis; 400,000 because of traumas and fractures leading to pelvic fractures or spinal cord injuries; and another 650,000 as a result of radical surgery, including prostatectomies, colostomies, and cystectomies. In addition, the clinician should be aware of the possible pharmacological effects of medication on sexual functioning. The increased incidence of organic causes for erectile dysfunction in the past 15 years may partly reflect the increased use of psychotropic and antihypertensive medications. Statistics indicate that, depending on age, a relatively high percentage of men with erectile dysfunction may have a medical basis for their problem. However, in young and middle-aged men, the cause is usually psychological.

21.17 The answer is C

In premature ejaculation, the man recurrently achieves orgasm and ejaculates before he wishes to do so. *There is no definite time frame within which to define the dysfunction.* The diagnosis is made when the man regularly ejaculates before or immediately after entering the vagina or following minimal sexual stimulation. The clinician should consider factors that affect duration of the excitement phase, such as age, novelty

TABLE 21.3

Diseases and Other Medical Conditions Implicated in Male Erectile Disorder

Infectious and parasitic diseases
  Elephantiasis
  Mumps
Cardiovascular disease[a]
  Atherosclerotic disease
  Aortic aneurysm
  Leriche's syndrome
  Cardiac failure
Renal and urological disorders
  Peyronie's disease
  Chronic renal failure
  Hydrocele and varicocele
Hepatic disorders
  Cirrhosis (usually associated with alcohol dependence)
Pulmonary disorders
  Respiratory failure
Genetics
  Klinefelter's syndrome
  Congenital penile vascular and structural abnormalities
Nutritional disorders
  Malnutrition
  Vitamin deficiencies
Endocrine disorders[a]
  Diabetes mellitus
  Dysfunction of the pituitary-adrenal-testis axis
  Acromegaly
  Addison's disease
  Chromophobe adenoma
  Adrenal neoplasia
  Myxedema
  Hyperthyroidism
Neurological disorders
  Multiple sclerosis
  Transverse myelitis
  Parkinson's disease
  Temporal lobe epilepsy
  Traumatic and neoplastic spinal cord diseases[a]
  Central nervous system tumor
  Amyotrophic lateral sclerosis
  Peripheral neuropathy
  General paresis
  Tabes dorsalis
Pharmacological factors
  Alcohol and other dependence-inducing substances (heroin, methadone, morphine, cocaine, amphetamines, and barbiturates)
  Prescribed drugs (psychotropic drugs, antihypertensive drugs, estrogens, and antiandrogens)
Poisoning
  Lead (plumbism)
  Herbicides

TABLE 21.3

Diseases and Other Medical Conditions Implicated in Male Erectile Disorder

Surgical procedures[a]
  Perineal prostatectomy
  Abdominal-perineal colon resection
  Sympathectomy (frequently interferes with ejaculation)
  Aortoiliac surgery
  Radical cystectomy
  Retroperitoneal lymphadenectomy
Miscellaneous
  Radiation therapy
  Pelvic fracture
  Any severe systemic disease or debilitating condition

[a]In the United States an estimated 2 million men are impotent because they suffer from diabetes mellitus; an additional 300,000 are impotent because of other endocrine diseases; 1.5 million are impotent as a result of vascular disease; 180,000 because of multiple sclerosis; 400,000 because of traumas and fractures leading to pelvic fractures or spinal cord injuries; and another 650,000 are impotent as a result of radical surgery, including prostatectomies, colostomies, and cystectomies.

of the sexual partner, and the frequency and duration of coitus. Masters and Johnson conceptualized the disorder in terms of the couple and consider a man a premature ejaculator if he cannot control ejaculation long enough during intravaginal containment to satisfy his partner in at least half of their episodes of coitus. That definition assumes that the female partner is capable of an orgasmic response. As with other dysfunctions, the disturbance is diagnosed only if it is not caused exclusively by medical factors or is not symptomatic of any other Axis I syndrome.

Premature ejaculation is *more common (not less common) today among college-educated men* than among men with less education and is thought to be related to their concern for partner satisfaction. It is estimated that about 35 to 40 percent of men treated for sexual disorders have premature ejaculation as the chief complaint.

Difficulty in ejaculatory control may be associated with anxiety regarding the sex act. Both anxiety and ejaculation are *mediated by the parasympathetic nervous system.* Other psychological factors that have been noted include sexual guilt, a history of parent–child conflict, interpersonal hypersensitivity, and perfectionism or unrealistic expectations about sexual performance.

Current research also suggests that a subgroup of premature ejaculators (particularly those with a lifelong history of the dysfunction) may be biologically predisposed to this problem. Some researchers believe that certain males are constitutionally more vulnerable to sympathetic stimulation, hence they ejaculate rapidly. Other workers have found a shorter bulbocavernosus reflex nerve latency time in men with lifelong premature ejaculation than in men who had acquired the dysfunction.

Premature ejaculation also may result from negative cultural conditioning. The man who has most of his early sexual contacts with prostitutes who demand that the sex act proceed quickly or in situations in which discovery would be embarrassing, such as in an apartment shared with roommates or in the parental home, may become conditioned to achieving orgasm rapidly. *In ongoing relationships* the partner has been found to have great influence on the premature ejaculator. A stressful marriage exacerbates the disorder.

21.18 The answer is E (all)
Some medical conditions—specifically such endocrine diseases as hypothyroidism, diabetes mellitus, and primary hyperprolactinemia—can affect a woman's ability to have orgasms. Also, a number of drugs affect women's ability to have orgasms. Antihypertensive medications, *CNS stimulants*, *tricyclic drugs*, *serotonin reuptake inhibitors*, and frequently *monoamine oxidase inhibitors (MAOIs)* have interfered with female orgasmic capacity. However, one study of women taking MAOIs found that after 16 to 18 weeks of pharmacotherapy, that adverse effect of the medication disappeared, and the women could reexperience orgasms, even though they continued taking an undiminished dosage of the drug.

21.19 The answer is C
Most antipsychotic drugs are dopamine receptor antagonists that also block adrenergic and cholinergic receptors, which accounts for their adverse sex effects. Chlorpromazine (Thorazine), *thioridazine (Mellaril)*, *trifluoperazine (Stelazine)*, and *haloperidol (Haldol)* are potent anticholinergic agents that impair erection and ejaculation in men and inhibit vaginal lubrication and orgasm in women. *Thioridazine has the particular adverse effect of causing retrograde ejaculation*, in which the seminal fluid backs up into the bladder rather than being propelled through the penile urethra. Patients still have a pleasurable sensation of orgasm, but it is dry. When urinating after orgasm, the urine may be milky white since it contains the ejaculate. The condition is startling but harmless and may occur in up to 50 percent of patients taking the drug. Paradoxically, rare cases of priapism have been reported with antipsychotics.

21.20 The answer is E (all)
A variety of drugs has been explored in the treatment of sexual dysfunction. One of the major new medications is *sildenafil.*

Sildenafil is a nitric oxide enhancer that facilitates the inflow of blood to the penis necessary for an erection. The physiological mechanism of penile erection involves release of nitric oxide in the corpus cavernosum during sexual stimulation. Nitric oxide activates the enzyme guanylate cyclase, which increases cyclic guanosine monophosphate concentration and produces smooth muscle relaxation in the corpus cavernosum that allows the penile vessels to dilate and admit blood. Sildenafil enhances the effect of nitric oxide by inhibiting the enzyme that degrades cyclic guanosine monophosphate. In short, sildenafil augments the natural process involved in gaining and maintaining an erection during sexual stimulation. The drug takes effect about 1 hour after ingestion, and its effect can last up to 4 hours. Sildenafil has no effect in the absence of sexual stimulation.

The most common adverse events associated with sildenafil are headaches, flushing, and dyspepsia. Some sildenafil users see things in a blue tint for several hours after taking the medication; because of this, airline pilots have been prohibited from taking the drug, so that this visual artifact does not interfere with safe landings. The use of sildenafil is contraindicated for people taking organic nitrates. The concomitant action of the two drugs can result in large, sudden, and sometimes fatal drops in systemic blood pressure. The U.S. Food and Drug Administration (FDA) has posted 130 deaths in which sildenafil was listed as an associated medication and advises caution in prescribing sildenafil to men with a recent (6 month) history of myocardial infarction, stroke, life-threatening arrhythmia, significant hypotension or hypertension, cardiac failure, angina, or retinitis pigmentosa.

Sildenafil is not effective in all cases of erectile dysfunction. It fails to produce an erection rigid enough for penetration in about 50 percent of men who have had radical prostate surgery or in those with longstanding insulin-dependent diabetes. It is also ineffective in certain cases of nerve damage.

The use of sildenafil in women is being researched, but no significant studies have been published. Anecdotal reports describe individual women who have experienced intensified excitement when they have tried sildenafil.

Dopaminergic agents have been reported to increase libido and improve sexual functioning. Those drugs include L-dopa, a dopamine precursor, and *bromocriptine*, a dopamine agonist. The antidepressant *bupropion* has dopaminergic effects and has increased sex drive in some patients. *Selegiline*, an MAOI, is selective for MAO_B and is dopaminergic. It may improve sexual functioning in some older persons.

21.21 The answer is E (all)
The majority of gay men and lesbians report *being in a committed romantic relationship*, with some surveys indicating that 45 to 80 percent of lesbians and 40 to 60 percent of gay men are currently in such relationships. From 8 to 14 percent of lesbian couples and from 18 to 25 percent of gay male couples report that they have lived together for more than 10 years. While same-sex marriage is still legally prohibited, many same-sex couples live in relationships that are as enduring and emotionally significant as any heterosexual relationship, in spite of discrimination against these relationships, the absence of rituals and laws that support them, and the denial of equal protection and benefits to these couples.

Findings from the limited but growing research on gay and lesbian couples reveal that *lesbian couples tend more frequently to be sexually exclusive* than male couples. In addition, *gay male and, particularly, lesbian couples*, in comparison with heterosexual couples, generally have *more equality in their relationships* and do not differentiate household functions according to gender-based categories of work. Gay men and lesbians report the *same degree of global satisfaction in their relationships* as heterosexual men and women. However, undoubtedly as a result of gender socialization, women tend to appraise the value of and rewards from their relationships more highly than men, but gay and heterosexual men and lesbian and heterosexual women describe similar levels of valuing and rewards.

Empirical research by David McWhirter and Andrew Mattison led to the description of six stages in the development of male–male relationships: blending, nesting, maintaining, building, releasing, and renewing. Each stage is marked by specific characteristics and a time span, although the stages may overlap and occur in a different sequence for some couples and the characteristics may appear in more than one stage. The relevance of this stage model for lesbians has not been determined, but some variation from the gay male experience should be expected.

21.22 The answer is D

Many lesbians and gay men have had children, historically most often within heterosexual marriages and more recently through other avenues as well, including adoption, artificial insemination, and co-parenting arrangements outside of marriage. Numerous studies since the late 1970s have demonstrated the characteristics of gay and lesbian families and the impact of having a gay or lesbian parent on children. A significant change in recent years has been the greater visibility of families with gay and lesbian parents and the increased viability for gay men and lesbians to be involved in childrearing.

Research on gay and lesbian families was initially undertaken to disprove psychological and judicial assumptions about the harm that might be done to children raised by gay and lesbian parents. The findings resulting from such research have confirmed that lesbian and gay parents neither affect their children in a negative way psychologically nor produce *significantly different outcomes* in the *gender identity*, *gender role*, or *sexual orientation* of their children when compared with the children of heterosexual parents. Children with gay and lesbian parents *may have to struggle with their difference from heterosexual families* and may have difficulty overcoming the possible stigma associated with this situation. The first era of research into the effects of gay and lesbian parents on their children has now yielded to a period of greater emphasis on understanding the dynamics of and determining the potential differences between families with heterosexual, gay, and lesbian parents. Future studies may involve greater methodological precision, focusing more on family process than on structure alone and allowing for improved understanding of differences between gay and lesbian families, derived from religion, age, class, race, and other characteristics, as well as sex and sexual orientation.

The emergence of families with openly gay, lesbian, and bisexual parents and children since the 1970s represents one of the most significant shifts in the structure of the family during the latter part of the 20th century. The psychiatrist must recognize and validate the importance of this phenomenon in the lives of millions of men, women, and children and not confound the clinical evaluation and approach to treatment of patients from these families with negative portrayals derived from political, religious, or psychological biases.

21.23 The answer is E (all)

The revised fourth edition of *Diagnostic and Statistical Manual of Mental Disorders* (DSM-IV-TR) recognizes the paraphilias as consisting of recurrent, intensely sexually arousing fantasies, sexual urges, or sexual behaviors that involve either nonhuman objects, the suffering of the self or partner, or children, or nonconsenting persons. To qualify as a diagnosis, however, these patterns must have existed for at least 6 months and they have to cause clinically significant distress or impairment in social, occupational, or some other important area, such as sexual function.

DSM-IV-TR specifies nine paraphiliac diagnoses: exhibitionism or genital exposure; voyeurism or clandestine observation of another person's undressing, toileting, or sexual behavior; sadism or causing suffering during sexual behavior; masochism or being humiliated during sexual behavior; pedophilia or sexual behavior with prepubescent or peripubertal children; fetishism or use of nonliving objects for sexual behavior; frotteurism or rubbing against or touching a nonconsenting person; transvestic fetishism or use of clothing of the opposite sex for arousal; and paraphilia not otherwise specified for other observed atypical sexual patterns such as dressing in diapers, requiring a partner who has an amputated limb, and others.

All paraphilia behaviors are rehearsed repeatedly in fantasy; often these unusual fantasies have been present since childhood or puberty. Some persons with paraphilias *never experience any sexual behavior with partners*. The shame of the paraphilia interest and the fear of negative consequences may contribute to a lifelong avoidance of intimate contact. Sexual behaviors consist entirely of masturbation, often with magazine or Internet pictures and bulletin boards, videotapes, reading material, clothing, or mechanical props. People in this category are the most psychologically unprepared for sexual expression within an ordinary relationship.

While the usual functional significance of any paraphilia is that the person needs to use the paraphiliac fantasy or behavior in order to desire a partner, obtain arousal, and reach orgasm, the degree to which this occurs varies within most of the categories of paraphilia.

In the most severe forms of paraphilia, the *specific paraphiliac imagery or activity is absolutely necessary* for any sexual function. Without it, the person is always sexually apathetic—there is no desire for sexual behavior with the partner, no sustainable arousal, or no orgasmic attainment. When embarrassment prevents the paraphiliac from sharing the secret, the relationship may never be consummated and the partner is either baffled or settles on a wrong explanation. If the paraphiliac is able to integrate the paraphiliac requirements into the lovemaking, either by engaging in the behavior or imagining it, sexual functioning may even be normal.

The final parameter of severity is the degree of drivenness to masturbate or act out the fantasy with a partner.

The most severe form of compulsivity is the loss of autonomy. The loss of autonomy has three characteristics: (1) the *need for sexual behavior* consumes so much money, time, concentration, and energy that the patient describes himself as out of control; (2) intrusive, unwanted paraphiliac thoughts prevent concentration on other life demands and are the source of anxiety; and (3) *orgasm does not produce satiety* in the way it typically does for age mates. Thus, a man may masturbate six times a day, visit a prostitute twice in a day, or spend hundreds of dollars on phone sex. Although such drivenness may exist for long periods of time and is presented to the clinician as uncontrollable, a careful history often reveals that both the thoughts and the behaviors can be interrupted by other life demands.

21.24 The answer is C

Of the terms used to describe those who have genital contacts with young adolescents and children who are at least 5 years their junior—child molester, incest offender, sex offender, child rapist, statutory rapist, sexual abuser, sexual deviant, serial child molester, ephebophile, and pedophile—only the last is a formal diagnosis. Its criteria, however, do not cover all those who are arrested for child molestation. *The term pedophile has two meanings*: (1) a person who fulfills the DSM-IV-TR criteria for the diagnosis and (2) a person with a lifelong erotic preference for children.

Child molesters are subdivided in four ways. First, by age of the perpetrators: a large minority of molestations are committed by adolescents seemingly in their attempt to learn about sex with naive and accessible children; young and middle-aged adults who molest their own children, stepchildren, or friends' children; and elderly men who may be organically impaired, isolated, or lonely. Second, by sex of the offender: *Females are found to molest children far less frequently than males.* When they are discovered, *they are often deteriorated by substance abuse, major mental illness, major organic illness*, or thought to be *coerced into the behavior* by a dominant man. However, many adolescent sex offenders claim to have been abused by women in their prepubertal period. Third, by orientation: Men who have been sexually aroused by children all their lives have the largest numbers of child victims. The most destructive of these individuals find work or recreational opportunities to be in the company of children and young adolescents. They are synonymously labeled as having an anomalous orientation or a preference for children or as fixated pedophiles. Pedophiliac orientation is often seen in pure form. When it coexists with an adult heterosexual or homosexual orientation, the person may be called a regressed pedophile who under extenuating circumstances has sex with children. Fourth, *by victim characteristics*: boys versus girls (androphilic versus gynephilic); infants and toddlers, preschoolers, grade schoolers, or adolescents; and *indiscriminant*. Although these four categories are not mutually exclusive, they suggest that children are molested under such a wide array of circumstances that clinicians should not seek a single explanation for pedophiliac offenses.

Within each of these categories, however, child molesters display a startling set of rationalizations for their behavior. These include: (1) "I was educating the child about sex to learn the right way"; (2) the child initiated the behavior; (3) the child readily consented to it; (4) it was merely a caring act to provide pleasure; (5) it caused no harm whatsoever; and (6) it was less problematic than having an affair with an adult. These notions are referred to as cognitive distortions that demonstrate the molesters' lack of empathy for their victims. While children of many ages are subjectively attractive to many adults who never behave sexually with children, the compelling question about child molesters is what accounts for their behavior. Since the answer seems to vary significantly from case to case, the clinician should formulate an individualized answer with each perpetrator.

21.25 The answer is E (all)

Five types of psychiatric interventions are used to assist the paraphilia patient to rebalance internal control mechanisms, cease victimization of others, and enhance the capacities to relate to others: *external control*, reduction of sexual drives, *treatment of comorbid conditions, cognitive-behavioral therapy*, and *dynamic psychotherapy*. The art of therapy is to select and modify these various elements for the individual patient.

When sexual victimization of others has occurred, new external controls should be instituted. Prison is an external control for sexual crimes that usually does not contain a treatment element. All relevant persons in the environment need to know what the person has done and is capable of doing again under opportune conditions. For intrafamilial abuse of children, for instance, the adults and other children in the family are informed of the abuse. The children in the family are not permitted to be alone with the

offender again as long as they are unable to adequately protect themselves. With such controls implemented, those who victimize girls in their own home have recidivism rates of less than 5 percent. The more socially, economically, and psychologically disruptive alternative is to remove the offender from the home. When professionals who have sexually offended return to their work settings, external controls take the form of restricting access to potential victims and monitoring by administration, co-workers, and sometimes by patients with the use of exit questionnaires. Perpetrators and their professional colleagues can be educated about boundary crossings. When a therapist agrees to keep the knowledge of the patient's victimizing sexual patterns from family members, administrators, or colleagues on the basis of confidentiality, the single most effective psychiatric intervention is removed from the treatment plan. The therapist will probably be the last to know of the resumption of victimizing behaviors.

Psychiatrists need to consider the role of inadequately treated comorbid states when planning to treat sexual compulsivity or impulsivity. Alcohol and substance abuse, major depressive disorder, grief, psychotic disorder, attention-deficit/hyperactivity disorder, bipolar II disorder, and others may be the co-factor that enables a compensated sexual pattern to deteriorate and come to clinical attention.

It is frequently observed that sex offenders lack the social skills necessary to live effectively and create nonproblematic sexual relationships. Correcting some of these deficits is a goal of most cognitive-behavioral treatment programs for sexually offending paraphiliac individuals. Each intervention is an aspect of a therapy approach that assumes that a paraphiliac lifestyle is learned and can be significantly modified. The specific techniques can be implemented in individual or group settings.

The nonviolent paraphilias and the paraphilia-related disorders are often treated with traditional individual or group therapies using a combination of supportive, growth-promoting tactics. Such therapies aim at creating an evolving hypothesis about the unique developmental origin of the patient's eroticism. The defensive function of the impulse to act out (the anxiety reduction function) is defined so that the person can deal directly with the unpleasant feelings that trigger the impulses. Hypotheses get more complex as more developmental details emerge. The vast majority of patients need many therapeutic opportunities to work through the paraphiliac defense so that they can simply feel and cope with their particular life issue. Dynamic psychotherapy approaches emphasize the importance of the trusting relationship with the therapist to enable the work to occur. Therapists often face a delicate situation because most paraphilia embodies the capacity to transform the pain of childhood misery—for instance, "Mother didn't love me" into the pleasure of sexual arousal—"I'll exhibit myself to a teenager." Although the patient may no longer want to act out sexually, his desire to avoid reexperiencing his painful past may be greater. When the therapist decides to assist the patient in working through some of his distressing memories, a great deal of support may be needed. Generally speaking, the more globally impaired the paraphiliac is, the less likely it is that he (or she) can be treated in a dynamic psychotherapy.

21.26 The answer is C

A 1994 study, which was based on a representative United States population between the ages of 18 and 59, found the following:

1. Eighty-five percent of married women and 75 percent of married men are *faithful to their spouses.*

2. Forty-one percent of married couples have sex twice a week or more, compared with 23 percent of single persons.

3. Cohabiting single persons have the most sex of all, twice a week or more.

4. The median *number of sexual partners* over a lifetime for men is 12 (not six) and for women, six (not two).

5. A homosexual orientation was reported by 2.8 percent of men and 1.4 percent of women, with 9 percent of men and 5 percent of women reporting that they had at least one homosexual experience after puberty.

6. *Vaginal intercourse* is considered the most appealing type of sexual experience by the majority of both men and women.

7. Among married partners, 93 percent are of the same race, 82 percent are of similar educational level, 78 percent are within 5 years of each other's age, and 72 percent are of the same religion.

8. Both men and women who as children had been sexually abused by an adult were more likely as adults to have had more than ten sex partners, to engage in group sex, to report a homosexual or bisexual identification, and to be unhappy.

9. Fewer than 8 percent of the participants reported having sex more than four times a week; about two-thirds said they had sex a few times a month or less, and about three in ten have sex a few times a year or less.

10. About one man in four and one woman in ten masturbates at least once a week, and *masturbation* is less common (not more common) among those 18 to 24 years of age than among those 24 to 34 years old.

11. Three-quarters of the married women said "they usually or always" had an *orgasm during sexual intercourse,* compared with 62 percent of the single women. Among men, married or single, 95 percent said they usually or always had an orgasm.

12. More than half of the men said that they thought about sex every day or several times a day, compared with only 19 percent of the women.

Answers 21.27–21.31

21.27 The answer is B

21.28 The answer is B

21.29 The answer is B

21.30 The answer is C

21.31 The answer is D
The fourth revised edition of *Diagnostic and Statistical Manual of Mental Disorders* (DSM-IV-TR) defines a four-phase sexual response cycle: phase 1, desire; phase 2, excitement; phase 3, orgasm; phase 4, resolution.

The *desire phase* is distinct from any phase identified solely through physiology, and it reflects the psychiatrist's fundamental interest in motivations, drives, and personality. It is characterized by sexual fantasies and the desire to have sexual activity. The *excitement phase* is brought on by psychological stimulation (fantasy or the presence of a love object) or physiological stimulation (stroking or kissing) or a combination of the two. It consists of a subjective sense of pleasure. The excitement phase is characterized by penile tumescence leading to erection in the man and by *vaginal lubrication* in the woman. Initial excitement may last several minutes to several hours. With continued stimulation, the woman's vaginal barrel shows a characteristic constriction along the outer third, known as the *orgasmic platform*, and the man's *testes increase in size 50 percent* and elevate.

The *orgasm phase* consists of a peaking of sexual pleasure, with the release of sexual tension and the rhythmic contraction of the perineal muscles and the pelvic reproductive organs. A subjective sense of ejaculatory inevitability triggers the man's orgasm. The forceful emission of semen follows. The male orgasm is also associated with four to five rhythmic spasms of the prostate, seminal vesicles, vas, and urethra. In the woman, orgasm is characterized by three to 15 involuntary contractions of the lower third of the vagina and by strong sustained contractions of the uterus, flowing from the fundus downward to the cervix. Blood pressure rises 20 to 40 mm (both systolic and diastolic), and the heart rate increases up to 160 beats a minute. Orgasm lasts 3 to 25 seconds and is associated with a *slight clouding of consciousness.*

The *resolution phase* consists of the disgorgement of blood from the genitalia *(detumescence),* and that detumescence brings the body back to its resting state. If orgasm occurs, resolution is rapid; if it does not occur, resolution may take 2 to 6 hours and may be associated with irritability and discomfort. Tables 21.4 and 21.5 describe the male and female sexual response cycles.

Answers 21.32–21.34

21.32 The answer is C

21.33 The answer is K

21.34 The answer is J
In fetishism the sexual focus is on objects (such as shoes, gloves, pantyhose, and stockings) that are intimately associated with the human body. The particular fetish may be linked to someone involved closely with the patient during childhood, and has some quality associated with that loved, needed, or even traumatizing person. Voyeurism is the recurrent preoccupation with fantasies and acts that involve observing people who are naked or engaging in sexual activity. It is also known as scopophilia. Masturbation to orgasm usually occurs during or after the event.

Frotteurism is usually characterized by the male's *rubbing up against a fully clothed woman to achieve orgasm.* The acts usually occur in crowded places, particularly subways and buses. Exhibitionism is the recurrent urge to expose one's genitals to a stranger or an unsuspecting person. Sexual excitement occurs in anticipation of the exposure, and orgasm is brought about by masturbation during or after the event.

Persons with sexual masochism have a recurrent preoccupation with sexual urges and fantasies involving the act of being humiliated, beaten, bound, or otherwise made to suffer. Persons with sexual sadism have fantasies involving harm to others. According to psychoanalytic theory, sexual sadism is a defense against fears of castration—the persons with sexual sadism do to others what they fear will happen

TABLE 21.4

Male Sexual Response Cycle[a]

Organ	Excitement Phase	Orgasmic Phase	Resolution Phase
	Lasts several minutes to several hours; heightened excitement before orgasm, 30 seconds to 3 minutes	3 to 15 seconds	10 to 15 minutes; if no orgasm, $1/2$ to 1 day
Skin	Just before orgasm: sexual flush inconsistently appears; maculopapular rash originates on abdomen and spreads to anterior chest wall, face, and neck and can include shoulders and forearms	Well-developed flush	Flush disappears in reverse order of appearance; inconsistently appearing film of perspiration on soles of feet and palms of hands
Penis	Erection in 10 to 30 seconds caused by vasocongestion of erectile bodies of corpus cavernosa of shaft; loss of erection may occur with introduction of asexual stimulus, loud noise; with heightened excitement, size of glans and diameter of penile shaft increase further	Ejaculation; emission phase marked by three to four 0.8-second contractions of vas, seminal vesicles, prostate; ejaculation proper marked by 0.8-second contractions of urethra and ejaculatory spurt of 12 to 20 inches at age 18, decreasing with age to seepage at 70	Erection: partial involution in 5 to 10 seconds with variable refractory period; full detumescence in 5 to 30 minutes
Scrotum and testes	Tightening and lifting of scrotal sac and elevation of testes; with heightened excitement, 50 percent increase in size of testes over unstimulated state and flattening against perineum, signaling impending ejaculation	No change	Decrease to baseline size because of loss of vasocongestion; testicular and scrotal descent within 5 to 30 minutes after orgasm; involution may take several hours if no orgasmic release takes place
Cowper's glands	2 to 3 drops of mucoid fluid that contain viable sperm are secreted during heightened excitement	No change	No change
Other	Breasts: inconsistent nipple erection with heightened excitement before orgasm Myotonia: semispastic contractions of facial, abdominal, and intercostal muscles Tachycardia: up to 175 beats a minute Blood pressure: rise in systolic 20 to 80 mm; in diastolic 10 to 40 mm Respiration: increased	Loss of voluntary muscular control Rectum: rhythmical contractions of sphincter Heart rate: up to 180 beats a minute Blood pressure: up to 40 to 100 mm systolic; 20 to 50 mm diastolic Respiration: up to 40 respirations a minute	Return to baseline state in 5 to 10 minutes

[a]A desire phase consisting of sex fantasies and desire to have sex precedes excitement phase.

to them. Pleasure is derived from expressing the aggressive instinct.

Transvestic fetishism is marked by fantasies and sexual urges by heterosexual men to dress in female clothes for purposes of arousal and as an adjunct to masturbation or coitus. Transvestic fetishism begins typically in childhood or early adolescence. As years pass, some men with transvestic fetishism want to dress and live permanently as women. Such persons are classified as persons with transvestic fetishism, with gender dysphoria.

Sexual desire disorders are divided into two classes: hypoactive sexual desire disorder, characterized by a deficiency or the absence of sexual fantasies and of desire for sexual activity, and *sexual aversion disorder*, characterized by an aversion to and avoidance of genital sexual contact with a sexual partner. Hypoactive sexual desire disorder is more common than sexual aversion disorder. An estimated 20 percent of the total population have hypoactive sexual desire disorder.

Dyspareunia is recurrent or *persistent genital* pain occurring before, during, or after intercourse in either the man or the woman. Dyspareunia should not be diagnosed when an organic

basis for the pain is found or when, in a woman, it is caused exclusively by vaginismus or by a lack of lubrication.

Vaginismus is an *involuntary muscle constriction* of the outer third of the vagina that interferes with penile insertion and intercourse.

Answers 21.35–21.39

21.35 The answer is B

21.36 The answer is C

21.37 The answer is A

21.38 The answer is A

21.39 The answer is D

Sexuality depends on four interrelated psychosexual factors: sexual identity, gender identity, sexual orientation, and sexual behavior. These factors affect personality, development, and functioning.

Sexual identity is the pattern of a person's biological sexual characteristics: *chromosomes*, external and internal genitalia,

TABLE 21.5

Female Sexual Response Cycle[a]

Organ	Excitement Phase	Orgasmic Phase	Resolution Phase
	Lasts several minutes to several hours; heightened excitement before orgasm, 30 seconds to 3 minutes	3 to 15 seconds	10 to 15 minutes; if no orgasm, $\frac{1}{2}$ to 1 day
Skin	Just before orgasm: sexual flush inconsistently appears; maculopapular rash originates on abdomen and spreads to anterior chest wall, face, and neck; can include shoulders and forearms	Well-developed flush	Flush disappears in reverse order of appearance; inconsistently appearing film of perspiration on soles of feet and palms of hands
Breasts	Nipple erection in two-thirds of women, venous congestion and areolar enlargement; size increases to one fourth over normal	Breasts may become tremulous	Return to normal in about $\frac{1}{2}$ hour
Clitoris	Enlargement in diameter of glans and shaft; just before orgasm, shaft retracts into prepuce	No change	Shaft returns to normal position in 5 to 10 seconds; detumescence in 5 to 30 minutes; if no orgasm, detumescence takes several hours
Labia majora	Nullipara: elevate and flatten against perineum Multipara: congestion and edema	No change	Nullipara: increase to normal size in 1 to 2 minutes Multipara: decrease to normal size in 10 to 15 minutes
Labia minora	Size increased 2 to 3 times over normal; change to pink, red, deep red before orgasm	Contractions of proximal labia minora	Return to normal within 5 minutes
Vagina	Color change to dark purple; vaginal transudate appears 10 to 30 seconds after arousal; elongation and ballooning of vagina; lower third of vagina constricts before orgasm	3 to 15 contractions of lower third of vagina at intervals of 0.8 second	Ejaculate forms seminal pool in upper two thirds of vagina; congestion disappears in seconds or, if no orgasm, in 20 to 30 minutes
Uterus	Ascends into false pelvis; labor-like contractions begin in heightened excitement just before orgasm	Contractions throughout orgasm	Contractions cease, and uterus descends to normal position
Other	Myotonia A few drops of mucoid secretion from Bartholin's glands during heightened excitement Cervix swells slightly and is passively elevated with uterus	Loss of voluntary muscular control Rectum: rhythmical contractions of sphincter Hyperventilation and tachycardia	Return to baseline status in seconds to minutes Cervix color and size return to normal, and cervix descends into seminal pool

[a]A desire phase consisting of sex fantasies and desire to have sex precedes excitement phase.

hormonal composition, *gonads, and secondary sex characteristics.* In normal development, these characteristics form a cohesive pattern that leaves persons in no doubt about their sex.

Gender identity is a person's *sense of maleness or femaleness.* By the age of 2 or 3 years, almost everyone has a firm conviction that "I am male" or "I am female." Gender identity results from an almost infinite series of clues derived from experiences with family members, peers, and teachers and from cultural phenomena. For instance, male infants tend to be handled more vigorously and female infants to be cuddled more. Fathers spend more time with their infant sons than with their daughters, and they also tend to be more aware of their sons' adolescent concerns than of their daughters' anxieties. Boys are more likely than girls to be physically disciplined. A child's sex affects parental tolerance for aggression and reinforcement or extinction of activity and of intellectual, aesthetic, and athletic interests. Physical characteristics derived from a person's biological sex (e.g., physique, body shape, and physical dimensions) interrelate with an intricate system of stimuli, including rewards, punishment, and parental gender labels, to establish gender goals.

Sexual orientation describes the *object of a person's sexual impulses:* heterosexual (opposite sex), homosexual (same sex), or bisexual (both sexes). In the United States, research indicates that 2.8 percent of men and 1.4 percent of women identify themselves as homosexual. These numbers are compatible with figures from Western European countries as well. However, a higher percentage of persons have had at least one same-sex experience in their lives. Additionally, gay people more typically settle in urban areas, so the incidence of homosexuality in some large cities is as high as 9 or 10 percent.

Sexual behavior includes *desire, fantasies,* pursuit of partners, autoeroticism, and all the activities engaged in to express and gratify sexual needs. It is an amalgam of psychological and physiological responses to internal and external stimuli.

Answers 21.40–21.42

21.40 The answer is A

21.41 The answer is B

21.42 The answer is A

Treatment of sexual dysfunction tends to be short term and behaviorally oriented. Specific exercises are prescribed to help the couple with their particular problem. Sexual dysfunction often involves a fear of inadequate performance. Thus, couples are specifically prohibited from any sexual play other than that prescribed by the therapist. Initially, *intercourse is interdicted*, and couples learn to give and receive bodily pleasure without the pressure of performance. Beginning exercises usually focus on heightening sensory awareness to touch, sight, sound, and smell.

During those exercises, called *sensate focus exercises,* the couple is given much reinforcement to lessen anxiety. They are urged to use fantasies to distract them from obsessive concerns about performance, which is termed *spectatoring*. The needs of both the dysfunctional partner and the nondysfunctional partner are considered. If either partner becomes sexually excited by the exercises, the other is encouraged to bring him or her to orgasm by manual or oral means. That procedure is important to keep the nondysfunctional partner from sabotaging the treatment. Open communication between the partners is urged, and the expression of mutual needs is encouraged. Resistances, such as claims of fatigue or not enough time to complete the exercises, are common and must be dealt with by the therapist. Genital stimulation is eventually added to general body stimulation. The couple is taught sequentially to try various positions for intercourse without necessarily completing the act, and to use varieties of stimulating techniques before they are permitted to proceed with intercourse.

The specific exercises vary with differing presenting complaints, and special techniques are used to treat the various dysfunctions. In cases of vaginismus, for instance, the woman is advised to dilate her vaginal opening with her fingers or with size-graduated vaginal dilators as part of the therapy. In cases of premature ejaculation, an exercise known as the *squeeze technique* is used *to raise the threshold of penile excitability*. In that exercise the man or the woman stimulates the erect penis until the earliest sensations of impending orgasm and ejaculation are felt. Penile stimulation is then stopped abruptly, and the coronal ridge of the penis is squeezed forcibly for several seconds. The technique is repeated several times. A variation is the stop–start technique in which stimulation is interrupted for several seconds but no squeeze is applied. Masturbation to the point of imminent orgasm raises the threshold of excitability to a more tolerant stimulation level. The man is encouraged to focus on sensations of excitement rather than distract himself from them. This makes him more familiar with his excitement pattern and lets him feel in control rather than overwhelmed by sensations of arousal. Communication between the partners is improved, because the man must let his partner know his level of sexual excitement so that she can squeeze his penis before the ejaculatory process has started. Sex therapy has been successful with some premature ejaculators; however, a subgroup of dysfunctional men may need pharmacotherapy as well.

A man with sexual desire disorder or erectile disorder is sometimes told to masturbate to demonstrate that full erection and ejaculation are possible. A woman with lifelong female orgasmic disorder is directed to masturbate, sometimes using a vibrator. Kegel's exercises may be introduced to strengthen the pubococcygeal muscles; that is, the woman is encouraged to contract her abdominal and perineal muscles at various times, including during masturbation and coitus. When a man has erectile disorder, the woman may be instructed to stimulate or tease his penis. The same technique is used with men who suffer from retarded ejaculation, with stimulation sometimes involving a vibrator. Retarded ejaculation is managed by extravaginal ejaculation initially, and gradual vaginal entry after stimulation to the point of near ejaculation.

22 ▲

Gender Identity Disorders

Gender identity is the basic, firm sense that one is male or female. For most people this is not even remotely an issue. One is clearly either male or female, and this recognition is irrefutable from about the age of 3 on. However, for those individuals with gender identity disorder, this bedrock sense of oneself is profoundly altered. People with gender identity disorders frequently describe themselves as being "trapped in the wrong body," have an all-consuming need to belong to the opposite sex, and usually report that these feelings have been present from childhood.

The revised fourth edition of the *Diagnostic and Statistical Manual of Mental Disorders* (DSM-IV-TR) describes gender identity disorder as having two components: a strong cross-gender identification, and a persistent sense of discomfort with the person's own sex. Persons with a disorder have a pervasive sense that they are of the opposite sex and do not accept the fact of their own sex.

It is important to differentiate sexual orientation from gender identity. Orientation refers to the object of a person's sexual feelings and behavior: hetero-, homo-, or bisexual orientations. Gender identity is a person's inner conviction of being male or female. Many times male to female transsexuals define themselves as heterosexual because they experience themselves as females attracted to males. Another important term is transgender, which refers to an individual who has sexual characteristics of both male and female (i.e., breasts and a penis). Transvestism refers to the dressing in the opposite sex's clothing and presenting as the opposite sex, but still having a clear sense of one's original gender. For instance, a man who knows he is a man dressing as a woman. Transvestism is not considered a gender identity disorder.

Gender identity disorders are reported to occur more often in men than in women, but this may reflect an increased sensitivity to the disorder in boys. The causes of gender identity disorders are not yet known. Research has focused both on biological forces, and psychosocial and developmental ones.

The student should study the questions and answers below for a useful review of these disorders.

HELPFUL HINTS

The student should know the gender identity syndromes and terms listed below.

- adrenogenital syndrome
- agenesis
- ambiguous genitals
- androgen insensitivity syndrome
- asexual
- assigned sex
- Barr chromatin body
- bisexuality
- buccal smear
- cross-dressing
- cross-gender
- cryptorchid testis
- dysgenesis
- effeminate boys and masculine girls
- gender confusion
- gender identity
- gender identity disorder not otherwise specified
- gender role

- genotype
- hermaphroditism
- heterosexual orientation
- homosexual orientation
- hormonal treatment
- intersex conditions
- Klinefelter's syndrome
- male habitus
- phenotype
- prenatal androgens
- pseudohermaphroditism
- rough-and-tumble play
- sex of rearing
- sex-reassignment surgery
- sex steroids
- sexual object choice
- testicular feminization syndrome
- transsexualism
- transvestic fetishism
- Turner's syndrome
- virilized genitals
- X-linked

▲ QUESTIONS

DIRECTIONS: Each of the incomplete statements or questions below are followed by five suggested completions or responses. Select the *one* that is *best* in each case.

22.1 True statements about the epidemiology of gender identity disorders include

A. As many as five boys are referred for each girl referred.

B. Among a sample of 4- to 5-year-old boys referred for a range of clinical problems, the reported desire to be the opposite sex was 15 percent.

C. Most parents of children with gender identity disorder report that cross-gender behaviors were apparent before age 3.

D. The prevalence rate of transsexualism is estimated to be about 1 case per 10,000 males.

E. All of the above

22.2 Gender-dysphoric adults may be

A. homosexual

B. heterosexual

C. bisexual

D. asexual

E. all of the above

22.3 Nonhomosexual gender-dysphoric adults

A. are equally divided between males and females

B. typically seek help for their disorders in their early 20s

C. typically seek help for their disorder at the same age as homosexual gender-dysphoric adults

D. most often have prodromes of the disorder present before puberty

E. generally qualify for a DSM-IV-TR diagnosis of gender identity disorder in childhood

22.4 Most empirical evidence suggests that

A. The three main types of nonhomosexual gender identity disorder in males are superficially variant forms of the same condition.

B. Nonhomosexual and homosexual gender identity disorders are etiologically different conditions.

C. Nonhomosexual gender identity disorder is related etiologically to transvestic fetishism.

D. Homosexual gender identity disorder is related etiologically to typical homosexuality.

E. All of the above

DIRECTIONS: Each set of lettered headings below is followed by a list of numbered phrases. For each numbered, select

A. if the item is associated with *A only*

B. if the item is associated with *B only*

C. if the item is associated with *both A and B*

D. if the item is associated with *neither A or B*

Questions 22.5–22.8

A. Ethel Person and Lionel Ovesey

B. Robert Stoller

C. Both

D. Neither

22.5 Transexualism in males originates from unresolved separation anxiety during the separation-individuation phase of infantile development

22.6 Developmental theory begins with the grandmother of the future transsexual

22.7 Biological males who fall within the DSM-IV-TR category of gender identity disorder and are sexually attracted to males are true transsexuals

22.8 Psychoanalytic theorists of gender identity disorder

Questions 22.9–22.11

A. Homosexual gender identity disorder

B. Nonhomosexual gender identity disorder

C. Both

D. Neither

22.9 Surreptitious cross-dressing in childhood

22.10 Most establish relationships with women at some point and many marry and father children

22.11 More likely to pursue sex-reassignment surgery

DIRECTIONS: Each group of questions below consists of lettered headings followed by a list of numbered statements or descriptions. For each numbered statement or description, select the *one* lettered heading that is most closely associated with it. Each heading can be used once, more than once, or not at all.

Questions 22.12–22.15

A 25-year-old patient called Charles requested a sex-change operation. Charles had for 3 years lived socially and been employed as a man. For the past 2 years, Charles had been the housemate, economic provider, and husband-equivalent of a bisexual woman who had fled from a bad marriage. Her two young children regarded Charles as their stepfather and they had a strong affectionate bond.

In social appearance, the patient passed as a not very virile man whose sexual development in puberty could be conjectured to have been delayed or hormonally deficient. Charles's voice was pitched low but was not baritone. Charles wore bulky clothing to camouflage tightly bound, flattened breasts. A strap-on penis produced a masculine-looking bulge in the pants; it was so constructed that in case of social necessity, it could be used as a urinary conduit in the standing position. Without success the patient had tried to obtain a mastectomy so that in summer only a T-shirt could be worn while working outdoors as a heavy construction machine operator. Charles had also been unsuccessful in trying to get a prescription for testosterone to produce male secondary sex characteristics and to suppress menses. The patient wanted a hysterectomy and an oophorectomy and looked forward to obtaining a successful phalloplasty.

The patient's history was straightforward in its account of progressive recognition in adolescence of being able to fall in love only with a woman, following a tomboyish childhood that had finally consolidated into the transsexual role and identity.

A physical examination revealed normal female anatomy, which the patient found incongruous and a source of continual distress. The endocrine laboratory results were within normal limits for a woman.

    A. Gender identity
    B. Gender role
    C. Sexual identity
    D. Sexual orientation

22.12 Charles recognized in adolescence that she could fall in love only with a woman.

22.13 Charles was regarded by the two young children of her housemate as their stepfather.

22.14 The physical examination revealed normal female anatomy, and the endocrine laboratory results were within normal limits for a woman.

22.15 In a subsequent interview, Charles stated that she viewed herself as a man.

Questions 22.16–22.20

    A. Klinefelter's syndrome
    B. Turner's syndrome
    C. Congenital virilizing adrenal hyperplasia
    D. True hermaphroditism
    E. Androgen insensitivity syndrome

22.16 A 17-year-old girl presented to a clinic with primary amenorrhea and no development of secondary sex characteristics. She was short in stature and had a webbed neck.

22.17 A baby was born with ambiguous external genitalia. Further evaluation revealed that both ovaries and testes were present.

22.18 A baby was born with ambiguous external genitalia. Further evaluation revealed that ovaries, a vagina, and a uterus, were normal and intact.

22.19 A buccal smear from a phenotypically female patient revealed that the patient was XY. A further workup revealed undescended testes.

22.20 A tall, thin man presented for infertility problems was found to be XXY.

DIRECTIONS: Select the *one* that is *best* in each case.

22.21 A boy with gender identity disorder

    A. usually begins to display signs of the disorder after age 9
    B. experiences sexual excitement when he cross-dresses
    C. has boys as his preferred playmates
    D. is treated with testosterone
    E. may say that his penis or testes are disgusting

22.22 Girls with gender identity disorder in childhood

    A. regularly have male companions
    B. may refuse to urinate in a sitting position
    C. may assert that they have or will grow a penis
    D. may give up masculine behavior by adolescence
    E. all of the above

22.23 Which of the following statements does *not* apply to the treatment of gender identity disorder?

    A. Adult patients generally enter psychotherapy to learn how to deal with their disorder, not to alter it.
    B. Before sex-reassignment surgery, patients must go through a trial of cross-gender living for at least 3 months.
    C. A one-to-one play relationship is used with boys in which adults role-model masculine behavior.
    D. Hormonal therapy is not required as a preceding event in sex-reassignment surgery.
    E. During hormonal treatments, both males and females need to be watched for hepatic dysfunction and thromboembolic phenomena.

ANSWERS

Gender Identity Disorders

22.1 The answer is E (all)

The prevalence of the gender identity disorder of childhood can only be estimated because no epidemiological studies have been published. A rough estimate can be obtained from two items on Thomas Achenbach's Child Behavior Checklist that are consistent with components of the diagnosis: behaves like opposite sex and wishes to be of opposite sex. In one study, among *a sample of 4- to 5-year-old boys* referred for a range of clinical problems, the reported desire to be of the opposite sex was 15 percent. Among 4- to 5-year-old boys not referred for behavioral problems, it was only 1 percent. For ages 6 to 7, the rates were 2.7 and 0 percent; for ages 8 to 9, 5.1 and 0 percent; and for ages 10 to 11, 1.1 and 2.3 percent. For clinically referred girls, there was more uniformity across the ages, with the highest being 8 percent at age 9 and the lowest being 4 percent. For nonreferred girls, the highest rate was 5 percent at ages 4 to 5 and less than 3 percent for other ages.

As many as five boys are referred for each girl referred, for which several explanations are possible. First, there is greater parental concern with sissiness than with tomboyishness and greater peer group stigma attaches to substantial cross-gender behavior in boys. Thus, there may be an equal prevalence of gender identity disorder in boys and girls but a differential referral rate. Another possibility is that a genuine disparity results from the male's more perilous developmental course. The fundamental mammalian state is female. No sex hormones are required for prenatal female anatomical development (XO children with gonadal dysgenesis [Turner's syndrome] appear female at birth). Sex hormones are required at critical developmental times for male anatomical differentiation. If the mechanisms of behavioral development track anatomical development, the masculine behavioral system requires adequate levels of hormones at the appropriate time for normative expression. Finally, the psychodynamic developmental model explaining the disparate referral rates views both boys and girls as initially identifying with the female parent, with only boys needing to make the developmental shift for later normative male identification.

Most children with a gender identity disorder are referred for clinical evaluation in early grade school. Parents typically report that *cross-gender behaviors were apparent before age 3.*

There is no basis for estimating the proportion of adults who would qualify for a DSM-IV-TR diagnosis of gender identity disorder. The only relevant data are for transsexuals, who comprise only a subgroup of gender-dysphoric adults, and even those figures may be underestimates. The available data (from the United Kingdom, the Netherlands, Sweden, and Australia) place *the prevalence rate of transsexualism* at about 1 case per 10,000 males and 1 in 30,000 females.

22.2 The answer is E (all)

Following a long tradition of classifying cross-gender syndromes according to the patient's sexual orientation, DSM-III and DSM-III-R listed three subtypes of gender identity disorder. The *heterosexual* subtype is attracted to members of the opposite genetic sex, the *homosexual* subtype to members of their own genetic sex, and the *asexual* subtype to neither. DSM-IV-TR continues the tradition while avoiding the customary labels for those orientations. It also added a fourth subtype, bisexual, based on evidence that among gender-dysphoric men, the *bisexual* subtype is at least as common as the heterosexual or asexual subtypes. DSM-IV-TR subtypes are (1) sexually attracted to males, (2) sexually attracted to females, (3) sexually attracted to both, and (4) sexually attracted to neither.

22.3 The answer is D

Most gender-dysphoric adults of the homosexual subtype would have qualified for a DSM-IV-TR diagnosis of gender identity disorder in childhood, with their adult behavior simply being a continuation of their childhood disorder. Both males and females of that subtype tend to present for clinical attention for the first time in their mid-20s.

Nonhomosexual gender-dysphoric adults (*the great majority of whom are males*) *typically seek help for their disorder in their mid-30s—a* striking *difference from the homosexual subtype.* If the age of onset is considered to be the point at which they first qualify for a DSM-IV-TR diagnosis of gender identity disorder, they *generally have an adolescent or adult onset.* However, *in most cases prodromes of the disorder were present before puberty.*

22.4 The answer is E (all)

Most empirical evidence suggests that *the three main types of nonhomosexual gender identity disorder in males* (heterosexual, bisexual, and asexual) are superficially variant forms of the same condition; that *nonhomosexual and homosexual gender identity disorder are etiologically different conditions;* that *nonhomosexual gender identity disorder is related etiologically to transvestic fetishism;* and that *homosexual gender identity disorder is related etiologically to typical homosexuality.*

The conclusion that heterosexual, bisexual, and asexual gender identity disorders are superficially variant forms of the same condition is based on a wide variety of evidence. Similar majorities of men with heterosexual, bisexual, and asexual gender identity disorder acknowledge some history of transvestic fetishism; such self-reports are rare in men with homosexual gender identity disorder. Men with heterosexual, bisexual, and asexual gender identity disorder are also similar to each other and dissimilar to men with homosexual gender identity disorder with regard to their degree of recalled childhood femininity, age at clinical presentation, extent of interpersonal heterosexual experience, and a history of erotic arousal in association with thoughts of being a woman.

It is possible that the common denominator linking transvestic fetishism and heterosexual, bisexual, and asexual gender identity disorder is autogynephilia, a male's tendency to be sexually aroused by the thought or image of himself as a woman. Autogynephilia is highly variable in its manifestations. It may be expressed in fantasies of dressing as a woman (transvestic fetishism); in (masturbatory) fantasies of engaging in stereotypically feminine behavior like knitting; in fantasies of gestating, lactating, or menstruating; in fantasies of being treated by other people as a woman; or in fantasies of possessing a woman's body. When an autogynephilic man's favorite sexual fantasy is that of possessing a vagina, he is very likely to develop cross-gender wishes that persist even when he is not sexually aroused, along with a desire for surgical sex-reassignment.

Autogynephilia may be conceived as a modified form of heterosexuality, in which a man's sexual approaches are directed not at external women but at a feminized version of himself. It seems to involve some developmental anomaly in the learning of sexual behavior, because the man's principal erotic object in many cases—for example, the thought or image of himself wearing pantyhose, applying make-up, or knitting—cannot be innate but must have been assembled from experiences. It remains to be discovered whether some men are relatively prone to such developmental anomalies for neurological reasons. The conclusion that homosexual gender identity disorder and typical homosexuality (i.e., homosexuality without gender identity disorder) have etiological commonalities is based on two lines of evidence. The first is that the early manifestations of homosexuality and homosexual gender identity disorder appear rather similar. Research has consistently shown that at least 50 percent of adult homosexual men with no gender identity problems nonetheless recall significant amounts of cross-gender behavior in childhood. Similar, although somewhat less striking, findings were obtained for homosexual women. These observations suggest that the difference between ordinary homosexuality and homosexual gender identity disorder may begin as a difference in degree, which develops during adolescence into a difference in kind.

Answers 22.5–22.8

22.5 The answer is A

22.6 The answer is B

22.7 The answer is B

22.8 The answer is C

As in other areas of psychopathology, *psychoanalytic theories* about gender identity disorders constitute a tradition distinct from biological and other nonbiological approaches. One influential theory is that of Ethel Person and Lionel Ovesey, who advanced the hypothesis that *transsexualism in males originates from unresolved separation anxiety during the separation-individuation phase* of infantile development. To cope with this anxiety, the child resorts to a reparative fantasy of symbiotic fusion with his mother. Adult transsexualism may be understood as an attempt to master that anxiety through sex reassignment surgery, through which the transsexual acts out his unconscious fantasy and symbolically becomes his mother.

According to this hypothesis, male transsexuals vary in the directness with which they proceed to the transsexual resolution. Some individuals never develop any other psychosexual phenomena as defenses against separation anxiety, and they proceed to the transsexual outcome in a straightforward manner. Others develop transvestism or effeminate homosexuality as initial defenses. When those defenses fail in the face of various stressors, the individual regresses to the primitive fantasy of symbiotic fusion with his mother and begins to experience transsexual impulses.

The other major psychoanalytic theory was developed by Robert Stoller to explain the etiology of transsexualism in a specific group of biological males, who would fall within the DSM-IV-TR category of gender identity disorder, sexually attracted to males. Stoller called those males *"true transsexuals."*

The developmental theory begins with the grandmother of the future transsexual who treats her daughter coldly and neither encourages nor models femininity for her. The grandfather has a closer relationship with the daughter, but he encourages masculinity in her. In consequence, the mother of the future transsexual develops a mild gender identity disorder of her own. In adolescence, however, she abandons her conscious transsexual wishes of someday being male and adopts a heterosexual facade. According to this theory, at the unconscious level she nevertheless retains a strong penis envy.

The transsexual's mother eventually enters an empty marriage with a passive and withdrawn husband who is psychologically, if not physically, absent from the household. The final pathogenic process becomes operative when the mother gives birth to an infant son whom she perceives as particularly beautiful and graceful. The boy, who represents her feminized phallus, fulfills her lifelong wish for a penis. The mother–son interaction, described by Stoller as a blissful symbiosis, includes excessively close and prolonged body contact, sometimes with the infant's nude body cradled against the mother's nude body. The mother's behavior expresses her need to treat her son as an extension of her own body.

The transsexual's early experiences, especially the continuous skin-to-skin contact, produce an overidentification with his mother, a blurring of ego boundaries, and eventually a feminine gender identity. The transsexual boy never develops a "heterosexual" relationship with his mother and therefore never develops an oedipal conflict. His femininity is produced nonconflictually and remains a nonconflictual, autonomous form of behavior. This theory does not account for "secondary" transsexuals, notably those who evolve through a transvestite, heterosexual pattern.

Answers 22.9–22.11

22.9 The answer is C

22.10 The answer is B

22.11 The answer is A

Adult homosexual gender-dysphoric persons primarily represent that fraction of gender identity disorder children who did not normalize in gender identity by the end of adolescence. The course of the disorder is continuous, although certain manifestations of it may be driven underground in late childhood or the early teens. *A feminine boy, for example, may cross-dress frequently in connection with fantasy play;* cease cross-dressing entirely from junior high school to early adulthood as he attempts to fit into society or at least to minimize conflicts with family and peers; and then resume cross-dressing in his 20s with the possible ultimate intention of pursuing sex-reassignment surgery.

Homoerotic feelings begin at least by puberty. Some adolescents label themselves initially as homosexual and seek companionship with gay contemporaries. They find they do not really fit in there either, although some adolescent male transsexuals continue to socialize in the homosexual drag circuit because it offers the only available supportive environment. Eventually, homosexual gender-dysphoric persons of both sexes begin to label their erotic attractions in terms of their subjective gender identity. Thus, for example, a female-to-male transsexual will assert that her romantic interest in another woman is heterosexual not lesbian because inside she is really a man.

In young adulthood there is often an increase in cross-dressing and in attempts to pass as the opposite sex. Some patients have already moved into the cross-gender role full-time by the time they present for clinical attention. These developments reflect freedom from parental controls and increased opportunities for self-expression more than intensification of the gender dysphoria. The homosexual type (biological male sexually attracted to males, and biological female sexually attracted to females) of gender identity disorder does not have the character of a progressive disorder. In young males, adoption of the female role is sometimes accompanied by withdrawal from society at large into a subculture consisting mostly of other male-to-female transsexuals.

At initial presentation female patients more often than males are involved in love relationships with same-sex partners. The female partner typically concurs with the patient's self-evaluation that she is really a man and reports that she perceives her lover as a man without a penis. Such partners are often anxious to be part of the transsexual's evaluation.

In terms of observable symptoms, nonhomosexual gender identity disorders may be characterized as progressive disorders with an insidious onset. The course is fairly continuous in some cases; in others, the intensity of symptoms fluctuates to the point that the course might be called episodic. The subjective experience is of a lifelong struggle with feminine longings that change their focus from time to time and may temporarily recede in the face of conflicting desires, but which have always been present in one form or another from the early years.

In most cases the first outward manifestation of the disorder is *surreptitious cross-dressing in childhood* (e.g., in mother's or sister's clothing). Many men also report that they initially began wishing they were female during that period. The boyhood behavior does not, however, exhibit the pervasive pattern of effeminacy required for a childhood diagnosis of gender identity disorder. At puberty, cross-dressing begins to elicit penile erection, and for the next few years or decades, the individual may qualify for a diagnosis of transvestic fetishism. In his 20s or 30s, the person's penile response to cross-dressing begins to wane while at the same time his desire to have a woman's body grows stronger and more insistent. In general, the cross-gender wishes attain the highest intensity by the mid-

30s and remain about the same thereafter. It must be emphasized, however, that the course is highly variable.

Most men with gender identity disorder, sexually attracted to females, sexually attracted to both, or sexually attracted to neither *establish relationships with women at some point in their lives and many marry and father children.* Those who fall in love with a woman often report that, during the early days of the romance, they lose their interest in cross-dressing or surgical sex reassignment. When the relationship becomes routine and the initial excitement subsides, however, the desire to dress or live as a woman reasserts itself.

The course of nonhomosexual gender identity disorders may also be punctuated by periods of increased symptomatology. Men of that type occasionally present during an episode of intensified gender dysphoria, with anguished longings to be female accompanied by frustration and despair at their male state. The disorder tends to be chronic. Its tendency towards cyclical variation in many cases may mislead the patient or his therapist into thinking that the patient has been cured when he would be better regarded as in remission. As a group, *nonhomosexual gender-dysphoric patients are less likely (not more likely) than homosexual gender-dysphoric patients to pursue surgical sex reassignment* to completion. Many simply learn to live with their feelings. Acute episodes of intensified gender dysphoria usually resolve to the pre-episode level after a few months, and patients should be discouraged from taking steps toward establishing themselves as females during such periods.

Answers 22.12–22.15

22.12 The answer is D

22.13 The answer is B

22.14 The answer is C

22.15 The answer is A

Sexual identity (also known as biological sex), is strictly limited to the anatomical and physiological characteristics that indicate whether one is male or female.

Sexual orientation is a person's erotic-response tendency toward men or women or both. Sexual orientation takes into account one's object choice (man or woman) and one's fantasy life—for example, erotic fantasies about men or women or both.

Gender identity is a psychological state that reflects the inner sense of oneself as being male or female. Gender identity is based on culturally determined sets of attitudes, behavior patterns, and other attributes usually associated with masculinity or femininity. The person with a healthy gender identity is able to say with certainty, "I am male" or "I am female."

Gender role is the external behavioral pattern that reflects the person's inner sense of gender identity. It is a public declaration of gender; it is the image of maleness versus femaleness that is communicated to others.

When Charles stated that *she viewed herself as a man,* that was a statement of her gender identity. Since *Charles was regarded by the two young children of her housemate as their stepfather*, that revealed her masculine *gender role.* Charles's sexual identity was confirmed when the *physical examination revealed normal female anatomy*, and the endocrine laboratory results were within normal limits for a woman. Charles's expressed sexual orientation was toward the same sex, as was shown when she stated that she *recognized in adolescence that she could fall in love only with a woman.*

Answers 22.16–22.20

22.16 The answer is B

22.17 The answer is D

22.18 The answer is C

22.19 The answer is E

22.20 The answer is A

In *Turner's syndrome* (see Figure 21.5), one sex chromosome is missing (XO). The result is an absence (agnesis) or minimal development (dysgenesis) of the gonads; no significant sex hormones, male or female, are produced in fetal life or postnatally. The sexual tissues remain in a female resting state. Because the second X chromosome, which seems to be responsible for full femaleness, is missing, the girls have an incomplete sexual anatomy and, lacking adequate estrogens, have *amenorrhea and* develop *no secondary sex characteristics* without treatment. They often have other stigmata, such as a webbed neck, low posterior hairline margin, short stature, and cubitus valgus. The infant is born with normal-appearing female external genitals and so is unequivocally assigned to the female sex and is so reared. All the children develop as unremarkably feminine, heterosexually oriented girls.

True hermaphroditism is characterized by the presence of both ovaries and testes in the same person. The genitals' appearance at birth determines the sex assignment, and the core gender identity is male, female, or hermaphroditic, depending on the family's conviction about the child's sex. Usually, a panel of experts determines the sex of rearing; they base their decision on buccal smears, chromosome studies, and parental wishes.

Congenital virilizing adrenal hyperplasia results from an excess of androgen acting on the fetus. When the condition occurs in girls, excessive fetal androgens from the adrenal gland cause *ambiguous external genitals, ranging from mild clitoral enlargement to* external genitals that look like *a normal scrotal sac, testes, and a penis*; but they also have *ovaries, a vagina, and a uterus* (Figure 22.1).

Androgen insensitivity syndrome, a congenital X-linked recessive-trait disorder, results from an inability of the target tissues to respond to androgens. Unable to respond, the fetal tissues remain in their female resting state, and the central nervous system is not organized as masculine. The infant at birth *appears to be female*, although she is later found to have *undescended testes*, which produce the testosterone to which the tissues do not respond, and minimal or absent internal sexual organs. Secondary sex characteristics at puberty are female because of the small but sufficient amounts of estrogens typically produced by the testes. The patients invariably sense themselves to be female and are feminine. They are clinically considered to be female. Intersex conditions, such as androgen insensitivity syndrome and congenital adrenal hyperplasia, are diagnosed as gender identity disorders not otherwise specified.

In *Klinefelter's syndrome* the person (usually *XXY*) has a male habitus, under the influence of the Y chromosome, but the effect is weakened by the second X chromosome. Although the patient is born with a penis and testes, the testes are small and *infertile*, and the penis may also be small. Beginning in adolescence, some patients develop gynecomastia and other feminine-appearing contours. Their sexual desire is usually weak. Sex assignment and rearing should lead to a clear sense of male-ness, but the patients often have gender disturbances, ranging from transsexualism to an intermittent desire to put on women's clothes. As a result of lessened androgen production, the fetal hypogonadal state in some patients seems to have interfered with the completion of the central nervous system organization that should underlie masculine behavior. In fact, patients may have any of a wide variety of neuro- and psychopathologies, ranging from emotional instability to mental retardation.

22.21 The answer is E

A boy with gender identity disorder *may say that his penis or testes are disgusting* and that he would be better off without them. Persons with this disorder *usually begin to display signs of the disorder before age 4 (not after age 9),* although it may present at any age. Cross-dressing may be part of the disorder, but boys *do not experience sexual excitement when they cross-dress.* A boy with a gender identity disorder is generally preoc-cupied with female stereotypical activities and usually *has girls (not boys) as his preferred playmates.* Gender identity disorder *is not treated with testosterone.*

22.22 The answer is E (all)

Girls with gender identity disorder in childhood *regularly have male companions* and an avid interest in sports and rough-and-tumble play; they show no interest in dolls and playing house. In a few cases a girl with this disorder *may refuse to urinate in a sitting position, may assert that she has or will grow a penis,* does not want to grow breasts or men-struate, and that she will grow up to become a man. Girls with gender identity disorder in childhood *may give up masculine behavior by adolescence.*

22.23 The answer is D

Hormone treatment is required and must be received by patients for about a year prior to sex-reassignment surgery, with estradiol and progesterone in male-to-female changes and testosterone in female-to-male changes. Many transsexuals like the changes in their bodies that occur as a result of that treatment, and some stop at that point, not progressing on to surgery. Another requirement before sex-reassignment surgery is that patients *must go through a trial of cross-gender living for at least 3 months* and in many cases up to 1 year. *Adult patients* generally *enter psychotherapy to learn how to deal with their condition, not to alter it.* In boys with

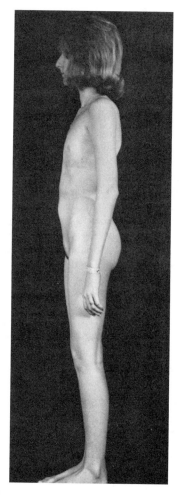

FIGURE 22.1

A phenotypic female with XY karyotype. The vaginal canal was normal without clitoral enlargement. At laparotomy, dysgenetic gonads and a uterus with Fallopian tubes were present. On cyclic estrogen-progestogen therapy, menses were induced at regular intervals and good breast development resulted.

gender identity disorder, a one-to-one play relationship is used, in which *adults or peers role-model masculine behavior. During hormonal treatments,* both males and females need to be watched for hepatic dysfunction and thromboembolic phenomena.

23 ▲

Eating Disorders

Severe disturbances in eating behavior, defined as eating disorders in the revised fourth edition of the *Diagnostic and Statistical Manual of Mental Disorders* (DSM-IV-TR), have been characterized as a cross-cultural syndrome associated with highly developed countries, especially the United States.

Anorexia nervosa is defined as occurring at onset in a person, usually an adolescent girl, who refuses to maintain a minimally normal body weight, fears gaining weight, and has a disturbed perception of body shape and size. Bulimia nervosa is characterized by a person engaging in binge eating and using inappropriate and dangerous compensatory methods, such as induced vomiting or use of laxatives, to prevent weight gain. Besides those who clearly fit diagnostic criteria for these disorders, there are many others who may exhibit various aspects and degrees of them. Bulimia nervosa is more common than anorexia nervosa.

Patients tend to be female (although there is increasing evidence of these disorders in males) who are highly achieving and perfectionistic and come from families with similar characteristics. Psychological struggles center around issues of autonomy and control, as well as on conflicts surrounding sexual maturation. Frequently, parents of these patients have histories themselves of similar behaviors and struggles. There is often a family history of depression. Biological treatments for both disorders may involve the use of antidepressant medications, with serotonin and norepinephrine neurotransmitters being particularly implicated.

Anorexia nervosa and bulimia nervosa are strikingly similar in some regards but differ dramatically in others. The student needs to be aware of these differences as well as of the various treatments available. Treatment strategies usually involve a combination of biological, psychosocial, and psychological approaches. Family therapy has traditionally been considered a mainstay of treatment, especially with younger anorexic patients. Treatment in some severe cases of both disorders is ineffective, and death can result. In fact, eating disorders have one of the highest mortality rates of all psychiatric illnesses.

The student should study the questions and answers below for a useful review of these disorders.

HELPFUL HINTS

The student should know and be able to define these terms.

- ACTH
- amenorrhea
- anorexia nervosa
- aversive conditioning
- binge eating
- borderline personality disorder
- bulimia nervosa
- compulsive eating
- cyproheptadine (Periactin)
- denial
- eating disorder not otherwise specified
- ECT
- edema
- family therapy
- fluoxetine
- geophagia
- hyperphagia
- hypersexuality
- hypersomnia
- hypokalemic alkalosis
- hypothermia
- imipramine (Tofranil)
- Kleine-Levin syndrome
- Klüver-Bucy syndrome
- lanugo
- laxative and diuretic abuse
- LH
- MHPG
- obsessive-compulsive disorder
- postbinge anguish
- purging
- psychodynamic factors
- pyloric stenosis
- satiety
- self-stimulation
- ST segment depression
- T waves

▲ QUESTIONS

DIRECTIONS: Each of the incomplete statements below is followed by five suggested completions. Select the *one* that is *best* in each case.

23.1 Studies suggest that

    A. The overall incidence of anorexia nervosa has decreased in the last 50 years.

    B. The overall incidence of bulimia nervosa has increased in the last 50 years.

    C. The incidence rate of anorexia nervosa in industrialized countries is approximately 20 per 100,000 population per year.

    D. The lifetime prevalence rate of anorexia nervosa in the United States has been estimated to be 5 percent.

    E. Bulimia nervosa has a prevalence rate of about 10 percent in adolescents and young adult women.

23.2 Anorexia nervosa patients have been reported to have a high rate of

A. major depression
B. anxiety disorders
C. obsessive-compulsive disorder
D. social phobia
E. all of the above

23.3 Neuroendocrine changes caused by anorexia nervosa include

A. decreased CRH (corticotrophin-releasing hormone)
B. increased LH (luteinizing hormone)
C. increased FSH (follicle stimulating hormone)
D. hyperreactivity of the hypothalamic-pituitary-adrenal axis
E. all of the above

23.4 The binge-eating/purging type of anorexia nervosa when compared to the restricting type is more often associated with

A. suicide attempts
B. drug abuse
C. premorbid obesity
D. familial obesity
E. all of the above

23.5 Biological complications of eating disorders may include

A. salivary gland and pancreatic inflammation
B. gastric or esophageal tearing or rupture
C. cardiac arrhythmias, loss of cardiac muscle, and cardiomyopathy
D. leukopenia
E. all of the above

23.6 Medical complications of eating disorders related to weight loss include all of the following *except*

A. erosion of dental enamel with corresponding decay
B. bradycardia
C. constipation and delayed gastric emptying
D. abnormal taste sensation
E. osteoporosis

23.7 Ipecac intoxication is associated with

A. pericardial pain and cardiac failure
B. dyspnea
C. generalized muscle weakness
D. hypotension
E. all of the above

23.8 Characteristic laboratory test results in anorexia nervosa include

A. ST-segment and T-wave changes on ECG
B. decreased serum cholesterol levels
C. increased fasting serum glucose concentrations
D. decreased serum salivary amylase concentrations
E. all of the above

DIRECTIONS: The questions below consist of lettered headings followed by a list of numbered phrases. For each numbered phrase, select

A. if the item is associated with *A only*
B. if the item is associated with *B only*
C. if the item is associated with *both A and B*
D. if the item is associated with *neither A nor B*

Questions 23.9–23.16

A. Anorexia nervosa
B. Bulimia nervosa
C. Both
D. Neither

23.9 Severe weight loss and amenorrhea

23.10 Visual agnosia, compulsive licking and biting, hypersexuality

23.11 After 5 to 10 years, at least 50 percent will be markedly improved

23.12 Higher fatality rate

23.13 Family therapy is not widely used

23.14 Cognitive-behavioral therapy is the benchmark, first-line treatment

23.15 Decreased appetite only occurs in the most severe stages

23.16 Body weight of less than 85 percent of the patient's expected weight

DIRECTIONS: Select the most appropriate lettered response for each of the following numbered questions or statements.

23.17 According to DSM-IV-TR, which of the following laboratory findings is *not* associated with anorexia nervosa?

A. arrhythmias
B. thrombocytopenia
C. metabolic alkalosis
D. elevated liver function tests
E. increased ventricular-brain ratio

23.18 Which of the following features can be associated with bulimia nervosa?

A. undeveloped breasts
B. abnormal insulin secretion
C. widespread endocrine disorder
D. a previous episode of anorexia nervosa
E. body weight at least 15 percent below normal

DIRECTIONS: Each of the incomplete statements below is followed by five suggested completions. Select the *one* that is *best* in each case.

23.19 Anorexia nervosa occurs

A. ten to 20 times more often in females than in males
B. five times more often in males than in females
C. in 4 percent of adolescent girls
D. predominantly in the upper economic classes
E. with greatest frequency among young women in professions associated with food preparation

23.20 Anorexia nervosa has a mortality rate of up to approximately

A. 1 percent
B. 18 percent
C. 30 percent
D. 42 percent
E. 50 percent

23.21 Treatments that have shown some success in ameliorating anorexia nervosa include

A. cyproheptadine
B. electroconvulsive therapy (ECT)
C. chlorpromazine
D. fluoxetine
E. all of the above

23.22 Characteristics of binge-eating disorder include

A. recurrent episodes of binge eating
B. inappropriate compensatory behaviors characteristic of bulimia nervosa
C. binge eating that occurs at least twice a week for less than 6 months
D. fixation on body weight
E. all of the above

Question 23.23

Mary was a gaunt 15-year-old high-school student evaluated at the insistence of her parents, who were concerned about her weight loss. She was 5 feet 3 inches tall and had reached her greatest weight, 100 pounds, a year earlier. Shortly thereafter she decided to lose weight to be more attractive. She felt "chubby" and thought she would be more appealing if she were thinner. First she eliminated all carbohydrate-rich foods, and gradually intensified her dieting until she was eating only a few vegetables a day. She also started a vigorous exercise program. Within 6 months, she was down to 80 pounds. She then became

preoccupied with food and started collecting recipes from magazines in order to prepare gourmet meals for her family. She had difficulty sleeping and was irritable and depressed, having several crying spells every day. Her menses started the previous year, but she had only a few normal periods.

Mary had always had high grades in school and had spent a great deal of time studying. She had never been active socially and had never dated. She was conscientious and perfectionistic in everything she undertook. She had never been away from home as long as a week. Her father was a business manager. Her mother was a housewife who for the past 2 years had a problem with hypoglycemia and was on a low-carbohydrate diet.

During the interview, Mary said she felt fat, even though she weighed 80 pounds, and she described a fear of losing control and eating so much food that she would become obese. She did not feel she was ill and thought that hospitalization was unnecessary.

23.23 The diagnosis of anorexia nervosa can be made on the basis of Mary's

A. 20-pound weight loss
B. feeling fat at a weight of 80 pounds and a height of 5 feet 3 inches
C. having had only a few normal periods
D. fear of becoming obese
E. all of the above

23.24 Features associated with anorexia nervosa include

A. normal hair structure and distribution
B. the fact that 7 to 9 percent of those affected are male
C. onset between the ages of 10 and 30
D. mortality rates of 20 to 25 percent
E. all of the above

ANSWERS

Eating Disorders

23.1 The answer is B

Incidence rates are commonly expressed with eating disorders as the rate per 100,000 of a population per year. One of the major problems in studying the epidemiology of eating disorders over time is the change in criteria for these syndromes since the late 1960s. Despite this problem, studies suggest that *the overall incidence of both anorexia nervosa and bulimia nervosa has increased in the past 50 years.* There was a consistent increase in the registered incidence of anorexia nervosa from 1931 to 1986 in cases presenting to the health care system in several industrialized countries. A study in northeastern Scotland showed that between 1965 and 1991 there was almost a sixfold increase in the incidence of anorexia nervosa—from 3/100,000 to 17/100,000. A study conducted in southwest London between July 1991 and June 1992 showed an incidence of anorexia nervosa to be 2.7 cases per 100,000 total population. In females aged 15 to 29 years, the incidence was 19.2 cases

per 100,000. In Rochester, Minnesota a recent study found an overall adjusted incidence for females of 14.6 per 100,000; for men, the corresponding figure was 1.8. When estimates are based on the population at large, *the incidence rate of anorexia nervosa in industrialized countries is estimated at 8.1 (not 20.1) per 100,000 population per year.* A recent prevalence study of anorexia nervosa was found to be 20.2 cases per 100,000 population (0.02 percent total population) in the United Kingdom. In a recent study conducted *in the United States, lifetime prevalence rates for anorexia nervosa were found to be 0.51 percent (narrowly defined) and 3.7 percent (not 5 percent) (broadly defined).* A summary of numerous prevalence studies across European countries reported an average prevalence of anorexia nervosa, using strict diagnostic criteria, of 0.28 percent of young females.

There are very few studies of the incidence of bulimia nervosa. A large representative sample of the Dutch population in Holland showed an incidence of bulimia nervosa at 11.4 per 100,000 population per year during the period from 1985 through 1989.

A review of over 50 prevalence studies of bulimia nervosa conducted from 1981 through 1989 in Europe and the United States showed a remarkable consistency in finding that *bulimia nervosa* had *a prevalence rate of about 3 percent (not 10 percent) in adolescents and young adult women*. Partial or subthreshold eating disorders occur at a far greater frequency in the general community—in about 5 to 10 percent of young women. In a recent Canadian study the lifetime prevalence rate for bulimia nervosa was 1.1 percent for females and 0.1 percent for males. In industrialized countries the prevalence is about 1 percent for bulimia nervosa.

23.2 The answer is E (all)

Anorexia nervosa patients had *a high rate of major depression* (68 percent), *anxiety disorders* (65 percent), *obsessive-compulsive disorder* (26 percent), and *social phobia* (34 percent) in one large study. About one-fourth of patients with the restricting type of anorexia nervosa have a Cluster C (anxious) personality disorder. About 40 percent of patients with the binge eating/purging type of anorexia nervosa have a Cluster B (impulsive) personality disorder diagnosis. They also have a high prevalence (32 percent) of the anxious cluster of personality disorders. Bulimia nervosa patients have considerable comorbidity: with major depressive disorder, varying from 36 to 70 percent; substance abuse, from 18 percent to 32 percent; and Axis II personality disorders, from 28 percent to 77 percent, with a predominance of Cluster B (impulsive) personality disorders.

23.3 The answer is D

Corticotrophin-releasing factor (CRF) is a potent inhibitor of feeding. Emaciated patients with anorexia nervosa have increased concentrations of CSF and CRF, which return to normal range with weight gain. The increased CRF may be one of the physiological mechanisms that maintains the anorexia and abnormal eating behavior in patients with anorexia nervosa. Neuropeptide Y, which stimulates feeding behavior, was found to be elevated in the CSF of underweight and recently weight-restored anorexia nervosa patients. However, in long-term weight-restored anorexia nervosa patients these concentrations return to normal. A reduction of food intake may produce a homeostatic increase in neuropeptide secretion that should serve to stimulate feeding, but this mechanism seems to be ineffective in the anorectic patient. Decreased secretion of gonadotrophin-releasing hormone (GnRH) is the cause of amenorrhea in anorexia nervosa. The secretion of GnRH is highly influenced by the neurotransmitters norepinephrine and serotonin, which help to regulate eating behavior and to influence mood. The relation of these neurotransmitters to GnRH, neuropeptide Y, and CRF secretion in anorexia nervosa is an area of ongoing research and may help to reveal biological risk factors. Amenorrhea is due to diminished secretion of GnRH, which in turn *diminishes (not increases) the pituitary secretion of follicle-stimulating hormone (FSH)* and *luteinizing hormone (LH)*; this in turn is responsible for abnormally low levels of estrogen. Starvation-induced changes such as reduced norepinephrine turnover, *hyperactivity of the hypothalamic-pituitary-adrenal axis*, diminished thyroid-stimulating hormone (TSH) response to thyrotrophin-releasing hormone (TRH), low plasma triiodothyronine (T3) concentrations, and increased basal growth hormone concentrations revert to within the normal range with nutritional rehabilitation.

Because of the role of serotonin in producing satiety or fullness and in regulating impulsive behaviors, a dysfunction of the serotonergic neurotransmitter system has been suspected in bulimia. Normal-weight bulimic patients have decreased prolactin response to the pharmacological challenge test of fenfluramine and methchlorophenylpiperazine (mCPP) compared with controls. High binge frequency in bulimia patients is significantly related to lower CSF5 HIAA than is present in controls. This is some evidence for a cerebral-CNS serotonergic deficiency in bulimia nervosa patients. Table 23.1 presents neuroendocrine changes caused by anorexia nervosa.

23.4 The answer is E (all)

DSM-IV-TR divides anorexia nervosa into two subtypes: the restricting type and the binge-eating/purging type. There are significant differences between anorexia nervosa patients who engage in bulimic or purging behaviors and those who consistently restrict their dietary intake. Impulsive behaviors such as stealing, *drug abuse, suicide attempts*, and self-mutilations are significantly more prevalent in the binge-eating/purging type compared with the restricting type. The bulimic group of anorexia nervosa patients also has a higher prevalence of *premorbid obesity, familial obesity*, mood lability, and debilitating personality characteristics; the latter are often in the context of a Cluster B (impulsive) personality disorder cluster. The binge-eating/purging type of patients are similar to persons with bulimia nervosa in behaviors and characteristics. They are not classified as having bulimia nervosa because they have lost large amounts of weight and meet the criteria for anorexia nervosa. The specific mechanisms by which the binge-eating/purging type patients are able to obtain and maintain large weight losses are still unknown to researchers and are being investigated.

23.5 The answer is E

Most of the physiological and metabolic changes in anorexia nervosa are secondary to the starvation state or purging behaviors. These changes usually revert to normal with nutritional rehabilitation or cessation of the purging behavior (see Table 23.2).

23.6 The answer is A (all)

Erosion of dental enamel with corresponding decay is associated with the purging behavior of eating disorders, not to the weight loss of eating disorders. Table 23.2 lists medical complications related to weight loss and purging in eating disorders. Among these complications are *bradycardia, delayed gastric emptying*, disturbed *taste sensation*, and *osteoporosis*.

23.7 The answer is E (all)

Bulimia nervosa patients who engage in self-induced vomiting and who abuse purgative or diuretic medications are susceptible to the same complications as anorexia nervosa patients involved in this behavior. Exposure to gastric juices through vomiting can cause severe erosion of the teeth, pathological pulp exposures, diminished masticatory ability, and an unaesthetic facial appearance. Parotid gland enlargement is associated with elevated serum amylase concentrations and is commonly observed in patients who binge and vomit. Acute dilatation of the stomach is a rare emergency condition for patients who binge eat, and esophageal tears can occur in the process of self-induced vomiting. Severe abdominal pain in the bulimia nervosa patient should alert the physician to a diagnosis of gastric dilatation

Table 23.1
Neuroendocrine Changes in Anorexia Nervosa and Experimental Starvation

Hormone	Anorexia Nervosa	Weight Loss
Corticotropin-releasing hormone (CRH)	Increased	Increased
Plasma cortisol levels	Mildly increased	Mildly increased
Diurnal cortisol difference	Blunted	Blunted
Luteinizing hormone (LH)	Decreased, prepubertal pattern	Decreased
Follicle-stimulating hormone (FSH)	Decreased, prepubertal pattern	Decreased
Growth hormone (GH)	Impaired regulation	Same
	Increased basal levels and limited response to pharmacological probes	
Somatomedin C	Decreased	Decreased
Thyroxine (T_4)	Normal or slightly decreased	Normal or slightly decreased
Triiodothyronine (T_3)	Mildly decreased	Mildly decreased
Reverse T_3	Mildly increased	Mildly increased
Thyrotropin-stimulating hormone (TSH)	Normal	Normal
TSH response to thyrotropin-releasing hormone (TRH)	Delayed or blunted	Delayed or blunted
Insulin	Delayed release	—
C-peptide	Decreased	—
Vasopressin	Secretion uncoupled from osmotic challenge	—
Serotonin	Increased function with weight restoration	—
Norepinephrine	Reduced turnover	Reduced turnover
Dopamine	Blunted response to pharmacological probes	—

and the need for nasal gastric suction, X-rays, and surgical consultation. Cardiac failure caused by cardiomyopathy from ipecac toxication is a medical emergency that usually results in death. Symptoms of *pericardial pain, dyspnea,* and *generalized muscle weakness* associated with *hypotension,* tachycardia, and electrocardiogram (ECG) abnormalities should alert medical personnel to possible ipecac intoxication.

23.8 The answer is A

There are no laboratory tests that can provide a diagnosis of anorexia nervosa. The medical phenomena present in this disorder result from the starvation or purging behaviors. There are several relevant laboratory tests that should be obtained in these patients. A complete blood count will often reveal a leukopenia with a relative lymphocytosis in emaciated anorexia nervosa patients. If binge eating and purging are present, serum electrolytes will reveal a hypokalemic alkalosis. *Fasting serum glucose concentrations are often low (not increased)* during the emaciated phase, and *serum salivary amylase concentrations are often elevated (not decreased)* if the patient is vomiting. An *electrocardiogram may show ST-segment and T-wave changes,* which are usually secondary to electrolyte disturbances; emaciated patients will have hypotension and bradycardia. Adolescents may have an *elevated (not decreased) serum cholesterol level.* All these values revert to normal with nutritional rehabilitation and cessation of purging behaviors. Endocrine changes that occur, such as amenorrhea, mild hypothyroidism, and hypersecretion of corticotrophin-releasing hormone, are due to the underweight condition and revert to normal with weight gain.

Answers 23.9–23.16

23.9 The answer is A

23.10 The answer is D

Table 23.2
Medical and Biological Complications of Eating Disorders

Related to weight loss

Cachexia: Loss of fat, muscle mass, reduced thyroid metabolism (low T_3 syndrome), cold intolerance, and difficulty in maintaining core body temperature

Cardiac: Loss of cardiac muscle; small heart; cardiac arrhythmias, including atrial and ventricular premature contractions, prolonged His bundle transmission (prolonged QT interval), bradycardia, ventricular tachycardia; sudden death

Digestive-gastrointestinal: Delayed gastric emptying, bloating, constipation, abdominal pain

Reproductive: Amenorrhea, low levels of luteinizing hormone (LH) and follicle-stimulating hormone (FSH)

Dermatological: Lanugo (fine baby-like hair over body), edema

Hematological: Leukopenia

Neuropsychiatric: Abnormal taste sensation (?zinc deficiency), apathetic depression, mild cognitive disorder

Skeletal: Osteoporosis

Related to purging (vomiting and laxative abuse)

Metabolic: Electrolyte abnormalities, particularly hypokalemic, hypochloremic alkalosis; hypomagnesemia

Digestive-gastrointestinal: Salivary gland and pancreatic inflammation and enlargement with increase in serum amylase, esophageal and gastric erosion, dysfunctional bowel with haustral dilation

Dental: Erosion of dental enamel, particularly of front teeth, with corresponding decay

Neuropsychiatric: Seizures (related to large fluid shifts and electrolyte disturbances), mild neuropathies, fatigue and weakness, mild cognitive disorder

Reprinted with permission from Yager I. Eating disorders. In: Stoudemire A, ed. *Clinical Psychiatry for Medical Students.* Philadelphia: JB Lippincott; 1990:324.

23.11 The answer is C

23.12 The answer is A

23.13 The answer is B

23.14 The answer is B

23.15 The answer is A

23.16 The answer is A

If bingeing and purging behaviors are occurring in a person who meets diagnostic criteria for anorexia nervosa, bulimia nervosa cannot be the diagnosis. *Severe weight loss and amenorrhea* are two features differentially distinguishing anorexia nervosa from bulimia nervosa.

On rare occasions a central nervous system tumor may be associated with bulimic behaviors. Overeating episodes also occur in the Klüver-Bucy syndrome, which consists of *visual agnosia, compulsive licking and biting,* inability to ignore any stimulus, *and hypersexuality.* Another uncommon syndrome associated with hyperphagia is the Kleine-Levin syndrome, which is characterized by periodic hypersomnia lasting for several weeks.

Ten-year outcome studies in the United States have shown that about one-fourth of anorexic patients recover completely and another *one-half are markedly improved* and functioning fairly well. The other one-fourth includes an overall 7 percent mortality rate and those who are functioning poorly with a chronic underweight condition. Swedish and English studies over a 20- and 30-year period have a mortality rate of 18 percent. Good prognostic indicators across studies include an earlier age of onset (under age 18), no previous hospitalization for the illness, and no purging behaviors. Some factors such as parental conflict, degree of denial, immaturity, and self-esteem have been related to outcome in some studies but not others. Importantly, about half of anorexia nervosa patients will eventually have the symptoms of bulimia, usually within the first year after the onset of anorexia nervosa, which has a higher *fatality rate.*

After between 5 and 10 years about 50 percent of bulimic patients will be fully recovered; 20 percent will continue to meet diagnostic criteria for bulimia nervosa. About one-third of recovered bulimic patients will relapse within 4 years of presentation. Patients with personality disorders marked by problems with impulse control generally have a worse prognosis compared with bulimia nervosa patients with no personality disorder problems.

The severity of illness will determine the intensity of treatment required for the anorexia nervosa patient. Treatment levels can range from an inpatient specialized and multimodal eating disorder unit, to a partial hospitalization or day program, to outpatient care depending on the weight, medical status, and other psychiatric comorbidity of the patient. Decisions about particular treatment modalities and strategies must be based on the needs of the individual patients as well as the capabilities of the treatment setting. Understandably, it has been extremely difficult to subject severely medically ill patients with anorexia nervosa to controlled treatment studies during the emaciated state of the illness. Since patients with anorexia nervosa are resistant to, uninterested in, and fearful of treatment, there are very few (outpatient) controlled treatment studies. Open stud-

ies have indicated that a multifaceted treatment approach is the most effective, which includes medical management, psychoeducation, and one-to-one therapy utilizing cognitive and behavior therapy principles. Controlled studies have shown that youth under the age of 18 do better if they participate in family therapy.

In contrast to the relatively *few outpatient treatment studies of anorexia nervosa,* treatment outcome studies of bulimia nervosa have proliferated since the late 1980s.

Family therapy is not widely used in the treatment of bulimia nervosa, as it is for anorexia nervosa, because most patients with bulimia nervosa are in their 20s or older and live away from their family of origin. There is a consensus that families of younger patients should be involved with their treatment; however, controlled studies are needed to prove this.

A family analysis should be done on all anorexia nervosa patients who are living with their families. On the basis of this analysis, a clinical judgment can be made as to what type of family therapy or counseling is advisable. In some cases family therapy is not possible. However, in those cases, issues of family relationships can be addressed in individual therapy. In some cases, brief counseling sessions with immediate family members may be the extent of family therapy required.

Cognitive-behavioral therapy should be considered the benchmark, first-line treatment for bulimia nervosa. It has been found to be the most effective treatment in over 35 controlled psychosocial studies. About 40 to 50 percent of patients are abstinent from both binge eating and purging at the end of treatment (16 to 20 weeks). Altogether, improvement by a reduction in binge eating and purging occurred in a range from 70 to 95 percent of patients. Additionally, another 30 percent of those who did not show improvement immediately posttreatment nevertheless showed improvement to full recovery 1 year after treatment. In patients with a depressive disorder and bulimia nervosa, cognitive-behavioral therapy was also found to decrease depression.

Cognitive and behavior therapy principles can be applied in both inpatient and outpatient settings in anorexia nervosa, but there are no large-sample-size controlled studies of formal cognitive-behavioral therapy with anorexia nervosa patients.

Generally, a patient with a depressive disorder has a decreased appetite, whereas an anorexia nervosa patient may deny the existence of, yet still have, an appetite. It is *only in the most severe stages of anorexia nervosa that the patient actually has a decreased appetite.*

The diagnostic criteria of anorexia nervosa include a persistent refusal to maintain body weight at or above a minimum expected weight (for example, loss of weight leading to a *body weight of less than 85 percent of the patient's expected weight*) or a failure to gain the expected weight during a period of growth, leading to a body weight less than 85 percent of the expected weight.

23.17 The answer is C

According to DSM-IV-TR, *metabolic alkalosis* (elevated serum bicarbonate) is most often a symptom of bulimia nervosa (not anorexia nervosa) caused by the loss of stomach acid through vomiting. *Arrhythmias,* although rare, and sinus bradycardia are findings discovered on electrocardiography. *Thrombocytopenia* is occasionally seen in bloodwork of patients with anorexia nervosa. *Elevated liver function tests* are common results, and patients often show an *increased ventricular-brain ratio* in brain imaging.

23.18 The answer is D

A previous episode of anorexia nervosa is often associated with bulimia nervosa. This episode may have been fully or only moderately expressed.

Undeveloped and underdeveloped breasts, *abnormal insulin secretion*, widespread *endocrine disorder*, and *body weight at least 15 percent below normal* are all associated with anorexia nervosa, not bulimia nervosa.

23.19 The answer is A

Anorexia nervosa occurs *10 to 20 times more often in females than in males*. Anorexia nervosa is estimated to occur *in about 0.5 percent (not 4 percent) of adolescent girls*. Although the disorder was *initially reported predominantly in the upper economic classes*, recent epidemiological surveys do not show that distribution. The disorder may be seen with *greatest frequency* among young women *in professions that require thinness*, such as modeling and ballet, *not in professions associated with food preparation*.

23.20 The answer is B

Most studies show that anorexia nervosa has a range of mortality rates from 5 percent to *18 percent*.

23.21 The answer is E (all)

Medications can be useful adjuncts in the treatment of anorexia nervosa. The first drug used in treating anorectic patients was *chlorpromazine*. This medication is particularly helpful for severely ill patients who are overwhelmed with constant thoughts of losing weight and behavioral rituals for losing weight. There are few double-blind controlled studies to defini-tively prove this drug's effectiveness for calming such patients and inducing needed weight gain. *Cyproheptadine (Periactin)* in high dosages (up to 28 mg a day) can facilitate weight gain in anorectic restrictors and also has an antidepressant effect. Some recent studies indicate that *fluoxetine* may be effective in pre-venting relapse in patients with anorexia nervosa.

Amitriptyline (Elavil) has been reported to have some benefit in patients with anorexia nervosa, as have imipramine (Tofranil) and desipramine (Norpramin). There is some evidence that *electroconvulsive therapy (ECT)* is beneficial in certain cases of anorexia nervosa associated with major depressive disorder.

23.22 The answer is A

Binge-eating disorder is characterized by *recurrent episodes of binge eating in the absence of the inappropriate compensatory behaviors* characteristic of bulimia nervosa. The binge eating occurs, on average, *at least twice a week for at least (not less than) 6 months*. Patients with this eating disorder are *not fixated on body weight*. Binge-eating disorder is an example of an eating disorder not otherwise specified.

23.23 The answer is E (all)

The diagnosis of anorexia nervosa can be made on the basis of Mary's *20-pound weight loss*, her *feeling fat* at a weight of 80 pounds and a height of 5 feet 3 inches, her having had *only a few normal periods*, and her *fear of becoming obese*.

23.24 The answer is C

Features associated with anorexia nervosa include *onset between the ages of 10 and 30; lanugo* (neonatal-like body hair), not normal hair structure and distribution; *mortality rates of 5 to 18 percent (not 20 to 25 percent); and the fact that 4 to 6 percent (not 7 to 9 percent) of those affected are male*.

Normal Sleep and Sleep Disorders

To understand sleep disorders one must first have a solid understanding of the processes involved in normal sleep. Normal sleep has two essential phases: nonrapid eye movement sleep (NREM) and rapid eye movement sleep (REM). Sleep disorders are often characterized as being either NREM or REM disorders.

NREM sleep is composed of stages 1 through 4, and is characterized as the phase of sleep associated with a strong reduction in physiological functioning. REM sleep, on the other hand, is characterized by a highly active brain with physiological levels similar to the awake state.

REM sleep is associated with dreaming and is characterized by low-voltage random fast activity with sawtooth waves. The four stages of NREM sleep are qualitatively different from REM sleep. Stage 1, the lightest stage, is characterized on an electroencephalogram (EEG) by low-voltage regular activity at three to seven cycles per second. Stage 2 shows a pattern of spindle-shaped tracings at 12 to 14 cycles a second, with slow triphasic waves called K complexes. In stages 3 and 4, delta waves (high voltage activity at 0.5 to 2.5 cycles per second) appear, increasing from less than 50 percent of the tracing in Stage 3 to more than 50 percent in stage 4.

NREM sleep normally changes over to the first REM episode about 90 minutes after a person falls asleep. In disorders such as depression or narcolepsy, this 90-minute latency period is often markedly shortened, meaning that REM sleep begins much sooner in these disorders. Many antidepressants act to suppress REM sleep, thus effectively increasing this latency period back toward normal. The first REM period is usually the shortest, typically lasting less than 10 minutes, with later periods lasting from 15 to 40 minutes each. Most REM sleep normally occurs in the last third of the night, with most of stage 4 sleep occurring in the first third.

Sleep and dreaming appear to be essential to normal functioning, although the necessary amount of sleep can vary greatly from person to person. Many factors interfere with sleep, from emotional or physical stress, to multiple substances and medications. Sleep deprivation can lead to ego disorganization, hallucinations, and delusions, and has been shown to lead to death in animals.

Sleep disorders are very common, with insomnia being the most frequently reported. The revised fourth edition of the *Diagnostic and Statistical Manual of Mental Disorders* (DSM-IV-TR) organizes the disorders first as primary ones (dyssomnias and parasomnias), then as those related to another mental disorder (such as anxiety, depression, or mania), as due to a general medical condition (the physiological effects of the condition on the sleep–wake cycle), and as substance-induced—either due to intoxication or withdrawal, and from either recreational drugs or medications. Dyssomnias are disturbances in the amount, quality, or timing of sleep, and parasomnias are abnormal or physiological events that occur in connection with various sleep stages or during the sleep–wake transition.

Students should be aware of how biological rhythms can affect sleep, and how the 24-hour clock affects the natural body clock of 25 hours. Treatments of sleep disorders, such as the antidepressants mentioned above, as well as many other biological, psychological, and environmental interventions, are based on knowledge of normal sleep anatomy and physiology. To effectively treat sleep disorders, the clinician must have a firm understanding of normal sleep and the factors that interfere with it.

The student should study the questions and answers below for a useful review of these disorders.

HELPFUL HINTS

The student should know and be able to define each of these terms.

- ► acetylcholine
- ► advanced sleep phase syndrome
- ► alveolar hypoventilation syndrome
- ► circadian rhythm sleep disorder
- ► delayed sleep phase syndrome
- ► dysesthesia
- ► dyssomnias
- ► EEG
- ► familial sleep paralysis
- ► hypersomnia
- ► idiopathic CNS hypersomnolence
- ► insomnia:
  nonorganic
  organic
  persistent
  primary
- secondary
  transient
- ► jactatio capitis nocturna
- ► K complexes
- ► Kleine-Levin syndrome

- ▶ melatonin
- ▶ microsleeps
- ▶ narcolepsy
- ▶ nightmare disorder
- ▶ nightmares
- ▶ normal sleep
- ▶ paradoxical sleep
- ▶ parasomnias
- ▶ paroxysmal nocturnal hemoglobinuria
- ▶ *pavor nocturnus, incubus*
- ▶ poikilothermic
- ▶ REM, NREM
- ▶ REM latency
- ▶ sleep apnea
- ▶ sleep deprivation, REM-deprived
- ▶ sleep drunkenness
- ▶ sleep paralysis, sleep attacks
- ▶ sleep patterns
- ▶ sleep-related abnormal swallowing syndrome
- ▶ sleep-related asthma
- ▶ sleep-related bruxism
- ▶ sleep-related cardiovascular symptoms
- ▶ sleep-related cluster headaches and chronic paroxysmal hemicrania
- ▶ sleep-related epileptic seizures
- ▶ sleep-related gastroesophageal reflux
- ▶ sleep-related (nocturnal) myoclonus syndrome
- ▶ sleep spindles
- ▶ sleep terror disorder
- ▶ sleepwalking disorder
- ▶ slow-wave sleep (SWS)
- ▶ somniloquy
- ▶ somnolence
- ▶ L-tryptophan
- ▶ variable sleepers

▲ QUESTIONS

DIRECTIONS: Each of the questions or incomplete statements below is followed by five suggested responses or completions. Select the *one* that is *best* in each case.

24.1 In REM sleep

A. there is infrequent genital tumescence
B. cardiac output is decreased
C. cerebral glucose metabolism is decreased
D. respiratory rate is decreased
E. brain temperature is decreased

24.2 True statements about circadian processes include all of the following *except*

A. It is easier to shift sleep–wake rhythms to earlier rather than later.
B. Circadian rhythms are endogenously regulated.
C. Slow-wave activity is driven mainly through homeostatic processes, whereas REM sleep is driven by the circadian system.
D. A circadian clock may be located in the retina.
E. Exposure to bright light in the evening and darkness in the morning may help with jet lag when traveling westward.

24.3 True statements about sleep in the elderly include all of the following *except*

A. After the age of 65, one-third of women and one-fifth of men report that they take over 30 minutes to fall asleep.
B. The incidence of nocturnal myoclonus increases with age.
C. Average daily total sleep time decreases after the age of 65 .
D. Death rates are higher in the elderly both in people who sleep more than 9 hours and those who sleep fewer than 5 hours.
E. Individuals with periodic limb movements sleep about an hour less per night than controls.

24.4 Anatomical sites implicated in the generation of NREM sleep include

A. basal forebrain area
B. thalamus and hypothalamus
C. dorsal raphe nucleus
D. medulla
E. all of the above

24.5 Depression is associated with

A. increased REM latency
B. decreased REM sleep
C. decreased REM sleep density
D. loss of stages 3 and 4 sleep
E. all of the above

24.6 Antidepressant effects have been linked to

A. total sleep deprivation
B. selective REM sleep deprivation
C. sleep deprivation in the last half of the night
D. all of the above
E. none of the above

24.7 Dyssomnias include all of the following *except*

A. narcolepsy
B. breathing-related sleep disorders
C. circadian rhythm sleep disorder
D. nightmares
E. primary hypersomnia

24.8 Many benzodiazepine hypnotic medications cause

A. profound hypersomnia during withdrawal
B. increases in slow wave sleep
C. reductions in REM sleep
D. abnormally decreased EEG beta and sleep spindle activity
E. all of the above

24.9 Which of the following features is *not* typical of REM sleep?

A. Dreams are typically concrete and realistic.
B. Polygraph measures show irregular patterns.
C. The resting muscle potential is lower in REM sleep than in a waking state.
D. Near-total paralysis of the postural muscles is present.
E. A condition of temperature regulation similar to that in reptiles occurs.

24.10 Which of the following statements does *not* correctly describe sleep regulation?

A. Melatonin secretion helps regulate the sleep–wake cycle.

B. Destruction of the dorsal raphe nucleus of the brainstem reduces sleep.

C. L-Tryptophan deficiency is associated with less time spent in NREM sleep.

D. REM sleep can be reduced by increased firing of noradrenergic neurons.

E. Disrupted REM sleep patterns in patients with depression show shortened REM latency.

24.11 The characteristic 4-stage pattern of electroencephalographic (EEG) changes from a wakeful state to sleep are

A. regular activity, delta waves at three to seven cycles a second, sleep spindles and K complexes

B. regular activity at three to seven cycles a second, delta waves, sleep spindles and K complexes

C. regular activity, sleep spindles and K complexes, delta waves at three to seven cycles a second

D. regular activity, delta waves, sleep spindles and K complexes at three to seven cycles a second

E. regular activity at three to seven cycles a second, sleep spindles and K complexes, delta waves

24.12 During rapid eye movement (REM) sleep

A. the pulse rate is typically five to ten beats below the level of restful waking

B. a poikilothermic condition is present

C. frequent involuntary body movements are seen

D. dreams are typically lucid and purposeful

E. sleepwalking may occur

24.13 The symptoms of narcolepsy include all of the following *except*

A. catalepsy

B. daytime sleepiness

C. hallucinations

D. sleep paralysis

E. cataplexy

24.14 All of the following disorders can take place during deep sleep (stages 3 and 4) *except*

A. enuresis

B. somnambulism

C. nightmare disorder

D. somniloquy

E. sleep terror disorder

24.15 Which of the following statements about the sleep stage histograms shown in Figure 24.1 is true?

A. *A* is characteristic of obstructive sleep apnea syndrome.

B. Both are normal.

C. *B* is characteristic of major depressive disorder.

D. *A* is characterized by an abnormal latency to REM sleep.

E. Both are within normal limits.

24.16 Figure 24.2 illustrates the stages of a patient's sleep pattern. Which of the following statements regarding this sleep pattern is true?

A. The sleep pattern is abnormal because of the shortened latency of REM sleep.

B. The sleep pattern represents human sleep between the ages of newborn and young adult.

C. The sleep pattern is consistent with that found in a patient with depression.

D. The sleep pattern is consistent with that found in a patient with narcolepsy.

E. The sleep pattern is normal.

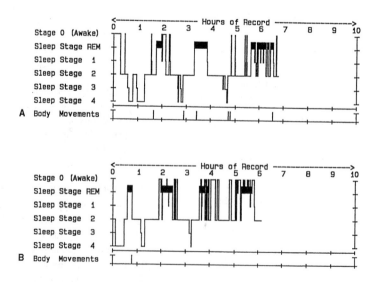

FIGURE 24.1

Reproduced with permission from Hauri P. *The Sleep Disorders.* Current Concepts, Kalamazoo, MI: Upjohn; 1982:82.

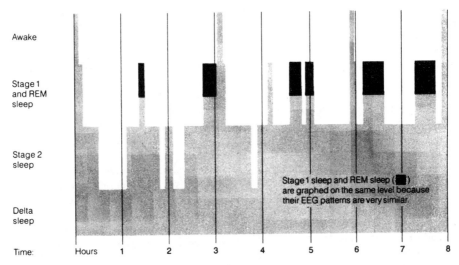

FIGURE 24.2
Reproduced with permission from Hauri P. *The Sleep Disorders*. Current Concepts, Kalamazoo, MI: Upjohn; 1982:82.

24.17 An 11-year-old girl asked her mother to take her to a psychiatrist because she feared she was going crazy. Several times during the past 2 months she had awakened confused about where she was until she realized that she was on the living room couch or in her little sister's bed, even though she went to bed in her own room. When she woke up in her older brother's bedroom, she became concerned and felt guilty about it. Her younger sister said that she had seen the patient walking during the night, looking like "a zombie," that she did not answer when called, and that she had walked at night several times but usually went back to her bed. The patient feared she had amnesia because she had no memory of anything happening during the night.

Which of the following statements about the patient's disorder is *false*?

A. Usually the disorder begins between the ages of 4 and 8 and peaks at age 12.
B. Patients often have vivid hallucinatory recollections of an emotionally traumatic event with no memory upon awakening.
C. There is no impairment in consciousness several minutes after awakening.
D. The disorder is more commonly seen in girls than in boys.
E. There is a tendency for the disorder to run in families.

DIRECTIONS: Each group of questions below consists of lettered headings followed by a list of numbered words or phrases. For each numbered word or phrase, select the *one* lettered heading that is most closely associated with it. Each lettered heading may be selected once, more than once, or not at all.

Questions 24.18–24.22

A. Sleep terror disorder
B. Nocturnal myoclonus
C. Jactatio capitis nocturnus
D. Sleep-related hemolysis
E. Sleep-related bruxism

24.18 Urge to move the legs
24.19 Brownish-red morning urine
24.20 Patient wakes up screaming
24.21 Head banging
24.22 Damage to the teeth

Questions 24.23–24.32

A. REM sleep
B. NREM sleep

24.23 Sleepwalking
24.24 Bed-wetting (enuresis)
24.25 Paroxysmal hemicrania
24.26 Erections
24.27 D sleep
24.28 Paradoxical sleep
24.29 Slow wave sleep (SWS)
24.30 EEG synchronized sleep
24.31 Most occurs in the last half of the night
24.32 Autonomic functioning is usually slow and steady

Questions 24.33–24.35

A. Delayed sleep phase syndrome
B. Advanced sleep phase syndrome

24.33 Drowsy in evening, more alert in morning
24.34 More tired in morning, stay up later
24.35 Greater difficulty adjusting to eastward travel

ANSWERS

Normal Sleep and Sleep Disorders

24.1 The answer is B

Figure 24.1 lists sleep patterns of a young adult showing NREM and REM sleep. In REM sleep, *there may be genital tumescence, cardiac output is decreased, cerebral glucose metabolism is unchanged or increased (not decreased), respiratory rate is variable (not decreased), and brain temperature is increased (not decreased).*

24.2 The answer is A

The daily sleep–wake cycle is an example of a circadian rhythm (from the Latin *circa*, meaning "about," and *dies*, meaning "day"). *Circadian rhythms are endogenously regulated* by a biological clock located in the suprachiasmatic nuclei of the anterior hypothalamus, which in turn is synchronized with the environment by visual or other, nonphotic time clues (*Zeitgebers*, meaning "time givers"). For example, if humans and animals are kept in an environment devoid of time clues, the period length of the sleep–wake cycle and other biological rhythms, such as core body temperature or cortisol, increases from about 24 hours to about 24.2 hours; this condition is called free-running. If, however, a 24-hour light–dark cycle of sufficient amplitude is imposed on this environment, subjects revert to a 24-hour sleep–wake cycle, that is, the subjects and their rhythms are entrained to the 24-hour day.

Sleep and wakefulness are influenced strongly by two separate processes: (1) an endogenous biological clock, which drives the circadian rhythm of the propensity for sleep and the characteristics of sleep across the 24-hour day; and (2) a homeostatic process that increases sleep propensity the longer the period of wakefulness prior to sleep.

Studies have supported the hypothesis that *slow-wave activity is driven mainly through homeostatic processes* whereas REM sleep as well as sleep spindles are driven by the circadian system. Humans appear to have two peaks of daytime sleepiness. The first, and obvious, one is at night in the normally entrained individual; the second is in midafternoon ("siesta hour"). Not surprisingly, automobile accidents, in which the driver falls asleep at the wheel, peak during the last half of the night and in the midafternoon. If the circadian temperature curve is used to index the phase position of the circadian pacemaker, it is seen that the major period of sleepiness occurs near the nadir of temperature, that is, at about 3:00 to 5:00 AM in normal circumstances. Both the duration of sleep and the type of sleep are influenced strongly by the phase position of sleep onset. People tend to awaken on the rising limb of the temperature curve; thus, sleep tends to be longest when it starts near the peak of the temperature curve. Furthermore, REM sleep is most likely to occur near the temperature nadir; thus, REM latency is shorter and REM time higher during morning naps compared with afternoon or evening naps.

The 24-hour sleep–wake rhythm is driven by the suprachiasmatic nuclei synchronized to the environmental light–dark cycle by *Zeitgebers*. Lesions of the suprachiasmatic nuclei in animals result in arrhythmic rest-activity patterns, which no longer follow a circadian rhythm but are distributed in numerous short bouts of sleep and wakefulness during the 24-hour period. Despite the dramatic alteration of the temporal organization of sleep and wakefulness the total amount of sleep and wakefulness in 24 hours remains fairly constant in the suprachiasmatic nuclei-lesioned animal. Indeed, a suprachiasmatic nuclei-lesioned animal deprived of sleep shows the normal compensatory increase in sleep during the recovery period, thereby demonstrating that the homeostatic and circadian processes can be separated. Although the major circadian pacemaker in mammals is the suprachiasmatic nuclei, a second *circadian clock may be located in the retina.*

Because the endogenous period in humans is slightly longer than 24 hours, *it is easier to shift sleep–wake rhythms to later rather than earlier.* For example, most individuals cope with jet lag more easily when traveling west than when traveling east. It usually takes about 1 day to accommodate for each time zone traveled when moving in an easterly direction, somewhat faster in a westerly direction. In addition, shift workers seem to feel better and perform better when going from a day to an evening to a night shift (forward shifting) than from a day to a night to an evening shift (backward shifting). Appropriate administration of bright light and darkness may ameliorate jet lag and shift-work problems by hastening the resynchronization of the endogenous clock modulating sleep–wakefulness and controlling temperature and other psychobiological rhythms. For example, *exposure to bright light in the evening and darkness in the morning* may help with jet lag when traveling westward or shifting from an evening to a night schedule of work. In addition, the administration of exogenous melatonin may shift the phase position of the clock and offers hope for treating jet lag, shift work, and other circadian sleep–wake disorders in which rapid resynchronization of the internal clock with the sleep–wake cycle is required. At this time, however, neither the efficacy nor the safety of melatonin administration for more than very short-term use has been demonstrated.

24.3 The answer is C

After the age of 65, about one-third of women and one-fifth of men report that they take *over 30 minutes to fall asleep.* Wake time after sleep onset (WASO) tends to increase with age, perhaps because of the greater incidence of sleep-related breathing disorders (i.e., mild apnea) and *nocturnal myoclonus.* In general, the severity of apnea in older persons is mild compared with that seen in patients with clinical sleep apnea. *Periodic limb movements* during sleep are also common in the elderly, with prevalence rates ranging from 25 to 60 percent in various studies of the healthy elderly. Individuals with periodic limb movements are reported to sleep about an hour less per night than controls without periodic limb movements. Perhaps as a result, napping also increases with age, although it rarely accounts for a large proportion of total sleep time in healthy individuals.

Average daily total sleep time actually increases slightly (rather than decreases) after the age of about 65. Greater numbers of elderly individuals fall into either long-sleeping (>9 hours) or short-sleeping (<5 hours) subgroups. It is noteworthy that *death rates are higher both in long-sleeping and excessively short-sleeping individuals.* The reasons for that are still unknown, although there has been speculation that sleep apnea might contribute to increased mortality in the long-sleeping group.

Although the incidence of insomnia and certain other sleep–wake disorders tends to increase with age, clinicians should not assume that age explains these complaints. Rather, the clinician must search for underlying conditions that can be treated, such as medical, neurological, psychiatric, situational, pharmacological, or circadian factors.

24.4 The answer is E (all)

At least five anatomical sites have been implicated in the generation of NREM sleep: the *basal forebrain area, thalamus, hypothalamus, dorsal raphe nucleus, and* nucleus tractus solitarius of the *medulla.* For example, lesions of the preoptic basal forebrain area produce hyposomnia lasting 4 to 6 weeks in rats and cats, whereas electrical stimulation and local warming of this region elicit both EEG and behavioral signs of sleep. In addition, some noncholinergic neurons in the basal forebrain discharge selectively during NREM sleep. The thalamus in general and the reticular nucleus of the thalamus in particular appear to play an important role in the generation of cortical sleep spindles (12 to 14 Hz) and delta waves (0.5 to 3 Hz, 75 mV or greater in humans) during NREM sleep. Recently, Mircea Steriade and colleagues hypothesized that thalamocortical cells are hyperpolarized by corticothalamic cells and are depolarized by cholinergic input from basal forebrain and the lateral dorsal tegmental and pedunculopontine tegmental, as well as through noradrenergic, serotonergic, and excitatory amino-acid input. The thalamocortical cells, which drive and synchronize the ensembles of cortical cells to produce the major EEG rhythms, change their rhythms from spindle frequencies to delta frequencies as they hyperpolarize. This theory also explains why immediately prior to and during REM sleep, when cholinergic activity in the lateral dorsal tegmental and pedunculopontine tegmental is high, the EEG becomes gradually desynchronized. While histaminergic cells in the posterior hypothalamus maintain arousal, ventrolateral preoptic neurons in the anterior hypothalamus may be involved in the induction of slow-wave sleep. The dorsal tegmental, the origin of the serotonergic projections of the brain, may be involved in the induction of sleep, at least insofar as either selective lesions or depletion of serotonin induce a dramatic insomnia lasting several days. Finally, the nucleus tractus solitarius was implicated by experiments in which medullary anesthesia or cooling of the fourth ventricular floor caused EEG activation. Low-frequency stimulation of this region produced EEG synchronization and behavioral sleep while cells in this region increase their discharge rate during NREM sleep. These regions appear to facilitate sleep; however, none have been found to be essential.

24.5 The answer is D

The neurobiology of sleep has important implications for depression, some types of alcoholism and schizophrenia, eat-

ing disorders, borderline personality disorder, and other clinical conditions associated with *short (not increased) REM latency, increased (not decreased) REM sleep, increased (not decreased) REM sleep density,* and *loss of stages 3 and 4 sleep.*

The emerging concepts of sleep neurophysiology are consistent with the cholinergic-aminergic imbalance hypothesis of mood disorders, which proposes that depression is associated with an increased ratio of central cholinergic to aminergic neurotransmission. The characteristic sleep abnormalities of depression may reflect a relative predominance of cholinergic activity, originating within the lateral dorsal tegmental and pedunculopontine tegmental, in relationship to noradrenergic and serotonergic activity, originating within the locus ceruleus, and the dorsal raphe nucleus (DRN), respectively. Cholinergic projections from dorsal tegmentum or basal forebrain to thalamus may also suppress delta sleep. Consistent with the role of cholinergic mechanisms, depressed patients are significantly more sensitive, compared with normal controls, to the REM-sleep–inducing effects of muscarinic agonists, such as arecoline or RS 86 (but not of pilocarpine, another selective muscarinic agonist). On the other hand, central depletion of either serotonin or catecholamines shortens REM latency and increases REM sleep. Antidepressant medications presumably reduce REM sleep by either their anticholinergic properties or by enhancing aminergic neurotransmission. Intense and prolonged dreams often accompany abrupt withdrawal from antidepressant drugs, a reflection of an REM rebound following drug-induced REM deprivation.

24.6 The answer is D (all)

Although the morbidity associated with sleep deprivation has been emphasized, the paradoxical finding that *total sleep deprivation,* partial *sleep deprivation* (especially in the last half of the night), and *selective REM sleep deprivation* have antidepressant effects in depressed patients must not be overlooked; unfortunately, the beneficial effect of total and partial sleep deprivation only lasts until the next sleep period, after which the patient typically awakens depressed again. Hence, sleep may be depressogenic in some patients. There is some evidence suggesting that selective REM sleep deprivation repeated over about 2 weeks, or a continued sleep-phase advance protocol after total sleep deprivation, might result in a sustained antidepressant effect. However, so far the latter treatment modes have scientific rather than practical implications because these protocols are extremely costly and time-consuming.

Many of the following observations suggest that some depressed patients are overaroused, at least in some areas of the brain: the antidepressant effects of sleep deprivation, loss of delta sleep and sleep continuity, and increased core body temperature during sleep. Moreover, a preliminary PET study showed that cerebral glucose metabolism during the first NREM period was significantly elevated in depressed patients compared with normal controls and that depressed patients had some of the abnormalities during sleep that had previously been reported in other patients while awake, such as decreased relative metabolic activity in the anterior cingulate and ventral-medial prefrontal cortex. Consistent with the overarousal hypothesis, depressed patients who responded to sleep deprivation showed significantly elevated metabolic rates within the anterior cingulate gyrus before sleep deprivation as compared with nonresponders and normal controls. After clinical improvement, metabolic activity normalized in responders, but did not change in the two other groups.

24.7 The answer is D

Primary sleep disorders are dichotomized into dyssomnias and parasomnias. Dyssomnias include insomnias and hypersomnias. DSM-IV-TR defines insomnia as difficulty initiating sleep or maintaining sleep. Many sleep specialists also would include nonrestful or poor-quality sleep. Hypersomnia is excessive sleepiness. Dyssomnias can be characterized by disturbance in amount, quality, or timing of sleep. By contrast, parasomnias are characterized by abnormal behaviors or physiological events associated with sleep. These events can occur during specific sleep states, during any stage of sleep, or at the transition between sleep and wakefulness.

Dyssomnias are thought of as disturbances involving sleep–wake generating or timing mechanisms. Parasomnias, however, involve inappropriately timed activation of (or failure to suppress) behavioral or physiological systems or both during sleep and sleep–wake transitions.

DSM-IV-TR lists five specified classifications for primary dyssomnias: primary insomnia, *primary hypersomnia, narcolepsy, breathing-related sleep disorders*, and *circadian rhythm sleep disorder* as well as a not otherwise specified category. *Nightmares* are anxiety-provoking dreams that occur during REM sleep, and are classified as a parasomnia. Narcolepsy is an abnormal manifestation of REM sleep characterized by recurrent sleep attacks. Breathing-related sleep disorders are characterized by sleep disruption secondary to a sleep-related breathing condition. Circadian rhythm sleep disorder includes a number of conditions involving a misalignment between desired and actual sleep periods. Primary hypersomnia is characterized by excessive time spent sleeping.

24.8 The answer is C

Alcohol, anxiolytics, opioids, and sedative-hypnotics all promote sleep by sedation. However, the resulting sleep, while apparently of greater quantity, is of poorer quality. Many benzodiazepine hypnotic medications alter the basic architecture of sleep. Most *reduce (rather than increase) slow-wave sleep*, and *some reduce REM sleep. Abnormally increased (not decreased) EEG beta and sleep spindle activity* result from ingesting some hypnotic drugs. Alcohol may relax a tense person and thereby decrease latency to sleep; however, sleep later in the night is fragmented by arousals. As tolerance develops to chronic drug and alcohol use, increased dosage is needed to sustain effects; lower dosage produces an abstinence syndrome, and sleep regresses to its initial abnormal pattern. Furthermore, during withdrawal of hypnotic medication or after tolerance has developed, the sleep disturbance can rebound to a more severe level than the initial problem leading to insomnia.

By contrast, psychostimulant use poses a different problem. Cocaine, amphetamine and related stimulants, caffeine, and theobromine all produce CNS arousal that may persist into the sleep period and produce insomnia. Especially in cases of stimulant abuse, an individual usually becomes severely sleep deprived. Over time a massive sleep debt accu-

mulates, and upon substance discontinuation, *profound hypersomnia* results. This compensatory sleep, or sleep rebound, continues for an extended time (several weeks or more in some instances).

24.9 The answer is A

In REM sleep, *dreams are typically abstract and surreal, not concrete and realistic*. People report dreaming 60 to 90 percent of the time during REM sleep. Dreaming also occurs during NREM sleep, but these dreams are lucid and purposeful.

During REM sleep, *polygraph measures show irregular patterns*, sometimes close to waking patterns. Aside from measures of muscle tone, physiological measures during REM periods could be inferred as those of a person in a waking state. Pulse, respiration, and blood pressure are all high during REM sleep, higher than during NREM sleep, and sometimes higher than during waking.

The *resting muscle potential is lower in REM sleep* than in a waking state. *Near-total paralysis of the postural muscles* is present during REM sleep, so that the body cannot move. This motor inhibition is sometimes thought to be associated with dreams of being unable to move. Also during REM sleep, a condition of *temperature regulation* similar to that in reptiles occurs; in this condition (poikilothermia) body temperature varies with the temperature of the environment.

24.10 The answer is C

L-*Tryptophan deficiency* is associated with less time spent in REM sleep, not in NREM sleep. Ingestion of large amounts of L-tryptophan reduces sleep latency and nocturnal awakening.

Melatonin secretion helps regulate the sleep–wake cycle; melatonin secretion is inhibited by bright light, so that the lowest concentrations occur during the day. A circadian pacemaker in the hypothalamus may regulate melatonin secretion. *Destruction of the dorsal raphe nucleus of the brainstem* reduces sleep, as nearly all of the brain's serotonergic cell bodies are located there. Reduced REM sleep can also be caused by *increased firing of noradrenergic neurons*.

Disrupted REM sleep patterns in patients with depression show shortened REM latency. As compared with normal sleep patterns, those of people with depression also show an increased percentage of REM sleep and a shift of REM sleep from the last to the first half of the night.

24.11 The answer is E

The characteristic sequential pattern of electroencephalographic (EEG) changes from a wakeful state to sleep are *regular activity at 3 to 7 cycles a second, sleep spindles and K complexes, and delta waves*—not *regular activity, delta waves,* and *sleep spindles and K complexes* in other configurations. The waking EEG is characterized by alpha waves of 8 to 12 cycles a second and low-voltage activity of mixed frequency. As the person falls asleep, alpha activity begins to disappear. Stage 1, considered the lightest stage of sleep, is characterized by low-voltage regular activity at three to seven cycles a second. After a few seconds or minutes, that stage gives way to stage 2, a pattern showing frequent spindle-shaped tracings at 12 to 14 cycles a second (sleep spindles) and slow triphasic waves known as K complexes. Soon thereafter, delta waves—high-voltage activity at 0.5 to 2.5 cycles a second—make their appearance and occupy less than 50 percent of the tracing (stage 3). Eventually, in stage 4, delta waves occupy more than 50 percent of the record. It is common practice to describe stages 3 and 4 as delta sleep or slow-wave sleep because of their characteristic appearance on the EEG record.

24.12 The answer is B
During rapid eye movement (REM) sleep *a poikilothermic condition is present*. Poikilothermia is a state in which body temperature varies with the temperature of the surrounding medium. In contrast, a homeothermic condition is present during wakefulness and nonrapid eye movement (NREM) sleep; in that condition the body temperature remains constant regardless of the temperature of the surrounding medium.

In REM sleep *the pulse rate is not typically five to ten beats below the level of restful waking;* that is characteristic of NREM sleep. In fact, pulse, respiration, and blood pressure in humans are all high during REM sleep—much higher than during NREM sleep and often higher than during waking. Because of motor inhibition, *body movement is absent (not frequent)* during REM sleep. *Dreams* during REM sleep *are typically abstract and unreal (not lucid and purposeful).* Dreaming does occur during NREM sleep, but is typically more realistic. *Sleepwalking does not occur* in REM sleep but does occur during stages 3 and 4 of NREM sleep.

24.13 The answer is A
Catalepsy is a condition in which a person maintains the body position in which it is placed. It is a symptom observed in severe cases of catatonic schizophrenia. Excessive *daytime sleepiness,* naps, and the accessory symptoms of *cataplexy, sleep paralysis,* and hypnagogic *hallucinations* are the classically recognized symptoms of narcolepsy. Patients generally report the onset of daytime sleepiness before the accessory symptoms are noted.

The sleepiness may persist throughout the day, but more often it is periodic and may be relieved by a sleep attack or by a nap from which the patient characteristically awakens refreshed. Thus, there are often refractory periods of 2 or 3 hours of almost normal alertness. The sleep attacks are usually associated with characteristic times of the day, such as after meals, when some degree of sleepiness is quite normal. The attacks are typically irresistible and may even occur while eating, riding a bicycle, or actively conversing and also during sexual relations.

Cataplexy, which occurs in 67 to 95 percent of the cases, is paralysis of the antigravity muscles in the awake state. A cataplectic attack often begins during expressions of emotion, such as laughter, anger, and exhilaration. The attacks vary in intensity and frequency; they can consist of a weakening of the knees, a jaw drop, a head drop, or a sudden paralysis of all of the muscles of the body—except for the eyes and the diaphragm—leading to a complete collapse.

Sleep paralysis is a neurological phenomenon that is most likely due to a temporary dysfunction of the reticular activating system. It consists of brief episodes of an inability to move or speak when awake or asleep.

Hypnagogic hallucinations are vivid perceptual, dream-like experiences occurring at sleep onset. They occur in about 50 per-

cent of patients. The accompanying affect is usually fear or dread. The hallucinatory imagery is remembered best after a brief narcoleptic sleep attack, when it is often described as a dream.

24.14 The answer is C
Nightmare disorder consists of repeated awakenings from long, frightening dreams. The awakening usually occurs during the second half of the sleep period, during rapid eye movement (REM) sleep. *Enuresis,* the involuntary loss of urine, can occur during all stages of sleep, but usually occurs during NREM sleep. *Somnambulism,* also known as sleepwalking disorder, takes place during the first third of the night during stages 3 and 4. *Sleep terror disorder* is characterized by terrified arousal in the first third of the night during deep NREM stages (stages 3 and 4). *Somniloquy*—talking in one's sleep—occurs in all stages of sleep but is more common in NREM stages.

24.15 The answer is C
The sleep stage histograms demonstrate *normal sleep* in A and that found in a patient with *major depressive disorder* in B. As shown in histogram A, *REM sleep normally has a latency (time between sleep onset and first REM episode) of about 90 minutes.* In contrast, REM latency is shortened to 60 minutes or less in major depressive disorder, as shown in histogram B. Other findings in *B* consistent with major depressive disorder include disruption of sleep continuity and early morning awakenings.

Obstructive sleep apnea syndrome is characterized by repetitive episodes of upper airway obstruction that occur during sleep, usually associated with a reduction in blood oxygen saturation. Sleep is disturbed by frequent awakenings, while REM and slow-wave (stages 3 and 4) sleep are nearly absent.

24.16 The answer is E
Figure 24.1 represents a *normal sleep pattern* of a young human adult. The periods of REM sleep shown are consistent with that found in a normal young adult, occurring every 90 to 100 minutes during the night, with most REM sleep occurring in the last third of the night.

Depressed patients, in contrast, experience *shortened REM latency* (60 minutes or less), an increased percentage of REM sleep (over the normal 25 percent), and a shift in REM distribution from most occurring in the last half (normal) to most occurring in the first half of the night (abnormal).

Narcolepsy is characterized by abnormal manifestations of REM sleep, including the appearance of REM sleep within 10 minutes of sleep onset (sleep-onset REM periods), as well as hypnagogic and hypnopompic hallucinations, cataplexy, and sleep paralysis.

Sleep patterns change over the life span. In the neonatal period, REM sleep occurs during more than 50 percent of total sleep time, whereas in *young adulthood*, REM sleep occurs during 25 percent of total sleep time. In addition, the EEG pattern of *newborns* goes from the alert state directly to the REM state without going through stages 1 through 4.

24.17 The answer is D
The patient's diagnosis is sleepwalking disorder. This disorder is *more commonly seen in boys than in girls*. Patients often have *vivid hallucinatory recollections* of emotionally traumatic events with *no memory upon awakening*. Sleepwalking disorder consists of a sequence of complex behaviors initiated in the first

third of the night during deep nonrapid eye movement (NREM) sleep (stages 3 and 4). It consists of arising from bed during sleep and walking about, appearing unresponsive during the episode, amnestic for the sleepwalking on awakening, and with *no impairment in consciousness several minutes after awakening*. Sleepwalking usually begins *between ages 6 and 12* and *tends to run in families.*

Answers 24.18–24.22

24.18 The answer is B

24.19 The answer is D

24.20 The answer is A

24.21 The answer is C

24.22 The answer is E

Nocturnal myoclonus consists of highly stereotyped contractions of certain leg muscles during sleep. Though rarely painful, the syndrome causes an almost irresistible *urge to move the legs*, thus interfering with sleep. *Sleep-related hemolysis* (paroxysmal nocturnal hemoglobinuria) is a rare acquired chronic hemolytic anemia in which intravascular hemolysis results in hemoglobinemia and hemoglobinuria. Accelerated during sleep, the hemolysis and consequent hemoglobinuria color the *morning urine a brownish red.* Sleep-related hemolysis is diagnosed as sleep disorder due to a general medical condition.

In *sleep terror disorder* the patient typically sits up in bed with a frightened expression and *wakes up screaming*, often with a feeling of intense terror; patients are often amnestic for the episode. Sleep-related *head banging (jactatio capitis nocturnus)* consists chiefly of rhythmic to-and-fro head rocking, and less commonly of total body rocking, occurring just before or during sleep, rarely persisting into or occurring in deep nonrapid eye movement (NREM) sleep. According to dentists, 5 to 10 percent of the population suffers from *sleep-related bruxism* (tooth grinding) severe enough to produce noticeable *damage to the teeth.* Although the condition often goes unnoticed by the sleeper, except for an occasional feeling of jaw ache in the morning, the bed partner and roommates are acutely cognizant of the situation, as they are awakened repeatedly by the sound.

Answers 24.23–24.32

24.23 The answer is B

24.24 The answer is B

24.25 The answer is A

24.26 The answer is A

24.27 The answer is A

24.28 The answer is A

24.29 The answer is B

24.30 The answer is B

24.31 The answer is A

24.32 The answer is B

Sleepwalking occurs during the first third of the night during NREM sleep, stages 3 and 4. Bed-wetting (*enuresis*), a repetitive and inappropriate passage of urine during sleep, is usually associated with NREM sleep, stages 3 and 4, but may occur during any stage of sleep. *Paroxysmal hemicrania* is a type of unilateral vascular headache that is exacerbated during sleep and that occurs only in association with REM sleep. Erections are associated with REM sleep. Almost every REM period is accompanied by a partial or full penile *erection* or clitoral erection in women.

Most mammals have two major phases of sleep: rapid eye movement (REM) sleep and nonrapid eye movement (NREM) sleep. REM sleep is sometimes called *dreaming or D sleep* insofar as it is associated with dreaming, or *paradoxical sleep*, because the electroencephalogram (EEG) becomes activated during this state of sleep. NREM sleep, on the other hand, conforms to traditional concepts of sleep as a time of decreased physiological and psychological activity; it is therefore sometimes called orthodox sleep or *slow wave sleep (SWS), EEG synchronized sleep*, or S sleep.

NREM sleep is further divided into four sleep stages on the basis of visually scored EEG patterns.

Sleep normally begins with stage 1, a brief transitional phase, before progressing successively into stages 2 through 4. Stage 2 sleep is defined by the presence of sleep spindles and K-complexes in the EEG. Stage 3 and stage 4 sleep, or delta sleep, are defined by the presence of delta waves in the EEG, a moderate (20 to 50 percent) and large (>50 percent) proportion of an epoch (usually 30 seconds long) of sleep, respectively.

REM sleep is characterized by an activated EEG, loss of tone in the major antigravity muscles, and periodic bursts of rapid eye movements. The REM latency is usually about 70 to 100 minutes in normal subjects but may be shortened significantly in some patients with depressive disorder, eating disorders, borderline personality disorder, schizophrenia, alcohol use disorder, or other psychiatric disorders. Thereafter, NREM and REM sleep oscillate with a cycle length of roughly 90 to 100 minutes. When it does occur, delta sleep is highest in the first NREM period of the night and declines with each successive NREM period. Most of the delta sleep occurs in the first half of the night and *most of the REM sleep occurs in the last half of the night.*

REM sleep and NREM sleep differ from each other in many psychological and physiological domains. On a psychological level, REM sleep is associated with dreaming mentation, while NREM sleep is more likely to be associated with abstract thinking. *Autonomic functioning* is often highly variable during REM sleep; it is usually slow and steady in NREM sleep.

Answers 24.33–24.35

24.33 The answer is B

24.34 The answer is A

24.35 The answer is A

In an optimal schedule, hours in bed must coincide with the sleepy phase of the circadian cycle. When the circadian sleep–wake cycle lags behind the desired schedule, the mismatch is called phase delay. Individuals with a delayed sleep phase are more alert in the evening and early nighttime, *stay up later*, and are *more tired in the morning*. These individuals are characterized as "owls." When this desynchrony is severe enough to interfere with daily living, delayed sleep phase syndrome is diagnosed.

In contrast to delayed sleep phase, individuals *with advanced sleep phase are drowsy in the evening*, want to retire to bed earlier, awaken earlier, and are *more alert in the early morning*. Individuals with this pattern of advanced sleep phase are sometimes called "larks." When severity impairs routine daily function, the diagnosis is made.

With the advent of high-speed air travel, an induced desynchrony between circadian and environmental clocks became possible. Thus, the term *jet lag* came into use. Individuals who rapidly cross many time zones induce either a circadian phase advance or a phase delay, depending upon the direction of travel. Typically, a one– or two–time-zone translocation does not produce a sustained problem; however, overseas travel can be marked by great difficulty in adjusting one's sleep–wake routine. Individuals who frequently travel for business can find themselves quite impaired at the time they need to make important decisions. Owls experience *greater difficulty adjusting to eastward travel* because resynchronization requires phase advance. Similarly, larks theoretically have more difficulty with westward travel. The number of time zones crossed is a critical factor. Normally, healthy individuals can adapt easily to one to two time-zone changes per day; therefore, natural adjustment to an 8-hour translocation may take 4 or more days.

25 ◢

Impulse-Control Disorders Not Elsewhere Classified

Giving into an impulse that one regrets is a familiar experience for most people. However, giving into the impulses characterized by disorders in impulse control is a qualitatively different matter. The revised fourth edition of the *Diagnostic and Statistical Manual of Mental Disorders* (DSM-IV-TR) lists several impulse-control disorders that are not classified under any other diagnostic heading in DSM-IV-TR, but are nonetheless serious enough to be highlighted. These are intermittent explosive disorder, kleptomania, pyromania, pathological gambling, trichotillomania, and impulse-control disorder not otherwise specified. All are quite different in their epidemiology, etiology, psychodynamic formulation, course, prognosis, and treatment, but all share the characteristic of persons failing to resist an impulse to perform an act that is harmful to themselves or others. The subjective description of experiencing such an impulse and then giving into it has the quality of an almost sexual experience for many of those diagnosed with the disorder: a rising sense of tension before giving into the impulse, associated with a sense of pleasure and relief once the impulse is acted on.

Intermittent explosive disorder is characterized by impulsive episodes of aggression leading to assaults or property destruction. Kleptomania is characterized by an inability to control the impulse to steal, usually objects that the person does not need. Pyromania is associated with the uncontrollable urge to set fires. Trichotillomania involves the irresistible urge to pull out one's own hair, often to the point of baldness or to removing eyebrows and lashes. Impulse-control disorder not otherwise specified includes all other impulsive disorders that human beings can imagine and then act upon that do not meet the criteria for another disorder in DSM-IV-TR.

As with most psychiatric disorders, both biological and psychological components contributing to the etiology of these disorders have been studied and identified. Biological investigations have been particularly relevant to the understanding of violent impulse–control disorders. Studies include investigations of the limbic system of the brain, the effects of testosterone, histories of head trauma and childhood abuse, childhood histories of

attention-deficit/hyperactivity disorder, and CSF levels of 5-hydroxyindoleacetic acid (5-HIAA), a metabolite of serotonin. Alcohol abuse has been associated with some of the more violent impulse-control disorders and can act as a facilitator to losing control. Identified psychosocial factors are extensive and vary depending on the diagnosis. Unfulfilled narcissistic, dependency, and self-object needs are implicated, as are exposure to parental impulse-control problems during development.

The student should study the questions and answers below for a useful review of these disorders.

HELPFUL HINTS

These terms relate to impulse-control disorders and should be defined by the student.

- ► alopecia
- ► anticonvulsants
- ► attention-deficit/ hyperactivity disorder
- ► behavior therapy
- ► benzodiazepines
- ► biofeedback
- ► desperate stage
- ► enuresis
- ► epileptoid personality
- ► 5-HIAA
- ► hydroxyzine hydrochloride
- ► hypnotherapy
- ► impulse-control disorder
- ► impulse-control disorder not otherwise specified
- ► intermittent explosive disorder
- ► kleptomania
- ► limbic system
- ► lithium
- ► lust angst
- ► multidetermined
- ► oniomania
- ► parental factors
- ► pathological gambling
- ► pleasure principle, reality principle
- ► progressive-loss stage
- ► psychodynamics
- ► pyromania
- ► social gambling
- ► SSRIs
- ► testosterone
- ► trichophagy
- ► trichotillomania
- ► winning phase

▲ QUESTIONS

DIRECTIONS: Each of the questions or incomplete statements below is followed by five suggested responses or completions. Select the *one* that is *best* in each case.

25.1 Impulse-control disorders are thought to be closely related to obsessive-compulsive spectrum disorders, based on which of the following?

A. epidemiological data
B. clinical presentation
C. proposed causes
D. response to common treatments
E. all of the above

25.2 True statements about kleptomania include

A. The majority of identified shoplifters have kleptomania.
B. Women tend to be older at first presentation compared to men.
C. Impulsive stealing has been characterized as an attempt to restore early childhood losses.
D. A low rate of pathological stealing appears among patients with eating disorders.
E. None of the above

25.3 True statements about pathological gambling include

A. Rates of pathological gambling are lower in locations where gambling is legal.
B. Rates of pathological gambling are lower among the poor and minorities.
C. Rates of pathological gambling have been shown to be lower in high school students than in the general population.
D. The natural history of the illness has been divided into four phases: winning, losing, desperation, and hopelessness.
E. All of the above

25.4 People with trichotillomania

A. often have family histories of tics
B. often respond preferentially to serotonergic agents
C. have an increased prevalence of mood and anxiety disorders
D. often require a biopsy to confirm the diagnosis
E. all of the above

25.5 Intermittent explosive disorder

A. is relatively common
B. is characterized by discrete periods of aggressive episodes
C. is associated with lower than expected rates of depressive disorders in first-degree relatives of patients
D. is typically seen in small men with avoidant personality features
E. none of the above

25.6 Examples of impulse control disorders not otherwise specified include

A. compulsive sexual behavior
B. compulsive face picking
C. self-mutilation
D. compulsive buying
E. all of the above

25.7 Which of the following selections is *not* associated with intermittent explosive disorder?

A. Patients may feel helpless before an episode.
B. The disorder usually grows less severe with age.
C. A predisposing factor in childhood is encephalitis.
D. Dopaminergic neurons mediate behavioral inhibition.
E. Neurological examination can show left-right ambivalence.

25.8 Biological factors involved in the causes of impulse-control disorders include all the following *except*

A. limbic system
B. testosterone
C. tyrosine levels
D. temporal lobe epilepsy
E. mixed cerebral dominance

25.9 Which of the following drugs has been found to cause a paradoxical reaction of dyscontrol in some cases of impulse-control disorder?

A. lithium
B. phenytoin
C. carbamazepine
D. trazodone
E. benzodiazepines

25.10 The estimated number of pathological gamblers in the United States is

A. fewer than 100,000
B. 250,000
C. 500,000
D. 750,000
E. 1 million or more

25.11 All of the following have been identified as predisposing factors for the development of pathological gambling *except*

A. loss of a parent before the child is 15 years old
B. childhood enuresis
C. attention-deficit/hyperactivity disorder
D. inappropriate parental discipline
E. family emphasis on material symbols

DIRECTIONS: Each set of lettered headings below is followed by a list of numbered words or phrases. For each numbered word or phrase, select

    A. if the item is associated with *A only*
    B. if the item is associated with *B only*
    C. if the item is associated with *both A and B*
    D. if the item is associated with *neither A nor B*

Questions 25.12–25.17

    A. Trichotillomania
    B. Pyromania
    C. Both
    D. Neither

25.12 More common in females than in males

25.13 Onset generally in childhood

25.14 Sense of gratification or release during the behavior

25.15 Treated with lithium

25.16 Associated with truancy

25.17 May be a response to an auditory hallucination

Questions 25.18–25.22

    A. Compulsive buying
    B. Kleptomania
    C. Both
    D. Neither

25.18 Chronic condition

25.19 Recognized as a discrete disease entity by DSM-IV-TR

25.20 Preponderance in women

25.21 Increased lifetime rate of major mood disorders

25.22 Treatment has included both psychological and pharmacological modalities

---

ANSWERS

Impulse-Control Disorders Not Elsewhere Classified

25.1 The answer is E (all)

Controversy continues about whether these disorders should be placed in a distinct category or should be listed as variations of other Axis I or Axis II disorders. Those who argue that impulse-control disorders are subgroups of other psychiatric disorders point to similarities with obsessive-compulsive disorder, mood disorders, substance dependence, paraphilias, and mental disorders due to a medical condition. Others suggest that impulse-control disorders share features with certain personality disorders such as antisocial personality disorder or borderline personality disorder. DSM-IV-TR, however, emphasizes that the category of impulse-control disorders is a residual group separate from all others.

Recently, investigators have proposed that the impulse-control disorders are more aptly included in an entity that has been called obsessive-compulsive spectrum disorders. Included within this category are the disorders involving preoccupation with bodily appearance or sensations such as the somatoform disorders (i.e., body dysmorphic disorder and hypochondriasis), eating disorders, dissociative disorders, and neurological disorders (Tourette's disorder, Sydenham's chorea, parkinsonism, and autistic disorder). Features proposed to be common to these disorders include *epidemiological data* (age of onset, family history, and clinical course), *clinical presentation* (repetitive thoughts or behaviors), *proposed causes* (serotonin alterations and modified frontal lobe activity), and *response to common treatments* such as selective serotonin reuptake inhibitors (SSRIs) and behavior therapy.

25.2 The answer is C

Because of the absence of studies, little is known about kleptomania. An estimated six out of 1,000 individuals in the general population suffer from kleptomania. According to DSM-IV-TR *fewer than 5 percent of identified shoplifters (not the majority)*

actually have kleptomania. However, many factors that influence these data result in an underestimated rate of kleptomania. Persons with kleptomania are ashamed and rarely report their behavior. Since kleptomania is a recurrent disorder, individuals apprehended multiple times are often viewed as recidivist criminals and thus not referred for psychiatric evaluation. Furthermore, some apprehended shoplifters are misdiagnosed as having an antisocial personality.

Information from case reports points to a preponderance of kleptomania in women. Recent studies show that approximately three-quarters of reported cases meeting DSM-IV-TR criteria for kleptomania were in women. However, women are more likely to present for psychiatric evaluation than men. Similarly, they are more likely to be referred by the courts for psychiatric evaluations, whereas male shoplifters are more likely to be sent to prison. *Men (not women) tend to be older at first presentation, approximately 50 years old, compared with 35 years old for women.* The time between onset of symptoms and presentation may be years to several decades.

No definitive cause for kleptomania is known. It appears that rates of shoplifting, in general, increase when the availability of goods increases. Psychodynamic theories center on the concept of pathological stealing as a defense against forbidden unconscious impulses, wishes, conflicts, or needs. These impulses or wishes may reflect sexual or masochistic themes, and the act of stealing may represent a mechanism whereby a narcissistically vulnerable individual prevents a fragmentation of the self by carrying out the impulse. Most studies suggest that persons with kleptomania have typically had a stormy and dysfunctional childhood; this history is used to support the analytic premise that *impulsive stealing is an attempt to restore early childhood losses.*

Phenomenological theories suggest that kleptomania may in fact be part of a larger spectrum disorder. Studies have demonstrated a high comorbidity with mood disorders, both major depressive disorder and bipolar disorders. A higher rate of mood disorders is reported in the families of these patients as well, which suggests that pathological stealing may be part of affective spectrum disorders. However, many individuals with kleptomania demonstrate obsessive and compulsive symptoms including compulsive hand washing, cleaning, checking, hoarding, collecting, and buying. In one study of 20 patients with kleptomania, 7 percent of first-degree relatives met criteria for obsessive-compulsive disorder. This supports the idea of pathological stealing as part of obsessive-compulsive spectrum disorders. *A high rate (not a low rate) of pathological stealing also appears among patients with eating disorders (particularly bulimia nervosa).* Given that kleptomania is at least partially responsive to serotonergic agents, these conditions may well have a common pathophysiological link. Further definitive studies are necessary to determine the viability of this hypothesis.

25.3 The answer is D

Up to 3 percent of adults in the general population may be classified with probable pathological gambling. Based on treatment samples, the typical pathological gambler is an upper-middle-class or middle-class white man between the ages of 40 and 50. However, pathological gamblers in treatment may differ significantly from those in the general population. Surveys demonstrate that *rates of pathological gambling are higher (not lower) among the poor and minorities* and that these individuals are underserved by current treatment resources. Although male pathological gamblers outnumber women, the previous ratio of 2 to 1 may be high. Individuals under the age of 30 are probably underrepresented in treatment centers, and data suggest that the prevalence of pathological gambling among adolescents is increasing. Some surveys have shown *higher (not lower) rates of pathological gambling among high school students* than in the general population. Pathological gamblers tend to have had an alcohol- or other substance-abusing parent, and approximately 25 percent had a parent who was probably a pathological gambler. Surveys also demonstrate that *rates of pathological gambling are considerably higher (not lower) in locations where gambling is legal.*

The course of pathological gambling is insidious, and conversion to pathological gambling probably is precipitated either by increased exposure to gambling or by the occurrence of a psychological stressor or significant loss. In males, the onset of pathological gambling begins in adolescence; in females the onset occurs later in life.

The *natural history of the illness has been divided into four phases*. In the *first (winning)* phase, a big win stimulates feelings of omnipotence. Women do not generally experience a big win initially. They may see gambling as a means of escaping overwhelming problems in their environment or in their past. Thus, there are apparently two possible motivators for ongoing gambling activity: action seeking (characterized by the big win) or escape seeking. In the *second (losing)* phase, the person either has a string of bad luck or begins to find losing intolerable. Gamblers then alter their strategy in an attempt to win back everything at once (chasing). Debts accrue, and there is a sense of urgency and an attempt to cover up both the behavior and the losses by lies. Relationships suffer as the gambler becomes irritable and secretive. In the *third (desperation)* phase gamblers engage in uncharacteristic, often illegal behaviors. Bad checks are written, funds are embezzled, and they desperately seek ways to obtain money to continue gambling, both to recoup

losses and to regain the feeling of arousal characteristic of the initial phase. Relationships deteriorate further. Symptoms of depression appear, including neurovegetative signs, suicidal ideation, and suicide attempts. The fourth and *final phase (hopelessness)* involves an acceptance that losses can never be made good. Nevertheless, gambling continues, with the main motivator being the attainment of arousal or excitement.

Although a few gamblers seek help while in the winning phase, most seek help much later, generally because their relationships are threatened or they have committed illegal acts.

The course of the disorder is accelerated by the use of alcohol or drugs, the death or loss (possibly through divorce) of a significant other, the birth of a child, physical illness, a job or career disappointment, or increasing interpersonal difficulties. Job promotion or success may also hasten the course of the disorder.

25.4 The answer is E (all)

The cause of trichotillomania remains unclear and both psychological and biological mechanisms have been proposed. Psychodynamic explanations suggest that the disorder is a response to loss or separation in childhood. Mothers of patients are often characterized as critical, and fathers are frequently passive or emotionally weak. Alternatively, behaviorists point out that the disorder is common in children and adolescents, and when it persists, it takes on the characteristics of a habit that remits with behavioral techniques. Biochemical explanations stem from the finding that patients have *an increased prevalence of both mood and anxiety disorders* and some symptoms of obsessive-compulsive disorder. The *family history* of patients with trichotillomania often *includes tics*, habits, and obsessive-compulsive symptoms. This disorder *responds preferentially to serotonergic agents*, which lends credence to a biochemical relation to either mood or anxiety disorders. However, since serotonergic agents are not always effective, the disorder most likely has more than one cause. Another biochemical theory points to the potential role of the opiate system, largely on the basis of the response of dogs with canine acral lick dermatitis to opioid antagonists. It was proposed that patients with trichotillomania have a general hypoalgesia that allows them to continue plucking hair without the perception of pain, but a recent study found no difference in pain perception thresholds.

Trichotillomania can be quite difficult to diagnose for a number of reasons. Although this disorder disrupts most patients' lives, they tend to deny the illness and frequently disguise it successfully for decades. Most often, people with this disorder pull hair from the scalp, most commonly the vertex, though people also pull frequently from the temporoparietal, occipital, and frontal regions. Generally, hair plucking involves multiple sites on the scalp or other body regions such as the eyebrows, eyelashes, facial hair, and the pubic area. The average dermatologist sees three to seven cases of trichotillomania a year. The affected site usually shows a mixture of short and long hairs in a linear or circular pattern. *A biopsy is often necessary* to confirm the diagnosis and distinguish it from alopecia areata or tinea capitis.

25.5 The answer is B

The notion that explosive violence may be linked to a discrete diagnosable condition is controversial. In DSM-IV-TR intermittent explosive disorder is characterized by aggressive impulses out of proportion to any precipitating psychosocial stressor. In the intervals between episodes there is no sign of impulsiveness or aggressiveness.

The existence of intermittent explosive disorder as a unique entity remains controversial. Many have difficulty with the idea of *a normal baseline with superimposed periods of aggressive episodes*. In addition, anger outbursts are a part of many other disease entities.

Intermittent explosive disorder is thought to be rare (not common) and occurs more frequently in males. High rates of fire-setting behavior in persons with the disorder have been reported. Recent studies suggest higher than normal rates of intermittent explosive disorder in families of patients with the diagnosis. *First-degree relatives of patients with the disorder appear to have higher (not lower) than expected rates of depressive disorders* and alcohol and substance abuse.

Hypotheses about the cause of impulsive aggression derive from both psychological and biological perspectives. Psychoanalytic reports suggest that such outbursts occur in response to narcissistic injurious events. Rage outbursts serve as defenses that regulate interpersonal distance and protect against further narcissistic wounding. *Typical patients appear to be large (not small) men with dependent (not avoidant) personality features* who respond to feelings of uselessness or impotence with violent outbursts.

25.6 The answer is E (all)

Impulse-control disorder not otherwise specified is a diagnosis reserved for disorders that involve the inability to resist an impulse but are not described by any of the other five categories. Examples include *compulsive sexual behavior, compulsive face picking,* and *self-mutilation.* Recently it was suggested that *compulsive buying* also falls in this category.

Although little attention has been paid, until recently, to compulsive buying, the entity was recognized by both Emil Kraepelin and Eugen Bleuler. It was originally referred to as oniomania and categorized as one of the "reactive impulses" or "impulsive insanities." Although not recognized by DSM-IV-TR or ICD-10 as a unique subcategory of the impulse-control disorders, some attempt has been made to develop a formal definition and diagnostic criteria of compulsive buying for both research and clinical purposes, based on the phenomenology of cases in the literature to date.

25.7 The answer is D

Serotonergic neurons (not dopaminergic neurons) mediate behavioral inhibition. Decreases in serotonergic transmission can reduce the effect of punishment as a deterrent of behavior, and the restoration of serotonin activity restores the behavioral effect of punishment. Researchers have suggested a connection between low levels of CSF 5-HIAA and impulsive behavior. Patients with intermittent explosive disorder are typically large, dependent men with a poor sense of masculine identity. *Patients may feel helpless* before an episode. A predisposing factor in childhood is *encephalitis,* as are perinatal trauma, minimal brain dysfunction, and hyperactivity. A patient's childhood was often violent and traumatic. Neurological examination can show *left-right ambivalence* and perceptual reversal. The disorder *usually grows less severe with age,* but heightened organic impairment can lead to frequent and severe episodes.

25.8 The answer is C

Tyrosine levels have not been implicated in impulse-control disorders. Specific brain regions, such as the *limbic system,* are associated with impulsive and violent activity; other brain regions are associated with the inhibition of such behaviors. Certain hormones, especially *testosterone,* have been associated with violent and aggressive behavior. Some reports have described a relationship between *temporal lobe epilepsy* and certain impulsive violent behaviors, an association of aggressive behavior in patients with histories of head trauma, increased numbers of emergency room visits, and other potential organic antecedents. A high incidence of *mixed cerebral dominance* may be found in some violent populations.

25.9 The answer is E

Anticonvulsants have long been used in treating explosive patients, with mixed results. *Phenothiazines* and antidepressants have been effective in some cases. *Benzodiazepines have been reported to produce a paradoxical reaction of dyscontrol* in some cases. *Lithium (Eskalith)* has been reported to be useful in generally lessening aggressive behavior, as have *carbamazepine (Tegretol)* and *phenytoin (Dilantin).* Propranolol (Inderal), buspirone (BuSpar), and *trazodone (Desyrel)* have also been effective in some cases. Reports increasingly indicate that fluoxetine (Prozac) and other serotonin-specific reuptake inhibitors are useful in reducing impulsivity and aggression.

25.10 The answer is E

Estimates place the number of pathological gamblers in the United States at *1 million or more*—not *750,000, 500,000, 250,000,* or *fewer than 100,000.* The disorder is thought to be more common in men than in women. Males whose fathers have the disorder and females whose mothers have the disorder are more likely to gamble pathologically than the population at large.

25.11 The answer is B

Childhood enuresis is the involuntary loss of urine (sometimes the condition is seen as voluntary). It is not a predisposing factor for the development of pathological gambling. *Loss of a parent* by death, separation, divorce, or desertion before the child is 15 years old may be a predisposing factor. Other possible factors include *attention-deficit/hyperactivity disorder, inappropriate parental discipline, family emphasis on material symbols,* and a lack of family emphasis on saving, planning, and budgeting.

Answers 25.12–25.17

25.12 The answer is A

25.13 The answer is C

25.14 The answer is C

25.15 The answer is D

25.16 The answer is B

25.17 The answer is D

Both pyromania and trichotillomania have their *onset in childhood* and are characterized by a *sense of gratification or release during the act.* Trichotillomania is apparently *more common in females than in males.* Pyromania is associated with antisocial traits, such as *truancy,* running away from home, and delinquency. *Neither disorder is treated with lithium (Eskalith), and according to the DSM-IV-TR diagnostic criteria, neither can be a response to an auditory hallucination.*

Table 25.1
Diagnostic Criteria for Compulsive Buying

A. Maladaptive preoccupation with buying or shopping, or maladaptive buying or shopping impulses or behavior, as indicated by at least one of the following:

  1. Frequent preoccupation with buying or impulses to buy that are experienced as irresistible, intrusive, and/or senseless.

  2. Frequent buying of more than can be afforded, frequent buying of items that are not needed, or shopping for longer periods of time than intended.

B. The buying preoccupations, impulses, or behaviors cause marked distress, are time consuming, significantly interfere with social or occupational functioning, or result in financial problems (e.g., indebtedness or bankruptcy).

C. The excessive buying or shopping behavior does not occur exclusively during periods of hypomania or mania.

Reprinted with permission from McElroy SL, Keck PE Jr, Pope HG Jr, Smith JM, Strakowski SM. Compulsive buying: a report of 20 cases. *J Clin Psychiatry.* 1994;55:242.

Answers 25.18–25.22

25.18 The answer is C

25.19 The answer is B

25.20 The answer is C

25.21 The answer is C

25.22 The answer is C

Kleptomania is a chronic illness, generally beginning in late adolescence and continuing over many years. The spontaneous remission rate and long-term prognosis are unknown.

Compulsive buying is a chronic condition that can have devastating financial, marital, and vocational consequences. Though individuals frequently attempt to stop the behavior on their own, they are usually unsuccessful. Limiting access to shopping, including credit cards, home catalogs, the Internet, and the home shopping network, has met with some success for this disorder.

Kleptomania has been recognized as a discrete disease entity by DSM-III, DSM-III-R, DSM-IV, and DSM-IV-TR. The disorder was excluded from the second edition of DSM (DSM-II) and was mentioned in the first edition of DSM (DSM-I) as an accessory term only. Features include a recurrent impulse to steal objects that are not needed for personal use or monetary value. DSM-IV-TR diagnostic criteria stipulate that the stealing is not an expression of anger or revenge, is not associated with a delusion or hallucination, and is not due to a conduct disorder, manic episode, or antisocial personality disorder.

Compulsive buying is not recognized by DSM-IV-TR as a unique subcategory, but some attempts have been made recently to develop a more formal definition of diagnostic criteria. Table 25.1 lists some proposed diagnostic criteria for compulsive buying.

Current estimates of the prevalence of compulsive buying range from 1.1 to 5.9 percent of the general population. *General population surveys of people meeting criteria for compulsive buying have shown that 80 to 92 percent are women.* The onset of the disorder appears to be approximately 18 years of age, though frequently a decade passes before the buying pattern is recognized as a problem. Information from case reports points to a *preponderance of kleptomania in women,* although women are more likely to present for psychiatric evaluation than men.

Patients with kleptomania have an increased lifetime rate of major mood disorders, anxiety disorders, and eating disorders. They frequently have a history of sexual dysfunction. Persons with kleptomania do not meet the criteria for antisocial personality disorder. Those with a psychiatric disorder in addition to kleptomania generally state that of all their difficulties, stealing causes them the greatest grief.

Compulsive buying must be distinguished from spending that occurs exclusively during a hypomanic or manic period. Compulsive shoppers demonstrate a more enduring pattern of behavior that is not limited to episodes in which other symptoms of mania can be observed.

These individuals show a high comorbidity with other Axis I conditions. In one study of 20 patients, all met criteria for two or more Axis I conditions, and 13 met criteria for four or more conditions. *All of these patients met criteria for some form of mood disorder,* most commonly bipolar I or bipolar II disorder. Symptoms seemed to increase when individuals felt more dysphoric and to decrease when patients were hypomanic. Many of these individuals stated that buying relieved their depressive symptoms.

Other disorders comorbid with compulsive buying include anxiety disorders such as obsessive-compulsive disorder, panic disorder, and phobias. Substance abuse and dependence, eating disorders, and other impulse-control disorders are frequently seen in these patients.

Information regarding treatment of compulsive buying is based on case reports; no formal, rigorously controlled treatment studies exist for compulsive shopping. *Treatment of compulsive buying has included both psychological and pharmacological modalities,* though information is based upon case reports rather than clinical trials. Some patients receiving cognitive-behavioral, supportive, or insight-oriented therapy report gaining some control over their buying compulsions. Others have been helped by supportive self-help groups like Debtors Anonymous. Pharmacological data are limited, with mixed results. In one series, 9 of 20 patients receiving pharmacological interventions had complete or partial remission of symptoms. Medications that were at least somewhat effective included antidepressants, mood-stabilizing agents, anxiolytics, and antipsychotics used singly or in conjunction with other agents. Some individuals who did not improve had discontinued pharmacotherapy early in treatment because of adverse effects or induction of hypomania.

The *literature describes the use of psychodynamic psychotherapy, behavioral techniques, and somatic interventions in the treatment of kleptomania, with variable outcomes.* However, there are no controlled studies in the treatment of kleptomania. The use of long-term, insight-oriented psychotherapy is of questionable value to this patient population. Behavioral techniques have met with some success. Effective pharmacological interventions have been described in case reports, including the use of fluvoxamine (Luvox), amitriptyline (Elavil), imipramine (Tofranil), nortriptyline (Pamelor), trazodone (Desyrel), fluoxetine (Prozac), lithium (Eskalith), and valproate (Depakote). The use of electroconvulsive therapy (ECT) has also met with some success in case reports.

26 ▲

Adjustment Disorders

Adjustment disorders are defined in the revised fourth edition of the *Diagnostic and Statistical Manual of Mental Disorders* (DSM-IV-TR) as the clinically significant behavioral and emotional reactions that occur in response to a particular stress. These reactions are further classified as an adjustment disorder with depressed mood, with anxiety, with mixed anxiety and depressed mood, with a disturbance in conduct, with a mixed disturbance of emotions and conduct, or as unspecified. The clinically significant reactions take on characteristics of the specifiers (i.e., anxiety or depression or disturbance in conduct) without rising to the levels of specific anxiety, depression, or conduct disorders.

Adjustment disorders are among the very few diagnoses in DSM-IV-TR that have an implied etiology in their definition; that is, the symptoms must occur in response to a psychosocial stressor.

Per DSM-IV-TR, the symptoms must occur within 3 months of the stress occurring, and there must be marked distress or impairment in social or occupational functioning. The symptoms must resolve within 6 months of the resolution of the stress, unless the stress is defined as chronic or with ongoing consequences.

Treatment depends on the symptom presentation, and may even require brief pharmacotherapy. By and large, treatment strategies involve crisis intervention, supportive therapies, and environmental manipulations.

The student should study the questions and answers below for a useful review of these disorders.

HELPFUL HINTS

The student should know these terms and types (including case examples) of adjustment.

- ▶ acute stress reaction
- ▶ adjustment disorder:
  - with anxiety
  - with depressed mood
  - with disturbance of conduct
  - with mixed anxiety and depressed mood
  - with mixed disturbance of emotions and conduct
- ▶ adolescent onset
- ▶ bereavement
- ▶ crisis intervention
- ▶ good-enough mother
- ▶ maladaptive reaction
- ▶ mass catastrophes
- ▶ posttraumatic stress disorder
- ▶ psychodynamic factors
- ▶ psychosocial stressor
- ▶ recovery rate
- ▶ resilience
- ▶ secondary gain
- ▶ severity of stress scale
- ▶ vulnerability
- ▶ Donald Winnicott

▲ QUESTIONS

DIRECTIONS: Each of the statements or questions below is followed by five suggested responses or completions. Select the *one* that is *best* in each case.

26.1 Adjustment disorders

- A. must remit within 6 months following the cessation of the stressor
- B. are in response, most often, to everyday events rather than rare, catastrophic events
- C. have subtypes indicating that almost any subthreshold condition associated with a psychosocial stressor may meet criteria for the disorder
- D. as a diagnosis may be used excessively and incorrectly by clinicians
- E. all of the above

26.2 The rate of reliability in the diagnosis of adjustment disorders is

- A. considered good
- B. improved by the variability produced by cultural expectations regarding reactions to and management of stressful events
- C. increased by the absence of any impairment criteria in the diagnostic algorithm that defines maladaption to stress
- D. consistent with the fact that measurement of psychosocial stress on Axis IV has been found to be questionable
- E. none of the above

26.3 Factors affecting the relationship of stress to the development of psychopathology include

- A. preexisting mood symptomatology
- B. preexisting adaptive skills
- C. genetic influence
- D. the nature of the preexisting event
- E. all of the above

26.4 The symptomatic profile and level of impairment in adjustment disorders with depressed mood has been found to be quite similar to

    A. dysthymic disorder
    B. major depressive disorder
    C. bipolar I disorder
    D. all of the above
    E. none of the above

DIRECTIONS: The lettered headings below are followed by a list of numbered phrases. For each numbered phrase, select

    A. if the item is associated with *A only*
    B. if the item is associated with *B only*
    C. if the item is associated with *both A and B*
    D. if the item is associated with *neither A nor B*

Questions 26.5–26.7

    A. Posttraumatic stress disorder
    B. Adjustment disorder
    C. Both
    D. Neither

26.5 Unusually high levels of stress
26.6 Patients are thought to be unusually sensitive to psychosocial events that are not likely to cause disturbances in others
26.7 Pharmacological interventions are most often used to augment psychosocial strategies

DIRECTIONS: Each of these statements or questions is followed by five suggested responses or completions. Select the *one* that is *best* in each case.

26.8 According to DSM-IV-TR, which of the following conditions need *not* be considered when diagnosing adjustment disorder?

    A. bereavement
    B. panic disorder
    C. personality disorder
    D. acute stress disorder
    E. posttraumatic stress disorder

26.9 For a diagnosis of adjustment disorder, the reaction to a psychosocial stressor must occur within

    A. 1 week
    B. 2 weeks
    C. 1 month
    D. 2 months
    E. 3 months

26.10 Adjustment disorder

    A. correlates with the severity of the stressor
    B. occurs more often in males than in females
    C. is a type of bereavement
    D. usually requires years of treatment
    E. occurs in all age groups

26.11 Adjustment disorder is

    A. an exacerbation of a preexisting mental disorder
    B. a normal response to a nonspecific stressor
    C. a normal response to a clearly identifiable event
    D. a maladaptive reaction to an identifiable stressor
    E. a type of brief psychotic disorder

26.12 Regarding the treatment of an adjustment disorder, which of the following is *incorrect*?

    A. Patients with clearly delineated stressors do not require psychotherapy, since their disorder will remit spontaneously.
    B. Crisis intervention is a brief type of therapy that may involve the use of hospitalization to resolve the disorder.
    C. A brief period of pharmacotherapy with antidepressants or antianxiety agents may benefit some patients.
    D. Patients may attempt secondary gains through the use of the illness role.
    E. Psychotherapy remains the treatment of choice for adjustment disorder.

ANSWERS

Adjustment Disorders

26.1 The answer is E
Adjustment disorders is one of the most problematic diagnostic categories in DSM-IV-TR. The fact that the relationship between stress and psychiatric disorder is both complex and uncertain has caused many to question the theoretical basis of adjustment disorders. In addition, the absence of operationalized, symptom-based criteria and a threshold level of symptomatology required for diagnosis has resulted in the use of this category for patients who might otherwise fulfill criteria for another, more specific mental disorder. Since incorrect diagnosis may result in inadequate treatment, inappropriately conceptualizing a patient's problem as constituting an adjustment disorder may result in delays or errors in treatment planning. Misdiagnosis of other, more specific

disorders when an adjustment disorder should be diagnosed is also a problem. For example, in one study, medical residents frequently diagnosed major depressive disorder when adjustment disorder with depressed mood was considered the correct diagnosis by an attending psychiatrist.

Problems with the use of the adjustment disorders category among child and adolescent psychiatrists were highlighted in a survey conducted as a means of informing the DSM-IV-TR work groups about the use of psychiatric disorders in clinical practice. Of those who responded to the survey, 55 percent indicated that they used adjustment disorders to avoid stigmatization of patients. Many of those who favored the use of this category were not trained formally in the revised third edition of DSM (DSM-III-R) and were not inclined to use not otherwise specified categories. Over half of these psychiatrists did not consider the temporal-onset criterion for adjustment disorders or the relevant exclusionary criteria in applying this diagnosis.

The survey results indicate that adjustment disorders diagnoses may be used excessively and incorrectly by some clinicians.

Adjustment disorders are characterized in DSM-IV-TR by the development of emotional or behavioral symptoms in the context of one or more identified psychosocial stressors. The resultant symptomatology is deemed to be clinically significant by virtue of either impairment in social, occupational, or educational function or the subjective experience of distress in excess of what would normally be expected for the given stressors. The nature and severity of the stressors are not specified. *However, the stressors are more often everyday events that are ubiquitous* (e.g., loss of a loved one, change of employment or financial situation) *rather than rare, catastrophic events,* such as natural disasters or lethal crimes. The symptomatology must, by definition, occur within 3 months of the occurrence of the stressor and *must remit within 6 months following the cessation of the stressor.* Finally, the disturbance must not fulfill the criteria for another major psychiatric disorder or bereavement (not considered a mental disorder, although it may be a focus of clinical attention). A variety of symptomatic presentation subtypes of adjustment disorders are identified. The scope of symptomatology covered by these subtypes indicates that *virtually any subthreshold condition deemed to be associated with a psychosocial stressor may potentially meet the criteria for adjustment disorders.*

26.2 The answer is D

The few extant *studies of reliability in adjustment disorders have produced unimpressive (not good) results.* One study determined the inter-rater agreement (κ) for adjustment disorders to be 0.05 (P = not significant) in a survey of psychiatrists and psychologists using 27 case histories of child and adolescent cases. The κ for the DSM-II category transient situational disorder was somewhat higher in this study (κ = 0.28; P <0.05). The results of the United Kingdom World Health Organization (UK-WHO) study of reliability of the ninth revision of *International Statistical Classification of Disease* (ICD-9) categories in children and adolescents were consistent with these findings. The κ for adjustment disorders was 0.23, which was considerably lower than for many other categories. Reclassification using a glossary improved reliability to 0.33, suggesting that structured assessment can at least partially ameliorate the limited reliability of adjustment disorders.

There are many potential sources of poor reliability, although the lack of an operationalized symptom checklist and a threshold level of symptoms that demarcate entrance into the diagnosis seem paramount. *Other sources of poor (not improved) reliability include* (1) difficulties in determining when subjective distress or observable symptomatology exceeds what would normally be expected for a given stressor in an "average" individual; (2) *the absence of any impairment* criterion in the diagnostic algorithm that defines maladaptation to stress; and (3) *the variability produced by cultural expectations* regarding the reaction to and management of stressful events. The low reliability of adjustment disorders is consistent with the fact that *measurement of psychosocial stress on Axis IV* has repeatedly been found to be *questionable.*

26.3 The answer is E (all)

The results of studies that have examined the relationship of stress to the development of psychopathology provide addi-

tional information to be considered in evaluating the model of stress–disease interaction in adjustment disorders. Several studies have found that individuals with and without preexisting symptoms respond differently to the presence of stressful events. This has been observed both in samples with adjustment disorders and in other conditions. *Preexisting mood symptomatology* was the only factor that predicted a prolonged course of adjustment disorders following cardiac surgery. In Israeli children who suffered the loss of their fathers in war, preexisting conduct symptoms were correlated highly with poor adjustment (although not necessarily adjustment disorders).

Other studies have focused on those factors that protect individuals from developing stress-related symptoms. For example, *preexisting adaptive skills* decrease the likelihood of symptoms developing in the face of stress. In child and adolescent populations, a warm and supportive relationship with the primary caregiver, easy and adaptable child temperament, and healthier adjustment of the family to stress all predict a more positive response to stress within the child. Finally, *the nature of preexisting life events* has important implications for the level of adjustment. Control over life events has generally been associated with improved adjustment even though it may increase stress. Similarly, pleasurable events are on the whole linked to psychological well-being, even though they may be stressful. In contrast, life events of a more dependent nature, which are undesirable and outside the control of the affected individual, are more likely to produce psychiatric symptoms.

The relationship of family, environmental, and genetic factors to adverse life events must also be considered. Findings from a study of over 2,000 twin pairs indicate that life events are correlated modestly in twin pairs, with monozygotes showing greater concordance than dizygotes. Family-environmental and genetic factors each accounted for approximately 20 percent of the variance in that study. Another twin study that examined *genetic contributions* to the development of symptoms of posttraumatic stress disorder (not necessarily at the level of full disorder, and therefore relevant to adjustment disorders) similarly concluded that the likelihood of developing symptoms in the context of traumatic life events is partially under genetic control. The findings of these studies suggest that the occurrence of adverse life events and their consequences are not necessarily random. Certain individuals appear to be at increased risk both for the occurrence of these events and for the development of pathology once they occur.

26.4 The answer is A

Adjustment disorders has been described as a transitional diagnostic category because the level of symptomatology and impairment in adjustment disorders was found to be intermediate between that observed in comparison groups who only had a DSM-IV-TR problem-level diagnosis and patients with specific, above-threshold diagnoses. The symptomatic profile and level of impairment in patients with adjustment disorders with depressed mood was quite *similar to that found in dysthymic disorder* and atypical (minor) depression, although it was *distinct from major depressive disorder* and *bipolar I disorder,* suggesting poor discriminate validity of adjustment disorders with depressed mood with respect to minor depressive disorders. Adjustment disorders has also been described as an admission diagnosis or initial diagnosis for many adolescent and adult psychiatric inpatients. In one study, a large number (40 percent) of patients given this preliminary diagnosis were assigned a different diagnosis at the time of discharge. An even smaller number (18 percent) of those who were subsequently readmitted to the hospital were again diagnosed as having adjustment disorders.

Answers 26.5–26.7

26.5 The answer is A

26.6 The answer is B

26.7 The answer is C
The linear model of stress–disease interaction, which has served as the model for adjustment disorders in DSM, has been criticized by several authors. This model presupposes that a direct and clearly identifiable pathological reaction follows a stressful event. However, there are many possible ways in which stress may be related to psychiatric illness that are not adequately taken into account by this model. For example, there may be multiple stressors or insidious or chronic circumstances, as opposed to discrete events. Recent studies suggest that pathology is more often associated with an accumulation of stressors over time, rather than the occurrence of any one stressor. Classification of individuals with chronic disturbance, chronic stress, or both, may be difficult to achieve using the DSM model of adjustment disorders. The development of psychopathology in individuals exposed to chronic stress is not always direct, and relatively minor precipitating events may generate symptomatology in individuals who have previously been sensitized to stress.

The stressor criterion in adjustment disorders has also been criticized for its lack of specificity. Several authors note that there is no mechanism to measure the stressors in adjustment disorders and, as a result, their clinical implications are often uncertain. These authors question whether *patients with adjustment disorders are unusually sensitive to psychosocial events* that are not likely to cause disturbance in others, or whether these individuals have been exposed to high levels of stress, the severity or accumulation of which would likely produce negative consequences in most people. The current DSM definition clearly favors the former explanation because *unusually high levels of stress are* more *characteristic of posttraumatic stress disorder (PTSD) and acute stress disorders* than adjustment disorders.

There are no studies assessing the efficacy of pharmacological interventions in individuals with adjustment disorders; however, it may be reasonable to consider the judicious use of medication to treat specific symptoms associated with adjustment disorder. One report presented a rationale for the use of benzodiazepines in the treatment of adjustment disorder with anxious mood. Selective serotonin reuptake inhibitors have been found to be useful in treating symptoms of traumatic grief and may be useful for other groups with subthreshold depressive symptoms. Indeed, a recent survey of prescribing practices among outpatient physicians indicated a robust increase in antidepressant use in individuals with adjustment disorder. It should be stressed, however, that *pharmacological intervention in this population is most often used to augment psychosocial strategies* rather than serving as the primary modality. Controlled clinical trials are needed to more accurately specify the

role of pharmacotherapy in adjustment disorder and other minor disorders.

One view of medication use in anxiety disorders posits that anxiety disorders result from underlying cognitive, behavioral, or psychodynamic abnormalities and that the role of medications is to allow the patient to participate in appropriate psychotherapeutic work. The knowledge base is evolving rapidly, but it will be many years before definitive statements can be made and causal relationships among neurophysiology, psychopathology, drugs, specific psychotherapeutic interventions, and behavioral outcome can be established. However, medication management of most anxiety disorders with or without psychotherapy is one of the most successful treatments in healthcare today. Treatment response rates can reach 80 percent in panic disorder, with steadily improving rates for many other anxiety disorders. Nevertheless, a nonpharmacological treatment will almost always be preferable if comparable efficacy can be established. Even at their most benign and tolerable, medications usually entail some adverse effects. Medications may also be contraindicated because of underlying medical conditions or pregnancy. Additionally, psychotherapy should always be part of the management of PTSD.

26.8 The answer is B
Panic disorder is not considered when diagnosing adjustment disorder. All of the other conditions—*bereavement, personality disorder, acute stress disorder,* and *posttraumatic stress disorder*—are possible diagnoses when considering adjustment disorder. To diagnose adjustment disorder, there must be an external stressor producing the symptoms, and the patient must show considerable social dysfunction. Panic disorder occurs without a stressor.

26.9 The answer is E
According to the revised fourth edition of *Diagnosis and Statistical Manual of Mental Disorders* (DSM-IV-TR), symptoms of adjustment disorder must occur within *3 months* of the onset of the stressor. If a longer time intervenes between the onset of the psychiatric symptoms and an identifiable psychosocial stressor, the clinician should not make a diagnosis of adjustment disorder. Symptoms can occur as early as *1 week, 2 weeks, 1 month,* or *2 months,* but DSM-IV-TR allows more time between the stressor and the onset of the symptoms.

26.10 The answer is E
Adjustment disorder *occurs in all age groups*. It *does not always correlate with the severity of the stressor* and *appears to occur more often in females than in males*. Adjustment disorder *is not a type of bereavement*. The overall prognosis for a person with adjustment disorder is generally favorable with appropriate treatment. Most patients return to their previous level of functioning within 3 months and *do not require years of therapy*.

26.11 The answer is D
According to DSM-IV-TR, adjustment disorder is a *maladaptive reaction to an identifiable stressor. It is not an exacerbation of a preexisting mental disorder*. The patient's response is to an identifiable stressor rather than to a nonspecific stressor. The response must be identified by significant impairment in social or occupational functioning or by symptoms that are in marked excess of a normal and expectable reaction to the stressor. Thus, adjustment disorder is *not a normal response to either a non-*

specific stressor or to a clearly identifiable event. Adjustment disorder is *not a type of brief psychotic disorder.* Even if a precipitant stressor can be identified, the diagnosis of brief psychotic disorder is assigned only if the patient shows evidence of psychotic thinking, speech, or behavior.

26.12 The answer is A

Regarding the treatment of an adjustment disorder, *it is often believed that patients with clearly delineated stressors do not require psychotherapy*, since their disorder will remit spontaneously. However, such thinking fails to consider that many persons exposed to the same stressor do not experience similar symptoms and that the response is pathological. Psychotherapy can help the person adapt to the stressor if it is not reversible or time-limited and can serve as a preventive intervention if the stressor does not remit. *Crisis intervention* is a brief type of therapy that may involve the use of hospitalization to resolve the disorder. A course of *brief pharmacotherapy* using antidepressants or antianxiety agents may benefit some patients if used, especially in conjunction with psychotherapy. Patients may attempt *secondary gains* through the use of the illness role's capacity to remove them from responsibility. *Psychotherapy* remains *the treatment of choice for adjustment disorder.*

27

Personality Disorders

People who are diagnosed with personality disorders frequently are among the most difficult, perplexing, and frustrating of all patients for clinicians to treat. This is particularly true, perhaps, for nonpsychiatric doctors who are trying to manage medical problems in the context of someone who may, often seemingly inexplicably, work against everything the clinician is trying to accomplish. Psychiatrists have an advantage here, in that at least in psychiatry the patient's personality can become the object of treatment. However, as all psychiatrists are well aware, the personality-disordered patient, if mismanaged, can lead to treatment nightmares. These may include repeated suicide attempts, sexually inappropriate behavior, boundary crossing, and angry recriminations. Despite this, the effective and appropriate treatment of people with personality disorders can be fascinating, challenging, and gratifying.

People with personality disorders have chronic problems with interpersonal relations, although they may be at a loss to explain them. Often, they externalize internal problems, leading them to blame others for their unhappiness and conflicts. There are several different and varied presentations of the personality disorders. Individuals may be isolated and introverted, or exhibitionistic and dramatic. They may have ongoing problems with impulse control and substance abuse, or they may be rigid and controlling. They may be suspicious and hostile, or overly intimate and sexualized. They may be timid and pathologically self-effacing, or contemptuous and arrogant. The common thread is that the person's characteristic style of relating to others has been present since at least the age of 18 and is pervasive, inflexible, and tenacious. Individuals may or may not be aware of how their relatedness style affects others, but they are generally aware of problems in social and occupational functioning, and these can lead to subjective distress.

The revised fourth edition of the *Diagnostic and Statistical Manual of Mental Disorders* (DSM-IV-TR) specifies 11 personality disorders. These include paranoid, schizoid, schizotypal, antisocial, borderline, histrionic, narcissistic, avoidant, dependent, and obsessive-compulsive personality disorders as well as personality disorder not otherwise specified. These are further grouped informally into three clusters—A, B, and C—according to predominant personality traits. Cluster A includes paranoid, schizoid, and schizotypal personality disorders, all of which are characterized to some degree by odd, reclusive, or eccentric behavior. Cluster B includes borderline, histrionic, antisocial, and narcissistic disorders, characterized by more dramatic and interpersonally abrasive presentations, and Cluster C includes the avoidant, dependent, and obsessive-compulsive disorders, characterized by more inhibited and anxious behaviors.

The study of personality disorders is a rich field of psychiatric research. Biological aspects include the impact of genetics and temperament on personality development as well as the common comorbidity of other psychiatric conditions such as mood disorders. Interesting findings include the fact that more people with schizotypal personality disorder are found in families of people with schizophrenia than in control groups, suggesting that perhaps the two disorders are related, and that there may be a genetic influence in the development of antisocial personality disorder. Psychosocial factors are complex and multiple, from the impact of early childhood abuse to the abnormal development of object constancy. Treatments are correspondingly multifactorial, involving pharmacotherapy, behavioral and cognitive approaches, psychodynamic formulations, and analytic understanding as well as controlled hospitalizations, 12-step support groups, and individual and family therapies.

The student should study the questions and answers below for a useful review of these disorders.

HELPFUL HINTS

The student should be able to define the terms that follow.

- acting out
- alloplastic
- ambulatory schizophrenia
- anankastic
- antisocial
- as-if personality
- autoplastic
- avoidant
- borderline
- Briquet's syndrome
- castration anxiety
- chaotic sexuality
- character armor
- Stella Chess, Alexander Thomas
- clusters A, B, and C
- counterprojection
- denied affect
- dependence
- dependent
- depressive
- dissociation
- ego-dystonic
- ego-syntonic
- emotionally unstable personality
- endorphins

- ▶ Erik Erikson
- ▶ extroversion
- ▶ fantasy
- ▶ free association
- ▶ genetic factors
- ▶ goodness of fit
- ▶ histrionic
- ▶ hypochondriasis
- ▶ idealization/devaluation
- ▶ ideas of reference
- ▶ identity diffusion
- ▶ inferiority complex
- ▶ internal object relations
- ▶ introversion
- ▶ isolation
- ▶ Carl Gustav Jung

- ▶ Heinz Kohut
- ▶ *la belle indifférence*
- ▶ macropsia
- ▶ magical thinking
- ▶ mask of sanity
- ▶ micropsychotic episodes
- ▶ narcissistic
- ▶ object choices
- ▶ obsessive-compulsive
- ▶ oral character
- ▶ organic personality disorder
- ▶ panambivalence
- ▶ pananxiety

- ▶ panphobia
- ▶ paranoid
- ▶ passive-aggressive
- ▶ personality
- ▶ platelet MAO
- ▶ projection
- ▶ projective identification
- ▶ psychotic character
- ▶ Wilhelm Reich
- ▶ repression
- ▶ saccadic movements
- ▶ Leopold von Sacher-Masoch
- ▶ Marquis de Sade

- ▶ sadistic personality
- ▶ sadomasochistic personality
- ▶ schizoid
- ▶ schizotypal
- ▶ secondary gain
- ▶ self-defeating personality
- ▶ self-mutilation
- ▶ splitting
- ▶ three Ps
- ▶ timid temperament
- ▶ turning anger against the self

▲ QUESTIONS

DIRECTIONS: Each of the questions or incomplete statements below is followed by five suggested responses or completions. Select the *one* that is *best* in each case.

27.1 True statements about the aspects of personality called "temperament" include all of the following *except*

  A. They are heritable.
  B. They are observable early in childhood.
  C. They are relatively stable in time.
  D. They are inconsistent in different cultures.
  E. They are predictive of adolescent and adult behavior.

27.2 Individuals high in novelty seeking are most likely

  A. impulsive
  B. disorderly
  C. easily bored
  D. extravagant
  E. all of the above

27.3 True statements about diagnosing specific personality disorders include

  A. Diagnosis may not be made in children.
  B. Antisocial personality disorder may be diagnosed in individuals under 18.
  C. There is a potential sex bias in diagnosing personality disorders.
  D. Real gender differences do not exist in the prevalence of personality disorders.
  E. All of the above

27.4 True statements about paranoid personality disorder include

  A. Patients are at decreased risk for major depression.
  B. It may be a prepsychotic antecedent of delusional disorders, paranoid type.
  C. Impairment is frequently severe.
  D. The disorder is not complicated by brief psychotic disorder.
  E. All of the above

27.5 Antisocial personality disorder is associated with an increased risk for

  A. major depressive disorder
  B. anxiety disorders
  C. somatization disorder
  D. borderline personality disorder
  E. all of the above

27.6 Borderline personality disorder is associated with

  A. decreased risk for psychotic symptoms
  B. increased risk for premature death
  C. decreased risk for other coexisting personality disorders
  D. decreased risk for bulimia
  E. decreased risk for posttraumatic stress disorder

27.7 The etiology of borderline personality disorder involves

  A. childhood trauma
  B. vulnerable temperament
  C. biological vulnerabilities
  D. familial aggregation
  E. all of the above

27.8 Basic rules with regard to the treatment of patients with personality disorders include all of the following *except*

  A. a passive therapist
  B. use of pharmacotherapy
  C. supervision and a support network for therapists
  D. rare use of pure supportive psychotherapy
  E. frequent sessions

DIRECTIONS: Each group of questions consists of lettered headings followed by a list of numbered statements. For each numbered phrase or statement, select the *one* lettered heading that is most closely associated with it. Each lettered heading may be selected once, more than once, or not at all.

Questions 27.9–27.13

    A. Schizoid personality disorder
    B. Schizotypal personality disorder

27.9 Strikingly odd or eccentric behavior
27.10 Magical thinking
27.11 Ideas of reverence
27.12 Formerly called latent schizophrenia
27.13 Suspiciousness or paranoid ideation

Questions 27.14–27.21

    A. Cluster A
    B. Cluster B
    C. Cluster C

27.14 Borderline personality disorder
27.15 Avoidant personality disorder
27.16 Narcissistic personality disorder
27.17 Obsessive-compulsive personality disorder
27.18 Paranoid personality disorder
27.19 Reward dependence
27.20 Novelty seeking
27.21 Harm avoidance

DIRECTIONS: Each of these questions or incomplete statements is followed by five suggested responses or completions. Select the *one* that is *best* in each case.

27.22 Leon was a 45-year-old postal service employee who was evaluated at a clinic specializing in the treatment of depression. He claimed to have felt constantly depressed since the first grade, without a period of normal mood for more than a few days at a time. His depression was accompanied by lethargy, little or no interest or pleasure in anything, trouble in concentrating, and feelings of inadequacy, pessimism, and resentfulness. His only periods of normal mood occurred when he was home alone, listening to music or watching TV.

    On further questioning, Leon revealed that he could never remember feeling comfortable socially. Even before kindergarten, if he was asked to speak in front of a group of family friends, his mind would go blank. He felt overwhelming anxiety at children's social functions, such as birthday parties, which he either avoided or attended in total silence. He could answer questions in class only if he wrote down the answers in advance; even then, he frequently mumbled and could not get the answer out. He met new children with his eyes lowered, fearing their scrutiny, expecting to feel humiliated and embarrassed. He was convinced that everyone around him thought he was "dumb or a jerk."

    During the past several years, he had tried several therapies to help him get over his shyness and depression. Leon had never experienced sudden anxiety or a panic attack in social situations or at other times. Rather, his anxiety built gradually to a constant level in anticipation of social situations. He had never experienced any psychotic symptoms.

    The *best* diagnosis is

    A. avoidant personality disorder
    B. schizoid personality disorder
    C. schizotypal personality disorder
    D. social phobia
    E. adjustment disorder with anxiety

27.23 Which of the following statements about borderline personality disorder is *false*?

    A. Patients with borderline personality disorder have more relatives with mood disorders than do control groups.
    B. Borderline personality disorder and mood disorders often coexist.
    C. First-degree relatives of persons with borderline personality disorder show an increased prevalence of alcohol dependence.
    D. Smooth-pursuit eye movements are abnormal in borderline personality disorder.
    E. Monoamine oxidase inhibitors are used in the treatment of borderline personality disorder patients.

27.24 The defense mechanism most often associated with paranoid personality disorder is

    A. hypochondriasis
    B. splitting
    C. isolation
    D. projection
    E. dissociation

27.25 A pervasive pattern of grandiosity, lack of empathy, and need for admiration suggests the diagnosis of which of the following personality disorders?

    A. schizotypal
    B. passive-aggressive
    C. borderline
    D. narcissistic
    E. paranoid

27.26 A 34-year-old single man who lives with his mother and works as an accountant is seeking treatment because he is very unhappy after having just broken up with his girlfriend. He feels trapped and forced to choose between his mother and his girlfriend, and because "blood is thicker than water," he has decided not to go against his mother's wishes. Nonetheless, he is angry at himself and at her and believes that she will never let him marry and is possessively hanging on to him. His mother "wears the pants in the family" and is used to getting her way. He is afraid of disagreeing with his mother for fear that she will not be supportive of him and then he will have to fend for himself. He feels that his own judgment is poor.

    He has lived at home his whole life except for 1 year of college, from which he returned because of homesickness. Heterosexual adjustment has been normal except for his inability to leave his mother in favor of another woman.

Based on this patient's clinical presentation, what is the *least likely* diagnosis?

A. Adjustment disorder
B. Dependent personality disorder
C. Narcissistic personality disorder
D. Schizoid personality disorder
E. Borderline personality disorder

27.27 The same patient provides you with additional personal information. At his accounting job, he has on several occasions turned down promotions because he didn't want the responsibility of having to supervise other people or make independent decisions. He has worked for the same boss for 10 years, gets on well with him, and is in turn highly regarded as a dependable and unobtrusive worker. He has two very close friends whom he has kept since early childhood. He has lunch with one of them every workday and feels lost if his friend is sick and misses a day.

He is the youngest of four children and the only boy. He was "babied and spoiled" by his mother and elder sisters. He had considerable separation anxiety as a child—he experienced difficulty falling asleep unless his mother stayed in the room, mild school refusal, and unbearable homesickness when he occasionally tried sleepovers.

Based on the additional information provided, what is the *most likely* diagnosis for this patient?

A. adjustment disorder
B. dependent personality disorder
C. narcissistic personality disorder
D. schizoid personality disorder
E. borderline personality disorder

27.28 People who are prone to dependent personality disorder include all of the following *except*

A. men
B. younger children
C. persons with chronic physical illness in childhood
D. persons with a history of separation anxiety disorder
E. children of mothers with panic disorder

27.29 Which statement concerning antisocial personality disorder is *false*?

A. The prevalence of antisocial personality disorder is 3 percent in men and 1 percent in women.
B. A familial pattern is present.
C. The patients commonly show abnormalities in their electroencephalograms and soft neurological signs.
D. Antisocial personality disorder is synonymous with criminality.
E. The patients appear to lack a conscience.

ANSWERS

Personality Disorders

27.1 The answer is D

Pioneering work by Alexander Thomas and Stella Chess conceptualized temperament as the stylistic component (how) of behavior, as differentiated from motivation (why) and content (what) of behavior. Modern concepts of temperament, however, emphasize its emotional, motivational, and adaptive aspects. Specifically, four major temperament traits have been identified: harm avoidance, novelty seeking, reward dependence, and persistence.

Temperament traits of harm avoidance, novelty seeking, reward dependence, and persistence are defined as *heritable differences* underlying one's automatic response to danger, novelty, and various types of reward, respectively. These four temperament traits are associated closely with the four basic emotions of fear (harm avoidance), anger (novelty seeking), attachment (reward dependence), and mastery (persistence). Individual differences in temperament and basic emotions modify the processing of sensory information and critically shape early learning characteristics, especially associative conditioning of unconscious behavior responses. In other words, temperament is conceptualized as heritable biases in emotionality and learning that underlie the acquisition of emotion-based, automatic behavior traits and habits *observable early in life and that are relatively stable over one's life span*.

Each of the four major dimensions is a normally distributed quantitative trait. The four dimensions were shown to be genetically homogeneous and independently inherited from one another in large, independent twin studies in the United States

and Australia. Temperamental differences, which are not very stable initially, tend to stabilize during the second and third years of life. Accordingly, ratings of these four temperament traits at age 10 years predicted personality traits at ages 15, 18, and 27 years in a large sample of Swedish children. The four dimensions have been shown repeatedly to be *universal across different cultures*, ethnic groups, and political systems on five continents. In summary, these aspects of personality are called "temperament" because they are heritable, observable early in childhood, relatively stable in time, *moderately predictive of adolescent and adult behavior*, and consistent in different cultures.

27.2 The answer is E (all)

Novelty seeking reflects a heritable bias in the initiation or activation of appetitive approach in response to novelty, signals of reward, avoidance of conditioned signals of punishment, and skilled escape from unconditioned punishment. All four of these behaviors are hypothesized to co-vary as part of one heritable system of learning. They are observed as exploratory activity in response to novelty, impulsiveness, extravagance in approach to cues of reward, and active avoidance of frustration. Individuals high in novelty seeking are quick-tempered, curious, *easily bored, impulsive, extravagant*, and *disorderly*. Adaptive advantages of high novelty seeking are enthusiastic explorations of new and unfamiliar stimuli, leading potentially to originality, discoveries, and reward. The disadvantages include frequent and easy boredom, excessive impulsivity and angry outbursts, potential fickleness in relationships, and impressionism in efforts. Persons low in novelty seeking are slow tempered, stoic, reflective, frugal, reserved, and orderly. Their reflectiveness, stoic resilience, systematic efforts, and meticulous approach are clearly advantageous when these features are needed adaptively. The disadvantages include an uninquiring attitude, lack of enthusiasm, and tolerance of monotony, potentially leading to prosaic routinization of activities.

Mesolimbic and mesofrontal dopaminergic projections have a crucial role in incentive activation of each aspect of novelty seeking in animals. For example, dopamine-depleting lesions in the nucleus accumbens or the ventral tegmentum lead to neglect of novel environmental stimuli and reduce both spontaneous activity and investigative behavior. Behavioral activation by dopaminergic agonists depends on integrity of the nucleus accumbens but not the caudate nucleus. In human studies, individuals at risk for Parkinson's disease have low premorbid scores in novelty seeking but not other dimensions of personality, supporting the importance of dopamine in incentive activation of pleasurable behavior. The initiation and frequency of hyperactivity, binge eating, sexual hedonism, drinking, smoking, and other substance abuse (especially stimulants) are each associated with high scores in novelty seeking.

27.3 The answer is C

Diagnosis of specific personality disorders may be made in children or adolescents when observed maladaptive personality traits are pervasive, persistent, and unlikely to be limited to a particular developmental stage or an episode of an Axis I disorder. Diagnosis of a personality disorder in an individual under 18 years of age requires that the features be present for more than 1 year. The only exception to this *is antisocial personality disorder, which cannot be diagnosed in individuals under 18 years of age.*

Clinical experience points to *a potential sex bias in diagnosing personality disorders.* Certain personality disorders are diagnosed more frequently in men (e.g., antisocial and schizoid), whereas some disorders are diagnosed more frequently in women (e.g., borderline, histrionic, and dependent). Even though *real gender differences likely exist* in the prevalence of these disorders, clinicians are cautioned not to overdiagnose or underdiagnose certain personality disorders in males and females because of social stereotypes about typical gender roles and behaviors.

27.4 The answer is B

The hallmarks of paranoid personality disorder are excessive suspiciousness and distrust of others expressed as a pervasive tendency to interpret actions of others as deliberately demeaning, malevolent, threatening, exploiting, or deceiving. *Frequently, impairment is mild, not severe,* but the disorder typically includes occupational and social difficulties.

These patients are at *increased (not decreased) risk for major depressive disorder,* obsessive-compulsive disorder, agoraphobia, and substance abuse or dependence. The most common co-occurring personality disorders are schizotypal, schizoid, narcissistic, avoidant, and borderline personality disorders. The disorder *may be complicated by brief psychotic disorder,* particularly in response to stress. Paranoid personality disorder has been *postulated to be a prepsychotic antecedent of delusional disorder, paranoid type.*

27.5 The answer is E (all)

Antisocial patients are at increased risk for impulse control disorders, *major depression,* substance abuse or dependence, patho-

logical gambling, *anxiety disorders,* and *somatization disorder.* The most common co-occurring personality disorders are narcissistic, *borderline,* and histrionic.

27.6 The answer is B

The hallmarks of borderline personality disorder are pervasive and excessive instability of affects, self-image, and interpersonal relationships as well as marked impulsivity.

The disorder may be complicated by *psychotic-like symptoms* (hallucinations, body image distortions, hypnagogic phenomena, ideas of reference) in response to stress, and an increased risk for *premature death* (or physical handicap) from suicide and suicidal gestures, failed suicide, and self-injurious behavior. Frequent and severe impairment may lead to job losses, interrupted education, and broken marriages.

These patients are at *increased (not decreased) risk* for major depression, substance abuse or dependence, *eating disorders (notably bulimia), posttraumatic stress disorder,* and attention-deficit/hyperactivity disorder. Borderline personality disorder *co-occurs with most other personality disorders.*

27.7 The answer is E (all)

Numerous studies have pointed to *early traumatic experiences* as a cause of this personality disorder. Recently, a tripartite etiological model, including childhood trauma, *vulnerable temperament,* and a series of triggering events has been formulated. Dynamic and biological psychiatry agree that a combination of early traumatic events and *certain biological vulnerabilities* (mostly in the emotional domain) represent primary etiological factors. Physical and sexual abuse, neglect, hostile conflict, and early parental loss or separation are common in childhood histories of patients with this disorder. *Familial aggregation* of borderline personality disorder has been demonstrated repeatedly. Borderline personality disorder is five times more common among relatives of probands with this disorder than in the general population. The disorder is also associated with increased familial risk for antisocial personality disorder, substance abuse, and mood disorders.

27.8 The answer is A

As a rule, combinations of various orientations and formats along with emphasis on teamwork are optimal in the psychotherapy of personality disorders. Some basic guidelines and values are, nevertheless, strictly observed. Probably most crucial is having a stable therapeutic framework with consistent and reliable care. Next, behavior and feelings are used as the principal mode of communication. *The therapist is active, not passive,* and uses high-energy confrontation and care (so-called therapeutic pressing). The central message is "do something with the patient, not something to the patient." This way, patients feel more in control, which might keep them in treatment. Reflecting their splitting mechanism, these patients alternately feel inferior and omnipotent, angry at others and self-destructive, sensitive to rejection but usually provoking it. Flexibility in therapeutic *approach* but firmness in core values, with creativity and readiness to step away from the rules to get beyond "no way out" situations, is essential. Many of these patients cannot tolerate feeling better, as this means, at least in part, that the therapist is successful. These and similar frustrating situations cause countertransference problems, with a potential loss of professional objectivity; *constant supervision and a support network* are therefore necessary for the therapist treating borderline patients. Remember, these patients are almost never as good as they look when they are doing well, and almost never as bad as they look when they are not doing well.

Pure supportive psychotherapy is rarely used for personality disorders. Pure support, aimed at strengthening existing coping styles (which are, by definition, maladaptive in personality disorders), often reinforces the problems of these patients.

The psychobiological approach incorporates these psychodynamic strategies into a comprehensive treatment plan aimed at stimulating character development, primarily self-directedness and cooperativeness. The main focus is to change internalized conceptual representations of the self and the external objects (i.e., concepts about self, society, and the world as a whole). This is attempted either with cognitive methods (aimed at revising these concepts), with dynamic methods (aimed at generating maturation of internalized object relations), or, most frequently, with a combination of the two. Cognitive methods use emotions as the royal road to cognition. Also, object relations are a special kind of internalized concept about self and others associated with either positive or negative affects, depending on the nature of the relation. In other words, both cognitive and psychodynamic methods address emotional and conceptual aspects of deviant behaviors. Dynamic and cognitive methods are complemented by behavioral and experiential techniques, which are efficient in transforming concepts and insights into everyday life.

During therapy, as character matures and new concepts and their associated secondary emotions develop, they neutralize extreme temperament traits and their related basic emotions of fear and anger. Behaviors change accordingly, from being primarily reactive (i.e., steered by basic emotions and automatic responses regulated by temperament) to being primarily proactive (i.e., steered predominantly by secondary emotions and active symbolic constructs regulated by character traits).

Psychotherapy of personality disorders is a strategy rather than a strictly defined method because the therapy takes place constantly (during any contact with the patient), not only during the psychotherapy sessions proper. In fact, what is happening between sessions may be critical for the outcome of the treatment as a whole. With these patients, psychotherapy essentially means reparenting, which, although sometimes demanding, leaves space for various types of interventions, such as education, help with real-life problems, and encouragement. *Frequent sessions* (at least once a week) are needed to develop reasonably complex interactions in the relationship, for diagnostic and (especially) treatment purposes.

Increasing evidence shows *pharmacotherapy* to be at least as important as psychotherapy in the overall treatment of personality disorders. Pharmacotherapy is either (1) causal, aimed at correcting neurobiological dispositions underlying deviant traits; or (2) symptomatic, aimed at correcting target behaviors and symptoms of personality disorders. The third approach, based on the expectation that the treatment of diagnosable comorbid Axis I disorders might improve personality symptoms indirectly, receives least support in the literature.

Answers 27.9–27.13

27.9 The answer is B

27.10 The answer is B

27.11 The answer is B

27.12 The answer is B

27.13 The answer is B

Unlike schizoid personality disorder, *schizotypal personality disorder* manifests with *strikingly odd or eccentric behavior. Magical thinking, ideas of reference*, illusions, and derealization are common; their presence formerly led to defining this disorder as borderline, *or latent schizophrenia. Suspiciousness or paranoid ideation* occurs in schizotypal personality disorder, not schizoid personality disorder.

Answers 27.14–27.21

27.14 The answer is B

27.15 The answer is C

27.16 The answer is B

27.17 The answer is C

27.18 The answer is A

27.19 The answer is A

27.20 The answer is B

27.21 The answer is C

DSM-IV-TR arranges categorical personality disorders into three clusters, each sharing some clinical features: Cluster A includes three disorders with odd, aloof, and eccentric features (*paranoid*, schizoid, and schizotypal); *Cluster B* includes four disorders with dramatic, impulsive, and erratic features (*borderline*, antisocial, *narcissistic*, and histrionic); and *Cluster C* includes three disorders sharing anxious and fearful features (*avoidant*, dependent, and *obsessive-compulsive*). Several studies have supported the construct validity of these clusters except that the symptoms for compulsive disorder sometimes tend to form a fourth cluster. Note that the three dimensions underlying Clusters A, B, and C (i.e., detachment, impulsivity, and fearfulness) correspond closely to normal temperament traits (*reward dependence, novelty seeking, and harm avoidance,* respectively), suggesting that variation in these temperament traits might be significant in distinguishing among the three clusters of disorders.

Patients with *obsessive-compulsive personality disorder* are preoccupied with orderliness and perfectionism and are rigid and stubborn. In ICD-10 it is called anankastic personality disorder. Patients with *avoidant personality disorder* are unwilling to be involved with people unless certain of being liked. In ICD-10 this is called anxious personality disorder. *Borderline personality disorder* is characterized by identity disturbance, impulsivity, and recurrent suicidal behavior. In ICD-10 the disorder is called emotionally unstable personality disorder. Patients with *paranoid personality disorder* read hidden demeaning or threatening meanings into benign events and comments.

27.22 The answer is A

The best diagnosis is *avoidant personality disorder.* Although feeling constantly depressed caused him to seek treatment, the pervasive pattern of social avoidance, fear of criticism, and lack of close peer relationships was of equal importance. Persons with avoidant personality show an extreme sensitivity to rejection, which may lead to social withdrawal. They are not asocial but are shy and show a great desire for companionship; they need unusually strong guarantees of uncritical acceptance. In the case presented, the patient exhibited a longstanding pattern of difficulty in relating to others. Persons with *schizoid personality disorder* do not evince the same strong desire for affection and acceptance; they want to be alone. *Schizotypal personality disorder* is characterized by strikingly odd or strange behavior, magical thinking, peculiar ideas, ideas of reference, illusions, and derealization. The patient described did not exhibit those characteristics. *Social phobia* is an irrational fear of social or performance situations such as public speaking and eating in public. A social phobia is anxiety concerning socially identified situations, not relationships in general.

A person with a personality disorder can have a superimposed adjustment disorder, but only if the current episode includes new clinical features not characteristic of the individual's personality. No evidence in the case described indicated that the anxiety was qualitatively different from what the patient always experienced in social situations. Thus, an additional diagnosis of *adjustment disorder with anxiety* is not made.

27.23 The answer is D

Smooth pursuit eye movements are normal (not abnormal) in borderline personality disorder. They are abnormal in schizophrenic patients and patients with schizotypal personality disorder.

Patients with borderline personality disorders have *more relatives with mood disorders* than do members of control groups, and *borderline personality disorder and mood disorders often coexist.* First-degree relatives of persons with borderline personality disorder show an *increased prevalence of alcohol dependence* and substance abuse. *Monoamine oxidase inhibitors* are used in the treatment of borderline personality disorder patients and have been effective in modulating affective instability and impulsivity in a number of patients. However, due to the high incidence of impulsivity, substance abuse, and eating disorders in borderline patients, MAOIs must only be used in selective patients, and even then with great restraint.

27.24 The answer is D

The defense mechanism most often associated with paranoid personality disorder is *projection.* The patients externalize their own emotions and attribute to others impulses and thoughts that they are unable to accept in themselves. Excessive fault finding, sensitivity to criticism, prejudice, and hypervigilance to injustice can all be understood as examples of projecting unacceptable impulses and thoughts onto others.

Hypochondriasis is a defense mechanism in some personality disorders, particularly in borderline, dependent, and passive-aggressive personality disorders. Hypochondriasis disguises reproach; that is, the hypochondriac complaint that others do not provide help often conceals bereavement, loneliness, or unacceptable aggressive impulses. The mechanism of hypochondriasis permits covert punishment of others with the patient's own pain and discomfort.

Splitting is used by patients with borderline personality disorder in particular. With splitting, the patient divides ambivalently regarded people, both past and present, into all-good or all-bad, rather than synthesizing and assimilating less-than-perfect caretakers.

Isolation is the defense mechanism characteristic of the orderly controlled person, often labeled an obsessive-compulsive personality. Isolation allows the person to face painful situations without painful affect or emotion and thus to remain always in control.

Dissociation consists of a separation of consciousness from unpleasant affects. It is most often seen in patients with histrionic or borderline personality disorder.

27.25 The answer is D

A pervasive pattern of grandiosity (in fantasy or behavior), lack of empathy, and need for admiration suggests the diagnosis of *narcissistic* personality disorder. The fantasies of narcissistic patients are of unlimited success, power, brilliance, beauty, and ideal love; their demands are for constant attention and admiration. Narcissistic personality disorder patients are indifferent to criticism or respond to it with feelings of rage or humiliation. Other common characteristics are a sense of entitlement, surprise and anger that people do not do what the patient wants, and interpersonal exploitiveness.

Schizotypal personality disorder is characterized by various eccentricities in communication or behavior coupled with defects in the capacity to form social relationships. The term emphasizes a possible relation with schizophrenia. The manifestation of aggressive behavior in passive ways—such as obstructionism, pouting, stubbornness, and intentional inefficiency—typify *passive-aggressive* personality disorder. *Borderline* personality disorder is marked by instability of mood, interpersonal relationships, and self-image. *Paranoid* personality disorder is characterized by rigidity, hypersensitivity, unwarranted suspicion, jealousy, envy, an exaggerated sense of self-importance, and a tendency to blame and ascribe evil motives to others.

27.26 The answer is C

The *least likely diagnosis is narcissistic personality disorder* because the patient exhibits no signs of a heightened sense of self importance, grandiose feelings of uniqueness, lack of empathy, and need for admiration. *Adjustment disorder* is a more likely diagnosis based on the patient's mood from his recent break-up with his girlfriend. *Dependent personality disorder* is a possible diagnosis because the patient shows a lack of self-confidence and has difficulty expressing disagreement with others because of fear of loss of support or approval. *Schizoid personality disorder* is another possibility based on the patient's seemingly lifelong pattern of social withdrawal. Finally, *borderline personality disorder* is considered because the patient shows unstable mood and self-image.

27.27 The answer is B

Based on the additional information provided, *dependent personality disorder* is the most likely diagnosis for this patient. The patient states he turned down promotions at work to avoid the responsibility of supervising others and to avoid making independent decisions. The patient feels uncomfortable or helpless when alone because of exaggerated fear of being unable to care for himself. The patient exhibits no *narcissistic personality disorder* traits. *Adjustment disorder* cannot be applied to this patient's case because his symptoms are lifelong symptoms, and not just related causally to his recent break-up. The patient does not wish to be alone, as seen in *schizoid personality disorder,* and in fact, desires affection and acceptance. He shows no signs of impulsivity, recurrent suicidal behavior, or chronic feelings of emptiness, as seen in *borderline personality disorder.*

27.28 The answer is A

People who are prone to dependent personality disorder include *women (who are more commonly affected than men, not vice versa), younger children,* and *persons with chronic physical illness in childhood.* Some workers believe that *a history of separation anxiety disorder* predisposes to the development of dependent personality disorder. Separation anxiety disorder has its onset before the age of 18 and is characterized by excessive anxiety concerning separation from people to whom the child is attached. Separation anxiety disorder itself may be frequent in *children of mothers with panic disorder,* and that factor may predispose to the development of dependent personality disorder.

27.29 The answer is D

Antisocial personality disorder is characterized by continual antisocial or criminal acts, but it *is not synonymous with criminality.* Rather, it is a pattern of irresponsible and antisocial behavior that pervades the patient's adolescence and adulthood. The prevalence of antisocial personality disorder is *3 percent in men and 1 percent in women. A familial pattern is present* in that it is five times more common among first-degree relatives of males with the disorder than among controls. A notable finding is a lack of remorse; that is, *patients often appear to lack a conscience.* In addition, patients commonly *show abnormalities in their electroencephalograms and soft neurological signs,* suggestive of minimal brain damage in childhood.

28

Psychological Factors Affecting Medical Condition

It is well established that psychological and behavioral factors can affect medical conditions. Noncompliance with treatment and continuing to smoke in the face of pulmonary disease are probably two of the most obvious. However, almost all medical conditions have associated psychological or behavioral factors that can affect their course. The revised fourth edition of the *Diagnostic and Statistical Manual of Mental Disorders* (DSM-IV-TR) includes a classification specifically for psychological factors affecting medical condition, and characterizes the factors as having to have a significant effect on the course or outcome of the condition, or place the patient at significantly higher risk for an adverse outcome. The factors may influence its course, interfere with treatment, constitute an additional risk, or precipitate the symptoms. The nature of the various psychological factors are delineated in DSM-IV-TR and include mental disorder, psychological symptoms, personality traits or coping styles, maladaptive health behaviors, and unspecified psychological factors. DSM-IV-TR does not stipulate that these factors must directly cause the medical condition, but it does specify that there must be a close temporal relationship between the factors and the condition.

Consultation-liaison (C-L) psychiatrists work with nonpsychiatric clinicians to better understand, manage, and treat patients whose psychology and behavior are adversely affecting their medical condition. Psychological factors affecting medical condition have been well studied in a number of disorders, and C-L psychiatrists are frequently called upon to assist in the management of these patients. Virtually every major system of the body has been investigated with regard to the relationship between psychological factors and disease. Psychological factors affecting the cardiovascular, respiratory, immune, endocrine, gastrointestinal, and dermatologic systems are well-known. Responses to and recovery from major surgery, hemodialysis treatments, or any major medical procedure can be compromised by adverse psychological or behavioral reactions. The apparently simple act of correctly following a medication regimen can be complicated, and even undermined, by unaddressed or unrecognized psychological factors.

The emotional and physical stress of medical illness can trigger underlying conflicts or exacerbate preexisting personality problems that can then profoundly affect the proper management of the illness. Increasing investigation of the complex relationship between mind and body, and the interrelationship of stress, illness, and outcome, is assisting clinicians in recognizing and treating the psychological and behavioral factors that can thwart successful medical treatment.

The student should study the questions and answers below for a useful review of these factors.

HELPFUL HINTS

These terms relating to psychophysiological medicine should be defined.

- AIDS
- Franz Alexander
- alexithymia
- allergic disorders
- analgesia
- atopic
- autoimmune diseases
- behavioral medicine
- behavior modification deconditioning program
- biofeedback
- bronchial asthma
- bulimia nervosa and anorexia nervosa
- C-L psychiatry
- cardiac arrhythmias
- cell-mediated immunity
- chronic pain
- climacteric
- command hallucination
- compulsive personality traits
- congestive heart failure
- conversion disorder
- coronary artery disease
- crisis intervention
- Jacob DaCosta
- diabetes mellitus
- dialysis dementia
- Flanders Dunbar
- dysmenorrhea
- dysthymic disorder
- essential hypertension
- fibromyalgia
- Meyer Friedman and Roy Rosenman
- general adaptation syndrome
- giving up–given up concept
- gun-barrel vision
- hay fever
- hemodialysis units
- Thomas Holmes and Richard Rahe
- humoral immunity
- hyperhidrosis
- hyperthyroidism

- ▶ hyperventilation syndrome
- ▶ hypochondriasis
- ▶ ICUs
- ▶ idiopathic amenorrhea
- ▶ IgM and IgA
- ▶ immediate and delayed hypersensitivity
- ▶ immune disorders
- ▶ immune response
- ▶ life-change units
- ▶ low back pain
- ▶ menopausal distress
- ▶ migraine
- ▶ myxedema madness
- ▶ neurocirculatory asthenia
- ▶ obesity

- ▶ obsessional personalities
- ▶ oral-aggressive feelings
- ▶ organ transplantation
- ▶ pain clinics
- ▶ pain threshold and perception
- ▶ pancreatic carcinoma
- ▶ Papez circuit
- ▶ peptic ulcer
- ▶ personality types
- ▶ pheochromocytoma
- ▶ PMS
- ▶ postcardiotomy delirium
- ▶ premenstrual dysphoric disorder
- ▶ propranolol (Inderal)

- ▶ pruritus
- ▶ psyche and soma
- ▶ psychogenic cardiac nondisease
- ▶ psychophysiological
- ▶ psychosomatic
- ▶ Raynaud's phenomenon
- ▶ relaxation therapy
- ▶ rheumatoid arthritis
- ▶ Hans Selye
- ▶ skin disorders
- ▶ social readjustment rating scale
- ▶ somatization disorder
- ▶ specific versus nonspecific stress

- ▶ specificity hypothesis
- ▶ surgical patients
- ▶ systemic lupus erythematosus
- ▶ tension headaches
- ▶ tension myositis syndrome (TMS)
- ▶ thyrotoxicosis
- ▶ type A and type B personalities
- ▶ ulcerative colitis
- ▶ undermedication
- ▶ vasomotor syncope
- ▶ vasovagal attack
- ▶ Wilson's disease

▲ QUESTIONS

DIRECTIONS: Each of the questions or incomplete statements below is followed by five responses or completions. Select the *one* that is *best* in each case.

28.1 The Social Readjustment Rating Scale (or Schedule of Recent Experience Scale) is associated with

  A. Thomas Holmes and Richard Rahe
  B. Hans Selye
  C. John Mason
  D. Richard Lazarus
  E. Harold Wolff and Stewart Wolf

28.2 True statements about research in psychocardiology include

  A. The most consistent psychological correlates of hypertension are inhibited anger expression and excessive anger expression.
  B. Stress leads to excess secretion of epinephrine, which raises cardiac contractility and conduction velocity.
  C. Cardiac surgery patients at greatest risk for complications are depressed and in denial about their anxiety.
  D. Mental stress leads to diminished cardiac perfusion.
  E. All of the above

28.3 True statements about type A behavior include

  A. Once coronary artery disease is present, global type A behavior appears to increase the risk of subsequent cardiac morbidity.
  B. Of all the elements of the syndrome, hostility has been found to be the most toxic element.
  C. Global type A behavior consistently predicts risk of coronary artery disease.
  D. Expressive hostility and antagonistic interactions appear to be least strongly related to the risk of coronary artery disease in women.
  E. Lifestyle modification has little effect on revascularization.

28.4 Evidence suggesting a linkage between major depression and increased morbidity in patients with coronary artery disease (CAD) includes

  A. The point prevalence of major depression in patients with CAD is twice that in primary care patients.
  B. The 30-day point prevalence of major depression in patients with CAD is three to four times that in the general population.
  C. A major depressive episode is the best predictor of major cardiac events during the 12 months after cardiac catheterization.
  D. The impact of depressive disorders on poor outcome of CAD appears to equal or exceed that of other well-known cardiovascular risk factors.
  E. All of the above

28.5 True statements about the effects of psychosocial interventions in cancer outcomes and prognosis include

  A. There is no evidence that psychotherapy influences the outcome of metastatic breast cancer.
  B. The mortality rates and recurrence rates in patients with malignant melanoma have been shown to be greater in patients who did not receive a structured group intervention than in those who did.
  C. Group behavioral intervention in patients with breast cancer does not appear to have any effect on lymphocyte mitogen responses.
  D. Lack of social support and depression have not been shown to be linked to diminished immune responses in women with breast cancer.
  E. Hypothalamic-pituitary-adrenal axis hyperactivity induced by exposure of rats to stress is associated with increased tumor growth.

28.6 Exposure of rats to stress reliably

A. decreases plasma concentrations of ACTH
B. decreases plasma concentrations of corticosterone
C. increases secretion of growth hormone
D. increases secretion of CRF in locus ceruleus
E. all of the above

28.7 The most frequent functional gastrointestinal disorder is

A. functional abdominal bloating
B. functional chest pain
C. functional heartburn
D. irritable bowel syndrome
E. globus

28.8 True statements about obesity include

A. The number of obese Americans is less than that of nonobese Americans.
B. The prevalence of obesity in America has doubled since the early 1900s.
C. Higher rates of obesity are linked with lower socioeconomic and educational levels and type of diet.
D. Its prevalence in children appears to be stabilized and even decreasing.
E. All of the above

28.9 Psychiatric forces may affect the clinical expression of asthma by

A. suggestibility to airway constriction
B. altered awareness of airway resistance
C. comorbidity with panic disorder
D. comorbidity with depression
E. all of the above

28.10 Psoriasis has been shown to be

A. unaffected by such psychosocial interventions as meditation or relaxation
B. associated with lower levels of anxiety and depression than in the general population
C. triggered by external factors such as cold weather and physical trauma
D. rarely associated with personality disorders
E. none of the above

28.11 Antidepressants have been shown to be helpful in the treatment of

A. idiopathic pruritus
B. urticaria
C. vulvodynia
D. glossodynia
E. all of the above

28.12 Medical patients have a much higher morbidity, when compared with the general population, for

A. delirium
B. depression
C. panic
D. substance abuse
E. all of the above

28.13 A review of the impact of biobehavioral factors on adult cancer pain concluded that

A. there was a consistent role of personality factors
B. the relationship to affective states was major
C. environmental influences were strong
D. all of the above
E. none of the above

DIRECTIONS: The questions below consist of five lettered headings followed by a list of numbered phrases. For each numbered item, select the *one* lettered heading that is most closely associated with it. Each lettered heading may be selected once, more than once, or not at all.

Questions 28.14–28.18

A. Wilson's disease
B. Pheochromocytoma
C. Systemic lupus erythematosus
D. Acquired immune deficiency syndrome (AIDS)
E. Pancreatic cancer

28.14 Dementia syndrome with global impairment and seropositivity
28.15 Resemblance to steroid psychosis
28.16 Explosive anger and labile mood
28.17 Symptoms of a classic panic attack
28.18 Sense of imminent doom

DIRECTIONS: Each of the questions or incomplete statements below is followed by five responses or completions. Select the *one* that is *best* in each case.

28.19 A major advance in the revised fourth edition of *Diagnostic and Statistical Manual of Mental Disorders* (DSM-IV-TR) in regard to the diagnostic criteria for psychological factors affecting medical condition is that DSM-IV-TR allows for emphasis on

A. environmental stimuli
B. psychological stimuli
C. somatoform disorders
D. conversion disorder
E. all of the above

28.20 A decrease in T lymphocytes has been reported in all of the following *except*

A. bereavement
B. caretakers of patients with dementia of the Alzheimer's type
C. women who are having extramarital affairs
D. nonpsychotic inpatients
E. medical students during final examinations

28.21 The major worker in the application of psychoanalytic concepts to the study of psychosomatic disorders was

A. George Mahl
B. Harold Wolff
C. Franz Alexander
D. Robert Ader
E. Meyer Friedman

28.22 Which of the following statements about psycho-neuroimmunology is true?

A. Immunological reactivity is not affected by hypnosis.
B. Lymphocytes cannot produce neurotransmitters.
C. The immune system is affected by conditioning.
D. Growth hormone does not affect immunity.
E. Marijuana does not affect the immune system.

28.23 Symptoms of mood disorder and psychotic disorder are found most often with the use of

A. hexamethylmelamine
B. steroids
C. interferon
D. hydroxyurea
E. L-asparaginase

28.24 Disorders in which autoimmune diseases have been implicated include all of the following *except*

A. Graves' disease
B. rheumatoid arthritis
C. peptic ulcer
D. regional ileitis
E. pernicious anemia

28.25 Phantom limb occurs after leg amputation in what percentage of patients?

A. 98 percent
B. 90 percent
C. 80 percent
D. 50 percent
E. 10 percent

28.26 In the psychotherapeutic treatment of patients with psychosomatic disorders, the most difficult problem is patients'

A. resistance to entering psychotherapy
B. erotic transference to the psychotherapist
C. positive response to the interpretation of the physiological meaning of their symptoms
D. recognition of the psychological correlation with their physiological symptoms
E. none of the above

28.27 A 53-year-old male patient is found to have an occipital lobe tumor. He would be *least likely* to exhibit which of the following symptoms and complaints?

A. paranoid delusions
B. visual hallucinations
C. headache
D. papilledema
E. homonymous hemianopsia

28.28 A patient presenting with mood disturbances, psychoses, fever, photosensitivity, butterfly rash, and joint pains is *most likely* to be given a diagnosis of

A. acute intermittent porphyria
B. hypoparathyroidism
C. systemic lupus erythematosus
D. hepatic encephalopathy
E. pheochromocytoma

28.29 In evaluating patients with complaints of chronic pain of whatever cause, the physician must be alert to

A. use of over-the-counter medications
B. alcohol dependence
C. withdrawal symptoms during the evaluation
D. an underlying medical illness
E. all of the above

28.30 Dialysis dementia is characterized by all of the following *except*

A. disorientation
B. loss of memory
C. seizures
D. dystonias
E. delusions

28.31 A highly emetogenic anticancer agent is

A. cisplatin
B. doxorubicin
C. vincristine
D. vinblastine
E. bleomycin

28.32 The percentage of cancer patients who later have mental disorders is

A. 1 to 10 percent
B. 15 to 20 percent
C. 25 to 30 percent
D. 35 to 40 percent
E. 45 to 50 percent

ANSWERS

Psychological Factors Affecting Medical Condition

28.1 The answer is A
A major area of psychosomatic research involving social stress is based on the work of *Thomas Holmes and Richard Rahe*, using the Schedule of Recent Experience (SRE). Recent life events (e.g., the death of a close relative, a job change, or a divorce) are assigned life change units. An expanded and revised version of the SRE, the Recent Life Change Questionnaire, also asks subjects to score recent life changes on the degree of perceived adjustment. Both instruments are designed to measure recent life stress and to correlate the degree of life stress with subsequent illness. The basic hypothesis is that stressful life occurrences are risk factors for the development of physical illness. Numerous studies demonstrate a probability relation between stressful life events and one's

Table 28.1
Social Readjustment Rating Scale

Life Event	Mean Value
1. Death of spouse	100
2. Divorce	73
3. Marital separation from mate	65
4. Detention in jail or other institution	63
5. Death of a close family member	63
6. Major personal injury or illness	53
7. Marriage	50
8. Being fired at work	47
9. Marital reconciliation with mate	45
10. Retirement from work	45
11. Major change in the health or behavior of a family member	44
12. Pregnancy	40
13. Sexual difficulties	39
14. Gaining a new family member (through birth, adoption, elder moving in, etc.)	39
15. Major business readjustment (merger, reorganization, bankruptcy, etc.)	39
16. Major change in financial state (a lot worse off or a lot better off than usual)	38
17. Death of a close friend	37
18. Changing to a different line of work	36
19. Major change in the number of arguments with spouse (either a lot more or a lot less than usual regarding child rearing, personal habits, etc.)	35
20. Taking on a mortgage greater than $10,000 (purchasing a home, business, etc.)[a]	31
21. Foreclosure on a mortgage or loan	30
22. Major change in responsibilities at work (promotion, demotion, lateral transfer)	29
23. Son or daughter leaving home (marriage, attending college, etc.)	29
24. In-law troubles	29
25. Outstanding personal achievement	28
26. Wife beginning or ceasing work outside the home	26
27. Beginning or ceasing formal schooling	26
28. Major change in living conditions (building a new home, remodeling, deterioration of home or neighborhood)	25
29. Revision of personal habits (dress, manners, associations, etc.)	24
30. Troubles with the boss	23
31. Major change in working hours or conditions	20
32. Change in residence	20
33. Changing to a new school	20
34. Major change in usual type or amount of recreation	19
35. Major change in church activities (a lot more or a lot less than usual)	19
36. Major change in social activities (clubs, dancing, movies, visiting, etc.)	18
37. Taking on a mortgage or loan less than $10,000 (purchasing a car, TV, freezer, etc.)	17
38. Major change in sleeping habits (a lot more or a lot less sleep or change in part of day when asleep)	16
39. Major change in number of family get-togethers (a lot more or a lot less than usual)	15
40. Major change in eating habits (a lot more or a lot less food intake or very different meal hours or surroundings)	15
41. Vacation	15
42. Christmas	12
43. Minor violations of the law (traffic tickets, jaywalking, disturbing the peace, etc.)	11

[a]This figure no longer has any relevance in the light of inflation; what is significant is the total amount of debt from all sources.
Reprinted with permission from Holmes T. Life situations, emotions, and disease. *Psychosom Med.* 1978;9:747.

chances of having a physical illness. Epidemiological research involving other types of stressful life events (e.g., natural disasters, social disruption, social changes, poor social support, and work-related stress) has shown similar trends toward an increased probability of physical illness and relatively poor medical outcome. Current models of psychosomatic research integrate the interaction of psychological variables, stressful social situations, and biological vulnerability with latent physical disease. Table 28.1 provides the Social Readjustment Rating Scale.

The concept of stress has been central in the development of psychosomatic theory. Walter Cannon conducted the first systematic study involving stress paradigms relevant to psychosomatic medicine. His model of stress was derived from the idea that under certain circumstances, physical or emotional stimuli can strain an animal beyond its ability to adapt successfully.

The research of *Harold Wolff* and *Stewart Wolf* continues to serve as a model for scientific investigations of stress. One of Wolff's fundamental premises was that disease is a failure or inability to adapt to life stress. Wolff's theory heralded the concept that the way in which a person copes with a stressful event is critical in determining the magnitude of subsequent physiological effects. Events are deemed stressful only if the person perceives the stress as threatening to life, well-being, or emotional security.

Wolff and Wolf also observed that the physiological states of the gastrointestinal tract appear to correlate with specific emotional states (hyperfunction with hostility and hypofunction with sadness). Nevertheless, they regarded such reactions as relatively nonspecific, believing that the patient's reaction is determined by the general life situation and perceptual appraisal of the stressful event. Wolff also emphasized that the capacity to adapt to a threatening event (e.g., familial discord, emotional deprivation, goal frustration, object loss, separation, and unemployment) determines the nature and severity of psychophysiological response patterns.

Hans Selye's model of stress was based on experiments in which toxic substances were injected into animals and the subsequent reactions observed. Selye outlined the general adaptation syndrome as consisting of three phases: (1) the alarm reaction; (2) the stage of resistance, in which adaptation is ideally achieved; and (3) the stage of exhaustion, in which acquired adaptation or resistance may be lost. Selye's concept of stress was originally used to describe the effects of a force acting against an organism's innate resistance. He considered stress a nonspecific bodily response to any demand caused by either pleasant or unpleasant conditions. Selye's basic theory that physical and emotional stressful stimuli can produce relatively predictable responses formed a fundamental model for much of the behaviorally oriented stress experimentation in psychosomatic research that followed.

Selye's concept of a single nonspecific physiological response to stressors was superseded by experiments demonstrating complex adaptational reactions to stress. For example, *John Mason* performed elegant research in psychoendocrinology demonstrating that in experimental stress situations, physiological reactions are largely influenced by the emotional response to the stimuli—that is, not determined just by the nature of the stimulus itself. Mason focused on intervening psychological variables that determine both acute hormonal reactions to stressful stimuli and the effects of psychological variables on long-term adaptational responses.

Richard Lazarus elaborated the concept of individualized stress responses, which are determined by cognitive factors. He proposed that responses are determined by the manner in which a person cognitively appraises and copes with stressful events. Hence, persons' reactions to stress depend on their appraisal of the event and their belief in their ability to cope with the stress; their attitude regarding the significance of the outcome of the event is also considered important. The reality of the stress is of less importance than an individual's subjective cognitive assessment of it in determining the subsequent emotional and physiological reactions.

28.2 The answer is E (all)

Psychocardiology encompasses the spectrum of interactions of psychiatric disorders, cardiac symptoms, and cardiac disease, including associated complicating health behavior. For the past several decades, attention to the psychosocial and behavioral factors in cardiovascular disease has increased significantly. The research has taken two primary pathways: one has examined hypertension and the other has looked generally at coronary artery disease, including myocardial infarction and sudden cardiac death.

Hypertension, one of the originally hypothesized psychosomatic illnesses, is a major risk factor for coronary artery disease and cerebral vascular disease. Psychological factors have been studied closely as part of the pathogenesis of the condition; these factors have been categorized as pressure reactivity and personality and behavioral factors. Physiological hyperactivity to environmental stimuli (pressure reactivity) has been studied many times, and although results are contradictory, some specific commonalities appear. Relatively strong evidence indicates that some persons have greater blood pressure reactivity than do others to a variety of stressors, ranging from experimental stress induced in the laboratory to such social and societal stressful conditions as racism. However, the evidence linking reactivity in normotensive persons with hypertension is equivocal. Perhaps most important, pressure reactivity in hypertensive individuals may exacerbate and even accelerate the disease process.

Other research examining *psychological aspects of hypertension* has focused on personality traits or coping styles. Traits such as submissiveness and distorted expression of anger have emerged as correlates of hypertension. The most consistent correlates have involved anger-coping styles, both *inhibited anger expression and excessive anger expression.* Epidemiological researchers have noted that persons using an active coping style under environmental conditions that are not conducive to success (e.g., low education and socioeconomic status) may be predisposed to hypertension.

As evidence has clarified how psychological factors affect hypertension, investigators have focused on treatment interventions. Various behavioral procedures including biofeedback, relaxation training, and psychotherapy have been used as interventions. Some investigators have reported clinically significant success in controlled studies. For example, studies that used 24-hour monitoring of blood pressure to examine the effects of combined relaxation therapy and medication found the combination to be more effective in controlling blood pressure than medication alone.

Stress causes a sympatheticoadrenal medullary alarm reaction characterized by excess catecholamine secretion. Specifically, excess epinephrine is secreted under what the body interprets as stressful conditions. The *outpouring of epinephrine* raises blood pressure and heart and respiratory rates, enhances neuromuscular transmission, elevates the concentration of blood sugar by glycogenolysis, mobilizes fat, redirects hemodynamic patterns to suit muscular activity, and while increasing blood oxygenation, increases oxygen consumption. More specific β-adrenergically mediated cardiac effects include increased heart rate, *contractility*, and *conduction velocity* and a short arteriovenous refractory period. These catecholamine-mediated cardiac effects are thought to be pathogenically related to adverse cardiac events.

Studies of stress-induced cardiac changes and studies examining stress, arrhythmias, and sudden cardiac death suggest a significant relation in the pathophysiology of coronary artery disease. Early researchers examined temporally related stressful life experiences including stressful states described among patients who had experienced sudden death attributed to arrhythmias. One study found that the *cardiac surgery patients at greatest risk for complications*, including arrhythmias and sudden death, were depressed, anxious, and in denial of their anxiety, or both.

Recent research has examined the direct cardiac effect of controlled stress. For example, in a study of the effects of psychological stress on patients with ventricular arrhythmias, the stress of mental arithmetic and recalling past traumatic events increased the ventricular premature beat frequency in most patients. Other studies have *documented diminished cardiac perfusion during mental stress* via positron emission tomography and radionucleotide ventriculography in patients with coronary artery disease.

28.3 The answer is B

Most of the studies examining the influence of psychosocial and behavioral risk factors in the etiology of coronary artery disease have focused on type A behavior (Fig. 28.1). Individuals with type A behavior exhibit enhanced aggressiveness, ambitiousness, competitive drive, impatience, and a chronic sense of time urgency. Associated speech and motor characteristics are rapid body movements, tense facial and body musculature, explosive conversational speech, and hand or teeth clenching. Three major prospective studies have found the type

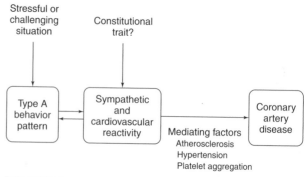

FIGURE 28.1

Conceptual model of type A behavior and the development of coronary artery disease. (Adapted from Goldstein MG, Niaura R. Cardiovascular disease, Part 1: Coronary artery disease and sudden death. In Stoudemire A, ed. *Psychological Factors Affecting Medical Conditions.* Washington DC: American Psychiatric Press; 1995:117.)

A behavior pattern to be a risk factor for clinical coronary artery disease; *however, once the disease is present, global type A behavior does not appear to increase the risk of subsequent cardiac morbidity.*

The initial enthusiasm for the global type A concept waned in the middle 1980s, as *hostility was found to be the most toxic element of the syndrome.* Whereas *global type A behavior does not always predict risk* of coronary artery disease, hostility is consistently linked to coronary artery diseases and appears to be pathophysiologically related to the disease by numerous mechanisms. *Expressive hostility and antagonistic interactions* appear to be the subcomponents of type A behavior that *are most strongly (not least strongly) related to the risk of coronary artery disease, especially among female patients* and middle-aged male patients.

Physiological correlates of type A behavior have also been studied with regard to cardiac morbidity. Type A behavior is believed to be part of a stress paradigm. Numerous studies report that persons with type A behavior patterns display large, episodic increases in blood pressure, heart rate, and catecholamine concentrations when confronted by stressful tasks. Interestingly, evidence from primate studies links atherosclerosis in coronary disease and sympathetic nervous system activation. Findings suggest a link between psychological states, physiological activity, and subsequent cardiovascular disease.

A metaanalysis of 18 controlled studies examining effects of psychological treatment on type A behavior concluded that psychological treatment aimed at reducing the behavior had a positive outcome. When type A behavior decreased, treatment had a significant improved effect on coronary events and mortality at 1-year follow-up.

A recent study by Dean Ornish revealed that *lifestyle modification* (e.g., aerobic exercise, stress management, group therapy) *actually promoted revascularization* and improved the prognosis of patients with cardiac disease.

28.4 The answer is E (all)

A number of mood states have been linked with cardiovascular disease, and an increasing body of literature links major depression to increased morbidity and mortality in individuals with coronary artery disease. Recent investigations using standardized instruments and current diagnostic categories have found the *point prevalence of major depression* in patients with coronary artery disease to be between 17 and 22 percent—approximately *twice that in primary care patients* and *three to four times the 30-day point prevalence in the general population.* One study showed that *a major depressive episode was the best predictor of major cardiac events* during the 12 months after cardiac catheterization; the events were independent of such variables as severity of cardiac disease, left ventricular function, and smoking. In a recent prospective study of patients hospitalized following a myocardial infarction, major depressive disorder was found to be an independent risk factor for mortality at 6 months. The risk was at least equivalent to that of left ventricular dysfunction and previous myocardial infarction. When these patients were studied 18 months after their hospitalization for myocardial infarction, depression was a significant predictor of cardiac mortality, particularly among patients with ten or more premature ventricular contractions per hour.

Increasing evidence of an association between depressive disorders and coronary artery disease makes it important to ascertain the strength of this association because of the important practical health implications. Therefore, researchers have assessed both the persistence of this relation over time and its magnitude. In most patients with coronary artery disease, depressive disorders do not appear to be a transient adjustment to a major illness but rather a clinically significant comorbid disorder that is often chronic. Moreover, recent studies have shown that among individuals with coronary artery disease, women appear to have a higher prevalence of depressive disorders than men. The *impact of depressive disorders on poor outcome* of coronary artery disease *appears to equal or exceed that of other well-known cardiovascular risk factors.* Current explanations for this relation include biological correlates linked to sympathetic activity and autonomic dysregulation, neuroendocrine-immunological interactions producing cytokine-mediated coronary artery occlusion including serotonin-mediated platelet aggregation, and behavioral factors associated with the effect of depression on cardiac treatment adherence. The importance of aggressive treatment of depression in coronary artery disease is clear, and research examining treatment benefits and prevention strategies is under way.

A convincing body of literature focuses on the mood states related to acute situational disturbances. A number of studies have demonstrated a connection between sudden death and acutely disturbing life events. One study found that the onset of malignant ventricular arrhythmia was associated with identifiable emotional triggers in 21 percent of patients referred for antiarrhythmic treatment. Finally, such sociological factors as work overload and life stress in the face of a lack of social support enhance general coronary risk (Table 28.2). Research is increasing into the possibility that central or autonomic nervous system events, or both, mediate the increase in cardiovascular morbidity and mortality.

28.5 The answer is B

The growing interface between the social sciences and oncology between the 1930s and 1950s was the foundation for the emergence of the subspecialty called psychosocial oncology or psycho-oncology. This area, which has become a major contender in psychosomatic medicine research, seeks to study both the impact of cancer on psychological functioning and the role that psychological and behavioral variables may play in cancer risk and survival. A hallmark of psycho-oncology research has been intervention studies that attempt to influence the course of illness in patients with cancer. While most psychosocial interventions are aimed at providing psychological support rather than direct treatment of comorbid conditions such as major depressive disorder, important clinical observations have emerged that focus on such variables as cancer outcome and psychoneuroimmunology. For example, one landmark study demonstrated that *women with metastatic breast cancer* who received weekly group psychotherapy survived an average of 18 months longer than control patients randomly assigned to routine care. In their study of *patients with malignant melanoma,* one group of investigators found that control patients who did not receive a structured group intervention had a statistically significant recurrence of cancer and a greater mortality rate than patients who did receive such therapy. The malignant melanoma patients who received the group intervention also exhibited a significant increase in the number of large granular

Table 28.2
Psychological Factors Related to Coronary Artery Disease

Risk Factor	Cardiac Effects
Stressful life experiences	Sudden death, myocardial ischemia, arrhythmias
Type A behavior pattern	
Expressive hostility	
Antagonistic interactions	Risk of coronary artery disease; episodic increases in blood pressure, heart rate, and catecholamine levels (linked to atherosclerosis in primates)
Cynicism	
Hostile affect	
Aggressive responding	Significant relationships to cardiac mortality
Psychiatric diagnosis	
Major depression	Significant predictor of morbidity after cardiac catheterization; significant predictor of cardiac mortality up to 18 months following myocardial infarction may increase platelet aggregation and thrombus formation
Anxiety	Enhanced risk of cardiac morbidity
Sociocultural factors	
Work overload and life stress	
Lack of social support	Enhanced risk of cardiac morbidity

lymphocytes and NK cells as well as indications of increased NK cell activity. Another group of investigators used a *group behavioral intervention* (relaxation, guided imagery, and biofeedback training) *in patients with breast cancer* to demonstrate increased NK cell activity and lymphocyte mitogen responses in patients receiving treatment compared with controls.

Increasingly, intervention studies in psycho-oncology are focusing on complex variables of disease outcome including neuroendocrine and immune parameters. Investigators have found that psychosocial variables such as *lack of social support and depressive symptoms* may be linked to reduced NK cell activity in women with breast cancer and that more metastatic nodes and decreased NK cell activity are associated with depressive symptoms, emphasizing the need for more research in the area. Addressing psychoneuroimmunological aspects of depression in patients with cancer may have important treatment implications, particularly regarding hypothalamic-pituitary-adrenal axis hyperactivity associated with depression. In fact, hypothalamic-pituitary-adrenal hyperactivity in depressed cancer patients may have important prognostic implications, particularly since *hypothalamic-pituitary-adrenal hyperactivity* induced by exposure of rats to stress is associated with increased tumor growth, especially in older rats. Psychosocial treatment of patients with malignant melanoma has been shown by Fawzy to improve prognoses and enhance certain immune parameters.

28.6 The answer is D

Hans Selye first described the adaptation syndrome in rats exposed to chronic stress, a response characterized by adrenal

hypertrophy, gastric ulcers, and thymus and lymph node involution. Since then, psychoneuroendocrinology, the subspecialty that addresses the relationship between hormones and behavior, has continued as an area of study. While earlier researchers in psychosomatic medicine were more interested in endocrine disturbances that produce psychiatric syndromes (Cushing's syndrome, hyperthyroidism, hypothyroidism), exogenous hormone–induced syndromes (glucocorticoid administration), and psychiatric aspects of other endocrine abnormalities (diabetes mellitus), more recent research has focused on the multifaceted role of neuroendocrine modulation and its relation to behavioral disturbances and psychiatric symptomatology.

For example, exposure of rats to stress reliably *increases (not decreases) plasma concentrations of ACTH* and *corticosterone* and *decreases (not increases) secretion of growth hormone* and gonadotropins. Increased secretion of CRF from the hypothalamic-hypophysial portal system mediates a complex cascade. Within the CNS, CRF activates the sympathetic nervous system, raising plasma concentrations of epinephrine and norepinephrine, thereby increasing heart rate, blood pressure, and plasma glucose concentrations. Stress-induced alterations in immune function may also be mediated by increased CRF secretion. *The CRF concentration in the locus ceruleus increases markedly after acute stress.*

When administered directly into the CNS of laboratory animals, CRF produces a number of physiological and behavioral changes similar to the physiological changes observed in stressed animals, which resemble signs and symptoms of depression and anxiety disorders. Centrally administered CRF increases mean arterial pressure, heart rate, oxygen consumption, and plasma glucose and catecholamine concentrations. It also alters locomotor activity, decreases sexual activity, diminishes food consumption, increases emotionality, and induces sleep disturbances.

28.7 The answer is C

Functional gastrointestinal disorders are common syndromes associated with significant subjective distress and abnormalities of bowel function, without evidence of structural abnormalities. Functional gastrointestinal disorders frequently have high rates of psychiatric comorbidity.

Functional heartburn is the most common functional gastrointestinal disorder. Functional heartburn needs to be distinguished from gastroesophageal reflux disease. In functional heartburn, symptoms of acid reflux are present (i.e., heartburn, regurgitation of food), but there is no evidence of anatomical abnormality or esophagitis on endoscopy or radiography.

Emotional distress and anxiety disorders can result in abnormal respiration and air swallowing or aerophagia. Swallowed air produces distension of the stomach and feelings of *abdominal* fullness or *bloating* along with belching.

Chest pain frequently prompts attention for potential cardiac causes. However, functional esophageal motility disorders can produce chest pain and need to be considered in patients with chest pain and no evidence of cardiac abnormalities. Pain related to esophageal motility disturbances can be described as angina-like in location and character. High-amplitude esophageal contractions in the distal esophagus, "nutcracker esophagus," can produce significant pain.

Referral to gastroenterology for evaluation of gastrointestinal causes of chest pain frequently occurs after cardiac causes have been ruled out. It is not unusual for several specialists to see the chest pain patient prior to appropriate psychiatric referral. However, at times psychiatrists may be involved before a comprehensive medical evaluation has been completed. Psychiatrists need to be aware of the possible gastrointestinal causes for chest pain, particularly when there is limited evidence for a psychiatric disorder in an unexplained chest pain presentation (Table 28.3).

Irritable bowel syndrome is the prototypical functional gastrointestinal disorder characterized by abdominal pain and diarrhea or constipation. The International Congress of Gastroenterology has developed a standardized set of criteria for irritable bowel syndrome:

1. Abdominal pain relieved by defecation or associated with change in frequency or consistency of stool.
2. Disturbed defecation involving two or more of the following:

   ▶ altered stool frequency
   ▶ altered stool form (hard or loose and watery)
   ▶ altered stool passage (straining or urgency, feeling of incomplete evacuation)
   ▶ passage of mucus

Irritable bowel syndrome can often be categorized into diarrhea-predominant, constipation-predominant, and mixed subtypes. Medical treatment often targets the predominant symptom. Some studies suggest that irritable bowel syndrome accounts for up to 50 percent of all outpatient evaluations done by gastroenterologists. Comorbid psychiatric disorders appear to increase the likelihood of health-care-seeking behavior for people with symptoms of irritable bowel syndrome.

Some patients with irritable bowel syndrome may demonstrate physiological abnormalities including abnormal intestinal myoelectric activity, gastrointestinal hormonal abnormalities, or allergic responses to some foods. Most clinicians agree that both physiological and psychological factors contribute to the clinical picture of irritable bowel syndrome in most patients.

Globus, the Latin word for lump, indicates a sensation of having a lump in the throat. Alternate terms for globus include *globus pharyngeus, globus hystericus*, and *globus syndrome*. Globus must be distinguished from *dysphagia*, or difficulty swallowing. Patients complaining of globus may also report dysphagia and fear of choking, but most patients with globus endorse neither of these other symptoms. Historically, globus constituted one of the symptoms of hysteria and was described by Hippocrates as a symptom related to the wandering uterus putting pressure on the neck. Approximately half of patients complaining of globus have no medical diagnosis after extensive testing. Acid reflux can produce globus and is the most common medical cause of the sensation. Other pharyngeal disorders including pharyngeal cancer can also produce globus.

28.8 The answer is C

Obesity refers to an excess of body fat. In healthy individuals body fat accounts for approximately 25 percent of body weight in women and 18 percent in men. Estimating body fat accurately is expensive, although advances in the assessment of body composition may change this picture. Overweight refers to elevated weight above some reference norm, typically standards derived from actuarial or epidemiological data. In most cases, increasing weight reflects increasing obesity, but not always. Muscular individuals may be overweight (weight may

Table 28.3
Common Gastrointestinal Diseases

Disorders of the esophagus
  Reflux esophagitis (GERD)
  Infectious esophagitis
  Esophageal motility disorders
Disorders of the stomach and intestines
  Peptic ulcer disease
  Gastroparesis
  Malabsorption and maldigestion
  Inflammatory bowel disease
    Crohn's disease
    Ulcerative colitis
  Diverticular disease
Diseases of the anorectum
  Hemorrhoids
  Anal fissures
  Perirectal abscess
Diseases of the pancreas
  Acute pancreatitis
  Chronic pancreatitis
Diseases of the liver and gallbladder
  Infectious hepatitis
  Toxic and drug-induced hepatitis
  Primary biliary cirrhosis
  Primary sclerosing cholangitis
  Metabolic liver disease
  Gallstones and cholecystitis
Cancer of the gastrointestinal tract
  Colon and rectal cancer
  Pancreatic cancer
  Esophageal cancer
  Stomach cancer
  Liver cancer

be elevated given height) but not obese, and a person might have normal weight but have excess body fat.

Indexes have been developed using height and weight to estimate levels of obesity. The most common of these is the body mass index (BMI). BMI is calculated by dividing weight in kilograms by height squared in meters. Although there is debate about the ideal BMI, it is generally thought that a BMI of 20 to 25 kg/m² represents healthy weight; a BMI of 25 to 27 kg/m² is associated with somewhat elevated risk; a BMI of above 27 kg/m² is where the increase in risk is clear; and a BMI above 30 kg/m² is where there is greatly increased risk.

The prevalence of obesity varies greatly by nation, by social groups within nations, and in some cases, within a given nation over time. In the United States approximately 35 percent of women and 31 percent of men are significantly overweight (BMI 27 or above—about 20 percent overweight). If one defines obesity as BMI over 25, *there are now more obese (not fewer) than nonobese Americans.* Using BMI over 31 (approximately 40 percent overweight), 11 percent of women and 8 percent of men are severely overweight. *The prevalence of obesity in America has tripled (not doubled) since the early 1900s.* Through the 1960s, 1970s, and early 1980s there was a steady rise in prevalence, but the dramatic changes occurred in subsequent years; there has been a 25 percent increase since the 1980s alone.

The prevalence of obesity is highest in minority populations, particularly among women. Fully 60 percent of African-American women ages 45 years and older are overweight, as defined by a BMI of 27 or greater. The high prevalence of *obesity among minorities appears attributable primarily to lower income, type of diet, and educational attainment*. Obesity is six times more prevalent in women of low socioeconomic status than in women of high socioeconomic status.

Weight gain is most pronounced in both sexes between the ages of 25 and 44. During this time, men gain an average of 4 kg and women 7 kg. Pregnancy probably contributes to the greater increase in women, who, on average, begin each successive pregnancy approximately 2.5 kg heavier than at the last. After age 50, weights of men stabilize, and even decline slightly between ages 60 and 74. Women, in contrast, continue to increase in weight until age 60, at which time weight begins to decline.

Obesity is a massive public health problem by any standard. *The prevalence* is extreme, is increasing rather than decreasing, and in what speaks to a bleak future, is *especially high and growing (not stabilized or decreasing) in children*. Obesity rivals the most serious illnesses in the public health toll it takes.

28.9 The answer is E (all)

Research suggests that psychiatric forces may affect the clinical expression of asthma in several ways: altered awareness of airway resistance, suggestibility to airway constriction, and comorbidity with panic disorder and depression.

The assumption that *suggestibility to airway constriction* confirms the presence of psychopathology or psychosomatic vulnerability is weak but pervasive. Suggestible patients are more likely to be anxious and to feel physically vulnerable than nonsuggestible patients, but their actual comparative risk for more asthma episodes or symptoms as a result of stressful life events is unknown.

Perception of changes in airway resistance appears to be an important event in asthma self-care. The patient's timely reports of dyspnea can also help to initiate an appropriate medical response. From patient to patient there is considerable variability in reported breathlessness for a given degree of experimentally induced airway obstruction.

Coexisting anxiety or panic disorder probably worsens the course of asthma, and the prevalence of panic disorder and agoraphobia among asthma patients is higher than in the general population. Up to 30 percent of persons with asthma meet the criteria for panic disorder or agoraphobia. Panic disorder appears to be underrecognized in asthma patients, and its symptoms may be misunderstood by both the patient and physician as arising from an exacerbation of asthma. Hyperventilation, a common symptom of both anxiety and panic disorder, may trigger a worsening of a pulmonary illness.

Repeated experience with severe dyspnea or near-suffocation provides little in the way of cognitive or emotional protection for future episodes. Such events often seem only to traumatize patients and may lead to the development of anxiety disorders or panic disorders. Cohorts of panic disorder patients are more likely than patients with other anxiety disorders to have an antecedent history of lung disease.

Patients with both asthma and panic disorder seem to have greater anticipatory anxiety about both dyspnea and anxiety itself than patients who are not comorbid. The fear of dyspnea may directly trigger asthma attacks. An extremely high level of anxiety predicts increased rates of hospitalization and asthma-associated mortality. Certain personality traits in asthma patients appear to be associated with greater use of corticosteroids and bronchodilators, as well as longer hospitalizations than would be predicted from pulmonary function alone. Such traits include intense fear, emotional lability, sensitivity to rejection, and lack of persistence in difficult situations.

Many researchers suggest that *depression has a meaningful and negative effect* on the course of asthma. Shame and low self-esteem, two common symptoms of depression, are seen in many chronically ill patients and are risk factors for a severe course. Patients who feel they are worth little tend to manage their asthma poorly, and compliance with a medication regimen may suffer. The sleep disturbances of depression could affect self-care adversely, as could the concentration and attention deficits of the mood disorder. Sleep deprivation may reduce a patient's proprioceptive capacity to detect changes in airway resistance and can erode daytime cognitive performance. In a severely depressed patient, unconscious suicidal wishes may find expression in self-neglect. In addition to these behavioral manifestations, the hypothetical parasympathetic dominance of depression could contribute to airway reactivity and constriction.

28.10 The answer is C

Psoriasis is a chronic, relapsing disease of the skin with variable clinical features. Characteristic lesions involve both the vasculature and the epidermis and have clear-cut borders and noncoherent silvery scales with a glossy, homogeneous erythema under the scales. Some patients also develop nail dystrophy and arthritis. It affects 1 to 2 percent of the United States' general population and is equally common in women and men, with most developing initial lesions in the third decade of life.

Common triggers of psoriasis include cold weather, physical trauma, acute bacterial and viral infections, and drug-related effects associated with corticosteroid withdrawal and with the use of β-adrenergic receptor antagonists and lithium. Lithium-induced psoriasis typically occurs within the first few years of treatment, is resistant to treatment, and resolves after discontinuation of lithium treatment.

The adverse effect of psoriasis on the quality of life can lead to stress that may in turn trigger more psoriasis. In a recent survey of psoriatic patients, 46 percent reported daily problems secondary to psoriasis. The 40 to 80 percent of patients who reported that stress triggered psoriasis often described disease-related stress, resulting mainly from the cosmetic disfigurement and social stigma of psoriasis, rather than stressful major life events. Psoriasis-related stress may have more to do with psychosocial difficulties inherent in the interpersonal relationships of patients with psoriasis than with the severity or chronicity of psoriasis activity. The mechanism of stress-induced exacerbations is unknown but may involve the nervous, endocrine, and immune systems in such a way that descending autonomic information from the CNS is transmitted to sensory nerves in the skin, resulting in relapse of neuropeptides such as substance

P into the skin. These neuropeptides help initiate and maintain the inflammatory response in psoriatic lesions.

Controlled studies have found psoriatic *patients to have high (not low) levels of anxiety and depression* and *significant comorbidity with a wide array of personality disorders* from DSM-IV-TR, including schizoid, avoidant, and obsessive-compulsive personality disorders, as well as tendencies toward passive-aggressive traits. Patients' self-reports of psoriasis severity correlated directly with depression and suicidal ideation, and comorbid depression reduced the threshold for pruritus in psoriatic patients. Heavy alcohol drinking (>80 grams of ethanol daily) by male psoriatic patients may predict a poor treatment outcome.

These possible links between mental state and psoriasis have led to the development of *psychosocial interventions* in its treatment. Controlled studies have shown *meditation*, hypnosis, *relaxation training*, cognitive-behavioral stress management, and symptom control imagery training to be *effective in reducing psoriasis activity.*

28.11 The answer is E (all)
Pruritus, or itching, is the most common symptom of dermatological disorders and of several systemic diseases including chronic renal disease, hepatic disease, hematopoietic disorders, endocrine disorders, malignant neoplasms, drug toxicity, and neurological syndromes (e.g., multiple sclerosis). Other problems such as advanced age, infections with internal parasites, and viremia can also be associated with pruritus.

Chronic *idiopathic pruritus* and idiopathic pruritus ani (itching in the anal area), vulvae (itching in the vaginal area), and scroti (itching in the scrotum) frequently have been called psychogenic, but more study is needed to determine how psychiatric and other CNS disorders contribute to the development of pruritus. *Antidepressant medications, particularly the tricyclic drugs, can relieve pruritus of many origins.*

Urticaria (also known as hives) is characterized by circumscribed, raised, erythematous, usually pruritic areas of edema that involve the superficial dermis.

Glossodynia (also called burning mouth syndrome) is an unexplained, prolonged sensation of pain, burning, or both inside the oral cavity, most frequently at the tip and lateral borders of the tongue, and often accompanied by other symptoms such as dryness, paresthesia, and changes in taste and smell.

Vulvodynia is chronic vulvar and perineal discomfort of variable severity with burning, stinging, irritation, or rawness.

28.12 The answer is E (all)
Psychosocial disability and psychiatric disorders are prevalent in the population and more often encountered in medical inpatient and outpatient settings than in psychiatric settings. One-month and point-prevalence studies found that 16 percent of community cohorts exhibited psychiatric morbidity. It is estimated that 21 to 26 percent of medical outpatients have psychiatric disorders. The age- and sex-adjusted prevalence of mental disorders was 25 percent in patients with a chronic medical condition and 17.5 percent in those without. Lifetime prevalence of a mental disorder in chronically physically ill patients reached 42 percent (most often substance abuse and mood or anxiety disorders) compared to 33 percent in those who did not have long-term physical disability. Finally, 30 to 60 percent of those in short-term general medical or surgical inpatient settings have significant psychosocial or psychiatric morbidity.

Medical patients have a much higher morbidity for specific mental disorders than those in the general population: *delirium* in 15 to 30 percent of those hospitalized; *depression* (two to three times higher); *panic* and somatization (10 to 20 times higher); *and substance abuse* (three to five times higher). Thus, the medical setting—where patients have already put themselves within a healthcare facility—is an excellent venue for screening, triage, and confronting psychiatric morbidity. In fact, the medical setting is an important de facto mental health setting from which to launch an effort to ameliorate mental suffering. Table 28.4 lists some common consultation-liaison problems.

28.13 The answer is E (none)
Patients with pain have a significantly higher incidence of depression and anxiety. It has been suggested that chronic pain may be a depressive equivalent, that pain may cause psychiatric syndromes, and that pain may coexist with psychopathology in vulnerable subjects. In cancer patients, the evidence suggests that these emotional reactions both result from and contribute to the experience of pain, and that treatment of one improves the other. However, *a review of the impact of biobehavioral factors on adult cancer pain concluded that the role of personality factors was inconsistent (not consistent), the relationship to affective states minimal (not major), the environmental influences were weak (not strong)*, and the role of cognitive factors was unexplored. Hence, the psychiatric consultant is wise to avoid diagnostic inferences that minimize the patient's complaints. Patients with significant psychopathology are indeed more difficult to evaluate, so the consultant must help the staff make the same aggressive efforts at symptom relief for these patients as for other patients. The incidence of psychiatric complications is particularly high when pain is underestimated and undermedicated by caretakers, an event that recurs with a regularity that cries out for explanations.

Answers 28.14–28.18

28.14 The answer is D

28.15 The answer is C

28.16 The answer is A

28.17 The answer is B

28.18 The answer is E
Wilson's disease, hepatolenticular degeneration, is a familial disease of adolescence that tends to have a long-term course. Its cause is defective copper metabolism leading to excessive copper deposits in tissues. The earliest psychiatric symptoms are *explosive anger and labile mood*—sudden and rapid changes from one mood to another. As the illness progresses, eventual brain damage occurs with memory and intelligence quotient (IQ) loss. The lability and combativeness tend to persist even after the brain damage develops.

Pheochromocytoma is a tumor of the adrenal medulla that causes headaches, paroxysms of severe hypertension, and the physiological and psychological *symptoms of a classic panic attack*—intense anxiety, tremor, apprehension, dizziness, palpitations, and diaphoresis. The tumor tissue secretes catecholamines that are responsible for the symptoms.

Table 28.4
Common Consultation-Liaison Problems

Reason for Consultation	Comments
Suicide attempt or threat	High-risk factors: men over 45, no social support, alcohol dependence, previous attempt, incapacitating medical illness with pain, and suicidal ideation; if risk is present, transfer to psychiatric unit or start 24-h nursing care
Depression	Suicidal risks must be assessed in every depressed patient (see above); presence of cognitive defects in depression may cause diagnostic dilemma with dementia; check for history of substance abuse or depressant drugs (e.g., reserpine, propranolol); use antidepressants cautiously in cardiac patients because of conduction side effects, orthostatic hypotension
Agitation	Often related to cognitive disorder, withdrawal from drugs (e.g., opioids, alcohol, sedative-hypnotics); haloperidol most useful drug for excessive agitation; use physical restraints with great caution; examine for command hallucinations or paranoid ideation to which patient is responding in agitated manner; rule out toxic reaction to medication
Hallucinations	Most common cause in hospital is delirium tremens; onset 3 to 4 days after hospitalization; in intensive care units, check for sensory isolation; rule out brief psychotic disorder, schizophrenia, cognitive disorder; treat with antipsychotic medication
Sleep disorder	Common cause is pain; early morning awakening associated with depression; difficulty falling asleep associated with anxiety; use antianxiety or antidepressant agent, depending on cause (those drugs have no analgesic effect, so prescribe adequate painkillers); rule out early substance withdrawal
No organic basis for symptoms	Rule out conversion disorder, somatization disorder, factitious disorder, and malingering; glove and stocking anesthesia with autonomic nervous system symptoms seen in conversion disorder; multiple body complaints seen in somatization disorder; wish to be hospitalized seen in factitious disorder; obvious secondary gain in malingering (e.g., compensation case)
Disorientation	Delirium versus dementia; review metabolic status, neurological findings, substance history; prescribe small dose of antipsychotics for major agitation; benzodiazepines may worsen condition and cause sundowner syndrome (ataxia, confusion); modify environment so patient does not experience sensory deprivation
Noncompliance or refusal to consent to procedure	Explore relationship of patient and treating doctor; negative transference is most common cause of noncompliance; fears of medication or of procedure require education and reassurance; refusal to give consent is issue of judgment; if impaired, patient can be declared incompetent, but only by a judge; cognitive disorder is main cause of impaired judgment in hospitalized patients

Systemic lupus erythematosus is an autoimmune disorder in which the body makes antibodies against its own cells. The antibodies attack cells as if the cells were infectious agents, and depending on which cells are being attacked, give rise to various symptoms. Frequently, the arteries in the cerebrum are affected, causing a cerebral arteritis, which alters the blood flow to various parts of the brain. The decreased blood flow can give rise to psychotic symptoms, such as a thought disorder with paranoid delusions and hallucinations. The symptoms can *resemble steroid psychosis* or schizophrenia.

The diagnosis of *acquired immune deficiency syndrome* (AIDS) includes a *dementia syndrome with global impairment and seropositivity*. The dementia can be caused by the direct attack on the central nervous system by the human immunodeficiency virus (HIV) or by secondary infections, such as toxoplasmosis.

Although any chronic illness can give rise to depression, some diseases, such as *pancreatic cancer*, are more likely causes than are others. The depression of pancreatic cancer patients is often associated with a *sense of imminent doom*.

28.19 The answer is B

A major advance in the revised fourth edition of *Diagnostic and Statistical Manual of Mental Disorders* (DSM-IV-TR) from the third edition (DSM-III-R) is that DSM-IV-TR allows clinicians to specify the *psychological stimuli* that affect the patient's medical condition. In DSM-III-R, psychologically meaningful *environmental stimuli* were temporally related to the physical disorder. Excluded in DSM-III-R were *somatoform disorders*, such as *conversion disorder*, in which the physical symptoms are not based on organic pathology. The DSM-IV-TR emphasis on psychological factors permits a wide range of psychological stimuli to be noted (for example, personality traits, maladaptive health behaviors).

28.20 The answer is C

There are no studies on the T cells of *women who are having extramarital affairs*. Investigators have found a decrease in lymphocytic response in *bereavement* (conjugal and anticipatory), the *caretakers of patients with dementia of the Alzheimer's type*, in *nonpsychotic inpatients*, in resident physicians, in *medical students during final examinations*, in women who were separated or divorced, in the elderly with no social support, and in the unemployed. Table 28.5 lists some of the common behavioral states associated with in vitro immune suppression.

28.21 The answer is C

Franz Alexander applied psychoanalytic concepts to the study of peptic ulcers, bronchial asthma, and essential hypertension. He studied specific repressed unconscious conflicts that he believed were associated with those diseases. *George Mahl* was an experimental psychologist who studied ulcer development in animals. He concluded that chronic anxiety provoked by any conflict is causally important. *Harold Wolff* and Stewart Wolf attempted to correlate life stress with physiological protective human responses. *Robert Ader* studied the immune response and psychoneuroimmunology in psychosomatic disorders. *Meyer Friedman* correlated personality types (type A and type B) with certain psychosomatic disorders, such as coronary heart disease.

28.22 The answer is C

The immune system is affected by *conditioning*. According to Ader, immunological reactivity is affected by *hypnosis, lymphocytes* can

**Table 28.5
Behavioral States Associated with
In Vitro Immune Suppression**

Disturbed sleep function
Examination stress
Loneliness
Unemployment
Marital discord
Divorce
Alzheimer's disease—caregivers' stress
Bereaved spouses (including anticipatory bereavement)
Clinical anxiety
Major depressive disorder

**Table 28.6
Summary of Psychoneuroimmunology
Factors by Robert Ader**

Nerve endings have been found in the tissues of the immune system. The central nervous system is linked to both the bone marrow and the thymus, where immune system cells are produced and developed, and to the spleen and the lymph nodes, where those cells are stored.

Changes in the central nervous system (the brain and the spinal cord) alter immune responses, and triggering an immune response alters central nervous system activity. Animal experiments dating back to the 1960s show that damage to different parts of the brain's hypothalamus can either suppress or enhance the allergic-type response. Recently, researchers have found that inducing an immune response causes nerve cells in the hypothalamus to become more active and that the brain cell anxiety peaks at precisely the same time that levels of antibodies are at their highest. Apparently, the brain monitors immunological changes closely.

Changes in hormone and neurotransmitter levels alter immune responses, and vice versa. The stress hormones generally suppress immune responses. But other hormones, such as growth hormone, also seem to affect immunity. Conversely, when experimental animals are immunized, they show changes in various hormone levels.

Lymphocytes are chemically responsive to hormones and neurotransmitters. Immune system cells have receptors—molecular structures on the surface of their cells—that are responsive to endorphins, stress hormones, and a wide range of other hormones.

Lymphocytes can produce hormones and neurotransmitters. When an animal is infected with a virus, lymphocytes produce minuscule amounts of many of the same substances produced by the pituitary gland.

Activated lymphocytes—cells actively involved in an immune response—produce substances that can be perceived by the central nervous system. The interleukins and interferons—chemicals that immune system cells use to talk to each other—can also trigger receptors on cells in the brain, more evidence that the immune system and the nervous system speak the same chemical language.

Psychosocial factors may alter the susceptibility to or the progression of autoimmune disease, infectious disease, and cancer. Evidence for those connections comes from many researchers.

Immunological reactivity may be influenced by stress. Chronic or intense stress, in particular, generally makes immune system cells less responsive to a challenge.

Immunological reactivity can be influenced by hypnosis. In a typical study, both of a subject's arms are exposed to a chemical that normally causes an allergic reaction. But the subject is told, under hypnosis, that only one arm will show the response—and that, in fact, is often what happens.

Immunological reactivity can be modified by classical conditioning. As Ader's own key experiments showed, the immune system can learn to react in certain ways as a conditioned response.

Psychoactive drugs and drugs of abuse influence immune function. A range of drugs that affect the nervous system—including alcohol, marijuana, cocaine, heroin, and nicotine—have all been shown to affect the immune response, generally suppressing it. Some psychiatric drugs, such as lithium (prescribed for bipolar I disorder), also modulate the immune system.

Adapted from Goleman D, Guerin J. *Mind Body Medicine.* Yonkers, NY: Consumer Reports; 1993.

produce neurotransmitters, *growth hormone* does affect immunity, and *marijuana* does affect the immune system. Robert Ader has summarized the psychoneuroimmunology factors (Table 28.6).

28.23 The answer is B
Steroids produce marked alterations of the patient's mental status, particularly from mania to depression—even to a suicidal degree. Psychotic symptoms are not an uncommon negative consequence of steroid use. Dacarbazine produces depression, especially when used with *hexamethylmelamine. Interferon* may produce anxiety and depression with suicidal ideation. Hallucinations have been reported with *hydroxyurea.* L-*Asparaginase* produces reversible depression. Table 28.7 lists chemotherapy agents with mood and psychotic symptoms.

28.24 The answer is C
Peptic ulcer is not considered an autoimmune disease. Disorders in which an autoimmune component has been implicated include *Graves' disease*, Hashimoto's disease, *rheumatoid arthritis*, ulcerative colitis, *regional ileitis*, systemic lupus erythematosus, psoriasis, myasthenia gravis, and *pernicious anemia.*

28.25 The answer is A
Phantom limb occurs in *98 percent* of patients—not 10 percent, 50 percent, 80 percent, or 90 percent—who have undergone leg amputation. The experience may last for years. Sometimes the sensation is painful, and a neuroma at the stump should be ruled out. The condition has no known cause or treatment and usually stops spontaneously.

28.26 The answer is A
The most difficult problem in the treatment of psychosomatically ill patients is patients' *resistance to entering psychotherapy* and to recognizing the psychological factors in their illness. Generally, clinicians have difficulty in forming a positive transference with the patients. *An erotic transference to the psychotherapist* usually does not develop, nor is it relevant to the treatment of these patients. The patients *usually react negatively to the interpretation of the physiological meaning of their symptoms* and *do not recognize the psychological correlation with their physiological symptoms.*

28.27 The answer is A
A patient with an occipital lobe tumor would be least likely to exhibit *paranoid delusions. Visual hallucinations, headache, papilledema, and homonymous hemianopsia* are all reported symptoms and complaints of occipital lobe tumors. Papille-

Table 28.7
Chemotherapy Agents with Mood and Psychotic Symptoms

Dacarbazine: depression and suicide reported, especially when used with hexamethylamine

Vinblastine: frequent reversible depression

Vincristine: 5 percent incidence of hallucinations; depression noted

L-Asparaginase: reversible depression noted

Procarbazine: MAOI; concurrent tricyclic drugs are contraindicated; associated with mania and depression; potentiates alcohol, barbiturates, phenothiazines

Hydroxyurea: hallucinations reported

Interferon: anxiety, depression with suicidal ideation common at doses above 40 million units

Steroids: frequent alterations of mental state ranging from emotional lability through mania or severe, suicidal depression to frank psychosis

Courtesy of Marguerite S. Lederberg, M.D., and Jimmie C. Holland, M.D.

Table 28.9
Suicide Vulnerability Factors in Cancer Patients

Depression and hopelessness

Poorly controlled pain

Mild delirium (disinhibition)

Feeling of loss of control

Exhaustion

Anxiety

Preexisting psychopathology (substance abuse, character pathology, major psychiatric disorder)

Family problems

Threats and history of prior attempts of suicide

Positive family history of suicide

Other usually described risk factors in psychiatric patients

Adapted from Breitbart W. Suicide in cancer patients. *Oncology.* 1987;1:49.

---

dema (edema of the optic disk) may be caused by increased intracranial pressure. Homonymous hemianopsia is blindness in the corresponding (right or left) field of vision of each eye.

28.28 The answer is C

Although the psychological symptoms are similar in all of the conditions listed, a medical workup would reveal that fever, photosensitivity, butterfly rash, and joint pains are diagnostic of *systemic lupus erythematosus.*

In *acute intermittent porphyria,* abdominal pain, fever, peripheral neuropathy, and elevated porphobilinogen are significant. In *hypoparathyroidism* the patient has constipation, polydipsia, and nausea with increased calcium and variable parathyroid hormone (PTH) levels. In *hepatic encephalopathy* the patient has asterixis, spider angioma, and abnormal liver function test results. In *pheochromocytoma* the patient has par-

Table 28.8
Emetogenic Potential of Some Commonly Used Anticancer Agents

Highly emetogenic	Cisplatin
	Dacarbazine
	Streptozocin
	Actinomycin
	Nitrogen mustard
Moderately emetogenic	Doxorubicin
	Daunorubicin
	Cyclophosphamide
	Nitrosoureas
	Mitomycin-C
	Procarbazine
Minimally emetogenic	Vincristine
	Vinblastine
	5-Fluorouracil
	Bleomycin

Courtesy of Marguerite S. Lederberg, M.D., and Jimmie C. Holland, M.D.

oxysmal hypertension, headache, elevated vanillylmandelic acid (VMA), and tachycardia.

28.29 The answer is E (all)

Most chronic pain patients attempt to treat themselves before resorting to medical help. Billions of dollars are spent annually by people seeking relief through *over-the-counter preparations* or other nonmedical means. Those persons often have *alcohol dependence* and other substance-related disorders. Therefore, the physician should be alert for substance toxicity (especially overmedication) and *withdrawal symptoms during the evaluation* and treatment of chronic pain patients. Explaining to the patient and family that sensitivity to pain may greatly increase during substance withdrawal may partially decrease anxiety and increase pain sensitivity. A physician should always remember that a psychiatric diagnosis does not preclude the existence of *an underlying medical illness.* Finally, the clinician should recognize that the patient's pain is not imaginary. It is real and cannot be "willed away."

28.30 The answer is E

Delusions are not usually a characteristic of dialysis dementia. Dialysis dementia is a rare condition characterized by *loss of memory, disorientation, dystonias, and seizures.* The dementia occurs in patients who have been receiving dialysis treatment for many years. The cause is unknown.

28.31 The answer is A

Cisplatin (Platinol) is highly emetogenic. *Doxorubicin* (Adriamycin) is moderately emetogenic, and *vincristine* (Oncovin), *vinblastine* (Velban), and *bleomycin* (Blenoxane) are minimally emetogenic. Table 28.8 summarizes the emetogenic problems with various chemotherapeutic agents.

28.32 The answer is E

About *50 percent* of cancer patients later have mental disorders; 68 percent of these disorders are adjustment disorder; 15 percent of those with psychiatric symptoms have major depressive disorder; and 8 percent have delirium. Although cancer patients may express suicidal wishes, the actual suicide incidence is only 1.4 to 1.9 times that of the general population. Vulnerability to suicide is increased by the factors listed in Table 28.9.

29 ▲

Alternative Medicine and Psychiatry

Alternatives to traditional psychiatric and medical treatments have always been available and are increasingly so today. Many people who are concerned about the powerful chemicals and side effects of traditional treatments look for what they hope will be gentler, more natural treatments. Sometimes these alternatives are able to provide treatment that is less toxic and still effective. Unfortunately, alternative methods are not always without their own risk, ranging from simple ineffectiveness to actual harm.

The National Institutes of Health (NIH) established an Office of Alternative Medicine (OAM) in 1991, to attempt to evaluate and test many nontraditional, alternative treatments. In 1995, the OAM published a classification of alternative medical practices. (For a full listing, see Table 29.1.)

The power of suggestion has been shown to play a significant role in both alternative and more traditional medical and psychiatric treatments. One major difference between traditional and nontraditional methods, however, is that most alternative treatments have not been extensively tested or subjected to controlled studies. Thus, the mechanisms of action, the role of psychology in their effectiveness, and their systemic impact and long-term effects have not been identified adequately. Clinicians may keep an open mind about these treatments until such studies can be performed, but should also refrain from endorsing or recommending treatments with which they are unfamiliar.

In psychiatry, patients often ask questions about alternative treatments, ranging from St. John's Wort to acupuncture. Psychiatrists should feel comfortable indicating which treatments they are familiar with and which they are not, and which treatments they feel comfortable accepting and which they do not. If they are knowledgeable about particular alternative treatments and feel that they might be effective in a specific patient, then this can be discussed. Patients are always free to seek care from practitioners who use alternative methods, and no physician should feel pressured to recommend or support any treatments outside their area of expertise, or that they feel are not indicated, effective, or evaluated sufficiently.

The student should study the questions and answers below for a useful review of this field.

HELPFUL HINTS

Students should know the following terms.

- ▶ acupressure
- ▶ acupuncture
- ▶ Alexander technique
- ▶ allopathy
- ▶ aromatherapy
- ▶ Ayurveda
- ▶ Bates method
- ▶ bioenergetics
- ▶ biofeedback
- ▶ chelation therapy
- ▶ chiropractic
- ▶ color therapy
- ▶ complementary medicine
- ▶ dance therapy
- ▶ diet and nutrition
- ▶ endorphins
- ▶ environmental medicine
- ▶ essential oils
- ▶ Moshe Feldenkrais
- ▶ Max Gerson, M.D.
- ▶ Samuel Hahnemann, M.D.
- ▶ herbal medicine
- ▶ holistic medicine
- ▶ homeopathy
- ▶ hypnosis
- ▶ light therapy
- ▶ macrobiotics
- ▶ massage
- ▶ meditation
- ▶ moxibustion
- ▶ naturopathy
- ▶ nutritional supplements
- ▶ Office of Alternative Medicine (OAM)
- ▶ osteopathy
- ▶ ozone therapy
- ▶ past life
- ▶ prana
- ▶ psychosomatic approach
- ▶ reflexology
- ▶ Reiki
- ▶ Ida Rolf
- ▶ scientific method
- ▶ shamanism
- ▶ sound therapy
- ▶ Rudolf Steiner
- ▶ yin and yang
- ▶ yoga

Table 29.1

Classification of Alternative Medical Practices from the NIH Office of Alternative Medicine

Diet, nutrition, lifestyle changes
- Changes in lifestyle
- Diet
- Nutritional supplements
- Gerson therapy
- Macrobiotics
- Megavitamin

Mind/body control
- Art therapy, relaxation techniques
- Biofeedback
- Counseling and prayer therapies
- Dance therapy
- Guided imagery
- Humor therapy
- Psychotherapy
- Sound, music therapy
- Support groups
- Yoga, meditation

Alternative systems of medical practice
- Acupuncture
- Anthroposophically extended medicine
- Ayurveda
- Community-based health care practices
- Environmental medicine
- Homeopathic medicine
- Latin American rural practices
- Native American
- Natural products
- Naturopathic medicine
- Past life therapy
- Shamanism
- Tibetan medicine
- Traditional oriental medicine

Manual healing
- Acupressure
- Alexander technique
- Aromatherapy
- Biofield therapeutics
- Chiropractic medicine
- Feldenkrais method
- Massage therapy
- Osteopathy
- Reflexology
- Rolfing
- Therapeutic touch
- Trager method
- Zone therapy

Pharmacological and biological treatments
- Antioxidizing agents
- Cell treatment
- Chelation therapy
- Metabolic therapy
- Oxidizing agents (ozone, hydrogen peroxide)

Bioelectromagnetic applications
- Blue light treatment and artificial lighting
- Electroacupuncture
- Electromagnetic fields
- Electrostimulation and neuromagnetic stimulation devices
- Magnetoresonance spectroscopy

Herbal medicine
- *Echinacea* (purple coneflower)
- *Ginkgo biloba* extract
- Ginger rhizome
- Ginseng root
- Wild chrysanthemum flower
- Witch hazel
- Yellowdock

This classification was developed by the ad hoc Advisory Panel to the Office of Alternative Medicine (OAM), National Institutes of Health (NIH), and further refined by the Workshop on Alternative Medicine as described in the report *Alternative Medicine: Expanding Medical Horizons*. This classification was designed to facilitate the grant review process and should not be considered definitive.

▲ QUESTIONS

DIRECTIONS: Each of the questions or incomplete statements below is followed by five responses or completions. Select the *one* that is *best* in each case.

29.1 Acupuncture is reported to be useful in the treatment of

   A. addiction
   B. stroke rehabilitation
   C. low back pain
   D. asthma
   E. all of the above

29.2 Hypericum extracts (St. John's Wort) have potential side effects that include

   A. photodermatitis
   B. dizziness
   C. restlessness
   D. all of the above
   E. none of the above

29.3 True statements about eye movement desensitization and reprocessing include all of the following *except*

A. It is a form of exposure therapy.
B. It has been used in treatment of people with posttraumatic stress disorder.
C. It is expected to reduce levels of distress associated with traumatic memories.
D. As the quality of research increases, there is more support for the efficacy of the treatment.
E. Increased activation of traumatic memories may be associated with increased shame, guilt, and anger.

DIRECTIONS: Each of the three incomplete statements below refers to one of the six lettered terms. Choose the most appropriate term for each statement.

Questions 29.4–29.6

A. Allopathy
B. Homeopathy
C. Osteopathy
D. Biomedicine
E. Technomedicine
F. Herbal medicine

29.4 The medicine taught in U.S. schools
29.5 Similar methods of practice to those of allopathy
29.6 A term coined by Samuel Hahnemann, M.D.

ANSWERS

Alternative Medicine and Psychiatry

29.1 The answer is E (all)

Acupuncture describes a family of procedures involving stimulation of anatomical locations on or beneath the skin by a variety of techniques. The most studied mechanism of stimulation of acupuncture points employs penetration of the skin by extremely thin, solid, metallic needles that are manipulated manually or stimulated by electrical impulses.

Over the years, the United States Public Health Service and National Institutes of Health have funded a variety of research projects on acupuncture, including studies on the mechanisms by which acupuncture may have its effects, as well as clinical trials and other studies. There is also a considerable body of international literature on the risks and benefits of acupuncture, and the World Health Organization lists a variety of medical conditions that may benefit from the use of acupuncture or moxibustion. Such applications include prevention and treatment of nausea and vomiting; treatment of pain and addictions to alcohol and illicit drugs; treatment of pulmonary problems such as asthma and bronchitis; and rehabilitation from neurological damage such as that caused by stroke.

The report concludes that positive results have been obtained regarding adult postoperative and chemotherapy nausea and vomiting and postoperative dental pain. Acupuncture may be a useful adjunct treatment or an acceptable alternative or be included in a comprehensive management program for conditions such as *addiction, stroke rehabilitation,* headache, menstrual cramps, tennis elbow, fibromyalgia, myofascial pain, osteoarthritis, *low back pain,* carpal tunnel syndrome, and *asthma.* Plausible mechanisms of action for acupuncture include the release of endogenous opioids and other neuropeptides in the central nervous system and the periphery and changes in neuroendocrine function.

29.2 The answer is D (all)

There are many herbal products that have been used legally or illegally for their mood-altering or sedative effects. Examples include the opium poppy (opium), *Atropa belladonna* (deadly nightshade), Indian hemp (hashish), hyoscyamine (henbane),

scopolamine (thorn apple), and hypericum (St. John's Wort). Of these, St. John's Wort has received the greatest recent research attention and is currently the subject of an NIH-funded multisite trial of its effects on depression. Prior research with St. John's Wort has used a variety of methods including comparison with placebo controls, comparison with imipramine (Tofranil), large-scale postmarket reporting, and animal research. Metaanalysis of 23 randomized trials that included a total of 1,757 outpatients with mainly mild or moderate depressive disorders concluded that hypericum extracts were significantly superior to placebo and may be as effective as standard antidepressants. The individual research studies reported very low (in most studies, none) rates of adverse effects, and fewer and milder adverse effects compared with imipramine. Criticism of the research includes concerns regarding heterogeneity of patients, interventions, dosage levels, extract preparations, and diagnostic classification.

There has been some concern regarding longer-term effects and possible enhancement of photosensitivity. In particular, it has been suggested that the use of St. John's Wort should not be combined with use of a selective serotonin reuptake inhibitor (SSRI) (e.g., paroxetine [Paxil]). This example of potential undesirable consequences resulting from combinations of herbal and standardized pharmaceuticals is emblematic of a larger concern regarding all the known and unknown side effects of drug and herbal product combinations.

A recent review of St. John's Wort included a detailed discussion of the several proposed mechanisms of action and added concerns regarding adverse effects and drug interaction effects. Generally, the authors felt that there were fewer adverse effects with hypericum than with conventional antidepressants. Potential adverse effects that were listed included *photodermatitis,* delayed hypersensitivity, gastrointestinal tract upset, *dizziness,* dry mouth, sedation, *restlessness,* and constipation. Contraindications for the use of St. John's Wort included pregnancy, lactation, exposure to strong sunlight, and pheochromocytoma. The potential for monoamine oxidase inhibitor–like drug interactions cannot be excluded since appropriate drug interaction studies are not available.

29.3 The answer is D

Eye movement desensitization and reprocessing is a method discovered by Francine Shapiro, who reported *reduced levels of distress associated with traumatic memories* if the recall of these memories could be accompanied with a certain form of rapid and rhythmic eye movements. While the nature of the research and the necessary components of the treatment are controversial, it is generally conceded that the procedure is useful in the treatment of traumatic stress reactions in some patients. Criticisms largely concern the fidelity to standards of treatment; the necessity of eye movements; the use of appropriate control groups, research designs, and measures; consideration of comorbidity; and consideration of other concurrent treatment. It has been suggested that *as the quality of the research increases, there is less (not more) support for the efficacy of the technique* beyond its imaginal exposure component. While initial reports concerning this technique have been encouraging, additional research is recommended. However, the current popularity of the method is notable.

In recent years the technique, *a form of exposure therapy*, has been shown to help desensitize patients with *posttraumatic stress disorder* without fully engaging them in a verbal reliving of the traumatic experience. Although exposure therapy can help overcome traumatic intrusions, it needs to be applied cautiously. Some patients recalling their trauma may become flooded with both the traumatic memories and memories of previously forgotten trauma. *Increased activation of traumatic memories may be associated with increased shame, guilt, anger,* and alcohol and drug use. Patients with posttraumatic stress disorder are a particularly avoidant group that presents a number of treatment obstacles, especially for exposure techniques.

29.4 The answer is A

29.5 The answer is C

29.6 The answer is B

Allopathy, from the Greek *Allos* ("other"), is the term for traditional medicine of the kind taught in U.S. medical schools. It is based on the scientific method, the use of experiments to validate a theory or to determine the validity of a hypothesis. In allopathy, the body is a biological and physiological system, and disorders have causes that can be treated with medications, surgery, and other complex methods to produce cures. Other terms for traditional medicine are *biomedicine* and *technomedicine*. Allopathy refers to the use of medicine to counteract signs and symptoms of diseases; it remains the most prevalent form of medicine in the Western world.

Homeopathy was derived from the Greek *homos* ("same"); it refers to a form of medicine in which special medicinal remedies, different from allopathic remedies, are used. Homeopathic healing was developed in Germany in the early 1800s by Samuel Hahnemann, M.D., who coined the term *homeopathy*. It is based on the concept that the medicine whose effects in normal people most closely resemble the illness being treated is the one most likely to cure the illness. Although traditional medical practitioners doubt its efficacy, homeopathy is increasingly used in this country, in Europe, and throughout the world.

Osteopathy is similar to traditional medicine; doctors of osteopathy are licensed to practice in every state, are qualified to practice in every branch of clinical medicine, and take the same licensure examinations as do medical doctors. Their medical education is identical, except that doctors of osteopathy have additional training in musculoskeletal system disorders.

30

Psychiatry and Reproductive Medicine

There are many potential psychiatric issues related to reproductive medicine, and the psychiatrist often has a major role to play in assisting patients and their doctors diagnose, treat, and manage problems related to the reproductive system in both men and women.

These issues can include the role of psychogenic stress in reproductive dysfunction, changes in sexuality associated with aging, psychological repercussions of infertility, possible psychogenic causes of pelvic pain, premenstrual dysphoric disorder, and psychological and physiologic responses to menopause. Psychiatry may be helpful in addressing a range of issues related to pregnancy, from the impact of emotional support during labor, to the phenomenon of hyperemesis gravidarum, to the safe utilization of psychiatric medications during pregnancy.

Clinicians must be aware of various postpartum conditions, such as postpartum depression and psychosis, and how to distinguish these very serious and potentially life-threatening disorders from the normal "baby blues" that many women experience.

Disorders of sexual development, such as adrenogenital syndrome, testicular feminization, and Turner's syndrome (XO gonadal dysgenesis), are fascinating and unusual conditions that can raise a number of complex and painful parental and physician decisions, which may include psychiatric consultation.

The student should study the questions and answers below for a useful review of these issues.

▲ QUESTIONS

DIRECTIONS: Each of the questions or incomplete statements below is followed by five suggested responses or completions. Select the *one* that is *best* in each case.

30.1 Fetal sex steroid exposure exerts primarily organizational effects upon the fetal

A. central nervous system (CNS)
B. testes
C. ovary
D. neuromuscular system
E. cardiovascular system

30.2 Functional hypothalamic anovulation (FHA) is

A. a diagnosis of exclusion

B. a consequence of structural abnormalities of the thyroid, adrenal, pituitary, or brain

C. a result of increased pituitary secretion of gonadotropins

D. the result of ovaries that are incapable of responding to appropriate gonadotropin input

E. often the result of drug use suppressing GnRH

30.3 True statements about the relationship between psychogenic stress and reproductive dysfunction include

A. In women with functional amenorrhea, the activity of the hypothalamic-pituitary-adrenal axis is increased.

B. There appears to be a dose-response relationship between the severity and number of stressors and the proportion of women who develop anovulation.

C. Various personality characteristics such as perfectionism and unrealistic expectations have been linked to the development of anovulation.

D. In FHA, pharmacological intervention alone does not lead to spontaneous recovery.

E. All of the above

30.4 Changes in male sexuality associated with aging include

A. More stimulation is required to achieve an erection.

B. The plateau phase of sexual excitement is longer and may not end in ejaculation.

C. The force of expulsion of semen during ejaculation is lower.

D. After ejaculation the erection resolves more quickly and the refractory period increases.

E. All of the above

30.5 According to the FDA rating of drug safety in pregnancy, which of the following is listed as having no indication for use even in life-threatening situations (category X)?

A. Lithium

B. Valproic acid

C. Tetracycline

D. Ethanol

E. None of the above

30.6 Long-term follow-up studies of children of lesbian mothers reveal that the children

A. differ from children of heterosexual mothers in emotional health

B. differ from children of heterosexual mothers in interpersonal relationships

C. are more likely to be gay or lesbian themselves

D. all of the above

E. none of the above

30.7 Continuous emotional support during labor reduces

A. the rate of cesarian section

B. the duration of labor

C. the use of anesthesia

D. the use of oxytocin

E. all of the above

30.8 Hyperemesis gravidarum

A. may be associated with women who have histories of anorexia nervosa or bulimia nervosa

B. has a poor prognosis for mother and fetus

C. is rarely chronic or persistent

D. is caused by psychological factors

E. none of the above

30.9 True statements about infertility include

A. In the United States, about 5 percent of married couples are unable to have children.

B. Causes of infertility are attributed to disorders in women in about 75 percent of cases.

C. Causes are attributable to disorders in men in about 10 percent of cases.

D. Causes are attributable to disorders in both in about 20 percent of cases.

E. Fifty percent of couples have no identifiable etiology.

30.10 Causes of pelvic pain include

A. bowel or rectal disease

B. hernias

C. emotional disturbances associated with ongoing or past incest or sexual abuse

D. infertility fears

E. all of the above

30.11 Premenstrual dysphoric disorder

A. is associated with hormonally abnormal menstrual cycles

B. is associated with changing levels of sex steroids that accompany an ovulatory menstrual cycle

C. is seen in approximately 50 percent of women

D. is not treated with SSRIs

E. all of the above

DIRECTIONS: Each group of questions below consists of lettered headings followed by a list of numbered statements. For each numbered statement, select the *one* lettered heading that is most closely associated with it. Each lettered heading may be used once, more than once, or not at all.

Questions 30.12–30.18

A. Postpartum depression

B. "Baby blues" (normal sadness)

C. Both

D. Neither

30.12 10 percent of women who give birth

30.13 Can last months to years if untreated

30.14 No association with history of a mood disorder

30.15 Tearfulness

30.16 Often associated with thoughts of hurting the baby

30.17 Often associated with anhedonia

30.18 Suicidal thoughts

Questions 30.19–30.22

A. Adrenogenital syndrome

B. Turner's syndrome (XO gonadal dysgenesis)

C. Testicular feminization

D. XY gonadal dysgenesis

E. Hermaphroditism

30.19 Masculinized genitalia are usually recognized in the delivery room; however, the internal reproductive tract is normal and puberty usually occurs at the expected time with adequate treatment

30.20 Ovaries do not contain responsive oocytes because of premature atresia of oocytes or failure of germ cell migration

30.21 Gonads are testes but the fetus is phenotypically female

30.22 Caused by a gonad that fails to secrete testosterone; generally the uterus, tubes, and vagina are present

---

ANSWERS

Psychiatry and Reproductive Medicine

30.1 The answer is A

Sexual differentiation of the central nervous system (CNS) is believed to depend on the presence or absence of circulating levels of testosterone. The *fetal testes* begin to secrete testosterone in the late first trimester in response to placental human chorionic gonadotropin (hCG), while the *fetal ovary* does not. The organizational effects of testosterone on the developing CNS are thought to depend primarily upon in situ aromatization (the conversion of androgens to estrogens by the enzyme aromatase) of testosterone to estradiol. In contrast, estrogens from fetal or placental sources do not cross the blood–brain barrier and are not thought to imprint the developing CNS. Also, testosterone may bind directly (without conversion to estradiol) to androgen receptors in the CNS. The behavioral consequences that early exposure to testosterone has upon the developing brain are not clear, but brain areas with high aromatase activity (which thus can convert testosterone to estradiol) and androgen receptors in the nonhuman primate brain include the hypothalamus, amygdala, prefrontal visual, and somatosensory cortices. The asymmetry in exposure to testosterone also is present in early neonatal life. In late pregnancy, gonadotropin secretion is restrained by placental steroid production; when that restraint is lost at the time of birth, gonadotropin secretion rises dramatically in both sexes. In boys but not in girls, the gonadotropin rise is followed by an elevation of testosterone concentrations to adult levels. Thus, by 2 years of age, the brains and bodies of girls and boys have been exposed to dramatically different patterns of sex steroid secretion. The degree to which gender-related behavioral asymmetries are accounted for by those differences in hormone exposure is open to debate, but clearly a mechanism for inducing differences exists. In summary, the *fetal sex steroid exposure exerts primarily organizational effects upon the fetal CNS,* not the neuromuscular or cardiovascular systems.

30.2 The answer is A

Functional hypothalamic anovulation or amenorrhea (FHA) is a consequence of a nonorganic reduction in GnRH secretion that *results in reduced (not increased) pituitary secretion of gonadotropins* and subsequent anovulation. Previously referred to as idiopathic or psychogenic amenorrhea in the psychiatric literature, *FHA is a diagnosis of exclusion.* This implies that the *ovaries are capable (not incapable) of responding to appropriate gonadotropin input* of either endogenous or exogenous origin; that there are *no structural abnormalities of the thyroid, adrenal, pituitary, or brain;* that the *use of drugs, including antipsychotic medications, does not account for the suppression of GnRH;* and that the patient is not pregnant. Neuroimaging may be needed to establish that there are no significant anatomical lesions of the brain or pituitary. Two major areas concerning the pathogenesis of FHA remain unresolved. First, the peripheral and central signals that disrupt GnRH pulsatility are poorly understood. Second, how do behavioral, cognitive, and personality variables activate the neural systems to disrupt GnRH secretion? Physicians and patients alike wonder what lifestyle variables provoke or contribute to this type of ovulatory dysfunction and what pharmacological and nonpharmacological treatment interventions should be considered.

30.3 The answer is E (all)

The concept that psychogenic stress can induce reproductive dysfunction in women was introduced formally in 1946. The best biochemical evidence in support of the concept that stress impairs GnRH release in women with functional hypothalamic amenorrhea is the consistent demonstration that the *activity of the hypothalamic-pituitary-adrenal axis is increased.* Further, a prospective study found that young American women who developed transient amenorrhea while studying in Israel had higher urinary cortisol concentrations upon arrival than those whose menses remained regular.

There appears to be *a dose-response relationship* between the type, severity, and number of stressors on one hand and the proportion of women who develop anovulation. Biological and psychological predispositions may confer resistance or sensitivity to various stressors. Exercise, low weight and weight loss, affective and eating disorders, *personality characteristics* such as perfectionism and unrealistic expectations, drug use, and a variety of external and intrapersonal stresses *have been linked to the development of anovulation.* Most women with FHA, when carefully evaluated, display more than one of these traits or behaviors. Recent evidence suggests synergism between metabolic stressors, such as excessive exercise and nutritional restriction, which suppress the hypothalamic-pituitary-thyroidal axis, and psychosocial challenges that activate the hypothalamic-pituitary-adrenal axis.

Recovery is possible if women with FHA develop response patterns to ongoing psychosocial demands that are less likely to activate the central and metabolic processes that disrupt pulsatile GnRH release. The current standard of practice, other than observation, is to offer pharmacological interventions such as oral contraceptives or hormonal replacement if fertility is not desired, and pharmacological ovulation induction if fertility is sought. However, *pharmacological intervention alone does not lead to spontaneous recovery* and cannot be expected to ameliorate stress-induced alterations in central neurotransmission and hypothalamic function, or to reverse ongoing metabolic derangements secondary to exercise or weight loss. For instance, bone accretion does not proceed apace, even if exogenous hormone replacement is given in supraphysiological doses, in the face of metabolic compromise. Although women with FHA frequently do not meet DSM-IV-TR criteria for eating disorders or depressive disorders, all of these states are characterized by increased cortisol secretion, which alone can alter thyroid hormone secretion and action and induce metabolic adjustments. Thus, it is not surprising to find that women with amenorrhea due to decreased GnRH drive, regardless of cause, have lower bone mineral density. Further, pharmacological intervention alone may mask recognition of psychological dysfunction and forestall the development of more effective response patterns. Also, ovulation induction may place low-weight women with functional hypothalamic amenorrhea who conceive at risk for premature labor and intrauterine growth retardation. If the parenting skills of women with the disorder are impaired by ongoing stress, their children may be at risk for poor psychosocial development. Clearly, treatment strategies need to consider that stress and mild psychological dysfunction can play an important role in the genesis of this form of anovulation. If an eating disorder is recognized, specialized psychiatric treatment is indicated.

30.4 The answer is E (all)

Aging may be associated with changes in sexuality. While sexual interest declines to some degree with aging, older men and women who live together are more sexually active than those who are not in a relationship. Because women tend to live longer than men, many elderly women will be without partners and will have limited opportunities for sexual expression, even if sexual drive is present. In men, significant changes in erections and ejaculation occur with aging. Usually it takes *more stimulation to achieve an erection* as a male ages. *The plateau phase of sexual excitement* is longer and may not end in ejaculation. When ejaculation occurs, *the force of expulsion of semen and the intensity of ejaculation are lower. After ejaculation, the erection resolves more quickly* and the refractory period increases. Many of these changes start to occur when men are in their 20s, and age-associated changes should be anticipated and viewed as normal.

30.5 The answer is B

In many instances the risk of psychiatric illness (e.g., depression or psychosis) is much worse for the brain and the interaction of mother and child than the potential adverse effects of psychotropic medication. If a woman becomes pregnant, however, medications should be evaluated immediately. The hormonal effects of pregnancy may change the course of her illness. However, it is not necessary to induce unwarranted guilt or to have the woman consider aborting if she does become pregnant while on psychotropic medications.

Definitive answers to the question of which psychotropic medications are safest during pregnancy and lactation are unlikely. While ethical considerations limit performing randomized, prospective interventional trials, observational data can and should be collected in registries. In patients with worsening psychiatric illness during pregnancy, outpatient psychotherapy, hospitalization, and milieu therapy should be attempted before routine use of psychotropic medication. Before a planned pregnancy, if possible, withdrawal of psychotropic medications

Table 30.1
FDA Rating of Drug Safety in Pregnancy

Category	Definition	Drug Examples
A	No fetal risks in controlled human studies	Iron
B	No fetal risk in animal studies and no risk in well-controlled human studies	Acetaminophen
C	Adverse fetal effects in animals and no human data available	Aspirin, haloperidol, chlorpromazine
D	Human fetal risk seen (may be used in life-threatening situation)	Lithium, tetracycline, ethanol
X	Proved fetal risk in humans (no indication for use, even in life-threatening situations)	Valproic acid, thalidomide

should be attempted under close supervision. The importance of close rapport between the treating physician and the pregnant or breastfeeding patient cannot be overstated and will obviate or decrease reliance on psychotropic medication in some cases. The Food and Drug Administration (FDA) rates drugs in five categories of safety for use in pregnancy (Table 30.1). Of *lithium, tetracycline, ethanol,* and *valproic acid,* only valproic acid is listed as having no indication for use in pregnancy.

30.6 The answer is E (none)

Some lesbian couples may decide that one partner should become pregnant through artificial (or natural) insemination. Societal attitudes may create stresses to this arrangement, but if the two women have a secure relationship, they tend to bond strongly together as a family unit. Long-term follow-up studies have shown that children of lesbian mothers *do not differ from children of heterosexual mothers in emotional health* or *interpersonal relationships,* and the children *are not more likely to be gay or lesbian themselves.* Also, men in committed gay relationships are fathering children through artificial (or natural) insemination with surrogate mothers. The long-term effects on children reared by gay men have not been determined; however, preliminary findings are similar to those pertaining to children who are raised in lesbian homes.

30.7 The answer is E (all)

Fears regarding pain and bodily harm during delivery are universal and to some extent, warranted. Preparation for childbirth affords a sense of familiarity and can ease anxieties, which facilitates delivery. Continuous emotional support during labor *reduces the rate of cesarean section* and forceps deliveries, *the need for anesthesia, the use of oxytocin, and the duration of labor.* A technically difficult delivery, however, does not appear to influence the decision to bear additional children.

30.8 The answer is A

Hyperemesis gravidarum is differentiated from morning sickness in that vomiting *is chronic, persistent*, and frequent, leading to ketosis, acidosis, weight loss, and dehydration. The *prognosis is excellent* for both mother and fetus with prompt treatment. Most women can be treated as outpatients with change to smaller meals, discontinuation of iron supplements, and avoidance of certain foods. In severe cases hospitalization may be necessary. Although the cause is unknown, *there may be a psychological component. Women with histories of anorexia nervosa or bulimia nervosa may be at risk.*

30.9 The answer is D

Infertility is the inability of a couple to conceive after 1 year of coitus, without the use of a contraceptive. *In the United States, about 15 percent (not 5 percent) of married couples are unable to have children.* Until recently, women were blamed when couples did not have children, and feelings of guilt, depression, and inadequacy frequently accompanied this perception. *Today, causes of infertility are attributed to disorders in women in 40 percent (not 75 percent) of cases, disorders in men in 40 percent (not 10 percent) of cases, and disorders of both in 20 percent of cases.* Tests in an infertility workup usually reveal the specific cause; *however, 10 to 20 percent (not 50 percent) of couples have no identifiable etiology.*

30.10 The answer is E (all)

Pelvic pain can have many causes, including endometriosis, pelvic adhesions, ovarian or adnexal masses, *hernias, and bowel or rectal disease.* Pelvic pain can also be secondary to psychogenic causes, such as guilt, *infertility fears,* and the *emotional disturbances associated with ongoing or past incest or sexual abuse.* Pelvic pain should not be attributed to psychogenic causes unless a thorough evaluation has excluded organic causes. In most instances, the evaluation should include a diagnostic laparoscopy. Likewise, dyspareunia or pain with intercourse should not be assumed to have a psychogenic origin unless all anatomical causes have been excluded.

30.11 The answer is B

Premenstrual syndrome (PMS), termed *premenstrual dysphoric disorder* in the revised fourth edition of the *Diagnostic and Statistical Manual of Mental Disorders* (DSM-IV-TR), is a somatopsychic illness *triggered by the expected excursions in sex steroids* that accompany *a hormonally normal (not abnormal) ovulatory menstrual cycle.* These somatic changes disturb psychological functioning in predisposed women.

It occurs about one week prior to the onset of menses and is characterized by irritability, emotional lability, headache, anxiety, and depression. Somatic symptoms include edema, weight gain, breast pain, syncope, and paresthesias. *Approximately 5 percent (not 50 percent) of women have the disorder.* Treatment is symptomatic and includes analgesics for pain and sedatives for anxiety and insomnia. *Some cases respond to short courses of SSRIs.* Fluid retention is relieved with diuretics.

Answers 30.12–30.18

30.12 The answer is A

30.13 The answer is A

30.14 The answer is B

30.15 The answer is C

30.16 The answer is A

30.17 The answer is A

30.18 The answer is A

About 20 to 40 percent of women report some emotional disturbance or cognitive dysfunction in the postpartum period. Many experience so-called *"baby blues,"* a normal state of sadness, dysphoria, frequent *tearfulness,* and clinging dependence. These feelings, which may last several days, have been ascribed to rapid changes in women's hormonal levels, the stress of childbirth, and the awareness of the increased responsibility that motherhood brings.

Postpartum depression is characterized by a depressed mood, *anhedonia,* excessive anxiety, and insomnia. The onset is within 3 to 6 months after delivery. Table 30.2 differentiates postpartum "baby blues" from postpartum depression.

In rare cases (1 to 2 in 1,000 deliveries), a woman's postpartum depression is characterized by depressed feelings and *suicidal ideation.* In severe cases, the depression may reach psychotic proportions, with hallucinations, delusions, and

Table 30.2
Comparison of "Baby Blues" and Postpartum Depression

Characteristic	"Baby Blues"	Postpartum Depression
Incidence	50% of women who give birth	10% of women who give birth
Time of onset	3–5 days after delivery	Within 3–6 months after delivery
Duration	Days to weeks	Months to years, if untreated
Associated stressors	No	Yes, especially lack of support
Sociocultural influence	No; present in all cultures and socio-economic classes	Strong association
History of mood disorder	No association	Strong association
Family history of mood disorder	No association	Some association
Tearfulness	Yes	Yes
Mood lability	Yes	Often present, but sometimes mood is uniformly depressed
Anhedonia	No	Often
Sleep disturbance	Sometimes	Nearly always
Suicidal thoughts	No	Sometimes
Thoughts of harming the baby	Rarely	Often
Feelings of guilt, inadequacy	Absent or mild	Often present and excessive

Reproduced with permission from Miller LJ. How "baby blues" and postpartum depression differ. *Women's Psychiatric Health.* 1995:13. © 1995, The KSF Group.

thoughts of infanticide. Although *previous psychiatric problems put women at risk for postpartum disturbances,* there is evidence to suggest that postpartum mood disorder is a specific concept, distinct from other psychiatric diagnoses. Others argue that these mood disorders are not a distinct entity but are part of a bipolar spectrum as reflected in the DSM-IV-TR classification. Women with severe postpartum depressions are at high risk for future episodes, and *failure to treat may contribute to long-term, treatment-refractory mood disorders.*

Answers 30.19–30.22

30.19 The answer is A

30.20 The answer is B

30.21 The answer is C

30.22 The answer is D

Disorders of sexual development in phenotypic girls generally present at birth or at the time of expected puberty. *Adrenogenital syndrome* can be caused by congenital adrenal hyperplasia in female fetuses; the fetal adrenal secretes excess androgens, which then masculinize the external genitalia and possibly the brain. In female infants, the *masculinized genitalia usually are recognized in the delivery room.* Surgery to reduce clitoral size and create or widen the vaginal introitus may be necessary at a later date to restore the external appearance. *However, the internal reproductive tract is normal and puberty generally occurs around the expected time if adrenal replacement therapy is adequate.* Despite medical and surgical interventions, concerns over capacity for sexual function may emerge, particularly in late adolescence or young adulthood.

Turner's syndrome (XO gonadal dysgenesis) may be recognized at birth because of the associated physical stigmata, while XX gonadal dysgenesis usually presents at puberty. From a reproductive perspective, the two conditions are similar in that the *ovaries do not contain responsive oocytes* because of premature atresia of oocytes or failure of germ cell migration. Donor oocytes allow the option of pregnancy.

Other disorders of sexual development include *testicular feminization* and its variants; the *gonads in that condition are testes,* but the fetus is phenotypically female in that a defect in the androgen receptor confers androgen insensitivity. Because the testes are normal, they secrete testosterone and müllerian regression occurs (regression of the anlage that would develop into the uterus and tubes). The vagina ends blindly, and the presenting complaint is usually primary amenorrhea. Thelarche (onset of breast development) occurs at the normal time because at puberty the testes secrete testosterone, which then is aromatized to estradiol, which stimulates the growth of breast tissue. Orchiectomy (removal of the testes) is recommended after puberty to avoid the risk of gonadoblastoma, unless there is partial androgen sensitivity, in which case it is performed earlier to prevent the pubertal development of hirsutism and partial masculinization. .

There are many types of androgen receptor defects and a spectrum of clinical presentations. Some individuals look phenotypically like men and may present with infertility secondary to azoospermia or oligospermia. A related disorder occurs when there is an inefficiency of the enzyme 5α-reductase, which converts testosterone to dihydrotestosterone (DHT); DHT, in turn, masculinizes the external genitalia. Boys with a deficiency of that enzyme may look phenotypically female or incompletely masculinized at birth. At puberty, further masculinization, including phallic enlargement, may develop, as the increased testicular secretion of testosterone partially overcomes the enzyme deficiency and more dihydrotestosterone is made. Fertility is preserved in this condition, so it is prudent to rear the child as a male if possible. Neonatal treatment with dihydrotestosterone may help to masculinize the external genitalia.

XY gonadal dysgenesis is caused by a gonad that fails to secrete testosterone and MIS; generally the uterus, tubes, and vagina are present. This condition is detected when the menarche does not occur. A karyotype can confirm the XY chromosomal status. Because the gonads are inactive hormonally, they should be removed before puberty to avoid the risk of malignant degeneration. Exogenous hormone replacement is required to stimulate puberty and cause the development of secondary sexual characteristics. If donor oocytes are available, pregnancy is possible following in vitro fertilization and embryo transfer. Telling a young adolescent and her parents about the diagnosis can be difficult, particularly since surgery may be required to remove the gonads.

31

Relational Problems

People in intimate relationships with each other often experience problems. This may especially be the case when the relationships are affected by the presence of a mental disorder or medical condition. The revised fourth edition of the *Diagnostic and Statistical Manual of Mental Disorders* (DSM-IV-TR) attempts to formally classify problems in relationships, and this classification is meant to be employed when the focus of clinical attention is the impaired relationship. The specific relational problems indicated in DSM-IV-TR are those between parents and children, and between partners or siblings, as well as those seen in the context of a mental disorder or general medical condition. There is also a category for relational problems not otherwise specified.

An example of a relational problem related to a mental disorder might be the impaired interaction between a mother and her schizophrenic daughter, or the interaction between a brother of normal intelligence and his developmentally delayed sibling. An example of a relational problem related to a general medical condition might be the inability of a husband and wife to have sexual relations because of the husband's diabetes, and the wife's subsequent extramarital affair. A parent–child relational problem might arise in the context of divorce and remarriage, when the child must adjust to a new stepparent or to living for periods of time with each parent.

The student should study the questions and answers below for a useful review of these problems.

HELPFUL HINTS

Each of the following terms should be defined by the student.

- ▶ communication problems:
    negative
    distorted
    noncommunication
- ▶ day care centers
- ▶ divorce and remarriage
- ▶ dual obligation
- ▶ environmental factors
- ▶ family characteristics
- ▶ family system
- ▶ family therapy
- ▶ marital roles
- ▶ parent–child problem
- ▶ partner relational problem
- ▶ physician marriages
- ▶ physician's responsibility
- ▶ polysomnographic findings
- ▶ premature child
- ▶ prevention
- ▶ psychotherapy
- ▶ psychotic symptoms
- ▶ racial and religious prejudice
- ▶ relational problem due to mental disorder or medical condition
- ▶ sibling relational problem
- ▶ sibling rivalry

▲ QUESTIONS

DIRECTIONS: The questions below consist of lettered headings followed by a list of numbered statements. For each numbered statement, select the *one* lettered heading that is most closely associated with it. Each lettered heading may be used once, more than once, or not at all.

Questions 31.1–31.4

    A. Anxious-ambivalent attachment style
    B. Avoidant attachment style
    C. Both
    D. Neither

31.1 Tendency to be obsessed with romantic partners
31.2 Breakup rates are high
31.3 Tendency to behave without much fear of rejection
31.4 Extreme jealousy

Questions 31.5–31.8

    A. Relational problem linked to a mental disorder or general medical condition

    B. Parent–child relational problem

    C. Partner relational problem

    D. Sibling relational problem

    E. Relational problem not otherwise specified

31.5 A man with multiple sclerosis resents being taken care of by his wife

31.6 A 60-year-old married woman has problems with her neighbor, and because of differences between the two, the police have been called numerous times; otherwise, the woman has many good friends

31.7 The oldest daughter in a family of four siblings refuses to come home for any family gatherings if her oldest brother also comes home

31.8 An adopted child continually feels that the family who adopted him pays more attention to their biological daughter than to him; he is becoming increasingly withdrawn and irritable

---

ANSWERS

Relational Problems

Answers 31.1–31.4

31.1 The answer is A

31.2 The answer is C

31.3 The answer is D

31.4 The answer is A

A core issue in all close personal relationships is the establishment and regulation of the affiliative connection between the participants. In a typical attachment interaction, one person seeks more proximity and affection and the other either reciprocates, rejects, or disqualifies the request. A pattern is shaped through repeated exchanges. Attachment behavior between an infant and its primary caregiver will lead to the development of an *attachment style*, which is a relatively stable communication pattern exhibited in close relationships. Distinct attachment styles have been observed in children and adults. Adults with an *anxious-ambivalent attachment style tend to be obsessed with romantic partners*, suffer from *extreme jealousy*, and have a *high divorce rate*. People with a secure attachment style are highly invested in relationships and tend to *behave without much possessiveness or fear of rejection*. People with an avoidant attachment style tend to ignore or disqualify conflict, often leading to frustration in a partner, which can result in high breakup rates. Their avoidance of conflict may be secondary to a fear of rejection, but, paradoxically, their style often ends in rejection by the partner.

Answers 31.5–31.8

31.5 The answer is A

31.6 The answer is E

31.7 The answer is D

31.8 The answer is B

The *man with multiple sclerosis*, who resents being taken care of by his wife, is classified as *having a relational problem related to a mental disorder or general medical condition*. The 60-year-old *woman who has problems with her neighbor* but gets along well with other people is classified as having *relational problem not otherwise specified*. The classification of *sibling relational problem* is best for the *daughter who refuses to attend family gatherings* if her oldest brother is also present. *Parent–child relational problem* is the appropriate diagnosis for the *adopted child* who feels slighted by his family's attention to their biological daughter.

32

Problems Related to Abuse or Neglect

Abuse and neglect of children and adults are major public health concerns in the United States. For instance, the National Center on Child Abuse and Neglect in Washington, D.C., has estimated that there are more than 300,000 instances of child maltreatment reported to central registries throughout the country every year. It is estimated that 2,000 to 4,000 deaths of children from abuse occur annually. Problems related to abuse and neglect are defined as physical or sexual abuse of a child or adult, and neglect of a child.

More than 50 percent of abused or neglected children were born prematurely or had low birth weight. Many abused children are perceived by their parents as difficult, slow in development or mentally retarded, bad, selfish, or hard to discipline. More than 80 percent of abused children are living with married parents at the time of the abuse and 90 percent of abusing parents were abused by their own parents.

The only sure way of proving infant abuse or neglect, other than catching the perpetrator in the act, is to show that significant recovery occurs when the caretaking is altered. All markedly deprived infants should warrant an investigation of the social and environmental conditions of the family and the psychological status of the parent in order to determine the factors responsible for inadequate and destructive treatment. Parents who abuse substances, who suffer from psychotic or pronounced mood disorders, or who are severely personality disordered are at higher risk for impaired judgment and potentially abusive behavior.

Child abuse and neglect may be suspected when a child appears unduly afraid (especially of the parents), the child is kept confined for overly long periods of time, the child shows evidence of repeated skin or other injuries, the child is undernourished, the child is dressed inappropriately for the weather, the child cries often, and the child has bruising/pain/itching in the genital or anal region or repeated urinary tract infections and vaginal discharges. Unusually precocious knowledge of sexual acts may indicate sexual abuse. Clinicians are required to report suspected cases of child abuse or neglect and must be familiar with the current laws and regulations in their individual states.

Sexual or physical abuse of adults, including the elderly, is also a major problem in the United States. Spouse abuse, for example, is thought to occur in as many as 12 million families in this country, and there are estimated to be almost 2 million battered wives.

The age range for rape cases in the United States is reported to be from infancy to the 80s and 90s, and the FBI reports that there are more than 80,000 rapes each year. It has been estimated that only 10 to 25 percent of rapes are ever reported to the proper authorities. About 10 percent of rapes are perpetrated by close relatives, and 50 percent are committed by men known to varying degrees by the victim. Elder abuse is seen in nursing homes and other institutions, as well as in some private households where the demands of caring for a frail, helpless, or demented person can lead individuals to commit acts of physical or sexual abuse.

The student should study the questions and answers below for a useful review of these problems.

HELPFUL HINTS

The student should know the following words and terms.

- ▶ annual deaths
- ▶ child abuse
- ▶ child pornography
- ▶ dysthymic disorder
- ▶ emotional deprivation
- ▶ environmental factors
- ▶ family characteristics
- ▶ functional impairment
- ▶ genetic factors
- ▶ hyperactivity
- ▶ incest:
  - father–daughter
  - mother–son
- ▶ irritable versus depressed mood
- ▶ learning disability
- ▶ low-birth-weight child
- ▶ major depressive disorder
- ▶ mania
- ▶ mood disorders
- ▶ National Committee for the Prevention of Child Abuse
- ▶ physician's responsibility
- ▶ polysomnographic findings
- ▶ precocious sexual behavior
- ▶ premature child
- ▶ prevention
- ▶ psychotic symptoms
- ▶ retinal hemorrhages
- ▶ secondary complications
- ▶ suicide
- ▶ symmetrical injury patterns

▲ QUESTIONS

DIRECTIONS: Each of the questions or incomplete statements below is followed by five suggested responses or completions. Select the *one* that is *best* in each case.

32.1 True statements about the epidemiology of child abuse include

A. Many child fatalities are linked to parental substance abuse.
B. The median age of victims of maltreatment has been reported to be 2 years.
C. The vast majority of victims are girls.
D. About five of every 1,000 children have been reported as—and verified to be—victims of maltreatment.
E. All of the above

32.2 Child maltreatment is correlated strongly with

A. less parental education
B. underemployment
C. poor housing
D. welfare reliance
E. all of the above

32.3 Psychological symptoms considered pathognomonic for sexual abuse in children include

A. periods of amnesia
B. imitating intercourse
C. touching the genitals of others
D. masturbating with an object
E. none of the above

32.4 True statements about typical physical injuries related to abuse include all of the following *except*

A. Less than 50 percent of serious intracranial injuries sustained in the first year of life result from physical abuse.
B. Subdural bleeding ranks among the most dangerous inflicted injuries.
C. Retinal tearing can be caused by shaking injuries.
D. Falls from 1 to 3 feet rarely result in subdural hematomas or clavicle fractures.
E. Bilateral black eyes immediately following facial trauma generally indicates intentional injury.

32.5 A false allegation of abuse may occur

A. in child custody disputes
B. due to leading or suggestive questions by an interviewer
C. to protect the actual offender
D. as a result of parental misinterpretation of innocent remarks or behaviors
E. all of the above

DIRECTIONS: The questions below consist of lettered headings followed by a list of numbered phrases or statements. For each numbered phrase or statement, select

A. if the item is associated with *A only*
B. if the item is associated with *B only*
C. if the item is associated with *both A and B*
D. if the item is associated with *neither A nor B*

Questions 32.6–32.8

A. Neglect
B. Abuse
C. Both
D. Neither

32.6 Failure to feed the child adequately
32.7 Failure to provide medical care
32.8 Verbal assaults, such as belittling, threats, blaming

DIRECTIONS: Each of the questions or incomplete statements below is followed by five suggested responses or completions. Select the *one* that is *best* in each case.

32.9 Which of the following statements about rape is *incorrect*?

A. Rapes are usually premeditated.
B. Rape most often occurs in a woman's own neighborhood.
C. Fifty percent of all rapes are perpetrated by close relatives of the victim.
D. The age range reported for rape cases in the United States is 15 months to 82 years.
E. According to the Federal Bureau of Investigation, more than 100,000 rapes are reported each year.

32.10 Which of the following statements about rape is *false*?

A. About 10 to 25 percent of rapes are reported to authorities.
B. The greatest danger of rape exists for women aged 16 to 24.
C. Most men who commit rape are between 25 and 44 years of age.
D. Alcohol is involved in at least 75 percent of forcible rapes.
E. About 50 percent of rapes are committed by strangers.

32.11 Spouse abuse is

A. carried out by men who tend to be independent and assertive
B. a recent phenomenon
C. least likely to occur when the woman is pregnant
D. directed at specific actions of the spouse
E. an act that is self-reinforcing

32.12 Rape is predominantly used to express power and anger in all of the following cases *except*

A. rape of elderly women
B. homosexual rape
C. rape of young children
D. statutory rape
E. date rape

32.13 Which of the following statements about incest is *true*?

    A. About 15 million women in the United States have been the victims of incestuous attacks.

    B. One-third of incest cases occur before the age of 9.

    C. It is most frequently reported in families of low socioeconomic status.

    D. Father–daughter incest is the most common type.

    E. All of the above

ANSWERS

Problems Related to Abuse or Neglect

32.1 The answer is A

The National Committee to Prevent Child Abuse collects data each year on the incidence of child maltreatment. The committee estimated that in 1997 almost 3.2 million alleged victims were reported to child protective services. Of those reports, about 1 million were substantiated; this represents *about 15 of every 1,000 (not five of every 1,000) children.* The substantiated cases were distributed as follows: neglect, 54 percent; physical abuse, 22 percent; sexual abuse, 8 percent; emotional abuse, 4 percent; and other or unspecified cases, 12 percent.

The committee reported that in 1996 over 1,000 children died as the result of maltreatment. About 38 percent of these deaths were children under age 1. *Many child fatalities were linked to parental substance abuse.* A large number (41 percent) of the deaths were children who were current, open cases or previous clients of a child protection service agency.

The National Center on Child Abuse and Neglect also collects data each year on child maltreatment. The center estimated that in 1995 the *median age of victims of child maltreatment was 7 (not 2) years.* Of the victims, *about 53 percent were girls* and 47 percent were boys. It was reported that approximately 80 percent of the victims were abused by parents; 10 percent by other relatives; 5 percent by noncaregivers; and 2 percent by foster parents, facility staff, or child-care providers.

These figures are only estimates because the actual amount of abuse is unclear. The reporting of abuse has mounted in recent years. In large part, this increase in reported abuse is the result of greater public awareness and willingness to report child abuse, as well as improved data collection techniques in individual states. As for the rise in child abuse itself, it can be attributed, at least in part, to local economic conditions that place a larger number of families under stress.

32.2 The answer is E (all)

Although child abuse occurs at all socioeconomic levels, it is highly associated with poverty and psychosocial stress, especially financial stress. *Child maltreatment is* strongly correlated with *less parental education, underemployment, poor housing, welfare reliance,* and single parenting. Child abuse tends to occur in multiproblem families, that is, families characterized by domestic violence, social isolation, parental mental illness, and parental substance abuse, especially alcoholism. The probability of maltreatment may be increased by risk factors such as prematurity, mental retardation, and physical handicap.

32.3 The answer is E (none)

Abused children manifest a variety of emotional, behavioral, and somatic reactions. *These psychological symptoms are nei-* *ther specific nor pathognomonic;* the same symptoms may occur without any history of abuse.

A variety of symptoms, behavioral changes, and diagnoses sometimes occur in sexually abused children. These include:

1. Anxiety symptoms such as fearfulness, phobias, insomnia, nightmares that directly portray the abuse, somatic complaints, and posttraumatic stress disorder.
2. Dissociative reactions and hysterical symptoms such as *periods of amnesia,* daydreaming, trance-like states, hysterical seizures, and symptoms of dissociative identity disorder.
3. Depression manifested by low self-esteem and suicidal or self-mutilative behaviors.
4. Disturbances in sexual behaviors, including sexual hyperarousal. Some sexual behaviors are particularly suggestive of abuse, such as *masturbating with an object, imitating intercourse,* inserting objects into the vagina or anus; other sexual behaviors are less specific, such as showing genitals to other children and *touching the genitals of others*; a younger child may manifest age-inappropriate sexual knowledge; sexually abused children may display sexually aggressive behavior toward others; in contrast to these overly sexualized behaviors, the child may avoid sexual stimuli through phobias and inhibitions.
5. Somatic complaints, such as enuresis, encopresis, anal and vaginal itching, anorexia, obesity, headache, and stomachache.

Nonabused children may exhibit any of these symptoms and behaviors. For example normal, nonabused children commonly exhibit sexual behaviors such as *masturbating,* displaying their genitals, and trying to look at people who are undressing. Further, approximately one-third of sexually abused children have no symptoms. On the other hand, the following factors have been associated with more severe symptoms in the victims of sexual abuse: greater frequency and duration of abuse, sexual abuse that involves force or penetration, and sexual abuse perpetrated by the child's father or stepfather.

32.4 The answer is A

More than 95 percent (not less than 50 percent) of serious intracranial injuries sustained in the first year of life result from physical abuse. The cause of injury, typically, is violent shaking to-and-fro whiplash, or slamming. *Subdural bleeding ranks among the most dangerous inflicted injuries,* often resulting in death or serious crippling sequelae. *Retinal tearing* and hemorrhage *may be caused by shaking injuries.* Falls are often blamed for injuries, and *a fall from 1 to 3 feet* can result in linear skull fracture and epidural hematoma. *Such falls, however, rarely result in subdural hematomas or clavicle* or humerus *fractures.*

Inflicted black eyes are more common than serious eye injuries. Victims smacked about the eyes with an open or closed hand have both eyelids swollen, with massive bruising. Generally, black eyes sustained from accidents involve trauma to one eye. Although other scenarios are possible, the *onset of bilateral black eyes immediately following facial trauma* generally indicates intentional injury.

Traumatic alopecia and subgaleal hematomas are caused by pulling the hair. Alopecia areata (noninflammatory hair loss) is characterized by loose hairs at the periphery of the bald area and is easily distinguished from inflammation or boggy swelling of the scalp caused by violent lifting of the child by the hair. Subgaleal hematomas may result when the aponeurosis connection between the occipital and frontalis muscles is wrenched off the calvarium, permitting rapid filling of the remaining space with blood.

32.5 The answer is E (all)

A false allegation of abuse may occur for several reasons. Sometimes a false allegation arises in the mind of a parent or other adults and is imposed on the child. *The parent may have misinterpreted an innocent remark*, a neutral piece of behavior, or a benign physical condition as evidence of abuse and induced the child to endorse this interpretation. This happens in *child custody disputes* as well as other settings. Sometimes the parent and child share a *folie à deux* or the pressured child may give in and agree with a delusional parent. A parent may have fabricated the story and induced the child to collude in presenting it to authorities.

A false allegation may result from *an interviewer's suggestion,* or previous interviewers may have asked leading *or suggestive questions.* An interviewer who believes abuse occurred may unwittingly shape a child's responses until the child validates the interviewer's assumptions.

Group contagion may lead to false allegations. In epidemic hysteria, people modify what they have heard to meet their own emotional needs. Thus, rumors may become more convincing as they are retold.

A younger child may confuse fantasy with reality, and although rare, older children and adolescents may experience delusions about sexual activities in the context of a psychotic illness. Sometimes children misunderstand what happened and report it inaccurately, or they may misunderstand an adult's question and the adult may later misinterpret or take the child's statement out of context. In confabulation, children fill gaps in their memory with whatever information makes sense to them and others at the time.

The child may have been sexually abused and exhibit symptoms consistent with abuse yet the child identifies the wrong person as the perpetrator, resulting in a false allegation. The child may do this *to protect the actual offender* or to displace the memories and accompanying affects onto another individual.

Answers 32.6–32.8

32.6 The answer is A

32.7 The answer is A

32.8 The answer is B

The most prevalent form of child maltreatment, *neglect* is the failure to provide sufficient care and protection for children. Children can be harmed by malicious or ignorant withholding of physical, emotional, and educational necessities. Neglect includes *failure to feed children adequately* and protect them from danger. Physical neglect includes abandonment, expulsion from home, disruptive custodial care, inadequate supervision, and reckless disregard for a child's safety and welfare. Medical neglect includes refusal, delay, or *failure to provide medical care.* Educational neglect includes failure to enroll a child in school and allowing chronic truancy.

Physical abuse may be defined as any act that results in a nonaccidental physical injury, such as beating, punching, kicking, biting, burning, and poisoning. Some physical abuse is the result of unreasonably severe corporal punishment or unjustifiable punishment. Physical abuse may be organized by the site of injury; damage to skin and surface tissue, damage to the head, damage to internal organs, and skeletal damage.

Psychological abuse occurs when a person conveys to a child that he or she is worthless, flawed, unloved, unwanted, or endangered. The perpetrator may spurn, terrorize, isolate, or berate the child. Emotional abuse includes *verbal assaults* (e.g., belittling, screaming, threats, blaming, or sarcasm), unpredictable responses, persistent negative moods, constant family discord, and double-message communications. Some authors feel that the terms "psychological" or "emotional abuse" should not be used and that "verbal abuse" more accurately describes the pathological behavior of the caregiver.

Sexual abuse of children refers to sexual behavior between a child and an adult or between two children when one of them is significantly older or uses coercion.

32.9 The answer is C

About 10 percent, not 50 percent, of rapes are perpetrated by close relatives. About half of rapes are committed by strangers and half by men known in varying degrees (but unrelated) to the victim. *Rapes are usually premeditated,* although rape often accompanies another crime such as mugging. A rapist frequently threatens a victim with his fists or a weapon and often harms her in nonsexual as well as sexual ways. *Rape most often occurs in a woman's own neighborhood.* It may take place inside or near her home. *The age range reported for rape cases* in the United States is 15 months to 82 years. According to the Federal Bureau of Investigation, *more than 80,000 rapes are reported each year.* The incidence is declining slightly.

32.10 The answer is D

Alcohol is involved in about 35 percent, not 75 percent, of forcible rapes. *The greatest danger of rape exists for women aged 16 to 24,* although victims of rape can be any age. Most men who commit rape are *between the ages of 25 and 44 years old.* It has been estimated that *10 to 25 percent of rapes are reported* to authorities. *About 50 percent of rapes are committed by strangers to the victims,* and the remaining 50 percent are committed by men known to them by varying degrees.

32.11 The answer is E

Spouse abuse is an *act that is self-reinforcing*; once a man has beaten his wife, he is likely to do so again. Abusive husbands *tend to be* immature, *dependent, and nonassertive,* and to suffer from strong feelings of inadequacy. Spouse abuse is *not a recent phenomenon*; it is a problem of long standing that is *most likely (not least likely) to occur when the woman is pregnant.*

Fifteen to 25 percent of women are physically abused while pregnant, and the abuse often results in birth defects. The *abuse is not directed at specific actions of the spouse;* rather, impatient and impulsive abusive husbands physically displace aggression provoked by others onto their wives.

32.12 The answer is D

Statutory rape deviates dramatically from the other kinds of rape in being nonassaultive and a sexual act, not a violent act. Statutory rape is intercourse that is unlawful because of the age of the participants. Intercourse is unlawful between a male older than 16 years of age and a female under the age of consent, which ranges from 14 to 21 years, depending on the jurisdiction.

Other types of rape—including *the rape of elderly women, homosexual rape, date* or acquaintance *rape,* and *the rape of young children*—are used predominantly to express power and anger. Studies of convicted rapists suggest that the crime is committed to relieve pent-up aggressive energy against persons of whom the rapist is in some awe. Although the objects of awe are usually men, the retaliatory violence is displaced toward women.

32.13 The answer is E (all)

About 15 million women in the United States have been the victims of incestuous attacks, and *one-third of incest cases occur before the age of 9.* Incest is *most frequently reported in families of low socioeconomic status.* That finding may be the result of these families' greater than usual contact with welfare workers, public health personnel, law enforcement agents, and other reporting officials; it may not be a true reflection of higher incidence in that demographic group. *Father–daughter incest* is the most common type.

33

Additional Conditions That May Be a Focus of Attention

As any experienced clinician well knows, there are numerous conditions that are not diagnosable mental disorders, but nonetheless can be very much the focus of clinical attention. These conditions may or may not cause severe distress and dysfunction in those experiencing them, but all of them interfere—to varying degrees—with optimal functioning and may represent just the most visible manifestations of some real, underlying mental disorder. The revised fourth edition of the *Diagnostic and Statistical Manual of Mental Disorders* (DSM-IV-TR) lists and describes 13 such conditions that may or may not be associated with mental disorders, and may or may not be precursors of mental disorders. However, all of these conditions can be identified only when they are not directly attributable to a specific mental or neurological disorder. These 13 conditions are noncompliance with treatment, malingering, adult antisocial behavior, child or adolescent antisocial behavior, borderline intellectual functioning, age-related cognitive decline, bereavement, academic problem, occupational problem, identity problem, religious or spiritual problem, acculturation problem, and phase-of-life problem.

Malingering, for instance, is the conscious and intentional feigning of physical or psychological symptoms for some clearly definable goal, such as to avoid responsibilities or to receive free compensation. Clinically, it is often crucial to distinguish malingering from true mental illnesses such as factitious, somatoform, or dissociative disorders. Isolated, trivial incidents of malingering (e.g., calling in sick when one really isn't) occur frequently and are not usually the focus of clinical attention. More serious or extensive incidents (for example, feigning illness or injury to obtain psychoactive drugs or to defraud insurance or social service agencies) may reflect genuine underlying psychopathology. Malingering may be associated with child, adolescent, or adult antisocial behavior, which is characterized by engaging in illegal or immoral activities. However, the antisocial behavior in these conditions never reaches the level necessary to diagnose an antisocial personality disorder.

Bereavement is a condition that can become the focus of clinical attention, even if it does not progress to the outright actual mental disorder of depression. The clinician must be aware of the difference between normal bereavement and depression and be alert for the development of more serious symptoms. A bereaved person may view what he or she is experiencing as normal but still seek treatment for an associated symptom such as insomnia. Bereavement is not associated typically with such signs and symptoms as active suicidal ideation, prolonged or marked functional impairment, prominent hallucinations, or with delusional guilt.

Examples of an occupational problem include job dissatisfaction and uncertainty about career choices. A phase-of-life problem might be associated with such major life-cycle changes as starting college, getting married, or having children. Stress during times of cultural transitions, such as moving to a new country or entering the military, can lead to an acculturation problem. Young people who join cults might provide examples of a religious or spiritual problem. Age-related cognitive decline must be distinguished from dementia, while borderline intellectual functioning must be distinguished from diagnosable developmental delays or specific learning disorders. Academic problem, identity problem, and noncompliance with treatment are the remaining conditions addressed in this chapter and the student should be able to describe and recognize their characteristics.

The student should study the questions and answers below for a useful review of these conditions.

HELPFUL HINTS

The students should know the following terms.

- acculturation problem
- adherence
- adoption studies
- age-associated memory decline
- antisocial behavior
- bereavement
- brainwashing
- compliance
- conditioning
- coping mechanisms
- cults
- cultural transition
- culture shock
- doctor–patient match
- dual-career families
- job-related stress
- kleptomania
- malingering
- marital problems
- mature defense mechanisms
- medicolegal context of presentation
- noncompliance
- noncustodial parent
- normal grief
- occupational problem
- phase-of-life problem
- religious or spiritual problem
- sociopathic
- stress
- superego lacunae

▲ QUESTIONS

DIRECTIONS: Each of the questions or incomplete statements below is followed by five suggested responses or completions. Select the *one* that is *best* in each case.

33.1 True statements about compliance include

A. Noncompliance is more common and roughly double among inpatients than among outpatients.

B. Modification in lifestyles is more easily achieved than medication compliance.

C. Compliance is a particular problem in disorders such as glaucoma.

D. Compliance is improved if patients view their disease as not terribly serious.

E. None of the above

33.2 Acculturation problems, as defined by DSM-IV-TR, may include effects related to

A. joining the military

B. moving across country

C. brainwashing

D. prisoner-of-war experiences

E. all of the above

33.3 Malingered amnesia is

A. probably the least common clinical presentation of malingering

B. difficult to feign

C. easy to detect

D. more convincing when global rather than spotty and episode-specific

E. none of the above

33.4 Borderline intellectual functioning

A. is defined as an IQ below 70

B. is essentially the same as mental retardation

C. is usually diagnosed after completion of school

D. is present in approximately 14 percent of the general population

E. none of the above

33.5 Academic problems

A. cannot be diagnosed if due to a mental disorder

B. can be diagnosed only if they are the result of factors external to the student, such as family difficulties or social stressors

C. are evidenced by a pattern of academic underachievement or a decline from a previous level of functioning

D. intelligence tests are rarely useful in making the diagnosis

E. none of the above

33.6 Occupational problems as defined by DSM-IV-TR can be associated with

A. suicide risk

B. domestic violence

C. working teenagers

D. loss of a job

E. all of the above

33.7 Persons best able to cope with phase-of-life problems appear to be those with

A. good verbal communication skills

B. capacity for sublimation

C. flexibility

D. adequate financial status

E. all of the above

DIRECTIONS: The questions below consist of lettered headings followed by a list of numbered phrases. For each numbered phrase, select

A. if the item is associated with *A only*

B. if the item is associated with *B only*

C. if the item is associated with *both A and B*

D. if the item is associated with *neither A nor B*

Questions 33.8–33.10

A. Adult Antisocial Behavior

B. Antisocial Personality Disorder

C. Both

D. Neither

33.8 Previous diagnosis of conduct disorder with onset before age 15

33.9 Mental disorder

33.10 Occurs more often in males than in females

DIRECTIONS: Each of the questions or incomplete statements below is followed by five suggested responses or completions. Select the *one* that is *best* in each case.

33.11 Exit therapy is designed to help people

A. with adult antisocial behavior

B. with acculturation problems

C. who are involved in cults

D. with occupational problems

E. in bereavement

33.12 A person who malingers

A. often expresses subjective, ill-defined symptoms

B. should be confronted by the treating clinician

C. is usually found in settings with a preponderance of women

D. rarely seeks secondary gains

E. can achieve symptom relief by suggestion or hypnosis

33.13 Antisocial behavior is generally characterized by

A. poor intelligence

B. heightened nervousness with neurotic manifestations

C. often successful suicide attempts

D. lack of remorse or shame

E. all of the above

33.14 Which of the following statements involving women in the work force is *false*?

    A. More than 50 percent of all mothers in the work force have preschool-aged children.

    B. Specific issues that should be addressed are provisions for child care or for care of elderly parents.

    C. Managers are more sensitive to crises in women employees' lives than in men employees' lives.

    D. Ninety percent of women and girls alive today in the United States will have to work to support themselves.

    E. Managers often ignore the stress placed on a worker by the illness of a child.

33.15 Which of the following is *not* considered a mental disorder?

    A. Factitious disorder

    B. Antisocial personality disorder

    C. Malingering

    D. Hypochondriasis

    E. Somatization disorder

ANSWERS

Additional Conditions That May Be a Focus of Attention

33.1 The answer is C

The determinants of compliance are kaleidoscopic and ever-changing. There is no stereotypical noncompliant person or situation. Nonetheless, there are areas of consensus.

Noncompliance is more common and *roughly double among outpatients than among inpatients (not vice versa). Medication compliance is more (not less) readily achieved than modification in lifestyle.*

Compliance is a particular problem in disorders that have no symptoms, are persistent, and have no method for self-monitoring such as hypertension, diabetes, and glaucoma. Glaucoma presents the most difficult problem because, currently, there is no home tonometer to measure intraocular pressure corresponding to the sphygmometer and glucometer that measure blood pressure and blood sugar concentrations, respectively.

Compliance diminishes across time in disorders that are chronic or long lasting. Compliance generally improves when patients' expectations are met, when they are satisfied, and when they are supervised. *It helps if patients view their disease as a serious one* to which they are susceptible and if they have developed compliance strategies of their own. Supportive family members or friends are important. Factors that generally impede compliance are complicated regimens, troublesome adverse effects, social stress, isolation, and alcohol dependence.

33.2 The answer is E (all)

In DSM-IV-TR the following statement about the acculturation problem appears:

"This category can be used when the focus of clinical attention is a problem involving adjustment to a different culture (e.g., following migration)."

Major cultural change can evoke severe distress, termed culture shock. This condition arises when individuals suddenly find themselves in a new culture in which they feel completely alien. They may also feel conflict over which lifestyles to maintain, change, or adopt. Children and young adult immigrants often adapt more easily than middle-aged and elderly immigrants. They learn the new language with less difficulty, and they continue to mature in the new culture, whereas those more senior have had more stability and unchanging routines in their former culture. Culture shock

from immigration clearly differs from psychiatric patients' restless and continuous moving secondary to their illness.

Culture shock may occur within one's own country with geographical, school, and work changes such as *joining the military*, experiencing school busing, or *moving across country* or to a vastly different neighborhood, or from a rural area to a very urban one. Reactive symptoms are understandable and include anxiety, depression, isolation, fear, and a sense of loss of identity as one adjusts. If the person is part of a family or group making the transition together, and the move is positive and planned, stress can be lower. Furthermore, if selected cultural mores can be safely maintained as persons integrate into the new culture, stress is also minimized.

The constant geographical moves because of work opportunities and necessity involve a large proportion of U.S. workers. Joining activities in the new community and actively trying to meet neighbors and coworkers can lessen the culture shock.

First practiced on American prisoners during the Korean War by the Chinese Communists, *brainwashing* is the deliberate creation of culture shock. Victims are isolated, intimidated, and made to feel different and out of place in an attempt to break their spirits and destroy their coping skills. Once the isolated victims appear mentally weak and helpless, new ideas that they would never have accepted in their normal state are imposed upon them by the aggressors. As with cult victims, upon release and return to their homes, brainwashed individuals with posttraumatic stress disorder require deprogramming treatment, including reeducation and ongoing supportive psychotherapy both on a one-to-one and group basis. Treatment is usually long term in order to rebuild healthy self-esteem and restore coping skills.

Prisoners who survive war or torture experiences withstand the ordeal because of personal inner strengths developed in their earlier lives, beginning within their emotionally strong and caring families; if from troubled families, they may more likely take their own lives. Such prisoners must cope continuously with anxiety, fear, isolation from others they know, and loss of all control. Those who appear to cope best believe they must survive for a reason (e.g., to tell others what they experienced or to return to loved ones). Prisoners who cope best describe living simultaneously on two levels: living in the "here-and-now" to survive the immediate situation while maintaining constant mental connections to their past values and experiences and to those important to them.

Beyond the surviving prisoner's personal difficulties, including posttraumatic stress disorder, if and when their survival behavior continues, it can affect their consequent families, with inordinate fear of police and strangers, overprotection and overburdening of children to replace those lost, lack of sharing of the past, continued isolation from their current communities, or inappropriately expressed anger. Another generation can thus be affected in their personal development and psychological functioning, and they may require psychiatric evaluation and treatment.

33.3 The answer is D

Amnesia, probably the most (not the least) common clinical presentation of malingering, is claimed by 30 to 55 percent of perpetrators of homicide. *It is easy (not difficult) to feign and is particularly difficult (not easy) to detect.*

At least six possible causes have been suggested for amnesia: (1) conversion disorder; (2) psychosis; (3) alcoholism; (4) head injury; (5) epilepsy; and (6) malingering. Before malingering is ascribed, the clinician should review and eliminate the other five potential causes. A good diagnostic battery would include negative results on skull X-ray, head computed tomography or magnetic resonance imaging, and electroencephalography; normal findings on a neurological examination; a life history inconsistent with either conversion disorder or alcoholism (or other causes of intoxication); and a clinical examination and history inconsistent with either alcoholic amnesia (alcohol-induced persisting amnestic disorder) or psychosis (alcohol-induced psychotic disorder).

If the preceding tests are negative, the clinician faces the difficult task of amassing evidence, albeit inferential, of malingering. Motivation is a key indicator. Previous amnestic episodes without apparent motivational precursors lower the likelihood that the patient is malingering. Similarly, a patient with histrionic personality traits is more likely to be experiencing true dissociative amnesia than one with primarily antisocial traits.

The timing of onset and recovery, and correlation of the alleged amnestic episode with convenience, are other clues to the presence of malingering. *Global amnesia is somewhat more convincing than spotty,* patchy, *episode-specific,* and self-serving amnesia. There have been several reported epidemics of copy-cat amnesias following famous or highly publicized cases; an eye to recent sensational litigation is prudent. Table 33.1 summarizes some guidelines on detecting malingered amnesia.

33.4 The answer is D

DSM-IV-TR describes borderline intellectual functioning as follows:

"This category can be used when the focus of clinical attention is associated with borderline intellectual functioning, that is, *an IQ in the 71–84 range (not an IQ below 70).* Differential diag-

Table 33.1
Clues to the Detection of Malingered Amnesia

1. No history of amnestic episodes
2. Antisocial personality traits more prominent than histrionic personality traits
3. Spotty, episode-specific amnesia rather than global amnesia
4. Self-serving timing of onset and recovery
5. Recent, widely publicized, suspiciously familiar cases involving amnesia

nosis between Borderline Intellectual Functioning and *Mental Retardation (an IQ of 70 or below)* is especially difficult when the coexistence of certain mental disorders (e.g., schizophrenia) is involved. Coding note: This is coded on Axis II."

The 1959 edition of *Classification in Mental Retardation* defined anyone with an IQ greater than one standard deviation below the mean (IQ below 85) as mentally retarded. This definition was applied without regard to functional impairment, and many individuals who fell within this range had no discernible adaptive difficulties. The 1973 edition of *Classification in Mental Retardation* redefined mental retardation as an IQ greater than two standard deviations below the mean (70 or below) with associated impairments in adaptive functioning. This definition of mental retardation has been retained in subsequent editions and is adhered to in DSM-IV-TR and the 10th revision of *International Statistical Classification of Diseases and Related Health Problems* (ICD-10). An IQ between 71 and 84 was "declassified" as mentally disordered and redefined as borderline intellectual functioning. Because individuals within this IQ range tend to have little impairment outside of educational settings, *the diagnosis is often overlooked after completion of school.* The condition may continue to be a focus of clinical attention if it compromises social functioning, vocational adjustment, or compliance with medical management. *Approximately 14 percent of the general population* has an IQ within this range; borderline intellectual functioning is similarly named and defined in ICD-10.

33.5 The answer is C

DSM-IV-TR describes academic problems as follows:

"This category can be used when the focus of clinical attention is an *academic problem that is not due to a mental disorder or, if due to a mental disorder,* is sufficiently severe to warrant independent clinical attention. An example is a pattern of failing grades or of significant underachievement in a person with adequate intellectual capacity in the absence of a Learning or Communication Disorder or another mental disorder that would account for the problem."

Academic problems can result from factors intrinsic as well as external to the student. Psychiatric conditions such as anxiety or mood disorders can impair learning or lead to performance decline. Attention-deficit/hyperactivity disorder, chronic illness, and identity problems can lead to demoralization in school studies apart from any diagnosable mental condition. Family difficulties, social stressors, cultural deprivation, or poor fit between a student and a teacher's temperamental style can also adversely affect scholastic performance.

Academic problems are evidenced by a pattern of *academic underachievement or a decline* from a previous level of functioning. A comprehensive biopsychosocial assessment is fundamental to identification of causal factors. Particular focus should be given to past academic functioning and family and social stressors; concurrent psychopathology must be ruled out. *Intelligence tests,* measures of academic achievement, or language evaluation *may be useful in differentiating academic problems from specific learning or communication disorders.* Review of the medical history and physical examination may be of value in identifying general medical conditions, such as hearing loss, poor vision, and chronic illness, that may adversely affect academic performance.

33.6 The answer is E (all)

DSM-IV-TR includes the following statement about occupational problem:

"This category can be used when the focus of clinical attention is an occupational problem that is not due to a mental disorder or, if it is due to a mental disorder, is sufficiently severe to warrant independent clinical attention. Examples include job dissatisfaction and uncertainty about career choices."

Occupational psychiatry and its expansion to include organizational psychiatry are focused specifically on the psychiatric aspects of work problems, including vocational maladjustment. Symptoms of employment dissatisfaction are varied and include blatant work errors, perceived and verbalized unhappiness and disinterest, absenteeism and tardiness, and passive-aggressive behaviors including accidents and uncooperativeness. Psychiatric symptoms include general signs of distress, anger, resentment about most work assignments, lack of confidence, and lack of interest in carrying out agreed upon and expected work responsibilities.

Occupational problems often arise during stressful changes in work, namely, at initial entry into the work force or when making job moves within the same organization to a higher position because of good performance or to a parallel position because of corporate need. Distress occurs particularly if these changes are not sought and no preparatory training has taken place, as well as during layoffs and at retirement, especially if retirement is mandatory and the person is unprepared for it. Work distress can result if initially agreed-to conditions change to work overload or lack of challenge and opportunity to experience work satisfaction, if persons feel unable to fulfill conflicting expectations or feel that work conditions prevent accomplishing assignments because of lack of legitimate power, and finally if persons believe they work in a hierarchy with harsh and unreasonable superiors.

Some occupations both attract persons with a high *suicide risk* and involve increased chronic distress that may lead to higher suicide rates. Included are health professionals, financial service workers, and police, the first and latter groups because of easier access to lethal drugs and weapons.

Many teenagers work part-time while attending high school. Stress can arise because of reduced parent–teenager interaction and constructive parental control issues about use of earnings and time spent away from home and consequent behaviors in as well as outside the home. When each parent or a single parent works outside the home, as does the teenager, verbal communication must be proactive and clear.

Although occurring in the home, signs and symptoms that interfere with work often trigger identification of *domestic violence* victims. All employees experiencing work distress must be questioned about domestic violence by trained professionals.

Regardless of the reason *for job loss,* most people experience distress, including symptoms of normal grief, loss of self-esteem, anger, and reactive depressive and anxiety symptoms, as well as somatic symptoms and possibly substance abuse and increased (or the onset of) domestic violence. Timely education, support programs, and vocational guidance should be instituted.

33.7 The answer is E (all)

The DSM-IV-TR description of phase-of-life problem includes the following:

"This category can be used when the focus of clinical attention is a problem associated with a particular developmental phase or some other life circumstance that is not due to a mental disorder or, if it is due to a mental disorder, is sufficiently severe to warrant independent clinical attention. Examples include problems associated with entering school, leaving parental control, starting a new career, and changes involved in marriage, divorce, and retirement."

Although on some level adults recognize that in the course of a lifetime, life events will intrude on expected plans, experiencing unexpected, multiple, and major negative occurrences, especially if they are chronic, may overwhelm a person's ability to recover and function constructively. Common phase-of-life problems include changes in significant personal relationships, job crises, and parenthood.

Major life changes precipitate distress in the form of anxiety and depressive symptoms, inability to express reactive emotions directly, and difficulties in coping with life responsibilities.

Persons best able to cope with phase-of-life problems appear to be those with positive attitudes and mature defense mechanisms and coping styles, including basic trust in self and others, *good verbal communication skills,* a capacity for creative and positive thinking, and the ability to be *flexible,* reliable, and energetic, with strong family and personal relationships. Furthermore, a *capacity for sublimation, adequate financial* and work *status,* solid values, and healthy, feasible goals can enable people to face, accept, and deal realistically with life problems and changes.

Answers 33.8–33.10

33.8   The answer is B

33.9   The answer is B

33.10 The answer is C

The diagnosis of *antisocial personality disorder,* in contrast to *adult antisocial behavior,* requires evidence of preexisting psychopathology, such as *previous diagnosis of conduct disorder with onset before age 15,* and a long-standing pattern of irresponsible and antisocial behavior since the age of 15. Illegal behavior is not considered the equivalent of psychopathology, and without evidence of preexisting psychological disturbance is not deemed secondary to antisocial personality disorder.

Adult antisocial behavior is not considered a *mental disorder,* but antisocial personality disorder is. Both adult antisocial behavior and antisocial personality disorder *occur more often in males than in females.* Familial patterns for each of the two diagnostic classes have also been reported.

33.11 The answer is C

Exit therapy is designed to help people *who are involved in cults;* it works only if their lingering emotional ties to persons outside the cult can be mobilized. Most potential cult members are in their adolescence or otherwise struggling with establishing their own identities. The cult holds out the false promise of emotional well-being and purports to offer the sense of direction for which the persons are searching. Cult members are encouraged to proselytize and to draw new members into the group. They are often encouraged to break with family members and friends and to

Table 33.2
Malingering Features Usually Not Found in Genuine Illness

Symptoms are vague, ill-defined, overdramatized, and not in conformity with known clinical conditions.

The patient seeks addicting drugs, financial gain, the avoidance of onerous (e.g., jail) or other unwanted conditions.

History, examination, and evaluative data do not elucidate complaints.

The patient is uncooperative and refuses to accept a clean bill of health or an encouraging prognosis.

The findings appear compatible with self-inflicted injuries.

History or records reveal multiple past episodes of injury or undiagnosed illness.

Records or test data appear to have been tampered with (e.g., erasures, unprescribed substances in urine).

Courtesy of Arthur T. Meyerson, M.D.

socialize only with other group members. Cults are invariably led by charismatic personalities, who are often ruthless in their quest for financial, sexual, and power gains and in their insistence on conformity to the cult's ideological belief system, which may have strong religious or quasi-religious overtones.

Exit therapy is not designed to help people with *adult antisocial behavior*, with *acculturation* or *occupational* problems, or in *bereavement*. Occupational problems may bring a person into contact with the mental health field, and psychotherapy may aid in working through some occupational problems.

33.12 The answer is A

A person who malingers *often expresses subjective, ill-defined symptoms*—for example, headache; pains in one's neck, lower back, chest, or abdomen; dizziness; vertigo; amnesia; anxiety; and depression—and the symptoms often have a family history, in all likelihood not organically based but extremely difficult to refute. A patient suspected of malingering should be thoroughly and objectively evaluated, and the physician should refrain from showing any suspicion. The patient *should not be confronted by the treating clinician*. If the clinician becomes angry (a common response to malingerers), a confrontation may occur, with two likely consequences: (1) The doctor–patient relationship is disrupted, and no further positive intervention is possible; and (2) the patient is even more on guard, and obtaining proof of deception may become virtually impossible. Preserving the doctor–patient relationship is often essential to accurate diagnosis and effective long-term treatment. Careful evaluation usually reveals the relevant issue without the need for a confrontation.

Malingering *is usually found in settings with a preponderance of men (not women)*, such as the military, prisons, factories, and other industrial settings. The malingerer *always (not rarely) seeks secondary gains*, such as money, food, and shelter. The malingerer *cannot usually achieve symptom relief by suggestion or hypnosis*. Table 33.2 lists malingering features not found in genuine illness.

33.13 The answer is D

Antisocial behavior is generally characterized by *lack of remorse or shame*. Other characteristics are *(not heightened) good (not poor) intelligence, an absence of nervousness and neurotic manifestations, and rarely (not often) successful suicide attempts.*

33.14 The answer is C

Studies reveal that managers are more sensitive to crises in men's than in women's lives (not vice versa). Managers respond to such major events as divorce and death of a family member but *ignore the stress placed on a worker by the illness of a child* or a school closing because of a snow day. *More than 50 percent of mothers* in the work force have preschool-aged children. *Specific issues* that should be addressed are *provisions for child care or for the care of elderly parents. Ninety percent of women and girls* alive today in the United States *will have to work to support themselves* and probably one or two other people.

33.15 The answer is C

Malingering is not considered a mental disorder; it is characterized by the voluntary production and presentation of false or grossly exaggerated physical or psychological symptoms. The patient always has an external motivation, which falls into one of three categories: (1) to avoid difficult or dangerous situations, responsibilities, or punishment; (2) to receive compensation, free hospital room and board, drugs, or haven from the police; and (3) to retaliate when one feels guilt or suffers a financial loss, legal penalty, or job layoff or termination.

Factitious disorder, antisocial personality disorder, hypochondriasis, and *somatization disorder* are all considered mental disorders. The presence of a clearly definable goal is the main factor that differentiates malingering from factitious disorder. Antisocial personality disorder requires evidence of conduct disorder that began before the age of 15. Hypochondriasis and somatization disorder are both somatoform disorders, which are characterized by physical symptoms that suggest physical disease, although no demonstrable organ pathology or pathophysiological mechanism can usually be identified. In hypochondriasis the patient is excessively concerned about disease and health. In somatization disorder, multiple somatic symptoms cannot be explained medically and are associated with psychosocial distress and medical help seeking.

34

Emergency Psychiatric Medicine

Emergencies occur in psychiatry just as they do in every field of medicine. However, psychiatric emergencies are often particularly disturbing because they do not just involve the body's reactions to an acute disease state, as much as actions directed against the self or others. These emergencies, such as suicidal acts, homicidal delusions, or a severe inability to care for oneself, are more likely than medical ones to be sensationalized when they are particularly dramatic or bizarre. A mother killing her five children in the belief that they are inhabited by Satan, a famous poet killing herself, the delusional murder of a legendary musician, the son of a prominent family found wandering confused and malnourished in a city park, all of these are psychiatric emergencies that can and do end up on the front pages of newspapers.

Of course, psychiatric emergencies occur everyday to people who do not make the evening news. Psychiatric emergencies arise when mental disorders impair people's judgment, impulse control, or reality testing. Such mental disorders include all the psychotic disorders, manic and depressive episodes in mood disorders, substance abuse, borderline and antisocial personality disorders, and dementias. There may also be emergencies related to particularly severe reactions to psychiatric medications, such as neuroleptic malignant syndrome or acute agranulocytosis, that must be recognized, diagnosed, and treated immediately.

The most common psychiatric emergency is suicide, which is reported to be the eighth leading cause of death in the United States. Clinicians must be aware of the relevant risk factors for suicide (such as age, sex, race, marital status, occupation, family history, physical and mental health, and past suicidal behavior), but must also be aware that the suicidal patient they are evaluating in the emergency room may not necessarily have any of them.

Major depressive disorder, alcohol abuse, and schizophrenia are all associated with a higher than usual risk for suicide, as is a positive family history for suicide. Genetic influence in the expression of suicidal behavior has been postulated, and there appears to be substantiating evidence for this in twin and adoption studies. There is also speculation that a genetic transmission of a tendency toward impulsive behavior (associated with a deficiency in cerebral serotonin) is also implicated. However, a behavior as complex as suicide cannot be reduced to any simplistic biological formulation.

Emile Durkheim in the 1800s approached suicide from a sociological perspective, studying how suicide is perceived differently in various cultural groups. He described three types of suicide: egoistic, altruistic, and anomic. Per Durkheim, egoistic suicide occurs in people who are not strongly integrated into a social group. This might be reflected in the higher suicide risk for unmarried people over married, and in city dwellers over those living in rural environments. Altruistic suicide might be reflected in military situations, where soldiers sacrifice themselves in battle. Anomic suicide might be represented in people whose social integration is sufficiently disturbed or fragile, such as an apparently upstanding person who suddenly faces exposure as a criminal.

Psychiatrists must learn how to evaluate a suicidal or homicidal patient and must learn how to ask the questions that will help reveal suicidal or homicidal plan and intent. A skilled clinician will combine this information with a sense of the person's overall risk, based on detailed knowledge of the person's history as well as overall knowledge of suicidal and homicidal behaviors in the context of mental impairment.

The student should study the questions and answers below for a useful review of this subject.

HELPFUL HINTS

These terms relate to psychiatric emergencies and should be defined.

- ▶ acute intoxication
- ▶ adolescent suicide
- ▶ age of suicide
- ▶ akinetic mutism
- ▶ alcohol dependence
- ▶ alcohol withdrawal
- ▶ alkalosis
- ▶ amnesia

- ▶ anniversary suicide
- ▶ anorexia nervosa
- ▶ bulimia nervosa
- ▶ copycat suicides
- ▶ delirious state
- ▶ delirium
- ▶ dementia
- ▶ drugs and suicide

- ▶ DTs
- ▶ Emile Durkheim
- ▶ dysmenorrhea
- ▶ ECT
- ▶ exhaustion syndrome
- ▶ grief and bereavement
- ▶ headache
- ▶ 5-HIAA in CSF

- ▶ hyperthermia
- ▶ hypertoxic schizophrenia
- ▶ hyperventilation
- ▶ hypnosis
- ▶ hypothermia
- ▶ inpatient vs. outpatient treatment

- ▶ insomnia
- ▶ lethal catatonia
- ▶ method
- ▶ miosis
- ▶ mood disorders
- ▶ "Mourning and Melancholia"
- ▶ mydriasis
- ▶ nystagmus
- ▶ opioid withdrawal: anxiolytic

- hypnotic sedative
- ▶ panic disorder
- ▶ platelet MAO activity
- ▶ posttraumatic stress disorder mania
- ▶ premenstrual dysphoric disorder
- ▶ prevention center
- ▶ psychiatric interview

- ▶ psychotic disorders
- ▶ psychotic withdrawal
- ▶ restraints
- ▶ suicidal depression
- ▶ suicidal thoughts
- ▶ suicidal threats
- ▶ suicide: altruistic anomic egoistic

- ▶ suicide belt
- ▶ suicide rate
- ▶ Thanatos
- ▶ violence and assaultive behavior
- ▶ Wernicke's encephalopathy
- ▶ Werther's syndrome

▲ QUESTIONS

DIRECTIONS: Each of the questions or incomplete statements below is followed by five suggested responses or completions. Select the *one* that is *best* in each case.

34.1 Suicide rates

- A. have remained relatively stable except for 15- to 24-year-olds, whose rates have decreased two- to threefold
- B. have averaged five per 1,000,000 in the 20th century
- C. make suicide the eighth leading cause of death in the United States
- D. reflect about 10,000 suicides each year in the United States
- E. none of the above

34.2 Suicide among schizophrenic patients

- A. is low
- B. is approximately 10 percent
- C. occurs most often in the later years of the illness
- D. occurs most often in older, women patients
- E. is most frequently secondary to command hallucinations

34.3 Increased rates of suicide attempts occur in patients with

- A. panic disorder
- B. social phobia
- C. personality disorders
- D. substance abuse
- E. all of the above

34.4 True statements about suicide in the elderly include

- A. Compared to other age groups, those 65 and older have the highest risk of committing suicide.
- B. The suicide rate for the elderly is more than ten times that of young persons.
- C. The least frequent means of committing suicide in the elderly is with a firearm.
- D. Alcoholism is less likely to be associated with suicide in the elderly than in younger people.
- E. All of the above

34.5 True statements about patients with parasuicidal behavior include

- A. About 50 percent are found to have a personality disorder at psychiatric assessment.
- B. About 40 percent have made previous attempts.
- C. About 1 percent of persons who attempt suicide will commit suicide during the following year.
- D. Suicide risk is particularly high during the first year after a suicide attempt.
- E. All of the above

34.6 The presence of medical illness should be strongly considered when

- A. Psychiatric symptoms appear suddenly in a previously well-functioning person.
- B. There is a reported personality change or marked lability of mood.
- C. Psychotic symptoms appear for the first time after the age of 30.
- D. Temperature, pulse, or respiratory rate are increased.
- E. All of the above

34.7 Basic principles of emergency psychiatry include

- A. availability of a seclusion room
- B. availability of four-point leather restraints
- C. rapid tranquilization
- D. presence of uniformed city police and hospital security personnel
- E. all of the above

34.8 Suicidal behavior

- A. tends not to be familial
- B. is not associated with a family history of suicide
- C. has been found to have the same concordance rate in dizygotic as in monozygotic twins
- D. occurs more frequently in the biological relatives of adoptees who commit suicide than in the adoptive relatives
- E. none of the above

DIRECTIONS: Each group of questions below consists of lettered headings followed by a list of numbered phrases or statements. For each numbered phrase or statement, select the *one* lettered heading that is most closely associated with it. Each lettered heading may be selected once, more than once, or not at all.

Questions 34.9–34.11

    A. Emile Durkheim
    B. Sigmund Freud
    C. Karl Menninger

34.9 Divided suicide into three social categories: egoistic, altruistic, and anomic

34.10 Described three components of hostility in suicide: the wish to kill, the wish to be killed, and the wish to die

34.11 Wrote that suicide represents aggression turned inward

Questions 34.12–34.17

    A. Opioid OD
    B. Barbiturates
    C. Phencyclidine (PCP) OD
    D. Monoamine oxidase inhibitors (MAOIs)
    E. Acetaminophen (Tylenol) OD

34.12 Treated with propranolol (Inderal)
34.13 Toxic interaction with meperidine hydrochloride (Demerol)
34.14 Phenothiazines contraindicated
34.15 Fever, pancytopenia, hypoglycemic coma, renal failure
34.16 Pale, cyanotic, respiratory depression, pinpoint pupils
34.17 Seizure with withdrawal

DIRECTIONS: Each of the questions or incomplete statements below is followed by five suggested responses or completions. Select the *one* that is *best* in each case.

34.18 The patient was a 25-year-old female graduate student in physical chemistry who was brought to the emergency room by her roommates, who found her sitting in her car with the motor running and the garage door closed. The patient had entered psychotherapy 2 years before, complaining of long-standing unhappiness, feelings of inadequacy, low self-esteem, chronic tiredness, and a generally pessimistic outlook on life. While she was in treatment, as before, periods of well-being were limited to a few weeks at a time. During the 2 months before her emergency room visit, she had become increasingly depressed, had had difficulty in falling asleep and trouble in concentrating, and had lost 10 pounds. The onset of those symptoms coincided with a rebuff she had received from a chemistry instructor to whom she had become attracted.

The treatment of the patient could include

    A. hospitalization
    B. outpatient psychotherapy
    C. antidepressants
    D. electroconvulsive therapy
    E. all of the above

34.19 Suicide rates

    A. are equal among men and women
    B. decrease with age
    C. are higher among blacks than among whites
    D. increase during December and other holiday periods
    E. are lower among Catholics than the rates among Protestants and Jews

34.20 Which of the following neurobiological findings is associated with suicide?

    A. increased 5-hydroxyindoleacetic acid (5-HIAA) levels in the cerebrospinal fluid (CSF)
    B. changes in the dopaminergic system
    C. serotonin deficiency
    D. increased levels of platelet monoamine oxidase (MAO)
    E. normal findings on electroencephalogram (EEG)

34.21 Among men, suicide peaks after age 45; among women, it peaks after age

    A. 35
    B. 40
    C. 45
    D. 50
    E. 55

34.22 Figure 34.1 shows the U.S. distribution, according to race and sex, of which of the following?

    A. the prevalence of schizophrenia
    B. rates of alcohol-related disorders
    C. Rates of suicide attempts (successful and unsuccessful)
    D. death rates for suicide
    E. prevalence of bipolar disorder

34.23 Commonly cited predictors of dangerousness to others include

    A. chronic anger or hostility
    B. early loss of parent
    C. prior violent acts
    D. frequent threats
    E. all of the above

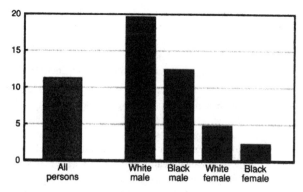

FIGURE 34.1
Reprinted with permission from National Center for Health Statistics. *Health, United States, 1991.* Hyattsville, MD: Public Health Service; 1992.

DIRECTIONS: For each of the four numbered syndromes below, select the letter of the most appropriate set of emergency manifestations.

Questions 34.24–34.27

    A. Delirium, mania, depression, psychosis
    B. Marked aggressive and assaultive behavior
    C. Alcohol stigmata, amnesia, confabulation
    D. Mental confusion, oculomotor disturbances, cerebellar
       ataxia
    E. None of the above

34.24 Bromide intoxication
34.25 Korsakoff's syndrome
34.26 Idiosyncratic alcohol intoxication
34.27 Wernickes's encephalopathy

ANSWERS

Emergency Psychiatric Medicine

34.1 The answer is C

Suicide is a major public health problem: approximately 0.9 percent of all deaths are the result of suicide. About 1,000 persons are estimated to commit suicide each day worldwide. *In the United States suicide ranks as the eighth leading cause of death*, and there are approximately 75 suicides per day, or one every 20 minutes, and *more than 30,000 (not 10,000) each year.* The suicide rate in the United States has *averaged 12.5 per 100,000 (not 5 per 1,000,000) in the 20th century,* with a high of 17.4 per 100,000 during the Great Depression. From 1983 to 1998 the overall suicide rate has remained relatively stable whereas the rate *for 15- to 24-year-olds has increased (not decreased) two to threefold.* The number one suicide site in the world is the Golden Gate Bridge in San Francisco.

34.2 The answer is B

The suicide risk is high (not low) among schizophrenia patients: *up to 10 percent die by committing suicide.* Most persons with schizophrenia who commit suicide do so *during the first few years of their illness.* Thus, schizophrenic *suicides tend to be relatively young (not old), and about 75 percent are unmarried males (not older women);* approximately 50 percent have made a previous suicide attempt. Depressive symptoms are closely associated with their suicide; studies have reported that depressive symptoms were present during the last period of contact in up to two-thirds of schizophrenia patients who committed suicide; *only a small (not a high) percent commit suicide because of hallucinated instructions* or in order to escape persecutory delusions. Up to a third of schizophrenic suicides occur during the first few weeks and months following discharge from hospital; another third commit suicide while they are inpatients.

34.3 The answer is E (all)

Alcoholic persons have an increased risk of suicide, with a lifetime suicide risk of 2.2 to 3.4 percent. More men than women are found among alcoholic suicide victims. Alcoholic persons usually commit suicide after years of alcohol abuse. Comorbidity plays an important role; persons with alcoholism who have comorbid depressive disorders are at particularly high risk. Workers in St. Louis examined the relationship of alcoholic suicide to specific life events. Among 31 alcoholic suicides, 48 percent had lost a loved one during the year before they committed suicide, and 32 percent had experienced such a loss during their last 6 weeks. The St.

Louis group examined the lives of 50 other alcoholic suicide victims. Based on the hypothesis that suicide among alcoholics may represent a reaction to life events, the researchers recorded their opinions about the most important reason for suicide in each case (Table 34.1). Loss of a close relationship was the most frequently cited precipitating event; other events included job trouble, financial difficulties, and being in trouble with the law. For only 1 of the 50 suicide victims could no precipitating event be identified.

There is an *increased risk of suicide among substance abusers.* For example, the suicide rate of heroin addicts is about 20 times greater than that of the general population. The availability of lethal amount of drugs, intravenous use, associated antisocial personality disorder, chaotic lifestyle, and impulsivity are some of the factors that predispose drug-dependent persons to suicidal behavior, particularly when they are dysphoric, depressed, or intoxicated.

It is recognized that patients with borderline personality disorders have an increased risk of suicide. Recently one group reported a psychological autopsy study of suicide victims with

Table 34.1
Presumed Most Important Reason for Suicide Among 50 Alcoholic Suicide Victims

Presumed Reason	Number
Marital separation/divorce	8
Friction with spouse/lover	9
Expectation of loss (realistic)	5
Estrangement from family	2
Bereavement	2
Friction with family	1
Job trouble	4
Financial trouble	3
Trouble with the law	2
Depressed (as principal or only reason)	6
Feeling of disgrace	2
Feared rehospitalization	2
Inability to control drinking	1
Other	2
No provocation identified	1
Total	50

Reprinted with permission from Murphy G. Suicide in alcoholism. In: Roy A, ed. *Suicide.* Baltimore: Williams & Wilkins; 1986.

personality disorders and found that they were almost always (95 percent) associated with current Axis I depressive disorders, substance use disorders, or both.

The group also reported that *67 of a random sample of 229 suicide victims had an Axis II personality disorder.* About one-fifth (N = 43, 29 percent) of all the 229 suicides had a Cluster B diagnosis (dramatic, emotional, or erratic), compared to the estimated prevalence of 4 to 5 percent in the general population. Ten percent of the sample (N = 23) had a Cluster C diagnosis (anxious or fearful), and only one person had a Cluster A diagnosis (odd or eccentric).

The next compared the personality-disorder suicide victims with sex- and age-matched suicide victims without personality disorder. Suicides with Cluster B personality disorders were more likely than comparison subjects to have substance-use disorders (79 percent versus 40 percent) and previous nonfatal suicide attempts (70 percent versus 37 percent) and were less likely to have Axis III physical disorders (29 percent versus 50 percent). Suicide victims in Cluster B almost always had (98 percent) either comorbid depressive disorders (74 percent), substance-use disorders (79 percent), or both (55 percent). They found no evidence of impulsive suicides that would have occurred without Axis I disorders. In contrast, subjects with Cluster C personality disorders did not differ from their controls on any variable.

Data from the National Institute of Mental Health (NIMH) Epidemiologic Catchment Area (ECA) Study showed that *20 percent of individuals with panic disorder had made a suicide attempt at some time.* This high rate was similar to the rate for individuals with major depression. When patients with panic disorder without comorbidity were examined, the lifetime rate of suicide attempts remained raised at 7 percent. Similarly, individuals *with social phobia have increased rates of suicidal ideation and suicide attempts.* One group found that current panic disorder was rare among completed suicides, being found in only 1.2 percent of all suicides. However, panic disorder suicide victims had superimposed major depression and substance abuse, and associated personality disorders. Thus, clinical assessment of suicide risk in panic and phobia patients should include determination of the presence or absence of major depressive disorder, substance abuse, and personality disorder.

34.4 The answer is A

Compared to other age groups, *those 65 years and older have the highest risk* of committing suicide. For example, the suicide rate for the *elderly is* more than three (not ten) times that of young persons. In the United States, 18 elderly persons commit suicide each day, one every 80 minutes. The majority of elderly suicides are *committed using a firearm.* Some older individuals have a higher suicide risk than others: most at risk are males, whites, the recently widowed, and those aged 75 years or more.

The two psychiatric conditions most associated with suicide in the elderly are depression and alcoholism. Psychological autopsy studies show that approximately 70 percent of elderly suicide victims suffered from depression in the weeks and months before their suicide. Approximately 20 percent of elderly suicides meet the criteria for a substance abuse disorder, usually alcohol abuse or dependence.

Studies show that loss and stress are major etiologic factors in the depression and alcohol abuse found among elderly sui-

cide victims. These include physical losses resulting from poor health, painful illness, sensory deficits, and cognitive decline; social losses like death of a spouse and loss of the work role; and income losses associated with retirement and medical expenses. Such losses may lead to reduced social networks and social isolation, and can produce feelings of despair, loneliness, demoralization, dependency on others, helplessness and hopelessness, as well as suicidal ideation.

34.5 The answer is E (all)

Persons who attempt suicide also pose a major health problem. *Attempted suicide* is in many ways an unsatisfactory term. For example, most attempters do not actually wish to commit suicide; their motives are different. Thus, the Edinburgh group introduced the term parasuicide in an effort to signify that suicide attempts are not just failed suicides but are a very different behavior.

Hospital studies show that about 40 percent of those who attempt suicide have a history of psychiatric treatment. Psychiatric assessments reveal that about *50 percent have a personality disorder*, and up to 40 percent have other psychiatric disorders. The most common diagnoses that are not personality disorders are depressive disorders (up to 40 percent of women and 30 percent of men).

Studies using observer-rated instruments find that although symptoms like tension, depressed mood, hopelessness, irritability, worrying, and poor concentration are present in 40 to 75 percent of attempters, a definite psychiatric disorder can be diagnosed at admission in only about 30 percent of attempters; this percentage decreases rapidly over subsequent weeks. However, workers in Christchurch, New Zealand, have shown that among serious suicide attempters 90 percent had a psychiatric disorder with high rates of mood disorder, substance abuse, and antisocial personality disorder. The incidence of comorbidity was high: 56 percent had two or more disorders. The risk of a serious suicide attempt increased with increasing psychiatric comorbidity.

About 40 percent of attempters have made a previous attempt. Follow-up studies show that between 13 and 35 percent will repeat the attempt during the next 2 years. During this time up to 7 percent will make two or more attempts, 2.5 percent three or more attempts, and 1 percent five or more attempts. Thus, there appear to be three subgroups of repeaters: the very occasional repeater, the person who repeats several times within a short period, and the chronic or habitual repeater.

There are seven main items that may be helpful in identifying the patient at risk of making another suicide attempt: problems with alcohol, antisocial or borderline personality disorder, impulsivity, previous inpatient psychiatric treatment, previous outpatient psychiatric treatment, previous attempt that led to admission, and living alone.

It is recognized that those who attempt and those who commit suicide represent different populations with some overlap. *Approximately 1 percent of persons who attempt suicide will commit suicide during the following year.* For 8 to 50 suicide attempters, one will eventually commit suicide. The risk of subsequent suicide varies with sex and age. For example, at the Karolinska Hospital in Stockholm the suicide risk over the next 5 years after attempting suicide among men (8.3 percent) was nearly twice the suicide risk among women. Both older and younger male suicide attempters are at high risk of suicide (7 percent and 10 percent, respectively), and older women are at higher risk than younger women (6 percent versus 2 percent). The *suicide risk* was *particularly high during the first year after the suicide attempt.*

Follow-up studies show that other factors associated with subsequent suicide include being unemployed or retired; being separated, divorced, or widowed; living alone; having poor physical health; having received medical treatment within the last 6 months; having a psychiatric disorder, including alcoholism; having made many previous attempts by violent methods; the presence of a suicide note; and a history of previous attempts. A subgroup of suicide attempters who have severe personality disorder and interpersonal conflicts, and who often had alcohol or other substance dependence, commit suicide while acutely depressed.

34.6 The answer is E (all)
The presence of medical illness should be strongly considered when *psychiatric symptoms appear suddenly in a previously well-functioning person. A patient over the age of 30 with psychotic symptoms appearing for the first time,* an awareness or conviction that these symptoms are foreign, and especially with concomitant symptoms of cognitive dysfunction should be considered to have a possible organic illness. Clinicians should consider medical and substance-related causes when a patient has a history of a recently diagnosed medical illness, a new prescription, or a change in dosage. *A personality change or marked lability of mood* noticed by friends or relatives also suggest the onset of a serious medical condition.

Vital signs should be obtained on admission to the emergency department, even when the patient appears physically healthy or is intimidating because of disturbed behavior. Psychiatric disorders do not affect vital signs to a significant degree; therefore, abnormal vital signs must be further evaluated by a history, physical examination, and appropriate laboratory tests. *Elevation of temperature, pulse, or respiratory rate* suggests an underlying medical condition. Certain physical findings strongly suggest an organic disorder, including lateralizing neurological symptoms, confusion, and incontinence. Table 34.2 lists common medical conditions that frequently present as psychiatric emergencies and may be marked by abnormal vital signs. Table 34.3 lists those conditions that, although not common, may also appear initially as psychiatric problems. Delay in recognizing them can be life threatening.

34.7 The answer is E (all)
In the emergency department the physician frequently has to evaluate an unwilling or uncooperative patient, in contrast to the private practice of psychiatry, where considerations such as holding a patient for an adequate evaluation are rare; even if the patient should decide to walk out of an evaluation prematurely, the obligation of the physician is minimal. In addition, the stimulation of a busy emergency department can escalate the patient's symptoms. Environmental controls may be needed to protect the other patients as well as to ensure that the patient does not leave the emergency department unnoticed before the evaluation is complete.

Table 34.2
Common Medical Illnesses That Often Present as Psychiatric Emergencies

Hypothyroidism
Hyperthyroidism
Diabetic ketoacidosis
Hypoglycemia
Urinary tract infection
Pneumonia
Myocardial infarction
Alcohol intoxication
Alcohol withdrawal
Chronic obstructive pulmonary disease
Acute liver disease
Substance withdrawal

Decreasing the noise, the activity, and the anxiety exhibited by other patients or by medical personnel who are uncomfortable around psychiatric patients can reduce the patient's symptoms. *A "quiet room" or a seclusion room is useful* in this regard. The patient's vital signs should be obtained before he or she is placed in a quiet room, and then the patient should be monitored visually and checked regularly. *Restraints may be needed* to hold a patient long enough for a proper evaluation, particularly when the patient is unknown to the staff and the cause of the symptoms is uncertain, the patient is unable to cooperate with the examination, the patient needs a secure environment, or if the patient cannot be left unattended safely. When a disturbed patient leaves the emergency department before an adequate assessment can be done, malpractice actions can ensue, especially if it can be shown that the patient was in an altered mental state when he or she left. In national surveys on the use of restraint in psychiatric facilities, *four-point leather restraints remain the most used method of containing an out-of-control patient.* Their advantage over medication is that they are immediately reversible, and are an obvious

Table 34.3
Less Common but Potentially Life-Threatening Conditions That Present Frequently with Psychiatric Symptoms

Myocardial infarction
Pulmonary embolism
Subarachnoid hemorrhage
Epidural hemorrhage
Cocaine intoxication
Amphetamine intoxication
Encephalitis
Malignant hypertension
Hypokalemia
Hypercalcemia
Hypocalcemia
Splenic rupture
Subacute bacterial endocarditis
Steroid-induced psychotic disorder
Phencyclidine-induced psychotic disorder

reminder of the patient's condition. Once a diagnosis is clearer, pharmacological management may be used to control the patient's symptoms and behavior and to initiate or resume treatment. Emergency department staff should regularly practice using restraints, and the restraints should be maintained and reviewed regularly, much as the hospital crash cart. Seclusion, restraints, and psychopharmacologic management should not be construed as sufficient treatment, nor should these measures ever be regarded as punitive.

There is a growing literature on identification of the potentially violent patient, on staff training in the management of violent or disruptive patients, and on the social network and environment that increases or decreases violent behavior. In most studies, substance abuse, severe psychiatric disorders, and especially the combination of the two are disproportionately disruptive, and such patients are more likely to become violent in the emergency department. *The presence of uniformed city police and hospital security personnel* stationed in the emergency department appears to reduce the incidence of violence and of harm to health care workers. It is not clear how helpful metal detectors are. Willingness to use physical restraints for the patient who has been identified as potentially violent is reassuring to the staff, which in turn sets an atmosphere of calm and a sense that things are under control, which also decreases the incidence of patient outbursts. Other measures that increase the safety and effectiveness of staff are self-defense courses, a protocol for handling violent patients, good lighting, video monitoring of all areas of the emergency department, panic buttons, and secure handling of addictive drugs, syringes, and needles.

An acutely agitated or psychotic patient can be calmed in a very short period of time. For several years various protocols for *rapid neuroleptization* were promulgated; however, it was never demonstrated that rapid relief of acute psychosis led to shorter hospitalizations or that it was in the best interests of the patient to use this treatment. A common practice in the United States is to administer high-potency dopamine receptor antagonists, intramuscularly if necessary, and a benzodiazepine concurrently. This allows for a lower dose of the antipsychotic, and a decreased likelihood of extrapyramidal adverse effects. Although there are as yet no controlled studies regarding the use of the newer serotonin-dopamine antagonists or anticonvulsants in emergency room settings, their efficacy and relative lack of extrapyramidal symptoms make them potentially useful alternatives.

34.8 The answer is D
Suicidal behavior, like other psychiatric disorders, tends to run in families. For example, Margaux Hemingway's 1997 suicide was the fifth suicide among four generations of Ernest Hemingway's family. *In psychiatric patients a family history of suicide increases the risk both of attempted suicide and of completed suicide in most diagnostic groups.* In medicine the strongest evidence for the possibility of genetic factors comes from twin and adoption studies and from molecular genetics.

In 1991, 176 twin pairs in which one twin had committed suicide were investigated. In nine of these twin pairs, both twins had committed suicide. Seven of these nine pairs concordant for suicide were found among the 62 monozygotic pairs, while two pairs concordant for suicide were found among the 114 dizygotic twin pairs. *This twin-group difference for concordance for suicide (11.3 percent versus 1.8 percent) is statistically significant (P <.01).*

In another study a group of 35 twin pairs of which one twin had committed suicide was collected and the living co-twin was interviewed. It was found that 10 of the 26 living monozygotic co-twins had themselves attempted suicide, compared with zero of the nine living dizygotic co-twins (P <.04). Although monozygotic and dizygotic twins may have some differing developmental experiences, these results show that monozygotic twin pairs have significantly greater concordance for both suicide and attempted suicide, which suggests that genetic factors may play a role in suicidal behavior.

The strongest evidence suggesting the presence of genetic factors in suicide comes from the adoption studies carried out in Denmark. A screening of the registers of causes of death revealed that 57 of 5,483 adoptees in Copenhagen eventually committed suicide. They were matched with adopted controls. Searches of the causes of death revealed that 12 of the 269 biological relatives of these 57 adopted suicide victims had themselves committed suicide, compared with only 2 of the 269 biological relatives of the 57 adopted controls. This is a highly significant difference for suicide between the two groups of relatives. *None of the adopting relatives of either the suicide or control group had committed suicide.*

In a further study of 71 adoptees with mood disorder, adoptee suicide victims with a situational crisis, impulsive suicide attempt, or both particularly had more biological relatives who had committed suicide than controls. This led to the suggestion that a genetic factor lowering the threshold for suicidal behavior may lead to an inability to control impulsive behavior. Psychiatric disorder or environmental stress may serve as potentiating mechanisms which foster or trigger the impulsive behavior, directing it toward a suicidal outcome.

Answers 34.9–34.11

34.9 The answer is A

34.10 The answer is C

34.11 The answer is B
The first major contribution to the study of the social and cultural influences on suicide was made at the end of the 19th century by the French sociologist *Emile Durkheim*. In an attempt to explain statistical patterns, Durkheim *divided suicides into three social categories: egoistic, altruistic, and anomic.* Egoistic suicide applies to those who are not strongly integrated into any social group. The lack of family integration can be used to explain why the unmarried are more vulnerable to suicide than are the married and why couples with children are the best-protected group of all. Rural communities have more social integration than do urban areas and thus less suicide. Protestantism is a less cohesive religion than Catholicism is, and so Protestants have a higher suicide rate than do Catholics. Altruistic suicide applies to those whose proneness to suicide stems from their excessive integration into a group, with suicide being the outgrowth of that integration—for example, the Japanese soldier who sacrifices his life in battle. Anomic suicide applies to persons whose integration into society is disturbed, depriving them of the customary norms of behavior. Anomie can explain why those whose economic situation has changed drastically are more vulnerable than they were before their change in fortune. Anomie also refers to social instability, with a breakdown of society's standards and values.

The first important psychological insight into suicide came from *Sigmund Freud.* In his paper "Mourning and Melancholia," Freud *wrote that suicide represents aggression turned inward* against an introjected, ambivalently cathected love object. Freud doubted that there would be a suicide without the repressed desire to kill someone else.

Building on Freud's concepts, *Karl Menninger* in *Man Against Himself* conceived of suicide as a retroflexed murder, inverted homicide as a result of the patient's anger toward another person, which is either turned inward or used as an excuse for punishment. He also described a self-directed death instinct (Freud's concept of Thanatos). He *described three components of hostility in suicide: the wish to kill, the wish to be killed, and the wish to die.*

Answers 34.12–34.17

34.12 The answer is C

34.13 The answer is D

34.14 The answer is C

34.15 The answer is E

34.16 The answer is A

34.17 The answer is B

Substance abuse is one of the many reasons for visits to the psychiatric emergency room. Patients who take overdoses of *opioids* (for example, heroin) tend *to be pale and cyanotic* (a dark bluish or purplish coloration of the skin and mucous membranes), with *pinpoint pupils* and absent reflexes. After blood is drawn for a study of drug levels, those patients should be given intravenous naloxone hydrochloride (Narcan), a narcotic antagonist that reverses the opiate effects, *including respiratory depression*, within 2 minutes of the injection.

The use of *barbiturates* and anxiolytics is widespread, and withdrawal from sedative-hypnotic drugs is a common reason for psychiatric emergencies. The first symptom of withdrawal can start as soon as 8 hours after the last pill has been taken and may consist of anxiety, confusion, and ataxia. *As withdrawal progresses the patient may have seizures;* occasionally, a psychotic state erupts, with hallucinations, panic, and disorientation. Barbiturates are cross-tolerant with all antianxiety agents, such as diazepam (Valium). In the treatment of sedative, hypnotic, or anxiolytic withdrawal, one must take into account the usual daily substance intake.

Phencyclidine (PCP or angel dust) is a common cause of psychotic drug–related hospital admissions. The presence of dissociative phenomena, nystagmus (ocular ataxia), muscular rigidity, and elevated blood pressure in a patient who is agitated, psychotic, or comatose strongly suggests PCP intoxication. In the treatment of PCP overdose, the patient should have gastric lavage to recover the drug, diazepam to reduce anxiety, an acidifying diuretic program consisting of ammonium chloride and furosemide (Lasix), which will enhance PCP excretion, and the treatment of hypertension with *propranolol (Inderal).* Acidification is not recommended with hepatic or renal failure or when barbiturate use is suspected. *Phenothiazines are contraindicated,* because muscle rigidity and seizures, side effects of PCP, can be exacerbated by phenothiazines, as can the anticholinergic effects of PCP.

Monoamine oxidase inhibitors (MAOIs) are useful in treating depression, but a hypertensive crisis can occur if patients have eaten food with a high tyramine content while on their medication.

Hypertensive crisis is characterized by severe occipital headaches, nausea, vomiting, sweating, photophobia, and dilated pupils. When a hypertensive crisis occurs, the MAOI should be discontinued, and therapy should be instituted to reduce blood pressure. Chlorpromazine (Thorazine) and phentolamine (Regitine) have both been found useful in those hypertensive crises. MAOIs have *a toxic interaction with meperidine hydrochloride (Demerol)*, which can be fatal. When patients combine the two drugs, they become agitated, disoriented, cyanotic, hyperthermic, hypertensive, and tachycardic.

Acetaminophen (Tylenol) is an analgesic and antipyretic. Overdose with acetaminophen is characterized *by fever, pancytopenia, hypoglycemic coma, renal failure,* and liver damage. Treatment should begin with the induction of emesis or gastric lavage, followed by the administration of activated charcoal. Early treatment is critical to protect against hepatotoxicity.

34.18 The answer is E (all)

The treatment of the depressed, suicidal 25-year-old female graduate student described could include *hospitalization or outpatient treatment, antidepressants, or electroconvulsive therapy* (ECT). Whether to hospitalize the patient with suicidal ideation is a crucial clinical decision. Not all such patients require hospitalization; some may be treated as outpatients. Indications for hospitalization include the lack of a strong social support system, a history of impulsive behavior, and a suicidal plan of action. Most psychiatrists believe that the young woman described should be hospitalized because she had made a suicide attempt and so was clearly at increased risk. Other psychiatrists believe that they could treat the patient on an outpatient basis provided certain conditions were met, such as (1) reducing the patient's psychological pain by modifying her stressful environment through the aid of a friend, a relative, or her employer; (2) building realistic support by recognizing that the patient may have legitimate complaints and offering alternatives to suicide; (3) securing commitment on the part of the patient to agree to call when she reached a point beyond which she was uncertain of controlling further suicidal impulses; and (4) assuring commitment on the part of the psychiatrist to be available to the patient 24 hours a day until the risk has passed. Because it is difficult to meet many of those conditions, hospitalization is often the safest route.

Many depressed suicidal patients require treatment with antidepressants or ECT. The young woman described had a recent sustained and severely depressed mood that was associated with insomnia, trouble in concentrating, weight loss, and a suicide attempt. Those factors indicate a major depressive episode. There was also evidence of long-standing mild depressive symptoms (pessimism, feelings of inadequacy, and low energy level) that although insufficient to meet the diagnostic criteria for a major depressive episode, do meet the criteria for dysthymic disorder. With those clinical features, the indication for the use of antidepressants is clear; ECT may be necessary if the patient was unresponsive to antidepressants or so severely depressed and suicidal that she required faster-acting treatment than is possible with antidepressants. ECT is a safe and effective procedure that is often misunderstood and even attacked by antipsychiatry forces in society.

34.19 The answer is E

Suicide rates *among Catholics are lower than the rates among Protestants and Jews.* A religion's degree of orthodoxy and integration may be a more accurate measure of risk for suicide than is religious affiliation.

Suicide rates *are not equal among men and women*. Men commit suicide more than three times as often as do women. Women, however, are four times as likely to attempt suicide as are men. The higher rate of completed suicide for men is related to the methods they use. Men use firearms, hanging, or jumping from high places. Women are likely to take an overdose of psychoactive substances or a poison, but they are beginning to use firearms more than previously. The use of guns has decreased as a method of suicide in states with gun control laws.

Suicide rates *increase (not decrease) with age*. The significance of the midlife crisis is underscored by suicide rates. Rates of 40 suicides per 100,000 population are found in men aged 65 and older. The elderly attempt suicide less often than do younger people but are successful more often. The elderly account for 25 percent of suicides, although they make up only 10 percent of the total population. The rate for those 75 or older is more than three times the rate among the young.

Suicide rates *are higher among whites than among blacks*. In 1989 the suicide rate for white males (19.6 per 100,000 persons) was 1.6 times that for black males (12.5), four times that for white females (4.8), and 8.2 times that for black females (2.4). Among ghetto youth and certain Native American and Alaskan Indian groups, suicide rates have greatly exceeded the national rate. Suicide among immigrants is higher than in the native-born population. Two of every three suicides are white males. Contrary to popular belief, suicide rates *do not increase during December and other holiday periods*.

34.20 The answer is C

A serotonin deficiency, as measured by *decreased (not increased) 5-hydroindoleacetic acid (5-HIAA) levels in the cerebrospinal fluid* (CSF), has been found in some patients who attempted suicide. In addition, some postmortem studies have reported *changes in the noradrenergic system (not dopaminergic system). Decreased (not increased) levels of platelet monoamine oxidase (MAO)* have been discovered in some suicidal patients. When blood samples from normal volunteers were analyzed, it was found that those with the lowest level of MAO in their platelets had eight times the prevalence of suicide in their families. *Abnormal findings on electroencephalograms (EEGs) (not normal findings)* and ventricular enlargement have been found in a few studies of suicidal patients.

34.21 The answer is E

Among women suicide peaks after age 55. Rates of 40 per 100,000 population are found in men age 65 and older; the elderly attempt suicide less often than do younger people but are successful more frequently. A decline in suicide in men begins between the ages of 75 and 85. A peak risk among males is also found in late adolescence, when death by suicide is exceeded only by death attributed to accidents and cancer.

34.22 The answer is D

Figure 34.1 represents *death rates for suicide* in the United States according to race and sex. The rate of suicide among whites is nearly twice that among nonwhites, but the figures are being questioned, as the suicide rate among blacks is increasing. In 1989, the suicide rate for white males was 1.6 times that of black males, four times that for white females, and 8.2 times that for black females. Two out of every three suicides are white males. Women are four times as likely to attempt suicide as are men, while overall, men commit suicide more than three times as often as do women.

Schizophrenia is equally prevalent in men and women. *Bipolar I disorder* also has a prevalence that is equal for men and women. The ratio of *alcohol-related disorder* diagnoses for men to women is about 2 to 1 or 3 to 1. Although the rate of alcohol-related disorders has traditionally been highest among young white men, evidence now indicates that young black men and young Hispanic men may have surpassed young white men in their rates of alcohol-related disorders.

34.23 The answer is E (all)

When a patient has exhibited violent behavior in the past or threatens violence, a decision must be made about the risk of violent behavior in the future. Decisions must be made about whether to hospitalize a potentially violent patient, when to discharge a previously violent patient, and whether to warn a potential victim. As with the evaluation of suicide potential, evaluation of violence potential includes assessment of how well planned the threat or violent ideation is. Vague threats of killing someone are not as serious as well-formulated threats against a specific person. As with suicide, the availability of means of inflicting injury is important. If the patient has recently purchased or owns a gun, the clinician should take the threat more seriously.

A history of violence or other impulsive behavior often predicts future violence. The clinician should assess the degree of past injuries, the person toward whom violence was directed, and the circumstances. Often there is a repetitive pattern of violent behavior and escalation. Alcohol and drug abuse should be assessed. Central nervous system disorders have been associated with violent behavior, as have some systemic disorders affecting the central nervous system. As with suicide, the clinician should take seriously threats of violence by a psychotic person and assess the potential for violence. Compliance with treatment, for example, in a paranoid schizophrenia patient receiving depot antipsychotic agents or an alcoholic patient receiving disulfiram (Antabuse), is reassuring. All of those factors are weighted in the final assessment of whether the patient poses enough risk to others to require some action.

Answers 34.24–34.27

34.24 The answer is A

34.25 The answer is C

34.26 The answer is B

34.27 The answer is D

Delirium, mania, depression, and psychosis are manifestations of bromide intoxication. If a patient's serum levels are above 50 mg a day, bromide intake should be discontinued; if the patient is agitated, lorazepam (Ativan) may be given for sedation. For severe agitation or psychotic syndromes an antipsychotic dopamine receptor antagonist may be necessary.

Alcohol stigmata, amnesia, and *confabulation* are manifestations of Korsakoff's syndrome. Because this disorder has no effective treatment, the patient must often be institutionalized in a protective environment.

Marked aggression and assaultive behavior are manifestations of idiosyncratic alcohol intoxication. Generally no treatment other than a protective environment is required.

Mental confusion, oculomotor disturbances, and *cerebellar ataxia* are manifestations of Wernicke's encephalopathy.

35

Psychotherapies

Psychiatry attempts to address and understand human behavior and emotion. Part of this involves formulating theories about the etiology of disturbances in behavior and emotion. As would be expected in a field that deals with such a complex and at times mysterious subject, there are many different etiologic theories, some contradictory, some intersecting. This is why the revised fourth edition of the *Diagnostic and Statistical Manual of Mental Disorders* (DSM-IV-TR) is largely atheoretical in terms of etiology: obviously not because there are no theories to explain the causes of mental disorders, but because not everyone in the field agrees on a central, organizing theoretical framework. The most sophisticated theories recognize that human behavior and emotion cannot be reduced to a simple biological versus psychological equation, and that a true understanding of human functioning begins with the acceptance of a biopsychosocial etiologic model.

The variety of available psychotherapies reflects the multi-etiologic theoretical basis of psychiatry. Skilled clinicians are aware of all available therapies, but some may choose to focus their treatment of patients on just one. Others will utilize aspects of different therapies, depending on the problem or the patient. Many clinicians combine the use of psychotherapy with the prescription of medication. Students need to be aware of the theories that underlie the different psychotherapies, as well as the proposed indications for each. The most prominent therapies with which students should be familiar include psychoanalytic, cognitive, behavioral, family, and group.

The psychoanalytic therapies are based on freudian principles of a dynamic unconscious and psychic determinism. Many modifications have been made in the practice of modern psychoanalytic therapies since Freud's time, but all remain insight-oriented. Psychoanalysis differs from psychoanalytic psychotherapy and brief dynamic psychotherapies in such parameters as the frequency of treatments (up to five sessions a week in psychoanalysis), whether the patient sits up or lies on the couch (the couch in psychoanalysis), and the scope of the issues addressed (deep and open-ended in psychoanalysis). Brief dynamic psychotherapies focus on one specific, delineated problem and are time-limited in their course.

Cognitive therapies (or cognitive-behavioral therapies) are short-term structured treatments aimed at correcting irrational and illogical thinking, which can lead to dysfunctional attitudes and behavior. The therapies involve an active collaboration between therapist and patient, as well as numerous homework assignments. These therapies have been shown to be helpful in the treatment of certain depressive disorders, as well as others such as obsessive-compulsive and panic disorders.

Behavioral therapies focus on overt, observable behaviors and are unconcerned with underlying causes. These therapies are based on learning theory, which posits that learned behavior is reinforced and conditioned in a variety of ways. The therapies are based on the belief that learned behavior can be unlearned through techniques of deconditioning and changing reinforcements, such as systematic desensitization, flooding, positive or negative reinforcement, and extinction. The indications for this type of therapy tend to be very specific, delineated problems, such as phobias and compulsions.

Family therapies are based on general systems theory and focus on the patterns of family communication and interaction. Family therapists focus on the family as a homeostatic operating system and attempt to understand how the individual family members maintain this system, even at the cost of dysfunction.

Group therapies run the theoretical gamut and may be supportive, psychoanalytic, cognitive, or behavioral in their orientation. Twelve-step support groups have been shown to be effective in the treatment and management of substance-abuse disorders.

There are many other available therapies, from dialectical-behavioral therapy, to biofeedback, to hypnosis, to interpersonal therapy. Students should be knowledgeable about all of these different treatments, their indications, theoretical underpinnings, strengths, and weaknesses.

The student should study the questions and answers below to test his or her knowledge of the subject.

HELPFUL HINTS

The names of the workers, their theories, and the therapy techniques should be known to the student.

- ▶ AA, GA, OA
- ▶ abreaction
- ▶ analyst incognito
- ▶ Anna O.
- ▶ assertiveness
- ▶ authority anxiety
- ▶ autogenic therapy
- ▶ aversive therapy
- ▶ Michael Balint
- ▶ Aaron Beck
- ▶ behavioral medicine
- ▶ bell and pad

- Hippolyte Bernheim
- Murray Bowen
- cognitive rehearsal
- cognitive triad of depression
- cohesion
- combined individual and group psychotherapy
- confidentiality
- countertransference
- crisis intervention
- crisis theory
- day's residue
- disorders of self-control
- disulfiram (Antabuse) therapy
- double and multiple double
- dyad
- early therapy
- ego psychology
- eye-roll sign
- H. J. Eysenck
- family group therapy

- family sculpting
- family systems
- family therapy
- flexible schemata
- flooding
- galvanic skin response
- genogram
- Gestalt group therapy
- graded exposure
- group psychotherapy
- guided imagery
- hierarchy construction
- homogeneous versus heterogeneous groups
- hypnosis
- hypnotic capacity and induction
- hysteria
- identified patient
- implosion
- insight-oriented psychotherapy
- intellectualization, interpretation
- interpersonal psychotherapy

- Jacobson's exercise
- Daniel Malan
- mental imagery
- mirror technique
- Jacob Moreno
- operant conditioning
- parapraxes
- participant modeling
- patient–therapist encounter
- peer anxiety
- positive reinforcement
- psychodrama
- psychodynamic model
- psychotherapeutic focus
- psychotherapy
- reality testing
- reciprocal inhibition
- relaxation response
- resistance
- reward of desired behavior
- Carl Rogers
- role reversal
- rule of abstinence

- schemata
- Paul Schilder
- self-analysis
- self-help groups
- self-observation
- Peter Sifneos
- B. F. Skinner
- splitting
- structural model
- structural theory
- *Studies on Hysteria*
- supportive therapy
- systematic desensitization
- tabula rasa
- testing automatic thoughts
- token economy
- transactional group therapy
- transference, transference neurosis, negative triangulation
- universalization
- ventilation and catharsis

▲ QUESTIONS

DIRECTIONS: Each of the questions or incomplete statements below is followed by five suggested responses or completions. Select the *one* that is *best* in each case.

35.1 Intersubjectivity

- A. is a form of short-term psychodynamic therapy
- B. implies two psychologies in mutual interaction with one another
- C. describes the concept that the analyst is a "blank screen"
- D. refers to the idea that psychoanalysis is a one-person psychology
- E. none of the above

35.2 Contraindications to psychoanalytic treatment include

- A. elderly patients
- B. personality disorders
- C. history of unsuccessful previous treatments
- D. history of sexual abuse or assault
- E. none of the above

35.3 Contemporary views of transference include the idea that it

- A. occurs only in psychoanalytic treatment
- B. is considered solely a reenactment of a past relationship with a significant childhood figure
- C. does not involve the therapist as an active participant in the therapeutic relationship
- D. is shaped by the therapist's real personal characteristics
- E. none of the above

35.4 All of the following are considered to be possible flexible boundary issues in psychotherapy *except*

- A. self-disclosure by the therapist
- B. physical contact between therapist and patient
- C. sexual contact between therapist and patient
- D. gift-giving and receiving
- E. extra-analytic contacts

35.5 True statements about the efficacy of psychotherapy include

  A. Abundant evidence indicates that psychotherapy is effective.

  B. Psychodynamic psychotherapy, overall, is equivalent in efficacy to cognitive-behavior therapy, behavior therapy, and other standardized modalities.

  C. Psychodynamic therapy is equally effective in the treatment of depressed patients as cognitive-behavior therapy.

  D. There is increasing evidence that considerable cost savings occur when regular therapy is provided over an extended period of time.

  E. All of the above

35.6 Concepts associated with dialectical behavior therapy include

  A. validation

  B. therapy-interfering behaviors

  C. consequences implemented by the therapist in response to impulsive behaviors

  D. withdrawal of attention as a time-out from positive reinforcement of parasuicidal behavior

  E. all of the above

35.7 Interpersonal psychotherapy has been shown in efficacy trials to be indicated for

  A. delusional depression

  B. opioid dependence

  C. cocaine abuse

  D. anxiety disorders

  E. none of the above

35.8 Psychotherapy research has shown a consistent relationship between research outcome and

  A. age

  B. gender

  C. education

  D. race

  E. none of the above

DIRECTIONS: The questions below consist of five lettered headings followed by a list of numbered statements. For each numbered statement, select the *one* lettered heading that is most closely associated with it. Each lettered heading may be selected once, more than once, or not at all.

Questions 35.9–35.13

  A. Arbitrary inference

  B. Overgeneralization

  C. Personalization

  D. Selective abstraction

  E. Dichotomous thinking

35.9 Drawing a general conclusion across all situations on the basis of a single incident

35.10 Occurs when a patient tends to make interpretations on an either-or, black-or-white basis

35.11 Focusing on a detail taken out of context, ignoring other more salient features of the situation, and conceptualizing the whole experience on the basis of this extraneous element

35.12 Process of drawing a conclusion in the absence of evidence supporting it or even in the face of evidence to the contrary

35.13 Tendency to relate external events to oneself when there is no basis for making such a connection

DIRECTIONS: The lettered headings below are followed by a list of numbered statements. For each numbered statement, select

  A. if the item is associated with *A only*

  B. if the item is associated with *B only*

  C. if the item is associated with *both A and B*

  D. if the item is associated with *neither A nor B*

Questions 35.14–35.17

  A. Behavioral techniques

  B. Cognitive techniques

  C. Both

  D. Neither

35.14 Track automatic thoughts

35.15 Testing dysfunctional beliefs

35.16 Graded task assignment

35.17 Identifying imperatives—"shoulds"

DIRECTIONS: Each of the questions or incomplete statements below is followed by five suggested responses or completions. Select the *one* that is *best* in each case.

35.18 A patient with a fear of heights is brought to the top of a tall building and is required to remain there until the anxiety dissipates. That is an example of

  A. graded exposure

  B. participant modeling

  C. aversion therapy

  D. flooding

  E. systematic desensitization

35.19 Which of the following conditions is *not* amenable to hypnosis?

  A. Paranoia

  B. Pruritus

  C. Alcohol dependence

  D. Obesity

  E. Asthma

35.20 Which of the following methods is *not* used in biofeedback?

  A. Electromyography

  B. Electroencephalography

  C. Galvanic skin response

  D. Strain gauge

  E. All of the above

35.21 The cognitive therapy approach includes

    A. eliciting automatic thoughts
    B. testing automatic thoughts
    C. identifying maladaptive underlying assumptions
    D. testing the validity of maladaptive assumptions
    E. all of the above

35.22 The therapeutic factors in group therapy include

    A. multiple transferences
    B. collective transference
    C. universalization
    D. cohesion
    E. all of the above

35.23 Systematic desensitization is applicable in the treatment of

    A. obsessive-compulsive disorder
    B. sexual disorders
    C. stuttering
    D. bronchial asthma
    E. all of the above

35.24 Which of the following is *not* a psychotherapeutic intervention?

    A. Affirmation
    B. Verification
    C. Clarification
    D. Confrontation
    E. Interpretation

35.25 Patients with poor frustration tolerance and poor reality testing are best treated with

    A. supportive psychotherapy
    B. insight-oriented psychotherapy
    C. expressive therapy
    D. intensive psychoanalytic psychotherapy
    E. all of the above

ANSWERS

Psychotherapies

35.1 The answer is B

A major theoretical trend in recent years that has profoundly affected psychoanalytic technique is the growing recognition that psychoanalysis is both a two-person psychology and a *one-person psychology*. The image of the *analyst as a detached "blank screen"* figure dispassionately observing the patient is regarded largely as a mythical construct that is misleading in terms of the realities of psychoanalytic work. In fact, the analyst's own subjectivity has a continuing influence on the patient, just as the patient's subjectivity influences the analyst's perceptions in an ongoing way. This recognition of *two psychologies in mutual interaction with one another* is often subsumed under the term *intersubjectivity,* which is not per se a form of *short-term psychodynamic therapy.*

35.2 The answer is E (none)

Adult developmental studies indicate that significant changes in defenses, internal object relations, and self-representations occur throughout the adult life cycle. *Analysts now treat older and even elderly patients—in their 50s, 60s, 70s, and beyond.*

Conditions considered amenable to analysis today include, in addition to the symptomatic neuroses, certain anxiety disorders; highly perfectionistic depressed individuals; some sexual disorders; *certain personality disorders*, including obsessive-compulsive, histrionic, avoidant, and narcissistic; selected patients at the upper end of the spectrum of borderline personality disorder; and many cases of mixed personality disorder. In addition, many patients who do not fit the revised fourth edition of *Diagnostic and Statistical Manual of Mental Disorder* (DSM-IV-TR) categories may experience significant distress and frequently seek psychoanalytic treatment. Common problems that bring such individuals to analysis include difficulties with intimacy, relatedness, and commitment; lack of assertiveness; avoidant tendencies; self-defeating behavior; problems with authority; shyness; unresolved grief; or problems related to separation or rejection.

One broadly based indication for psychoanalysis *is a history of unsuccessful previous treatments.* A survey of 580 analytic patients found that 82 percent of the patients currently in psychoanalysis had undergone other forms of psychotherapy in the past. The mean age at the beginning of the analysis of the sample was 36.2 years, and 59 percent of the patients were female. Of the 580 patients, 71.4 percent had at least one personality disorder diagnosis. Of the Axis I diagnoses, a mood disorder was the most common, and anxiety disorder was second. A significant number of the patients, 27 percent of the total, had been *sexually abused or assaulted.* High levels of sexual dysfunction, 43.4 percent of the total, were also found in the group.

35.3 The answer is D

Transference refers to the displacement onto the analyst of attitudes and feelings experienced originally in relationships with people from the past. Transference patterns appear automatically and unconsciously in the analytic relationship. Analysands suddenly find themselves reacting to the analyst with intense feelings that are inappropriate, at least in part, to the current situation. Patients unconsciously reenact a past relationship instead of remembering and verbalizing it. Transference is *not unique to the analytic setting.* Every significant relationship in adult life is a new addition of the original attachments of childhood. The chief difference between transference in the analytic relationship and transference as it occurs in outside relationships is that transference is analyzed in the analytic setting.

In the contemporary view, transference is regarded as *a mixture of the new relationship with the analyst and a reenactment of a past relationship with a significant childhood figure. The analyst is regarded as an active participant* in the therapeutic relationship. In the current conceptual framework, *the analyst's personal characteristics exert a powerful influence* on the specific shape and intensity of the patient's transference. The notion of opacity is considered a myth by contemporary analysts, and the analyst's real characteristics must be taken into account when the analyst formulates therapeutic interventions.

35.4 The answer is C

Analytic boundaries must build in flexibility. They provide an envelope that creates an optimal environment for the emergence of the analytic process. They must be flexible because different patients require adjustments in the boundaries. Similarly, different patient–analyst dyads find their own optimal conditions under which analysis can be conducted. The relative degree of gratification versus frustration varies given the subjectivities of the two parties. Some patients may benefit from direct *self-disclosure* of the analyst's feelings about a specific situation, while others may deeply resent it and close down as a result. Nevertheless, a variety of boundary considerations serve as guidelines to assist the analyst in maintaining a professional rather than a personal relationship.

Lavish or expensive *gifts from analyst to patient or from patient to analyst* may also violate a professional boundary. Such gifts may serve as an unconscious bribe designed to suppress anger in either party. Small and inexpensive gifts may be accepted by the analyst when the analyst feels that the acceptance might enhance the process. Even when such gifts are accepted, however, the meaning of the gift to the patient may be analyzed as an important part of the work.

As noted previously, self-disclosure is a significant boundary issue that analysts must attend to in their decisions about interventions. Analysis is by nature asymmetrical. Although two subjectivities are in the room and strong feelings are stirred in both parties, the process is designed to focus primarily on the person who is paying for the service. Self-disclosure by the analyst is inevitable, of course, and the analyst is always making decisions about how useful it would be to disclose certain aspects of the analyst's subjectivity to the patient. It may be extraordinarily useful in some cases to talk about areas of common interest with the patient in the service of building a therapeutic alliance. However, self-disclosure of one's personal problems may unduly burden the patient. Analysts who talk about their own problems misuse the patient's time and money. In some cases, the disclosure of here-and-now countertransference feelings may advance the process in a constructive way. However, telling patients, "I have sexual feelings for you" shuts down the process and makes patients feel that they must be the ones to set the boundaries in the relationship. Similarly, disclosing that one hates a patient or is bored by a patient is not useful.

Sexual contact of any form between analyst and patient is unacceptable. This constitutes a firm, inflexible boundary. In the transference the analyst becomes a parent to the patient so that any form of sexual relations is symbolically incestuous. Moreover, because of the transference and the power differen-

tial, the patient cannot provide informed consent to such a relationship, even if the patient is an adult and consciously attracted to the analyst. This absolute abstinence regarding sexual contact facilitates frank and detailed discussion of the patient's sexual desires in a safe environment.

Physical contact such as hugs or pats on the back may also be problematic. In general, a handshake is probably the ordinary limit of physical contact between analyst and analysand. An occasional hug in the midst of a personal tragedy, such as the loss of a child, spouse, or parent, might be appropriate if initiated by the patient. However, when the analyst initiates a hug, the patient may readily misconstrue the analyst's motives. Another basic guideline regarding touch is that the impact of such behavior on the patient may be dramatically different from the analyst's intent. Patients may ask for hugs or even demand them, but psychoanalysis is about the wish to be held or hugged rather than the concrete enactment of such wishes. The patient must be engaged in a mourning process to deal with the grief and resentment about the deprivations of childhood, the frustrations in the present, and the insistence of the analyst that the relationship remain an analytic one. When actual physical contact occurs, especially on a regular basis, the distinction between the symbolic and the concrete is lost, and the patient may feel that powerful childhood longings will finally be satisfied by the person of the analyst. This situation will likely evoke false hopes in the patient that can never be gratified. Table 35.1 lists some of the dimensions of analytic boundaries and boundary violations.

35.5 The answer is E (all)

Abundant evidence indicates that psychotherapy is effective. At the end of psychotherapy, the average treated patient is better off than 80 percent of untreated patients. Moreover, the magnitude of the effect of psychotherapy is equivalent to a level that justifies the interruption of clinical trials on the grounds that it would be unethical to withhold such a valuable treatment from patients.

When the efficacy of psychodynamic therapies is compared with that of other forms of psychotherapy, the results

Table 35.1
Analytic Boundaries and Boundary Violations

Dimensions of analytic boundaries	Professional role, time, place and space, money, gifts, business transactions, clothing, language, confidentiality, excessive self-disclosure of personal problems, physical contact, sexual relations
Boundary violations	Egregious enactments that are often repetitive, not subject to analytic scrutiny, pervasive, and harmful to the patient while also destroying the viability of the analysis
Boundary crossings	Benign, and even helpful, countertransference enactments that are attenuated, occur in isolation, are subject to analytic scrutiny, and extend the analytic work in a positive direction

Data from T. Gutheil, M.D., G. Gabbard, M.D., and J. Lester, M.D.

are generally comparable. In other words, *overall, psychodynamic psychotherapy is equivalent in efficacy* to cognitive-behavior therapy, behavior therapy, and other standardized modalities. *Dynamic therapy of depressed patients* has been tested in direct comparisons with *cognitive-behavior therapy* and has been found *equally effective.* Expressive-supportive therapy of opiate-dependent methadone-maintenance patients has been compared with standard drug counseling. At 6-month follow-up, patients who received the expressive-supportive therapy were doing better on all outcome measures than those with standard drug counseling. Specifically, the psychotherapy patients maintained gains that had been established during the therapy, while those who had standard drug counseling had lost many of those gains.

In an Australian study of 30 patients with borderline personality disorder, the 12-month period prior to psychotherapy was compared with the 12-month period after the patients received psychotherapy. The psychotherapy itself consisted of twice-weekly psychodynamic treatment for 12 months. There was marked clinical improvement following the psychotherapy period. Medical visits dropped from 3.5 visits per patient per month to 0.5 visits. Incidents of self-harm fell from 3.8 episodes per year to 0.8 episodes. Hospital admissions fell from 1.8 per year to 0.7, while months spent as an inpatient dropped from 2.9 to 1.5 months.

While psychoanalytic psychotherapy is often thought to be prohibitively expensive, this study of patients with borderline personality disorder suggests that in many cases providing such treatment is notably cost-effective. Borderline patients tend to use up a great many health care dollars in visits to emergency rooms, visits to other medical specialists, psychiatric hospitalizations, and various diagnostic workups. There is considerable *cost saving in providing regular therapy over an extended period* of time. Almost all of the outcome measures included a reduction in total expense as well.

35.6 The answer is E (all)

A systematic behavioral analysis of borderline personality disorder began as an analysis of suicidal behaviors and evolved into a treatment called dialectical behavior therapy. The term dialectic was chosen to reflect the approach of finding a third way (synthesis) to resolve opposing contingencies affecting these patients. Problems in the development of a sense of self can arise when other persons assume control over children's labeling of their private events. This reasoning has led to the inclusion of the important therapeutic *principle of validation* into dialectical behavior therapy and other recently developed treatments.

Besides the basic problem with invalidation, patients may have been raised in either chaotic, abusive families or in families that had low tolerance for emotional, expressive behaviors. Expecting more or different behaviors than a child can emit, the parent resorts to coercive control. This leads to problems inherent in such control, including diminished exploratory behaviors, restricted problem-solving abilities, and skills deficits. In addition, unavoidable punishment leads to learned helplessness, anxiety depression, and post-traumatic stress symptoms.

Behavioral deficits in regulating emotional behaviors, tolerating distress, interacting with others, and problem solving reduce access to positive reinforcers. This contributes to a lean reinforcement environment that increases dependency on the few reinforcers available to the patient. Consequently, the patient may be unable to leave current chaotic or abusive relationships.

A history of physical abuse establishes rewarding consequences for avoidance and escape behaviors. Self-mutilatory behaviors may function as escape behaviors. For example, physical abuse administered on a noncontingent time schedule (e.g., whenever the parent is drunk) may establish "passage of time without punishment" as a conditional aversive establishing stimulus. In such a schedule, the lowest probability of punishment occurs immediately after an abusive episode. In adult life, the patient may functionally "reset" the clock with an episode of self-mutilatory behavior, thus shortening the agony of "waiting for the other shoe to drop."

Parasuicidal behaviors, unsafe sexual behaviors, and aggressive behaviors are impulsive behaviors. Such behaviors are maintained by certain immediate reinforcers and are insufficiently affected by undesirable but delayed consequences. In addition, the patient may respond to idiosyncratic, verbally constructed future realities that serve as reinforcers for avoidance or escape behaviors.

Consequences implemented by the therapist become an important countermeasure. *Withdrawal of attention can serve as a time-out* from positive reinforcement. This can be applied contingent on a parasuicidal behavior; such withdrawal also is a useful strategy to counteract the therapist's natural tendency to increase attention for (and thus reinforcing) such behaviors. On the other hand, positive reinforcement is needed to retain the patient in treatment. Validation by the therapist is an important positive reinforcer.

Dialectic behavior therapy begins with efforts to address current problems, and among these, the first efforts are focused on behaviors that interfere directly with further treatment. Such *therapy-interfering behaviors* include suicidal behaviors, substance abuse, high-risk sexual behaviors, criminal behaviors, dysfunctional relationship behaviors, vocational behaviors, and housing-related behaviors (e.g., living in shelters).

35.7 The answer is E (none)

Interpersonal psychotherapy, a time-limited treatment for major depressive disorder, was developed in the 1970s, defined in a manual, and tested in randomized clinical trials by the late Gerald L. Klerman and collaborators.

Interpersonal psychotherapy was formulated initially as a time-limited, weekly, outpatient treatment for depressed patients. Based on the ideas of Harry Stack Sullivan and the interpersonal school, interpersonal psychotherapy makes no etiological assumptions but uses the connection between onset of depressive symptoms and current interpersonal problems as a treatment focus. Interpersonal psychotherapy generally deals with current rather than past interpersonal relationships, focusing on the patient's immediate social context. It attempts to intervene in symptom formation and social dysfunction associated with depression rather than addressing enduring aspects of personality, which are difficult to assess during an episode of an Axis I disorder.

Indications for interpersonal psychotherapy have been defined by efficacy trials. Interpersonal psychotherapy has been one of the most carefully studied psychotherapies for mood disorders and the only psychotherapy tested in a maintenance treatment study. Its efficacy has been established for various subtypes of nonpsychotic depressive disorders and for bulimia nervosa.

Interpersonal psychotherapy showed no benefit in two studies of patients with substance abuse. It has not yet been definitively tested for other psychiatric disorders, such as *anxiety disorders* and borderline personality disorder, although studies are planned or under way.

Interpersonal psychotherapy is not intended to be a treatment for *delusional depression.* It showed no benefit in two studies of patients with *opioid dependence and cocaine abuse.*

35.8 The answer is E (none)

Despite numerous studies, *research has not shown a consistent relationship between treatment outcome and patient age, gender,* or sociodemographic variables. A meta-analysis of over 500 studies found no correlation between age and psychotherapy outcome, and patient gender has also been shown to be unrelated to treatment effectiveness. As noted, other sociodemographic variables, such as *education and race,* are related to the probability both of seeking and obtaining psychotherapy, but there is no clear relationship between socioeconomic status and treatment outcome.

Answers 35.9–35.13

35.9 The answer is B

35.10 The answer is E

35.11 The answer is D

35.12 The answer is A

35.13 The answer is C

Logical errors in thinking, which are addressed in cognitive-behavioral therapy, include: *Arbitrary inference,* i.e., the process of drawing a conclusion in the absence of evidence supporting it or even in the face of evidence to the contrary; *selective abstraction,* which refers to focusing on a detail taken out of context, ignoring other more salient features of the situation, and conceptualizing the whole experience on the basis of this element; *overgeneralization,* referring to drawing a general conclusion across all situations on the basis of a single incident; magnification and minimization, representing distorted evaluations of the relative importance of particular events; *personalization,* which describes the tendency to relate external events to oneself when there is no basis for making such a connection; and *dichotomous thinking,* which occurs when the patient makes interpretations on an either-or, black-or-white basis.

Answers 35.14–35.17

35.14 The answer is C

35.15 The answer is C

35.16 The answer is A

35.17 The answer is B

As in other therapies, the therapist–patient relationship is important in cognitive therapy and provides the medium for improve-

ment. Therapists function as guides to enable their patients to acquire the understanding that will help them to cope better with their problems—the process of guided discovery—and also as catalysts to promote the kind of corrective experiences outside of therapy that will enhance the patients' adaptive skills.

The proximal goal is to promote behavioral activation and cognitive restructuring, which involves modification of the patient's systematic bias in interpreting personal life experiences and making future predictions. In sum, cognitive therapy is a learning experience in which the therapist plays an active role in *helping the patient to uncover and modify cognitive distortions and dysfunctional beliefs.*

Behavioral and cognitive techniques are prominently used at the beginning of therapy with profoundly depressed patients who have a limited capacity for the introspection and abstraction needed to *identify and evaluate automatic thoughts* or assumptions.

Initially, therapist and patient agree on scheduling activities that help to mobilize the patient and counteract the inertia often present, especially in depression. Because most patients need to proceed in small steps, *a graded-task assignment* is developed to enable them to have progressively greater success experiences without overextending themselves. Typical behavioral techniques are listed in Table 35.2.

When the patient is already active, more purely cognitive procedures may be used. The patients *track their automatic thoughts,* particularly when they precede or accompany a negative feeling. An automatic thought occurs spontaneously, is very rapid, and represents an immediate interpretation of a situation. A depressed patient, for example, on seeing a close friend, had the automatic thought, "She won't want to talk to me." These patients are asked to fill out the Daily Record of Dysfunctional Thoughts and are trained to give reasonable or rational responses to their negative automatic thoughts.

During the course of cognitive therapy the therapist and patient review the relationship between the automatic thoughts and an objective description of a disturbing event. Logical errors are identified and more realistic interpretations of the event are considered, thereby correcting the automatic thoughts.

Reality testing of automatic thoughts and assumptions is carried out by treating the belief or thought as a hypothesis to be tested; for example, discussion of its validity with the therapist using information already provided by the patient in prior

Table 35.2
Behavioral and Cognitive Techniques

Behavioral Techniques	Cognitive Techniques
Mastery and pleasure ratings	Identifying automatic thoughts
Activity scheduling	Testing and correcting automatic thoughts
Graded task assignment	Reattribution techniques
Behavioral rehearsal	Identifying and testing imperatives—"shoulds"
Role-playing	Cognitive rehearsal through imagery
Testing dysfunctional beliefs	Imaginal recreation of pathogenic events

sessions or through prior homework assignments. Alternatively, the therapist and patient may design a homework assignment ("experiment") to more directly test the notion in question by gathering new evidence.

As therapy progresses, attention is focused on the patient's underlying beliefs, such as "If I'm not successful, then I am a failure" or "If somebody doesn't like me, it means I'm socially undesirable." These beliefs are reevaluated in the same way as automatic thoughts; namely, in terms of the evidence supporting them, the logical basis on which they rest, and empirical testing.

Cognitively oriented techniques are applied as patients become less symptomatic and thereby become more objective about themselves and their thinking. As patients are able to view their thoughts objectively, these thoughts become hypotheses that are amenable to experimental testing and revision using cognitive techniques. They thereby unravel, clarify, and modify the meanings they have assigned to upsetting events. Cognitive techniques, such as identifying automatic thoughts *or imperatives (such as "shoulds")*, recognizing and correcting cognitive distortions, and identifying broad beliefs and assumptions that underlie the dysfunctional thoughts, are used to clarify patients' problems.

35.18 The answer is D
Flooding is a technique in which, for example, a patient with a fear of heights is brought to the top of a tall building and is required to remain there until the anxiety dissipates. Flooding is based on the premise that escaping from an anxiety-provoking experience reinforces the anxiety through conditioning. Thus, if the person is not allowed to escape, anxiety can be extinguished, and the conditioned avoidance behavior can be prevented. In clinical situations, flooding consists of having the patient confront the anxiety-inducing object or situation at full intensity for prolonged periods of time, resulting in the patient's being flooded with anxiety. The confrontation may be done in imagination, but results are better when real-life situations are used.

In *graded exposure,* the patient is exposed over a period of time to objects that cause increasing levels of anxiety. It is similar to flooding except that the phobic object or situation is approached through a series of small steps, rather than all at once. *Participant modeling* is based on imitation, whereby patients learn to confront a fearful situation or object by modeling themselves after the therapist's behavior in response to the situations. *Aversion therapy* involves the presentation of a noxious stimulus immediately after a specific behavioral response, leading to the response's being inhibited and extinguished. The negative stimulus (punishment) is paired with the undesired behavior, which is thereby, theoretically, suppressed. *Systematic desensitization*, like graded exposure, is based on the concept that a person can overcome maladaptive anxiety elicited by a situation or object by approaching the feared situation gradually and in a psychophysiological state that inhibits anxiety. The patient attains a state of complete relaxation and then is exposed to the anxiety-producing stimulus. The negative reaction of anxiety is inhibited by the relaxed state. Systematic desensitization differs from graded exposure in two respects: (1) systematic desensitization uses relaxation training, whereas graded exposure does not, and (2) systematic desensitization uses a graded list or hierarchy of anxiety-provoking scenes that

the patient imagines, as opposed to graded exposure, in which the treatment is carried out in a real-life context.

35.19 The answer is A
Paranoia is not amenable to hypnosis, simply because paranoid patients are suspicious and usually avoid or resist efforts to be hypnotized. Any patient who has difficulty with basic trust or who has problems with giving up control is not a good candidate for hypnosis. However, a variety of conditions have been treated with varying degrees of success with hypnosis, including *pruritus, alcohol dependence, obesity, asthma,* substance-released disorders, smoking, warts, and chronic pain.

35.20 The answer is D
In *electromyography* (EMG), muscle fibers generate electrical potentials that can be measured on an electromyograph. Electrodes placed in or on a specific muscle group—for example, masseter, deltoid, or temporalis—can be monitored for relaxation training. In *electroencephalography* (EEG), the evoked potential of the EEG is monitored to determine relaxation. Alpha waves are generally indicative of meditative states, but wave frequency and amplitude are also measured. In *galvanic skin response* (GSR), skin conductance of electricity is measured as an indicator of autonomic nervous system activity. Stress increases electrical conduction and the GSR; conversely, relaxation is associated with lowered autonomic activity and changes in skin response. Similarly, skin temperature as a measure of peripheral vasoconstriction is decreased under stress and can be measured with thermistors (thermal feedback). A *strain gauge* is a device for measuring nocturnal penile tumescence that is used to determine whether erections occur during sleep. It has no biofeedback applications.

35.21 The answer is E (all)
The cognitive therapy approach includes four processes: (1) *eliciting automatic thoughts,* (2) *testing automatic thoughts,* (3) *identifying maladaptive underlying assumptions,* and (4) *testing the validity of maladaptive assumptions.* Automatic thoughts are cognitions that intervene between external events and the patient's emotional reaction to the event. An example of an automatic thought is the belief that "everyone is going to laugh at me when they see how badly I bowl"—a thought that occurs to someone who has been asked to go bowling and responds negatively. The therapist, acting as a teacher, helps the patient test the validity of automatic thoughts. The goal is to encourage patients to reject inaccurate or exaggerated automatic thoughts after careful examination. Patients often blame themselves for things that go wrong that may well have been outside their control. The therapist reviews with the patient the entire situation and helps to reattribute the blame or cause of the unpleasant events. Generating alternative explanations for events is another way of undermining inaccurate and distorted automatic thoughts.

35.22 The answer is E (all)
Many factors account for therapeutic change in group therapy. *Multiple transferences* are possible because a variety of group members stand for people significant in a patient's past or current life situation. Group members may take the roles of husband, wife, mother, father, siblings, and employer. The patient can then work through actual or fantasized conflicts with the surrogate figures to a successful resolution.

Collective transference is a member's personification of the group as a single transferential figure, generally the mother or the father. It is a phenomenon unique to group therapy. The therapist attempts to encourage the patient to respond to members of the group as individuals and to differentiate them. *Universalization* is the process by which patients recognize that they are not alone in having an emotional problem. It is one of the most important processes in group therapy. *Cohesion* is a sense of "we-ness," a sense of belonging. The members value the group, which engenders loyalty and friendliness among them. The members are willing to work together and take responsibility for one another in achieving their common goals. And they are willing to endure a certain degree of frustration to maintain the group's integrity. The more cohesion a group has, the more likely it is that it will have a successful outcome. Cohesion is considered the most important therapeutic factor in group therapy.

35.23 The answer is E (all)
Systematic desensitization is applicable in the treatment of *obsessive-compulsive disorder, sexual disorders, stuttering, bronchial asthma,* and other conditions. Joseph Wolpe first described systematic desensitization, a behavioral technique in which the patient is trained in muscle relaxation and then a hierarchy of anxiety-provoking thoughts or objects are paired with the relaxed state until the anxiety is systematically decreased and eliminated.

Obsessive-compulsive disorder (recurrent, intrusive mental events and behavior) is mediated by the anxiety elicited by specific objects or situations. Through systematic desensitization, the patient can be conditioned not to feel anxiety when around those objects or situations and thus to diminish the intensity of the obsessive-compulsive behavior. Desensitization has been used effectively with some stutterers by deconditioning the anxiety associated with a range of speaking situations. Some sexual disorders—such as male orgasmic disorder, female orgasmic disorder, and premature ejaculation—are amenable to desensitization therapy.

35.24 The answer is B
Verification (proving or documenting that something is true or actual) is not generally a psychotherapeutic intervention. *Affirmation* involves brief comments that support a patient's words or actions, such as "I see what you mean." In *clarification,* a therapist reformulates a patient's communication to express a coherent view of the content. Clarification helps patients articulate ideas that are difficult to put into words. *Confrontation* addresses something a patient does not want to accept or refers to a patient's avoidance or minimization. Confrontation need not be forceful or hostile and probably is more effective when phrased gently. *Interpretation* is considered a therapist's ultimate decisive instrument. When a therapist interprets something, he or she makes conscious that which was unconscious. Interpretation may associate a feeling, thought, behavior, or symptom with its unconscious significance.

35.25 The answer is A
Patients with poor frustration tolerance and poor reality testing are best treated with *supportive psychotherapy.* Supportive psy-

Table 35.3
Indications for Expressive or Supportive Emphasis in Psychotherapy

Insight-Oriented (Expressive)	Supportive
Strong motivation to understand	Significant ego defects of a long-term nature
Significant suffering	Severe life crisis
Ability to regress in the service of the ego	
Tolerance for frustration	Poor frustration tolerance
Capacity for insight (psychological-mindedness)	Lack of psychological-mindedness
Intact reality testing	Poor reality testing
Meaningful object relations	Severely impaired object relations
Good impulse control	Poor impulse control
Ability to sustain work	Low intelligence
Capacity to think in terms of analogy and metaphor	Little capacity for self-observation
Reflective responses to trial interpretations	Organically based cognitive dysfunction
	Tenuous ability to form a therapeutic alliance

Reprinted with permission from Gabbard GO. *Psychodynamic Psychotherapy in Clinical Practice.* 3rd ed. Washington, DC: American Psychiatric Press; 2000:108.

chotherapy (also called relationship-oriented psychotherapy) offers the patient support by an authority figure during a period of illness, turmoil, or temporary decompensation. It has the goal of restoring and strengthening the patient's defenses and integrating capacities that have been impaired. It provides a period of acceptance and dependence for a patient who is in need of help in dealing with guilt, shame, and anxiety and in meeting the frustrations or the external pressures that may be too great to handle. Supportive therapy uses a number of methods, either singly or in combination, including (1) warm, friendly, strong leadership; (2) gratification of some dependency needs; (3) support in the ultimate development of legitimate independence; (4) help in the development of pleasurable sublimations (for example, hobbies); (5) adequate rest and diversion; (6) the removal of excessive external strain, if possible; (7) hospitalization when indicated; (8) medication to alleviate symptoms; and (9) guidance and advice in dealing with current issues. It uses the techniques that help the patient feel secure, accepted, protected, encouraged, and safe and not anxious.

Insight-oriented psychotherapy (also called *expressive therapy* and *intensive psychoanalytic psychotherapy*) is not the best treatment for patients with poor frustration tolerance and poor reality testing. The psychiatrist's emphasis in insight-oriented therapy is on the value to patients of gaining a number of new insights into the current dynamics of their feelings, responses, behavior, and, especially, current relationships with other persons. Table 35.3 summarizes the indication for insight-oriented (expressive) therapy versus supportive therapy.

36 ▲
Biological Therapies

Psychopharmacologic advances continue to dramatically expand the parameters of psychiatric treatments today, 40 years after they began to revolutionize the field of psychiatry. Increasing understanding of how the brain functions has led to more effective, less toxic, better-tolerated, and more specifically targeted therapeutic agents. However, with the ever-increasing sophistication and array of treatment options, clinicians must still be fully aware of potential adverse effects, drug–drug (and drug–food or drug–supplement) interactions, and how to manage the emergence of unwanted or unintended consequences. Newer drugs may lead ultimately to side effects that are not recognized initially. Keeping up with the newest research findings is increasingly important as these findings proliferate. The management of medication-induced side effects (either through treating the effect with another agent or substituting another primary agent) must be understood thoroughly. Adverse, even life-threatening, reactions can still occur and clinicians must be able to recognize and manage these promptly and effectively.

Depression is one of the most common psychiatric disorders and there are multiple psychopharmacologic options for its treatment. Serotonin reuptake inhibitors, as well as newer agents, such as bupropion (Wellbutrin), venlafaxine (Effexor), nefazodone (Serzone), and mirtazapine (Remeron) offer a number of advantages over the older tricyclic drugs and monoamine oxidase inhibitors (MAOIs), particularly in terms of safety and side-effect profile. Unfortunately, many HMOs and other managed-care plans still cover only the older medications due to cost issues, severely limiting access for many people to the newer options. Patients with treatment-resistant depressions may respond to augmentation strategies with lithium, thyroid hormone, or combinations of differently acting antidepressants. In many cases, the combination of medication and psychotherapy is particularly helpful. The treatment of bipolar disorder has expanded beyond lithium to include other mood stabilizers, such as the anticonvulsants valproic acid (Depakote), carbamazepine (Tegretol), and gabapentin (Neurontin) and the calcium channel inhibitor, verapamil (Calan, Isoptin). Many of these medications have a number of potentially serious, even fatal, side effects and must be monitored closely. Verapamil, in particular, should be considered a fourth-line drug and should be very cautiously coadministered with other mood stabilizers, given its potential for serious toxicity.

For the treatment of psychotic disorders, the newer "atypical" serotonin-dopamine antagonists, such as olanzapine (Zyprexa) or risperidone (Risperdal), cause fewer extrapyramidal symptoms. They also appear to be more effective than the "typical" dopamine receptor antagonist antipsychotics, not only for positive symptoms but also for negative symptoms of psychosis. There are data that olanzapine has an antidepressant effect in patients with schizophrenia, and there are also indications that it is helpful in the treatment of mania and suicidality. Recent data have suggested the possibility of a higher incidence for the development of drug-induced diabetes with olanzapine, although this potential risk is present in other psychiatric medications as well. Weight gain is a potential adverse effect in many of the newer as well as the older psychopharmacologic agents.

The treatment of the spectrum of anxiety disorders has been enhanced by the addition of such agents as the serotonin reuptake inhibitors, which provide a number of advantages over the use of benzodiazepines and older sedatives. To a lesser degree, agents such as buspirone (BuSpar) and the β-adrenergic receptor antagonists (e.g. propranolol [Inderal]), also provide alternatives to the use of benzodiazepines and other sedatives. The serotonin agents have also been shown to be effective as part of the strategy of treating other mental conditions, such as eating disorders, compulsive behaviors, and paraphilias.

Among many other available psychopharmacologic options are the use of sympathomimetics such as methylphenidate (Ritalin) in the treatment of attention deficit/hyperactivity disorder, disulfiram (Antabuse) in the treatment of alcohol dependence, and anticholinesterase inhibitors, such as donepezil (Aricept), in the management of mild to moderate dementia of the Alzheimer's type.

Electroconvulsive therapy (ECT) continues to be refined, and to be an effective treatment for severe and tenacious depressions that are not optimally responsive to drug therapy. Transcranial magnetic stimulation (TMS) is an interesting technique with potential as both a research tool and a therapeutic modality. The electrical activity of the brain, which is registered by electroencephalography and is altered by ECT, is parallel to the magnetic activity of the brain. TMS can selectively inactivate or potentiate activity in discrete brain regions at subconvulsive doses. Although there are no established guidelines for its use outside research settings, a small number of depressed patients have experienced an improvement in mood following TMS treatments. Light therapy continues to be a treatment option in the management of some mood disorders.

The therapeutic bond between the clinician and the patient is very important to the successful response to psychiatric medications. A thorough diagnostic evaluation, including a medical evaluation where indicated, must be done prior to the administration of any psychoactive treatment. A discussion of expected benefits and risks, as well as potential side effects, must occur between physician/psychiatrist and patient before any treatment is initiated. A patient must feel comfortable in being able to ask questions about treatment at any time during its course. Regular laboratory and medical monitoring, as indicated, of drug levels, along with hematologic and systemic medication effects, must occur.

Students need to be aware of the pharmacokinetics and pharmacodynamics of psychiatric medications, including absorption, distribution, bioavailability, metabolism, and excretion, as well as receptor affinities, dose-response curves, therapeutic indices, the development of tolerance and withdrawal syndromes, therapeutic indications, adverse effects, drug–drug interactions, and signs and symptoms of overdose. Modifications of dosages or specific drug indications for special populations, such as children, the elderly, suicidal patients, and those with medical conditions, must be understood.

The student should study the questions and answers below for a useful review of these therapies.

HELPFUL HINTS

The student should know these terms and specific drugs.

- adjuvant medications
- adrenergic blockade
- akathisia
- allergic dermatitis
- amantadine (Symmetrel)
- anticholinergic side effects
- anticonvulsants
- antidepressants
- antipsychotics
- anxiolytics
- apnea
- artificial hibernation
- atropine sulfate
- benzodiazepine receptor agonists and antagonists
- Lucio Bini
- biotransformation
- bipolar I disorder, bipolar II disorder
- BPH
- bupropion
- buspirone (BuSpar)
- John Cade
- carbon dioxide therapy
- cardiac effects
- catatonia
- Ugo Cerletti
- cholinergic rebound
- clomipramine (Anafranil)
- clonazepam (Klonopin)
- clonidine (Catapres)
- CNS depression
- combination drugs
- continuous sleep treatment
- CYP enzymes
- D_2 receptors
- DEA
- demethylation

- depot preparations
- distribution volume
- dopamine receptor antagonists
- dose-response curve
- downregulation of receptors
- drug-assisted interviewing
- drug holidays
- drug-induced mania
- drug interactions
- drug intoxications
- drug selection
- dystonias
- eating disorders
- Ebstein's anomaly
- ECT
- ECT contraindications
- EEG, EMG
- electrolyte screen
- electrosleep therapy
- epileptogenic effects
- extrapyramidal side effects
- FDA
- fluoxetine (Prozac)
- fluvoxamine (Luvox)
- generalized anxiety disorder
- geriatric patients
- half-life
- haloperidol (Haldol)
- hematological effects
- hemodialysis
- hydroxylation and glucuronidation
- hypertensive crisis
- idiopathic psychosis
- impulse-control disorders
- informed consent
- insulin coma therapy
- intoxication and withdrawal syndromes

- jaundice
- light therapy
- lipid solubility
- lithium
- MAOIs
- medication-induced movement disorders
- megadose therapy
- megavitamin therapy
- melatonin
- mesocortical
- mesolimbic
- metabolic enzymes
- metabolites
- methadone
- Egas Moniz
- monoamine hypothesis
- mood stabilizers
- movement disorders
- mute patients
- narcotherapy
- narrow-angle glaucoma
- neuroendocrine tests
- neuroleptic malignant syndrome
- noncompliance
- noradrenergic, histaminic, cholinergic receptors
- obsessive-compulsive disorder
- oculogyric crisis
- orthomolecular therapy
- orthostatic (postural) hypotension
- overdose
- panic disorder with agoraphobia
- parkinsonian symptoms
- paroxetine (Paxil)
- pharmacodynamics
- pharmacokinetics
- phosphatidylinositol

- photosensitivity
- physostigmine
- pill-rolling tremor
- pilocarpine
- plasma levels
- positive and negative symptoms
- potency, high and low
- prolactin
- prophylactic treatment
- protein binding
- psychosurgery
- rabbit syndrome
- rapid neuroleptization
- Rauwolfia serpentina
- receptor blockade
- renal clearance
- retinitis pigmentosa
- retrograde ejaculation
- reuptake blockade
- schizoaffective disorder
- schizophrenia
- secondary depression
- secondary psychosis
- serotonin-dopamine antagonists
- sertraline (Zoloft)
- side-effect profile
- sleep deprivation
- SSRIs
- status epilepticus
- stereotactic
- sudden death
- sympathomimetic
- tapering
- tardive dyskinesia
- TD_{50}
- teratogenic
- TFT
- therapeutic index
- therapeutic trial
- tonic, clonic phase
- transcranial magnetic stimulation (TMS)

▶ treatment-resistant patients
▶ tricyclic and tetracyclic drugs
▶ L-triiodothyronine
▶ triplicate prescription
▶ use in pregnancy
▶ Julius Wagner-Jauregg
▶ weight gain
▶ Zeitgebers
▶ zolpidem

▲ QUESTIONS

DIRECTIONS: Each of the questions or incomplete statements below is followed by five suggested responses or completions. Select the *one* that is *best* in each case.

36.1 True statements about pharmacodynamics include

A. Haldol is less potent than chlorpromazine.
B. Haldol is more clinically effective than chlorpromazine.
C. The therapeutic index for Haldol is high.
D. The therapeutic index for lithium is high.
E. None of the above

36.2 Of the following biological treatments the most teratogenic is

A. Electroconvulsive therapy (ECT)
B. Haloperidol (Haldol)
C. Fluoxetine (Prozac)
D. Lithium (Eskalith)
E. Lorazepam (Ativan)

36.3 Blockade of muscarinic acetylcholine receptors causes all of the following side effects *except*

A. mydriasis
B. urinary retention
C. delayed ejaculation
D. photophobia
E. orthostatic hypotension

36.4 True statements about SSRI drug interactions include

A. SSRIs plus phenobarbital leads to increased SSRI concentration.
B. SSRIs plus codeine leads to decreased codeine concentration.
C. SSRIs plus clozapine lead to increased clozapine concentration.
D. Prozac plus alprazolam leads to decreased alprazolam concentration.
E. Prozac plus carbamazepine leads to decreased carbamazepine concentration.

36.5 Increased lithium concentrations are associated with all of the following drug interactions except

A. theophylline
B. furosemide
C. salt restriction
D. indomethacin
E. ibuprofen

36.6 Significant valproate interactions include

A. increased free valproate levels with aspirin
B. decreased concentration of phenobarbital with valproate
C. decreased lamotrigine levels with valproate
D. decreased valproate levels with fluoxetine
E. increased valproate levels with carbamazepine

36.7 True statements about neuroleptic malignant syndromes include

A. Mortality rates are reported in the 2 to 5 percent range.
B. Evidence implicates particular typical neuroleptic agents as more likely than others to cause the syndrome.
C. The syndrome is thought to be rare with clozapine.
D. The syndrome is less likely to develop when the dose is parenteral.
E. Rechallenge with a neuroleptic should not be considered until at least 2 months after resolution of the syndrome.

36.8 The risk of tardive dyskinesia is probably least associated with

A. Haloperidol (Haldol)
B. Chlorpromazine (Thorazine)
C. Thioridazine (Mellaril)
D. Perphenazine (Trilafon)
E. Clozapine (Clozaril)

36.9 Anticholinergic prophylaxis should be used routinely

A. past the second week of treatment with an antipsychotic medication
B. when the equivalent of greater than 12 mg a day of haloperidol is required of high-potency antipsychotics
C. in young women on low-potency antipsychotic medication
D. in elderly patients
E. prior to side effects such as parkinsonism activity

36.10 Which of the following psychotropic agents is *least* associated with significant weight gain?

A. Lithium (Eskalith)
B. Valproic acid (Depakene)
C. Carbamazepine (Tegretol)
D. Antihistaminergic agents, such as hydroxyzine or diphenhydramine
E. All of the above

36.11 Carbamazepine may decrease drug plasma concentrations of which of the following agents?

  A. Haloperidol (Haldol)
  B. Bupropion (Buspar)
  C. Birth control pills
  D. Methadone (Dolophine)
  E. All of the above

36.12 Factors associated with a more favorable antimanic response to valproate than to lithium include

  A. rapid cycling
  B. mixed or dysphoric mania
  C. mania associated with medical or neurological illness
  D. comorbid substance abuse or panic attacks
  E. all of the above

36.13 Of the following, the most common adverse effect of valproate is

  A. reversible thrombocytopenia
  B. hair loss
  C. diarrhea
  D. persistent elevation of hepatic transaminases
  E. ataxia

36.14 True statements about gabapentin include

  A. Gabapentin is metabolized almost exclusively in the liver.
  B. Gabapentin overdose is associated with serious toxicity.
  C. Studies suggest that gabapentin may be less useful in the treatment of bipolar II disorder than of bipolar I disorder.
  D. Abrupt discontinuation of gabapentin does not cause a withdrawal syndrome.
  E. Gabapentin interacts with hepatic enzymes and may both inhibit and induce them depending on dose.

36.15 The risk of a potentially life-threatening rash associated with the use of lamotrigine is increased

  A. in pediatric patients
  B. by combining lamotrigine with valproic acid
  C. by exceeding the recommended rate of dose escalation
  D. in the 2 to 8 weeks of the treatment initiation
  E. all of the above

36.16 Among the following benzodiazepines, which has antidepressant effects equal to those of tricyclic drugs in the treatment of mild to moderate depressions?

  A. Alprazolam (Xanax)
  B. Clonazepam (Klonopin)
  C. Triazolam (Halcion)
  D. Lorazepam (Ativan)
  E. Diazepam (Valium)

36.17 Zolpidem

  A. may be used as a muscle relaxant
  B. reaches peak plasma levels in about 4 to 6 hours
  C. is solely indicated as a hypnotic
  D. is generally associated with rebound insomnia after discontinuation of its use for short periods
  E. is not contraindicated for use by nursing mothers

36.18 Bupropion

  A. has efficacy comparable to conventional antidepressants
  B. demonstrates significant anticholinergic toxicity
  C. has shown major cardiovascular effects
  D. impairs psychosexual function
  E. causes appetite enhancement

36.19 Which of the following statements regarding transcranial magnetic stimulation is true?

  A. It does not require general anesthesia.
  B. Seizures do not appear to be required for therapeutic effects.
  C. Optimal stimulation patterns for TMS in psychiatric disorders are not yet known.
  D. It is a noninvasive CNS stimulant.
  E. All of the above

36.20 Which of the following drugs or foods is *not* contraindicated for concurrent administration with triazolobenzodiazepines such as alprazolam (Xanax), based on inhibition of the hepatic enzyme cytochrome P450 (CYP) 3A4?

  A. Cisapride (Propulsid)
  B. Grapefruit juice
  C. Nefazodone (Serzone)
  D. Venlafaxine (Effexor)
  E. All of the above

36.21 Carbamazepine affects each of the following organ systems *except*

  A. dermatological
  B. hematopoietic
  C. hepatic
  D. pulmonary
  E. renal

36.22 Which of the following dopamine receptor antagonists has more than 150 known metabolites?

  A. Chlorpromazine (Thorazine)
  B. Fluphenazine (Prolixin)
  C. Haloperidol (Haldol)
  D. Molindone (Moban)
  E. Trifluoperazine (Stelazine)

36.23 Which of the following is the most common adverse effect of valproate (Depakote)?

  A. Ataxia
  B. Nausea
  C. Sedation
  D. Vomiting
  E. Weight gain

36.24 Dantrolene is a potentially effective treatment for each of the following disorders *except*

  A. acute mania
  B. catatonia
  C. malignant hyperthermia
  D. neuroleptic malignant syndrome
  E. serotonin syndrome

36.25 Which of the following drugs is *least* likely to calm an acutely agitated patient?

A. Chlorpromazine (Thorazine)
B. Haloperidol (Haldol)
C. Olanzapine (Zyprexa)
D. Risperidone (Risperdal)
E. Trifluoperazine (Stelazine)

36.26 Data supporting the traditional dopamine hypothesis of schizophrenia include each of the following *except*

A. correlation of a decrease in plasma concentrations of homovanillic acid with improvement in symptoms
B. PET scan data correlating D_2 receptor occupancy with antipsychotic efficacy
C. precipitation of psychosis with amphetamines
D. the clinical efficacy of clozapine (Clozaril)
E. correlation of D_2 receptor affinity with the clinical efficacy of dopamine receptor antagonists

36.27 Which of the following statements about dexfenfluramine (Redux) is *false*?

A. It may deplete brain serotonin stores.
B. It may inhibit reuptake of serotonin.
C. It may result in activation of serotonin 5-HT_{2c} receptors.
D. It triggers release of dopamine.
E. It triggers release of serotonin.

36.28 Serotonin-specific reuptake inhibitors are generally *not* considered as monotherapy for which of the following indications?

A. Attention-deficit/hyperactivity disorder
B. Premature ejaculation
C. Schizophrenia
D. Syncope
E. Trichotillomania

36.29 Valproate (Depakote) may increase the tremor caused by which of the following drugs?

A. Amitriptyline (Elavil)
B. Diazepam (Valium)
C. Gabapentin (Neurontin)
D. Lithium (Eskalith)
E. Warfarin (Coumadin)

36.30 Of the following, β-adrenergic receptor antagonists are generally most effective in the treatment of

A. panic disorder
B. generalized anxiety disorder
C. alcohol withdrawal
D. akathisia
E. psychogenic seizures

36.31 Factors that predict a better response to carbamazepine (Tegretol) than to lithium (Eskalith) in bipolar I disorder include each of the following *except*

A. comorbid seizure disorder
B. dysphoric mania
C. first episode of mania
D. negative family history
E. rapid cycling

36.32 Which of the following drugs has the fastest onset of action against acute mania?

A. Carbamazepine (Tegretol)
B. Haloperidol (Haldol)
C. Lithium (Eskalith)
D. Risperidone (Risperdal)
E. Valproate (Depakote)

36.33 Which of the following is the most common adverse effect of olanzapine (Zyprexa)?

A. Constipation
B. Orthostatic hypotension
C. Sedation
D. Tardive dyskinesia
E. Weight gain

36.34 Potential treatments for the adverse sexual effects of the serotonin-specific reuptake inhibitors include each of the following drugs *except*

A. amantadine (Symmetrel)
B. bromocriptine (Parlodel)
C. cyproheptadine (Periactin)
D. liothyronine (Cytomel)
E. yohimbine (Yocon)

36.35 Which of the following is the most important factor determining a successful response to treatment with naltrexone (ReVia)?

A. Abstinence from opioids during therapy
B. Dosage
C. Duration of therapeutic trials
D. Ability to start and stop naltrexone without physical consequences
E. Psychosocial factors

36.36 Which of the following dopamine receptor antagonists would probably be the safest to use for psychotic symptoms due to a brain tumor?

A. chlorpromazine (Thorazine)
B. fluphenazine (Prolixin)
C. mesoridazine (Serentil)
D. sulpiride (Dogmatil)
E. thioridazine (Mellaril)

36.37 Anticholinergic drugs are indicated for treatment of all of the following *except*

A. neuroleptic-induced parkinsonism
B. Huntington's chorea
C. neuroleptic-induced acute dystonia
D. idiopathic Parkinson's disease
E. medication-induced postural tremor

36.38 Well-controlled studies have supported the use of carbamazepine (Tegretol) for which of the following disorders?

A. Anorexia nervosa
B. Insomnia
C. Neuroleptic-induced parkinsonism
D. Schizophrenia
E. Social phobia

36.39 Which of the following tricyclic drugs is *least* associated with anticholinergic effects?

A. Amitriptyline (Elavil)
B. Clomipramine (Anafranil)
C. Desipramine (Norpramin)
D. Imipramine (Tofranil)
E. Trimipramine (Surmontil)

ANSWERS

Biological Therapies

36.1 The answer is C

The major pharmacodynamic considerations include receptor mechanisms; the dose-response curve; the therapeutic index; and the development of tolerance, dependence, and withdrawal phenomena.

The dose-response curve plots the drug concentration against the effects of the drug (Fig. 36.1). The potency of a drug refers to the relative dose required to achieve certain effects. *Haloperidol (Haldol), for example, is more (not less) potent than chlorpromazine (Thorazine)* because approximately 5 mg of haloperidol is required to achieve the same therapeutic effect as 100 mg of chlorpromazine. However, both these drugs are equal in their clinical efficacy—that is, the maximum clinical response achievable by administration of a drug.

The adverse effects of most drugs are often a direct result of their primary pharmacodynamic effects. *Therapeutic index* is a relative measure of the toxicity or safety of a drug and is defined as the ratio of the median toxic dose to the median effective dose. The *median toxic dose* is the dose at which 50 percent of patients experience a specific toxic effect, and the *median effective dose* is the dose at which 50 percent of patients have a specified therapeutic effect. *The therapeutic index for haloperidol is high,* as evidenced by the wide range of dosages in which haloperidol is prescribed. Conversely, *the therapeutic index for lithium is low (not high),* thus requiring careful monitoring of serum lithium levels in patients for whom the drug is prescribed. Both interindividual and intraindividual variations can affect the response to a specific drug. An individual patient may be hyporeactive, normally reactive, or hyperreactive to a drug. For example, some patients require 150 mg a day of imipramine (Tofranil), whereas others may require 300 mg a day. Idiosyncratic drug responses occur when a patient experiences a particularly unusual or rare effect from a drug. For example, some patients become quite agitated when given a benzodiazepine, such as diazepam (Valium).

36.2 The answer is D

The basic rule is to avoid administering any drug to a woman who is pregnant (particularly during the first trimester) or who is breast-feeding a child. This rule, however, occasionally needs to be broken when the mother's psychiatric disorder is severe. Of the drug treatments listed (*Haldol, Prozac,* and *Ativan*), *lithium* would be considered the most potentially teratogenic due to its association with abnormalities such as Ebstein's malformation, a serious abnormality in cardiac development. Anticonvulsant agents, especially valproic acid, are also considered to

have high potential teratogenic effects. Other psychoactive drugs (antidepressants, antipsychotics, and anxiolytics) are less clearly associated with birth defects but should also be avoided during pregnancy if at all possible. The most common clinical situation occurs when a pregnant woman becomes psychotic. If a decision is made not to terminate the pregnancy, treatment with antipsychotic drugs or *electroconvulsive therapy (ECT)* may be preferable to lithium.

The administration of psychotherapeutic drugs at or near delivery may cause the baby to be overly sedated, thus requiring a respirator, or to be physically dependent on the drug, requiring detoxification and the treatment of a withdrawal syndrome. Virtually all psychiatric drugs are secreted in the milk of a nursing mother; therefore, mothers on those agents should be advised not to breast-feed their infants.

36.3 The answer is E

Most psychotherapeutic drugs neither affect a single neurotransmitter system nor are their effects localized to the brain. The effects of psychotherapeutic drugs on neurotransmitter systems result in a wide range of adverse effects associated with their use. For example, some of the most common adverse effects of psychotherapeutic drugs are caused by the blockade of muscarinic acetylcholine receptors (Table 36.1). Many psychotherapeutic drugs antagonize dopaminergic, histaminergic,

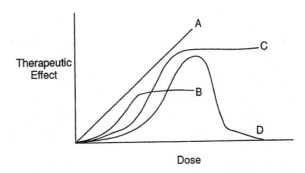

FIGURE 36.1

Dose-response curves plotting the therapeutic effect as a function of increasing the dose often calculated as the log of the dose. Drug A has a linear dose response, drugs B and C have sigmoidal curves, and drug D has a curvilinear dose-response curve. Although doses of drug B are more potent than are equal doses of drug C, drug C has a higher maximum efficacy than does drug B. Drug D has a therapeutic window, such that both low and high doses are less effective than are midrange doses.

Table 36.1
Potential Adverse Effects Caused by Blockade of Muscarinic Acetylcholine Receptors

Blurred vision
Constipation
Decreased salivation
Decreased sweating
Delayed or retrograde ejaculation
Delirium
Exacerbation of asthma (through decreased bronchial secretions)
Hyperthermia (through decreased sweating)
Memory problems
Narrow-angle glaucoma
Photophobia
Sinus tachycardia
Urinary retention

Table 36.2
Potential Adverse Effects of Psychotherapeutic Drugs and Associated Neurotransmitter Systems

Antidopaminergic
  Endocrine dysfunction
    Hyperprolactinemia
    Menstrual dysfunction
    Sexual dysfunction
  Movement disorders
    Akathisia
    Dystonia
    Parkinsonism
    Tardive dyskinesia
Antiadrenergic (primarily α_1)
  Dizziness
  Postural hypotension
  Reflex tachycardia
Antihistaminergic
  Hypotension
  Sedation
  Weight gain
Excessive serotonergic
  Akathisia and agitation
  Anxiety
  GI upset and diarrhea
  Headache
  Insomnia or somnolence
  Nausea and vomiting
  Sexual dysfunction
Multiple neurotransmitter systems
  Agranulocytosis (and other blood dyscrasias)
  Allergic reactions
  Anorexia
  Cardiac conduction abnormalities
  Nausea and vomiting
  Seizures

or adrenergic receptors, resulting in the adverse effects listed in Table 36.2.

Orthostatic hypotension is caused by the blockade of α_1-adrenergic receptors. It is necessary to warn patients of this possible adverse effect, particularly if patients are elderly. The risk of hip fracture from falls is significantly elevated in patients who are taking psychotropic drugs. With patients at high risk of experiencing orthostatic hypotension, the clinician should choose a drug with low α_1-adrenergic activity. The patient can be instructed to get up slowly and to sit down immediately if dizziness is experienced. The patient can also try support hose to help reduce venous pooling of blood.

The blockade of muscarinic acetylcholine receptors causes *mydriasis (pupillary dilation)* and cycloplegia (ciliary muscle paresis), resulting in presbyopia (blurred near vision). The symptom can be relieved by cholinomimetic eye drops. A 1-percent solution of pilocarpine can be prescribed as one drop in each eye four times daily; bethanechol can be used for dry mouth as an alternative. *Photophobia* is another side effect.

The anticholinergic activity of many psychiatric drugs can lead to *urinary hesitation, dribbling, and retention,* as well as an increased rate of urinary tract infections. Elderly male patients with enlarged prostate glands are at increased risk for such adverse effects; 10 to 30 mg of bethanechol three to four times daily is usually effective in the treatment of the adverse effects on urination.

The use of psychiatric drugs can be associated with sexual dysfunction—decreased libido, *impaired ejaculation* and erection, and inhibition of female orgasm. Although warning patients about these adverse effects may increase their concern, they are not likely to report sexual dysfunction spontaneously to the physician.

36.4 The answer is C
CYP 2D6 isoenzyme inhibition or induction can alter drug metabolism. This has taken on increased importance with the advent of potent inhibitors (e.g., fluoxetine and paroxetine [Paxil]) and potent inducers (e.g., carbamazepine), many of which are commonly used for various psychiatric disorders. Individuals can be genotyped for CYP 2D6 activity by use of polymerase chain reaction (PCR) techniques. *SSRIs plus cloza-*

pine lead to increased clozapine concentration. Table 36.3 lists selected SSRI drug interactions.

36.5 The answer is A
Increased lithium concentrations are associated with drug interactions including *furosemide, salt restriction, indomethacin,* and *ibuprofen,* but not *theophylline,* which decreases lithium concentrations. Table 36.4 lists some of the more common clinically relevant potential drug interactions with lithium.

36.6 The answer is A
Table 36.5 lists some of the important selected valproate interactions.

36.7 The answer is C
DSM-IV-TR defines this disorder as severe muscle rigidity, elevated temperature, and other related findings (e.g., diaphoresis, dysphagia, incontinence, changes in level of consciousness ranging from confusion to coma, mutism, elevated or labile blood pressure, elevated creatine phosphokinase [CPK]) developing in association with the use of neuroleptic medication.

Table 36.3
Selected SSRI Drug Interactions

Drug	Interaction	Type of Data[a]	Management
Alprazolam	Increased concentration of alprazolam with fluoxetine, nefazodone, and fluvoxamine	1	Monitor; may need to adjust dosage
Tricyclic drugs	Increased tricyclic drug concentration via CYP 2D6; fluvoxamine may also increase tricyclic drug concentrations via CYP 1A2	1	Use lower dosage of tricyclic drug
Warfarin	Increased warfarin concentrations with fluvoxamine; other SSRIs may cause idiosyncratic increased bleeding	1	Reduce dosage of anticoagulant with fluvoxamine; monitor prothrombin time and bleeding time with other SSRIs
MAOIs	Serotonin syndrome	1	Combination contraindicated
Phenytoin	Increased phenytoin concentration	2	Monitor phenytoin concentration; may need to adjust phenytoin dosage
Clozapine	Increased clozapine concentration	2	Monitor clinically and adjust dosage as needed
L-Tryptophan	Serotonin syndrome	2	Combination contraindicated
Carbamazepine	Increased concentration of carbamazepine with fluoxetine and fluvoxamine	2	Monitor and adjust dosage if needed
Hypoglycemic agents	Increased hypoglycemia, mostly with fluoxetine	2	Monitor; may need to adjust dosage
Theophylline	Increased theophylline concentration with fluvoxamine	2	Monitor; may need to decrease dosage of theophylline
Cimetidine	Increased SSRI concentration	2	Monitor clinically; may need to adjust dosage
Type 1C antiarrhythmic agents	Increased concentration of antiarrhythmic through CYP 2D6 inhibition	3	Use with caution or use drugs with lower CYP 2D6 inhibition
Thioridazine	Increased concentration of thioridazine through CYP 2D6 inhibition	3	Monitor clinically and decrease dosage if needed
β-Adrenergic receptor antagonists, (β-blockers) (e.g., metoprolol)	Increased β-adrenergic receptor antagonist concentrations	3	Monitor heart rate, blood pressure and adjust β-adrenergic receptor antagonist dosage
Phenobarbital	Decreased SSRI concentration	3	Monitor; may need to use higher SSRI dosage
Bupropion	Psychosis reported with fluoxetine	4	Concurrent use not well studied; use low dosage as appropriate
Codeine	Increased codeine concentrations	4	Use lower dosage
Terfenadine, astemizole, cisapride	Theoretical risks of ventricular arrhythmia	4	Contraindicated with fluvoxamine; use with caution with other SSRIs[b]
St. John's Wort	Serotonin syndrome	4	Avoid combination

[a]Type of data: 1, in vivo studies, well established; 2, multiple case reports and/or based on related compounds; 3, in vitro studies; 4, isolated case report.
[b]Preliminary in vitro data predict that paroxetine may have a relatively smaller effect on the clearance of terfenadine than fluoxetine or sertraline.
Adapted from Steffens DC, Krishnan RR, Doraiswamy PM. *Psychotropic Drug Interactions.* New York: MBL Communications; 1998.

Neuroleptic malignant syndrome has been reported since 1960, but it is still poorly defined. The syndrome may represent a heterogeneous group of neuroleptic-induced extrapyramidal adverse effects with concurrent fever. One should not automatically diagnose extrapyramidal adverse effects and fever as neuroleptic malignant syndrome. Estimates of the 1-year prevalence of this syndrome in individuals exposed to neuroleptic medications range from 0.02 to 2.4 percent. It is a rare but potentially fatal disorder; *mortality rates reported are in the 10 to 20 (not 2 to 5) percent range. No clear evidence implicates any particular typical neuroleptic agent* as more or less likely to cause neuroleptic malignant syndrome; atypical neuroleptics (e.g., clozapine and risperidone) have also been reported to be associated with neuroleptic malignant syndrome, but with *clozapine it is thought to be rare.*

The syndrome tends to develop when neuroleptic treatment is initiated or the dosage is increased, particularly when *the dose is* high or *parenteral.* Patients have been reported more likely to be agitated or dehydrated and often to need restraint or seclusion before development of neuroleptic malignant syndrome. The syndrome most often affects young males. Characteristic symptoms include muscular rigidity with elevated body temperature and serum CPK and, in severe cases, myoglobinuria and acute renal failure. The syndrome usually lasts 5 to 10 days after discontinuation of neuroleptic treatment. Differential diagnoses include catatonia, medical condition-induced movement disorders, malignant hyperthermia, and heat stroke.

Prevention is an essential part of managing this heterogeneous condition. The lowest dosage of neuroleptic is recommended, with monitoring of the onset of extrapyramidal adverse effects. Early detection and prompt intervention to eliminate extrapyramidal adverse effects, particularly severe muscular rigidity, may prevent its progress and development of neurolep-

Table 36.4
Selected Lithium Drug Interactions

Drug	Interaction	Type of Data[a]	Management
Thiazides	Increased lithium concentration	1	Avoid if possible; otherwise reduce dosage of lithium
Indomethacin	Increased lithium levels (as much as 60%)	1	Avoid if possible; consider aspirin or acetaminophen
Ibuprofen, diclofenac	15–30% increase in lithium concentration	1	Use lower dosage of lithium; consider aspirin or acetaminophen
Sodium chloride	Decreased lithium concentration	1	Monitor and increase dosage as needed
Sodium bicarbonate	Decreased lithium concentration	1	Monitor and adjust dosage as needed
Psyllium	Decreased lithium concentration	1	Monitor and adjust lithium concentration
Theophylline	Decreased lithium concentration (about 20%)	1	Adjust lithium concentration
Acetazolamide	Decreased lithium concentration	1	Monitor and adjust lithium concentration
Furosemide	Increased lithium concentration	2	Not as established as thiazides, but same considerations apply
Other NSAIDs	Increased lithium concentration	2	Use lower dosage of lithium; consider aspirin or acetaminophen
Salt restriction	Increased lithium concentration	2	Monitor and decrease dosage as needed
Angiotensin-converting enzyme	Increased lithium concentration	2	Monitor and decrease dosage as needed; be especially cautious in presence of renal disease
Calcium channel blockers (verapamil, diltiazem)	Unpredictable increase or decrease in lithium effect (rare)	2	Usually safe; increased awareness or monitoring prudent
Haloperidol	Neurotoxicity in rare cases	2	Awareness is needed
Iodides	Hypothyroidism (rare)	2	Avoid combination

[a]1, in vivo studies, well established; 2, multiple case reports and/or based on related compounds; 3, in vitro studies; 4, isolated case report.
Adapted from Steffens DC, Krishnan RR, Doraiswamy PM. *Psychotropic Drug Interactions.* New York: MBL Communications; 1998.

tic malignant syndrome and its serious complications. Once the syndrome is confirmed, initiate supportive measurements to stabilize autonomic dysfunction, discontinue neuroleptic treatment, continue administering an anticholinergic agent to alleviate muscle rigidity if cardiac status is stable, and institute necessary measurements to lower fever. β-Adrenergic receptor antagonists (β-blockers) or benzodiazepines may be indicated for akathisia or agitation if there is no clinical contraindication. Amantadine, bromocriptine (Parlodel), and dantrolene (Dantrium) have also been used in some cases. Dopamine agonists are important in patients with a fever over 103°F.

Two weeks (not 2 months) after the resolution of neuroleptic malignant syndrome, rechallenge with a neuroleptic may be considered. If a neuroleptic drug is clinically indicated, prescribe the

Table 36.5
Selected Valproate Interactions

Drug	Interaction	Type of Data[a]	Management
Phenobarbital	Increased concentration of phenobarbital	1	Reduce dosage of phenobarbital
Mg/Al hydroxide	Increased valproate levels	1	Reduce dosage of valproate if adverse effects occur
Carbamazepine	Decreased valproate levels and potential increased carbamazepine metabolites	1	Dosage adjustments as appropriate
Aspirin	Increased free valproate levels	2	High or chronic dosage of aspirin or naproxen should be used with prudence
Lamotrigine	Increased lamotrigine levels; increased incidence of Stevens-Johnson syndrome	2	Avoid, or use low doses of lamotrigine
Clonazepam	Increased sedation	2	Concurrent use usually uneventful
Fluoxetine	Increased valproate levels	4	Awareness and monitor

[a]1, in vivo studies, well established; 2, multiple case reports and/or based on related compounds; 3, in vitro studies; 4, isolated case report.
Adapted from Steffens DC, Krishnan RR, Doraiswamy PM. *Psychotropic Drug Interactions.* New York: MBL Communications; 1998.

lowest dosage with gradual incremental increases or prescribe a neuroleptic drug with more anticholinergic properties (e.g., an atypical neuroleptic agent). Adequate hydration and well-controlled ambient temperature are effective prophylactic measurements to lower the risks of recurrent neuroleptic malignant syndrome.

36.8 The answer is E

DSM-IV-TR defines tardive dyskinesia as involuntary choreiform, athetoid, or rhythmic movements (lasting at least a few weeks) of the jaw or extremities developing in association with the use of neuroleptic medication for at least a few months (may be for a shorter period of time in elderly persons).

Tardive dyskinesia is a well-recognized adverse effect associated with the long-term use of neuroleptic therapy and usually occurs insidiously, but early and more rapid onset sometimes occurs.

The disorder has expanded from the initial buccolingual-masticatory syndrome (pouting, puckering, and smacking of lips; tongue protrusion, curling worm-like movements and lateral movements of the tongue, which thrusts against the cheeks to produce the "bonbon" sign; plus chewing movement of the lower jaw) to include various additional abnormal movements and signs. These include facial grimacing; blinking of the eyes, movement of the eyelids; choreoathetoid movements of the fingers, wrists, ankles, and toes; axial hyperkinesia, rocking or torsion movement of the neck, trunk, or both; and diaphragmatic involvement resulting in grunting (glottal dyskinesia) and difficulty breathing.

The total cumulative dosage of neuroleptic drugs administered may relate to increased severity of tardive dyskinesia. All dopamine receptor antagonist have been associated with tardive dyskinesia. At present, there are insufficient data to affirm that serotonin-dopamine antagonist neuroleptic drugs are not associated with tardive dyskinesia. Clozapine, an atypical neuroleptic drug, may not cause tardive dyskinesia, and at the least, *the risk is likely to be lower with clozapine than with typical neuroleptic drugs.* Although the early findings with other atypical neuroleptic drugs suggest that these agents also possess a low risk, this needs to be evaluated in prospective studies.

36.9 The answer is B

The overuse of prophylactic anticholinergic medications has been the subject of numerous studies, prospective and retrospective. Recent prospective studies using lower doses of antipsychotics demonstrate a 20.9 to 33 percent incidence of acute dystonic reactions in patients receiving no prophylaxis. With increased dosages of higher-potency antipsychotics, the incidence of dystonia rose to 47 percent. Regardless of antipsychotic dosage, over 90 percent of all dystonic reactions reported in various studies occur within the first 3 days of treatment. The trends toward higher incidence among younger patients and those of male sex was observed in most studies. In particular, one retrospective study revealed a markedly higher incidence of acute dystonia in the 10- to 19-year-old group (65 percent) than in 20 to 29 year olds (46 percent) and 30 to 39 year olds (32 percent). These combined data suggest that *only when sufficient dosages* (>12 mg a day of haloperidol or its equivalent) of *high-potency antipsychotics are required* in a group at high risk by age and sex—neither *young women* nor *elderly patients*—should anticholinergic prophylaxis be entertained on a routine basis. *The anti-*

cholinergic dosage should be tapered during the second week of treatment (not used past the second week) unless the emergence of further extrapyramidal effects warrants continuation.

A consensus statement of the World Health Organization (WHO) published in 1990 summarizes this position:

> On the basis of these considerations, the prophylactic use of anticholinergics in patients on neuroleptic treatment is not recommended, and may be justified only early in treatment (after which it should be discontinued and its need should be reevaluated). As a rule, these compounds *should be used only when Parkinsonism has actually developed, (not prior to side effects such as Parkinsonism activity)* and when other measures, such as the reduction on neuroleptic dosage or the substitution of the administered drug by another less prone to induce Parkinsonism, have proven ineffective.

36.10 The answer is C

In contrast to other psychotropic agents used in the treatment of mood disorders, such as *lithium* and *valproic acid, carbamazepine does not appear to be associated with significant weight gain. Antihistaminergic agents* are associated with hypotension, sedation, and weight gain.

Weight gain accompanies the use of many psychotropic drugs as a result of retained fluid, increased caloric intake, decreased exercise, or altered metabolism. Weight gain is a very common reason for noncompliance with the drug treatment regimen. Edema can be treated by elevating the affected body parts or by administrating a thiazide diuretic. If the patient is taking lithium or cardiac medications, the clinician must monitor blood concentrations, blood chemistries, and vital signs carefully. The patient should also be instructed to minimize the intake of fats and carbohydrates and to exercise regularly. If patients have not been exercising, the clinician should recommend that they start an exercise program at a modest level of exertion.

36.11 The answer is E (all)

Carbamazepine may interfere with the dexamethasone-suppression test and with some pregnancy tests. Carbamazepine increases the metabolism of sex hormones used in birth control preparations, so higher-dose formulations of those preparations may be required for the oral contraceptives to maintain their efficacy.

As listed in Table 36.6, clinically meaningful drug interactions have occurred with concomitant medications. Most drug interactions result from carbamazepine's induction of hepatic microsomal CYP 2D6, 1A2, 3A4, and 2C9/10, which leads to an accelerated elimination of drugs normally metabolized by this system, including the barbiturates and oral contraceptives. Thus, carbamazepine may decrease the blood levels and efficacy of a variety of drugs. Most notably, *carbamazepine may interact with commonly prescribed agents, such as antidepressants (i.e., bupropion), antipsychotic drugs (i.e., haloperidol), oral contraceptives, methadone,* and anticoagulants. Plasma concentrations of these coprescribed agents may decrease to a clinically significant degree, requiring dosage adjustments to compensate for the lowered plasma concentrations. *Carbamazepine has been reported to decrease levels of haloperidol* by 40 to 60 percent. While administering carbamazepine to refractory excited psychotic patients taking neuroleptic drugs, such as haloperidol, is generally effective, occasional exacerba-

Table 36.6
Carbamazepine–Drug Interactions

Effect of Carbamazepine on Plasma Concentrations of Concomitant Agents		Agents That May Affect Carbamazepine Plasma Concentrations	
Carbamazepine may decrease drug plasma concentration of		*Agents that may increase carbamazepine plasma concentration*	
Acetaminophen	Haloperidol	Allopurinol	Itraconazole
Alprazolam	Hormonal contraceptives	Cimetidine	Lamotrigine
Amitriptyline	Imipramine	Clarithromycin	Loratadine
Bupropion	Lamotrigine	Danazol	Macrolides
Clomipramine	Methadone	Diltiazem	Nefazodone
Clonazepam	Methsuximide	Erythromycin	Nicotinamide
Clozapine	Methylprednisolone	Fluoxetine	Propoxyphene
Cyclosporine	Nimodipine	Fluvoxamine	Terfenadine
Desipramine	Pancuronium	Gemfibrozil	Troleandomycin
Dicumarol	Phensuximide	Itraconazole	Valproate[a]
Doxepin	Phenytoin	Ketoconazole	Verapamil
Doxycycline	Primidone	Isoniazid[a]	Viloxazine
Ethosuximide	Theophylline	*Drugs that may decrease carbamazepine plasma concentrations*	
Felbamate	Valproate	Carbamazepine (autoinduction)	Phenytoin
Fentanyl	Warfarin	Cisplatin	Primidone
Fluphenazine		Doxorubicin HCl	Rifampin[b]
Carbamazepine may increase drug plasma concentrations of		Felbamate	Theophylline
Clomipramine	Primidone	Phenobarbital	Valproate
Phenytoin			

[a]Increased concentrations of the active 10, 11-epoxide.
[b]Decreased concentrations of carbamazepine and increased concentrations of the 10, 11-epoxide.
Table by Carlos A. Zarate, Jr., M.D., and Mauricio Tohen, M.D.

---

tions may be associated with reduction of serum neuroleptic levels to the undetectable range.

36.12 The answer is E (all)
Several factors may be associated with a more favorable antimanic response to valproate than to lithium, including *rapid cycling* (the occurrence of four or more mood episodes in 1 year) and possibly ultrarapid cycling; mania accompanied by mild, moderate, or severe depressive symptoms, including *mixed or dysphoric mania;* and organic or complicated mania (*mania caused by, or associated with, medical or neurological illness* or drugs). Recent controlled data suggest that acutely manic patients with mixed features or rapid cycling are just as likely to display an antimanic response to valproate as patients with pure mania or slow cycling. Other possible predictors of a better response to valproate than to lithium include *comorbid substance abuse or panic attacks.* Prior response to lithium or other antiepileptic drugs is not associated with valproate response.

36.13 The answer is B
Bothersome side effects of valproate include *hair loss,* reported in 3 to 12 percent of patients. Although the hair loss is often transient, total alopecia has been reported in rare cases. Supplemental treatment with multivitamins containing zinc and selenium may minimize hair loss. The adverse effects of valproate are summarized in Table 36.7.

36.14 The answer is D
Case reports and uncontrolled trials suggest that gabapentin facilitates stabilization of mood cycling and helps control manic epi-

sodes. In almost all reports, gabapentin is used adjunctively. These reports involve patients with different bipolar disorders (bipolar I disorder, bipolar II disorder, cyclothymic disorder, and bipolar disorder not otherwise specified) who have failed to achieve adequate control with lithium (Eskalith, Lithobid), valproate, or carbamazepine. While there are reports that gabapentin may treat the depressive phase of bipolar disorder with a lower liability for induction of mania or mood cycling than with an antidepressant, apparent mania or cycling has been reported after initiation of gabapentin treatment. Some studies suggest that gabapentin *may be more (not less) useful in patients with bipolar II disorder than in those with bipolar I disorder.*

In contrast to an unusually large amount of highly positive open-label data and many spontaneous case reports, no placebo-controlled trials confirm the efficacy of gabapentin for bipolar disorders as either monotherapy or adjunctive therapy. It has been suggested that the observed benefits of gabapentin therapy in bipolar patients may differ qualitatively from those associated with conventional mood-stabilizing agents, perhaps reflecting secondary anxiolytic or antiagitation properties.

Gabapentin is mildly sedating and normalizes sleep. It can be given at bedtime as an alternative to benzodiazepine agonists or other hypnotic drugs. Withdrawal symptoms and craving that accompany discontinuation of benzodiazepines, alcohol, and cocaine may be helped by gabapentin. *Abrupt discontinuation of gabapentin does not cause a withdrawal syndrome.*

The most frequent side effects of gabapentin are sedation, dizziness, and ataxia, which tend to be mild and transient. Lower-extremity edema has been noted. Because gabapentin is

Table 36.7
Adverse Effects of Valproate

Common
  Gastrointestinal irritation
  Nausea
  Sedation
  Tremor
  Weight gain
  Hair loss
Uncommon
  Vomiting
  Diarrhea
  Ataxia
  Dysarthria
  Persistent elevation of hepatic transaminases
Rare
  Fatal hepatotoxicity (primarily in pediatric patients)
  Reversible thrombocytopenia
  Platelet dysfunction
  Coagulation disturbances
  Edema
  Hemorrhagic pancreatitis
  Agranulocytosis
  Encephalopathy and coma
  Respiratory muscle weakness and respiratory failure

almost exclusively eliminated through the kidneys, patients with renal impairment should be monitored closely. *There is no serious toxicity with gabapentin overdose.*

Gabapentin does not interact with hepatic enzymes and neither inhibits nor induces them.

36.15 The answer is E (all)
Lamotrigine, a phenyltriazine derivative, was approved for use in the United States in 1994. It is indicated for adjunctive treatment of partial seizures both with and without secondary generalization seizures in adults and adolescents. Anecdotal reports and controlled trials suggest that lamotrigine may possess activity in treating both mania and depression, suggesting that it may be a truly bimodal (i.e., effective in both depression and mania) mood stabilizer.

The most commonly observed adverse effects associated with use of lamotrigine are dizziness, ataxia, somnolence, headache, diplopia, blurred vision, nausea, vomiting, and rash. Approximately 10 percent of individuals in premarketing clinical trials discontinued treatment because of an adverse event. Lamotrigine therapy is not associated with changes in weight.

The frequency of adverse events in a placebo-controlled study of lamotrigine in bipolar disorder was similar for patients receiving lamotrigine or placebo. The only exception was headache, which occurred more frequently among patients taking lamotrigine.

The product information for lamotrigine contains a boxed warning about severe, potentially life-threatening rashes associated with use of the drug. These rashes occur in adults at an estimated rate of 1 in 1,000 and include Stevens-Johnson syndrome and toxic epidermal necrolysis. Rare deaths have been reported, but their numbers are too few to permit calculation of

risk. *In pediatric patients, the incidence of severe rash is very much higher than that reported in adults*, with reports from clinical trials suggesting an upper frequency estimate of 1 in 50 to 1 in 100 pediatric patients who may develop a potentially life-threatening rash.

Why age is a risk factor for rash is unknown. Other than age, *the risk of rash may be increased by* (1) *combining lamotrigine with valproic acid,* (2) exceeding the manufacturer's recommended starting dosage of lamotrigine, and (3) *exceeding the recommended rate of dose escalation* for lamotrigine. Nearly all life-threatening rashes associated with lamotrigine have occurred *within 2 to 8 weeks of treatment initiation.* Rash can occur after prolonged treatment (e.g., 6 months) as well. Lamotrigine should be discontinued at the first sign of rash, unless the rash is clearly not drug related. In some clinical trials the rate of rash has been significantly higher among placebo-treated patients than those being treated with lamotrigine. Routinely informing patients of the need to self-monitor for rash, while necessary, apparently leads to overrecognition in some instances.

36.16 The answer is A
Unique among the benzodiazepines, *alprazolam has antidepressant effects equal to those of the tricyclic drugs,* but alprazolam is not effective with seriously depressed inpatients. The efficacy of alprazolam in depressive disorders may reflect its potency; the antidepressant effects of other benzodiazepines (e.g., *clonazepam, triazolam, lorazepam,* and *diazepam*) may be evident only at doses that also induce sedation or sleep.

36.17 The answer is C
Zolpidem is a hypnotic that acts at the γ-aminobutyric acid (GABA)-benzodiazepine complex as the benzodiazepines do, but it is not itself a benzodiazepine. The drug *lacks the muscle-relaxant effects* that are common to the benzodiazepines. Zolpidem is an imidazopyridine, and its chemical structure is shown in Figure 36.2.

Zolpidem is rapidly and well absorbed after oral administration, and *it reaches peak plasma levels in about 2 to 3 hours (not 4 to 6 hours).* Zolpidem has a half-life of about 2½ hours and is metabolized primarily by conjugation.

The sole indication at this time for zolpidem is as a hypnotic. Several studies have found an absence of rebound REM after the use of the compound for the induction of sleep. The comparatively few data available indicate that *zolpidem may not be associated with rebound insomnia* after the discontinuation of its use for short periods.

FIGURE 36.2
Molecular structure of zolpidem.

Because of the short half-life of zolpidem, clinicians may reasonably evaluate a patient for the possibility of anterograde amnesia and anxiety the day after its administration, although neither of these adverse effects has been reported. Emesis and dysphoric reactions have been reported as adverse effects. Tolerance and dependence have been reported in less than 1 percent of patients, and the withdrawal symptoms are similar to those described for benzodiazepines. Zolpidem is secreted in breast milk and is, therefore, *contraindicated for use by nursing mothers.* The dosage of zolpidem should be reduced in patients with renal and hepatic impairment.

36.18 The answer is A

As predicted, early clinical trials demonstrated *that bupropion had efficacy comparable to that of conventional antidepressants* and an apparently more benign side-effect profile, with *a striking lack of significant anticholinergic toxicity* and *minimal (not major) effects on cardiovascular systems.*

Bupropion's adverse-effect profile is relatively mild and benign, and the medication is generally better tolerated than tricyclic drugs. While considerable attention has been focused on the issue of treatment-associated seizures, when bupropion is prescribed according to the current recommended guidelines regarding patient selection and dosage, the risk is similar to that of tricyclic and tetracyclic antidepressants.

In sharp contrast to selective serotonin reuptake inhibitors (SSRIs) and some other antidepressants, *bupropion does not appear to impair psychosexual function.* Bupropion does not seem to be associated with psychosexual dysfunction, including decreased libido, anorgasmia, and erectile problems. In fact, several published reports describe successful use of bupropion in patients who had stopped treatment with other antidepressants because of psychosexual adverse effects.

In contrast to tricyclic drugs and several other antidepressants, bupropion *causes appetite suppression more often than appetite enhancement.* Weight loss of more than 5 pounds occurred in 28 percent of patients treated with bupropion, about twice that seen with placebo or tricyclic antidepressants. In addition, less than 10 percent of bupropion-treated patients gained weight, versus nearly 35 percent of patients receiving tricyclic drugs.

36.19 The answer is E (all)

ECT has multiple effects on brain function that are responsible for both its therapeutic and adverse actions. If changes in only certain regions of the CNS are required for therapeutic benefits, it may be possible to develop stimulation paradigms that target these areas. Such treatments could have great advantages in avoiding many of the unwanted effects of ECT, perhaps including cognitive impairment. Transcranial magnetic stimulation (TMS) is one such treatment. In neurology, TMS has been *developed as a way to stimulate the CNS noninvasively* by application of a focal magnetic field over regions of the cortex. Refinements of magnetic stimulators, including the development of stimulators capable of discharging at frequencies up to 60 Hz (referred to as rapid-rate TMS [rTMS]) have allowed focal stimulation of the CNS to estimate motor thresholds and determine hemispheric language dominance. Interestingly, rTMS was found to benefit some patients with Parkinson's disease, and some Parkinson's disease patients exhibited improved

mood following rTMS. Additionally, subjects exposed to rTMS for purposes of determining hemispheric language dominance exhibited affective responses following stimulation of the left frontal cortex.

These observations suggest that rTMS may have therapeutic potential in psychiatry and may allow focal stimulation of areas most involved in affective states. While experience with rTMS in psychiatry is limited, some evidence suggests that depending on the placement of the magnetic coil, rTMS can improve or worsen affective state. In one of the best studies to date, left dorsolateral prefrontal cortex stimulation significantly improved depression ratings in 11 of 17 patients with psychotic major depression. rTMS appears to be well tolerated and *does not require general anesthesia. Seizures* may be a side effect in some patients but *do not appear to be required for therapeutic effects.*

TMS is performed using a high-speed magnetic stimulator that generates a 1.5 to 2.5 Tesla field for brief periods. This field is similar to that used for nuclear magnetic resonance imaging. rTMS stimulus is delivered at frequencies of 10 to 60 Hz using a figure-8–shaped coil that is placed over the desired region of the skull and cooled continuously with water to prevent overheating. Patients and staff usually wear earplugs because of the noise generated by the stimulator. Stimulation is typically given several times per session and is repeated over several days to weeks. *At present, optimal stimulation patterns for rTMS in psychiatric disorders are not known.*

36.20 The answer is D

Venlafaxine (Effexor) may be given with drugs such as alprazolam. An essential element of the ability of a chemical to act as a drug is that it can be metabolized by the body. Most psychotherapeutic drugs are oxidized by the hepatic cytochrome P450 (CYP) enzyme system.

The CYP genes may be induced by alcohol, certain drugs (barbiturates, anticonvulsants), or by smoking, which increases the metabolism of certain drugs and precarcinogens. Other agents may directly inhibit the enzymes and slow the metabolism of other drugs. In some cases, if one CYP enzyme is inhibited, once the precursor accumulates to a sufficiently high level within the cell, another CYP enzyme may begin to act. Cellular pathophysiology, such as that caused by viral hepatitis or cirrhosis, may also affect the efficiency of the CYP system. With the DNA sequence data available, several genetic polymorphisms in the CYP genes are now recognized, some of which are manifested in a decreased rate of metabolism. Patients with an inefficient version of a specific CYP enzyme are considered "poor metabolizers."

With respect to CYP 2D6, for which 7 percent of whites are poor metabolizers, tricyclic antidepressants, antipsychotics, and type 1C antiarrhythmics should be used cautiously or avoided with selective serotonin reuptake inhibitors (SSRIs). Because of inhibition of the CYP 3A4 enzyme, *nefazodone, cisapride, grapefruit juice,* and fluoxetine should not be used with terfenadine (Seldane), astemizole (Hismanal), carbamazepine (Tegretol), or the triazolobenzodiazepines alprazolam (Xanax) and triazolam (Halcion). Inhibition of CYP 2C9/10 and CYP 2C19 warrants caution for combinations such as fluoxetine plus phenytoin (Dilantin) and sertraline plus tolbutamide (Orinase). It is also important to consider the long half-lives of certain psychiatric drugs, especially fluoxetine, which may extend their inhibition of the CYP enzymes.

36.21 The answer is D

Carbamazepine has *no known effects* on the *pulmonary system*. Besides the effects on the CNS, carbamazepine has its most significant effects on the *hematopoietic* system. Carbamazepine is associated with a benign and often transient decrease in the white blood cell count, with values usually remaining above 3,000. The decrease is thought to be due to the inhibition of the colony-stimulating factor in the bone marrow, an effect that can be reversed by the coadministration of lithium (Eskalith), which activates the colony-stimulating factor. The benign suppression of white blood cell production must be differentiated from the potentially fatal adverse effects of agranulocytosis, pancytopenia, and aplastic anemia.

As reflected by its use to treat diabetes insipidus, carbamazepine apparently has a vasopressin-like effect on the *renal* vasopressin receptor, sometimes causing the development of water intoxication or hyponatremia, particularly in elderly patients. That side effect can be treated with demeclocycline (Declomycin) or lithium. Another endocrine effect associated with carbamazepine is an increase in urinary-free cortisol.

Carbamazepine induces several *hepatic* enzymes and may thus interfere with the metabolism of a variety of other drugs. The effects of carbamazepine on the cardiovascular system are minimal. It does decrease atrioventricular (A-V) conduction, so the use of carbamazepine is contraindicated in patients with A-V heart block.

Carbamazepine may cause a rash, which may be transient even if the drug is continued, but which rarely leads to serious and potentially life-threatening *dermatological* conditions. Other system-specific allergic reactions have been reported, and rarely a lupus-like disorder has been associated with the use of carbamazepine.

36.22 The answer is A

Chlorpromazine is notorious among psychopharmacologists for having more than 150 metabolites, some of which are active. The nonaliphatic phenothiazines, such *as fluphenazine* and *trifluoperazine*, the dihydroindole *molindone*, and the butyrophenone *haloperidol*, have few metabolites, and whether those metabolites are active remains controversial. The potential presence of active metabolites complicates the interpretation of plasma drug levels that report the presence of only the parent compound.

Peak plasma concentrations of dopamine receptor antagonists are usually reached 1 to 4 hours after oral administration and 30 to 60 minutes after parenteral administration. The half-lives of the butyrophenones and the diphenylbutylpiperidines are longer than for the phenothiazines, and the clinical effects are seen in the tendency of parkinsonism caused by the butyrophenones and the diphenylbutylpiperidines to linger longer than when parkinsonism is caused by other dopamine receptor antagonists. In addition, most dopamine receptor antagonist drugs have high binding to plasma proteins, volumes of distribution, and lipid solubilities. Dopamine receptor antagonist drugs are metabolized in the liver and reach steady-state plasma levels in 5 to 10 days. Some evidence indicates that after a few weeks of administration, chlorpromazine, thiothixene, and thioridazine induce metabolic enzymes, resulting in low plasma concentrations of the drugs.

Although the pharmacokinetic properties of the dopamine receptor antagonists vary widely (their half-lives range from 10 to 20 hours), the most important clinical generalization is that all of the antipsychotics currently available in the United States (with the exception of clozapine) can be given in one daily oral dose once the patient is in a stable condition and has adjusted to any adverse effects. Most dopamine receptor antagonists are incompletely absorbed after oral administration, although liquid preparations are absorbed more efficiently than are other forms. Many dopamine receptor antagonists are also available in parenteral forms that can be given intramuscularly in emergencies, resulting in a more rapid and reliable attainment of therapeutic plasma concentrations than is possible with oral administration.

In the United States, two dopamine receptor antagonists, *haloperidol* and *fluphenazine*, are available in long-acting depot parenteral formulations that can be given once every 1 to 4 weeks, depending on the dose and the patient. The depot formulation of haloperidol and fluphenazine consist of esters of the parent compound mixed in sesame seed oil. The rate of entry of the drug into the body is determined by the rate at which the esterified drug diffuses out of the oil into the body; then the esterified drug is hydrolyzed rapidly, releasing the active compound. Because of the long half-life of that formulation, it can take up to 6 months of treatment to reach steady-state plasma levels, indicating that oral therapy should perhaps be continued during the first months of depot antipsychotic treatment. The long half-life of the depot formulation also means that detectable concentrations of the antipsychotic are present long after the last administration of the drug.

36.23 The answer is B

Valproate treatment is generally well tolerated and safe, although a range of common mild adverse effects and serious and rare adverse effects have been associated with valproate treatment. The common adverse effects associated with valproate are those affecting the gastrointestinal system, such as *nausea* (25 percent of all patients treated), *vomiting* (5 percent of patients), and diarrhea. The gastrointestinal effects are generally most common in the first month of treatment but are also in evidence when the treatment is with valproic acid or sodium valproate, rather than enteric-coated divalproex sodium (Depakote), especially the sprinkle formulation. Some clinicians have treated gastrointestinal symptoms with histamine type 2 (H_2) receptor antagonists, such as cimetidine (Tagamet). Other frequently occurring adverse effects, such as *sedation, ataxia,* dysarthria, and tremor, affect the nervous system. Valproate-induced tremor has been reported to respond well to treatment with β-adrenergic receptor antagonists. Treatment of the other neurological adverse effects usually requires lowering of the valproate dosage. *Weight gain* is a common adverse effect, especially in long-term treatment, and can best be treated by a combination of a reasonable diet and moderate exercise. Hair loss has been reported to occur in 5 to 10 percent of all patients treated; rare cases of complete loss of body hair have been reported. Some clinicians have recommended treatment of valproate-associated hair loss with vitamin supplements that contain zinc and selenium. Another adverse effect that may occur in 5 to 40 percent of patients is a persistent elevation in liver transaminases to three times the upper limit of normal, which is usually asymptomatic and resolves after discontinuation of the drug. Other rare adverse events include effects on the hematopoietic system, including thrombocytopenia and platelet dysfunction, occurring most commonly at high dosages and resulting in the prolongation of bleeding times. Overdoses of valproate can lead to coma and death. There are reports that valproate-induced coma can be successfully treated with naloxone (Narcan) and reports that hemodialysis and hemoperfusion can be useful in the treatment of valproate overdoses.

The two most serious adverse effects of valproate treatment affect the pancreas and the liver. Rare cases of pancreatitis have been reported; they occur most often in the first 6 months of treatment, and the condition occasionally results in death. The most attention has been paid to an association between valproate and fatal hepatotoxicity. A result of that focus has been the identification of risk factors, including young age (less than 2 years), the use of multiple anticonvulsants, and the presence of neurological disorders, especially inborn errors of metabolism, in addition to epilepsy. The rate of fatal hepatotoxicity in patients who have been treated with only valproate is 0.85 per 100,000 patients. Therefore, the risk of that adverse reaction in adult psychiatric patients seems to be extremely low. Nevertheless, if symptoms of malaise, anorexia, nausea and vomiting, edema, and abdominal pain occur in a patient treated with valproate, the clinician must consider the possibility of severe hepatotoxicity. However, a modest change in liver function test results does not correlate with the development of serious hepatotoxicity.

Valproate should not be used by pregnant or nursing women. It has been associated with neural tube defects (such as spina bifida) in about 1 to 2 percent of babies of women who took valproate during the first trimester of pregnancy. Valproate is contraindicated in nursing mothers because it is excreted in breast milk. Clinicians should not administer it to patients with hepatic diseases.

36.24 The answer is A

Dantrolene (Dantrium) is a direct-acting skeletal muscle relaxant. The only indication for dantrolene in contemporary clinical psychiatry is as one of the potentially effective treatments for *neuroleptic malignant syndrome, catatonia,* and *serotonin syndrome.* It is also used to treat *malignant hyperthermia,* an adverse effect of general anesthesia that bears a clinical resemblance to neuroleptic malignant syndrome. Dantrolene has no other uses in psychiatry and *is not used to treat acute mania.*

Dantrolene produces skeletal muscle relaxation by directly affecting the contractile response of the muscles at a site beyond the myoneural junction. Specifically, dantrolene dissociates excitation-contraction coupling by interfering with the release of calcium from the sarcoplasmic reticulum. The skeletal muscle relaxant effect is the basis of its efficacy in reducing the muscle destruction and hyperthermia associated with neuroleptic malignant syndrome.

The primary psychiatric indication for intravenous (IV) dantrolene is muscle rigidity in neuroleptic malignant syndrome. Dantrolene is almost always used in conjunction with appropriate supportive measures and a dopamine receptor agonist such as bromocriptine (Parlodel). If all available case reports and studies

are summarized, about 80 percent of patients with neuroleptic malignant syndrome who received dantrolene apparently benefited clinically from the drug. Muscle relaxation and a general and dramatic improvement in symptoms can appear within minutes of IV administration, although in most cases the positive effects can take several hours to appear. Some evidence indicates that dantrolene treatment must be continued for a period of time, perhaps days to a week or more, to minimize the risk of the recurrence of symptoms, although the data for that clinical opinion are limited. Dantrolene has been used in efforts to treat other psychiatric conditions characterized by life-threatening muscle rigidity, such as catatonia and serotonin syndrome.

36.25 The answer is D

Risperidone is less likely than, *olanzapine*, and the dopamine receptor antagonists, such as *haloperidol* and *thioridazine*, to produce a calming effect acutely or in the first few days of use. This is due to risperidone's lack of anticholinergic and antihistaminergic effects. If risperidone is chosen for an acutely psychotic patient, addition of a benzodiazepine or a high-potency dopamine receptor antagonist may be necessary in the first 1 to 2 weeks. The benefit of risperidone is usually noted within 4 weeks.

36.26 The answer is D

The dopamine hypothesis of schizophrenia grew from the observations that drugs that block dopamine receptors (such as haloperidol) have antipsychotic activity and drugs that stimulate dopamine activity (such as *amphetamines*) can, when given in high enough doses, induce psychotic symptoms in nonschizophrenic persons. The dopamine hypothesis remains the leading neurochemical hypothesis for schizophrenia, but room is being made for a role for serotonin, based on the therapeutic success of the serotonin-dopamine antagonists, such as clozapine. Schizophrenia is now thought to result from misregulation of both dopamine and serotonin function. It is likely that the theories will have to be reconceived several times in the near future as agents become available for modification of particular receptor subtypes. Clozapine has relatively low potency as a dopamine type 2 (D_2) receptor antagonist. Clozapine has much higher potency as an antagonist at D_1, D_3, and D_4, serotonin type 2 (5-HT_2), and noradrenergic α-receptors (especially α_1). Clozapine also has intermediate antagonist activity at muscarinic and histamine type 1 (H_1) receptors. *Clozapine is one of the most effective antipsychotic drugs,* and its unique pharmacodynamic profile has indicated that dopamine is not the only neurotransmitter system involved in the etiology of schizophrenia. In animal models, clozapine appears more active in the mesolimbic system than in the striatonigral system, which correlates with the lack of parkinsonian side effects.

Evidence in support of the dopamine hypothesis of schizophrenia is as follows. The *potency of dopamine receptor antagonist drugs to reduce psychotic symptoms* is most closely correlated with the affinity of these drugs for D_2 receptors. The mechanism of therapeutic action for dopamine receptor antagonist drugs is hypothesized to be through D_2 receptor antagonism, thus preventing endogenous dopamine from activating the receptors. Neuroanatomists have defined two major dopamine tracts, the mesolimbic to cortical (mostly frontal lobe) projection and the substantia nigra to striatum projection. Studies using the *PET technique* in patients who were taking a variety of dopamine receptor antagonists in different dosages have produced data indicating that *occupancy of about 60 percent of the* D_2 *receptors* in the caudate-putamen is correlated with clinical response and that occupancy of more than 70 percent of the D_2 receptors is correlated with the development of extrapyramidal symptoms.

Another positive association between the clinical efficacy of dopamine receptor antagonists and their dopamine receptor activity is suggested by the effects of the drugs on the plasma concentrations of homovanillic acid, the major metabolite of dopamine. Several studies have reported that high pretreatment concentrations of plasma homovanillic acid are positively correlated with an increased likelihood of a favorable clinical response. Furthermore, *a decrease in plasma homovanillic acid concentrations* early in the course of treatment is correlated with a favorable clinical response.

36.27 The answer is D

Unlike its relatives amphetamine and racemic fenfluramine (Pondimin), dexfenfluramine *does not appear to be associated with a facilitation of dopamine release from neurons*. The major short-term effect of fenfluramine and dexfenfluramine is to *release neuronal stores of serotonin*. Some data indicate that fenfluramine and dexfenfluramine are also *inhibitors of serotonin reuptake*. It is possible that *stimulation of serotonin 5-HT$_{2c}$ receptors*, which results from increased synaptic concentrations of serotonin, may reduce the appetite. However, troubling questions remain about whether dexfenfluramine *may permanently deplete the brain of certain serotonin stores*. In 1997, both drugs were withdrawn from the market because they produced serious heart valve disorders in patients using these medications, which had wide distribution in the United States.

36.28 The answer is C

There have been case reports of fluoxetine monotherapy for *schizophrenia*, although *SSRIs are generally not considered for the treatment of psychotic symptoms*. Other indications for which there is preliminary evidence of efficacy for the SSRIs are dysthymic disorder, borderline personality disorder, panic disorder, hypochondriasis, *trichotillomania*, elective mutism, *attention-deficit/hyperactivity disorder*, obsessional jealousy, *premature ejaculation*, body dysmorphic disorder, autistic disorder in children and adults, Asperger's syndrome, augmentation of anticonvulsant for bipolar disorder, Tourette's disorder, self-injurious behavior, paraphilias, aggression in schizophrenia, *syncope*, neuropathic (diabetic, postherpetic) and non-neuropathic chronic pain, migraine and tension types of headache, and fibromyalgia.

36.29 The answer is D

Valproate is commonly coadministered with lithium and the antipsychotics. *The only consistent drug interaction with lithium is the exacerbation of drug-induced tremors,* which can usually be treated with β-adrenergic receptor antagonists or gabapentin. The combination of valproate and antipsychotics may result in increased sedation, as can be seen when valproate is added to any CNS depressant (such as alcohol), and increased severity of extrapyramidal symptoms, which usually respond to treatment with the antiparkinsonian drugs. The plasma concentrations of *diazepam, amitriptyline*, nortriptyline (Pamelor), and phenobarbital (Luminal) may be increased when those drugs are coadministered with valproate, and the plasma concentrations of phenytoin (Dilantin) and desipramine (Norpramin) may be decreased when phenytoin is combined with valproate. The plasma concentrations of valproate may be decreased when the drug is coadministered with carbamazepine and may be increased when coadministered with amitriptyline (Elavil) or fluoxetine (Prozac). Patients who are treated with anticoagulants, such as aspirin and *warfarin*, should also be monitored when valproate is initiated to assess the development of any undesired augmentation of the anticoagulation effects.

36.30 The answer is D

The use of the β-adrenergic receptor antagonists is best supported for neuroleptic-induced acute *akathisia*, lithium-induced postural tremor, and social phobia. The data on the use of these drugs as adjuncts to benzodiazepines for alcohol withdrawal and for the control of impulsive aggression or violence are also promising.

Neuroleptic-induced acute akathisia is recognized in the revised fourth edition of *Diagnostic and Statistical Manual of Mental Disorders* (DSM-IV-TR) as one of the medication-induced movement disorders. Many studies have shown that β-adrenergic receptor antagonists can be effective in the treatment of neuroleptic-induced acute akathisia. The majority of clinicians and researchers believe that β-adrenergic receptor antagonists are more effective for this indication than are anticholinergics and benzodiazepines, although the relative efficacy of those agents may vary among patients. However, the clinician must realize that the β-adrenergic receptor antagonists are not effective in the treatment of such neuroleptic-induced movement disorders as acute dystonia and parkinsonism. Propranolol has been most studied for neuroleptic-induced acute akathisia, and at least one study has reported that a less lipophilic compound was not effective in the treatment of the disorder. There does not appear to be a clear superiority of $β_1$-selective versus nonselective agents for this indication.

Propranolol has been reported to be useful as an adjuvant to benzodiazepines but not as a sole agent in the treatment of *alcohol withdrawal*. One study used the following dose schedule: no propranolol for a pulse less than 50; 50 mg propranolol for a pulse between 50 and 79; and 100 mg propranolol for a pulse equal to or greater than 80. The patients who received propranolol and benzodiazepines had less severe withdrawal symptoms, more stable vital signs, and a shorter hospital stay than did the patients who received only benzodiazepines.

Propranolol has been well studied for the treatment of social phobia, primarily of the performance type (for example, disabling anxiety before a musical performance), but data are also available for their use in treatment of social phobia, *panic disorder*, posttraumatic stress disorder, and *generalized anxiety disorder*. Use of β-adrenergic receptor antagonists for panic disorder, generalized anxiety disorder, and *psychogenic seizures* is less efficacious than the use of benzodiazepines or selective serotonin reuptake inhibitors.

36.31 The answer is C

Lithium is the most commonly used agent for treatment of a *first manic episode* because it is generally the most effective drug for this purpose. Almost two dozen well-controlled studies, however, have shown that carbamazepine is effective in the treatment of acute mania, with efficacy comparable to lithium and antipsychotics. About ten studies have also shown that carbamazepine is effective in the prophylaxis of both manic and depressive episodes in bipolar I disorder when it is used for prophylactic treatment. Carbamazepine is an effective antimanic agent in 50 to 70 percent of all patients. Additional evidence from those studies indicates that carbamazepine may be effective in some patients who are not responsive to lithium, such as patients with *dysphoric mania, rapid cycling,* or a *negative family history of mood disorders.* However, a few clinical and basic science data indicate that some patients may experience a tolerance for the antimanic effects of carbamazepine. Because lithium toxicity may produce convulsions, carbamazepine may be a preferred drug for patients with *comorbid seizure disorders.*

36.32 The answer is B

Dopamine receptor antagonists are often used in combination with antimanic drugs to treat psychosis or manic excitement in bipolar I disorder. Although *lithium, carbamazepine,* and *valproate* are the drugs of choice for that condition, these drugs generally have a slower onset of action than do dopamine receptor antagonists, such as *haloperidol,* in the treatment of the acute symptoms. Thus, the general practice is to use combination therapy at the initiation of treatment and to gradually withdraw the dopamine receptor antagonist after the antimanic agent has reached its onset of activity. *Risperidone* lacks the anticholinergic and antihistamine activities that contribute to the calming effects of the dopamine receptor antagonists, and it is not as effective as haloperidol for the treatment of acute mania.

36.33 The answer is C

The most common adverse effect of olanzapine is *sedation,* which may occur in 30 percent of patients on the usual maintenance dose (10 mg/day). Therefore, patients who take olanzapine should exercise caution when driving or operating dangerous machinery. This side effect may be minimized by giving the dose before sleep. Olanzapine-associated seizures are seen in less than 1 percent of patients. The D_2 receptor antagonism of olanzapine causes a modest rise in prolactin levels for the duration of the therapy. This is a theoretical concern in patients with a history of breast cancer, a tumor that may be dependent on prolactin for growth, although there are no human data establishing such a connection. Dizziness, akathisia, and nonaggressive objectionable behavior have also been reported at frequencies higher than those seen in placebo controls.

No cases of *tardive dyskinesia* have yet been reported in patients taking olanzapine, although experience is limited. No agranulocytosis was reported in more than 3,100 patients taking olanzapine, including 29 who previously had clozapine-induced agranulocytosis.

When olanzapine is first initiated, patients may develop signs and symptoms of *orthostatic hypotension,* such as dizziness, tachycardia, and syncope. The risk of these effects may be minimized by limiting the starting dose to 5 mg a day over a few weeks. Significantly, in 2 percent of patients taking olanzapine, serum ALT (SGPT) elevations more than three times normal were seen. None of these patients developed jaundice. The levels returned to normal whether or not the drug was discon-

tinued. These data indicate that olanzapine should be used with caution by patients with underlying liver disease. *Weight gain* and *constipation* have been associated with olanzapine use.

36.34 The answer is D

Serotonergic drugs may cause a reduction in libido, anorgasmia, inhibition of ejaculation, and/or impotence in up to 80 percent of patients. Many clinicians do not inquire about sexual adverse effects, yet these may be very troubling to patients. Some drugs that may be helpful in reducing these adverse are *amantadine, bromocriptine, cyproheptadine,* and *yohimbine.* Amantadine and bromocriptine have dopamine agonist effects; cyproheptadine is a serotonin antagonist; and yohimbine is an α_2-adrenergic antagonist that potentiates release of norepinephrine. Mirtazapine (Remeron), another α_2-adrenergic antagonist, and bupropion (Wellbutrin), an antidepressant with little serotonergic activity, are two antidepressants that are practically free of sexual adverse effects. *Liothyronine* is used as augmentation treatment for SSRI nonresponders, but it has no role in the treatment of sexual adverse effects.

36.35 The answer is E

The success of naltrexone drug and alcohol abstinence programs is more closely associated with *psychosocial factors,* such as educational level, motivation, family support, and continued behavioral therapy, than with factors associated directly with the use of naltrexone, such as *dosage* or *duration of therapeutic trials.*

Naltrexone is a pure opioid antagonist, effective in a once-a-day dose that has improved the success of existing behavioral approaches to the treatment of opioid and alcohol addiction. Naltrexone appears to reduce or eliminate the drug craving that torments former addicts by simply eliminating the subjective "high" associated with a return to drug abuse. *Abstinence from opioids during therapy* is therefore a secondary issue, because users do not experience the usual effects of opioids. Naltrexone must be initiated cautiously in individuals who may still be abusing opioids, because it may induce an acute withdrawal reaction, which may include life-threatening dehydration due to vomiting and diarrhea. It is therefore necessary to ensure an opioid-free state prior to use of naltrexone. Once in use, however, *naltrexone may be started and stopped, usually without physical consequence*s. This feature has unfortunately allowed many less motivated former addicts to withdraw from naltrexone treatment programs, which is an outcome in contrast to that usually seen in methadone programs, where stopping the drug precipitates an unpleasant withdrawal syndrome.

36.36 The answer is B

Secondary psychoses are psychotic syndromes that are associated with an identified organic cause, such as a brain tumor, a dementing disorder (such as dementia of the Alzheimer's type), or substance abuse. The dopamine receptor antagonist drugs are generally effective in the treatment of psychotic symptoms that are associated with those syndromes. The high-potency dopamine receptor antagonists, such as *fluphenazine,* are usually safer than the low-potency dopamine receptor antagonists, such as *chlorpromazine, mesoridazine, sulpiride,* and *thioridazine,* in such patients because of the high-potency drugs' lower cardiotoxic, epileptogenic, and anticholinergic activities. However, dopamine receptor antagonist drugs should not be used to treat withdrawal symptoms associated with ethanol or barbiturates because of the risk that such treatment will facilitate the development of withdrawal seizures. The drug of choice in such cases is usually a benzodiazepine. Agitation and psychosis associated with such neurological conditions as dementia of the Alzheimer's type are responsive to antipsychotic treatment; high-potency drugs and low dosages are generally preferable. Even with high-potency drugs, as many as 25 percent of elderly patients may experience episodes of hypotension. Low dosages of high-potency drugs, such as 0.5 to 5 mg a day of haloperidol, are usually sufficient for the treatment of those patients.

36.37 The answer is B

Anticholinergics have not been shown to be effective for treatment of *Huntington's chorea.* In the clinical practice of psychiatry, the anticholinergic drugs and amantadine (Symmetrel), like the antihistamines, have their primary use as treatments for medication-induced movement disorders, particularly *neuroleptic-induced parkinsonism, neuroleptic-induced acute dystonia,* and *medication-induced postural tremor.* The anticholinergic drugs and amantadine may also be of limited use in the treatment of neuroleptic-induced acute akathisia. Before the introduction of levodopa (Larodopa), the anticholinergic drugs were commonly used in the treatment of *idiopathic Parkinson's disease.* The antiparkinsonian effects of amantadine, which was initially developed as an antiviral compound, were discovered when its use improved the parkinsonian symptoms of a patient who was being treated with amantadine for influenza A2.

All of the available anticholinergics and amantadine are equally effective in the treatment of parkinsonian symptoms, although the efficacy of amantadine may diminish in some patients within the first month of treatment. Amantadine may be more effective than the anticholinergics in the treatment of rigidity and tremor. Amantadine may also be the drug of choice if a clinician does not want to add more anticholinergic drugs to a patient's treatment regimen, particularly if a patient is taking an antipsychotic or an antidepressant with high anticholinergic activity—such as chlorpromazine (Thorazine) or amitriptyline (Elavil)—or is elderly and therefore at risk for anticholinergic adverse effects.

Neuroleptic-induced acute dystonia is most common in young men. The syndrome often occurs early in the course of treatment and is commonly associated with high-potency antipsychotics, such as haloperidol. The dystonia most commonly affects the muscles of the neck, the tongue, the face, and the back. Opisthotonos (involving the entire body) and oculogyric crises (involving the muscles of the eyes) are examples of specific dystonias. Dystonias are uncomfortable, sometimes painful, and often frightening to the patient. The onset is often sudden and frequently results in patients complaining about having a thick tongue or difficulty in swallowing. Dystonic contraction can be powerful enough to dislocate joints, and laryngeal dystonias can result in suffocation if the patient is not treated immediately.

36.38 The answer is D

Several well-controlled studies have produced data indicating that carbamazepine is effective in the treatment of *schizophre-* nia and schizoaffective disorder. Patients with positive symptoms (such as hallucinations) and few negative symptoms (such as anhedonia) may be likely to respond, as are patients who have impulsive, aggressive outbursts as a symptom.

The available data indicate that carbamazepine is also an effective treatment for depression in some patients. About 25 to 33 percent of depressed patients respond to carbamazepine. That percentage is significantly smaller than the 60 to 70 percent response rate for standard antidepressants. Nevertheless, carbamazepine is an alternative drug for depressed patients who have not responded to conventional treatments, including electroconvulsive therapy (ECT), or who have a marked or rapid periodicity in their depressive episodes.

Several studies have reported that carbamazepine is effective in controlling impulsive, aggressive behavior in nonpsychotic patients of all ages, from children to the elderly. Other drugs for impulse control disorders, particularly intermittent explosive disorder, include lithium, propranolol (Inderal), and antipsychotics. Because of the risk of serious adverse effects with carbamazepine, treatment with these other agents is warranted before initiating a trial with carbamazepine.

According to several studies, carbamazepine is as effective as the benzodiazepines in the control of symptoms associated with alcohol withdrawal. It may also assist in withdrawal from chronic benzodiazepines in the control of symptoms linked to alcohol withdrawal. Similarly, it may aid in withdrawal from chronic benzodiazepine use, especially in seizure-prone patients. However, the lack of any advantage of carbamazepine over the benzodiazepines for alcohol withdrawal and the risk of adverse effects with carbamazepine limit the clinical usefulness of this application. Carbamazepine has not been shown to be useful in the treatment of *social phobia, insomnia, anorexia nervosa,* or *neuroleptic-induced parkinsonism.*

36.39 The answer is C

Clinicians should warn patients that anticholinergic effects of tricyclic drugs are common but that a patient may develop tolerance for them with continued treatment. *Amitriptyline, imipramine, trimipramine, clomipramine,* and doxepin are the most anticholinergic drugs; amoxapine, nortriptyline, and maprotiline are less anticholinergic; *desipramine* may be the least anticholinergic. Anticholinergic effects include dry mouth, constipation, blurred vision, and urinary retention. Sugarless gum, candy, or fluoride lozenges can alleviate the dry mouth. Bethanechol (Urecholine), 25 to 50 mg three or four times a day, may reduce urinary hesitancy and can be helpful in cases of impotence when the drug is taken 30 minutes before sexual intercourse. Narrow-angle glaucoma can be aggravated by anticholinergic drugs, and the precipitation of glaucoma requires emergency treatment with a miotic agent. Tricyclic and tetracyclic drugs should be avoided in patients with glaucoma, and an SSRI should be substituted. Severe anticholinergic effects can lead to a CNS anticholinergic syndrome with confusion and delirium, especially if tricyclic and tetracyclic drugs are administered with antipsychotics or anticholinergic drugs. Some clinicians have used intramuscular (IM) or intravenous (IV) physostigmine (Antilirium) as a diagnostic tool to confirm the presence of anticholinergic delirium.

37 ▲

Child Psychiatry: Assessment, Examination, and Psychological Testing

Just as in the assessment of adults, the assessment of children involves obtaining a thorough medical, psychiatric, and family history, performing indicated medical and laboratory evaluations, making direct observations, and implementing more standardized testing as indicated. A detailed developmental history is particularly crucial in the assessment of children, as delayed or missed developmental milestones are often what motivate parents to bring their child in, and may herald larger or more specific problems. The assessment process includes direct meetings with the child, the parents, and sometimes siblings. Collateral information may also be obtained from teachers, pediatricians, and school counselors. Standardized testing evaluates intellectual functioning, developmental level, and academic achievement. As with adults, biology and psychology interact in children in complex and profound ways, and clinicians must understand the impact of each on the other.

In order to interpret details from a developmental history, a clinician must have a firm grasp of normal development. Specific knowledge about the normative development of language, motor skills, interpersonal relatedness, academic achievement, and emotional regulation is crucial to recognizing, understanding, and managing deficits in any of these areas. For instance, appreciation of the range of normal activity levels and the relationship of activity to psychological and biological forces assist the clinician in making or ruling out a diagnosis of attention-deficit/hyperactivity disorder. Delayed language or motor skills development may reflect a temporary, self-remitting disturbance, or a more serious, pervasive disorder. Understanding the range and variations of normal development can assist the clinician in distinguishing the normal from the abnormal, and once abnormal signs and symptoms have been identified, this understanding can aid in tracking the evolution of psychiatric disorders.

Direct observation is especially important in the assessment of children, as language is not usually their most developed form of communication. Young children are often seen in a room that contains toys, dolls, puppets, and drawing supplies, to aid evaluation of their developmental level and disclosure of feelings. Children and adolescents may act out or draw feelings they cannot express verbally. Evaluation of an adolescent requires a different set of skills and developmental parameters, and treatment of adolescent problems demands very specific expertise. A mental status exam of children includes observation and assessment of physical appearance, activity level, parent–child interactions, separation and reunion behaviors, mannerisms, communication style, mood, cognitive functioning, levels of self-esteem, and the presence or absence of psychotic symptoms, among other areas. Diagnosing psychosis in a child or adolescent requires the clinician to be aware of normal and abnormal developmental as well as cultural variations in reality testing. An assessment of self-destructive behaviors and suicidal ideation should always be included in a comprehensive mental status assessment.

Students should be aware of the concept of temperament. Temperament defines a variety of dimensions that characterize the way a child interacts with the environment. Temperamental traits can influence behavior and emotional responsiveness throughout life. Temperamental categories include activity level, rhythmicity of biological function, approach to or withdrawal from new stimuli, adaptability to change, threshold of responsiveness, intensity of reaction, quality of mood, attention span, and persistence. Three common constellations of temperament have been described:

1. *Easy temperament* characterizes a child who tends to be adaptable, approaches new stimuli rather than withdraws, exhibits a generally positive mood of moderate intensity, and whose sleep–wake cycle, hunger levels, and activity seem to be internally regulated.

2. *Difficult temperament* characterizes a child irritated easily in response to change, demonstrating intense and negative reactions with withdrawal from new stimuli, and who is biologically irregular with regard to sleep–wake, hunger, activity, and mood.

3. *Slow-to-warm-up temperament* characterizes a child who may be more likely to withdraw initially from new stimuli, shows a slow adaptability to change, and demonstrates frequent negative emotional reactions of low intensity. These are the children who are often described as shy.

The student should study the questions and answers below for a useful review of this field.

HELPFUL HINTS

The student should define these terms.

- AAMD
- achievement tests
- adaptive functioning
- Bayley Infant Scale of Development
- borderline intellectual functioning
- Cattell Infant Scale
- Child Behavior Checklist
- chromosomal abnormality
- *cri-du-chat* syndrome
- developmental tests
- DISC-R (Diagnostic Interview Schedule for Children-Revised)
- Down's syndrome
- fragile X syndrome
- intelligence quotient (IQ)
- K-SADS (Kiddie Schedule for Affective Disorders and Schizophrenia)
- Lesch-Nyhan syndrome
- mental deficiency
- mental retardation
- neurofibrillary tangles
- neurofibromatosis
- nondisjunction
- PKU
- Prader-Willi syndrome
- prenatal exposure
- rubella
- Turner's syndrome
- Vineland Adaptive Behavior Scales
- WHO
- WISC-III (Wechsler Intelligence Scale for Children—Third Edition)

▲ QUESTIONS

DIRECTIONS: Each of the questions or incomplete statements below is followed by five suggested responses or completions. Select the *one* that is *best* in each case.

37.1 True statements about the distinctive features of child psychopathology include all of the following *except*

A. Disturbances usually consist of specific, pathognomonic symptoms.
B. In children, depression rarely presents with excessive guilt or depressive delusions.
C. Distressing emotions or impairing behavior may occur as part of a normal transition.
D. Fears, tantrums, or moodiness are relatively common in children and occur transiently at different stages.
E. Comorbidity is usually the rule, not the exception, in childhood disorders.

37.2 To facilitate the play component of an interview, which of the following tools are considered generally appropriate?

A. stock characters (such as Barbie or Disney characters)
B. elaborate toys
C. cards or board games
D. chess
E. all of the above

37.3 Projective techniques include

A. picture drawing
B. asking the child to disclose three wishes
C. asking the child to tell about a dream, a book, a movie, or a TV program
D. the Despert fables
E. all of the above

37.4 Structured assessment instruments for infants and young children

A. yield diagnoses
B. include the Denver Developmental Screening Test (Denver II) and the Bayley Scales
C. have a high degree of ability to predict later performances on IQ assessment
D. show only moderate reliability and validity
E. all of the above

37.5 Of the following diagnostic laboratory tests used in children who present with psychiatric problems, the most informative generally is

A. electroencephalograhy (EEG)
B. computed tomography (CT) scan
C. magnetic resonance imaging (MRI)
D. chromosomal analyses
E. thyroid function tests

DIRECTIONS: Each group of questions below consists of lettered headings followed by a list of numbered phrases or statements. For each numbered phrase or statement, select the *one* lettered heading that is most closely associated with it. Each lettered heading may be selected once, more than once, or not at all.

Questions 37.6–37.10

A. Vineland Adaptive Behavior Scales
B. Children's Apperception Test (CAT)
C. Wide-Range Achievement Test-Revised (WRAT-R)
D. Peabody Picture Vocabulary Test-Revised (PPVT-R)
E. Wechsler Intelligence Scale for Children—Third Edition (WISC-III)

37.6 Measures receptive word understanding, with resulting standard scores, percentiles, and age equivalents

37.7 Measures communication, daily living skills, socialization, and motor development, yielding a composite expressed in a standard score, percentile, and age equivalents

37.8 Generates stories from picture cards of animals that reflect interpersonal functioning

37.9 Measures functioning in reading, spelling, and arithmetic, with resulting grade levels, percentiles, and standard scores

37.10 Measures verbal, performance, and full-scale ability, with scaled subtest scores permitting specific skill assessment

Questions 37.11–37.13

Which test would usually be most helpful in the psychiatric evaluation of a child who presents with the described symptoms?

A. WISC-III
B. Child Behavior Checklist
C. Children's Apperception Test (CAT)

37.11 A 6 year old is highly aggressive and becomes very angry when he doesn't get his way. He has always been prone to severe tantrums and has difficulty with his behavior and mood in school. At home, he is considered manageable, although he seems to have a short attention span. He breaks new toys in a matter of minutes. He is unable to play with peers because of frequent fighting.

37.12 A 9 year old is clingy with her mother and will not speak to strangers. She is willing to answer specific questions but not to describe her thoughts or feelings. When she is stressed, she tends to withdraw and become tearful. She seems to be unusually sensitive to criticism and will not join in a group activity.

37.13 A 7 year old is reported to be unable to follow directions, is clumsy and slow, and has a poor vocabulary. Although he is friendly and good natured, he has been brutally picked on by peers, who say that he doesn't understand the rules of games. His teacher is concerned about his comprehension.

Questions 37.14–37.19

A. Structured interviews
B. Semistructured interviews
C. Both
D. Neither

37.14 Resemble clinical interviews more closely
37.15 Less costly to administer
37.16 K-SADS (Kiddie Schedule for Affective Disorders and Schizophrenia) and CAS (Child Assessment Scale)
37.17 Particularly appropriate for clinically based research in which subtle diagnostic distinctions may be critical for defining samples
37.18 Investigate issues of prevalence of disorders, developmental patterns of psychopathology, and psychosocial correlates designed to be used by highly trained clinical interviewers
37.19 Designed to be used by highly trained clinical interviewers

DIRECTIONS: Each of the questions or incomplete statements below is followed by five suggested responses or completions. Select the *one* that is *best* in each case.

37.20 Techniques that are helpful in eliciting information and feelings from a school-aged child include all of the following *except*

A. asking multiple-choice questions
B. asking the child to draw a family
C. using Donald Winnicott's squiggle game
D. using only open-ended questions
E. using indirect commentary

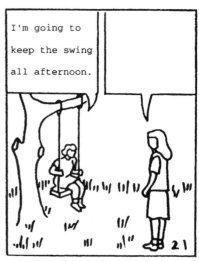

FIGURE 37.1
Courtesy of Saul Rosenzweig.

37.21 Which of the following statements about personality tests for children is true?

A. Personality tests and tests of ability have equal reliability and validity.
B. Both the Children's Apperception Test (CAT) and the Thematic Apperception Test (TAT) use pictures of people in situations.
C. The Rorschach test has not been developed for children or adolescents.
D. The Mooney Problem Check List is a self-report inventory.
E. None of the above

37.22 Figure 37.1 is part of a series of drawings used to test children for

A. depression
B. elation
C. frustration
D. anger
E. all of the above

37.23 Neurological soft signs include all of the following *except*

A. contralateral overflow movements
B. learning disabilities
C. asymmetry of gait
D. nystagmus
E. poor balance

37.24 Minor physical anomalies include all of the following *except*

A. multiple hair whorls
B. low-set ears
C. high-arched palate
D. partial syndactyly of several toes
E. Babinski reflex

ANSWERS

Child Psychiatry: Assessment, Examination, and Psychological Testing

37.1 The answer is A

The psychiatric assessment of the child requires a comprehensive approach that evaluates the child's developmental progress in various domains and positive adaptive capacities, as well as the presence of symptoms of specific disorders. A developmental approach to the assessment of the child is essential because children differ from adults in key respects.

First, psychiatric disturbances in children often consist of a lack of developmental progress in one or more domains, rather than the presence of specific symptoms that are pathognomonic of adult disorders. For example, a nursery school child's failure to develop useful social language or interactions or a school-aged child's inability to meet the developmental expectation of separating from parents and settling into the school day may prompt the parent, school, or both to request an assessment.

Second, the child's developmental status may affect the clinical presentation of various syndromes. For example, in children, *depression often presents with irritability and somatic complaints, while excessive guilt or depressive delusions are rare.*

Third, development brings expectable periods in which *distressing emotions or impairing behavior may occur as part of a normal transition,* for example, the separation anxiety of a child starting preschool or the oppositionality of the adolescent.

In many cases, clinical conditions represent severe forms of symptoms found in milder form in nonreferred children. *Fears, tantrums, moodiness,* or restlessness *are relatively common in childhood and occur transiently at different stages.* Assessment may be sought by concerned parents needing guidance on how to understand and manage these developmental manifestations. Thus, the clinician must judge whether the behavior is likely to resolve with time and without substantial deleterious impact on the child or family or whether, instead, the level of distress, compromised functioning, or symptom persistence indicates the need for clinical intervention.

To distinguish transient or normative difficulties from those that are more clinically worrisome, the evaluator must possess a solid knowledge of both normal and abnormal child development. This developmental frame of reference includes an understanding of what behaviors can be expected normally in children of different ages, the time frame within which various behaviors normally wax and wane, and the natural history of psychiatric disturbances at different stages in development, including knowledge of the ages at which particular syndromes are more or less likely to present.

Another difference in the adult and child psychiatric assessment is that many children coming to clinical attention have difficulties that cannot be subsumed neatly under the rubric of a single diagnostic label. *Thus, comorbidity is usually not the exception but the rule in childhood disorders.* Even in epidemiological studies of children and adolescents, as many as half of those who meet diagnostic criteria for one disorder also meet criteria for at least one other disorder. This high rate of comorbidity, found even in nonreferred populations, may have several sources. Many traditional nosological entities draw their definition from clinical experience with adults; although childhood analogues clearly exist, the appropriate descriptive boundaries may not be the same.

37.2 The answer is C

Children under 7 years of age have limited capacities to verbally recount their feelings or interpersonal interactions. For these younger children as well as a number of older ones, play is a useful adjunct to direct questioning and discussion and is often a less challenging mode for the child. Some children find it easier to communicate in displacement; thus, imaginative play with puppets, small figures, or dolls can provide the interviewer with useful inferential material about the child's concerns, perceptions, and characteristic modes of regulating affects and impulses.

The skilled interviewer will facilitate the child's engagement in play, without prematurely introducing speculations or reactions that might distort or cut short the presentation of certain types of material. During the course of play, the clinician follows the sequences of play content, noting themes that emerge, points at which a child backs away from the story line or shifts to a new sequence or activity, and situations in which the child gets stuck or falls into a repetitive loop. To facilitate the play component of an interview, the interview room should have a supply of human and animal figures or dolls and appropriate *props.* These *should be relatively simple, since elaborate toys can become distractions* rather than serve as vehicles for the expression of the child's fantasies. *Stock characters (such as Barbie or Disney characters) may impose their own specific story lines and thus limit access to the child's own concerns.*

Not only is the content of the child's play a rich source of information, careful observation of the form of play also provides important information for the mental status examination. During imaginative play, the clinician can observe the child's coordination and motor capacities, speech and language development, attention span, readiness to engage the interviewer, capacity for complex thought, and affective state. Absence of imaginative play or limited, concrete, noninteractive play may indicate a pervasive developmental disorder.

Games such as cards or board games are useful for putting the child at ease and developing rapport. These provide opportunities to observe the degree of the child's engagement in and enjoyment of the shared activity; how the child manages competition, including reactions to winning or losing; or whether the child is prone to cheating. Some play activities (e.g., throwing a ball back and forth or easy card games such as war) are simple enough to permit ongoing conversation, while helping to discharge tension and diminish the pressures of the interview situation. *As with toys, elaborate games (e.g., chess) should be avoided;* games that demand much cognitive energy and concentration usually preclude discussion of issues relevant to the assessment and may become a means of avoiding issues involved with the child's difficulties.

37.3 The answer is E (all)

In addition to imaginative play, projective techniques often help provide an indirect picture of concerns that the child may be reluctant or unable to report directly. These techniques can help the child feel more comfortable with the clinician, are often experienced as fun, and may provide access to concerns that are important to the diagnostic formulation.

One commonly used technique is picture drawing. The child can be asked to draw a picture, leaving the choice of subject up to the child or, alternatively, be given a specific suggestion (e.g., draw a person or the child's family doing something). When the picture is finished or nearly so, it is helpful to compliment the child's effort and express interest in what is happening in the drawing. The child's elaboration provides information that may not be readily apparent from the drawing itself. Both the content and form of the drawing offer a window on the child's emotional concerns and aspects of intellectual and visuomotor development. For example, the relative size and placement or omission of family members in a family drawing may be important nonverbal indicators of the child's perceptions or feelings about the family. Aggressive or sexual themes may be reflected more readily in drawings than in words. Self-image may be indicated through depiction of the child as nonhuman, grotesque, inconsequential, or of the opposite gender. The clinician should become familiar with the developmental progression and norms for human figure details, such as limbs, joints, facial features, and clothing, which can provide a useful rough estimate of intellectual maturity. Various systems have been developed for assessing the cognitive and emotional aspects of children's drawings. Also, the child's behavior and speech while drawing may yield valuable information (e.g., throwing the picture away unfinished and saying that it is no good).

Frequently used verbal projective techniques are asking what animal the child would most or least like to be or whom the child would pick to take along to a desert island. *It is useful to ask what the child would do with three magic wishes*; if elaboration is needed, the clinician can explain that the wishes could be to have anything, to have the world be any way, or to change oneself in any way. Children's responses are often revealing. Some may needily or impulsively wish for material possessions, such as a video game or a million dollars. Other responses may reveal longings to change distressing circumstances, such as "for my mom and dad to get back together again," "not to have tics anymore or get teased about them," or "to have a dad who doesn't yell at me all the time." Still other children appear uncomfortable wishing for something for themselves, preferring instead seemingly altruistic responses, such as "no more poverty or wars." Children's responses can be used as the starting point for further exploration. For example, the child who wishes for "a big house and lots of money," may be asked who else would live there and what they would do. Children who wish for "no more fighting in the world" can be asked if there are some particular fights that they would especially like to stop.

Some interactive imaginative techniques useful to interviewers comfortable with them provide elements of playing a game, which may appeal to the child. The squiggle drawing game developed by Donald Winnicott consists of the clinician drawing a curvy line and asking the child to turn it into a picture of something; the child then draws a curvy line that the therapist elaborates, and so on, taking turns. *The Despert fables* are a series of incomplete affectively evocative stories that the child is asked to complete.

Asking the child to tell about a dream, book, movie, or television program can provide information about the child's interests and preoccupations. (If the clinician is familiar with the plot, the distortions the child may introduce can be informative regarding the child's cognitive and emotional style.) Inquiring about what the child would like to do for a living when grown up can provide insight into the child's aspirations, values, and concerns as well as those of the child's family.

37.4 The answer is B

A variety of instruments exist for the structured assessment of infants and young children, and each has somewhat different goals, theoretical orientation, and psychometric properties. *These instruments do not yield diagnoses;* they detail the child's development in various areas relative to a normative population. For example, the *Denver Developmental Screening Test (Denver II)* is suitable for screening use by pediatricians or trained paraprofessionals to help identify children with significant motor, social, or language delays who need fuller evaluation. Population-specific norms are also available for assessing children from families of various ethnic or educational backgrounds. *The Bayley Scales of Infant Development II*, which are administered by a trained assessor, can be used to assess children 1 to 42 months of age; they include a mental scale (assessing information processing, habituation, memory, language, social skills, and cognitive strategies); a motor scale assessing gross and fine motor skills; and a Behavior Rating Scale for assessing qualitative aspects of the child's behavior during the assessment. This well-standardized instrument yields standard scores for a Mental Development Index and Psychomotor Development Index.

Although tests such as the Bayley Scales may show good (not moderate) reliability and concurrent validity, their ability to predict later performance on intelligence quotient (IQ) assessments or later adaptive functioning is highly variable. Among the reasons for this weakness of prediction are the intervening effects of social and family environment and the heavy emphasis infant tests place on perceptual and motor skills that may have relatively little to do with information-processing capacities.

The mental status examination of the infant and young child may be organized using a schema such that shown in Table 37.1.

37.5 The answer is D

The clinical utility and cost effectiveness of routine laboratory tests for children who present with psychiatric problems has not been thoroughly studied. Most guidelines for performing these tests for children have historically been developed using data from studies of adults. Adult studies generally suggest that routine laboratory tests are not clinically useful in such typical psychiatric settings as outpatient clinics and most inpatient units. Laboratory screening tests are of some use in psychiatric settings where patients are at high risk for medical illness, such as the emergency room, substance abuse treatment centers, acquired immune deficiency syndrome (AIDS) clinics, and geriatric clinics, as well as for patients who have new-onset psychosis, depression, or dementia. Similarly, routine screening laboratory measures are more likely to yield clinically significant information when clinical symptoms of physical illness are present.

The few studies of the use of routine laboratory tests in child psychiatry patient populations have yielded similar conclusions. One review of routine laboratory screenings (*thyroid function tests, electroencephalograms [EEG]*, chest X-ray, chemistry panel, urinalysis, complete blood count, electrocardiogram, and rapid plasma reagin) in 100 consecutive adolescent inpatient admissions reported variable rates of abnormal values, depending on the specific test, but in only 1 of these 100

Table 37.1
Infant and Toddler Mental Status Exam by Anne L. Benham, M.D.

I. Appearance

Size, level of nourishment, dress and hygiene, apparent maturity compared with age, dysmorphic features (e.g., facies, eye and ear shape and placement, epicanthal folds, digits), abnormal head size, cutaneous lesions.

II. Apparent Reaction to Situation

Note where evaluation takes place and with whom.

A. Initial reaction to setting and to strangers: explores; freezes; cries; hides face; acts curious, excited, apathetic, or anxious (describe).

B. Adaptation

1. Exploration: when and how child begins exploring faces, toys, stranger.

2. Reaction to transitions: from unstructured to structured activity; when examiner begins to play with infant; cleaning up; leaving.

III. Self-Regulation

A. State regulation: an infant's state of consciousness ranges from deep sleep through alert stages to intense crying. Predominant state and range of states observed during session; patterns of transition (e.g., smooth versus abrupt) capacity for being soothed and self-soothing; capacity for quiet alert state. (Some of these categories also apply to toddlers.)

B. Sensory regulation: reaction to sounds, sights, smells, light and firm touch; hyperresponsiveness or hyporesponsiveness (if observed) and type of response, including apathy, withdrawal, avoidance, fearfulness, excitability, aggression or marked behavioral change; excessive seeking of particular sensory input.

C. Unusual behaviors; mouthing after 1 year of age; head banging; smelling objects; spinning; twirling; hand-flapping; finger-flicking; rocking; toe-walking; staring at lights or spinning objects; repetitive, perseverative, or bizarre verbalizations or behaviors with objects or people; hair-pulling; ruminating; or breath-holding.

D. Activity level: overall level and variability (note that toddlers are often incorrectly called hyperactive). Describe behavior, e.g., squirming constantly in parent's arms; sitting quietly on floor or in infant seat; constantly on the go; climbing on desk and cabinets; exploring the room; pausing to play with each of six to eight toys.

E. Attention span: capacity to maintain attentiveness to an activity or interaction; longest and average length of sustained attention to a given toy or activity; distractibility. Infants: visual fixing and following at 1 month; tracking at 2 to 3 months; attention to own hands or feet and faces; duration of exploration of object with hands or mouth.

F. Frustration tolerance: ability to persist in a difficult task, despite failure; capacity to delay reaction if easily frustrated, e.g., aggression, crying, tantrums, withdrawal, avoidance.

G. Aggression: modes of expression; degree of control of or preoccupation with aggression; appropriate assertiveness.

IV. Motor

Muscle tone and strength; mobility in different positions; unusual motor pattern (e.g., tics, seizure activity), intactness of cranial nerves (e.g., movement of face, mouth, tongue, and eyes, including feeding, swallowing, and gaze [note excessive drooling]).

A. Gross motor coordination. Infants: pushing up; head control; rolling; sitting; standing. Toddlers: walking; running; jumping; climbing; hopping; kicking; throwing and catching a ball. (It is useful to have something for the child to climb on, such as a chair.)

B. Fine motor coordination. Infants: grasping and releasing; transferring from hand to hand; using pincer grasp; banging; throwing. Toddlers: using pincer grasp; stacking; scribbling; cutting. Both fine motor and visual-motor coordination can be screened by observing how the child handles puzzles, shape boxes, a ball and hammer toy, small cars, and toys with connecting parts.

V. Speech and Language

A. Vocalization and speech production: quality, rate, rhythm, intonation, articulation, volume.

B. Receptive language: comprehension of others' speech as seen in verbal or behavioral response (e.g., follows commands); points in response to "where is" questions; understands prepositions and pronouns (include estimate of hearing, especially in child with language delay, e.g., response to loud sounds and voice; ability to localize sound).

C. Expressive language; level of complexity (e.g., vocalization, jargon, number of single words, short phrases, full sentences); overgeneralization (e.g., uses "kitty" to refer to all animals); pronoun use including reversal; echolalia, either immediate or delayed; unusual or bizarre verbalizations. Preverbal children: communicative intent (e.g., vocalizations, babbling, imitation, gestures, such as head shaking and pointing; caregiver's ability to understand infant's communication; child's effectiveness in communication.

VI. Thought

The usual categories for thought disorder almost never apply to young children. Primary process thinking, as evidenced in verbalizations or play, is expected in this age group. The line between fantasy and reality is often blurred. Bizarre ideation; perseveration; apparent loose associations; and the persistence of pronoun reversals, jargon, and echolalia in an older toddler or preschooler may be noted in a variety of psychiatric disorders, including pervasive developmental disorders.

A. Specific fears: feared object; worry about being lost or separated from parent.

B. Dreams and nightmares: content is sometimes obtainable in children aged 2 to 3 years. Child does not always perceive it as a dream (e.g., "A monster came in the front door").

C. Dissociative state: sudden episodes of withdrawal and inattention; eyes glazed; "tuned out"; failure to track ongoing social interaction. Dissociative state may be difficult to differentiate from an absence seizure, depression, autism, or deafness. The context may be helpful (e.g., child with a history of neglect freezes in a dissociative state as mother leaves room). Neurological or audiological evaluation may be warranted.

D. Hallucinations: extremely rare, except in the context of a toxic or medical disorder, then usually visual or tactile.

(continued)

Table 37.1 (*continued*)

VII. Affect and Mood

The assessment of mood and affect may be more difficult in young children because of limited language; lack of vocabulary for emotions; and use of withdrawal in response to a variety of emotions from shyness and boredom to anxiety and depression.

A. Modes of expression: facial; verbal; body tone and positioning.

B. Range of expressed emotions: affect, especially in parent–child relationship.

C. Responsiveness: to situation, content of discussion, play, and interpersonal engagement.

D. Duration of emotional state: need history or multiple observations.

E. Intensity of expressed emotions: affect, especially in parent–child relationship.

VIII. Play

Play is a primary mode of information gathering for all sections of the Infant and Toddler Mental Status Exam. In very young children, play is especially useful in the evaluation of the child's cognitive and symbolic functioning, relatedness, and expression of affect. Themes of play are helpful in assessing older toddlers. The management and expression of aggression are assessed in play as in other areas of behavior. Play may be with toys or with child's own or another's body (e.g., peek-a-boo, roughhousing); verbal (e.g., sound imitation games between mother and infant); interactional or solitary. It is important to note how the child's play varies with different familiar caregivers and with parents versus the examiner.

A. Structure of play (ages approximate).

　1. Sensorimotor play:

　　a. (0–12 months): mouthing, banging, dropping and throwing toys or other objects.

　　b. (6–12 months): exploring characteristics of objects (e.g., moving parts, poking, pulling).

　2. Functional play.

　　a. (12–18 months): child's use of objects shows understanding and exploration of their use or function (e.g., pushes car, touches comb to hair, puts telephone to ear).

　3. Early symbolic play.

　　a. (18 months and older): child pretends with increasing complexity; pretends with own body to eat or sleep; pretends with objects or other people (e.g., "feeds" mother); child uses one object to represent another, e.g., a block becomes a car; child pretends a sequence of activities (e.g., cooking and eating).

　4. Complex symbolic play.

　　a. (30 months and older): child plans and acts out dramatic play sequences, uses imaginary objects. Later, child incorporates others into play with assigned roles.

　5. Imitation, turn taking, and problem solving as part of play.

B. Content of play. The toddler's choice and use of toys often reflect emotional themes. It is desirable to have on hand toys that tap different developmental and emotional domains. An overfull playroom may be overwhelming or overstimulating and reduce meaningful observations. Young toddlers of both sexes often gravitate to dolls, dishes, animals, and moving toys, such as cars. The examiner's choice of specific materials may facilitate the expression of pertinent emotional themes. For example, a child traumatized by a dog bite may more likely reenact the trauma if a dog and doll figures are available. The child's reaction to scary toys, such as sharks, dinosaurs, or guns, should be noted, especially if they are avoided or dominate the session. Does aggressive pretend play become "real" and physically hurtful? By age 2½ to 3 years, a child's animal or doll play can reveal important themes about family life, including reactions to separation, parent–child and sibling relationships, experiences at day care, quality of nurturance and discipline, and physical or sexual abuse. The examiner must use caution in interpreting play, viewing it as a possible combination of reenactment, fears, and fantasy.

IX. Cognition

Using information from all above areas, especially play, verbal and symbolic functioning, and problem-solving, roughly assess child's cognitive level in terms of developmental intactness, delays, or precocity.

X. Relatedness

A. To parents: how in tune do the child and parent seem? Does the child make and maintain eye, verbal, or physical contact? Is there active avoidance by child? Note infant's level of comfort and relaxation being held, fed, "molding" into caregiver's body. Does toddler move away from caregiver and check back or bring toys to show, to put into his or her lap, to play with together or near caregiver? Comment on physical or verbal affection, hostility, reaction to separation and reunion, and use of transitional objects (blanket, toy, caregiver's possession). Describe differences in relating if more than one caregiver is present.

B. To examiner: young children normally show some hesitancy to engage with a stranger, especially after 6 to 8 months of age. Appropriate wariness in young children may result in a period of watching the examiner; staying physically close to a familiar caregiver before engaging; or showing some constriction of affect, vocalization, or play. After initial wariness, does the child relate? Does the child engage too soon or not at all? How does relatedness with a stranger compare to that with a parent? Is the child friendly versus indiscriminately attention-seeking, guarded versus overanxious? Can examiner engage the child in play or structured activities to a degree not seen with caregiver? Does the child show pleasure in successes if the examiner shows approval?

C. Attachment behaviors: observe for showing affection, comfort-seeking, asking for and accepting help, cooperating, exploring, controlling behavior, and reunion responses. Describe age-related disturbances in these normative behaviors. Disturbances often are seen in abused and neglected children, e.g., fearfulness, clinginess, overcompliance, hypervigilance, impulsive overactivity, and defiance; restricted or hyperactive and distractible exploratory behavior; and restricted or indiscriminate affection and comfort-seeking.

Reprinted with permission from American Academy of Child and Adolescent Psychiatry. Practice parameter on psychiatric assessment of infants and toddlers (0–36 months). *J Am Acad Child Adolesc Psychiatry.* 1997;36(Suppl):21S.

patients did the tests produce a change in diagnosis from functional to organic—and even then the diagnostic information proved to have little clinical relevance. Most laboratory abnormalities in this study were regarded as minor and did not indicate a need for clinical follow-up.

More specialized diagnostic laboratory evaluations (EEG, *computed tomography [CT]* or *magnetic resonance imaging [MRI]*) also provide a relatively low yield of clinically useful information. In a study of 200 consecutive child psychiatric inpatients, these evaluations were done only when "clinically indicated"; despite their judicious use, the tests provided clinically relevant information in only 7 patients (3.5 percent of the total patient sample), or in 7 of 136 tests (5.1 percent of all tests performed). *Chromosomal analyses proved to be the most informative of all these tests,* yielding new medical diagnoses in 5 of 32 (15.6 percent of selected children for whom they were performed). A study of 111 putatively high-risk inpatients with new-onset adolescent psychoses produced similar conclusions. In this population, routine endocrine and neuroimaging screening evaluations failed to provide information of diagnostic utility in any patient (although inconsequential laboratory abnormalities were present in 15.4 percent of the neuroendocrine screens and 11 percent of the neuroimaging screening tests). More specialized neuroimaging technologies, such as positron emission tomography (PET), single photon emission computed tomography (SPECT), functional MRI (fMRI), and brain electrical activity mapping (BEAM) currently have no routine clinical or diagnostic utility in child and adolescent psychiatric populations.

Answers 37.6–37.10

37.6 The answer is D

37.7 The answer is A

37.8 The answer is B

37.9 The answer is C

37.10 The answer is E
The Vineland Adaptive Behavior Scales are used to measure communication, daily living skills, socialization, and motor development, yielding a composite expressed in a standard score, percentiles, and age equivalents. The scales are standardized for normal and mentally retarded people. A measure of adaptive function, as well as a standardized measure of intelligence, is a prerequisite when a diagnosis of mental retardation is being considered.

The *Children's Apperception Test* (CAT) is an adaptation for children of the Thematic Apperception Test (TAT). The CAT *generates stories from picture cards of animals that reflect interpersonal functioning.* The cards show ambiguous scenes related to family issues and relationships. The child is asked to describe what is happening and to tell a story about the outcome of the scene in the card. Animals are used because it was hypothesized that children respond more readily to animal images than to human figures.

The *Wide-Range Achievement Test-Revised (WRAT-R) measures functioning in reading, spelling, and arithmetic, with resulting grade levels, percentiles, and standard scores.* It can be used in children 5 years of age and older. It yields a score that is compared with the average expected score for the child's chronological age and grade level.

The Peabody Picture Vocabulary Test-Revised (PPVT-R) *measures receptive word understanding, with resulting standard scores, percentiles, and age equivalents.* It can be used for children 4 years of age and older. The *Wechsler Intelligence Scale for Children—Third Edition* (WISC-III), the most widely used test of intelligence for school-aged children, *measures verbal, performance, and full-scale ability, with scaled subtest scores permitting specific skill assessment.* In a full-scale intelligence quotient (IQ), 70 to 80 indicates borderline intelligence, 80 to 90 indicates low-average intelligence, 90–109 indicates average intelligence, and 110 to 119 indicates high-average intelligence. Table 37.2 lists some commonly used child and adolescent assessment instruments.

Answers 37.11–37.13

37.11 The answer is B

37.12 The answer is C

37.13 The answer is A
The *Child Behavior Checklist* can be very helpful in the evaluation of a 6-year-old child with multiple behavior problems, especially if the child presents with different symptoms in different settings, such as in school and at home. The Child Behavior Checklist provides a broad range of symptoms that relate to academic and social competence. There is a parent version and a teacher version so that the reports of these two observers may be compared. The child behavior checklist can help to systematically identify the problem symptoms related to mood, frustration tolerance, hyperactivity, oppositional behavior, and anxiety. For a child who has a variety of symptoms that span many diagnostic categories, a broad rating scale can be very helpful.

The *Children's Apperception Test (CAT)* consists of cards with pictures of animals in ambiguous situations that show scenes related to parent–child and sibling issues. The child is asked to describe what is happening in the scenes. Animals are felt to be less threatening to children who have difficulties speaking about emotional issues. For this 9-year-old girl who is inhibited and has difficulty disclosing her thoughts and feelings, the use of a projective but structured test such as the CAT can often be a conduit to helping these disclosures.

The *WISC-III (The Wechsler Intelligence Scale for Children—Third Edition) is the most widely used test of intellectual function.* Used in children from 6 to 17 years old, it provides information in a variety of verbal areas (vocabulary, similarities, general information, arithmetic, and comprehension), as well as testing abilities in the areas of performance (block design, picture completion, picture arrangement, object assembly, coding, and mazes). For a 7-year-old child who appears to be globally slow, unable to understand directions, follow rules, or comprehend tasks in the classroom, a test of intellectual function is indicated. The WISC-III will yield a full-scale IQ, a verbal IQ, and a performance IQ

Answers 37.14–37.19

37.14 The answer is B

37.15 The answer is A

37.16 The answer is B

37.17 The answer is B

Table 37.2
Commonly Used Child and Adolescent Psychological Assessment Instruments

Test	Age/Grades	Data Generated and Comments
Intellectual ability		
Wechsler Intelligence Scale for Children—Third Edition (WISC-III-R)	6–16	Standard scores: verbal, performance and full-scale IQ: scaled subtest scores permitting specific skill assessment.
Wechsler Adult Intelligence Scale—(WAIS-III)	16–adult	Same as WISC-III-R.
Wechsler Preschool and Primary Scale of Intelligence—Revised (WPPSI-R)	3–7	Same as WISC-III-R.
Kaufman Assessment Battery for Children (K-ABC)	2.6–12.6	Well grounded in theories of cognitive psychology and neuropsychology. Allows immediate comparison of intellectual capacity with acquired knowledge. Scores: Mental Processing Composite (IQ equivalent); sequential and simultaneous processing and achievement standard scores; scaled mental processing and achievement subtest scores; age equivalents; percentiles.
Kaufman Adolescent and Adult Intelligence Test (KAIT)	11–85+	Composed of separate Crystallized and Fluid scales. Scores: Composite Intelligence Scale; Crystallized and Fluid IQ; scaled subtest scores; percentiles.
Stanford-Binet, 4th Edition (SB:FE)	2–23	Scores: IQ; verbal, abstract/visual, and quantitative reasoning; short-term memory; standard age.
Peabody Picture Vocabulary Test—III (PPVT-III)	4–adult	Measures receptive vocabulary acquisition; standard scores, percentiles, age equivalents.
Achievement		
Woodcock-Johnson Psycho-Educational Battery—Revised (W-J)	K–12	Scores: reading and mathematics (mechanics and comprehension), written language, other academic achievement; grade and age scores, standard scores, percentiles.
Wide Range Achievement Test—3, Levels 1 and 2 (WRAT-3)	Level 1: 1–5 Level 2: 12–75	Permits screening for deficits in reading, spelling, and arithmetic; grade levels, percentiles, stanines, standard scores.
Kaufman Test of Educational Achievement, Brief and Comprehensive Forms (K-TEA)	1–12	Standard scores: reading, mathematics, and spelling; grade and age equivalents, percentiles, stanines. Brief Form is sufficient for most clinical applications; Comprehensive Form allows error analysis and more detailed curriculum planning.
Wechsler Individual Achievement Test (WIAT)	K–12	Standard scores: basic reading, mathematics reasoning, spelling (constituting Screener); reading comprehension, numerical operations, listening comprehension, oral expression, written expression. Conormal with WISC-III-R.
Adaptive behavior		
Vineland Adaptive Behavior Scales	Normal: 0–19 Retarded: All ages	Standard scores: adaptive behavior composite and communication, daily living skills, socialization and motor domains; percentiles, age equivalents, developmental age scores. Separate standardization groups for normal, visually handicapped, hearing impaired, emotionally disturbed, and retarded.
Scales of Independent Behavior—Revised	Newborn–adult	Standard scores: five adaptive (motor, social interaction, communication, personal living, community living) and three maladaptive (internalized, asocial, and externalized) areas; General Maladaptive Index and Broad Independence cluster.
Attentional capacity		
Trail Making Test	8–adult	Standard scores, standard deviations, ranges; corrections for age and education.
Wisconsin Card Sorting Test	6.6–adult	Standard scores, standard deviations, T-scores, percentiles, developmental norms for number of categories achieved, perseverative errors, and failures to maintain set; computer measures.
Behavior Assessment System for Children (BASC)	4–18	Teacher and parent rating scales and child self-report of personality permitting multireporter assessment across a variety of domains in home, school, and community. Provides validity, clinical, and adaptive scales. ADHD component avails.
Home Situations Questionnaire—Revised (HSQ-R)	6–12	Permits parents to rate child's specific problems with attention or concentration. Scores for number of problem settings, mean severity, and factor scores for compliance and leisure situations.
ADHD Rating Scale	6–12	Score for number of symptoms keyed to DSM cutoff for diagnosis of ADHD; standard scores permit derivation of clinical significance for total score and two factors (Inattentive-Hyperactive and Impulsive-Hyperactive).

(continued)

Table 37.2 (*continued*)

Test	Age/Grades	Data Generated and Comments
School Situations Questionnaire (SSQ-R)	6–12	Permits teachers to rate a child's specific problems with attention or concentration. Scores for number of problem settings and mean severity.
Child Attention Profile (CAP)	6–12	Brief measure allowing teachers' weekly ratings of presence and degree of child's inattention and overactivity. Normative scores for inattention, overactivity, and total score.
Projective tests		
Rorschach Inkblots	3–adult	Special scoring systems. Most recently developed and increasingly universally accepted is John Exner's Comprehensive System (1974). Assesses perceptual accuracy, integration of affective and intellectual functioning, reality testing, and other psychological processes.
Thematic Apperception Test (TAT)	6–adult	Generates stories which are analyzed qualitatively. Assumed to provide especially rich data regarding interpersonal functioning.
Machover Draw-A-Person Test (DAP)	3–adult	Qualitative analysis and hypothesis generation, especially regarding subject's feelings about self and significant others.
Kinetic Family Drawing (KFD)	3–adult	Qualitative analysis and hypothesis generation regarding an individual's perception of family structure and sentient environment. Some objective scoring systems in existence.
Rotter Incomplete Sentences Blank	Child, adolescent, and adult forms	Primarily qualitative analysis, although some objective scoring systems have been developed.
Personality tests		
Minnesota Multiphasic Personality Inventory-Adolescent (MMPI-A)	14–18	1992 version of widely used personality measure, developed specifically for use with adolescents. Standard scores: three validity scales, 14 clinical scales, additional content and supplementary scales.
Million Adolescent Personality Inventory (MAPI)	13–18	Standard scores for 20 scales grouped into three categories: Personality styles; expressed concerns; behavioral correlates. Normed on adolescent population. Focuses on broad functional spectrum, not just problem areas. Measures 14 primary personality traits, including emotional stability, self-concept level, excitability, and self-assurance.
Children's Personality Questionnaire	8–12	Generates combined broad trait patterns including extraversion and anxiety.
Neuropsychological screening tests and test batteries		
Developmental Test of Visual-Motor Integration (VMI)	2–16	Screening instrument for visual motor deficits. Standard scores, age equivalents, percentiles.
Benton Visual Retention Test	6–adult	Assesses presence of deficits in visual-figure memory. Mean scores by age.
Benton Visual Motor Gestalt Test	5–adult	Assesses visual-motor deficits and visual-figural retention. Age equivalents.
Reitan-Indiana Neuropsychological Test Battery for Children	5–8	Cognitive and perceptual-motor tests for children with suspected brain damage.
Halstead-Reitan Neuropsychological Test Battery for Older Children	9–14	Same as Reitan-Indiana.
Luria-Nebraska Neuropsychological Battery: Children's Revision (LNNB:C)	8–12	Sensory-motor, perceptual, cognitive tests measuring 11 clinical and two additional domains of neuropsychological functioning. Provides standard scores.
Developmental status		
Bayley Scales of Infant Development—Second Edition	16 days–42 months	Mental, motor, and behavior scales measuring infant development. Provides standard scores.
Mullen Scales of Early Learning	Newborn–5 years	Language and visual scales for receptive and expressive ability. Yields age scores and T scores.

Adapted from Racusin G, Moss N. Psychological assessment of children and adolescents. In: Lewis M, ed. *Child and Adolescent Psychiatry: A Comprehensive Textbook*. Baltimore: Williams & Wilkins; 1991.

37.18 The answer is A

37.19 The answer is B

Available diagnostic interviews differ from each other in several respects. A fundamental one is the degree of structure that is built into the interview. Interviews range from highly structured instruments that specify the exact order and wording of all components to semistructured interviews that delineate the symptoms to be covered and suggest phrases that may be used but permit much latitude in the order and phrasing of questions. The degree of structure reflects the intended use of the interview, the type of interviewer who will administer it, and the cost of using it in a study.

On a continuum of structure, *semistructured interviews resemble clinical interviews more closely than do structured interviews*, but they nevertheless differ substantially in style and content from a true clinical assessment. *Semistructured interviews are designed to be administered by interviewers with clinical training* or with very intensive training in the assessment of symptoms covered by the measure (e.g., the Child and Adolescent Psychiatric Assessment). The flexible structure of the interview allows the clinically informed interviewer some freedom in the manner of inquiry and permits judgments about whether a reported behavior or expression of distress is of the quality and severity required to be considered a symptom. Some structure is needed to ensure that symptom inquiry is complete, and the interviewer is also required to make specified ratings that can be compared and aggregated across the sample. *Interviews of this type include the many versions of the Kiddie Schedule for Affective Disorders and Schizophrenia (K-SADS), the Child Assessment Scale, (CAS)*, the Interview Schedule for Children (ISC), the Child and Adolescent Psychiatric Assessment (CAPA), and the recent forms of the Diagnostic Interview for Children and Adolescents (DICA). *Semistructured interviews are more costly to administer* than highly structured ones, but *they are particularly appropriate for clinically based research in which subtle diagnostic distinctions may be critical for defining samples* and where sample sizes are small enough to justify the expense of hiring interviewers trained to make these judgments.

Structured interviews, on the other hand, provide highly specified protocols that are particularly useful for epidemiological studies in which large sample sizes (i.e., in the thousands) require using many nonclinician interviewers. These studies *investigate issues of prevalence of disorders, developmental patterns of psychopathology, psychosocial correlates*, and risk and protective factors, topics that often require large samples to provide enough statistical power to examine study hypotheses. Because using highly trained interviewers often becomes prohibitively expensive, considerable effort has been devoted to the development of highly structured techniques. In recent years, the bulk of this work has focused on writing and testing the Diagnostic Interview Schedule for Children (DISC), which has proceeded through several rounds of methodological testing in clinical and community samples.

37.20 The answer is D

Open-ended questions can overwhelm a school-aged child and result in withdrawal or a shrugging of the shoulders; multiple-choice questions and partially open-ended questions may elicit more information from a school-aged child. If a child is not adept with verbal skills, *asking the child to draw a family* is often a way to break the ice. Activities such as *Donald Winnicott's squiggle game*, in which the examiner draws a curved line and then takes turns with the child in continuing the drawing, may also help open up communication with the child. *Using indirect commentary*, such as "I once knew a child about your age who felt very sad when he moved away from all his friends . . .," helps elicit feelings from the child, although the clinician must be careful not to lead youngsters into confirming what they think the clinician wants to hear.

37.21 The answer is D

The Mooney Problem Check List is basically a checklist of personal problems. It *is a self-report inventory*: a series of ques-

tions concerning emotional problems, worries, interests, motives, values, and interpersonal traits. The major usefulness of personality inventories is in the screening and identifying of children in need of further evaluation. *Personality tests and tests of ability do not have equal reliability and validity.* Personality tests are much less satisfactory with regard to norms, reliability, and validity. *The Children's Apperception Test (CAT) is different from the adult Thematic Apperception Test (TAT)* in that the TAT uses pictures of people, whereas the CAT uses pictures of animals on the assumption that children respond more readily to animal characters than to people. *The Rorschach test*, one of the most widely used projective techniques, *has been developed for children* between the ages of 2 and 10 years *and for adolescents* between the ages of 10 and 17.

37.22 The answer is C

Figure 37.1 is part of the Rosenzweig Picture-*Frustration* Study. The test presents a series of cartoons in which one person frustrates another. In the blank space provided, the child writes what the frustrated person replies. From that reply, the examiner determines the effect of frustration on the child; the effect can range from extreme passivity to extreme violence. The test is *not used to measure depression, elation*, or *anger*.

37.23 The answer is B

The term neurological soft signs was first used by Lauretta Bender in reference to nondiagnostic abnormalities that are seen in some children with schizophrenia. It is now evident that neurological soft signs do not indicate neurological disorders but are relatively common in children with a wide variety of developmental disabilities. *Learning disabilities* themselves are not neurological soft signs, although children with low intellectual function, learning disabilities, or brain damage are likely to show these signs. Soft signs refer to both behavioral findings, such as severe impulsivity or mood instability, and physical findings, such as persistence of infantile reflexes, mild incoordination, *poor balance, contralateral overflow movements, asymmetry of gait, nystagmus*, and mild choreiform movements. The Physical and Neurological Examination for Soft Signs (Paness), an instrument that is used for children up to 15 years, consists of 15 medical questions and 43 physical tasks such as touching a finger to the nose and hopping tasks. Neurological soft signs are important but are not specific in making a psychiatric diagnosis.

37.24 The answer is E

Minor physical anomalies or dysmorphic features are most frequently seen in children with developmental disabilities, speech and language disorders, learning disorders, and severe hyperactivity. As with neurological soft signs, they are rarely specific in determining a psychiatric diagnosis, but they are important to document in an examination of a child. Minor physical anomalies include *low-set ears, a high-arched palate*, epicanthal folds, hypertelorism, transverse palmar creases, *multiple hair whorls*, a large head, a furrowed tongue, *partial syndactyly of several toes*, and other facial asymmetries. The presence of the *Babinski reflex is a neurological sign rather than a minor physical anomaly*.

38 ▲

Mental Retardation

The revised fourth edition of the *Diagnostic and Statistical Manual of Mental Disorders* (DSM-IV-TR) categorizes mental retardation into four categories according to severity:

Mild: IQ 50–55 to approximately 70
Moderate: IQ 35–40 to 50–55
Severe: IQ 20–25 to 35–40
Profound: IQ below 20–25

Mental retardation, severity unspecified, is diagnosed when there is a strong presumption of mental retardation but the person has not been evaluated by standard intelligence tests. About 85 percent of people with mental retardation fall within the mild range.

Mental retardation must be diagnosed before the age of 18, and involves global deficits in intellectual capacity and functional levels. Similar deficits occurring after the age of 18 will more likely fall into the various categories of dementia. Mental retardation affects approximately 1 percent of the population and is estimated to be 1½ times as common in males as in females. In addition to deficits in intellectual, adaptive, and social functioning, people who are mentally retarded have higher-than-average rates of psychiatric disorders. These may include mood disorders, psychotic disorders, and behavioral disorders. An unresolved issue is the influence of severe parental mental disorders on the development of some mild cases of mental retardation.

There are multiple etiologies of mental retardation. The more severe or profound the deficits the more likely a specific etiology can be identified. For instance, about 75 percent of people with severe mental retardation have known causes for their condition, while no cause can be identified in 75 percent of individuals with borderline intellectual functioning. About half of those individuals with mild mental retardation have a known cause; overall, in up to two-thirds of all mentally retarded persons, a probable cause can be identified.

Established causative factors in mental retardation include genetic conditions (chromosomal and inherited), metabolic abnormalities, perinatal trauma, sociocultural factors, and prenatal exposure to toxins and infections. For instance, fetal alcohol syndrome, resulting from prenatal exposure to alcohol, is associated with microcephaly, cranial malformations, and limb and heart defects. Short adult stature and the development of a range of attention-deficit and learning disorders are present as well. Rubella (German measles) is the major cause of congenital malformations and mental retardation caused by maternal infection. Sociocultural factors that have been described as possibly contributing to the development of mild mental retardation include poverty, which can be associated with poor pre- and postnatal medical care and poor maternal nutrition. Exposure to such toxic substances as lead as well as physical trauma are more common in impoverished families. Teenage pregnancies are associated with obstetrical complications, prematurity, and low birth weight—all factors associated with a risk of mental retardation. More recently, researchers have increasingly recognized the likely contributions of an array of subtle biological factors in the development of mild mental retardation.

Examples of genetic conditions associated with mental retardation include Down's syndrome, fragile X syndrome, and Prader-Willi syndrome. Down's syndrome can be the result of any of three chromosomal aberrations: (1) trisomy 21, the most common abnormality, in which three of chromosome 21 are present; (2) nondisjunction, in which both normal and trisomic cells are found in various tissues; and (3) translocation, in which two chromosomes, usually 21 and 15, fuse. Babies with Down's syndrome are identified by the presence of oblique palpebral fissures, small flattened skull, single palmar crease, high cheekbones, and protruding tongue. Mental retardation is the overriding feature of Down's syndrome, with most affected people being moderately to severely retarded. The incidence of Down's syndrome is about 1 in every 700 births.

Fragile X syndrome is believed to occur in 1 in every 1,000 births. It results from a mutation on the X chromosome at the fragile site. Typically, these individuals have a large and long head, short stature, hyperextensible joints and macro-orchidism after puberty. The degree of mental retardation ranges from mild to severe. People with fragile X syndrome seem to have relatively strong skills in communications and socialization, with their intellectual functions declining in the pubertal period. Prader-Willi syndrome occurs in less than 1 in 10,000 births, and is the result of a small deletion involving chromosome 15. People with this syndrome exhibit compulsive eating behavior, hypogonadism, small stature, hypotonia, obesity, and often oppositional and defiant behavior.

Mental retardation and pervasive developmental disorders, such as autism, often coexist. Seventy to 75 percent of those with pervasive developmental disorders have an IQ of less than 70.

The student should study the questions and answers below for a useful review of this condition.

HELPFUL HINTS

The student should define these terms.

- adaptive functioning
- Bayley Infant Scale of Development
- borderline intellectual functioning
- Cattell Infant Scale
- causative factors
- chromosomal abnormality
- *cri-du-chat* syndrome
- CVS (chorionic villi sampling) and amniocentesis
- degrees of mental retardation (mild, moderate, severe, profound)
- Down's syndrome
- fetal alcohol syndrome
- fragile X syndrome
- intelligence quotient (IQ)
- Lesch-Nyhan syndrome
- mental deficiency
- mental retardation
- neurofibrillary tangles
- neurofibromatosis
- PKU
- Prader-Willi syndrome
- prenatal exposure
- primary, secondary, and tertiary prevention
- rubella
- Special Olympics
- Turner's syndrome
- Vineland Adaptive Behavior Scales
- WHO

▲ QUESTIONS

DIRECTIONS: Each of the questions or incomplete statements below is followed by five suggested responses or completions. Select the *one* that is *best* in each case.

38.1 DSM-IV-TR lists the prevalence of mental retardation in the United States as

A. 1 percent
B. 3 percent
C. 5 percent
D. 6 percent
E. none of the above

38.2 Using IQ as the sole criterion for mental retardation, the prevalence rate is estimated to be

A. 0.5 percent
B. 1 percent
C. 2 percent
D. 3 percent
E. none of the above

38.3 A decline in IQ begins at approximately 10 to 15 years in which of the following disorders?

A. Down's syndrome
B. fragile X syndrome
C. cerebral palsy
D. nonspecific mental retardation
E. none of the above

38.4 The most common inherited cause of mental retardation is

A. Down's syndrome
B. fragile X syndrome
C. fetal alcohol syndrome
D. Prader-Willi syndrome
E. none of the above

38.5 The *least* common disorder associated with fragile X syndrome is

A. autistic disorder
B. schizotypal disorder
C. attention-deficit/hyperactivity disorder
D. avoidant disorders
E. anxiety disorders

38.6 Compared to others with mental retardation, persons with which of the following disorders appear to be less prone to psychiatric disturbance?

A. Down's syndrome
B. Fragile X syndrome
C. Nonspecific type
D. Fetal alcohol syndrome
E. Prader-Willi syndrome

38.7 Mild mental retardation has been associated with

A. nonspecific causes
B. Prader-Willi syndrome
C. females with fragile X syndrome
D. poor socioeconomic background
E. all of the above

38.8 Moderate mental retardation

A. reflects an IQ range of 25 to 40
B. is seen in approximately 3 to 4 percent of persons with mental retardation
C. has an organic etiology in the vast majority of cases
D. usually is associated with the ability to achieve academic skills at the second to third-grade level
E. all of the above

38.9 Common symptoms of anxiety in persons with mental retardation include

A. aggression
B. agitation
C. compulsive or repetitive behaviors
D. self-injury
E. all of the above

DIRECTIONS: Each group of questions below consists of lettered headings followed by a list of numbered words or phrases. For each numbered word or phrase, select the *one* lettered heading that is most closely associated with it. Each lettered heading may be selected once, more than once, or not at all.

Questions 38.10–38.13

    A. Prader-Willi syndrome
    B. Down's syndrome
    C. Fragile X syndrome
    D. Phenylketonuria (PKU)

38.10 Theorized to be due to a deletion in chromosome 15

38.11 Autosomal recessive transmission, phenylalanine hydroxylase deficiency

38.12 Nondisjunction, translocation, or trisomy involving chromosome 21

38.13 Due to a mutation on the X chromosome at Xq27.3

Questions 38.14–38.17

    A. Unknown
    B. Trisomy 21
    C. Autosomal dominant
    D. Autosomal recessive
    E. X-linked semidominant

38.14 Neurofibromatosis

38.15 Tuberous sclerosis

38.16 Crouzon's syndrome

38.17 Cockayne's syndrome

Questions 38.18–38.22

    A. Phenylketonuria (PKU)
    B. Rett's disorder
    C. Acquired immune deficiency syndrome (AIDS)
    D. Rubella
    E. Cytomegalic inclusion disease

38.18 Mental retardation with intracerebral calcifications, jaundice, microcephaly, and hepatosplenomegaly

38.19 Progressive encephalopathy and mental retardation

38.20 An X-linked mental retardation syndrome that is degenerative and affects only females

38.21 Mental retardation, eczema, vomiting, and seizures

38.22 Mental retardation, microcephaly, microphthalmia, congenital heart disease, deafness, and cataracts

Questions 38.23–38.27

    A. Nonspecific (cultural-familial) mental retardation
    B. Boys with fragile X syndrome
    C. Down's syndrome
    D. Williams syndrome
    E. None of the above

38.23 May have particular weakness in expressive communication and special problems in grammatical abilities

38.24 Extra deficits in visuospatial processing skills

38.25 Highest IQ scores in first year of life

38.26 Weaker in sequential (serial) processing than in simultaneous (holistic) processing

38.27 Even or near-even performance across various intellectual domains

Questions 38.28–38.32

    A. Fetal alcohol syndrome
    B. Down's syndrome
    C. Lesch-Nyhan syndrome
    D. Prader-Willi syndrome
    E. Neurofibromatosis

38.28 High rates of temper tantrums, aggression, excessive daytime sleepiness, emotional lability, obsessions, and compulsions

38.29 Microcephaly, short stature, midface hypoplasia, mild to moderate mental retardation

38.30 Associated with increased incidence of thyroid abnormalities, congenital heart disease, leukemia, and early-onset Alzheimer's disease

38.31 Ataxia, chorea, kidney failure, gout, self-biting

38.32 Café-au-lait spots, short stature, macrocephaly

DIRECTIONS: Each of the questions or incomplete statements below is followed by five suggested responses or completions. Select the *one* that is *best* in each case.

38.33 All of the following chromosomal aberrations associated with Down's syndrome lead to a phenotypic expression of the disorder *except*
    A. Patients have 45 chromosomes.
    B. Patients have three of chromosome 21.
    C. Patients have 47 chromosomes with an extra chromosome 21.
    D. Patients have 46 chromosomes, but two, usually 21 and 15, are fused.
    E. Patients have mosaicism, with normal and trisomic cells in various tissues.

38.34 The genetic finding linked most closely to advancing maternal age is
    A. translocation between chromosome 14 and chromosome 21
    B. mitotic nondisjunction of chromosome 21
    C. partially trisomic karyotype
    D. meiotic nondisjunction of chromosome 21
    E. all of the above

38.35 Which of the following chromosomal abnormalities is most likely to cause mental retardation?
    A. extra chromosome 21 (trisomy 21)
    B. fusion of chromosomes 21 and 15
    C. XO (Turner's syndrome)
    D. XXY (Klinefelter's syndrome)
    E. XXYY and XXXY (Klinefelter's syndrome variations)

38.36 Mental retardation should be diagnosed when the intelligence quotient (IQ) is below
    A. 100
    B. 85
    C. 70
    D. 65
    E. 60

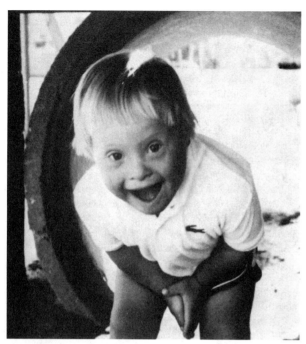

FIGURE 38.1
Courtesy of Ludwik S. Szymanski, M.D.

38.37 Fragile X syndrome
  A. has a phenotype that includes postpubertal micro-orchidism
  B. affects only males
  C. usually causes severe to profound mental retardation
  D. is associated with schizoid personality disorder in adulthood
  E. has a phenotype that includes a large head and large ears

38.38 The mentally retarded young child shown in Figure 38.1 demonstrates the characteristic facial features and high degree of social responsivity suggestive of which of the following etiologies?
  A. autosomal dominant inheritance
  B. prenatal substance exposure
  C. trisomy 21
  D. enzyme deficiency
  E. abnormality in sex chromosomes

38.39 Which of the following statements regarding the child with the karyotype shown in Figure 38.2 is true?
  A. The mother's karyotype is abnormal.
  B. The child's physical phenotype is likely to include microcephaly.
  C. The child's disorder is most likely the result of non-disjunction during mitosis.
  D. The child's IQ is likely to be in the range of 70 to 90.
  E. A minority of cases of the syndrome are the result of translocation involving fusion of two chromosomes.

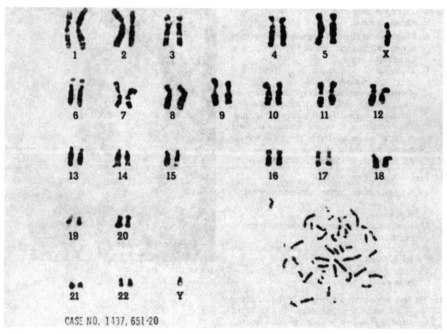

CASE NO. 1437, 651-20

FIGURE 38.2
Courtesy of the Department of Genetics, New York State Psychiatric Institute.

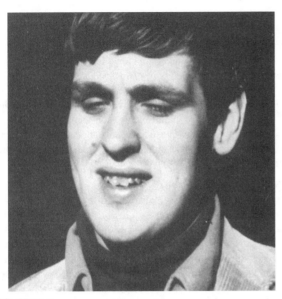

FIGURE 38.3
Courtesy of Ludwik. S. Szymanski, M.D.

38.40 The physical phenotype shown in Figure 38.3, including long facial contour, large anteverted ears, and macro-orchidism (not shown) in this young adult with mental retardation is consistent with which of the following diagnoses?

   A. Prader-Willi syndrome
   B. Down's syndrome
   C. Klinefelter's syndrome
   D. fetal alcohol syndrome
   E. fragile X syndrome

ANSWERS

Mental Retardation

38.1 The answer is A

According to some estimates, approximately *1 percent of the population* has mental retardation. *This 1 percent figure is cited by DSM-IV-TR* and is roughly the percentage found in most prevalence studies. Yet the widely cited 1 percent figure hides a variety of controversies within mental retardation. In particular, many have reasoned that mental retardation is more frequent—nearer to a 3 percent prevalence rate—while others question whether some categories of mental retardation are disappearing altogether. These controversies have enormous societal implications. Based on the current U.S. population, a difference of even 1 percent means that an extra 2.6 million Americans have mental retardation and may require services.

In 1967 Edward Zigler proposed that there are two groups of persons with mental retardation. Retardation in the first group was caused by the usual (and so far unidentified) factors that distinguish individuals across the normal range of intelligence. Researchers have variously referred to this group as having cultural-familial, familial, or nonspecific mental retardation. Many of these individuals come from poor, and low-educational backgrounds, and low IQ scores are also common in parents or siblings. Like variations across the entire IQ spectrum, some interplay of environmental and biological factors seems to be involved in this type of retardation.

Zigler referred to the second group as having "organic" mental retardation. The retardation of this group was caused by one of many different pre-, peri-, or postnatal causes. Over the years, increasing numbers of persons with organic mental retardation have been identified. Mental retardation has now been linked to approximately 750 different genetic causes, and other causes also exist. In all cases, however, these individuals have one or more organic insults associated with their mental retardation.

By summing percentages of the two groups, most workers of the 1960s and 1970s concluded that approximately 3 percent of individuals have mental retardation. In the early 1970s, however, Jane Mercer criticized the 3 percent figure and concluded that only 1 percent of the U.S. population *(not 3 percent, 5 percent, or 6 percent)* has mental retardation. Although the 1 percent versus 3 percent debate may be irresolvable, its details illustrate some of mental retardation's most complicated issues.

38.2 The answer is D

The 3 percent prevalence rate (not 0.5, 1, or 2 percent) considers IQ the sole criterion for mental retardation. That is, persons with an IQ below 70 are considered to have mental retardation, those with an IQ of 70 or above do not. Even considerations of the excess of individuals at the lowest IQ levels are based solely on the Gaussian distribution of IQ

But IQ is not the sole criterion of mental retardation. To be considered to have mental retardation, a person must have an IQ below 70 as well as deficits in adaptive behavior. If the two are perfectly correlated—if every person with a below-70 IQ also has deficits in adaptive behavior—then a 3 percent figure becomes tenable. If the two correlate weakly or not at all, much lower prevalence rates hold. Although strong IQ-adaptive correlations have been found for some organic groups and for individuals with severe and profound mental retardation, lower correlations probably hold for children with mild mental retardation. Throughout the entire population of persons with mental retardation, a moderate, but by no means perfect, correlation probably exists between IQ and adaptive behavior. To the extent that the two are uncorrelated for persons with an IQ falling below 70, less than 3 percent of individuals have mental retardation.

38.3 The answer is B

Children with *Down's syndrome* show their highest IQ (or DQ) scores during the first year of life, and then decline in IQ over the early and middle childhood years. *Boys with fragile X syndrome also decline in IQ, but their declines seem to begin at approximately 10 to 15 years.* Conversely, children with *cerebral palsy* (half of whom have mental retardation) remain remarkably stable in their IQ scores over time, much like groups with mixed or *nonspecific* etiologies of *mental retardation.* Thus, considering IQ alone, the age of the individual must be kept in mind when considering the prevalence rates of different degrees of mental retardation.

38.4 The answer is B

With advances in medicine generally and in molecular genetics in particular, new causes of mental retardation or the genetic causes of formerly unspecified syndromes are identified each year. John Opitz counts over 750 genetic causes of intellectual disability alone. Eleanor Feldman notes that some 95 mental retardation syndromes have been linked to the X chromosome. The most common causes of mental retardation are Down's syndrome, fragile X syndrome (accounting for 40 percent of all X-linked retardation), and fetal alcohol syndrome. Together, these three conditions are responsible for about 30 percent of all identified cases of mental retardation. Recently, early childhood anemia has been identified as a risk for mild to moderate mental retardation. *Down's syndrome* is the most common chromosomal abnormality leading to mental retardation. *Fetal alcohol syndrome* occurs in up to 15 percent of babies born to women who regularly ingest large amounts of alcohol. *Prader-Willi syndrome* is postulated to be the result of a small deletion in chromosome 15. Its prevalence is less than 1 in 10,000.

Fragile X syndrome, one of the most common inherited cause of mental retardation, results in a wide range of learning and behavioral problems, with males being more often and more severely affected than females. The recently discovered fragile X gene (FMR-1) represents a newly identified type of human disease, caused by amplification (or excessive repetition) of a three-nucleotide sequence (CGG) in deoxyribonucleic acid (DNA). Above a certain threshold of these triplet repeats (about 200), people are affected with the syndrome. Numbers of repeats between the normal threshold of 50, and below 200, are termed "premutations." As many as 1 in 259 women in the general population may carry the premutation, with 1 in 1,000 males and 1 in 2,000 females being fully afflicted with the syndrome.

38.5 The answer is A

Fragile X syndrome involves vulnerabilities toward shyness, gaze aversion, social *anxiety, avoidant disorders, schizotypal disorder, attention/deficit/hyperactivity disorder,* pervasive developmental disorder not otherwise specified and, *more rarely, autistic disorder.* These difficulties vary in severity but are typically found in persons across the IQ spectrum, from those with moderate mental retardation to those with mild learning disabilities.

38.6 The answer is A

Compared to others with mental retardation, *persons with Down's syndrome appear to suffer less often and less seriously from psychopathology.* Adults with Down's syndrome appear somewhat less prone to psychiatric disturbance than controls.

This trend seems to extend to children and adolescents as well; rates of psychiatric and behavioral problems exceed those in the general population but are appreciably lower than in persons in other groups with mental retardation—e.g., those with *fragile X syndrome, nonspecific type, fetal alcohol syndrome, and Prader-Willi syndrome.* Commonly noted problems include attention difficulties, impulsivity, hyperactivity, and aggression. In contrast to these problems, depression seems to be less common among children and adolescents than expected norms. Autism and pervasive developmental disorders appear to be relatively rare.

38.7 The answer is E (all)

Traditionally, individuals with mild mental retardation were thought to show relatively *few clear-cut organic causes (i.e., many nonspecific causes) for their delay.* While this may still be the case, recent years have seen an increase in the number of people with genetic syndromes who function in the mild range. Examples include most people with *Prader-Willi syndrome* and some males and *most females with fragile X syndrome.*

A more striking characteristic, however, is that more people with mild mental retardation come from minority groups and *low socioeconomic backgrounds* than would be expected from their percentages in the general population. This overrepresentation of minority groups has been used to criticize IQ tests and to highlight the importance of both environmental-cultural and genetic influences on mental retardation.

38.8 The answer is D

Mild mental retardation (IQ, 55 to 70) characterizes the largest group of persons with mental retardation, possibly as many as 85 percent of the total. These individuals appear similar to nonretarded individuals and often blend into the general population in the years before and after formal schooling. Many achieve academic skills at the sixth-grade level or higher, and some graduate from high school. As adults, many hold jobs, marry, and raise families—yet at times they may appear slow or need extra help negotiating life's problems and tasks.

Moderate mental retardation (IQ, 40 to 55, not 25 to 40) is seen in approximately 10 percent (not 3 to 4 percent) of those with mental retardation, including persons with more impaired cognitive and adaptive functioning. Individuals with moderate mental retardation typically receive their diagnosis in their preschool years, and *some (but not the majority) show a clear organic cause for their delay.* Persons with Down's syndrome often function in this range, as do many adolescents and adults with fragile X syndrome. *Most children with moderate mental retardation require special education services and achieve academic skills at the second- to third-grade level.* Supportive services are needed throughout life. With proper assistance, many live, work, and thrive in their local communities. A study by Ross and colleagues found that 20 percent of persons with an IQ from 40 to 49 lived independently, 60 percent were considered partially dependent, and 20 percent were totally dependent on others. Similarly, some individuals in this range are employed in the competitive job market and need minimal job supervision, whereas others require more extensive supervision on the job and may work in sheltered workshops or other, more segregated settings.

Severe mental retardation (IQ, 25 to 40) occurs in about 3 to 4 percent of persons with mental retardation. Individuals at this level often have one or more organic causes for their delay, and many show concurrent motor, ambulatory, and neurological problems as well as poorly developed communication skills. Most persons with severe mental retardation require close supervision and specialized care throughout their lives. Some individuals learn to perform simple tasks or routines that facilitate their self-care or their ability to perform in a sheltered workshop or preworkshop-type setting.

Profound mental retardation (IQ of 25 or below) affects relatively few individuals (1 to 2 percent) and involves pervasive deficits in cognitive, motor, and communicative functioning. Impaired sensory-motor functioning is often seen from early childhood on, and most individuals require extensive training to complete even the most rudimentary aspects of self-care, such as eating and toileting. The great majority of people with profound mental retardation have organic causes for their delay, and most require total supervision and care throughout life.

38.9 The answer is E (all)

Although common, anxiety disorders appear to be underdiagnosed in persons with mental retardation. Variability in prevalence rates, from 1 to 25 percent, is attributed to difficulty in making a diagnosis. Moreover, an individual with mental retardation may not be able to identify subjective anxiety as an underlying cause of distress, and a patient's aggression or agitation may suggest a disorder of impulse control rather than reflecting underlying anxiety. Common symptoms of anxiety in persons with mental retardation include *aggression, agitation, compulsive or repetitive behaviors, self-injury,* and insomnia. Panic may be expressed as agitation, screaming, crying, or clinging, which might even pass for delusional or paranoid behavior. Phobias also occur in this population and may even be more common in persons with developmental disabilities. Ruth Ryan has noted that persons with developmental disabilities are at high risk for abuse, which puts them at a greater risk for posttraumatic stress disorder. With data suggesting that it may be seen in nearly 8 percent of the general population, posttraumatic stress disorder is an important diagnosis to consider in individuals with mental retardation.

Answers 38.10–38.13

38.10 The answer is A

38.11 The answer is D

38.12 The answer is B

38.13 The answer is C

Prader-Willi syndrome, which appears to be the result of a small *deletion in chromosome 15,* usually occurs sporadically. Its prevalence is less than 1 in 10,000. It has predictable manifestations, including compulsive eating behaviors, obesity, often mental retardation, hypogonadism, hypotonia, and small stature. Disruptive behavior, including oppositional and defiant behavior and temper tantrums, are said to be common. Several chromosomal aberrations may result in *Down's syndrome. Trisomy 21* is the most frequent chromosomal aberration, believed to occur due to a *nondisjunction* during meiosis. Nondisjunction after fertilization in any cell division results in mosaicism, in which both normal and trisomic cells can be found. In *translocation,* mostly of chromosomes 15 and 21, there is a fusion of two chromosomes, resulting in a total of 46 chromosomes,

despite the presence of an extra chromosome 21. *Fragile X syndrome* is the second most common single cause of mental retardation. It results from a *mutation on the X chromosome* at the fragile site (Xq27.3). The fragile site is expressed in only some cells, and it may be absent in asymptomatic males and female carriers. There is much variation in both the genetic and phenotypic expression. It occurs in about 1 per 1,000 males and 1 per 2,000 females (but fully affected rates have been estimated to be 1 in 4,000 males and 1 in 8,000 females). Behaviorally, those with fragile X syndrome often have attentional problems, pervasive developmental disorders, and other learning disorders. Intellectual function seems to deteriorate in adolescence in persons with fragile X syndrome. *Phenylketonuria (PKU),* which is transmitted as an autosomal recessive trait, occurs in approximately 1 per 10,000 births. The defect transmitted is an inability to convert phenylalanine, an essential amino acid, to paratyrosine due to absence or *inactivity of the liver enzyme* phenylalanine hydroxylase. The majority of patients with PKU are severely retarded, but some have borderline or normal intelligence. Eczema, vomiting, and seizures are present in about one-third of cases. Early diagnosis is important, as a low-phenylalanine diet significantly improves both behavior and developmental progress.

Answers 38.14–38.17

38.14 The answer is C

38.15 The answer is C

38.16 The answer is C

38.17 The answer is D

Neurofibromatosis may manifest itself in the form of neurofibromas, café-au-lait spots, and seizures; optic and acoustic gliomas and bone lesions may also be present. Its form of genetic transmission is *autosomal dominant.*

Tuberous sclerosis manifests itself as seizures, intracranial calcification, pink to brownish skin lesions, and possibly bone lesions. Its form of transmission is *autosomal dominant.*

In *Crouzon's syndrome,* or craniofacial dysostosis, proptosis with shallow orbits, maxillary hypoplasia, and craniosynostosis are apparent. Its form of transmission is *autosomal dominant.*

Cockayne's syndrome is manifested by hypotrichosis, photosensitivity, thin skin, diminished subcutaneous fat, and impaired hearing. The craniofacial area may show pinched facies, sunken eyes, thin nose, prognathism, and retinal degeneration. Skeletal abnormalities include long limbs with large hands and feet and flexion deformities. Its form of transmission is *autosomal recessive.*

Cerebral gigantism, Noonan's syndrome, and Williams syndrome are examples of *disorders whose form of transmission is unknown.* Down's syndrome exhibits trisomy 21. Aarskog-Scott syndrome has an *X-linked semidominant* form of transmission.

Answers 38.18–38.22

38.18 The answer is E

38.19 The answer is C

38.20 The answer is B

38.21 The answer is A

38.22 The answer is D

Infants who are exposed to *cytomegalic inclusion disease* in utero may be stillborn; when they are born alive; they may have *mental retardation with intracerebral calcifications, jaundice, microcephaly, and hepatosplenomegaly.* Fetuses whose mothers have *acquired immune deficiency syndrome (AIDS)* often die in spontaneous abortions. Up to half of children born with AIDS have *progressive encephalopathy and mental retardation. Rett's disorder* is believed to be *an X-linked dominant mental retardation syndrome that is degenerative and affects only females. Phenylketonuria (PKU)* is a recessive autosomal disease in which the patient is unable to metabolize phenylalanine. Children with PKU often present with *mental retardation, eczema, vomiting, and seizures. Rubella* in a pregnant woman is a serious risk factor for the fetus. The risk of fetal impairment is greatest when the exposure is early in the first trimester. *Mental retardation, microcephaly, microphthalmia, congenital heart disease, deafness, and cataracts can result.*

Answers 38.23–38.27

38.23 The answer is C

38.24 The answer is D

38.25 The answer is C

38.26 The answer is B

38.27 The answer is A

Normal children have a specific, possibly universal, order to their development. For example, in Piagetian cognitive development, children proceed from sensorimotor, to preoperational, to concrete operational, to formal operational thought. Even within these four larger stages, smaller orderings hold; within sensorimotor development, normal infants proceed through Piaget's six substages in each of several subdomains.

Do children with mental retardation also follow a so-called similar sequence in development? For almost 30 years, parallel sequences have been found for a variety of children over many tasks. These sequences even hold for children with genetic or other organic causes for their retardation. The only possible exceptions include some children with uncontrollable seizures (which make accurate testing difficult) and some autistic children, who may show different orderings because of their particular disabilities on certain social tasks. Such sequences have been noted in many areas: in almost twenty Piagetian domains, in symbolic play, and in linguistic grammar and pragmatics. For almost all children and for a wide variety of behaviors, children with mental retardation and other children develop along similar pathways.

If children with retardation proceed in the same developmental ordering as other children, do they also show the even, or flat, profiles that groups of children without mental retardation show from one domain to another? Such a "similar structure" to development was proposed by Zigler in the late 1960s.

Unlike similar sequences—which hold for all children with mental retardation—cross-domain structures may differ, depending on which retarded group one considers. With a few exceptions, *children with cultural-familial mental retardation*

do show even or near-even performance across various intellectual domains.

In contrast, children with different organic forms of mental retardation show specific intellectual strengths and weaknesses. For example, three separate groups are *weaker in sequential* (i.e., bit-by-bit, serial) *processing than in simultaneous* (i.e., Gestalt, holistic) *processing* or achievement abilities. Such sequential deficits are found in *boys with fragile X syndrome*, children with Prader-Willi syndrome, and children with Smith-Magenis syndrome. *Children with Down's syndrome may have particular weaknesses in expressive* (versus receptive) *communication and special problems in grammatical abilities. Children with Williams syndrome show extra deficits in visuospatial processing skills*, and some subsets of these children show heightened abilities in language. Different causes of mental retardation thus result in different characteristic intellectual strengths and weaknesses.

Young children with Down's syndrome (who also show age-related slowings from 6 to 11 years) have difficulty with certain tasks of infant intelligence, even after one accounts for their already-slower rates of development. Toddlers lag in developing expressive skills in contrast to receptive language skills. As a result of both age- and task-related slowings, *children with Down's syndrome generally exhibit their highest IQ scores during the first year of life.*

Answers 38.28–38.32

38.28 The answer is D

38.29 The answer is A

38.30 The answer is B

38.31 The answer is C

38.32 The answer is E

Children with Down's syndrome appear to be *prone to heart problems, leukemia, thyroid abnormalities, and (by age 35)* the plaques and tangles of *Alzheimer's disease.* Similarly, *children with Prader-Willi syndrome* are prone to hyperphagia and obesity, and complications of obesity (e.g., diabetes, heart disease) remain the main cause of higher death rates for persons with Prader-Willi syndrome.

First identified 41 years ago, Prader-Willi syndrome affects about 1 in 15,000 births and is best known for its food-related characteristics. Babies invariably show hypotonia and pronounced feeding-sucking difficulties, while young children between 2 and 6 years of age develop hyperphagia and food-seeking behavior such as foraging and hoarding. Hyperphagia is probably associated with a hypothalamic abnormality resulting in a lack of satiety.

Although *people with Prader-Willi syndrome* invariably obsess about food, a *remarkably high proportion* also *show* nonfood *obsessions and compulsive behaviors.* These nonfood symptoms include skin picking; hoarding; needing to tell, ask, or say things; and having concerns with symmetry, exactness, ordering, arranging, cleanliness, and sameness in daily routine. Often these symptoms are associated with distress or adaptive impairment, suggesting a marked risk of obsessive-compulsive disorder in this population. Indeed, estimates are that obsessive-compulsive disorder is many times more likely in persons with

Prader-Willi syndrome than in the general population of persons with mental retardation.

In addition, even compared with others with mental retardation, children and *adults with Prader-Willi syndrome* display *high rates of temper tantrums, aggression, stubbornness,* underactivity, *excessive daytime sleepiness, and emotional lability.* Coupled with food seeking, these impulsive behaviors often lead those with Prader-Willi syndrome to need more restrictive care than would be assumed by their mild levels of mental retardation. Table 38.1 lists clinical features and behavioral phenotypes for *neurofibromatosis, Lesch-Nyhan syndrome,* and *fetal alcohol syndrome.*

38.33 The answer is A

Three types of chromosomal aberrations are recognized in Down's syndrome. First, patients with trisomy 21 (*three chromosome 21 instead of the usual two*) represent the overwhelming majority. They have *47 chromosomes with an extra chromosome 21.* The mother's karyotypes are normal. A nondisjunction during meiosis occurring for unknown reasons is held responsible.

Second, nondisjunction occurring after fertilization in any cell division results in *mosaicism, with both normal and trisomic cells found in various tissues.*

Third, in translocation, there is a fusion of two chromosomes, mostly 21 and 15, *resulting in a total of 46 chromosomes,* despite the presence of an extra chromosome 21. The disorder, unlike trisomy 21, is usually inherited and the translocated chromosome may be found in unaffected parents and siblings. *These asymptomatic carriers have only 45 chromosomes.*

38.34 The answer is D

Meiotic nondisjunction of chromosome 21 not only produces the majority of cases of Down's syndrome—almost 85 percent—*but also has been linked most closely to advancing maternal age.* Paternal age has also been implicated as a factor in some studies.

Translocation events, by contrast, constitute only 5 percent of Down's syndrome cases. Furthermore, in many cases in which an asymptomatic parent carries the aberrant chromosome in the genotype, the incidence of Down's syndrome is obviously unrelated to parental age. If the *translocation* occurs *between chromosome 14 and chromosome 21* (14/21), the proband carries 46 chromosomes, including two normal 21 chromosomes, one normal 14 chromosome, and the 14/21 translocation, which carries parts of both chromosomes. Any asymptomatic parent or sibling who is a carrier of the translocation has only 45 chromosomes, missing one chromosome 21, and is thus spared the excessive genetic complement.

Mitotic nondisjunction of chromosome 21, which occurs in 1 percent of all Down's syndrome cases, occurs after fertilization of a presumably healthy ovum and may therefore be considered independent of maternal age. *Partially trisomic karyotype* may refer to the mosaicism—some cells normal, others with trisomy 21—seen in mitotic nondisjunction or to the excessive complement of chromosome 21 produced by translocation. Neither case is as closely tied to maternal age as is meiotic nondisjunction.

38.35 The answer is A

An *extra chromosome 21 (trisomy 21)* is the most common genetic abnormality found in Down's syndrome and *the abnormality most likely to cause mental retardation.* Abnormalities in autosomal chromosomes are, in general, associated with mental retardation. The chromosomal aberration represented by 46 chromosomes with *fusion of chromosomes 21 and 15* produces a type of Down's syndrome that, unlike trisomy 21, is usually inherited. Aberrations in sex chromosomes are not always associated with mental retardation: for example, XO (*Turner's syndrome*), XXY (*Klinefelter's syndrome*) and XXYY and XXXY (*Klinefelter's syndrome variations*). Some children with Turner's syndrome have normal to superior intelligence.

In Turner's syndrome one sex chromosome is missing (XO). The result is an absence (agenesis) or minimal development (dysgenesis) of the gonads; no significant sex hormone, male or female, is produced in fetal life or postnatally. The sexual tissues thus retain a female resting state. Because the second X chromosome, which seems responsible for full femaleness, is

Table 38.1
Clinical Features and Behavioral Phenotypes for Neurofibromatosis, Lesch-Nyhan Syndrome, and Fetal Alcohol Syndrome

Disorder	Pathophysiology	Clinical Features and Behavioral Phenotype
Neurofibromatosis type 1 (NF1)	1/2,500–1/4,000; male = female; autosomal dominant; 50% new mutations; more than 90% paternal NF1 allele mutated; NF1 gene 17q11.2; gene product is neurofromin thought to be tumor suppressor gene	Variable manifestations; *café-au-lait spots,* cutaneous neurofibromas, Lisch nodules; *short stature and macrocephaly* in 30–45% Half with speech and language difficulties; 10% with moderate-to-profound mental retardation verbal IQ > performance IQ; distractable, impulsive, hyperactive, anxious; possibly associated with increased incidence of mood and anxiety disorders
Lesch-Nyhan syndrome	Defect in hypoxanthine guanine phosphoribosyltransferase with accumulation of uric acid; Xq26–27; recessive; rare (1/10,000–1/38,000)	*Ataxia, chorea, kidney failure, gout;* often severe *self-biting behavior;* aggression; anxiety; mild-to-moderate mental retardation
Fetal alcohol syndrome	Maternal alcohol consumption (trimester III>II>I); 1/3,000 live births in Western countries; 1/300 with fetal alcohol effects	*Microcephaly, short stature, midface hypoplasia,* short palpebral fissure, thin upper lip, retrognathia in infancy, micrognathia in adolescence, hypoplastic long or smooth philtrum *Mild-to-moderate mental retardation,* irritability, inattention, memory impairment

missing, the affected girls are incomplete in their sexual anatomy and, lacking adequate estrogens, develop no secondary sex characteristics without treatment. They often have other stigmata, such as web neck.

In Klinefelter's syndrome, the person (usually XXY) has a male habitus, under the influence of the Y chromosome, but that effect is weakened by the presence of the second X chromosome. Although born with a penis and testes, the child has small and infertile testes, and the penis may also be small. In adolescence, some patients begin to show gynecomastia and other feminine-appearing contours.

38.36 The answer is C

Mental retardation should be diagnosed when the intelligence quotient (IQ) falls below 70. According to the revised fourth edition of *Diagnostic and Statistical Manual of Mental Disorders* (DSM-IV-TR), the following classification of mental retardation is used: mild (IQ, 50–55 to approximately 70), moderate (IQ, 35–40 to 50–55), severe (IQ, 20–25 to 35–40), and profound (IQ, below 20 or 25).

38.37 The answer is E

Fragile X syndrome *has a phenotype that includes a large head and large ears*, long and narrow face, short stature, and postpubertal macro-orchidism*, not micro-orchidism*. The syndrome *affects both males and females.* Female carriers are usually less impaired than males but can manifest the typical physical characteristics and mild mental retardation. *In males* the syndrome usually causes low-average intelligence *to severe mental retardation (not severe to profound mental retardation).* The syndrome is *associated with antisocial (not schizoid) personality disorder in adulthood.* Those affected by the syndrome may also have attention-deficit/hyperactivity disorder and learning disorders.

38.38 The answer is C

Causative factors in mental retardation include genetic (chromosomal and inherited) conditions, prenatal exposure to infections and toxins, perinatal trauma (such as prematurity), acquired conditions, and sociocultural factors. The child in the photograph demonstrates the characteristic facial features (including slanted eyes, midface depression, and flat nose) and high degree of social responsivity characteristic of Down's syndrome. In the overwhelming majority of cases, the etiology of Down's syndrome is an abnormality of chromosome number 21 known as *trisomy 21* (three of chromosome 21 instead of the usual two).

Autosomal dominant inheritance as the etiology of mental retardation is demonstrated in tuberous sclerosis, characterized by a progressive mental retardation in up to two-thirds of cases, as well as seizures and other abnormalities. *Prenatal substance exposure* as the etiology of mental retardation is demonstrated in fetal alcohol syndrome, which occurs in up to 15 percent of babies born to women who regularly ingest large amounts of alcohol. *Enzyme deficiency* as the etiology of mental retardation

is demonstrated in phenylketonuria (PKU). The basic metabolic defect in PKU is an inability to convert phenylalanine, an essential amino acid, to paratyrosine because of absence or inactivity of the liver enzyme phenylalanine hydroxylase. *Abnormality in sex chromosomes* as the etiology of mental retardation is demonstrated in fragile X syndrome, the second most common cause of mental retardation, which results from a mutation on the X chromosome at what is known as the fragile site.

38.39 The answer is E

The figure shows the karyotype of a child with Down's syndrome. The overwhelming majority of cases of Down's syndrome are the result of trisomy 21 (three of chromosome 21 instead of the usual two). A *nondisjunction during meiosis (not mitosis)* is responsible for trisomy 21, and the *mother's karyotype is normal (not abnormal).* A minority of cases of Down's syndrome are the result of nondisjunction occurring after fertilization in any cell division, resulting in mosaicism, or of translocation involving fusion of two chromosomes, mostly 21 and 15.*

The overriding feature of Down's syndrome is mental retardation, which, according to the DSM-IV-TR diagnostic criteria, is characterized by an IQ of approximately 70 or below. The majority of patients with Down's syndrome belong to the moderately and severely retarded groups, with *only a minority having an IQ above 50 (and fewer still over 70).* Down's syndrome has a characteristic physical phenotype, which may include such features as upward slanting palpebral fissures, midface depression, epicanthic folds, and brachycephaly (a disproportionate shortness of the head), *not microcephaly.*

38.40 The answer is E

The figure shows a young adult with *fragile X syndrome*, the second most common single cause of mental retardation after trisomy 21, the predominant form of Down's syndrome. The physical phenotype of *Down's syndrome* includes oblique palpebral fissures, high cheekbones, protruding tongue, single palmar transversal crease, and a number of other associated features, such as congenital heart disease (40 percent) and gastrointestinal malformations (12 percent). *Prader-Willi syndrome*, postulated to be the result of a small deletion involving chromosome 15, is characterized by mental retardation, compulsive eating behavior, and often obesity, hypogonadism, small stature, hypotonia, and small hands and feet. *Fetal alcohol syndrome* consists of mental retardation and a typical phenotypic picture of facial dysmorphism that includes hypertelorism, microcephaly, short palpebral fissures, inner epicanthal folds, and a short, turned-up nose. *Klinefelter's syndrome* is an intersex condition with XXY genotype, characterized by a male habitus with a small penis and rudimentary testes because of low androgen production. Some patients develop gynecomastia in adolescence and many of them have a wide variety of psychopathology, ranging from emotional instability to mental retardation.

39 ▲

Learning Disorders

Learning disorders are diagnosed when standardized test achievements in reading, math, or written expression are substantially lower than expected for a particular age, school level, or intelligence. These disorders involve academic deficits and impairments in the specific areas of reading, math, spelling, and writing. About 5 percent of students in public schools in the United States are estimated to have a learning disorder, and up to 40 percent of these students drop out of school. The revised fourth edition of *Diagnostic and Statistical Manual of Mental Disorders* (DSM-IV-TR) describes demoralization, low self-esteem, and social skill deficits as associated features with learning disorders. Approximately 75 percent of children with learning disorders can be differentiated from comparison samples through lower levels of social competence. DSM-IV-TR also emphasizes that learning disorders must be distinguished from academic difficulties arising from lack of opportunity, poor teaching, cultural factors, and vision or hearing impairments. Learning disorders can be associated with other developmental disorders and with mood disorders and are frequently found in association with a number of medical conditions, such as lead poisoning or fetal alcohol syndrome; however, none of the disorders can be due to a known neurological deficit.

Reading disorder occurs in approximately 4 percent of school-aged children and is more common in boys than in girls. This disorder is characterized by low reading skill in the presence of normal intelligence and may involve impairments in the ability to recognize words, poor comprehension, and slow and inaccurate reading. Children with attention-deficit/hyperactivity disorders are at high risk for reading disorder. The term dyslexia was used for many years to describe a reading disability syndrome involving, among other features, right–left confusion. Since it has been better understood that reading disorders often occur in conjunction with other academic skill disorders, the term learning disorders has been more utilized.

Mathematics disorder involves an impairment in four basic arithmetic skills in children of normal intelligence. The four groups consist of linguistic skills (related to understanding mathematical terms and converting problems into mathematical symbols); perceptual skills (ability to recognize symbols and to order number clusters); mathematical skills (addition, multiplication, division, subtraction); and attentional skills (copying figures). It

is estimated to occur in about 6 percent of school-aged children, and is usually apparent by the age of 8. Mathematics disorder often occurs in conjunction with other learning disorders.

It was once felt that disorders of written expression, or dysgraphias, did not develop in the absence of a reading disorder. It is now known that disorders of written expression can occur on their own. Old terms to describe these disorders included spelling disorder and spelling dyslexia, while currently they are also known as developmental expressive writing disorders. Components of writing disabilities include poor spelling, errors in grammar and punctuation, and poor handwriting.

All of the learning disorders appear to have multifactorial causes and many of the disorders tend to be more prevalent among family members of affected individuals than in the general population. The disorders may represent one manifestation of developmental delay or maturational lag. Temperamental characteristics may play a role in the development of learning disorders, in particular those related to attention span and concentration.

DSM-IV-TR includes learning disorder not otherwise specified to cover those learning disorders that do not meet diagnostic criteria for the enumerated disorders. One example of an unspecified learning disorder might be in a child whose spelling skills alone are impaired significantly.

The student should study the questions and answers below for a useful review of these disorders.

HELPFUL HINTS

The student should define these terms related to learning disorders.

- ▶ academic skills disorders
- ▶ dyslexia
- ▶ hearing and vision screening
- ▶ phoneme
- ▶ right–left confusion
- ▶ spatial relations
- ▶ visual-perceptual deficits
- ▶ word additions
- ▶ word distortions
- ▶ word omissions

▲ QUESTIONS

DIRECTIONS: Each of the questions or incomplete statements below is followed by five suggested responses or completions. Select the *one* that is *best* in each case.

39.1 Common elements in the definition of reading disorder include

A. its underlying cause is central nervous system dysfunction
B. an uneven pattern of cognitive functioning
C. a discrepancy between learning potential and actual reading achievement
D. difficulty in single-word decoding
E. all of the above

39.2 A recently proposed definition of dyslexia includes which of the following components:

A. It is one of several distinct learning disabilities not characterized by difficulties in single-word decoding.
B. It does not usually reflect insufficient phonological processing.
C. It is not the result of sensory impairment.
D. It rarely includes a conspicuous problem with acquiring proficiency in writing and spelling.
E. None of the above

39.3 The psychiatric syndrome most often found in mathematical disorder is

A. anxiety
B. depression
C. reading disorder
D. attention-deficit/hyperactivity disorder
E. none of the above

DIRECTIONS: Each group of questions below consist of lettered headings followed by a list of numbered words or phrases. For each numbered word or phrase, select the *one* lettered heading that is most closely associated with it. Each heading may be selected once, more than once, or not at all.

Questions 39.4–39.7

A. Reading disorder
B. Mathematics disorder
C. Disorder of written expression
D. Learning disorder not otherwise specified

39.4 Used to be known as dyslexia
39.5 Spelling skills deficit is an example
39.6 Usually diagnosed later than the other learning disorders
39.7 Reported to occur frequently in children born in May, June, and July

Questions 39.8–39.12

A. Reading disorder
B. Mathematics disorder
C. Both
D. Neither

39.8 The study of this disorder has been neglected even though it appears to occur with the same frequency as learning disorders in other areas
39.9 The etiology is unknown
39.10 Higher monozygotic than dizygotic concordance rates
39.11 Diagnosis is generally not made until the second or third grade
39.12 Brain anomalies are inferred but not demonstrated conclusively

DIRECTIONS: Each of the questions or incomplete statements below is followed by five suggested responses or completions. Select the *one* that is *best* in each case.

39.13 Reading disorder is characterized by all of the following *except*

A. impairment in recognizing words
B. poor reading comprehension
C. increased prevalence among family members
D. occurrence in three to four times as many girls as boys
E. omissions, additions, and distortions of words in oral reading

39.14 Which of the following statements does *not* characterize mathematics disorder?

A. It is more common in boys than in girls.
B. The prevalence estimated to be about 6 percent in school-age children with normal intelligence.
C. It includes impairment in addition, subtraction, multiplication, and division.
D. It is usually apparent by the time a child is 8 years old.
E. It is often found in children with reading disorder.

39.15 Disorder of written expression

A. presents earlier than do reading disorder and communication disorders
B. occurs only in children with reading disorder
C. is not diagnosed until the teenage years
D. includes disability in spelling, grammar, and punctuation
E. is always self-limited

39.16 Janet, 13 years old, had a long history of school problems. She failed first grade, supposedly because her teacher was "mean," and was removed from a special classroom because she kept getting into fights with the other children. Currently in a normal sixth-grade classroom, she is failing reading, barely passing English and spelling, and doing satisfactory work in art and sports. Her teacher describes Janet as a "slow learner with a poor memory," and states that Janet does not learn in a group setting and requires a great deal of individual attention.

Janet's medical history was unremarkable except for a tonsillectomy at age 5 years and an early history of chronic otitis. She sat up at 6 months, walked at 12 months, and began talking at 18 months. An examination revealed an open and friendly girl who was nonetheless touchy about her academic problems. She stated that she was "bossed around" at school but had good friends in the neighborhood. Intelligence testing revealed a full-scale intelligence quotient of 97. Wide-range achievement testing produced grade-level scores of 4.8 for reading, 5.3 for spelling, and 6.3 for arithmetic.

The most likely diagnosis is

A. disorder of written expression
B. expressive language disorder
C. phonological disorder
D. reading disorder
E. none of the above

39.17 Disorder of written expression is often associated with
A. reading disorder
B. mixed expressive-receptive language disorder
C. developmental coordination disorder
D. mathematics disorder
E. all of the above

ANSWERS

Learning Disorders

39.1 The answer is E (all)
Despite over a century of research, the definition of a reading disorder remains controversial. A review of various definitions yields five common elements, each of which has generated considerable debate in the field. *The first element is that the underlying cause of reading disorder is central nervous system dysfunction.* Although neurological conditions often cannot be determined in individuals by external tests and medical examinations, it is presumed that dysfunction can be inferred from observation of behaviors.

The second element is an uneven pattern of cognitive functioning. In other words, although overall cognitive functioning is intact, specific areas (what one researcher calls "vertical modules" that are informationally encapsulated) are significantly degraded—in some instances to such an extent that the acquisition of basic decoding skills is extremely difficult. This uneven pattern of cognitive functioning has been referred to in the literature as the presence of a "psychological processing deficit" despite overall adequate cognitive functioning.

Most reading disorder definitions contain the third element, difficulty in single-word decoding. All 50 states have adopted definitions of specific learning disabilities that identify decoding skills as an area of academic achievement affected by reading disorder.

The *fourth element shared by most definitions* of reading disorder is *a discrepancy between learning potential and actual reading achievement.* This element has been a particular target of recent debate. It assumes that individuals are underachievers in the area of reading achievement, failing to exhibit decoding or comprehension skills or both, commensurate with their ability level.

The final definitional element is the exclusion of other causes of reading difficulty. Similar to the first, second, and fourth elements, pervasive disagreement exists about whether or not reading disorders can exist in combination with other disorders. Nonetheless, 48 of the 50 states have adopted this element in their definitions of specific learning disabilities. Inclusion of this fifth element reflects the need in the mid-1970s to establish specific learning disabilities, and thereby reading disorders, as discrete and separate entities for federal legislation.

39.2 The answer is C
Dyslexia is one of several distinct learning disabilities. It is a language-based disorder of constitutional origin *characterized by difficulties in single-word decoding, usually reflecting insufficient phonological processing.* These difficulties in single-word decoding are often unexpected in relation to age and other cognitive and academic abilities; *they are not the result of generalized developmental disability or sensory impairment.* Dyslexia is manifested by variable difficulty with different forms of language, *often (not rarely) including, in addition to problems with reading, a conspicuous problem with acquiring proficiency in writing and spelling.*

This recently proposed definition reflects two important advances. First, instead of defining reading disorders generically, it focuses on one type of reading disorder, dyslexia. Second, and for the first time, it localizes the difficulty associated with dyslexia at the single-word level and pinpoints the cause as insufficient phonological processing. Although this definition has not gained wide acceptance, it represents a significant first step in addressing some of the previous confusion and disagreement surrounding definitions of learning disabilities.

39.3 The answer is D
Other developmental learning disorders and difficulties are often linked with mathematics disorder. *Reading disorder,* disorder of written expression, expressive language disorder, mixed receptive-expressive language disorder, and developmental coordination disorder have all been reported in association with mathematics disorder. Specific cognitive processing difficulties (e.g., auditory-verbal deficits, visual-spatial deficits, motor deficits, memory deficits, and attention deficits) may be associated features.

Social immaturity, school and peer problems, social skills deficits, *anxiety,* and *depression* likewise have been reported as associated problems. *However, the psychiatric syndrome that is most often found is attention-deficit/hyperactivity disorder.* The precise nature of the relationship is unclear; however, three recent studies shed some light. One study compared mathematical underachievers with reading underachievers and found that the mathematically impaired youngsters had higher rates of inattention but not of hyperactivity or impulsivity. The second study examined children with attention-deficit/hyperactivity disorder and found correlations between measures of vigilance and distractibility and arithmetic test performance. The third study found that older children with attention-deficit/hyperactivity disorder were significantly more likely than younger children with the disorder to show a discrepancy between intelligence levels and mathematical achievement.

Answers 39.4–39.7

39.4 The answer is A

39.5 The answer is D

39.6 The answer is C

39.7 The answer is A

Reading disorder used to be known as dyslexia. It is *reported to occur frequently in children born in May, June, and July,* suggesting that reading disorder is linked to maternal winter infectious disease. *Disorder of written expression is usually diagnosed later than the other learning disorders,* since writing skills are acquired at a later age than are language reading skills. *Learning disorder not otherwise specified* is a category of learning disorders that covers disorders in learning that do not meet the criteria for any specific learning disorder. *Spelling skills deficit is an example.* Mathematics disorder includes deficits in linguistic skills related to understanding mathematical terms and converting written problems into mathematical symbols and perceptual skills (the ability to recognize and understand symbols and to order clusters of numbers).

Answers 39.8–39.12

39.8 The answer is B

39.9 The answer is C

39.10 The answer is C

39.11 The answer is C

39.12 The answer is C

Although the prevalence of mathematics disorder has not been studied in detail, several studies agree that approximately 6 percent of the school-aged population has serious arithmetic difficulties unexplained by cognitive or sensory functioning. *The study of mathematics disorder has been neglected even though it appears to occur with the same frequency as learning disorders in other academic areas.* Several researchers have asserted that this situation reflects cultural values that afford literacy skills (i.e., reading and writing) a higher status than mathematics skills.

The etiology of reading disorder is not known. The traditional view is that the disorder has multiple causes, most likely involving biological dysfunctions that result in a lag or impairment in the development of cognitive skills needed for learning to read. Numerous hypotheses exist regarding the types and sources of biological factors and cognitive impairments that may be involved.

Many of the theories of brain function in children with reading disorder are based on observations of associated symptoms. For example, because language and speech problems are often related, abnormalities in the left hemisphere and in the frontal speech regions in both hemispheres have been postulated. Similarly, insofar as motor problems with balance and equilibrium are frequently linked, abnormalities in cerebellar-vestibular function have been postulated. Thus, *brain anomalies are inferred but not demonstrated definitively.* Unfortunately, the types of neuroanatomical studies needed to demonstrate brain anomalies (e.g., computed tomography, electrophysiological

studies, or postmortem studies) are very limited and have produced contradictory results.

The cause of developmental mathematics disorder is also unknown. The earliest view of the disorder was derived from neurological studies of adults with acquired brain lesions that were accompanied by loss of arithmetical-mathematical skills. That early work implicated abnormalities in the cerebral right hemisphere (occipital) processing of visual-spatial stimuli. Subsequent work indicated that such lesions could not account for all cases of acalculia, either in children or adults. However, when children with developmental language disorders are excluded from consideration, symptom clusters of adults with acquired acalculia and children with mathematics disorder are markedly similar.

Twin studies have consistently found *higher concordance rates for dyslexia in monozygotic twin pairs than in dizygotic pairs.* An elevated concordance rate in monozygotic twins is generally accepted as proof of a genetic component. However, one investigator has argued that, owing to more cognitive or emotional similarity, the monozygotic twins might have created more similar environments for themselves, which in turn may have affected their reading acquisition. Nonetheless, the various twin studies that have looked at the heritability of reading disorder have attributed 30 to 60 percent of the similarity between monozygotic twins to genetic factors and the balance to environmental factors. The observation that some monozygotic twin pairs are discordant for reading disorder proves that genetics is not the only cause.

Some persons may have a genetic predisposition to mathematics disorder. Anecdotal and case history reports describe families with consistently high or low mathematical abilities. Furthermore, in the general population *monozygotic twins show a higher than chance correlation in mathematics test scores.*

Although symptoms of reading disorder may appear as early as age 5 years (e.g., inability to distinguish among common letters or to associate phonemes with letter symbols), referral and formal diagnosis may not occur until later. Many children are first diagnosed when they fail to respond to formal instruction in the second grade. Some, especially those with high intelligence, may not be diagnosed until the fourth or fifth grade.

Although difficulties with counting and number concepts may be apparent as early as kindergarten, *diagnosis is generally not made until the second or third grade.*

39.13 The answer is D

Reading disorder is reported *to occur in three to four times as many boys as girls (not vice versa).* The rate of reading disorder in boys may be inflated, since boys with reading disorder are more likely to have behavioral problems than are girls, and the boys may be identified initially for their behavioral problems. Reading disorder is characterized by *impairment in recognizing words,* slow and inaccurate reading, and *poor reading comprehension.*

Reading achievement is below that expected for the person's age, as measured by standardized tests. Although no unitary cause of reading disorder is known, it appears to have *increased prevalence among family members,* leading to the speculation that it has a genetic origin. Children with reading disorder make *omissions, additions, and distortions of words in oral reading.* They may have difficulty in distinguishing printed letter characters and sizes, especially letters that differ only in spatial orientation and length of line.

39.14 The answer is A

Unlike reading disorder, in which the rate in boys is reported to be three to four times the rate in girls, *the sex ratio for mathematics disorder has yet to be determined.* In fact, mathematics disorder *may be more common in girls than in boys.* The *prevalence* of mathematics disorder is *estimated to be about 6 percent* in school-aged children with normal intelligence. Mathematics disorder *includes impairment in addition, subtraction, multiplication, and division.* Mathematics disorder is *usually apparent by the time a child is 8 years old,* although in some children it may present as early as 6 years of age or as late as 10 years of age. Mathematics disorder is *often found in children with reading disorder.*

39.15 The answer is D

Disorder of written expression *includes disability in spelling, grammar, and punctuation marks.* The disorder is characterized by writing skills that are significantly below the expected level for the child's age and intelligence, as measured by a standardized test. Because a child normally speaks well in advance of learning to read and reads well in advance of learning to write, *disorder of written expression presents later (not earlier) than do reading disorder and communication disorders. Disorder of written expression can occur in children with—and without—* reading disorder. The disorder is *diagnosed in the early school years (not in the teenage years). It is not self-limited.*

39.16 The answer is D

The most likely diagnosis for Janet is *reading disorder.* Reading disorder is characterized by marked impairment in the development of word recognition skills and reading comprehension that cannot be explained by mental retardation, inadequate schooling, visual or hearing defect, or a neurological disorder. Reading-disordered children make many errors in their oral reading, including omissions, additions, and distortions of words. Janet's difficulties, apparently, were limited to reading and spelling. She had average intelligence and normal scores on achievement tests of arithmetic but markedly low scores for spelling and reading.

Disorder of written expression is characterized by poor performance in writing and composition. *Expressive language disorder* is characterized by serious impairment in age-appropriate expressive language. *Phonological disorder* is characterized by frequent and recurrent misarticulations of speech sounds, resulting in abnormal speech. The case described does not meet the criteria for any diagnosis other than reading disorder.

39.17 The answer is E (all)

Reading disorder, mixed expressive-receptive language disorder, developmental coordination disorder, mathematics disorder, and disruptive behavior disorders are often associated with disorder of written expression. The ability to transfer one's thoughts into written words and sentences requires multimodal sensorimotor coordination and information processing. Disorder of written expression is an academic skills disorder that presents during childhood and is characterized by poor performance in writing and composition (spelling words and expressing thoughts).

40 ◣▲

Motor Skills Disorder

Motor skills disorder is classified in the revised fourth edition of the *Diagnostic and Statistical Manual of Mental Disorders* (DSM-IV-TR) as developmental coordination disorder. It is characterized by imprecise or clumsy gross motor skills, and not infrequently is present in children who also exhibit language and other learning disorders, as well as problems in peer relations. Clumsiness has also been associated with attention-deficit/hyperactivity disorder and impulsive behavior disorders. Children with this disorder have normal intelligence but demonstrate markedly lower-than-expected performance in activities requiring motor coordination. Delays in such motor milestones as sitting up, crawling, and walking may occur, as well as deficits in such activities as writing. The child may be awkward and clumsy, slow to learn motor activities, or poor at drawing. The observed motor impairments cannot be due to a known medical or neuromuscular condition, such as cerebral palsy or muscular dystrophy, although subtle reflex abnormalities and other soft neurological signs may be present. Children with this disorder may be ostracized socially in that they may resemble younger children in their lagging motor abilities and are often poor in sports.

Developmental coordination disorder appears to be more common in boys than in girls and has been estimated to affect 6 percent of school-aged children. Specific causes, as with most such disorders, are unknown and assumed to be multifactorial. Risk factors include prematurity, hypoxia, perinatal malnutrition, and low birth weight. Suggestions of possible neurochemical abnormalities or parietal lobe lesions have been made to explain the presentation of this disorder, but there have been no definitive findings.

Depending on age, affected children may have trouble holding objects, may have an unsteady gait, may be unable to put together puzzles, or may not be able to participate in any type of ball game. Clumsiness usually persists into adolescence and adulthood. The diagnosis of the disorder involves taking a detailed history of a child's early motor development and is supported by investigations on standardized tests. Low-normal scores on performance subtests of standardized intelligence tests, in association with normal or above-normal scores on verbal tests, substantiate the diagnosis. Other specialized tests of motor coordination, such as the Bender Visual Motor Gestalt test, the Frostig Movement Skills test battery, and the Bruininks-Oseretsky Test of Motor Development, may be helpful in making the diagnosis. Informal screening can be done by asking the child

to demonstrate tasks involving gross and fine motor coordination and hand-eye coordination. These might include asking the child to stand on one foot, tie his or her shoelaces, or catch a ball.

More favorable outcomes seem to be associated with children who are able to compensate for their coordination difficulties with other valued activities that do not require motor coordination. Treatments of the disorder often include a global approach, addressing social skills training, as well as management of comorbid learning, communication, and behavior disorders. Modified physical education, perpetual motor training, and specific exercise techniques are employed. No single exercise or training method seems to be more effective than another. Supportive emotional counseling for both the child and parents may be helpful.

The student should study the questions and answers below for a useful review of this disorder.

HELPFUL HINTS

The student should know the terms listed here.

- ▶ attention-deficit/hyperactivity disorder
- ▶ Bender Visual Motor Gestalt test
- ▶ Bruininks-Oseretsky Test of Motor Development
- ▶ catching a ball
- ▶ cerebral palsy
- ▶ clumsiness
- ▶ conduct disorder
- ▶ deficits in handwriting
- ▶ delayed motor milestones
- ▶ expressive language disorder
- ▶ eye–hand coordination
- ▶ fine motor skills
- ▶ finger tapping
- ▶ Frostig Movement Skills Test Battery
- ▶ Gerstmann syndrome
- ▶ graphemes
- ▶ gross motor skills
- ▶ informal motor skills screening
- ▶ learning disorders
- ▶ linguistic, perceptual, mathematical, and attentional skills
- ▶ perceptual motor training
- ▶ psychoeducational tests
- ▶ remedial treatments
- ▶ shoelace tying
- ▶ social ostracism
- ▶ temperamental attributes
- ▶ unsteady gait

▲ QUESTIONS

DIRECTIONS: Each of the questions or incomplete statements below is followed by five suggested responses or completions. Select the *one* that is *best* in each case.

40.1 Manifestations of developmental coordination disorder include

A. delays in reaching motor milestones such as sitting and crawling
B. destructiveness
C. messy or illegible writing
D. difficulty learning feeding skills
E. all of the above

40.2 Which of the following tests is *not* helpful in demonstrating developmental coordination disorder?

A. Bender Visual Motor Gestalt test
B. Verbal subtests of the Wechsler Intelligence Scale for Children—Third Edition (WISC-III) (below-normal scores)
C. Bruininks-Oseretsky Test of Motor Development
D. Frostig Movement Skills Test Battery
E. None of the above

40.3 Which of the following is a risk factor for developmental coordination disorder?

A. Birth in May, June, or July
B. Borderline intellectual functioning
C. Female gender
D. Prematurity
E. Dysfunctional family

40.4 Which of the following statements is *false*?

A. Children with developmental coordination disorder may resemble younger children motorically.
B. Developmental coordination disorder is seen frequently in conjunction with a communication disorder.
C. The male-to-female ratio in developmental coordination disorder is estimated to be 2 to 1.
D. Prematurity, low birth weight, perinatal malnutrition, and hypoxia are all risk factors for developmental coordination disorder.
E. Developmental coordination disorder is usually due to a lesion in the parietal lobe of the brain.

DIRECTIONS: The group of questions below consists of lettered headings followed by a list of numbered words or statements. For each numbered word or statement, select the *one* lettered heading that is most closely associated with it. Each lettered heading may be selected once, more than once, or not at all.

Questions 40.5–40.7

A. dyspraxia
B. synkinesia
C. impersistence
D. asymmetries
E. hypertonus

40.5 Facial grimaces when child is asked to make hand movements
40.6 Clinician tracks how long a child can stick out his tongue
40.7 Child tends to throw a ball too hard and inaccurately at short distances

ANSWERS

Motor Skills Disorder

40.1 The answer is E (all)
Children with developmental coordination disorder perform motor coordination tasks at levels markedly below those of peers of the same chronological age and intellectual capacity. The motor performance deficits are sufficiently marked to interfere with academic achievement and activities of daily living. Specific manifestations of the disorder are described in Table 40.1. Many are age related, including delays in *achieving motor milestones* (walking, crawling, sitting), *difficulty learning to feed themselves*, dropping things, poor performance in sports, and *illegible handwriting*. Clumsiness can lead to unintentional *destructiveness*.

40.2 The answer is B
Children with developmental coordination disorder generally do not have below-normal scores on the *verbal subtest of the WISC-III*, but they sometimes have below-normal scores on the performance subtests of the WISC-III. *The Bender Visual Motor Gestalt test, the Bruininks-Oseretsky Test of Motor Development, and the Frostig Movement Skills Test Battery are all specialized batteries that detect motor coordination difficulties.*

40.3 The answer is D
Risk factors for developmental coordination disorder include *prematurity*. Reading disorder, not developmental coordination disorder, has been reported to be frequent in children *born in May, June, or July*, suggesting a link between winter maternal infectious illness and the development of reading disorder. *Borderline intellectual functioning* (an intelligence quotient [IQ] between 70 and 90) is not identified specifically as a risk factor for developmental coordination disorder. A *dysfunctional family* has not been pinpointed to date as a risk factor. The male-to-female ratio in developmental coordination disorder is about 2 to 1.

40.4 The answer is E
Developmental coordination disorder is not usually due to a lesion in the parietal lobe of the brain, although parietal lobe lesions have been suggested as causes of the disorder. *Children with developmental coordination disorder may resemble younger children motorically.* Developmental coordination disorder is *seen frequently in conjunction with a communication disorder. The male-to-female ratio* in developmental coordination disorder *is estimated to be 2 to 1* and occurs in

Table 40.1
Manifestations of Developmental Coordination Disorder

Gross motor manifestations

Preschool age

 Delays in reaching motor milestones such as sitting, crawling, walking

 Balance problems: falling, getting bruised frequently, poor toddling

 Abnormal gait

 Knocking over objects, bumping into things, destructiveness

Primary-school age

 Difficulty with riding bikes, skipping, hopping, running, jumping, doing somersaults

 Awkward or abnormal gait

Older

 Poor at sports, throwing, catching, kicking, hitting a ball

Fine motor manifestations

Preschool age

 Difficulty learning dressing skills (tying, fastening, zipping, buttoning)

 Difficulty learning feeding skills (handling knife, fork, or spoon)

Primary-school age

 Difficulty assembling jigsaw pieces, using scissors, building with blocks, drawing, or tracing

Older

 Difficulty with grooming (putting on makeup, blow-drying hair, doing nails)

 Messy or illegible writing

 Difficulty using hand tools, sewing, playing piano

approximately 6 percent of school-aged children of normal intelligence. *Prematurity, low birth weight, perinatal malnutrition, and hypoxia* are all *risk factors* for developmental coordination disorder.

Answers 40.5–40.7

40.5 The answer is B

40.6 The answer is C

40.7 The answer is E

The essential feature of developmental coordination disorder is poor motor coordination. The manifestations may include difficulties or delayed development in fine and gross motor coordination skills. However, motor skills tend to be imprecise or clumsy rather than globally impaired.

Coordination problems are diagnosed according to movement characteristics, generally observed while the person is

engaged in several different types of tasks requiring the use of different muscle groups. They are assigned clinically to one or more of seven diagnostic categories: dyspraxia, *synkinesia,* hypotonus, *hypertonus,* tremors, *impersistence,* and asymmetries. Dyspraxia describes the inability of the child to produce correctly sequenced, coordinated motor movements when presented with a demonstration or an oral request. Movements identified as *synkinesia* are best described as unintentional muscle movements, also termed muscle overflow. Mirror-movements such as finger twitching on the opposite hand when the child is asked to perform a finger opposition task, or *facial grimaces when the child is asked to make hand movements,* are examples of synkinetic motor actions.

 Two categories clinically describe tonus abnormalities: hypotonus and hypertonus. Hypotonus can be observed in all parts of the body and is characterized by a flaccid or sleepy quality in the child's facial expression and overall muscle tone. These children appear lazy and unfit; the condition is often accompanied by poor posture and obesity. *Hypertonus* describes generally high levels of muscle tone in a child. For example, a child with hypertonus movement cannot finish drawing a line at a given point, instead overshooting the intended stopping point. Another example is a *child who tends to throw a ball too hard and inaccurately at short distances.*

 The category of tremors is marked by irregular unsteadiness in motor movements observed in tasks requiring walking and/or drawing. For example, legibly formed letters might reveal, on closer inspection, rapid tremors in the actual lines themselves. Unsteadiness might be exhibited in the child's gait as high-amplitude fluctuations in leg muscle movement.

 The category of *impersistence* refers to the child's inability to sustain and maintain various body postures for reasonable periods of time. *Asking a child to "stick out your tongue"* is an example of a task used often to investigate impersistent motor movements. In this example, the clinician would keep track of how long the child could maintain this tongue position.

 The final movement category, asymmetries, describes motor behaviors that affect only one side of the body. This category includes unusual flexions, muscle weakness, or both, on one side of the body or general muscle weakness in the limbs on one side. These asymmetric muscle movements can be observed by instructing a child to move laterally in a rapid manner ("like a basketball player on defense, not crossing your feet"). If the child executes the movement more fluidly on one side than on the other, it might indicate an asymmetry.

 Specific manifestations vary across individuals; thus, there is no typical clumsy child. In some instances, presentations may be quite specific; one case report describes a child who could sew and do jigsaw puzzles without difficulty but could not write neatly. In fact, total disability in any one area of motor performance is rare.

41
Communication Disorders

Language disabilities, categorized in the revised fourth edition of the *Diagnostic and Statistical Manual of Mental Disorders* (DSM-IV-TR) as communication disorders, include disorders of expressive language and mixed receptive-expressive language, phonological disorder, and stuttering. These disorders can be acquired at any time in childhood, but most occur without a known etiology. There are two types of acquired language disorders: The first is associated with a known cerebral injury or trauma, and the second is characterized by a progressive loss of language due to a neurological disorder. Most childhood language disorders, however, are developmental deficits in language comprehension (receptive skills) or in the ability to express oneself through language (expressive skills). Expressive language impairments often stand alone, without comprehension or receptive difficulties, while receptive impairments usually affect language expression as well. Communication disorders interfere with academic, work, and social achievements, and the comorbidity, within the communication disorders category and with other types of learning disorders, is high. Many children with these disorders have family members with a higher rate of communication and other learning disorders than the general population. Males are affected three times as often as females. A significant number of language disorders improve spontaneously over time, but it seems that various remedial speech therapies are effective in facilitating improvement. Emotional problems associated with poor self-esteem, easy frustration, and mood disorders may occur in children struggling with these disorders. One recent study found that more than one-third of the youngsters referred to a psychiatric outpatient clinic had a language impairment. Early recognition is important.

Childhood expressive language disorder is characterized by a lower-than-expected ability in vocabulary, in the correct use of tenses, in the production of sentences, and in the recall of words. Language understanding (decoding) skills remain intact. In epidemiological studies, the prevalence of expressive language disorder ranges from 3 to 10 percent of all school-aged children, with most estimates between 3 and 5 percent. Subtle cerebral damage and maturational lags in cerebral development have been postulated as underlying causes, but no clear evidence supports these theories. Diagnosis is confirmed by testing with standardized expressive language and nonverbal intellectual tests. Close observation of language patterns in different settings and with a variety of people can help ascertain the severity of the impairment and assist in the early recognition of possible behavioral and emotional complications. An audiogram is often indicated to rule out impairments in hearing acuity.

Mixed receptive-expressive language disorder is characterized by impairments in both the expression and comprehension of language. Expressive language disorder alone is believed to be much more common than mixed receptive-expressive disorder, but both are more common in boys than in girls. With DSM-IV-TR it is impossible to code receptive language disorder in the absence of expressive language disorder, implying that clinically significant receptive language impairments are always accompanied by expressive language disorder. Early theories postulated a variety of subtle genetic, maturational, cerebral damage, and perceptual dysfunctions as probable causative factors, but no definitive evidence supports these theories. As with expressive language disorder, left-handedness and ambilaterality appear to increase the risk.

The essential feature of phonological disorder is a variety of developmentally inappropriate speech sounds, including misarticulations, sound substitutions, distortions of phonemes, and omissions of speech sounds, often giving the impression of baby talk. For instance, a child may use the sound "t" instead of "k" or may omit the final consonants of words. In severe cases the disorder is diagnosed by age 3, and in less severe cases the disorder may not be recognized until about age 6. The most common misarticulated speech sounds are those acquired later in development: the "r," "sh," "th," "f," "z," "l," and "ch" sounds. One or many speech sounds may be affected, but not vowel sounds. Omissions are felt to be the most serious type of misarticulation, with substitutions the next most serious, and distortions the least serious type. With omissions, the phonemes are absent entirely—for example, "bu" for "blue" or "ca" for "car." With distortions, the correct phoneme is approximated but is articulated incorrectly and results in a sound that is not part of the speaker's dialect. The most common distortions are lateral slips, in which a child pronounces "s" sounds with a whistling effect, and palatal lisps, in which the "s" sound produces a "ssh" effect.

Stuttering is a disturbance in the normal fluency and time patterning of speech. These disturbances include sound repetitions, prolongations, interjections, pauses within words, word substitutions to avoid blocking, and audible or silent blocking. Stuttering is much more common in boys than girls and, as with the other communication disorders, is more common in family members than in the general population. Chronic stuttering is often accompanied by emotional sequelae such as frustration, anxiety, and depression. Anxiety exacerbates stuttering, but there is no evidence that people who stutter have more psychiatric disturbances than do those with other forms of speech and language disorders. The precise cause of stuttering is unknown but is most likely multifactorial. In the general population the prevalence of stuttering is about 1 percent and is most common in young children, usually resolving in older children and adults. Treatment can involve breathing exercises, relaxation techniques, and speech therapy. Most modern treatments of stuttering are based on the view that stuttering is a learned behavior, with approaches aimed at minimizing the issues that maintain and exacerbate stuttering.

Communication disorder not otherwise specified is reserved for diagnoses that do not fall into the identified communication disorders. An example is a voice disorder in which a patient has abnormal pitch, loudness, quality, tone, or resonance of speech.

The student should study the questions and answers below for a useful review of these disorders.

HELPFUL HINTS

These terms relate to communication disorders and should be known by the student.

- ambilaterality
- articulation problems
- audiogram
- baby talk
- cluttering
- comprehension
- decoding
- developmental coordination disorders
- dysarthria
- encoding
- expressive language disorder
- fluency of speech
- language acquisition
- lateral slip and palatal lisp
- maturational lag
- misarticulation
- mixed receptive-expressive language disorder
- neurodevelopmental delays
- omissions
- phoneme
- phonological disorder
- semantogenic theory of stuttering
- sound distortion
- spastic dysphonia
- speech therapy
- standardized language test
- stuttering
- substitution
- time patterning of speech

▲ QUESTIONS

DIRECTIONS: Each of the incomplete statements below is followed by five suggested completions. Select the *one* that is *best* in each case.

41.1 Normal development in a child of 3 includes

    A. use of 900 to 1,000 words
    B. speech is usually understood by strangers
    C. follows three-step commands
    D. use of conjunctions (e.g., if, but, because)
    E. discusses feelings

41.2 True statements about diagnosis of communication disorders include

    A. Substantial deficits in receptive language do not preclude the diagnosis of expressive language disorder.
    B. Substantial deficits in nonverbal intelligence do not preclude the diagnosis of expressive language disorder.
    C. If both expressive and receptive deficits occur in the absence of nonverbal deficits, the diagnosis of mixed receptive-expressive language disorder is not appropriate.
    D. If language and nonverbal functioning are both substantially below age-level expectations, the diagnosis of mental retardation should be made.
    E. None of the above

41.3 True statements about developmental expressive language deficits include

    A. Only 25 percent of late talkers achieve language skills within the normal range during the preschool years.
    B. Most late talkers who recover during preschool appear to be at relatively high risk for severe learning and behavioral problems.
    C. As a group, children with mixed receptive-expressive disorder show a more favorable long-term outcome than those with persistent expressive disorders.
    D. Experts agree that intervention to improve expressive language should only be provided for children whose problems persist to age 4 or 5.
    E. None of the above

DIRECTIONS: Each group of questions below consist of lettered headings followed by a list of numbered words or phrases. For each numbered word or phrase, select the *best* lettered heading. Each lettered heading may be used once, more than once, or not at all.

Questions 41.4–41.8

    A. Expressive language disorder
    B. Phonological disorder
    C. Voice disorder
    D. Verbal apraxia
    E. None of the above

41.4 Disturbance in the programming of speech movements associated with a primary insult to the left cerebral hemisphere

41.5 Organic causes include endocrine dysfunction and laryngeal papillomas

41.6 Use of sentences that are short, incomplete, or ungrammatical

41.7 In DSM-IV-TR, this category encompasses speech sound problems that have no known cause and presumably reflect developmental difficulties in acquiring the sound system of a language

41.8 Associated with cleft lip and palate

Questions 41.9–41.11

    A. A child sings normally
    B. A child cannot understand language
    C. A child has an abnormally loud voice
    D. A child substitutes and omits speech sounds
    E. None of the above

41.9 Phonological disorder
41.10 Stuttering disorder
41.11 Mixed receptive-expressive language disorder

Questions 41.12–41.16

    A. Expressive language disorder
    B. Mixed receptive-expressive language disorder
    C. Phonological disorder
    D. Stuttering
    E. All of the above

41.12 When this disorder results from a neurological impairment, it may include dysarthria and apraxia
41.13 A child with this disorder may appear to be deaf
41.14 This disorder is most commonly seen in males
41.15 Cluttering, a dysrhythmic speech pattern with jerky spurts of words, is often an associated feature of this disorder
41.16 This disorder has two peaks of onset: between 2 and 3½ years and between 5 and 7 years

ANSWERS

Communication Disorders

41.1 The answer is A

Expressive language disorder is diagnosed when a selective deficit in expressive language development occurs in the presence of intact nonverbal intelligence and receptive language skills. Children with expressive disorders do acquire language, albeit at a slower rate than their peers. Accordingly, the specific manifestations of expressive language disorder change with maturation. Affected children often show expressive language characteristics that resemble those of younger children who are developing language at a normal rate. Table 41.1 provides an overview of typical milestones in language and nonverbal development—*for a child of 3, normal development includes use of 900 to 1,000 words.* Although milestones are listed only up to age 8, it is commonly recognized that substantial growth in vocabulary, grammar, and language use continues through adolescence.

41.2 The answer is D

Differential diagnosis of developmental expressive language disorder requires standardized evaluations of expressive language, receptive language, and nonverbal intellectual functioning. Expressive language development must fall significantly below (1) the range of normal expressive performance expected for a child's age, (2) receptive language performance, and (3) nonverbal intellectual performance. Further, the expressive language difficulties must be severe enough to impair academic performance or social communication. To help determine whether this clinical severity criterion is met, standardized testing is often supplemented with observational techniques and analysis of spontaneous language use.

    Substantial deficits in either *receptive language or nonverbal intelligence preclude the diagnosis of expressive language disorder* but may contribute to the diagnosis of other disorders that affect language growth. *If both expressive and receptive deficits occur in the absence of nonverbal deficits,* the diagnosis of mixed receptive-expressive language disorder is appropriate. However, if *language and nonverbal functioning are both sub-stantially below age-level expectations, the diagnosis of mental retardation should be made.*

41.3 The answer is E (none)

Developmental expressive language disorder is characterized by considerable variability in severity, course, and outcome. Recently, several research teams conducted prospective studies of late talkers (i.e., children with normal cognitive functioning who use fewer than 50 words and no word combinations at age 2). Experts disagree on whether late talkers actually meet criteria for the diagnosis of expressive language disorder. Nonetheless, their language delays often provoke parental concern and professional referral. The various studies of late talkers generally agree that *50 to 80 percent (not 25 percent) of these children achieve language skills within the normal range during the preschool years,* with vocabulary skills perhaps recovering more fully than grammatical abilities. *Most late talkers who recover during preschool appear to be at little (not high) risk for severe learning and behavioral problems,* at least through the early school years. Nonverbal intelligence scores, receptive language levels, the extent of initial expressive delay, and the amount and variety of early communicative intentions have been suggested as possible predictors of outcome in late talkers, but these suggestions require further empirical validation.

    Prognosis is generally less favorable for children whose expressive language disorders persist into the late preschool or early school-aged years. For these children, language growth proceeds but at a slower rate than for children who are developing typically. Children with persistent expressive disorders may also experience associated problems, particularly reading disorder and attention-deficit disorders. By adolescence, most children with expressive language disorder acquire sufficient language skill to function reasonably well in most daily communication activities. Subtle residual deficits may be apparent in more demanding speaking tasks, such as those that require precise vocabulary and complex explanations. As a group, however, *children with persistent expressive disorders show less (not more) favorable long-term outcomes than their counterparts with mixed receptive-expressive disorder.*

Table 41.1
Normal Development of Speech, Language, and Nonverbal Skills in Children

Speech and Language Development	Nonverbal Development
1 year	
Recognizes own name	Stands alone
Follows simple directions accompanied by gestures (e.g., bye-bye)	Takes first steps with support
Speaks one or two words	Uses common objects (e.g., spoon, cup)
Mixes words and jargon sounds	Releases objects willfully
Uses communicative gestures (e.g., showing, pointing)	Searches for object in location where last seen
2 years	
Uses 200–300 words	Walks up and down stairs alone but without alternating feet
Names most common objects	Runs rhythmically but is unable to stop or start smoothly
Uses two-word or longer phrases	Eats with a fork
Uses a few prepositions (e.g., in, on), pronouns (e.g., you, me), verb endings (e.g., -ing, -s, -ed), and plurals (-s), but not always correctly	Cooperates with adult in simple household tasks
Follows simple commands not accompanied by gestures	Enjoys play with action toys
3 years	
Uses 900–1,000 words	Rides tricycle
Creates three- to four-word sentences, usually with subject and verb but simple structure	Enjoys simple "make-believe" play
Follows two-step commands	Matches primary colors
Repeats five- to seven-syllable sentences	Balances momentarily on one foot
Speech is usually understood by family members	Shares toys with others for short periods
4 years	
Uses 1,500–1,600 words	Walks up and down stairs with alternating feet
Recounts stories and events from recent past	Hops on one foot
Understands most questions about immediate environment	Copies block letters
Uses conjunctions (e.g., if, but, because)	Role-plays with others
Speech is usually understood by strangers	Categorizes familiar objects
5 years	
Uses 2,100–2,300 words	Dresses self without assistance
Discusses feelings	Cuts own meat with knife
Understands most prepositions referring to space (e.g., above, beside, toward) and time (e.g., before, after, until)	Draws a recognizable person
Follows three-step commands	Plays purposefully and constructively
Prints own name	Recognizes part-whole relationships
6 years	
Defines words by function and attributes	Rides a bicycle
Uses a variety of well-formed complex sentences	Throws a ball well
Uses all parts of speech (e.g., verbs, nouns, adverbs, adjectives, conjunctions, prepositions)	Sustains attention to motivating tasks
Understands letter-sound associations in reading	Enjoys competitive games
8 years	
Reads simple books for pleasure	Understands conservation of liquid, number, length, etc.
Enjoys riddles and jokes	Knows left and right of others
Verbalizes ideas and problems readily	Knows differences and similarities
Understands indirect requests (e.g., "It's hot in here" understood as request to open window)	Appreciates that others have different perspectives
Produces all speech sounds in an adult-like manner	Categorizes same object into multiple categories

Adapted from Owens RE. *Language Development: An Introduction.* 4th ed. Needham Heights, MA: Allyn & Bacon; 1996.

Experts disagree on when intervention is warranted for expressive language disorder. Some suggest that a watch-and-see attitude is appropriate for young children with early expressive delays (late talkers) because most will acquire language functioning within the normal range during preschool. In this view, intervention to improve expressive language should only be provided for children whose problems persist to age 4 or 5. Others argue that this policy would deny children early help that might serve to prevent or minimize later language, academic, and behavioral difficulties. Unfortunately, no relevant data are available on the efficacy of early versus late language intervention.

Answers 41.4–41.8

41.4 The answer is D

41.5 The answer is C

41.6 The answer is A

41.7 The answer is B

41.8 The answer is B

Verbal apraxia (also referred to as apraxia of speech) *is a disturbance in the programming of speech movements.* It is differentiated from voice disorder by its association with a primary insult to the left cerebral hemisphere. Also, verbal output in apraxic patients is often easier or normal in automatic or overlearned speech output (e.g., automatic social greetings, the song "Happy Birthday"). In most voice disorders, particularly spasmodic dysphonia, struggle and the strained-strangled quality of production are relatively constant across communication contexts.

A voice disorder, as described in the revised fourth edition of *Diagnostic and Statistical Manual of Mental Disorders* (DSM-IV-TR), is any "abnormality of vocal pitch, loudness, quality, tone or resonance." Given the complexity and sensitivity of the process of voice production, it is not remarkable that these disorders may arise from a multiplicity of factors, including medical disease, emotional stress, psychological conflict, and environmental toxicity.

Voice disorders of organic cause among children and adolescents include laryngeal papillomas, vocal fold nodules, vocal hemorrhage, laryngomalacia, laryngeal webbing (congenital or traumatic), vocal polyps, vocal fold paralysis or paresis, *endocrine dysfunction,* and laryngeal cancer. Premature infants and children with a history of extended endotracheal intubation are at high risk for development of a number of laryngeal pathologies, including subglottic stenosis, arytenoid dislocation, vocal fold paralysis, and granuloma formation or loss of tissue of the vocal folds. Reflux esophagitis and irritation of the larynx are observed in anorexia nervosa and bulimia nervosa patients and are commonly accompanied by hoarseness and low-pitched voice. Because persistent hoarseness in a child or adolescent, as in an adult, may be a sign of malignancy or another serious medical condition, otolaryngological evaluation is warranted.

Children with *expressive language disorders* have difficulty communicating their needs, thoughts, and intentions via spoken language. They frequently (1) have speaking vocabularies that are limited in size and variety; (2) *use sentences that are short, incomplete, or ungrammatical*; and (3) relate stories and events in a disorganized, confusing, or unsophisticated manner. These communication problems are evident despite performance within the normal range on measures of hearing acuity, nonverbal intelligence, and understanding (comprehension, reception) of spoken language. As with many other childhood mental disorders, the definitional and diagnostic issues concerning expressive language disorders are complex and often controversial.

Children with phonological disorders have difficulties in correctly producing the speech sounds appropriate for their ages and dialects. They may omit sounds (e.g., saying "at" for hat or "bup" for bump), substitute sounds for other sounds (e.g., saying "tum" for come or "hewo" for hello), or distort sounds by producing them in an unusual manner (e.g., producing /sh/ while allowing too much air to flow noisily over the sides of the tongue or producing /s/ or /z/ while protruding the tongue). In many cases, the speech sound differences occur in systematic patterns. For example, consonants in the final position of words may be omitted (e.g., "fee" for feet, "no" for nose), or consonants that require a steady airflow may be produced with an interrupted airflow (e.g., "do" for zoo, "pan" for fan). Listeners may be unable to understand the speech of children with severe phonological disorders.

The revised fourth edition of *Diagnostic and Statistical Manual of Mental Disorders* (DSM-IV-TR) uses somewhat different terminology for speech sound production disorders than that commonly used in the clinical and scientific literature, which may cause a problem for diagnosticians. *In DSM-IV-TR, the category of phonological disorder is an inclusive one,* encompassing difficulties in speech sound production that have no known cause as well as those that arise from hearing impairment, structural abnormalities of the speech mechanism (e.g., *cleft lip or palate*), or neurological conditions (e.g., cerebral palsy, head injury). In the literature, the terms articulation disorder and speech sound production disorder are more often used to label such an inclusive category. The terms dysarthria and dyspraxia are typically used to refer to speech sound–production difficulties that have a neurological origin. The term phonological disorder is usually reserved for speech-sound problems that have no known cause and presumably reflect developmental difficulties in acquiring the regularities of phonology (the sound system of a language). In this section this more restrictive category is referred to as developmental phonological disorder to distinguish it from the larger DSM-IV-TR category of phonological disorder.

The speech of *children with cleft palate* may be characterized by excessive nasality and by inability to produce the many consonants that require the oral cavity to be closed off from the nasal passage by the palate. Children may develop unusual ways of articulating certain sounds in an attempt to compensate for structural deficiencies. Even after structural problems are corrected by surgical or prosthetic means, these unusual patterns may persist. Children with cleft palate are also at increased risk for upper respiratory infections and accompanying hearing losses, as well as developmental language and learning difficulties.

Answers 41.9–41.11

41.9 The answer is D

41.10 The answer is A

41.11 The answer is B

In *phonological disorder, a child substitutes and omits speech sounds.* The misarticulation of speech in this disorder may resemble baby talk. The omissions, substitutions, and distortions typically occur with late-learned phonemes.

A child who stutters may sing normally.

A child with *mixed receptive-expressive language disorder cannot understand language.* Although his or her nonverbal intellectual capacity is age appropriate, a child with this disorder neither speaks nor mimics others' sounds and may not play appropriately. A child who has an abnormally loud voice may have a communication disorder not otherwise specified. Other such disorders include severe abnormalities of pitch, quality, tone, or resonance.

Answers 41.12–41.16

41.12 The answer is C

41.13 The answer is B

41.14 The answer is E (all)

41.15 The answer is A

41.16 The answer is D

Phonological disorder is characterized by poor sound or articulation. There can be substitutions of one sound for another, omissions of some sounds, or inability to reproduce a sound correctly. Often children with phonological disorder give the impression of speaking baby talk. *In certain neurological conditions, dysarthria and apraxia (loss of movement) may occur.* Dysarthria results from impairment in the neural mechanisms regulating muscle control, whereas apraxia is an impairment in the muscles used for speech themselves. *Mixed receptive-expressive language disorder* is an impairment in both the understanding and the expression of language. It is generally believed that a deficit in receptive language always results in some impairment in expressive language. Children with mixed receptive-expressive language disorder show markedly delayed ability to comprehend verbal or sign language, despite normal intellectual capacity. *A child with this disorder often appears to be deaf*, since he or she does not respond normally to language sounds, except that such a child does respond to nonlanguage sounds in the environment. Usually, when these children begin to use language, their speech contains numerous articulation errors and substitutions of phonemes. *All of the communication disorders seem to be two to four times as common in males as in females.* This striking gender difference implies a genetic basis for the communication disorders. *Cluttering is a disordered speech pattern in which speech is erratic*, with bouts of rapid and jerky words or phrases. Commonly, a child with this speech pattern is unaware that the production of speech is abnormal. This differs from stuttering in that the disturbance in fluency in stuttering is characterized by sound repetitions, pauses within words, prolongations, and audible or silent word blocking. Stutterers are generally aware of their stuttering and many experience anxiety in anticipation of speaking and stuttering. *Cluttering is often an associated feature of an expressive language disorder. Stuttering* usually appears before the age of 12 years. There are *two peaks for its onset: 2 to 3½ years and 5 to 7 years.* In the preschool age group, children tend to stutter most often when they are excited or have a lot to say. Stuttering at this age may be a passing phase. In the elementary school years, stuttering may be more chronic and may characterize a child's everyday speech. Later in childhood, stuttering is often an intermittent event that manifests itself in the course of a specific situation. Stutterers often show fear, embarrassment, and anxious anticipation of speaking in public, or they avoid certain words or phrases that have become associated with their stuttering.

42

Pervasive Developmental Disorders

The revised fourth edition of the *Diagnostic and Statistical Manual of Mental Disorders* (DSM-IV-TR) includes the following disorders under the category of pervasive developmental disorders: autistic disorder, Rett's disorder, childhood disintegrative disorder, Asperger's disorder, and pervasive developmental disorder not otherwise specified. All of these disorders are characterized by profound impairments in social interactions and communications, often reflected in stereotyped, rigid, or ritualistic behavior, interests, and activities. In other words, in these disorders there are severe and pervasive deficits in reciprocal social skills, language development, and range of behavioral repertoire. In some cases (autistic disorder and Asperger's disorder) these skills do not develop normally, and in other cases (Rett's disorder and childhood disintegrative disorder) they develop but then diminish over time. The disorders are evident early in life and lead to persistent dysfunction. Some individuals with these disorders are mentally retarded (more than two-thirds of people with autistic disorder), and others have normal cognitive abilities (Asperger's disorder). Unusual or precocious cognitive or visuomotor abilities, called splinter functions or islets of precocity, occur in some autistic children, even in the context of overall retarded functioning. Fascinating examples of this include people who have been called "idiot savants," who, although otherwise impaired profoundly, may have extraordinary rote memories or calculating abilities, or may be exceptionally musically or artistically gifted. The movie *Rain Man* sought to depict such an individual.

Autistic disorder is the best known of the pervasive developmental disorders. The term infantile autism was coined by Leo Kanner in 1943, but the syndrome was not recognized as a distinct clinical diagnosis until later. Previously, children with characteristics of any of the pervasive developmental disorders were diagnosed with schizophrenia. Evidence has indicated that autistic disorder and schizophrenia are two separate psychiatric disorders, but a child with autistic disorder may develop a comorbid schizophrenic disorder.

Physical characteristics of children with autistic disorder include a failure of lateralization (remaining ambidextrous at ages when normal children establish cerebral dominance) and a higher incidence of upper respiratory infections, excessive burping, febrile seizures, constipation, and loose bowel movements than control groups. Autistic children may have a higher pain threshold than normal children, and their behavior and relatedness may improve noticeably when they are ill. They may be severely injured and not cry. Self-injurious behavior includes head banging, biting, scratching, and hair pulling.

Among behavioral characteristics are qualitative impairments in social interactions, disturbances of communication and language, stereotyped behavior, instability of mood and affect, abnormal responses to sensory stimuli, and other symptoms. Examples include a failure to develop empathy and gross deficits and deviances in language development, including echolalia and pronominal reversal. Ritualistic and compulsive activities including extreme attachment to inanimate objects, movement sterotypies, and resistance to change are frequent. Aggressiveness and temper tantrums are observed, often for no apparent reason or in response to even very small changes in routine.

Autistic disorder occurs in two to five per 10,000 children. In most cases, autism begins before age 3. The cause is unknown. The disorder was first thought to be psychosocial or psychodynamic in origin, but substantial evidence now indicates a complex biological etiology. Autistic children have significantly more minor physical anomalies than do normal children. Initially, it was thought that a high socioeconomic status was common in families with autistic children, but these findings were probably based on referral biases. Prognosis is considered best in autistic children with IQs above 70 who have communicative language skills by age 5 to 7 years.

Unlike autistic disorder, in Asperger's disorder there are no significant delays in language, cognitive development, or age-appropriate self-help skills. However, those with Asperger's disorder do show severe, pervasive impairments in social interactions and behavioral repertoires. Restricted interests and patterns of behavior are always present. Anecdotal reports of some adults diagnosed with Asperger's disorder as children describe them as verbal and intelligent but awkward, socially uncomfortable, and shy, and often with illogical thinking. Rett's disorder appears to occur only in girls and is estimated to occur in six to seven cases per 100,000 girls. The disorder is characterized by normal development for at least 5 months following birth. The onset of the disorder, occurring between 5 and 48 months after birth, manifests with a deceleration of head growth, the loss of previously acquired purposeful hand movements, and the appearance of stereotyped hand movements such as hand-wringing. A loss of social engagement early in the course is characteristic. Rett's disorder proceeds as a progressive encephalopathy, associated with seizures, irregular respiration, and muscle rigidity. Long-term receptive and expressive communication skills remain at a developmental level of less than 1 year.

Treatment of all these disorders is aimed at increasing socially acceptable and prosocial behavior, decreasing bizarre behavioral symptoms, and aiding in the development of verbal and nonverbal communication. Prognoses are variable depending on the severity of presentation, with Rett's disorder having the poorest prognosis.

The student should study the questions and answers below for a useful review of these disorders.

HELPFUL HINTS

The student should know the following terms related to pervasive developmental disorders.

- ▶ abnormal relationship
- ▶ acquired aphasia
- ▶ Asperger's disorder
- ▶ attachment behavior
- ▶ autistic disorder
- ▶ brain volume
- ▶ childhood disintegrative disorder
- ▶ childhood schizophrenia
- ▶ communication disorder
- ▶ concordance rate
- ▶ congenital deafness
- ▶ congenital physical anomaly
- ▶ congenital rubella
- ▶ CT scan
- ▶ dermatoglyphics
- ▶ disintegrative (regressive) psychosis
- ▶ dread of change
- ▶ echolalia
- ▶ echolalic speech
- ▶ educational and behavioral treatments
- ▶ EEG abnormalities
- ▶ ego-educative approach
- ▶ encopresis
- ▶ enuresis
- ▶ extreme autistic aloneness
- ▶ eye contact
- ▶ failed cerebral lateralization
- ▶ grand mal seizure
- ▶ haloperidol (Haldol)
- ▶ Heller's syndrome
- ▶ hyperkinesis
- ▶ hyperserotonemia
- ▶ hyperuricosuria
- ▶ "idiot savant"
- ▶ insight-oriented psychotherapy
- ▶ islets of precocity
- ▶ Leo Kanner
- ▶ language deviance and delay
- ▶ low-purine diet
- ▶ mental retardation
- ▶ monotonous repetition
- ▶ organic abnormalities
- ▶ pain threshold
- ▶ parental rage and rejection
- ▶ perinatal complications
- ▶ pervasive developmental disorder
- ▶ physical characteristics
- ▶ PKU
- ▶ play
- ▶ prevalence
- ▶ pronominal reversal
- ▶ psychodynamic and family causation
- ▶ Purkinje's cells
- ▶ Rett's disorder
- ▶ ritual
- ▶ rote memory
- ▶ seizures
- ▶ self-injurious behavior
- ▶ separation anxiety
- ▶ sex distribution
- ▶ social class
- ▶ splinter function
- ▶ stereotypy
- ▶ tardive and withdrawal dyskinesias
- ▶ temporal lobe
- ▶ tuberous sclerosis
- ▶ vestibular stimulation
- ▶ voice quality and rhythm

▲ QUESTIONS

DIRECTIONS: Each of the questions or incomplete statements below is followed by five suggested responses or completions. Select the *one* that is *best* in each case.

42.1 Which of the following features does *not* distinguish autistic disorder from mixed receptive-expressive language disorder?

A. echolalia
B. stereotypies
C. imaginative play
D. associated deafness
E. family history of speech delay

42.2 Neurological-biochemical abnormalities associated with autistic disorder include

A. grand mal seizures
B. ventricular enlargement on computed tomography (CT) scans
C. electroencephalogram (EEG) abnormalities
D. elevated serum serotonin levels
E. all of the above

42.3 True statements about autistic disorder include

A. Girls outnumber boys in individuals with autism without mental retardation.
B. There is an established and conclusive association between autism and upper socioeconomic status.
C. Prevalence rates may be as high as 1 in every 1,000 children.
D. Abnormalities in functioning must be present by age 2.
E. All of the above

42.4 True statements about the role of genetics in autistic disorder include

A. Early twin studies indicated only moderate concordance for monozygotes.
B. Family studies show a rate of recurrence of approximately 2 to 3 percent of autism among siblings.
C. Unaffected siblings are not at increased risk for language problems.
D. It is clear that what is inherited is a specific predisposition to autistic disorder.
E. The role of genetic factors in autistic disorder is not well established.

42.5 The most frequent presenting complaint of parents of autistic children is

A. their lack of interest in social interaction
B. their lack of usual play skills
C. their difficulty tolerating change and variations in routine
D. delays in the acquisition of language
E. stereotyped movements

42.6 Relative strengths of autistic children in psychological testing include

   A. block design and digit recall
   B. verbal concept formation
   C. integration skills
   D. similarities and comprehension
   E. abstract reasoning

42.7 What percentage of autistic individuals exhibit special abilities or splinter (savant) skills?

   A. less than 1 percent
   B. 5 percent
   C. 10 percent
   D. 25 percent
   E. 50 percent

42.8 Rett's disorder

   A. is seen only in boys
   B. does not involve motor abnormalities
   C. is associated with marked mental retardation
   D. shows no loss of social interactional skills
   E. none of the above

42.9 Childhood disintegrative disorder is

   A. relatively common
   B. also termed Heller's syndrome
   C. always characterized by a gradual onset
   D. similar to autistic disorder in that self-help skills do not deteriorate
   E. all of the above

42.10 Asperger's disorder is characterized by delays in

   A. self-help skills
   B. curiosity about the environment
   C. nonverbal communication
   D. receptive language
   E. none of the above

DIRECTIONS: Each group of questions below consists of lettered headings followed by a list of numbered statements. For each numbered word or statement, select the *one* lettered heading that is most closely associated with it. Each lettered heading may be selected once, more than once, or not at all.

Questions 42.11–42.15

   A. Autistic disorder
   B. Childhood disintegrative disorder
   C. Pervasive development disorder not otherwise specified
   D. Asperger's disorder
   E. Rett's disorder

42.11 Normal development for the first 5 months, followed by a progressive encephalopathy

42.12 A better prognosis than other pervasive developmental disorders because of the lack of delay in language and cognitive development

42.13 Some but not all of the features of autistic disorder

42.14 Several years of normal development followed by a loss of communication skills, a loss of reciprocal social interaction, and a restricted pattern of behavior

42.15 Occurrence at a rate of two to five cases per 10,000 and characterization by impairment in social interaction, communicative language, or symbolic play before age 3

Questions 42.16–42.20

   A. Risperidone (Risperdal)
   B. Haloperidol (Haldol)
   C. Naltrexone (ReVia)
   D. Fenfluramine (Pondimin)
   E. Selective serotonin reuptake inhibitors

42.16 This opiate antagonist is being investigated in the treatment of autism

42.17 This drug has both dopamine (D_2) and serotonin (5-HT) antagonist properties

42.18 This drug has been shown to reduce lability and stereotypic behaviors and is associated with withdrawal dyskinesias

42.19 This drug is used to decrease obsessive-compulsive and stereotypic behaviors

42.20 This drug increases brain serotonin levels and has not been shown to ameliorate behavioral problems of autistic children

Questions 42.21–42.24

   A. Autistic disorder
   B. Asperger's disorder
   C. Both
   D. Neither

42.21 Onset is usually later and outcome more positive

42.22 Motor clumsiness is more common

42.23 Qualitative impairments in social interaction and restricted patterns of interest

42.24 Withdrawn in the presence of others

ANSWERS

Pervasive Developmental Disorders

42.1 The answer is B

A *family history of speech delay* or language problems occurs in about 25 percent of children with autistic disorder as well as of those with mixed receptive-expressive language disorder. *Echolalia* occurs more commonly in children with autistic disorder and less commonly in those with the language disorder. The presence or absence of *stereotypies* helps to distinguish those with autistic disorder from those with mixed receptive-expressive language disorder. Stereotypies are more common and more severe among children with autistic disorder and absent or less severe among those with the language disorder. *Imaginative play* is absent or rudimentary in children with autistic disorder and usually present in some form in those with the language disorder. *Associated deafness* is very infrequent in children with autistic disorder and not infrequent in those with the language disorder.

42.2 The answer is E (all)

Current evidence indicates that significant neurological and biochemical abnormalities are usually associated with autistic disorder. *Grand mal seizures* develop at some time in 4 to 32 percent of autistic persons, and about 20 to 25 percent of autistic persons show *ventricular enlargement on computed tomography (CT) scans.* Various *electroencephalogram (EEG) abnormalities* are found in 10 to 83 percent of autistic children; although no EEG finding is specific in autistic disorder, there is some indication of failed cerebral lateralization. *Elevated serum serotonin levels* are found in about one-third of autistic children; however, the levels are also raised in about one-third of nonautistic children with severe mental retardation.

42.3 The answer is C

Autistic disorder, also known as childhood autism, infantile autism, or early infantile autism, is by far the best known of the pervasive developmental disorders. In this condition there is marked and sustained impairment in social interaction, deviance in communication, and restricted or stereotyped patterns of behavior and interest. *Abnormalities in functioning in each of these areas must be present by age 3 (not 2) years.* Approximately 70 percent of individuals with autistic disorder function at the mentally retarded level, and mental retardation is the most common comorbid diagnosis.

The first epidemiological study of autism was conducted by Victor Lotter in 1966, who reported a prevalence rate of 4.5 in 10,000 children among the entire 8- to 10-year-old population of Middlesex, a county northwest of London. Since then 23 epidemiological studies worldwide reported in the literature have surveyed over 4,000,000 children and identified 1,545 individuals thought to have autism. Prevalence rates ranged from 0.7 per 10,000 to 21.1 per 10,000. The median prevalence estimate of four to five per 10,000 is consistent with Lotter's initial value. Variability among studies reflects methodological issues such as sample size, syndrome definition, and aspects of screening and ascertainment. Recent studies have reported higher prevalence rates. Possible reasons for the increased rates involve (1) broader definitions of autism; (2) smaller target populations (since in general, smaller studies have yielded the higher rates); and (3) better detection of cases in the extreme ranges (i.e., severely mentally retarded children and nonretarded individuals with autism). Some studies have also included estimates of the wider spectrum of autistic conditions. Although the reliability for diagnostic ascertainment of these autistic-like conditions remains questionable, compelling evidence indicates that *perhaps 1 in every 1,000 children may exhibit* social disabilities consistent with the *autistic* spectrum of *disorders.*

Studies based on both clinical and epidemiological samples have suggested a *higher incidence of autistic disorder in boys than in girls (not vice versa),* with reported ratios averaging about 3.5 or 4.0 to 1.0. This ratio varies, however, as a function of intellectual functioning. *Some studies have reported ratios of up to 6 or more to 1 in individuals with autism without mental retardation,* whereas reported ratios within the moderately to severely mentally retarded range have been as low as 1.5 to 1.0. Why females are underrepresented in the nonretarded range remains unclear. One possibility is that males have a lower threshold for brain dysfunction than females or, conversely, that more severe brain damage is required to cause autism in a girl. According to this hypothesis, a girl with autism is more likely to be extremely cognitively impaired.

Although a few early studies supported Kanner's impression of *an association between autism and upper socioeconomic status,* epidemiological studies by L. Wing, Eric Schopler, and *others have failed to reveal the correlation.* In addition to the bias for more educated and successful parents to seek referral, families from disadvantaged backgrounds still seem to be underrepresented in clinically referred samples. Outreach initiatives are needed to give children from all socioeconomic backgrounds equal access to diagnostic and intervention services.

42.4 The answer is B

The early impression was that genetic factors had no role in the pathogenesis of autism. The condition is relatively rare and patients did not seem to reproduce. However, studies of twins indicated *high (not moderate) concordance, especially for monozygotic twin pairs,* with reduced concordance for fraternal, or dizygotic, same-sex twin pairs. Evidence also suggested that the high rates of cognitive difficulties in the unaffected monozygotic twin were associated with perinatal complications in the autistic co-twin, pointing to a perinatal insult related to autism in the face of some inherited liability for the disorder. In general, *family studies have shown a rate of recurrence of approximately 2 to 3 percent of autism among siblings.* This is 50 to 100 times the rate of autism in the general population. Parents who are given the diagnosis and presentation of autism in their child might decide against having additional children. If this phenomenon, "stoppage," is taken into account, the risk to siblings is even higher. *Even when not affected by autism, siblings are at increased risk for* various developmental difficulties, including *problems in language* and cognitive development. *It remains unclear whether what is inherited is a specific predisposition to autistic disorder or a more general predisposition to developmental difficulties.* Recent work on the family members of autistic persons finds higher rates of mood and anxiety problems and increased frequency of social difficulties. Although *the role of genetic factors in autistic disorder is now well established,* specific modes of inheritance remain unclear, and efforts are under way to identify potential genetic mechanisms. It is possible, and indeed even likely, that some genetic forms of autism will be identified over the next few years.

42.5 The answer is D

As many as 50 percent of individuals with autistic disorder never speak. *Delays in the acquisition of language* are the most frequent presenting complaint of parents. Usual patterns of language acquisition (e.g., playing with sounds and babbling) may be absent or rare. Infants and young children with autistic disorder may take the parent's hand to obtain a desired object without making eye contact (i.e., as if the hand, rather than the person, is obtaining the item). In contrast to children with language disorder, these children have no apparent motivation to engage in communication or attempt to communicate via nonverbal means.

When individuals with autistic disorder do speak, their language is remarkable in various ways. They may echo what they have heard (echolalia). Speech tends to be less flexible so that, for example, there is no appreciation that change in perspective or speaker requires pronoun change, which leads to pronoun reversal. Speech may be nonreciprocal (e.g., the child produces language that is not meant as communication). While the syntax and morphology of language are relatively spared, vocabulary and semantic skills may be slow to develop, and aspects of the social uses of language (pragmatics) are particularly difficult for individuals with autistic disorder. Thus, humor and sarcasm may confuse a person with autistic disorder who fails to appreciate the speaker's communicative intent—resulting in an overly literal interpretation of the utterance. Intonation is often monotonic and robotic.

Deficits in play may include a failure to develop usual patterns of symbolic-imaginative play. Children with autistic disorder may explore nonfunctional aspects of play materials (e.g., taste or smell) or use aspects of materials for self-stimulation (spinning the tires on a toy truck).

In autistic infants and young children, the human face holds little interest, and *disturbances are seen in* the development of joint attention, attachment, and other *aspects of social interaction.* For example, the child may not engage in the usual games of infancy, may have difficulties with imitation, and may *lack usual play skills.* These deficits are highly distinctive and do not just reflect associated developmental delay.

Children with autistic disorder often *have difficulty tolerating change and variations in routine.* For example, an attempt to alter the sequence of some activity may be met with what appears to be catastrophic distress on the part of the child. Parents may report that the child insists that they engage in activities in very particular ways. Changes in routine or in the environment may elicit great opposition or upset. The child may develop an interest in a repetitive activity such as collecting strings and using them for self-stimulation, memorizing numbers, or repeating certain words or phrases. In younger children, attachments to objects, when they occur, differ from usual transitional objects in that the objects chosen tend to be hard rather than soft, and often it is the class of object, rather than the particular object, that is important (e.g., the child may insist on carrying a certain kind of magazine around). *Stereotyped movements* may include toe walking, finger flicking, body rocking, and other mannerisms, which are engaged in as a source of pleasure, or self-soothing. The child may be intensely preoccupied with spinning objects, for example, spending long periods of time watching a ceiling fan rotate.

42.6 The answer is A

Approximately 75 to 80 percent of autistic children are mentally retarded, with about 30 percent falling within the mild-to-moderate range and about 45 percent being severely to profoundly mentally retarded. Low IQ is not simply a consequence of negativism or lack of motivation. The typical profile on psychological testing is marked by *significant deficits in abstract reasoning, verbal concept formation, and integration skills* and in tasks requiring social understanding. Therefore, on the Intelligence

Scale for Children, for example, weaknesses are usually obtained on the Similarities and Comprehension subtests. In contrast, relative strengths are usually observed in the areas of rote learning and memory skills and visual-spatial problem solving, particularly if the task can be completed piecemeal, that is, without having to infer the context, or gestalt, of the task. Therefore, *performance on the Block Design and Digit Recall subtests of the Wechsler scales usually corresponds to peak performances.* The typical preference for rote and sequential tasks rather than reasoning and integrative tasks carries the implication that individuals with autistic disorder fail to see "the trees for the leaves," a difficulty that cuts across functioning modalities, from cognitive testing to communication and social interaction. Given the ubiquity of verbal deficits in autistic disorder, individuals usually have higher performance than verbal scores, particularly in those scoring in the mentally retarded range. Interestingly, some studies have suggested the opposite pattern in individuals with Asperger's disorder.

42.7 The answer is C

One of the most fascinating cognitive phenomena in autistic disorder is the presence of so-called "islets" of special abilities, or splinter skills (i.e., preserved or very highly developed skills in specific areas, which contrast with the child's overall deficits in cognitive functioning). For example, autistic children frequently have great facility in decoding letters and numbers, at times precociously (hyperlexia), even though comprehension of what is read is much impaired. *Perhaps 10 percent of individuals with autistic disorder exhibit a form of savant skills*—high, sometimes prodigious, performance on a specific skill in the presence of mild or moderate mental retardation. This fascinating phenomenon usually relates to a narrow range of capacities—for example, memorizing lists or trivial information, calendar calculation, visual-spatial skills such as drawing, or musical skills involving perfect pitch or playing a piece of music after hearing it only once. Individuals with autistic disorder represent a disproportionate majority of all savants.

42.8 The answer is C

Rett's disorder is a progressive condition that develops after some months of apparently normal development. Head circumference at birth is normal, and early developmental milestones are unremarkable. Between 5 months and 48 months (usually between 6 months and 1 year), head growth begins to decelerate. *Among the motor abnormalities,* purposeful hand movements are lost, and characteristic midline hand-wringing or hand-washing stereotypies develop. Expressive and receptive language skills become severely impaired and are *associated with marked mental retardation.* Gait apraxia and truncal apraxia and ataxia develop in the preschool years. *A loss of social interactional skills is frequently observed during the preschool years,* but social interest often increases later. To date, the condition has been demonstrated convincingly *only in girls.*

42.9 The answer is B

Childhood disintegrative disorder is a rare (not relatively common) condition characterized by a marked regression in multiple areas of development after several years of normal development.

Childhood disintegrative disorder was first described by an educator, Theodore Heller, in 1908. He reported a series of patients who displayed a marked and persisting developmental regression after 3 or 4 years of normal development. Originally, he termed the condition dementia infantilis; subsequently it has *also* been *termed* disintegrative psychosis or *Heller's syndrome.* Over 100 cases have been reported in the years following Heller's report. While the condition is certainly rare, it is probably underrecognized nonetheless.

Early development must be normal for at least 2 years; this should include normal communication and social skills. Before age 10 years there is a regression in at least two (usually many) different areas (e.g., loss of previous skills in communication, social interaction, toileting, or motor abilities) and the development of symptoms similar to those seen in autistic disorder.

Onset is usually between the ages of 3 and 4 years and may be *either abrupt or gradual.* There may be nonspecific agitation or anxiety prior to developmental deterioration. The loss of social and communicative skills is (understandably) of great concern to parents. Stereotyped behaviors, problems with transitions and change, and nonspecific overactivity often develop. *Deterioration in self-help skills can be striking and is in contrast (not similar) to autistic disorder*, in which such skills are acquired somewhat later than usual but typically are not lost.

42.10 The answer is C

Asperger's disorder is characterized by impairments in social interaction and restricted interests and behaviors as seen in autism, but *its early developmental course is marked by a lack of* any clinically significant *delay in* spoken or *receptive language*, cognitive development, *self-help skills*, or *curiosity about the environment.* All-absorbing and intense circumscribed interests and motor clumsiness are typical of the condition but are not required for diagnosis.

In 1944, Hans Asperger, an Austrian pediatrician with an interest in special education, described four children who had difficulty integrating socially into groups. Unaware of Kanner's description of early infantile autism published just the year before, Asperger called the condition he described "autistic psychopathy," indicating a stable personality disorder marked by social isolation. Despite preserved intellectual skills, the children showed *marked paucity of nonverbal communication* involving both gestures and affective tone of voice; poor empathy and a tendency to intellectualize emotions; an inclination to engage in long-winded, one-sided, and sometimes incoherent speech; rather formalistic speech (Asperger called them "little professors"); all-absorbing interests involving unusual topics, which dominated their conversation; and motoric clumsiness.

Answers 42.11–42.15

42.11 The answer is E

42.12 The answer is D

42.13 The answer is C

42.14 The answer is B

42.15 The answer is A

Rett's disorder is characterized by normal development for the first 5 months, followed by a progressive deterioration. *Asperger's disorder* may have *a better prognosis than other pervasive developmental disorders* because of the lack of delay

in language and cognitive development. *Pervasive developmental disorder not otherwise specified* includes atypical autism— presentations that *include some but not all of the features of autistic disorder. Childhood disintegrative disorder* is characterized by *several years of normal development followed by a loss of communication skills,* a loss of reciprocal social interaction, and a restricted pattern of behavior. *Autistic disorder occurs at a rate of two to five cases per 10,000* and is characterized by impairment in social interaction, communicative language, or symbolic play before age 3.

Answers 42.16–42.20

42.16 The answer is C

42.17 The answer is A

42.18 The answer is B

42.19 The answer is E

42.20 The answer is D

Numerous drugs with various mechanisms are being investigated in the treatment of the pervasive developmental disorders. Symptoms being targeted include aggression, self-injurious behaviors, mood lability, irritability, obsessive-compulsive behaviors, hyperactivity, stereotypic behavior, and social withdrawal. *Naltrexone,* an opiate antagonist, has been tried with the hope that if endogenous opioids are blocked, there will be a decrease in stereotypic behaviors in autistic disorder. *Risperidone,* a high-potency antipsychotic with both dopamine (D_2) and serotonin (5-HT) blockade, appears to be somewhat efficacious in decreasing aggression and self-injurious behaviors. *Haldol* has been shown to reduce behavioral symptoms, reduce irritability, and improve sociability among autistic children. It has also been shown to promote learning of tasks. Approximately one-quarter of autistic children develop dyskinesias, however, when Haldol is withdrawn. This syndrome generally remits. The *selective serotonin reuptake inhibitors* have been shown to have positive effects on obsessive-compulsive symptoms among adults. They are now under investigation, and sertraline (Zoloft) has been approved as an effective drug for treating the obsessions, compulsions, and stereotypic symptoms among autistic children and adolescents. *Fenfluramine* results in an increase in brain serotonin level (and a reduction in blood serotonin levels). It has not been shown to ameliorate behavioral problems among autistic children. Fenfluramine was taken off the market in 1997 because of severe adverse effects, including mitral and aortic valve damage.

Answers 42.21–42.24

42.21 The answer is B

42.22 The answer is B

42.23 The answer is C

42.24 The answer is A

Unlike children with Asperger's disorder, the great majority of autistic children experience early delays and deviance in language acquisition and cognitive impairment. The differential diagnosis is more difficult when the comparison is made with children with autistic disorder without mental retardation.

Asperger's disorder differs from the latter in that the *onset is usually later and the outcome more positive*. In addition, social and communication deficits are less severe and motor mannerisms are usually absent, whereas circumscribed interest is more conspicuous, *motor clumsiness is more common*, and a family history of similar problems is more frequent.

Diagnosis of Asperger's disorder requires the demonstration of *qualitative impairments in social interaction and restricted patterns of interest*, criteria identical to those for autistic disorder. In contrast to autistic disorder, there are no criteria in the cluster of language and communication symptoms, and onset criteria differ in that there should be no clinically significant delay in language acquisition, cognitive, and self-help skills, symptoms that result in impairment in social and occupational functioning.

In contrast to the social presentation in *autistic disorder*, individuals with Asperger's disorder find themselves socially isolated but are not usually *withdrawn in the presence of others*; typically they approach others but in an inappropriate or eccentric fashion. For example, they may express interest in friendships and in meeting people, but their wishes are invariably thwarted by their awkward approaches and insensitivity to the other person's feelings, intentions, and nonliteral implied communications (e.g., signs of boredom, haste to leave, and need for privacy).

Their poor intuition and lack of spontaneous adaptation are accompanied by marked reliance on formalistic rules of behavior and unbending social conventions. This presentation is largely responsible for the impression of social naiveté and behavioral rigidity that these individuals convey so forcefully.

43 ▲

Attention-Deficit Disorders

In the 1960s, a heterogeneous group of children were described as having what was then called minimal brain damage and were characterized as being without specific neurological injury, but with poor coordination, learning disabilities, and emotional lability. Since then, diagnostic criteria have been sharpened and numerous theories have been postulated to explain the origin of the condition.

Attention-deficit/hyperactivity disorder (ADHD) is common and is associated with abnormal levels of arousal and inability to modulate emotions. It occurs up to three to five times more often in boys than girls and can cause tremendous chaos in school and at home. The characteristics of the disorder most often cited are, in order of frequency, hyperactivity, perceptual motor impairment, emotional lability, general coordination deficit, attention deficit, impulsivity, memory and thinking deficits, specific learning disabilities, speech and hearing deficits, and equivocal neurological and EEG irregularities. A high percentage of children with ADHD fairly consistently show behavioral symptoms of aggression and defiance, which seem to be more associated with adverse family relationships. Reports on the incidence of ADHD in the United States vary from 2 to 20 percent of grade-school children, although conservatively it is believed that about 3 to 5 percent of elementary school children meet criteria for the diagnosis. Siblings of children with ADHD are at higher risk to develop the disorder than children in the general population and are also more likely than others to develop anxiety and depressive disorders. Parents of children with ADHD show an increased incidence of sociopathy, alcohol-use disorders, conversion disorder, and hyperactivity. The causes of ADHD are unknown, although contributory factors seem to include prenatal toxic exposures, prematurity, and other prenatal insults to the fetal nervous system. No rigorous evidence thus far supports such factors as food additives, colorings, preservatives, or sugar as being causative factors. A genetic basis has been postulated. Most children with ADHD do not show evidence of gross structural central nervous system (CNS) damage. Children with ADHD are at high risk for learning disorders, communication disorders, and developmental coordination disorder. Generally, they have normal intelligence and are aware of their social difficulties, which include intrusive and impulsive behavior and poor peer relationships, and thus can develop a number of associated emotional problems.

According to the revised fourth edition of the *Diagnostic and Statistical Manual of Mental Disorders* (DSM-IV-TR), the disorder must cause impairment in academic or social functioning, must occur before the age of 7, and must be present in at least two settings (i.e., school and home) for at least 6 months. A child with the disorder must show "a persistent pattern of inattention and/or hyperactivity." The diagnosis is made by the observation of numerous symptoms either in the inattention domain or the hyperactivity-impulsivity domain, or both. A child may meet criteria for the disorder with only inattention symptoms or with only hyperactivity and impulsive symptoms, and some children exhibit multiple symptoms in both domains. DSM-IV-TR categorizes three subtypes of ADHD: the predominately inattentive subtype, the predominately hyperactive-impulsive subtype, and the combined type. Children with predominately hyperactive-impulsive symptoms are most likely to have an enduring syndrome and may be the ones most likely to develop comorbid conduct disorders.

Methylphenidate (Ritalin) has been approved in children 6 years of age and older. Dextroamphetamine is usually the second line of pharmacological treatment when methylphenidate is not effective, and it has been approved for children 3 years of age and older. No evidence indicates that medications improve learning impairments directly. Their effects seem to be more to diminish attention deficits, thus allowing children to learn more effectively. As helpful as medication can be, it is often insufficient to address the multiple problems and needs of children with ADHD. It can also be overused. Individual psychotherapy, behavioral treatments, parental counseling, and the treatment of any comorbid condition are essential.

The course of ADHD is variable. For instance, symptoms may persist into adolescence and adulthood or may remit at puberty. Hyperactivity may diminish but the distractibility and impulsivity may remain. Poorer prognosis has been associated with a positive family history for the disorder, stressful life events, and comorbidity with conduct and mood disorders. Remission is unlikely before age 12. Persistence of symptoms into adulthood is often associated with antisocial behaviors, substance abuse disorders, and mood disorders. About half of children with conduct disorder develop antisocial personality disorder in adulthood. More positive outcomes may be facilitated by improving a child's social functioning, decreasing aggressive behaviors, and improving extremely unstable family situations.

The student should study the questions and answers below for a useful review of these disorders.

▲ QUESTIONS

DIRECTIONS: Each of the questions or incomplete statements below is followed by five suggested responses or completions. Select the *one* that is *best* in each case.

43.1 ADHD

A. is a relatively uncommon disorder
B. is seen in approximately 0.5 to 1.0 percent of girls
C. prevalence rates are approximately 15 to 50 percent higher under DSM-IV-TR definitions than those determined by use of the earlier DSM-III-R criteria
D. remains one of the least-validated disorders in psychiatry
E. none of the above

43.2 Neuroimaging data in patients with ADHD has revealed

A. gender does not appear to influence regional cerebral blood flow
B. reduced perfusion in bilateral frontal areas
C. increased perfusion in the caudate nuclei
D. increased perfusion in additional basal ganglia areas, partially decreased by methylphenidate administration
E. all of the above

43.3 True statements about the genetics of ADHD include

A. There is little evidence that supports the view that ADHD is in large part genetic.
B. The risk of ADHD for a sibling of a child proband with ADHD increases up to five times in some studies.
C. Concordance rates for ADHD range from 25 to 40 percent for monozygotic twins.
D. Concordance rates for ADHD range from 5 to 10 percent for dizygotic twins.
E. The heritability of hyperactivity has been calculated in twin studies to be between 20 and 30 percent.

43.4 Possible acquired etiological influences in ADHD include

A. prenatal exposure to alcohol
B. prenatal exposure to nicotine
C. low birth weight
D. exposure to maternal toxemia
E. all of the above

DIRECTIONS: The questions below consist of lettered headings followed by numbered phrases or statements. For each numbered item, select the *one* lettered item that is most closely associated with it. Each lettered item may be used once, more than once, or not at all.

Questions 43.5–43.9

A. Methylphenidate (Ritalin)
B. Dextroamphetamine (Dexedrine)
C. Bupropion (Wellbutrin)
D. Clonidine (Catapres)
E. None of the above

43.5 This may become the drug of choice for children with ADHD and a history of severe tic disorders or increased difficulties in the late afternoon or evenings
43.6 This drug has the shortest half-life and has been shown to lead to improvement in about 75 percent of children with ADHD
43.7 This drug may be the drug of choice in children who cannot tolerate stimulants because of severe rebound reaction
43.8 This drug has a half-life of 8 to 12 hours, after which a rebound may be experienced
43.9 It has been shown that growth suppression occurring with this drug's use can be compensated for with "drug holidays" in the summer and weekends

Questions 43.10–43.13

A. ADHD, inattentive type
B. ADHD, hyperactive-impulsive type
C. ADHD, combined type
D. All of the above
E. None of the above

43.10 Most common
43.11 Least common
43.12 Most children identified as having this type were 3 to 4 years younger than children diagnosed with other subtypes
43.13 Sluggish, anxious, sleepy

DIRECTIONS: Each of the questions or incomplete statements below is followed by five suggested responses or completions. Select the *one* that is *best* in each case.

43.14 Which of the following statements about attention-deficit/hyperactivity disorder (ADHD) is *false*?

A. Children with ADHD can have inattention with no hyperactivity or impulsivity.

B. Children with ADHD may have symptoms of hyperactivity but no inattention.

C. The disturbance must be present in at least two settings.

D. Children can meet the criteria for ADHD with impulsive symptoms only.

E. Many children with ADHD have many symptoms of inattention, hyperactivity, and impulsivity.

43.15 The first symptom of ADHD to remit is usually

A. hyperactivity

B. distractibility

C. decreased attention span

D. impulse-control problems

E. learning problems

43.16 The hyperactive child is often

A. accident prone

B. explosively irritable

C. fascinated by spinning objects

D. preoccupied with water play

E. all of the above

ANSWERS

Attention-Deficit Disorders

43.1 The answer is C

Over the past 25 years, much research has attempted to (1) identify core deficits associated with ADHD; (2) develop empirically tested diagnostic criteria; and (3) further validate the diagnosis of ADHD by demonstrating the disorder's characteristic symptom profiles, natural history, family-genetic aspects, and response to treatment. Although emphasis has shifted somewhat from the importance of attention deficits to the current view of two primary dimensions of inattentive and hyperactive-impulsive behaviors, along the way *ADHD has become one of the best- (not the least-) validated disorders in psychiatry.* Furthermore, public acceptance of the need for treatment of the disorder is indicated by the increased number of children receiving stimulant treatment.

In general, a variety of epidemiological *data consistently finds ADHD to be a common (not a relatively uncommon) disorder* in community samples of children and adolescents (on average identified as 3 to 5 percent) and one of the most common disorders among children referred to child mental health services. However, as with most mental disorders, changes in definitions also influence estimates of prevalence, and some variability in rates of ADHD in nonreferred samples have been noted. Available large-scale epidemiological surveys using contemporary diagnostic criteria are summarized in Table 43.1.

These studies have found that prevalence rates of ADHD in nonreferred samples range between 2.0 and 9.5 percent. *Prevalence rates of ADHD under DSM-IV-TR definitions are 15 to 50 percent higher* than those determined by use of the earlier revised third edition of DSM (DSM-III-R) criteria. Despite these differences, some interesting consistencies are seen across studies. A strong male predominance of approximately 2 or 3 to 1 has been observed both for clinic samples of children with ADHD and school-aged children. *Rate estimates for ADHD in girls have been consistent at approximately 3 percent (not 0.5 to 1.0 percent),* in spite of study differences. The field awaits a large-scale epidemiological study applying DSM-IV-TR criteria to assess the full impact of this most recent criteria change on estimates of the prevalence of disorder, correlates, and comorbid difficulties.

43.2 The answer is B

Both structural and functional neuroimaging studies have contributed to elucidating the etiology of ADHD. Early studies using xenon-133 regional cerebral blood flow pointed to brain areas that form the crux of current neuroanatomical models of pathology in ADHD. Although complicated by the co-occurrence of specific developmental problems in some samples, *reduced perfusion in bilateral frontal areas, reduced (not increased) perfusion in the caudate nuclei, and reduced (not increased) perfusion in additional basal ganglia areas, partially increased (not decreased)* by methylphenidate administration, have been reported. The apparent *reductions in blood flow* in frontal and basal ganglia regions were consistent with the emerging view that many of the self-regulation difficulties seen in children with ADHD resembled the behavior seen in classic frontal lobe damage syndromes. The first positron emission tomography (PET) study of adults with familial ADHD also found both global and specific patterns of reduced metabolism in the brains of patients compared with controls. Compared with normal control adults, those with ADHD showed global reduced metabolism bilaterally, as assessed by a fluorodeoxyglucose (FDG) [18F] tracer. In addition, a survey of specific regions found

Table 43.1
Prevalence Estimates for ADHD in Community Samples

Author	ADD (%)	ADHD (%)
Anderson et al., 1987	6.7	5.7
Costello et al., 1988	2.2	2.0
Szatmari et al., 1989	—	6.3
Velez et al., 1989	12.6	—
Jensen et al., 1995	—	7.4
Costello et al., 1996	—	1.9
Shaffer et al., 1996	—	4.1
Wolraich, 1996	—	11.4

ADD, attention-deficit disorder; ADHD, attention-deficit/hyperactivity disorder; —, not reported.

significant metabolic reductions in superior prefrontal and premotor cortices. Attempts to replicate these findings in samples of adolescents with ADHD have found fewer differences; global metabolism did not differ, although metabolism in six specific regions (an equal number from right and left brain areas) was significantly lower than that in controls in one study. *Gender* apparently *strongly influences regional cerebral blood flow*, as only females with ADHD differed in group effects from controls in some studies. In general, the initial functional brain imaging studies indicate differences in brain activity associated with ADHD, which may vary with age. Reduced activity in brain areas associated with executive functions is consistent with the types of behavioral problems seen in the disorder.

43.3 The answer is B

Compelling (not little) evidence supports the view that ADHD is familial and *in large part genetic.* In spite of differences in diagnostic criteria, most published controlled family studies report a significantly higher relative risk of ADHD in first-degree and second-degree relatives of probands with ADHD than in normal controls. For example, the risk of ADHD for a sibling of a child proband with ADHD increases from 1.8 to 5 times, depending upon the study, the sample enrolled, and the gender of the probands. Comparisons of concordance rates for ADHD in monozygotic and dizygotic twins also strongly support genetic influence in ADHD and the core symptoms of hyperactivity and inattention. Concordance rates for ADHD have ranged from 51 to 80 percent *(not 25 to 40 percent)* for monozygotic twins versus 29 to 33 percent *(not 5 to 10 percent)* for dizygotic twins. Heritability estimates for individual symptom domains also support a genetic influence in producing hyperactive and inattentive behavior. *The heritability of hyperactivity has been calculated in twin studies to be between 64 and 77 percent (not 20 and 30 percent)* and that of inattention-related behaviors, between 76 and 98 percent. Therefore, from a dimensional perspective, these extremes along behavioral traits of activity and persistence appear to be influenced highly by genes.

43.4 The answer is E (all)

A variety of acquired influences has received support as etiologic factors for some children and adolescents with ADHD, including pregnancy and delivery complications, *low birth weight,* traumatic brain injury, and prenatal substance exposure. Although the strength and specificity of these influences appear to be more limited than familial factors within groups of subjects with ADHD, the risk factors may be critical forces in the genesis of nonfamilial forms of ADHD for individual children and adolescents.

Several studies have reported associations between ADHD, pregnancy, and delivery complications. Some, but not all, reports have noted *exposure to maternal toxemia* in children later diagnosed with ADHD. Other studies suggest that problems during labor, fetal distress, and other birth complications are associated with later disruptive behavior problems. Such experiences may be particularly germane to the etiology of ADHD in children who lack a family history of the disorder. Similarly, these adverse neonatal events may be associated with particular forms or subgroups of ADHD, such as ADHD with comorbid conduct disorder.

Low birth weight has been identified as a risk factor for disruptive behavior disorders, including ADHD in particular, in several studies. The relationship between low birth weight and risk

for ADHD does not appear to be due to other perinatal risk factors commonly associated with prematurity. However, not all studies of pre- or perinatal adversity have found associations with ADHD per se; therefore, these events appear to function usually as nonspecific risk factors for psychopathology in children.

While traumatic brain injury has been thought to represent a risk factor for later hyperactivity, support for this association has been mixed. Nevertheless, more recent studies of children and adolescents with carefully ascertained brain injury have uncovered a complex connection between severe brain injury and attentional and behavioral problems. The relationship between brain injury and ADHD symptoms is defined by several aspects, including severity of the injury, location of damage to brain tissue, and age at time of injury. The strongest relationship has been found for more severe injuries and younger age at the time of injury. In one prospective sample of children with severe head injury, 19 percent had developed new-onset ADHD at follow-up. An association between mesial frontal lobe lesions and postinjury ADHD has also been described. These findings have been interpreted to suggest that earlier injuries may compromise ongoing brain development and disrupt executive functions and that individuals who have achieved greater cognitive development prior to injury may adapt better to loss of skills.

Substance exposure in utero has long been believed to lead to problems of behavioral control and emotional regulation. *Prenatal exposure to alcohol and nicotine* has been strongly associated with later assessment of ADHD symptomatology. While these effects may be moderated in part by socioeconomic variables and other environmental features, for many children alcohol exposure represents a major etiologic factor associated with cognitive and behavioral problems. Similarly, prenatal nicotine exposure is also significantly associated with later development of disruptive behavior problems. Although the connection between prenatal nicotine exposure and ADHD has not always been consistent, there is general support for a relationship between nicotine exposure and later disruptive behavior problems, including overactivity.

Answers 43.5–43.9

43.5 The answer is D

43.6 The answer is A

43.7 The answer is C

43.8 The answer is B

43.9 The answer is A

The pharmacologic agents used most widely in the treatment of ADHD are the stimulants, including methylphenidate and dextroamphetamine. Cylert (pemoline) is also a stimulant and is used when methylphenidate or dextroamphetamine has not been effective. All of these drugs require close monitoring. Since tic disorders can be exacerbated by the use of the stimulants, in children with a history of troublesome tics, a drug from another category may be indicated. *Clonidine (Catapres)* has been chosen in some of these cases since it is *reported to diminish tic behaviors* as well as control hyperactivity and short attention span. Clonidine is also an antihypertensive, so that monitoring of blood pressure is necessary with its use. Clonidine can cause significant sedation for some children and this side effect *may be beneficial for children* with ADHD who become very *hyperaroused in the evening. Methylphenidate*

Table 43.2
Medications for the Treatment of ADHD and Suggested Monitoring

Medication	Preparation	Approximate Dosage Range
First-line agents		
Methylphenidate (Ritalin)	5-, 10-, and 20-mg scored tablets	0.3–1.0 mg/dose, t.i.d.; total daily dose <60 mg
	SR (sustained release): 20-mg tablet	
Dextroamphetamine (Dexedrine)	5- and 10-mg scored tablets	0.15–0.5 mg/kg/dose, b.i.d.; total daily
	Spansules (sustained release): 5-, 10-, and 15-mg capsules	dose <40 mg
Dextroamphetamine and amphet- amine salts (Adderall)	5-, 10-, 20-, 30-mg tablets	0.15–0.5 mg/kg dose, q.a.m. or b.i.d.; total daily dose <4 mg
Second-line agents		
Pemoline (Cylert)	18.75-, 37.5-, and 75-mg tablets; 37.5-mg chewable tablets	1–3 mg/kg/day
Bupropion (Wellbutrin; Zyban)	50-, 75-, 150-mg tablets, 150 mg	150–300 mg/day (3–6 mg/kg)
Venlafaxine (Effexor)	25-, 37.5-, 50-, 100-mg tablets	25–150 mg/day, b.i.d.
Clonidine (Catapres)	0.1-, 0.2-, and 0.3-mg scored tablets	3–10 μg/kg given t.i.d. or q.i.d. (average, 0.1 mg q.i.d.)
Monitoring		
Baseline	Physical examination within 6 months	
	Height, weight, blood pressure, and pulse	
Every 3–4 mo	Height, weight, blood pressure, and pulse	
Annual	Physical examination, laboratory studies as indicated	

(Ritalin) has its peak plasma level 1 to 2 hours after ingestion, and its *half-life* of 3 to 4 hours *is the shortest of the stimulant drugs.* Some children experience a rebound effect consisting of mild irritability and increased hyperactivity when the drug wears off. Studies with ADHD children have shown methylphenidate to have *an efficacy rate of about 75 percent.* Some children with ADHD *cannot tolerate either methylphenidate or Dexedrine* because of either severe rebound effects or an increased need for medication in the late afternoon and evening. *In this situation,* and especially for children who are also exhibiting symptoms of depression, *bupropion (Wellbutrin)* may be used. This drug is a unicyclic antidepressant whose half-life is approximately 12 hours. Thus, when it is given twice daily, a steady-state blood level can be achieved. Its efficacy for ADHD symptoms should be present throughout the day and evening evenly. *Dextroamphetamine (Dexedrine)* is approved by the U.S. Food and Drug Administration (FDA) for use in the treatment of ADHD in children 3 years old and older. Its *half-life is 8 to 12 hours,* after which a rebound may be experienced. Dextroamphetamine is an efficacious treatment for ADHD and is not infrequently found to be a drug of abuse among adolescents and adults with substance-use disorders. There has been concern over the years regarding the growth suppression that may occur in children during the course of *methylphenidate* use. While *growth may be suppressed* during the days that methylphenidate is being taken, there is *evidence that final height of children who have taken methylphenidate is not affected as long as "drug holidays" are given* on the weekends, summers, or during other periods. Table 43.2 describes commonly presented medications for ADHD and their approximate effective dosage ranges.

Answers 43.10–43.13

43.10 The answer is C

43.11 The answer is B

43.12 The answer is B

43.13 The answer is A
The DSM-IV-TR subtypes of ADHD describe some of the symptom variability in ADHD: ADHD, inattentive type; ADHD, hyperactive-impulsive type; or ADHD, combined type. Estimates of the frequency of subtypes in clinic-referred children suggests that the *combined type is most common,* followed by the inattentive type, *and finally by the hyperactive-impulsive type.* The average age at diagnosis of ADHD is approximately 7 to 9 years. In the field testing of the DSM-IV-TR ADHD categories, *most children identified as having ADHD, hyperactive-impulsive type, were 3 to 4 years younger* than children diagnosed with other subtypes. ADHD children with the inattentive subtype tend to have a later age of recognition, perhaps because they exhibit fewer of the oppositional, defiant, and aggressive behaviors that often spark referrals for evaluation. Although symptoms often overlap across subtypes of ADHD and hyperactivity-impulsivity and inattentive behaviors are significantly correlated, some prominent differences can be observed in individual cases. For example, *children with the inattentive subtype* are often described as *sluggish, anxious,* subject to daydreaming, and *sleepy*—if anything, hypoactive.

43.14 The answer is D
Children cannot meet the criteria for attention-deficit/hyperactivity disorder (ADHD) with impulsive symptoms only; hyperactivity or inattention symptoms are also needed. *Children with ADHD can have inattention with no hyperactivity or impulsivity* if they have at least six symptoms of inattention. *Children with ADHD may have symptoms of hyperactivity but no inattention,* but they must then have four symptoms of hyperactivity or at least four

symptoms of a combination of hyperactivity and impulsivity. *The disturbance must be present in at least two settings.* Many children with ADHD have *many symptoms of inattention, hyperactivity, and impulsivity.* Persons with adult manifestations of the disorder are maintained on sympathomimetic drugs.

43.15 The answer is A

Hyperactivity is usually the first symptom of ADHD to remit, and *distractibility* is the last. The course of the condition is highly variable: Symptoms may persist into adolescence or adult life, they may remit at puberty, or the hyperactivity may disappear but the *decreased attention span* and *impulse-control problems* persist. Remission is not likely before the age of 12. If remission does occur, it is usually between the ages of 12 and 20. Remission may be accompanied by a productive adolescence and adult life, satisfying interpersonal relationships, and few significant sequelae. The majority of patients with ADHD, however, undergo only partial remission and are vulnerable to antisocial and other personality disorders and mood disorders. *Learning problems* often continue.

43.16 The answer is E (all)

The hyperactive child is often *accident prone, explosively irritable, fascinated by spinning objects,* and *preoccupied with water play.* In school, hyperactive children may rapidly attack a test but answer only the first two questions, or they may be unable to wait to be called on. At home, they cannot be put off for even a minute. Irritability may be provoked by relatively minor stimuli, and the hyperactive child may seem puzzled and dismayed over that phenomenon. They are frequently emotionally labile and easily inspired to laughter—or tears. Their moods and performances are apt to be variable and unpredictable.

44

Disruptive Behavior Disorders

Learning to assert one's own will and oppose the will of others is an essential developmental task and is related to the establishment of autonomy and identity formation. One of the most familiar examples of this normal oppositional behavior is the "terrible twos," when children between the approximate ages of 18 and 24 months begin to express their growing individuation and autonomy. Another normal developmental oppositional phase occurs in teenagers as they struggle to establish an individual identity separate from their parents and embark on their entry into adulthood. Sometimes, environmental trauma of various kinds (illness, loss, abuse) may trigger oppositional behavior as a defense against feelings of helplessness and anxiety. Pathological signs and symptoms begin, and disruptive behavior disorders are diagnosed, if expected developmental phases persist or recur considerably more often or more intensely than in other children of the same age, and if significant impairments in social, work, or academic situations result. Oppositional defiant disorder, conduct disorder, and disruptive behavior disorder not otherwise specified are the three disruptive behavior disorders categorized in the revised fourth edition of the *Diagnostic and Statistical Manual of Mental Disorders* (DSM-IV-TR). Sometimes a child's temperament may predispose him or her to a personality characterized by strong preferences or great assertiveness. If the child's parents overreact to these characteristics (or have their own issues with power and control, leading them to inappropriately wield authority for their own needs), the resulting struggle can establish the foundation for the development of oppositional defiant disorder.

Oppositional defiant disorder is diagnosed when a child's tantrums, refusal to comply with rules, and annoying behaviors exceed the normal expectations for these behaviors in children of the same age. Oppositional defiant disorder is distinguished from conduct disorder in that in the defiant disorders there is an absence of the serious violations of social norms or of the rights of others that is seen in the conduct disorders. Oppositional defiant disorder presents with a persistent pattern of negativistic, disobedient, and hostile behavior toward authority figures. In DSM-IV-TR, the diagnosis is made if the behavior lasts at least 6 months and presents with the recurrence of such behaviors as temper tantrums, arguments with adults, defiance of rules, deliberately annoying behavior, blaming others for one's own problems, spiteful reactions, and touchiness, anger, and resentment. Despite normal intelligence, these children often perform poorly in school and have few friends. As a result of these difficulties, children with the disorder are at risk for low self-esteem and mood disorders. Typically, the disorder has an onset of between 8 years and adolescence, although it has been described as early as 3 years of age. While it seems that prepubertal boys with the disorder outnumber prepubertal girls, the sex ratio is estimated to be about equal after puberty. Some researchers have postulated that there may be something of a sex-ratio bias in diagnosis, with girls more often receiving the diagnosis of a defiant disorder and boys more often receiving diagnoses of conduct disorders. Often, symptoms of the disorder are most apparent in interactions with people the child knows well, which may mean that few or no signs of the disorder will be present when the child is examined clinically.

The course and prognosis of oppositional defiant disorder depend on its presenting severity, the existence of comorbid disorders (such as conduct, learning, mood, and substance abuse disorders), and the degree of family stability. Parental psychopathology, such as antisocial personality disorder and substance abuse, seems to be more common in families of children with the disorder than in the general population, a finding that creates increased risks and poorer prognosis. The primary treatment is individual psychotherapy for the child, with counseling and training in child management skills for the parents. Psychological and pharmacological treatment of associated comorbid conditions are also essential.

Conduct disorder is characterized most frequently by aggressive behavior and by violations of the rights of others. The four groups of characteristic behaviors described in DSM-IV-TR are aggressive conduct that can cause physical harm to people or animals, destruction of property, deceit or theft, and serious violations of rules. There are two subtypes: childhood onset, with at least one behavioral characteristic beginning before the age of 10 years, and adolescent onset, with behavioral characteristics beginning only after 10 years of age. DSM-IV-TR lists three degrees of intensity: mild, moderate, and severe. Conduct disorder is associated with many other disorders, including attention-deficit/hyperactivity, mood, and learning disorders. Associated psychosocial factors include harsh and punitive parenting, family instability, and low socioeconomic status. DSM-IV-TR lists 15 typical behaviors associated with conduct disorder, of which at least three are required to make the diagnosis. These include bullying, threatening, or intimidating others; physical cruelty to people or animals; deliberate fire-setting; frequent lying to or "conning" of others; and repeated truancy from school before the age of 13. Conduct disorder is estimated to occur in 6 to 16 percent of boys and 2 to 9 percent of girls under the age of 18. Conduct disorder is diagnosed 4 to 12 times as often in boys as in girls. Boys most commonly meet the diagnostic criteria by 10 to 12 years of age, while girls have a later age of onset (around 14 to 16 years of age). Parental histories of antisocial personality disorder and substance abuse are common. Aggressive children and their families show stereotyped patterns of impulsivity and hostility.

The younger the age of onset of conduct disorder, and the greater the number of symptoms, the poorer the prognosis. A good prognosis occurs more often with disorders characterized as mild in the presence of normal intelligence and in the absence of comorbidity. Multimodal treatment programs involving community and family resources are crucial. Medication may be a useful adjunctive treatment, especially in the management of overt, explosive aggression. Medications that have been used in the treatment of aggression, impulsivity, and lability include antipsychotics, lithium, and the selective serotonin reuptake inhibitors (SSRIs).

The student should study the questions and answers below for a useful review of these disorders.

HELPFUL HINTS

The student should be able to define the following terms.

- ADHD
- autonomy
- child abuse
- CNS dysfunction
- comorbid disorders
- harsh child-rearing structure
- issues of control
- mood disorders
- negativistic relationships
- normative oppositional stages
- parental psychopathology
- poor peer relationships
- poor self-esteem
- socioeconomic deprivation
- temperamental predispositions
- terrible twos
- truancy
- violation of rights

▲ QUESTIONS

DIRECTIONS: Each of the questions or incomplete statements below is followed by five suggested responses or completions. Select the *one* that is *best* in each case.

44.1 Oppositional defiant disorder

A. is associated with major antisocial violations
B. is defined as part of a developmental stage
C. is limited to a particular age group
D. most commonly emerges in late-preschool– or early school–aged children
E. diagnosis implies less circumscribed disturbances of greater severity than in conduct disorder

44.2 In oppositional defiant disorder

A. The average age of onset is 3 years.
B. Boys always outnumber girls, regardless of age range.
C. Occurrence is mostly in cohorts of middle to higher socioeconomic status.
D. Point prevalence has been reported to average around 6 percent.
E. All of the above

44.3 True statements about oppositional defiant disorder include

A. In one study, about one-third of boys with the disorder progress to develop conduct disorders.
B. Ninety percent of boys with conduct disorder have fulfilled criteria for oppositional defiant disorder previously in their lives.
C. The disorder has been linked to the presence of anxious-avoidant parental attachment.
D. Twenty-five percent of children with this disorder will have no further diagnosis.
E. All of the above

44.4 The most common comorbidity with oppositional defiant disorder is

A. attention-deficit/ hyperactivity disorder
B. dysthymic disorder
C. major depressive disorder
D. early-onset bipolar I disorder
E. anxiety disorders

44.5 In conduct disorder

A. Symptoms are clustered in two areas.
B. Subtyping is allowed based on the age of onset of symptoms.
C. At least five of a list of 15 antisocial behaviors must be present.
D. All behaviors must have been present in the last 6 months.
E. All of the above

44.6 Factors associated with conduct disorder include

A. chronic illness
B. disturbed laterality and language performance
C. viewing televised or other media violence
D. temperament
E. all of the above

44.7 The most virulent comorbid condition of conduct disorder is considered to be

A. paranoid psychotic disorders
B. substance-use disorders
C. oppositional defiant disorder
D. attention-deficit/hyperactive disorders
E. major depressive disorder

DIRECTIONS: These lettered headings are followed by a list of numbered statements. For each numbered statement, select the *one* lettered heading most closely associated with it. Each lettered heading may be used once, more than once, or not at all.

Questions 44.8–44.10

    A. Oppositional defiant disorder
    B. Conduct disorder

44.8 It may be diagnosed when symptoms occur exclusively with attention-deficit/hyperactivity disorder, learning disorders, and mood disorders

44.9 It may be equally prevalent in adolescent boys and adolescent girls

44.10 The patient often bullies, threatens, or intimidates others

DIRECTIONS: Match the statements with the appropriate medication.

Questions 44.11–44.15

    A. Haloperidol (Haldol)
    B. Lithium (Eskalith)
    C. Selective serotonin reuptake inhibitors
    D. Stimulants
    E. Carbamazepine (Tegretol)

44.11 This medication has recently been shown to work no better than placebo in decreasing aggression

44.12 This medication has been shown to be efficacious in the treatment of a disorder that commonly occurs with conduct disorder

44.13 This medication is under investigation as a treatment for irritability, mood disturbance, and mood lability among children with conduct disorder

44.14 This medication has been shown to produce withdrawal dyskinesias

44.15 This medication is used to stabilize mood as well as to diminish overt aggression

---

ANSWERS

Disruptive Behavior Disorders

44.1 The answer is D

Oppositional defiant disorder consists of negativistic, hostile, or defiant behavior creating disturbances in one of three domains of functioning (academic, occupational, or social) and lasting at least 6 months. The diagnosis also refers to angry and vindictive behavior and problems with control of temper. Most of the behaviors are directed at someone—that is, an authority figure. However, *there are no major antisocial violations*. The behavior is also *not part of a developmental stage* (i.e., oppositional behavior around ages 2 to 3 years and in early adolescence). The diagnosis is not limited to a particular age group, but *most commonly emerges in late-preschool– or early-school–aged children*. Exclusion criteria for other diagnoses (conduct disorder, antisocial personality disorder, psychotic disorder, or mood disorder) are added. *The diagnosis implies more (not less) circumscribed disturbances* of lesser (not greater) severity than in conduct disorder but represents more troublesome behavior than normative oppositionality. Behaviors of the oppositional defiant disorder type, on the average, appear 2 to 3 years earlier than those of conduct disorder. The latest factor analysis suggests that there is significant coherence of the oppositional defiant disorder behaviors as outlined in the diagnostic criteria. However, support for the diagnosis has not been uniform; some authors question its status as a separate diagnosis or even as any kind of taxonomy at all, and there have been some negative public reactions categorizing oppositional defiant disorder as an attempt to characterize normative behavior as pathological.

44.2 The answer is D

The epidemiological data for oppositional defiant disorder need to be regarded with some caution because of the recent modifications of the diagnostic criteria. *The point prevalence* of the disorder has been reported to vary between 1.7 to 9.9, with *a weighted average of around 6 percent. The average age of onset is about 6 (not 3) years. Boys outnumber girls in the prepubertal age range, after which the two genders are more equal. The disorder occurs mostly in cohorts of lower (not middle to higher) socioeconomic status.*

44.3 The answer is E (all)

Very little is known regarding the role of psychological factors in oppositional defiant disorder. Attachment theorists have noted the similarities between the behavioral manifestations of insecure attachment and disruptive behavior disorders. In their view, antisocial behavior is seen as a special signal to an unresponsive parent. Findings linking infant attachment status with problematic behavior in preschool have been inconsistent but interesting. Oppositional defiant disorder has been *linked to the presence of anxious-avoidant parental attachment* in particular. Insecure attachment also predicts aggression in elementary school in boys and multiple behavior problems in the classroom. Given the inconsistency in the data, most experts believe that multivariate transactional pathways will be found in this area of research. Another important research area includes the work of Kenneth Dodge, who focused on aggressive children's deficient information processing in regard to social stimuli. Aggressive children have shown deficits at every phase of this multistage process: They underutilize pertinent social clues, misattribute hostile intent to peers, generate fewer solutions to problems, and expect to be rewarded for aggressive responses.

One of the main explanatory problems in developmental psychopathology is the simultaneous existence of stability in behavior paired with its protean appearance. Nowhere is this as apparent as in the area of antisocial behavior and its syndromal disturbances. Models need to be developed that do justice to this heterotypic continuity. The underlying process may remain stable, but manifest disturbances can change, depending on the context of the situation and the developmental phase of a given individual. One of the crucial issues for the diagnostic category of oppositional defiant disorder is the demonstration of its continuity with conduct disorder and antisocial personality disorder. One longitudinal study establishes such a link: Researchers have demonstrated that *about one-third of boys* with oppositional defiant disorder *progress to suffer conduct disorders.* Conversely, *90 percent of boys with conduct disorder previously fulfilled criteria for oppositional defiant disorder.* Thus, the syndrome has considerable sensitivity for the prediction of conduct disorder from oppositional defiant disorder, but the positive predictive power is much less. One-half of the sample retained oppositional defiant disorder diagnoses while one-quarter desisted from oppositional defiant disorder at 3-year follow-up. It is an open issue whether children with oppositional defiant disorder who do not go on to develop conduct disorder will develop other psychiatric diagnoses.

With the exception of one 3-year prospective study there is no information about the naturalistic progression or response to treatment in these children. Most will not develop conduct disorders or antisocial personality disorder. One-half will show stable signs of oppositional defiant disorder after 3 years; *25 percent will have no further diagnosis.* Extrapolating from studies on conduct disorder and oppositional defiant disorder, about one-quarter of the initial total will go on to develop conduct disorders and about 10 percent will progress to antisocial personality disorder.

44.4 The answer is A

Differentiation of oppositional defiant disorder from normative oppositional behavior, transient antisocial acts, and conduct disorder is of paramount importance. Oppositional defiant disorder is not transient, leads to significant impairment, but does not involve major violations of the law and the rights of others. *Attention-deficit/hyperactivity disorder is the most common comorbidity*: Between 25 to 60 percent of children with oppositional defiant disorder also fulfill criteria for attention-deficit/hyperactivity disorder by parental report, and half of attention-deficit/hyperactivity disorder children have oppositional defiant disorder. As with conduct disorder, the association of oppositional defiant disorder and attention-deficit/hyperactivity disorder confers poor prognosis. Youngsters tend to be more aggressive, show a greater range and persistence of problem behaviors, are rejected at higher rates by peers, and underachieve more severely in the academic domain. Furthermore, attention-deficit/hyperactivity disorder facilitates the early appearance of oppositional defiant disorder and conduct disorder. Antagonistic behavior is commonly found in internalizing disorders in this age group: *dysthymic disorder, major depressive disorder*, and *early-onset bipolar I disorder* should be considered. *Anxiety disorders*, especially separation anxiety disorder, can present with predominant temper control problems. Pervasive developmental disorders also can demonstrate oppositionality, but the underlying bizarre problems with relating to others are usually absent in oppositional defiant disorder children.

44.5 The answer is B

Conduct disorder is a clinical term referring to the clustering of persistent antisocial acts of children and adolescents. The condition is thought to be due to underlying psychopathology lead-

ing to significant impairment in one or more domains of functioning. *The symptoms are clustered in four (not two) areas:* aggression to people and animals, destruction of property, deceitfulness and theft, and serious violations of rules. *Subtyping is allowed based on the age of onset of symptoms.* Severity can be specified as mild, moderate, or severe. The category is currently conceived of as a polythetic diagnosis in that no one specific criterion is necessary for and any combination of criteria will suffice to establish the diagnosis. There is no formal provision for evaluating the context in which these antisocial clusters occur. Both these features contribute to the fact that the category is inherently heterogenous. The current criteria require that *at least three (not five) of a list of 15 antisocial behaviors* be *present over a period of 12 months; one of them (not all) has to be present in the past 6 months.* Exclusion criteria for antisocial personality disorder are added. In epidemiological studies, this category has been robust, especially in its most recent, more stringent versions. Its inherent heterogeneity has made conduct disorder less useful for causal and treatment studies.

44.6 The answer is E (all)

One important model of conduct disorder posits that it is the gradual accumulation of risk as well as the absence or weak presence of protective factors and their interactions that lead ultimately to the conduct disorder, rather than single risk factors operating in isolation. Rolf Loeber has illustrated the gradual stacking of factors in the genesis of conduct disorder. An expanded model would include a parallel pyramid of resilience or protective factors, balancing the aggregation of risk as it accumulates over time. Figure 44.1 portrays the predominance of risks in ecological (e.g., poverty), constitutional (e.g., difficult temperament), and parenting (e.g., poor response to coercive behaviors, abuse) factors. This results in poor internal self-regulation, which becomes manifest especially during school age. School performance is also affected because these children lack skills needed to deal with authority and cannot fulfill their academic potential. Peer relationships suffer, as the child tends to find acceptance only from similarly socially inept peer groups. As there is an increasing aggregation of risk, it takes more and stronger protection to offset the risk, and more domains may be adversely affected. Empirical data also show that as risks accu-

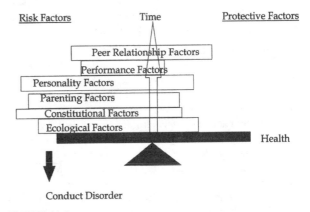

FIGURE 44.1
Developmental pathways to disruptive behavior disorders.

mulate in number, the greater is the chance that conduct disorder will develop via multiple interactive loops among risks.

Difficult *temperament has been repeatedly implicated* in the genesis of the disorder. It may work in at least two ways: It can make children more likely targets of parental anger and thus of poor parenting, or it may be linked directly to behavior problems later on. Inappropriate aggression at an early age, especially in combination with shyness, predicts later conduct disorder. *Chronic illness* and disability also have been known to increase the prevalence of conduct disorder, especially if the primary illness affects the central nervous system (CNS). Chronically ill children have three times the incidence of conduct problems of their healthy peers; if chronic illness affects the CNS, the risk is about five times as high.

Conduct disorder is more likely to be paired with diverse and complex disturbances in psychological domains. The origin of these disturbances is not clear, but their presence implies that many risks for conduct disorder are retained and internalized and independent of specific environments. Academic underachievement, learning disabilities, and problems with attention span and hyperactivity are all associated with conduct disorder. Hyperactivity, especially in the presence of poor parental functioning, is a risk; it seems to facilitate rapid development of conduct disorder. Neuropsychological deficits have been documented, implicating frontal and temporal lobe dysfunctions. *Laterality and language performance are disturbed.* Higher personality functions are also affected: In complex social situations, children with conduct disorder have been shown to perceive fewer appropriate responses, lack the skills to negotiate conflict, and lose their ability to restrain themselves when stressed emotionally.

Poor family functioning, familial aggregation of drug and alcohol abuse, psychiatric problems, marital discord, and especially poor parenting are all associated with conduct disorder. Abusive, neglectful parenting and child maltreatment is an unusually high risk factor for the development of conduct disorder. The specific parenting patterns contributing to the development of conduct disorder have been described as training in noncompliance by inconsistent responses to coercive behavior of the child, and by capitulating to demands in response to the child's coercion. There is substantial evidence that *viewing televised or other media violence* and violence in the child's community contributes to conduct disorder problems, especially in children who are at special risk for other reasons. Socioeconomic disadvantage as manifested in poor housing, crowding, and poverty all exert consistently negative influences.

44.7 The answer is D
Conduct disorder has to be distinguished, first and foremost, from antisocial behavior without underlying psychopathology, *oppositional defiant disorder*, antisocial personality disorder, and impulse-control disorders. *Substance-use disorders* are extremely common in conduct disorder and can be the primary diagnostic reason for antisocial conduct. *Attention-deficit/ hyperactivity disorder* is the next most common differential. The association with conduct disorder has been so frequent that there has been a debate over combining the diagnoses, but empirical data finds that the disorders differ in terms of premorbid risk and their respective predictive power for adult criminal outcomes. Divergent validity for conduct disorder from

attention-deficit/hyperactive disorders is generally considered as established. The latter disorder is *considered the most virulent comorbid condition*: It facilitates the early appearance of conduct disorder, which is a strong predictor of adverse outcome. *Psychotic disorders, especially those with paranoid processes,* can be mistaken for conduct disorder. Internalizing disorders, such as mood disorders, posttraumatic stress disorder, and dissociative disorder can be confused with conduct disorder, although less commonly. Age under 18 generally prevents the diagnosis of personality disturbances, but in some cases borderline, narcissistic, and antisocial personality disorders should be considered. DSM-IV-TR allows for extensive comorbidities, as no exclusion criteria are provided. Conduct disorder is usually accompanied by a wide range of comorbid conditions. These comorbidities contribute independently and interactively to prognosis and outcome. Internalizing and externalizing comorbidities become increasingly common as the disorder becomes more severe. Repeated studies have shown that complex diagnostic patterns are the rule in this population, resulting in compound psychopathology requiring special management and treatment. Loeber's data provide a unique opportunity to examine the developmental unfolding of various comorbid states: Prior to adolescence, attention-deficit/hyperactivity disorder is most frequently associated with conduct disorder, especially in boys, declining in importance thereafter. The typical sequence seems to be attention-deficit/hyperactivity disorder—opposition defiant disorder—conduct disorder; alcohol and substance abuse follow. Each additional comorbidity adds to the poor prognosis in boys. The picture is different for girls: They also have a greater chance of getting conduct disorder when they suffer from attention-deficit/hyperactivity disorder, but it is not clear that the prognostic implications are as grave. Internalizing disorders, most commonly mood and anxiety disorders, but also somatization disorders, seem to appear during adolescence when conduct disorder is firmly entrenched. *Depression* in particular affects both sexes but especially girls, especially after they have reached pubertal maturation. Evidence on the prognostic impact of internalizing comorbidity and conduct disorder is mixed.

Answers 44.8–44.10

44.8 The answer is B

44.9 The answer is A

44.10 The answer is B
Conduct disorder may be diagnosed when symptoms occur exclusively with attention-deficit/hyperactivity disorder, learning disorders, and mood disorders, whereas oppositional defiant disorder cannot be diagnosed when symptoms occur solely during a mood disorder. *Oppositional defiant disorder* may be equally prevalent in adolescent boys and adolescent girls, but conduct disorder is generally present more often in adolescent boys than adolescent girls. In *conduct disorder*, the patient often bullies, threatens, or intimidates others.

Answers 44.11–44.15

44.11 The answer is E

44.12 The answer is D

44.13 The answer is C

44.14 The answer is A

44.15 The answer is B

In controlled studies, *carbamazepine* was shown to be no better than placebo in decreasing overt aggression among children with conduct disorders. *Stimulants* have been used widely among children with conduct disorder who also have attention-deficit/hyperactivity disorder. There is some evidence that in these children, the stimulant medication diminishes aggression within the classroom setting. *Selective serotonin reuptake inhibitors,* for example, fluoxetine (Prozac), sertraline (Zoloft), and paroxetine (Paxil), are being investigated for treatment of the irritability, mood lability, and mood disorders among children with conduct disorder, with and without the full clinical picture of major depression. Haloperidol (Haldol), has been shown in studies to decrease explosive outbursts and assaultive behavior in children with conduct disorders. Haloperidol is known to produce *withdrawal dyskinesias* in approximately one-fourth of children who have been treated with it for the control of aggressive behavior. *Lithium* has also been shown to diminish aggression in children with rage outbursts, assaultive behavior, and unstable mood.

45

Feeding and Eating Disorders of Infancy or Early Childhood

Pica, rumination disorder, and feeding disorder of infancy or early childhood are the three disorders listed in the revised fourth edition of the *Diagnostic and Statistical Manual of Mental Disorders* (DSM-IV-TR) under the category feeding and eating disorders of infancy and early childhood. These disorders are characterized by persistent eating and feeding disturbances. Examples of culturally acceptable forms of pica are those that may occur in pregnant women who eat clay or starch. Pica can be diagnosed even if it occurs in the context of other mental disorders, such as autistic disorder or schizophrenia. Frequently, it occurs in people who are mentally retarded, and except in these people, usually remits by adolescence. The onset is typically between the ages of 1 and 2 years, and the incidence decreases with age. It is estimated to occur in 10 to 30 percent of children between the ages of 1 and 6 years. Etiologic theories have ranged from the postulation of nutritional deficiencies to parental neglect and deprivation. Cultural influences can be compelling, but if present, then the diagnosis of pica is not made.

Rumination disorder is characterized in DSM-IV-TR by a child's recurrent rechewing and regurgitation of food for a period of at least 1 month following a period of normal functioning. Partially digested food is brought up into the mouth without evidence of nausea, vomiting, or disgust. For the disorder to be diagnosed it must not be due to a gastrointestinal or other medical condition, and cannot occur exclusively during the course of anorexia or bulimia nervosa. The onset is usually between 3 months and 1 year of age, and infants appear to find the experience pleasurable. The disorder is rare, particularly in older children, but common in mentally retarded children and adults. Infants are most often brought for evaluation when they manifest signs of failure to thrive. In its most severe form, the disorder can be fatal.

The treatment of rumination disorder is often a combination of behavioral techniques, education, and support for the mother.

Feeding disorder of infancy and early childhood is characterized in DSM-IV-TR as a persistent failure to eat adequately, leading to significant failure to gain weight or significant loss of weight. The age of onset is defined as prior to age 6, and the disorder cannot be due to a medical condition, another mental condition (such as rumination disorder), or lack of food.

The student should study the questions and answers below for a useful review of these disorders.

HELPFUL HINTS

The student should know the following terms.

- amylophagia
- anemia
- behavioral interventions
- cultural practices
- esophageal reflux
- failure to thrive
- geophagia
- hiatal hernia
- impoverished environments
- intestinal parasites
- iron deficiency
- lead poisoning
- mental retardation
- nutritional deficiencies
- overstimulation
- parental neglect and deprivation
- positive reinforcement
- psychosocial dwarfism
- regurgitation
- self-stimulation
- spontaneous remission
- zinc deficiency

▲ QUESTIONS

DIRECTIONS: Each of the questions or incomplete statements below is followed by five suggested responses or completions. Select the *one* that is *best* in each case.

45.1 Feeding disorder of infancy or early childhood

A. has narrow DSM-IV-TR diagnostic criteria that address the specificity of various feeding disorders

B. has been reported in 1 to 2 percent of infants and toddlers

C. may have an age of onset after 6 years

D. does not necessarily result in significant failure to gain weight

E. none of the above

45.2 Pica

   A. is usually diagnosed most easily when the child is under 2 years of age

   B. decreases in prevalence with increasing severity of mental retardation

   C. is not diagnosed if symptoms occur in the context of another disorder (such as schizophrenia or autism)

   D. is diagnosed even if symptoms are culturally accepted

   E. none of the above

45.3 Pica may lead to or be related to

   A. toxoplasmosis

   B. bulimia nervosa

   C. thumb sucking

   D. delays in speech and psychosocial development

   E. all of the above

45.4 Rumination disorder

   A. is common in older children and adolescents

   B. has not been associated with death

   C. cannot be due to an associated gastrointestinal condition

   D. is common in infancy

   E. occurs more often in females than in males

DIRECTIONS: The questions below consist of lettered headings followed by a list of numbered phrases. For each numbered phrase, select

   A. If the item is associated with *A only*

   B. If the item is associated with *B only*

   C. If the item is associated with *both A and B*

   D. If the item is associated with *neither A nor B*

Questions 45.5–45.7

   A. Rumination disorder

   B. Feeding disorder of infancy or childhood

   C. Both

   D. Neither

45.5 Possibly related to a disturbed mother–infant relationship

45.6 In ICD-10 this disorder subsumes the other

45.7 The onset may occur at any age in life, including adolescence and adulthood

Questions 45.8–45.12

   A. Rumination disorder

   B. Pica

   C. Both

   D. Neither

45.8 High rate of spontaneous remission

45.9 Reinforcement by pleasurable self-stimulation

45.10 Associated with failure to thrive

45.11 Associated with adult eating disorders

45.12 Associated with pregnant women

ANSWERS

Feeding and Eating Disorders of Infancy or Early Childhood

45.1 The answer is B

According to DSM-IV-TR, feeding disorder of infancy or early childhood is a persistent failure to eat adequately, reflected in *significant failure to gain weight* or in significant weight loss over at least 1 month. The symptoms are not better accounted for by a medical condition or by another mental disorder and are not caused by lack of food. The *disorder has its onset before (not after) the age of 6 years.*

   The DSM-IV-TR diagnostic criteria are broad (not narrow) and do not address the specificity of various feeding disorders not included in DSM-IV or ICD-10.

   It is estimated that between 15 and 35 percent of infants and young children have feeding problems. The more common feeding difficulties include eating too little, refusing certain types of food, objectionable mealtime behaviors, and bizarre food habits. Severe feeding problems associated with poor weight gain, such as refusal to eat or vomiting, have been *reported in 1 to 2 percent of infants and toddlers.* A few studies found that about 70 percent of infants who exhibit food refusal in the first year of life continue to have feeding problems when followed up to school age. Picky eating and gastrointestinal symptoms in early childhood have been linked to anorexia nervosa, and pica and problem behaviors during

mealtime have been associated with bulimia nervosa during the adolescent years.

45.2 The answer is E (none)

In DSM-IV-TR, pica is described as the persistent eating of nonnutritive substances for at least 1 month. The behavior must be developmentally inappropriate, not culturally sanctioned, and sufficiently severe to merit clinical attention. *Pica is diagnosed even when these symptoms occur in the context of another disorder,* such as autistic disorder, schizophrenia, or Kleine-Levin syndrome.

   Pica appears much more frequently in young children than in adults; it also occurs more often in persons who are mentally retarded. Among adults, forms of pica, including geophagia (clay eating) and amylophagia (starch eating), have been reported to occur in pregnant women. In certain regions of the world and among various cultures, such as the Australian aborigines, rates of pica in pregnant women have been reported to be high. According to DSM-IV-TR, however, *if such practices are culturally accepted, the diagnostic criteria for pica are not met.*

   Since young infants mouthe objects quite commonly, *it is difficult (not most easily) to diagnose pica when the child is under the age of 2 years.* A survey of a large clinic population with wide-ranging ethnic backgrounds revealed that 75 percent of 12-month-old infants and 15 percent of 2- to 3-year-old toddlers were reported by their parents to put nonnutritive substances in their mouths. Among individuals with mental retardation, *the prevalence of pica appears to increase (not decrease) with the severity of the retardation.* The occurrence of pica among institutionalized mentally retarded individuals has been estimated to range from 10 to 33 percent.

45.3 The answer is E (all)
Young children with pica typically eat plaster, paper, paint, cloth, hair, insects, animal droppings, sand, pebbles, and dirt. Many of the children engage in other oral activities (e.g., *thumb sucking* or nail biting), which they seem to use for relief of tension and self-soothing. Pica may lead to anemia, diarrhea/constipation, worm infestation, *toxoplasmosis*, lead poisoning, and malnutrition. Intestinal obstruction may develop as the result of hair ball tumors.

Usually, pica lasts for several months and then remits. Occasionally, it may continue into adolescence or, less frequently, into adulthood. Several authors have pointed to the serious developmental impact of the disorder. The younger children showed *delays in speech and psychosocial development.* Half of the adolescents suffered from depression, personality disorders, or both; engaged in other forms of disturbed oral activities (e.g., thumb sucking and nail biting); and abused tobacco, alcohol, or drugs. More recently, some authors found a strong relation of pica during early childhood and *bulimia nervosa* during adolescence.

45.4 The answer is C
In DSM-IV-TR rumination disorder is described as an infant's or a child's repeated regurgitation and rechewing of food, after a period of normal functioning. The symptoms last for at least 1 month, are not caused by a medical condition, and are severe enough to merit clinical attention. The onset of the disorder generally occurs after 3 months of age. After regurgitation, the food may be swallowed or spit out. Infants who ruminate are observed to strain to bring the food back into their mouths and appear to find the experience pleasurable. The infants are often brought for evaluation because of failure to thrive. *The disorder is rare (not common) in older children, adolescents,* and adults. It varies in its severity, and *it is sometimes associated with* medical conditions, such as *hiatal hernia,* that result in esophageal reflux. *In its most severe form, the disorder can be fatal.*

Rumination disorder appears to occur more often in males than in females (not vice versa) and also in individuals with mental retardation. A few reports describe adults with eating disorders who developed rumination.

Answers 45.5–45.7

45.5 The answer is C

45.6 The answer is B

45.7 The answer is A
Various causes of rumination disorder have been proposed. *Several authors have attributed rumination to* separation or *a disturbed mother–infant relationships* (e.g., lack of responsiveness or neglect by the mother because of stressful family relationships or life events). Others consider rumination a symptom of gastroesophageal reflux. Several authors have postulated that rumination is a learned behavior that is maintained by special attention to the regurgitation. More recently, opiate receptor insensitivity

or reduced endorphinergic transmission have been implicated in rumination.

A biopsychosocial model has been proposed in which rumination is seen along a continuum in which an infant may have gastrointestinal pathology and little psychopathology at one end of the spectrum, and no organic pathology and severe psychopathology in the mother–infant relationship at the other. Frequently, vomiting secondary to gastroesophageal reflux or vomiting associated with an acute illness precedes the onset of rumination. Apparently, at some point the infant learns to initiate vomiting and rechew the food to relieve tension, self-soothe, or self-stimulate. When the infant fails to elicit or loses caring attention or tension-relieving responses from the mother, rumination seems to become a means of self-regulation. Once the infant has experienced rumination as a self-gratifying technique, the rumination develops into a habit that is difficult to break.

Unlike DSM-IV-TR, *ICD-10's feeding disorder of infancy or early childhood subsumes rumination disorder.* However, similar to DSM-IV-TR, the criteria are broad and do not delineate additional specific feeding disorders. This *disorder has also been associated with a possible disturbed mother–infant relationship.*

According to ICD-10, feeding disorder of infancy or childhood is "a feeding disorder of varying manifestations, usually specific in infancy and early childhood. It generally involves refusal of food . . . in the presence of an adequate food supply and a competent caregiver, and the absence of organic disease. There may or may not be associated rumination (repeated regurgitation without nausea or gastrointestinal illness)."

The onset of rumination is frequently in infancy, most commonly in the first year of life. However, *rumination may start at any point in life* and has been reported to start later in childhood in individuals with developmental delays and in adulthood in individuals with eating disorders.

According to DSM-IV-TR, feeding disorder of infancy and childhood has an age of onset before 6 years.

Answers 45.8–45.12

45.8   The answer is C

45.9   The answer is A

45.10 The answer is C

45.11 The answer is C

45.12 The answer is B
Both rumination disorder and pica seem to have *high rates of spontaneous remission. Rumination disorder* seems to be *reinforced by pleasurable self-stimulation. Pica* is sometimes *associated with failure to thrive,* notably psychosocial dwarfism, in which children have been reported to eat garbage and to drink out of the toilet. *Rumination disorder* also has been *associated with failure to thrive,* and in some cases life-threatening malnutrition may accompany rumination disorder in infants. *Both* rumination disorder and pica are *associated with adult eating disorders. Pica* is *associated with pregnant women* and is reported to be especially prevalent in certain cultures, such as among the Australian aborigines.

46 ▲

Tic Disorders

The revised fourth edition of the *Diagnostic and Statistical Manual of Mental Disorders* (DSM-IV-TR) defines a tic as a "sudden, rapid, recurrent, nonrhythmic, stereotyped motor movement or vocalization." DSM-IV-TR lists four different tic disorders: Tourette's disorder, chronic motor or vocal tic disorder, transient tic disorder, and tic disorder not otherwise specified. Tics are generally experienced as irresistible, but can be suppressed voluntarily from minutes to hours in various situations. They tend to be exacerbated by stress or anxiety and eased by concentration. They are often absent during sleep, but not always.

Motor and vocal tics are divided into simple and complex. Examples of simple motor tics include eye blinking, neck jerking, shoulder shrugging, and facial grimacing, and are composed of rapid contractions of functionally similar muscle groups. Examples of common simple vocal tics include throat clearing, barking, sniffing or snorting, coughing, and grunting. Complex tics appear to be more purposeful than simple ones, and the differentiation between these tics and compulsive rituals is not always easy to make. Common complex motor tics include echopraxia (the imitation of observed behavior) and copropraxia (the display of obscene gestures). They may also include grooming behaviors, smelling of objects, and touching behaviors, among others. Complex vocal tics may involve coprolalia (the use of obscene words or phrases), palilalia (the person repeating his or her own words), or echolalia (the repeating of the last word spoken by another person).

Tourette's disorder was first described in 1885 by Georges Gilles de la Tourette while he was studying with Jean-Martin Charcot in France. DSM-IV-TR describes the tics of Tourette's disorder as multiple motor tics and one or more vocal tics, occurring many times a day for more than 1 year, and causing significant disturbance in various areas of functioning. The onset of motor tics is usually by the age of 7 years; vocal tics generally develop by the age of 11 years. The disorder is diagnosed three times more often in boys than in girls, and the lifetime prevalence is estimated to be 4 to 5 per 10,000.

A genetic etiology is strongly suspected in Tourette's disorder, supported by evidence from twin, adoption, and segregation analysis studies. Tourette's disorder tends to occur in families in which chronic motor or vocal tic disorders also occur. Some evidence supports the theory that Tourette's disorder is inherited through an autosomal pattern intermediate between dominant and recessive. It has been estimated that up to 50 percent of Tourette's disorder patients have attention-deficit/hyperactivity disorder (ADHD), and that up to 40 percent of those with Tourette's disorder also have obsessive-compulsive disorder. First-degree relatives of people with Tourette's disorder have higher risk factors for a variety of tic disorders as well as obsessive-compulsive disorder. Strong evidence of dopamine system involvement is based on the efficacy of dopamine receptor blockers (i.e., haloperidol, pimozide, and fluphenazine) in suppressing tics, as well as the exacerbating effects of such dopaminergic agents as methylphenidate, amphetamines, pemoline, and cocaine. Interestingly, a recent study indicated that, in fact, methylphenidate (Ritalin) may reduce vocal tics in some children with hyperactivity and tic disorders. Untreated, Tourette's disorder can be chronic and lifelong, with intermittent remissions and exacerbations, but the treated disorder has a better prognosis.

Chronic motor or vocal tic disorder is defined in DSM-IV-TR as the presence of either motor tics or vocal tics but not both, thus distinguishing it from Tourette's disorder. The other criteria are the same as for Tourette's disorder. This disorder is considered much more common than Tourette's, with its rate estimated to be from 100 to 1,000 times greater than that of Tourette's. Both disorders aggregate in the same families. Transient tic disorder is defined in DSM-IV-TR as the presence of tics occurring many times a day for at least 4 weeks but for no longer than 1 year. The other features are the same as for Tourette's disorder. The disorder is considered common, with 5 to 24 percent of all school-aged children having a history of transient tics, which may be organic or psychologic in origin. Organic tics are more likely to progress to Tourette's disorder, and psychogenic tics are more likely to remit spontaneously. Most people with transient tic disorder do not progress to a more serious disorder.

The student should study the following questions and answers for a useful review of these disorders.

HELPFUL HINTS

The terms that follow relate to tic disorders and should be known by the student.

- ► attention-deficit/hyperactivity disorder
- ► barking
- ► behavioral treatments
- ► benztropine (Cogentin)
- ► Jean Charcot
- ► clonidine (Catapres)
- ► compulsions
- ► coprolalia
- ► dopamine antagonists and stimulants
- ► dystonia
- ► echokinesis
- ► echolalia
- ► echopraxia and copropraxia
- ► encephalitis lethargica
- ► eye blinking
- ► facial grimacing
- ► Gilles de la Tourette
- ► grunting
- ► Hallervorden-Spatz disease
- ► hemiballism
- ► Huntington's chorea
- ► hyperdopaminergia
- ► Lesch-Nyhan syndrome
- ► motor tic
- ► neck jerking
- ► obsessive-compulsive disorder
- ► palilalia
- ► Pelizaeus-Merzbacher disease
- ► pimozide (Orap)
- ► poststreptococcal syndromes
- ► shoulder shrugging
- ► simple or complex tic
- ► stereotypy
- ► Sydenham's chorea
- ► tardive dyskinesia
- ► torsion dystonia
- ► Tourette's disorder
- ► transient tic disorder
- ► tremor
- ► vocal tic
- ► Wilson's disease

▲ QUESTIONS

DIRECTIONS: Each of the questions or incomplete statements below is followed by five suggested responses or completions. Select the *one* that is *best* in each case.

46.1 In Tourette's disorder the initial tics are in the

- A. face and neck
- B. arms and hands
- C. body and lower extremities
- D. respiratory system
- E. alimentary system

46.2 True statements about Tourette's disorder include

- A. The most frequent initial symptom is mental coprolalia.
- B. Coprolalia usually begins around 6 to 8 years of age and occurs in about 5 percent of cases.
- C. Most complex motor and vocal symptoms emerge virtually simultaneously with the initial symptoms.
- D. The most frequent initial symptom is an eye-blink tic.
- E. Typically, behavioral symptoms, such as hyperactivity, are evident several years before or concurrent with the initial symptoms.

Question 46.3

A 49-year-old married man was referred to a psychiatrist for evaluation because of unremitting tics. At age 13 he developed a persistent eye blink, soon followed by lip smacking, head shaking, and barking noises. Despite these symptoms, he functioned well academically and graduated from high school with honors. He was drafted during the Vietnam War. While he was in the army his tics subsided significantly but were still troublesome; they resulted eventually in a medical discharge. He married, had two children, and worked as a semiskilled laborer and foreman. By age 30 his symptoms included tics of the head, neck, and shoulders; hitting his forehead with his hand and various objects; repeated throat clearing; spitting; and shouting out "Hey, hey, hey, la, la, la." Six years later, noisy coprolalia started: He would emit a string of profanities in the middle of a sentence and then resume his conversation.

Various treatments, all without benefit, were tried: administration of various phenothiazines and antidepressants, then electroconvulsive therapy. The patient's social life grew increasingly constricted. He was unable to go to church or to the movies because of the cursing and noises. He worked at night to avoid social embarrassment. His family and friends became less and less tolerant of his symptoms, and his daughters refused to bring friends home. He was depressed because of his enforced isolation and the seeming hopelessness of finding effective treatment. At 46, he sought a prefrontal lobotomy, but after psychiatric evaluation, his request was denied.

46.3 In this case example, the diagnosis is made on the basis of

- A. vocal tics
- B. coprolalia
- C. onset before age 18
- D. no known central nervous system disease
- E. all of the above

DIRECTIONS: Each of the questions or incomplete statements below is followed by five suggested responses or completions. Select the *one* that is *best* in each case.

Questions 46.4–46.5

46.4 If onset is after age 18, which of the following tic disorders may be diagnosed?

- A. Transient tic disorder
- B. Chronic motor or vocal tic disorder
- C. Tourette's disorder
- D. Tic disorder not otherwise specified
- E. All of the above

46.5 The dopamine system has been hypothesized to be involved in the development of tic disorders because

- A. haloperidol (Haldol) suppresses tics
- B. pimozide (Orap) suppresses tics
- C. methylphenidate (Ritalin) exacerbates tics
- D. pemoline (Cylert) exacerbates tics
- E. all of the above

46.6 Which of the following statements concerning evidence supporting genetic factors as likely to play a role in the development of Tourette's disorder is *false*?

A. Concordance for Tourette's disorder is significantly higher in monozygotic than dizygotic twins.

B. Tourette's disorder and chronic tic disorder tend to occur in the same family.

C. First-degree relatives of probands with Tourette's disorder are at higher-than-average risk for developing Tourette's disorder, chronic tic disorder, and obsessive-compulsive disorder.

D. Sons of men with Tourette's disorder are at highest risk for developing the disorder.

E. Concordance for Tourette's disorder or chronic tic disorder is high in monozygotic twins.

46.7 Which of the following distinguishes transient tic disorder from chronic motor or vocal tic disorder and Tourette's disorder?

A. age of onset
B. the presence of motor tics only
C. the presence of vocal tics only
D. the presence of both motor and vocal tics
E. progression of the tic symptoms over time

DIRECTIONS: Each group of questions below consists of lettered headings followed by a list of numbered phrases. For each numbered phrase, select the *one* lettered heading most associated with it. Each heading may be used once, more than once, or not at all.

Questions 46.8–46.10

A. Tonic tic
B. Dystonic tic
C. Clonic tic
D. Simple phonic tic
E. Complex tic

46.8 May be mistaken for volitional act
46.9 Sniffing, grunting, or yelping
46.10 Brisk movements

Questions 46.11–46.15

A. Tourette's disorder
B. Sydenham's chorea
C. Both
D. Neither

46.11 Associated with obsessive-compulsive behavior
46.12 Possible autoimmune response to streptococcal antigens
46.13 Self-limiting syndrome
46.14 Life-long illness with a waxing and waning course
46.15 More common in males

Questions 46.16–46.19

A. Tic disorders
B. Nontic movement disorders
C. Both
D. Neither

46.16 Repetitive vocalizations
46.17 Premonitory sensation
46.18 Description of movements as intentional in response to urges or sensations
46.19 Association with mental retardation or dementing process

---

ANSWERS

Tic Disorders

46.1 The answer is A

In *Tourette's disorder, the initial tics are in the face and neck.* Over time, the tics tend to occur in a downward progression or involve more complex movements of several muscle groups. The most commonly described tics are those affecting the face and head, the *arms and hands*, the *body and lower extremities*, and the *respiratory* and *alimentary systems*. In these areas, the tics take the form of grimacing; puckering the forehead; raising eyebrows; blinking eyelids; winking; wrinkling the nose; trembling nostrils; twitching mouth; displaying the teeth; biting the lips and other parts; extruding the tongue; protracting the lower jaw; nodding, jerking, or shaking the head; twisting the neck; looking sideways; head rolling; jerking the hands; jerking the arms; plucking fingers; writhing fingers; clenching fists; shrugging the shoulders; shaking a foot, knee, or toe; walking peculiarly; body writhing; jumping; hiccuping; sighing; yawning; snuffing; blowing through the nostrils; whistling inspiration; breathing exaggeratedly; belching; making sucking or smacking sounds; and clearing the throat.

46.2 The answer is D

Typically, prodromal *behavioral symptoms*—such as *hyperactivity*, attention difficulties, and poor frustration tolerance—*are evident before or concurrent with the onset of tics. The most frequent initial symptom is an eye-blink tic,* followed by a head tic or a facial grimace. Most *complex motor and vocal symptoms emerge several years after (not simultaneously with) the initial symptoms. Coprolalia usually begins in early adolescence (not between ages 6 and 8) and occurs in about 15 percent (not 5 percent) of all cases. Although it is not the most frequent initial symptom, mental coprolalia*—in which a patient thinks a sudden, intrusive, socially unacceptable thought or obscene word—*may also occur.* In some severe cases, physical injuries, including retinal detachment and orthopedic problems, have resulted from severe tics.

46.3 The answer is E (all)

In the case of this patient, the correct diagnosis is Tourette's disorder. He has both chronic motor tics and *vocal tics,* including *coprolalia.* The tics have occurred for more than a year. The disorder started when the patient was *under age 18.* He also has *no known central nervous system disease.* Obsessions and compulsions are often seen in persons with Tourette's disorder.

46.4 The answer is D

All tic disorders with onset after age 18 must be diagnosed as *tic disorder not otherwise specified,* a residual category for tics that do not meet the criteria for a specific tic disorder. *Transient tic disorder, chronic motor or vocal tic disorder,* and *Tourette's disorder* all specify onset before age 18.

46.5 The answer is E (all)

Supportive evidence of dopamine-system involvement in tic disorders includes the observations that pharmacologic agents that antagonize the dopamine system, such as *haloperidol (Haldol) and pimozide (Orap), suppress tics,* and observations that agents that increase central dopaminergic activity, such as cocaine, dextroamphetamine (Dexedrine), *methylphenidate (Ritalin), and pemoline (Cylert), exacerbate tics.*

46.6 The answer is D

Evidence that genetic factors are likely to play a role in the development of Tourette's disorder include the findings that *sons of mothers (not sons of fathers) with Tourette's disorder are at highest risk for developing the disorder.* Studies reveal that *concordance for Tourette's disorder is significantly higher in monozygotic twins* than in dizygotic twins. In addition, the findings that *Tourette's disorder and chronic tic disorder tend to occur in the same family* support the view that both disorders are part of a genetically determined spectrum. *First-degree relatives of probands with Tourette's disorder are at higher-than-average risk* for developing Tourette's disorder, chronic tic disorder, and obsessive-compulsive disorder, implying a genetic relationship among the three disorders. A genetic connection between Tourette's disorder and chronic tic disorder is also supported by findings that *concordance is high for Tourette's disorder or chronic tic disorder in monozygotic twins.*

46.7 The answer is E

Transient tic disorder can be distinguished from chronic motor or vocal tic disorder and Tourette's disorder only by following the *progression of the tic symptoms over time.* DSM-IV-TR emphasizes precise and specific symptom patterns, time framework, and age of onset in classifying the tic disorders. Transient tic disorder cannot be distinguished from chronic motor or vocal tic disorder and Tourette's disorder by *the age of onset, the presence of motor tics only, the presence of vocal tics only,* or *the presence of both motor and vocal tics.*

Answers 46.8–46.10

46.8 The answer is E

46.9 The answer is D

46.10 The answer is C

Tics are defined as rapid, repetitive muscle contractions or sounds that usually are experienced as outside volitional control and that often resemble aspects of normal movement or behavior. Tics can be elicited by stimuli or preceded by an urge or sensation. They are usually beyond attempts at suppression. Tics are classified as simple or complex tics and as motor or phonic or vocal tics. Simple motor tics involve one or a small number of muscle groups (e.g., eyeblinking tic, facial grimace, or shoulder shrug). Simple motor tics can be further subdivided into clonic, tonic, or dystonic types.

Clonic tics are *very brisk movements;* tonic and dystonic tics, on the other hand, can include more sustained muscle contractions, such as arm extension and muscle tensing. Other *dystonic tics* are very common among individuals with Tourette's disorder and can involve oculogyric movements or torticollis.

Complex motor tics, on the other hand, may come close to mimicking normal movements of various kinds, through the synchronous contraction of several muscle groups, as in hopping, or the simultaneous extension of arms and legs, in knee bends, and, rarely, obscene gesturing or copropraxia.

Phonic tics can also take simple or complex forms. *Simple phonic tics include sniffing, grunting, or yelping.* Examples of complex vocal tics include intelligible syllables or even phrases, such as "hi," "I love you, I love you," or (uncommonly) obscene utterances, defined as coprolalia. While simple tics are relatively easy to discern, *complex tics may be mistaken for volitional acts.*

Answers 46.11–46.15

46.11 The answer is C

46.12 The answer is C

46.13 The answer is B

46.14 The answer is A

46.15 The answer is A

Sydenham's chorea is a well-known *self-limiting syndrome* consisting of a variety of abnormal motor movements that can include tics, choreiform movements, and *compulsive behaviors caused by an autoimmune response to the streptococcal antigens.* Autoimmune processes related to streptococcal bacteria have been proposed as etiological components of some cases of obsessive-compulsive disorder, as well as some cases of *Tourette's disorder.* Such an autoimmune process may act synergistically with a genetic vulnerability for these disorders, or it may act without a prior vulnerability. Elevated titers of circulating autoantibodies can sometimes be detected in these cases. *The increased prevalence of Tourette's disorder* and other tic disorders *in males* may be related to high levels of gender-related hormones in the developing male central nervous system (Sydenham's chorea is more common in females.) *Obsessive-compulsive behaviors are associated with Tourette's disorder as well as with Sydenham's chorea.* One main differentiating feature between Tourette's disorder and Sydenham's chorea is that *Tourette's disorder is a lifelong illness* with a waxing and waning course, whereas *Sydenham's chorea usually is self-limiting.*

There are treatments for the core features of Tourette's disorder as well as for the associated syndromes. Dopamine blocking agents such as haloperidol (Haldol) and pimozide (Orap) have been shown to diminish tic behaviors. Conversely, agents that increase central dopaminergic activity, such as methylphenidate (Ritalin), may exacerbate tics. Selective serotonin reuptake inhibitors (SSRIs), such as fluoxetine (Prozac), sertraline (Zoloft), or paroxetine (Paxil), are sometimes used in patients with Tourette's disorder to treat associated obsessive-compulsive symptoms. Tourette's disorder appears to be transmitted via autosomal dominant genes in some family pedigrees. There seems to be variable penetrance, so that not every family member with the genetic contribution will exhibit the same number of symptoms or illness severity. Concordance for the disorder in monozygotic twins is significantly greater than in dizygotic twins. In other family pedigrees, Tourette's disorder may be transmitted in a bilinear mode—that is, a pattern intermediate between dominant and recessive.

Answers 46.16–46.19

46.16 The answer is A

46.17 The answer is A

46.18 The answer is A

46.19 The answer is B

Differentiating tics from other abnormal movements is generally straightforward by clinical history and examination. Although more complex tics, dystonic tics, and compulsive tics lack the rapidity of other tic movements, in general, patients exhibit a mixture of simple and more complex tics, enabling discrimination between tic disorders and other movement disorders. *Repetitive vocalizations,* while characteristic of tic disorders, *are rare in nontic movement disorders,* which also aids accurate classification. *Additional features more strongly associated with tics are premonitory sensations,* which are described by up to 80 to 90 percent of older patients. These sensations or experiences can take many forms, including an urge, an itch, a feeling of tightness, tingling, or the experience of irritation or worry. Other sub-jective features of tics include the experience of relief following the tic; conversely, some patients report a buildup of an urge or tension prior to the activity. Other features associated with compulsive tics involve the need to repeat behaviors until relief is achieved or the individual feels "just right." Similarly, the *description of tic movements as intentional,* or purposely performed, in response to an urge or sensation is uncommon among other types of abnormal movements. The complicated mental phenomena seen in some patients with tics often make the precise boundary between compulsive tics and obsessive-compulsive disorder difficult to delineate.

Other features that distinguish Tourette's disorder and the tic disorders from other movement disorders include differences in age of onset (younger in autistic disorder, athetoid cerebral palsy, Pelizaeus-Merzbacher disease, Lesch-Nyhan syndrome, and status dysmyelinatus; older in Huntington's disease, Wilson's disease, spastic torticollis) and the *lack of a frequent association of tic disorders with mental retardation or a dementing process* (in contrast to autistic disorder, cerebral palsy, Lesch-Nyhan syndrome, Wilson's disease, and Huntington's disease). Occasionally, tics are an adverse effect of commonly prescribed psychostimulants. Generally these tics resolve promptly with dosage reduction or drug discontinuation.

Elimination Disorders

The two elimination disorders described in the revised fourth edition of the *Diagnostic and Statistical Manual of Mental Disorders* (DSM-IV-TR) are encopresis and enuresis. Encopresis is defined as the "repeated passage of feces into inappropriate places (e.g., clothing or floor) whether voluntary or involuntary." Enuresis is defined as the "repeated voiding of urine into bed or clothes (whether involuntary or voluntary)." Encopresis must be present for at least 3 months and the child must be chronologically or developmentally at least 4 years of age. Enuresis must occur twice a week for at least 3 months, or must cause significant social or academic distress, and the child must be chronologically or developmentally at least 5 years of age. The implication of these disorders is that the affected child has the developmental ability to maintain bowel or bladder control. There is a significant relationship between encopresis and enuresis. Neither can be diagnosed if the behavior is due exclusively to substances such as laxatives or diuretics or to a general medical condition.

In Western cultures, 95 percent of children have established bowel control by the age of 4 years, and 99 percent by the age of 5 years. After the age of 4, encopresis is up to three to four times more common in boys than in girls. By the ages of 10 to 12, at least once a month, soiling occurs in about 1.3 percent of boys and in 0.3 percent of girls. Etiologic factors associated with encopresis include inadequate toilet training and inefficient sphincter control, as well as such emotional factors as anger, anxiety, and fear. Up to three-quarters of encopretic children suffer from constipation and have excessive fluid overflow. Power struggles between the child and parent over issues of autonomy and control often aggravate the condition. Behavioral problems may or may not be present, but when they do occur, they tend to be the social ramifications of soiling. Encopresis may be triggered by stressful life events such as the birth of a sibling, illness of a parent, parental conflict, or starting school. Encopretic children may retain feces and become constipated without evidence of preexisting anorectal dysfunction. This can lead to a chronic rectal distention, termed a megacolon, which in turn can lead to loss of tone in the rectum with pressure desensitization. These children become unaware of the need to defecate and overflow encopresis occurs. The outcome of encopresis depends on its cause as well as on coexisting behavioral problems. In most cases it is self-limiting, but outcome is affected by the family's ability to participate in treatment without shaming or punishing the child.

As with encopresis, enuresis decreases with increasing age. About 80 percent of 2 year olds are reported to be normally enuretic on a regular basis, while only 7 percent of 5 year olds have been similarly reported. Mental disorders in enuretic children are most common in girls, in children with both day and night symptoms, and in older children. Normal bladder control is influenced by neuromuscular and cognitive development, psychosocial factors, adequacy of toilet training, and possibly genetics. Developmental delays have been reported to be twice as common in enuretic children. Enuresis is usually self-limiting. Enuresis after at least 1 year of dryness usually begins between the ages of 5 and 8 years; organic causes must always be ruled out, but especially so if enuresis occurs at older ages. Treatment includes behavioral, psychological, and pharmacological interventions. A relatively high rate of spontaneous remission is common. Classical conditioning underlies the bell (or buzzer) treatment apparatus, which results in dryness in more than 50 percent of all cases. Medication is not the first line of treatment and often is not indicated. Even when it is indicated, symptoms may return as soon as the medication is withdrawn. Both imipramine (Tofranil) and desmopressin (DDAVP) have been used, and both have a number of adverse effects.

The student should study the following questions and answers for a useful review of these disorders.

HELPFUL HINTS

The student should know the following terms.

- ▶ abnormal sphincter contractions
- ▶ aganglionic megacolon
- ▶ behavioral reinforcement
- ▶ bell (or buzzer) and pad
- ▶ diurnal bowel control
- ▶ ego-dystonic enuresis
- ▶ fluid restriction
- ▶ functionally small bladder
- ▶ genitourinary pathology and other organic disorders
- ▶ Hirschsprung's disease
- ▶ imipramine
- ▶ intranasal desmopressin (DDAVP)
- ▶ laxatives
- ▶ low nocturnal antidiuretic hormone
- ▶ neurodevelopmental problems
- ▶ nocturnal bowel control
- ▶ obstructive urinary disorder abnormality
- ▶ olfactory accommodation
- ▶ overflow incontinence
- ▶ poor gastric motility
- ▶ psychosocial stressors
- ▶ rectal distention
- ▶ regression
- ▶ thioridazine
- ▶ toilet training

▲ QUESTIONS

DIRECTIONS: Each of the questions or incomplete statements below is followed by five suggested responses or completions. Select the *one* that is *best* in each case.

47.1 Enuresis can be defined as repeated voiding of urine into bed or clothes in children over the age of

A. 2 years
B. 3 years
C. 4 years
D. 5 years
E. 6 years

47.2 Nonretentive encopresis is associated with which of these features?

A. It corresponds to the DSM-IV-TR subtype, with constipation and overflow incontinence.
B. Feces are, characteristically, poorly formed.
C. Soiling and leakage are intermittent.
D. Only small amounts of feces are passed during toileting.
E. It occurs both during the day and during sleep.

47.3 True statements about enuresis include

A. The majority of enuretic children wet intentionally.
B. There is a correlation between enuresis and psychological disturbance that increases with age.
C. Children with enuresis have no more developmental delays than nonenuretic children.
D. Enuresis tends not to occur in family members.
E. Children living in socially disadvantaged situations do not have a greater frequency of enuresis.

47.4 In DSM-IV-TR, qualifiers to the diagnosis of enuresis include

A. primary vs. secondary enuresis
B. diurnal vs. nocturnal enuresis
C. combined nocturnal and diurnal pattern
D. physical causes such as bladder infection must be excluded
E. all of the above

47.5 The percent incidence of obstructive lesions in children with enuresis has been reported to be approximately

A. 1.5 percent
B. 3.5 percent
C. 10.0 percent
D. 15.0 percent
E. 25.0 percent

47.6 The primary differential diagnosis in enuresis is

A. anatomical malformations
B. obstructive lesions
C. urinary tract infection
D. underlying psychological disturbance
E. none of the above

47.7 True statements about enuresis include

A. The vast majority of enuretic children experience spontaneous resolution of the problem.
B. Psychotherapy is never the primary treatment modality.
C. The efficacy of psychotherapy for primary enuresis has been reported to be as high as 35 to 50 percent.
D. The success rate for behavioral interventions has been reported to be about 40 percent.
E. Classical conditioning treatments (bell and pad) are more effective in children without concomitant mental disorders.

DIRECTIONS: The lettered headings below are followed by a list of numbered phrases. For each numbered phrase, select

A. if the item is associated with *A only*
B. if the item is associated with *B only*
C. if the item is associated with *both A and B*
D. if the item is associated with *neither A nor B*

Questions 47.8–47.9

A. Primary encopresis
B. Secondary encopresis
C. Both
D. Neither

47.8 More likely to have developmental delays and associated enuresis

47.9 More often diagnosed with conduct disorder

Questions 47.10–47.16

A. Encopresis
B. Enuresis
C. Both
D. Neither

47.10 This disorder is seen more frequently in females

47.11 Psychopharmacological intervention for this disorder, such as desmopressin nasal spray (DDAVP), is limited in that relapse tends to occur as soon as medication is withdrawn

47.12 Physiological determinants are believed to be significantly contributory to this disorder, while structural abnormalities are rare

47.13 At age 7 years, approximately 1.5 percent of boys have this disorder

47.14 At age 5 years, approximately 7 percent of children have this disorder

47.15 To be diagnosed with this disorder, a child must have a chronological or developmental age of 5 years

47.16 To be diagnosed with this disorder, a child must have a chronological or developmental age of 4 years

ANSWERS

Elimination Disorders

47.1 The answer is D

Enuresis is manifested as a repetitive, inappropriate, involuntary passage of urine. Operationally, *enuresis* can be defined as repeated voiding of urine into bed or clothes in children *over the age of 5 years* (or equivalent developmental level) who fail to inhibit the reflex to pass urine when the impulse is felt during waking hours and in those who do not rouse from sleep of their own accord when the process is occurring during the sleeping state.

47.2 The answer is C

DSM-IV-TR currently defines encopresis with four related criteria: (1) the repeated inappropriate passage of feces, usually involuntarily; (2) occurrence at least once a month for at least 3 months; (3) a chronological or mental age of 4 years; and (4) exclusion of a substance or medical condition as a cause.

For several years the clinical and research literature concerning encopresis has distinguished between retentive and nonretentive encopresis. Accordingly, DSM-IV-TR lists two subtypes: with constipation and overflow incontinence and without constipation and overflow incontinence. The *subtype with constipation and overflow incontinence corresponds to retentive encopresis (not nonretentive encopresis)* and is described by DSM-IV-TR as follows: *"Feces are characteristically (but not invariably) poorly formed and leakage is continuous, occurring both during the day and during sleep. Only small amounts of feces are passed during toiletting* and the incontinence resolves after treatment of the constipation." *The subtype without constipation and overflow incontinence corresponds to nonretentive encopresis* and, as DSM-IV-TR notes, *"feces are likely to be of normal form* and consistency *and soiling is intermittent.* Feces may be deposited in a prominent location."

Some clinicians refer to a primary type in which the person has never established fecal continence and a secondary type in which the disturbance develops after a period of established fecal continence.

47.3 The answer is B

Inclusion in the DSM-IV-TR definition of enuresis of children who wet intentionally or involuntarily can be problematic. *The vast majority of enuretic children do not wet intentionally or even on a subconsciously motivated basis.* Increasingly, the research is pointing toward causal factors that may involve irregularities in physiological processes. Clearly, children who wet intentionally are in a different phenomenological grouping than those who do so involuntarily, even if they do meet the other diagnostic requirements. The most likely explanation for voluntary intentional wetting is either an oppositional defiant disorder or a psychotic disorder. A small number of children originally have enuretic events involuntarily and subsequently manifest the behavior on a voluntary learned basis as well.

There is a correlation between enuresis and psychological disturbance that increases with age. Children living in socially disadvantaged situations and experiencing psychosocial stress *have a greater frequency of enuresis than those who are not.* The type and range of behavioral disturbance seen in children with enuresis are broad, and no marker can reliably differentiate behaviorally disturbed from nondisturbed enuretic children. Thus, the associated behavioral disturbances are nonspecific and may represent a coincidental or secondary relationship rather than a causal correlation. Further supporting a secondary correlation are the repeated findings that *children with enuresis have significantly more developmental delays than nonenuretic children,* compared with both controls and other children attending a psychiatric clinic.

The observation that *enuresis tends to occur in family members* has been made for some time. A large Scandinavian study involving over 3,000 children found that a child's risk for being enuretic was 5.2 times greater if the mother was enuretic and 7.1 times greater if the father was enuretic, lending further support to a genetic influence. DSM-IV-TR notes that the concordance rate for the disorder is greater in monozygotic than in dizygotic twins, and 75 percent of children with enuresis have a similarly affected first-degree biological relative.

47.4 The answer is E (all)

The concreteness and simplicity of enuresis make the diagnosis relatively easy. As previously indicated, the diagnosis is not made in a child whose chronological or mental age is below 5 years. The wetting must occur at least twice a week for at least 3 consecutive months, or if less frequent, it must produce significant distress or *functional impairment. Physical causes such as a bladder infection must be excluded. Qualifiers* to the diagnosis indicate whether it *is primary or secondary enuresis. The other qualifiers refer to the timing of the enuretic event.* While most children exhibit only *nocturnal enuresis,* some have *daytime (diurnal) patterns* or a *combined nocturnal and diurnal pattern.*

47.5 The answer is B

Because urinary tract infections can produce enuresis, a urinalysis should be part of every evaluation. Using radiographic procedures with contrast media to detect an anatomical or physiological cause for the enuresis is more problematic, as the procedures are invasive and painful, and the diagnostic yield is low. A large study carried out in a pediatric primary care setting found *a 3.7 (not 1.5, 10.0, 15.0, or 25.0) percent incidence of obstructive lesions in children with enuresis.* Similar findings have been reported by others.

47.6 The answer is C

As suggested above, the *primary differential diagnosis is a urinary tract infection.* This is especially true for girls, who are more prone than boys to urinary tract infections. With a girl who has been continent for a considerable period and has recently begun wetting, a urinary tract infection should be the first consideration. Although the diagnostic yield is smaller with boys, urinalysis should still be carried out.

Enuresis can result from *anatomical malformations* or *obstructive lesions,* but the percentages are relatively low. If the history and interviews with the child suggest that the enuresis is intentional, then it is almost certainly related to *an underlying psychological disturbance.* The relationship between psychological disturbance and involuntary enuresis is less clear. The coexistence of another behavioral disturbance should be noted and attended to clinically.

47.7 The answer is A

The natural history of enuresis is significant because it figures prominently in treatment decisions insofar as enuresis is a self-limiting disorder that at some time will spontaneously remit. The fact that the diagnosis is not made until age 5 takes into account children who have delayed toilet training that is not outside the accepted range (between 2 and 5 years of age). The prevalence of enuresis is relatively high between the ages of 5 and 7 and then drops off substantially. *The vast majority of enuretic children experience spontaneous resolution of the problem* at some time, and only a few remain enuretic into adulthood. By age 14 years only 1.1 percent of boys wet once a week or more. The greatest rates of spontaneous remission occur after age 7 years and again after age 12 years.

The proven methods for the treatment of enuresis are primarily behavioral and pharmacological. Psychotherapy may be useful for ameliorating some of the associated behavioral problems that can be seen with enuresis, especially secondary enuresis. A particularly common clinical scenario for secondary enuresis is the development of *wetting in boys following the loss of their father* through death or divorce. *In these patients, psychotherapy is the primary treatment modality.* A review of the *efficacy of psychotherapy for primary enuresis* found *a 20 percent (not a 35 to 50 percent) success rate,* which is probably not significantly above what would be expected by spontaneous remissions and random chance.

A comprehensive review of several studies determined *the success rate for behavioral interventions* to be *75 percent (not 40 percent).* Recent studies have yielded comparable response rates. The primary behavioral intervention is the bell-and-pad method of conditioning. A pad is placed on the bed with a wire running to a bell. When the child wets, the moisture completes a circuit in the pad, ringing the bell and waking the child. With repeated use the child learns to awaken before wetting occurs. Buzzer ulcers were a potential adverse effect of the treatment, but the frequency has decreased considerably with improved technology. The treatment is *equally (not more) effective in children with and without concomitant mental disorders.*

Answers 47.8–47.9

47.8 The answer is A

47.9 The answer is B

As with enuresis, the distinction between primary and secondary encopresis relates to the issue of associated psychopathology. A study involving 63 boys with encopresis found that *boys with primary encopresis were more likely to have developmental delays and associated enuresis* while *those with secondary enuresis were more likely* to have experienced higher levels of psychosocial stressors and *to be diagnosed with conduct disorder.*

Answers 47.10–47.16

47.10 The answer is D

47.11 The answer is B

47.12 The answer is C

47.13 The answer is A

47.14 The answer is B

47.15 The answer is B

47.16 The answer is A

Bowel and bladder control appears to be more difficult for males than for females. *Both encopresis and enuresis are three to four times more common in males than in females.* At all ages, encopresis is three to five times more common in males than in females. Enuresis is also three to five times more common in males than in females. A variety of medications, such as imipramine and, more recently, desmopressin nasal spray, have been used with some success in the treatment of enuresis.

Imipramine has received FDA approval in the treatment of childhood enuresis on a short-term basis. Tolerance commonly develops, however, within 6 weeks of treatment, and relapse at former frequencies usually ensues when the drug is discontinued. *Desmopressin,* an antidiuretic compound that is available as an intranasal spray, *has been successful in treating some children with enuresis while it is being used,* but it does not seem to affect the condition after the medication is discontinued. The primary treatment of encopresis is a sensitively developed behavioral and family intervention. In order to do this, an accurate evaluation and understanding of a child's encopresis pattern are necessary. It is important to determine whether the child has chronic constipation with overflow incontinence. It is also necessary to determine whether the child is well aware of the passage of feces when it occurs. Furthermore, if encopresis is a behavior developed by a child to express anger or attract negative parental attention, this is also pertinent to the design of treatment. Psychopharmacological interventions are generally not a part of treatment of encopresis, although in cases of chronic constipation, medications are sometimes used to regulate fecal continence. Children with constipation who have difficulty with sphincter relaxation are among the more difficult to treat. *Physiological characteristics are believed to be important contributors to both encopresis and enuresis.* Abnormal sphincter contractions are very common in children with constipation and overflow incontinence. Enuresis tends to run in families (three-quarters of children with enuresis have a first-degree relative with enuresis), and children with enuresis are twice as likely to have concomitant developmental delay. Even when a structural anatomical defect is not obvious, evidence suggests that heritable physiological factors contribute to enuresis. Bowel control is established in 95 percent of the children by the fourth birthday and in 99 percent of children by the fifth birthday. *At age 7 to 8 years, the frequency of encopresis is 1.5 percent in boys* and 0.5 percent in girls. The *prevalence of enuresis* decreases with age; 82 percent of 2 year olds, 49 percent of 3 year olds, 26 percent of 4 year olds, and *7 percent of 5 year olds have enuresis* on a regular basis. *To be diagnosed as having encopresis,* a child must have a *chronological or developmental age of 4 years,* whereas *to be diagnosed as having enuresis,* a child must have *a chronological or developmental age of 5 years.*

48 ▲

Other Disorders of Infancy, Childhood, or Adolescence

The revised fourth edition of the *Diagnostic and Statistical Manual of Mental Disorders* (DSM-IV-TR) describes five disorders under the category of Other Disorders of Infancy, Childhood, and Adolescence. They are separation anxiety disorder; selective mutism; reactive attachment disorder of infancy and early childhood; stereotypic movement disorder; and disorder of infancy, childhood, or adolescence not otherwise specified.

Separation anxiety is a normal developmental experience, usually exhibited in the form of stranger anxiety around 1 year of age. It can also be seen as a normal phenomenon in some children when they are first entering school. The relationship between temperament and the development of anxiety symptoms has been explored. Children with a temperamental shyness, behavioral inhibition, or tendency to withdraw from unfamiliar situations have a higher risk than others for developing excessive and persistent anxiety. Genetic factors most likely contribute to this constellation of temperamental attributes. DSM-IV-TR describes separation anxiety disorder as "developmentally inappropriate and excessive anxiety concerning separation from home or from those to whom the individual is attached." At least three of a list of presenting behaviors must be evident to make the diagnosis. Among these behaviors are repeated physical complaints, such as head or stomach aches, surrounding separation issues; persistent and excessive worry about losing, or harm befalling, major attachment figures; refusal to go to sleep without a major attachment figure nearby; nightmares about separation; and persistent anxiety about going anywhere without the significant attachment figure. A child's anxiety can reach the level of panic or terror. Separation anxiety disorder is the only anxiety disorder specifically addressed in the child and adolescent section of DSM-IV-TR. Other DSM-IV-TR anxiety disorders that children experience, such as generalized anxiety disorder, posttraumatic stress disorder, or social phobias, have the same criteria as the adult disorders.

Separation anxiety disorder appears to be most common in 7 to 8 year olds, and the prevalence of the disorder has been estimated to be about 3 to 4 percent of school-aged children and 1 percent of adolescents. It seems to be equally common in boys and girls. Children whose parents have anxiety disorders (such as panic disorder or phobias) have a higher risk of developing the disorders themselves. In these situations it is difficult to distinguish the role of genetics from those of psychological and emotional factors. Anxiety can be communicated to a child through parental modeling. Environmental stressors, such as

the death of a relative, illness, or a move to a new neighborhood and school, may trigger development of the disorder. Treatment involves individual psychotherapy for the child, psychopharmacological approaches, family education, and family therapy. Selective serotonin reuptake inhibitors (SSRIs) are now used more often than tricyclic antidepressants, given the lower adverse-effect profile.

Selective mutism is described in DSM-IV-TR as the "consistent failure to speak in specific social situations (in which there is an expectation of speaking, e.g., at school) despite speaking in other situations." These children are able to speak fluently in situations in which they feel comfortable, and they have no significant biological disability. The disorder must last for at least 1 month and not be limited to the first month of school. Selective mutism is considered uncommon, with younger children being more vulnerable than older ones. Many children with the disorder have histories of delayed speech onset or speech abnormalities that may contribute to its onset, but the disorder is considered to be determined psychologically. A recent study indicated that 90 percent of children who met diagnostic criteria for selective mutism also met criteria for social phobia. The presence of parental anxiety, depression, and heightened dependency needs have been noted in families of children with selective mutism.

Pervasive inappropriate social relatedness, associated with pathogenic care taking, and beginning before the age of 5 years, defines reactive attachment disorder of infancy or early childhood. According to DSM-IV-TR, the disorder cannot be due solely to a developmental delay or a pervasive developmental disorder. The DSM-IV-TR disorder has two subtypes: the inhibited subtype, in which a child shows "predominately inhibited, hypervigilant, or highly ambivalent and contradictory responses"; and the disinhibited subtype, in which the child demonstrates "indiscriminate sociability with marked inability to exhibit appropriate selective attachment." The cause of this disorder is grossly pathogenic care of an infant of child, including maltreatment, neglect, or abuse. Repeated changes of a caretaker, such as those that can occur in frequent foster care moves, may lead to the disorder.

The clinical picture of stereotypic movement disorder varies considerably, in that affected individuals may suffer from one or more symptoms. Typically, one symptom predominates and may include hand shaking or waving, body rocking, head banging, self-biting and hitting, and skin or bodily orifice picking. The movements are repetitive and nonfunctional, and markedly interfere with normal activities. They can lead to self-inflicted injury if not prevented. According to DSM-IV-TR, stereotypic movement disorder can be dually diagnosed with mental retardation if the movements are severe enough to warrant treatment on their own. Stereotypic movements seem to be associated with dopamine in that dopamine antagonists generally decrease them, and dopamine agonists induce or exacerbate them. Disorder of infancy, childhood, or adolescence not otherwise specified is a residual category for disorders with onset in these age groups not meeting diagnostic criteria for any specific disorder.

The student should study the questions and answers below for a useful review of these disorders.

HELPFUL HINTS

The student should know the following terms.

- anticipatory anxiety
- behavioral inhibition
- delayed language acquisition
- desensitization
- driven, nonfunctional behavior
- dyskinetic movements
- emotional and physical neglect
- external life stressors
- failure to respond socially
- failure to thrive
- generalized anxiety
- head banging and nail biting
- indiscriminate familiarity
- inhibition to speak
- lack of stable attachment
- Lesch-Nyhan syndrome
- major attachment figure
- multimodal treatment approach
- nonverbal gestures
- panic disorder
- pathogenic caregiving
- psychopharmacologic interventions
- "psychosocial dwarfism"
- school phobia
- school refusal
- selective mutism
- self-injurious stereotypic acts
- sensory impairments
- separation anxiety
- shyness
- social anxiety
- social phobia
- specific phobia
- stereotypic movements
- stress anxiety
- temperamental constellation

▲ QUESTIONS

DIRECTIONS: Each of the questions or incomplete statements below is followed by five suggested responses or completions. Select the *one* that is *best* in each case.

48.1 Stereotypic movement disorder

A. includes trichotillomania
B. includes stereotypy that is part of pervasive developmental disorder
C. is not diagnosed if mental retardation is present
D. includes tics and compulsions
E. none of the above

48.2 Head banging

A. has a prevalence of approximately 1 percent in child populations
B. affects males three times more frequently than females
C. typically begins after the age of 12 months
D. is relatively common after the age of 3 years
E. is rarely self-limiting

48.3 The most widely used intervention for the treatment of stereotypic movements is

A. clomipramine (Anafranil)
B. desipramine (Norpramin)
C. haloperidol (Haldol)
D. chlorpromazine (Thorazine)
E. behavioral modification

48.4 Separation anxiety disorder

A. is a developmental phase
B. affects up to 4 percent of school-aged children
C. has its most common onset at 1 to 2 years of age
D. is less serious when it occurs in adolescence
E. always involves refusal to go to school

48.5 Selective mutism has been associated with

A. expressive language disorders
B. parental childhood shyness
C. parental public-speaking anxiety
D. children from multilingual homes
E. all of the above

48.6 A 16-year-old high school junior was referred by a teacher to the mental health clinic with the complaint that she was unable to make any verbal contribution in her classes. Her inability to speak had begun 1 year previously after the death of her mother. It took school personnel some time to realize that she did not speak in any of her classes. She had kept up with her assignments, handing in all her written work, and was receiving better-than-average grades on tests.

The patient's father was a janitor in a large apartment building. Because of his work, he usually came home late, and he was rather passive and indifferent toward the patient and her six younger siblings. He had never responded to school requests for visits to discuss his daughter's problems. Since her mother's death, the patient had assumed the mothering of the siblings: cooking the meals, cleaning, and listening to their wishes and complaints.

When seen, the patient was a thin, neatly dressed girl who was alert but responded at first only with brief nods of her head. With the clinician's reassurance, she began to whisper monosyllabic answers to questions. Her responses were rational and logical, but she denied that her failure to speak was a problem. A younger sibling reported that the patient had no difficulty in speaking at home.

As described, the patient's symptoms characteristic of selective mutism include all of the following *except*

A. no difficulty in speaking at home
B. difficulty speaking at school
C. communication by nodding
D. good school performance
E. onset following an emotional trauma

48.7 Figure 48.1A shows a 3-month-old baby boy whose weight is 1 ounce over birth weight. His history of care taking had been characterized by persistent disregard for his basic needs for comfort, affection, and stimulation.

Upon hospitalization, the infant's head circumference was normal, as was his bone age. While he failed to show proper spontaneous activity, his growth hormone levels were in the normal range.

This infant's symptoms typify a classic disorder of infancy. Which, if any, symptom is at odds with the diagnosed disorder?

A. insufficient spontaneous activity
B. normal head circumference vis-à-vis age
C. normal bone age
D. normal levels of growth hormone
E. none of the above

DIRECTIONS: Each group of questions below consists of lettered headings followed by a list of numbered phrases. For each numbered phrase, select the *best* lettered heading. Each heading may be used once, more than once, or not at all.

Questions 48.8–48.9

A. Reactive attachment disorder, inhibited type
B. Reactive attachment disorder, disinhibited type
C. Both
D. Neither

48.8 Linked to institutionalization or exposure to multiple caregivers before age 5 years
48.9 Linked to early childhood maltreatment

Questions 48.10–48.13

A. Separation anxiety disorder
B. Selective mutism
C. Reactive attachment disorder
D. Stereotypic movement disorder

48.10 Associated with grossly pathogenic caregiving
48.11 Difficult to treat when the major attachment figure also has the disorder
48.12 Often manifests only outside the home
48.13 Includes some symptoms, such as rocking or thumb sucking, that are considered developmentally normal, self-comforting behaviors in very young children

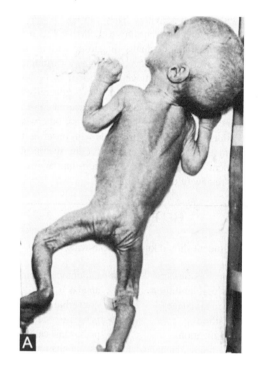

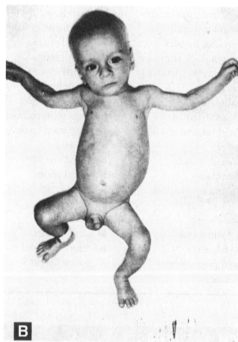

FIGURE 48.1

Reprinted with permission from Barton Schmitt, M.D., Children's Hospital, Denver, Co.

ANSWERS

Other Disorders of Infancy, Childhood, or Adolescence

48.1 The answer is E (none)

Stereotypic movement disorder has undergone some modification with the evolution of the DSM system. The third edition of DSM (DSM-III) contained a broader definition of the disorder than DSM-IV-TR contains. The DSM-III criterion describes voluntary, nondistressing, nonspasmodic movements and goes on to specify that the behaviors were more likely to be associated with extreme psychosocial deprivation, mental retardation, or pervasive developmental disorder but could occur independent of these conditions. Stereotypy/habit disorder, as it was called in the revised third edition of DSM (DSM-III-R), represented a broadened diagnostic category that included periodic and persistent nonfunctional behaviors such as nail biting. Also new in DSM-III-R was the inclusion of functional impairment in the diagnostic criteria; the behavior had to either cause physical injury or interfere with normal activities. DSM-III-R also added exclusions; the diagnosis could not be made if the movements occurred in the presence of a tic disorder or a pervasive developmental disorder. In addition to new criteria described above, *DSM-IV-TR* also *excludes* specific behaviors such as hair pulling *(trichotillomania), tics, and compulsions,* since they are thought to fit more coherently into other diagnostic categories.

When the movement occurs as a part of another general neurological, medical, or psychiatric condition (e.g., *pervasive developmental disorder* not otherwise specified or autism) *a* comorbid *diagnosis of stereotypic movement disorder is not deemed necessary.* Stereotypic movement disorder *can be diagnosed with mental retardation* when the stereotypic behaviors are severe enough to warrant treatment.

48.2 The answer is B

The prevalence of stereotyped movement disorders as a whole in the general population remains unknown; however, some data exist on the prevalence of individual stereotyped behaviors. The prevalence of self-injurious behaviors among individuals with mental retardation has been estimated to be between 2 and 3 percent in community samples of children and 25 percent among mentally retarded adults living in institutions. *Head banging has been estimated to have a prevalence of approximately 5 percent (not 1 percent) in child populations,* with *males affected three times more frequently than females. The behavior is usually (not rarely) self-limiting,* occurring in the first 3 years of life, *with typical age of onset between 5 and 11 months (not after 12 months). It is relatively rare (not relatively common) after age 3* but persists longer in about 5 percent of cases. Similar statistics are reported for head rolling, a behavior that can result in significant hair loss. Similarly, breath holding is also rare after the third birthday and occurs most commonly between 12 and 18 months of age. This behavior is also more common among boys than girls. Bruxism (teeth grinding) is estimated to occur in as much as 56 percent of the normal population in infancy, after eruption of the teeth.

48.3 The answer is E

No specific treatment has been shown to be effective for stereotypic movement disorder in general; however, a small number of double-blind studies have investigated the efficacy of pharmacological treatments for specific behaviors. For example, investigations have suggested the superiority of *clomipramine (Anafranil)* over *desipramine (Norpramin)* for severe nail biting. Although a wide variety of pharmacological agents have been used for stereotyped movements, with varying success, the standard neuroleptics are perhaps most frequently used and demonstrate superior clinical benefit. Both *haloperidol* (Haldol) and *chlorpromazine (Thorazine)* have demonstrated efficacy in placebo-controlled studies of patients with stereotyped movements associated with mental retardation and autistic disorder.

Behavioral modification techniques have been perhaps *the most widely used interventions* for the treatment of stereotypic movements. These techniques, which include both positive and negative reinforcement, have shown some success in diminishing the severity and frequency of the movements, and, in some cases, extinguishing the disorder.

48.4 The answer is B

Separation anxiety disorder *accounts for most of the anxiety in children,* affecting up to 4 percent of school-aged boys and girls. Unlike many other childhood psychiatric disorders, it has been reported to occur in boys and girls equally. While separation anxiety is a developmentally appropriate response to various situations, especially in young children, separation anxiety disorder *is not a developmental stage.* It is characterized by impaired function and *has its most common onset at 7 to 8 (not 1 to 2) years of age.* Separation anxiety disorder *is usually more serious (not less serious) in adolescence* than in childhood. Separation anxiety disorder consists of persistent worry about losing a parent or harm befalling a child's major attachment figure. Separation anxiety disorder *sometimes, but not always, involves refusal to go to school* to avoid separating from the parent.

48.5 The answer is E (all)

Various etiological explanations have been proposed. Historically, selective mutism has been seen as a child's response to family neurosis, believed to be characterized by overprotective or domineering mothers and strict or remote fathers. Unresolved psychodynamic conflicts, trauma, divorce, death of a loved one, and frequent moves have all been postulated to play a role in symptom development.

Recently, several investigators have likened children with selective mutism to socially phobic adults. Immense discomfort in social situations and chronic avoidance of interaction seen in socially phobic adults can be compared with selectively mute children's apprehension about speaking to people outside the immediate family or hearing their own voices. Furthermore, family histories were remarkable for the presence of anxiety disorders, *parental public-speaking anxiety*, and *parental childhood shyness*. Nearly all descriptions of selectively mute children have alluded to their shyness, inhibition, or anxiety. Reframing selective mutism as an anxiety disorder or as a symptom of social anxiety may be salient.

Although by definition the diagnosis of selective mutism cannot be made if the symptoms are better ascribed to developmental, organic, or sociocultural obstacles to adequate language acquisition, linguistic factors may be contributory. Despite the lack of systematic speech and language assessments, speech delays or difficulties in clinical samples have been reported. Delayed speech onset, articulation disorders, *expressive language disorders*, and mixed expressive-receptive language disorders are not uncommon in selectively mute children. The rates of speech and language disorders in this population and the impact of such problems merit further investigation.

Some children who have immigrated into a new linguistic environment have been reported to be selectively mute. Obviously, the diagnosis is precluded in children who have not yet attained fluency in their new language; however, selective mutism may result from resistance to the nondominant language or a sort of culture shock. *Children from multilingual homes* may display selectively mute behaviors upon starting in a school where a nondominant language is used exclusively. Familial and community isolation may play a role in such cases.

48.6 the answer is D

As described, the one symptom of the 16-year-old high school junior not characteristic of selective mutism is *her school performance.* She kept up with her assignments, handed in all of her written work, and received better-than-average grades. Children with selective mutism generally have *no difficulty in speaking at home,* but they do have problems elsewhere, especially *difficulty speaking at school.* Consequently, they often have significant academic difficulty and even failure. Some children with selective mutism *communicate by nodding* or saying "um-hum," which may be the entirety of their early responses to a therapist. In some children *the onset follows an emotional* or a physical *trauma.* As in this case, the inability to speak can begin after the death of a parent.

48.7 The answer is C

The infant suffers from *reactive attachment disorder of infancy,* presenting with the typical clinical picture of nonorganic failure to thrive. In such infants, hypokinesis, dullness, apathy, and *paucity of spontaneous activity* are usually seen. Most of the infants appear malnourished and many have protruding abdomens, as seen in the photograph. Although many such infants' weight is below the third percentile and markedly below the appropriate weight for the infants' height, *head circumference is usually normal for their age. Bone age is usually retarded (not normal). Growth hormone levels are usually normal or elevated,* suggesting that growth failure is secondary to caloric deprivation and malnutrition. The children improve physically and gain weight rapidly after they are hospitalized, as evident in Figure 48.1B.

Answers 48.8–48.9

48.8 The answer is B

48.9 The answer is A

Reactive attachment disorder of infancy and early childhood as described in DSM-IV-TR is characterized by "markedly dis-turbed and developmentally inappropriate social relatedness in most contexts." These findings must be consistent with "grossly pathogenic care." The disorder must begin before 5 years of age to meet criteria and cannot be accounted for "solely by developmental delay." Children who are mentally retarded are thus difficult to diagnose; those who meet criteria for pervasive development disorder are explicitly excluded from consideration for reactive attachment disorder.

Two subtypes are spelled out in the DSM-IV-TR criteria. The first pattern, generally *linked in the literature to early childhood maltreatment,* is characterized by inhibition of the normal developmental tendency to seek comfort from a select group of caregivers. Responses to social interactions are "excessively inhibited, hypervigilant, or highly ambivalent," reflecting the overall inhibition of the attachment system in affected children. The second pattern*, linked to institutionalization or exposure to multiple caregivers before age 5,* is characterized by a relative hyperactivation of the attachment system, resulting in "diffuse" and unselective attachments, and patterned behavior labeled "indiscriminate sociability."

Answers 48.10–48.13

48.10 The answer is C

48.11 The answer is A

48.12 The answer is B

48.13 The answer is D

Reactive attachment disorder is a disorder of social relatedness that is *associated with grossly pathogenic caregiving,* in the form of emotional or physical neglect or multiple caretakers precluding the development of attachments. *Separation anxiety disorder in children becomes difficult to treat* when the major attachment figure also has separation anxiety disorder. In such a case the attachment figure (usually the mother) exposes the child to her own anxiety, reinforcing the child's discomfort. Treatment for separation anxiety disorder includes the major attachment figure encouraging the child to separate and reinforcing a positive reunion after the separation. *Selective mutism* is a disorder that *often manifests only outside the home,* so that at home it is not apparent. In separation anxiety disorder, symptoms are not necessarily evident at home when the major attachment figure is home, yet they would emerge in the home if the mother were to leave and the separation occurred there. *In stereotypic movement disorder* some *symptoms, such as rocking or thumb sucking, are considered developmentally normal,* self-comforting behaviors when they occur in very young children. However, the symptoms can cause functional impairment if they continue into middle childhood and are displayed in socially unacceptable situations.

49 ◭

Mood Disorders in Children and Adolescents

There is considerable evidence that the mood disorders experienced by children and adolescents are essentially the same as those experienced by adults. The same fundamental genetic, other biological, and social factors influence the development and presentation of childhood mood disorders as adult ones. Although the diagnostic criteria in the revised fourth edition of the *Diagnostic and Statistical Manual of Mental Disorders* (DSM-IV-TR) for mood disorders are nearly identical across age groups, the expression of a specific mood disturbance will vary depending on age. Developmental issues influence the expression of all symptoms. Children are particularly vulnerable to social stressors, such as marital conflict, abuse and neglect, and school failures. Mood disorders in children and adolescents can lead to an accumulation of poorly accomplished or unaccomplished developmental tasks, which then can lead to further emotional and psychiatric problems.

Mood disorders in preschool-aged children are considered very rare—about 0.3 percent for major depression in community surveys—but the incidence of mood disorders increases with increasing age. About 2 percent of school-aged children in the community are estimated to meet criteria for major depression, as are about 5 percent of community adolescents. The prevalence in any age group is significantly higher in clinical settings than in community ones. For instance, among hospitalized children and adolescents, the rates of major depression skyrocket to about 20 percent of children and 40 percent of adolescents. Attention-deficit/hyperactivity disorder, oppositional defiant disorder, and conduct disorder may be present in children who later experience depression. Dysthymic disorder is reported to be more common than major depression in school-aged children, but less common in adolescents and adults. Dysthymia that persists for more than 1 year in school-aged children is most likely to progress to major depression. Bipolar I disorder occurs very rarely in prepubertal children, as manic symptoms usually first present in adolescence. The rate of bipolar I disorder in a community study of adolescents has been estimated to be about 0.6 percent, but if clinical variants of mania are included, the rates have been as high as 10 percent. Interestingly, depression is reported to be more common in boys than in girls, although boys also outnumber girls in clinical settings. Having two depressed parents has been estimated to quadruple the risk of a child developing a major mood disorder before the age of 18, when compared with the risk for children with two unaffected parents.

There are a few minor modifications of DSM-IV-TR diagnostic criteria for children and adolescents when compared to the criteria for adults. In major depressive disorder, irritability may be the presenting symptom rather than an overtly depressed mood, and the child or adolescent may fail to make expected weight gains rather than have significant weight changes. Symptoms that are more common among depressed adolescents than among younger children are pervasive anhedonia, severe psychomotor retardation, delusions, and a sense of hopelessness. Other symptoms, such as depressed or irritable mood, insomnia, and decreased concentration, appear to occur with the same frequency regardless of age. In dysthymic disorder, irritable mood may replace depressed mood, and the duration criterion is 1 year rather than the 2 years listed for adults. Criteria for bipolar I disorder are the same for children, adolescents, and adults. Treatment approaches are the same as with adults, including the options of hospitalization, psychotherapy, and pharmacotherapy. Family intervention must be a treatment component in addressing all childhood mood disorders.

Suicide is obviously one of the most severe and disturbing complications of the mood disorders in children and adolescents. Currently, suicide is the third leading cause of death among adolescents, after motor vehicle accidents and homicide. Recently, the rise in suicide rates among adolescents has been dramatic, although more so in the United States than in other countries. The rate among adolescents has quadrupled since 1950. In adolescents aged 15 to 19, the rate is about 13.6 per 100,000 for boys and 3.6 per 100,000 for girls. More than 12,000 children and adolescents are hospitalized each year following suicidal threats or behavior, although completed suicide is rare in children under 12 years of age. More than 5,000 adolescents commit suicide each year in the United States, with the most common method of completed suicide in both boys and girls being the use of a gun. The second most common method in boys is hanging and in girls is overdose on a toxic substance. Completed suicide occurs about five times more often in boys than in girls, but girls attempt suicide three times more often than boys. In adolescents younger than 14 years of age, suicide attempts are estimated to be at least 50 times more common than completed suicide, but among adolescents between 15 and 19 years of age, the ratio of attempted to completed suicides has dropped to 15 to 1. Suicidal risk factors in children and adolescents include a family history of suicidal behavior, exposure to violent and abusive homes, a history of impulsivity, substance abuse, and access to lethal methods. Children at the highest risk for suicide are those who have tried suicide before, especially with a lethal method; boys with histories of aggression or substance abuse; girls who have run away from home, are pregnant, or have made an attempt other than the ingestion of a toxic substance; and those with major depressive disorder characterized by social withdrawal, hopelessness, and anhedonia. Attempted suicide is a psychiatric emergency and must be treated as such, most often with hospitalization, but especially if the family is unable to adequately supervise the child or cooperate with outpatient strategies.

The student should study the questions and answers below for a useful review of these disorders.

HELPFUL HINTS

The student should study these terms.

- academic failure
- anhedonia
- antisocial behavior and substance abuse
- bereavement
- boredom
- copycat suicides
- cortisol hypersecretion
- developmental symptoms
- double depression
- environmental stressors
- family history
- hallucinations
- inpatient vs. outpatient treatment
- insidious onset
- irritable mood
- lethal methods
- poor concentration
- poor problem solving
- precipitants of suicide
- psychosocial deficits
- REM latency
- sad appearance
- social withdrawal
- somatic complaints
- temper tantrums
- toxic environments

▲ QUESTIONS

DIRECTIONS: Each of the questions or incomplete statements below is followed by five suggested responses or completions. Select the *one* that is *best* in each case.

49.1 The "cohort effect" is most evident in studies of

A. dysthymia
B. mild-to-moderate depression
C. more severe melancholic depressions
D. bipolar I disorder
E. none of the above

49.2 True statements about mood disorders in children and adolescents include

A. The incidence of a switch from depression to mania is significantly lower than it is for adults.
B. Among adolescents, severe depression associated with delusional symptoms and pervasive anhedonia is associated with a lower risk for future manic episodes.
C. Among young adults, the development of future hypomanic episodes (bipolar II disorder) has been associated with a history of atypical depression.
D. Adolescent bipolar I disorder patients appear to have a lower risk of experiencing psychotic symptoms than do patients who develop mania as adults.
E. All of the above

49.3 Adolescents who kill

A. are rarely suicidal
B. rarely warn adults or peers of their intent
C. report ease in obtaining firearms and are often expert in using them
D. have usually not explicitly displayed a fascination with violence
E. have a lower rate of major depression than same-aged peers

49.4 The antidepressant drugs of choice for mood disorders in children and adolescents are

A. selective serotonin reuptake inhibitors (SSRIs)
B. tricyclic drugs
C. bupropion (Wellbutrin)
D. monoamine oxidase inhibitors (MAOIs)
E. lithium (Eskalith)

49.5 Major depressive disorder in school-aged children

A. may present as irritable mood rather than depressed mood
B. usually includes pervasive anhedonia
C. is more common than dysthymic disorder
D. includes mood-congruent auditory hallucinations less often than in adults with this disorder
E. occurs more often in girls than in boys

49.6 Suicide in adolescents

A. decreases in frequency with increasing age
B. occurs more often in teenagers 12 to 14 years of age than in teenagers 14 to 16 years of age
C. is more common in girls than in boys
D. is almost always associated with a mood disorder
E. is often precipitated by arguments with family members, girlfriends, or boyfriends

49.7 Which of the following symptoms of major depressive disorder are equally common in all age groups?

A. Suicidal ideation
B. Somatic complaints
C. Mood-congruent auditory hallucinations
D. Pervasive anhedonia
E. All of the above

ANSWERS

Mood Disorders in Children and Adolescents

49.1 The answer is B

The epidemiology of mood disorders and suicide among children and adolescents is complicated by their increasing rates with increasing age. Also, over the last few decades, the criteria for diagnosing the disorders have changed. Finally, the reported incidence of mood disorders among youths over the last few decades has consistently increased, and the age of onset has decreased. This phenomenon has been called the cohort effect. It is most evident in studies of *mild-to-moderate depression*, but it has not been noted for *dysthymic disorder*. *More severe melancholic depressions* and *bipolar I disorder* are less affected by the cohort effect. Although the mechanism of the cohort effect is not clear, genetic anticipation, in which a genetic disorder tends to worsen in successive generations, has been suggested to explain it.

Prevalence rates for mood disorders and suicide are often reported separately for prepubertal children and for adolescents. Rates of completed suicide are separated by gender as well as age. Large differences in sampling and measurement instruments make it not surprising that a range of prevalence rates was found by different studies. There is also some variation in rates of depressive illness, depending on who the informant was. In most cases, patients reported higher rates of disorder than their parents. See Table 49.1 for prevalence rates.

49.2 The answer is C

An important possible sequela of major depression among children and adolescents is the development of mania and diagnosis of bipolar illness. *The incidence of a switch from depression to mania among children and adolescents is significantly higher (not lower) than it is for adults.* In the adult literature, between 5 and

**Table 49.1
Prevalence (Point or 1-year)**

Major depression	
Preschoolers	0.3%
Children	0.4–3.0%
Adolescents	0.4–6.4%
Dysthymic disorder	
Children	0.6–1.7%
Adolescents	1.6–8.0%
Bipolar I disorder	
Children	0.2–0.4%
Adolescents	1%
Attempted suicide	
Children	1%
Adolescents	1.7–5.9%
Completed suicide	
5–9-year-old boys	0.04/100,000
5–9-year-old girls	0
10–14-year-old boys	2.4/100,000
10–14-year-old girls	0.96/100,000
15–19-year-old males	18.25/100,000
15–19-year-old females	3.48/100,000

18 percent of patients with depression become manic. Among prepubertal children with severe major depression, the rates of eventual mania have been reported to be as high as 32 percent within a 2- to 5-year period. Among adolescents, rates of mania between 20 and 40 percent have been reported within 5 years of the index depression. *Among adolescents, severe depression characterized by* psychomotor retardation, *delusional symptoms, and pervasive anhedonia is associated with the highest risk (not a lower risk) for future manic episodes. Among young adults, the development of future hypomanic episodes (bipolar II disorder) has been associated with atypical depression,* early onset of depression, seasonal affective disorder, and comorbid substance abuse. Among adolescents, a switch to hypomania may sometimes be misconstrued as a disruptive behavior disorder.

Additional complications of major depressive disorder in children and adolescents are the persistence of social impairment and the perception of being socially isolated. While social disturbance is not unique to mood disorders, depression in youth is associated with increased risk of tobacco and substance use and continued negative attributions, all of which affect social functioning.

One recent study of depressed children followed up at 36 weeks found that 50 percent still met criteria for major depressive disorder; of those, 73 percent had remained depressed, and 27 percent had recovered and relapsed. In this sample, major depression at follow-up was predicted by more severe depression at intake, comorbid obsessive-compulsive disorder, and being older at the time of the index depression.

The course and prognosis of bipolar disorders are clearer in adolescents than in prepubertal children, since diagnosis is more clear-cut. A number of studies have indicated that an earlier age of onset (i.e., adolescent compared with young adult) of bipolar I disorder is associated with an increased frequency of cycles as well as an increased likelihood of mixed states. Other studies have suggested that the relapse rate for bipolar I disorder patients whose first episode is in their teens or early twenties is lower than that of bipolar I disorder patients who experienced a first episode in their thirties. *Adolescent bipolar I disorder patients appear to have a higher (not a lower) risk of experiencing psychotic symptoms* than patients who developed mania as adults. In a follow-up of adolescent bipolar I disorder patients, those whose index episode was purely manic or mixed recovered from the episode more rapidly than those whose index episode was depressive. Of this sample, 44 percent relapsed within 5 years and 21 percent of the sample manifested at least two relapses following recovery from the index episode. The likelihood of multiple relapses was highest for patients whose index feature was mixed episode or rapid cycling. Among adolescents who developed manic episodes, those with a premorbid history of psychiatric disorders, including disruptive behavior disorders, had significantly more first- and second-degree family members with a history of affective illness.

49.3 The answer is C

A disturbing number of reports over the last few years have depicted the tragic killings of both children and adults by adolescents. More than 200 deaths have occurred in schoolyards across the United States within the last decade. In more recent years, these killings have been more frequent in rural settings and have involved multiple victims. In the early 1990s many of the school-related killings were attributable to gang activities or disputes over money or romantic involvements. In the last few years, multiple homicides perpetrated by adolescents have related more to issues of revenge for being mercilessly teased or have been enactment scenarios of violence by adolescents who appear to be obsessed with violent destruction.

While no unifying profiles identify adolescents who may commit murder, some similarities can be noted retrospectively in the histories of adolescents who have killed. When pieces of the histories of adolescent murderers are disclosed, it appears that most of these adolescents had long-standing troubles, *some with major depression*; they were often socially isolated; and they *had explicitly displayed a fascination with violence*. Some of the adolescent killers disclosed their inner agony fueled by tormenting from peers who ridiculed and rejected them daily. Some had experienced clear family dysfunction or circumstances of abuse, neglect, or parental psychiatric history that influenced the adolescent negatively. Many of the adolescents who killed had expressed the desire for violent revenge to parents, teachers, or peers. All of the adolescent killers *reported ease in obtaining firearms, and many were expert in using them.* In most cases, adolescents acquired semiautomatic weapons that were unlocked and kept in their homes within easy reach. *Some of the adolescents gave literal warnings a day or a few weeks before the killings,* either stating that there would be a violent attack or warning certain peers to stay away from school on a certain day. Others wrote poems, compositions, or journal entries depicting the violent scenes. *Most of the adolescents who left notes at the time of the murders were suicidal* and assumed that they would also die during the attack.

Suicide rates among youths have been on the increase, and rates of depression have also increased in adolescents in younger age groups. A depressed, demoralized, socially rejected adolescent male preoccupied with violent fantasies, with easy access to semiautomatic weapons, is a potential disaster. Any violent threat must be taken seriously, and families must be taught to keep weapons away from these adolescents.

49.4 The answer is A

Current antidepressant treatment of mood disorders in children and adolescents is still in the early phases of being validated with double-blind efficacy studies. Thus far, no studies have supported the use of *tricyclic drugs* in children or adolescents. There are some published placebo-controlled double-blind studies comparing fluoxetine's efficacy for depressive symptoms in adolescents with that of placebo.

The tricyclic drugs have shown efficacy in multiple adult studies of mood disorder, but since the advent of antidepressants with safer adverse-effect profiles (i.e., minimal risk of cardiac arrhythmias and considerably lower lethal potential), the tricyclic drugs are usually not among the first-choice antidepressants for children and adolescents.

Selective serotonin reuptake inhibitors (SSRIs) have become the drugs of choice for mood disorders in children and adolescents because of promising research findings and the favorable drug profiles. Serotonin reuptake inhibitors include fluoxetine (Prozac), paroxetine (Paxil), sertraline (Zoloft), fluvoxamine

(Luvox), citalopram (Celexa), and nefazodone (Serzone). Nefazodone blocks norepinephrine receptors and serotonin receptors. These drugs all have a relatively mild adverse-effect profile, with low lethality after overdose. Dosage-related adverse effects include headache and nausea. Except nefazodone, all of these drugs can cause sexual dysfunction, including diminished libido, delayed ejaculation, or anorgasmia. There have been no indications thus far that plasma level can be correlated to expected response. In the double-blind study by Graham Emslie, response to the SSRIs seemed to be equivalent in children and older adolescents. Additional potential adverse effects of these drugs include insomnia and a syndrome of restlessness and agitation that can be ameliorated by decreasing the dosage.

Other antidepressants that can be used include bupropion (Wellbutrin), a dopaminergic drug; venlafaxine (Effexor), which blocks serotonin and norepinephrine reuptake; mirtazapine (Remeron), a serotonin-plus-norepinephrine reuptake inhibitor; and the monoamine oxidase inhibitors (MAOIs) phenelzine (Nardil) and tranylcypromine (Parnate). *Bupropion* is an antidepressant with stimulant properties that has few anticholinergic side effects, produces virtually no sedation, and is much safer in overdose than the tricyclic drugs. Because of its stimulant properties, it has also been used to treat attention-deficit/hyperactivity disorder. Venlafaxine is a relatively new antidepressant that largely shares an adverse-effect profile with the SSRIs; the most common adverse effects include nausea, anorexia, nervousness, and sexual dysfunction. Despite its potential to induce nervousness, there have been anecdotal reports of its efficacy in the treatment of anxiety. There have been no studies of mirtazapine, a new antidepressant similar to nefazodone in mechanism of action. Mirtazapine is significantly more sedating than nefazodone.

MAOIs have been sparsely studied in children and adolescents although they have been shown to be effective in adults with major depressive disorder and those with atypical depression. In one published open trial of phenelzine with adolescents who were refractory to treatment with tricyclic drugs, the treating physician judged that up to 60 percent of these adolescents were improved by the phenelzine treatment.

The MAOIs require strict adherence to a restricted diet (no cheese [except cottage cheese or cream cheese], processed meats, caviar, cured fish, overripe fruits, avocados, fava beans, yeast extracts, Chianti or burgundy wine, beers containing yeast, or over-the-counter cold preparations, especially decongestants and inhalers). Because of these prohibitions, MAOIs must be very cautiously and selectively used with children and adolescents. Aside from these restricted foods and drugs (which potentially result in hypertensive crises and death if ingested), other adverse effects of the drugs include orthostatic hypotension and sleep disturbances. The MAO type A inhibitor moclobemide (available in Canada but not in the United States) is a safer drug with a milder adverse-effect profile, but it has not yet been studied with children or adolescents. In children or adolescents with major depressive disorder, there is a risk of precipitating a hypomanic or manic episode during the course of any antidepressant treatment.

Although there has been only one double-blind placebo-controlled study showing the efficacy of *lithium* for bipolar children and adolescents, pharmacokinetic studies of lithium in children and adolescents with behavior disorders indicate that lithium can be used with the same safety precautions used for adults. As with adults, CBCs electrolytes, renal function tests, and thyroid function tests should be monitored closely. A baseline ECG is warranted. Lithium has a shorter half-life in children than in adults, consistent with a higher efficiency of the kidneys in children. Treating hypomania or mania in adolescents applies the same basic strategies used for adults. Initiation of a psychopharmacological treatment in a manic adolescent often requires hospitalization if the patient cannot be contained or follow directions reliably. For adolescent patients with pure mania, lithium is generally the drug of choice. It has demonstrated efficacy in the treatment of manic states in adults and has shown some prophylactic efficacy for future mood episodes in adults, more strongly for manic episodes than for depressed episodes. Since there is controversy regarding inclusion of a variety of cycling and non-cycling severe mood and behavioral disturbances in children and adolescents, the studies done in this age group have no doubt involved a heterogeneous diagnostic group. Nevertheless, in the published open-trial reviews of lithium treatment of youths, the efficacy of lithium for behavioral improvement has ranged from about 50 to 66 percent. This is substantially lower than reported lithium efficacy in manic adults. Clinical features that may predict poor responsivity to lithium include mixed mood states and atypical features.

49.5 The answer is A

Major depression in school-aged children is essentially the same disorder that occurs in adolescents and adults. One modification in the revised fourth edition of *Diagnostic and Statistical Manual of Mental Disorders* (DSM-IV-TR) criteria for major depressive disorder in children and adolescents is that it *may present as irritable mood rather than depressed mood*. Major depressive disorder in children *rarely (not usually) includes pervasive anhedonia*. It is *less common (not more common) than dysthymic disorder* in school-aged children, but it is more common than dysthymic disorder in adolescence. Major depressive disorder in children includes *mood-congruent*

auditory hallucinations more often (not less often) than in adults with this disorder. It *occurs more often in boys than in girls (not vice versa)* in this age group.

49.6 The answer is E

Suicide in adolescents *is often precipitated by arguments with family members, girlfriends, or boyfriends.* Completed suicide is rare in children under 12 years of age and *increases in frequency (rather than decreases) with increasing age.* Thus, suicide *occurs more often in teenagers 14 to 16 years of age than in teenagers 12 to 14 years of age* (not vice versa). Suicide attempts are about three times as common in adolescent girls as in boys, but completed suicide *is more common in boys than in girls* (not vice versa). That is primarily due to the greater lethality of the methods that adolescent boys use. The most common method of suicide in adolescent boys is the use of firearms, accounting for two-thirds of male suicides. Firearms account for half of completed suicides among adolescent girls. The second most common method of suicide in adolescent boys is hanging. Ingestions are an uncommon method of completed suicides in males, although they are common nonlethal methods used in suicide attempts by adolescent girls. Suicide *is not always (rather than almost always) associated with a mood disorder,* although the risk of suicide increases when there is a severe mood disorder.

49.7 The answer is A

Suicidal ideation occurs equally in patients with major depressive disorder in all age groups. Although the core features of major depressive disorder are essentially the same in children, adolescents, and adults, different specific symptoms predominate at different ages. In depressed school-aged children, *somatic complaints* and *mood-congruent auditory hallucinations* present more often than in depressed adolescents or adults. Mood congruent delusions and *pervasive anhedonia* increase with age and are more common in adolescents and adults than in young children.

Early-Onset Schizophrenia

Schizophrenia with onset in prepubertal children is extremely rare and is thought to be less common than autistic disorder. Schizophrenia is seldom diagnosed in children before the age of 5 years, while it is commonly diagnosed in adolescents older than 15 years of age. The characteristics of schizophrenia in children are the same as they are in adults, although in children delusions and hallucinations are usually less complex and visual hallucinations are more common. The frequency of delusions increases with increasing age, and a child's developmental level influences the presentation of delusional material. In the 1980s schizophrenia with childhood onset was formally separated from autistic disorder, reflecting accumulated evidence that the clinical picture, family history, age of onset, and course of the two disorders were different. In contrast to autistic disorder, children with schizophrenia are generally of normal intelligence, with a family history of schizophrenia, and manifest symptoms after the age of 5 years, demonstrating delusions, hallucinations, and thought disorder. The severe language impairments present in autistic disorder do not tend to occur in early-onset schizophrenia. However, complicating the diagnostic issues is research that suggests that a subgroup of autistic children will eventually develop schizophrenia, and that according to DSM-IV-TR, schizophrenia can be diagnosed in the presence of autistic disorder. Another complicating diagnostic issue is that normal developmental immaturities in language and in separating fantasy from reality can make diagnosing schizophrenia in children between the ages of 5 and 7 years difficult. The diagnostic criteria for children and adults with schizophrenia are identical except that instead of the deterioration in functioning seen in adults and older children, younger children will fail to meet the expected levels of social and academic achievement.

The prevalence of schizophrenia among the parents of children with schizophrenia is about 8 percent, nearly twice the prevalence in parents of patients with later-onset schizophrenia. The onset of symptoms is usually insidious, although it can also be sudden in a previously apparently normal child. The prevalence of schizophrenia in children is estimated to be nearly 50 times less than that in adolescents, with a slightly higher and earlier rate of occurrence in boys. Family and genetic studies provide substantial evidence of a biological etiology of schizophrenia. Higher-than-expected rates of neurological soft signs and impairments in attention and information processing have been described among high-risk children, associated with poor motor functioning, visuospatial impairments, and attention deficits. Children and adolescents with schizophrenia tend to have a greater premorbid history of social rejection, impaired social skills, clinginess and withdrawn behavior, and academic problems than those with adult-onset schizophrenia. Some children with schizophrenia show early histories of delayed motor and language milestones, similar to those seen in autistic disorder. Psychotic symptoms alone are not sufficient evidence of schizophrenia. In order to fulfill criteria for the diagnosis, the child must also show either a deterioration of function or a failure to meet expected levels of development.

Children with developmental delays, learning disorders, and premorbid behavioral disorders, such as attention-deficit/hyperactivity disorder and conduct disorder, seem to be poor responders to pharmacotherapy and tend to have the worst prognoses. In one long-term–outcome study of patients diagnosed with schizophrenia before the age of 14 years, the poorest prognosis was observed in children who were diagnosed before 10 years of age and who had preexisting behavioral disorders. In general, childhood-onset schizophrenia appears to be less medication-responsive than adult- and adolescent-onset schizophrenia, and the prognosis seems to be worse. Treatments include those utilized in adult patients: pharmacotherapy, family therapy, family education, plus a properly supportive and attuned academic setting.

The student should study the questions and answers below for a useful review of the condition.

HELPFUL HINTS

The student should understand these terms.

- ▶ agranulocytosis
- ▶ autistic disorder
- ▶ childhood psychosis
- ▶ clozapine (Clozaril)
- ▶ comorbidity
- ▶ delayed motor development
- ▶ developmental level and age-appropriate presentations
- ▶ diagnostic stability
- ▶ disturbed communication
- ▶ expressed emotion
- ▶ family support
- ▶ haloperidol (Haldol)
- ▶ high-risk children
- ▶ hypersalivation
- ▶ persecutory delusions
- ▶ pervasive developmental disorders
- ▶ premorbid disorders
- ▶ premorbid functioning
- ▶ risperidone (Risperdal)
- ▶ schizotypal personality
- ▶ sedation
- ▶ social rejection
- ▶ tardive dyskinesia
- ▶ transient phobic hallucinations
- ▶ visual hallucinations

▲ QUESTIONS

DIRECTIONS: The lettered headings below are followed by a list of numbered words or phrases. For each numbered word or phrase, select

    A. if the item is associated with *A only*
    B. if the item is associated with *B only*
    C. if the item is associated with *both A and B*
    D. if the item is associated with *neither A nor B*

Questions 50.1–50.3

    A. Early-onset schizophrenia
    B. Pervasive developmental disorders
    C. Both
    D. Neither

50.1 Prominent delusions or hallucinations
50.2 Language and communication deficits are common
50.3 Absence of a normal period of development

DIRECTIONS: Each of the incomplete statements below is followed by five suggested completions. Select the *one* that is *best* in each case.

50.4 Predictors of poor prognosis in schizophrenia with childhood onset include all of the following *except*

    A. misdiagnosed schizophrenia in a child with bipolar I disorder
    B. onset before 10 years of age
    C. premorbid diagnoses of attention-deficit/hyperactivity disorder and learning disorders
    D. lack of family support
    E. delayed motor milestones and delayed language acquisition

50.5 Schizophrenia with childhood onset differs from schizophrenia with adult onset in that

    A. schizophrenic children do not manifest command auditory hallucinations
    B. parents of patients with childhood-onset schizophrenia are less likely than parents of patients with adult-onset schizophrenia to be schizophrenic
    C. in children with schizophrenia there is often a premorbid history of behavior disorders, delayed motor milestones, and delayed language acquisition
    D. childhood schizophrenics respond more to medication than do adult schizophrenics
    E. childhood-onset schizophrenics are usually mildly mentally retarded

50.6 Schizophrenia

    A. is rare prior to age 12 years
    B. has a rate of onset that increases sharply in adolescence
    C. in children occurs predominantly in males
    D. appears to be essentially the same heterogeneous disorder in children as in adults
    E. all of the above

ANSWERS

Early-Onset Schizophrenia

Answers 50.1–50.3

50.1 The answer is A

50.2 The answer is C

50.3 The answer is B
Autism and other pervasive developmental disorders are distinguished from early-onset schizophrenia by the absence or transitory nature of the required positive psychotic symptomatology—that is, *hallucinations and delusions*—as well as by the predominance of the *characteristic deviant language patterns, aberrant social relatedness,* and other key symptoms that typify these disorders. The earlier age of onset and the *absence of a normal period of development* are also indicative, although some children with schizophrenia do have a lifelong history of developmental delays. However, compared to pervasive developmental disorders, the premorbid abnormalities in schizophrenia tend to be less pervasive and severe.

Approximately 10 to 20 percent of youths with schizophrenia have low intelligent quotient (IQ) scores. *Language and communication deficits* are common. Children with schizophrenia have deficits in their information-processing capacities, a finding also noted in adults.

Caution must be used in making the diagnosis of schizophrenia in children who have severe language impairments. Since the standard presentations of hallucinations and delusions involve language, assessing a child with severely impaired language for psychotic symptoms can be a diagnostic challenge. In these cases, the clinician is dependent on observations of behavior. Psychotic symptoms may be identified when their emergence is associated with a deterioration in mental status and global functioning.

If there is a history of autism or another pervasive developmental disorder, prominent delusions or hallucinations (for at least 1 month unless treated successfully) are required to make a diagnosis of schizophrenia.

50.4 The answer is A
Misdiagnosed schizophrenia in a child with bipolar I disorder is a factor indicative of a good prognosis, not a poor prognosis. Although prospective studies are needed, factors that seem to

predict poor prognosis in schizophrenia with childhood onset are *onset before age 10 years,* premorbid diagnoses *of attention-deficit/hyperactivity disorder and learning disorders, lack of family support,* and an early history of *delayed motor milestones and delayed language acquisition.*

50.5 The answer is C

Schizophrenia with childhood onset is recognized as the same disorder as is seen in adolescents and adults. But in children with schizophrenia, there is often a premorbid history of *behavior disorders, delayed motor milestones, and delayed language acquisition.* Schizophrenic children *do* manifest *command auditory hallucinations* similar to those of adult schizophrenia patients. There have been reports of increased genetic loading in childhood-onset schizophrenics. *Parents of patients with childhood-onset* schizophrenia are more likely (not less likely) than parents of patients with adult-onset schizophrenia to be schizophrenic; about 8 percent of first-degree relatives of childhood schizophrenics, as opposed to 4 percent of adult-onset schizophrenics, are affected. Although there have been no well-controlled studies, it appears that *childhood schizophrenics respond to medications less (not more) than do adult schizophrenics.* Epidemiological data indicate that *childhood-onset schizophrenics are usually not (rather than mildly) mentally retarded,* but rather function in the low-average to average range of intelligence.

50.6 The answer is E (all)

There is a paucity of research examining schizophrenia in youth. Treatment studies are generally lacking. Although the incidence of the disorder increases after the onset of puberty, much of the existing literature focuses on childhood onset. Other methodological problems include retrospective designs, lack of standardized assessment tools such as diagnostic interviews, small subject pools, and lack of comparison groups.

However, despite these limitations, reasonable conclusions can be drawn from the existing studies regarding the diagnosis of schizophrenia in youth. Furthermore, because *schizophrenia in youth appears to be essentially the same heterogeneous disorder as in adults*, the adult literature can generally be extrapolated to children and adolescents as long as developmental issues are taken into account.

Although schizophrenia in children under age 13 years has often been described as prepubertal, most studies have determined this by age, not by physical development. To avoid ambiguity, early-onset schizophrenia has been defined as onset prior to 18 years of age, with a subgroup of very-early-onset schizophrenia defined as onset before age 13 years.

The prevalence of schizophrenia in youth has not been established adequately. Clinical experience suggests that schizophrenia with *onset prior to age 12 years is rare.* It has been estimated that 0.1 to 1.0 percent of all schizophrenic disorders occur before age 10 years, with 4 percent presenting prior to 15 years of age. *The rate of onset increases sharply during adolescence,* with the peak ages of onset ranging from 15 to 30 years.

A study examining young adults during their first episode of schizophrenia (N = 232) found that 47 percent had displayed the first signs of their illness before age 21 years. However, only 21 percent developed psychotic symptoms prior to this age. There are reported cases of onset prior to age 6 years. However, a diagnosis of schizophrenia in young children must be scrutinized carefully.

Schizophrenia in youth, especially in children, occurs predominantly in males. As age increases, this ratio tends to even out. Since the adult literature suggests that the age of onset in males is significantly younger than that in females, the male predominance may be a cross-sectional effect.

51 ▲

Adolescent Substance Abuse

In the revised fourth edition of the *Diagnostic and Statistical Manual of Mental Disorders* (DSM-IV-TR), substance abuse is defined as a maladaptive pattern of substance use leading to clinically significant impairment or distress. Substance dependence is defined as a group of cognitive, behavioral, and physiological signs and symptoms, (such as tolerance, withdrawal, and compulsive drug-taking behavior) that indicate an individual is continuing the use of a substance despite significant (substance-related) problems. Problems associated with abuse and dependence can include recurrent use in situations that cause danger to the user, recurrent use leading to legal problems, and recurrent use leading to school or social impairments. Substance use can be viewed on a continuum, with experimentation at one end, leading gradually upward to mild use, then to regular use without obvious impairment, to actual abuse, and finally to dependence. Substances can include alcohol, marijuana, cocaine, methamphetamines, hallucinogens (such as lysergic acid diethylamide [LSD]), opiates, anxiolytics, and inhalants, among others. Substituted so-called designer amphetamines, such as methylenedioxymethamphetamine (MDMA or "ecstasy"), have generated much publicity lately and are widely available. Among adolescents enrolled in substance-abuse treatment programs, it has been estimated that 96 percent are polysubstance users. The use of inhalants (in the form of glue, aerosols, and gasoline) appears to be relatively more common among younger than older adolescents.

Over the last 10 years a number of risk factors have been identified for adolescent substance abusers, and the greater the number of risk factors, the greater the likelihood that an adolescent will be a substance abuser. These factors include high levels of family conflict, academic difficulties, comorbid psychiatric disorders such as conduct disorder and depression, parental and peer substance abuse, impulsivity, and early onset of cigarette smoking. Children in families with the lowest measure of parental supervision have been shown to initiate alcohol, tobacco, and other drug use earlier than children from families with greater supervision. The greatest risk was noted for children under 11 years of age. In the 1990s a downward trend in the prevalence of drug use has been reported, but substance abuse continues to be a problem for significant numbers of adolescents.

For instance, a recent survey indicates that alcohol abuse is a significant problem for 10 to 20 percent of adolescents. It has been estimated that in the United States, there are 3 million adolescent problem drinkers and 300,000 adolescents with alcohol dependence. Some studies have shown that by 13 years of age, one-third of boys and almost one-fourth of girls have tried alcohol. A large majority of adolescents report some alcohol use (up to 92 percent of males and 73 percent of females), and most of this use probably represents normal experimentation, not necessarily reflecting abuse or dependence. However, by 18 years of age, 4 percent of adolescents reported daily drinking, and 2 percent reported daily marijuana use, a better indicator of problem usage. Studies have shown a higher prevalence of substance abuse, particularly alcohol abuse and dependence, among biological children of alcoholics than among adopted youngsters. Rates of alcohol and drug use are reportedly higher in relatives of children with depression and bipolar disorder, and mood disorders are common among those with alcohol and drug abuse. In a recent survey of adolescents who used alcohol, more than 80 percent met criteria for another disorder. The most frequently noted comorbid conditions were depressive disorders, disruptive behavior disorders, and other drug-use disorders. These rates of comorbidity were noted to be higher than those for adults. There is a relationship between substance abuse and a number of high-risk behaviors, including the use of weapons, suicidal behavior, early sexual experimentation, and dangerous driving. It seems that most substance abusers have underlying deficits in social skills and may use substances as a way of feeling more comfortable and fitting in with peers.

Treatment of adolescents with substance-abuse disorders may include inpatient units, residential facilities, halfway houses, group homes, partial hospital programs, and outpatient settings. The basic components of adolescent substance abuse treatment mirror those utilized in the treatment of adults, including individual psychotherapy; 12-step and other self-help groups such as Alcoholics Anonymous (AA), Narcotics Anonymous (NA), Alateen, and Al-Anon; random urine testing; family therapy; and psychopharmacology. Determining coexisting psychiatric disorders is crucial. When mood disorders are present, antidepressants (usually the serotonin reuptake inhibitors are the first line of treatment) may be indicated. Other comorbid psychiatric disorders that may be amenable to pharmacologic interventions include anxiety disorders, conduct disorder, and attention-deficit/hyperactivity disorder.

The student should study the questions and answers below for a useful review of these abuses.

HELPFUL HINTS

The student should be able to define the following terms.

- aerosols
- Al-Anon
- Alateen
- Alcoholics Anonymous (AA)
- Antabuse
- cocaine
- comorbidity
- demographic drinking patterns
- gateway drug
- genetic contributions and adoption studies
- glue
- high-risk behaviors
- inhalants
- marijuana
- Narcotics Anonymous (NA)
- polysubstance abuse
- severity-oriented rating scales
- substance abuse
- substance dependence
- substance intoxication
- substance withdrawal
- 12-step program

▲ QUESTIONS

DIRECTIONS: Each of the questions or incomplete statements below is followed by five suggested responses or completions. Select the *one* that is *best* in each case.

51.1 The substance of choice for most adolescents is

A. marijuana
B. alcohol
C. cocaine
D. methylenedioxymethamphetamine (MDMA, "ecstasy")
E. lysergic acid diethylamide (LSD)

51.2 In general

A. male and female adolescents use substances equally
B. white and Hispanic students are less likely than African-American students to report lifetime alcohol use and heavy episodic use
C. white and Hispanic students are more likely than African-American students to report both lifetime and current marijuana use
D. rates of lifetime alcohol abuse or dependence are as high as 30 percent in 17 to 19 year olds
E. none of the above

51.3 The most common psychiatric disorder associated with substance-use disorders is probably

A. conduct disorder
B. attention-deficit/hyperactivity disorder
C. depressive disorders
D. anxiety disorders
E. none of the above

51.4 Psychiatric conditions that often present as comorbidities with substance-use disorders include

A. suicidal ideation and attempts
B. generalized anxiety disorder and panic disorder
C. posttraumatic stress disorder
D. learning disorders
E. all of the above

51.5 True statements about substance use and adolescents include

A. Use of marijuana is the strongest predictor of future cocaine use.
B. Prevalence rates for cocaine appear to be decreasing.
C. Children of alcohol abusers reportedly have a 25 percent chance of also abusing alcohol.
D. More than 17 percent of students in 8th, 9th, 10th, 11th, and 12th grades have used inhalants.
E. All of the above

51.6 Differences between adolescent and adult substance abusers include

A. Relapse in adolescents is more often associated with situations involving negative affect than social pressure for use, as is usually found in adult relapse.
B. Adolescents have a lower level of return to substance use after treatment when compared to adults.
C. Adolescents are more likely to experience more noxious or adverse reactions to substances than more experienced adult substance users.
D. Comorbid conduct disorder in adolescents is not correlated negatively with treatment completion and future abstinence.
E. None of the above

51.7 Successful substance-abuse prevention programs appear to be those that

A. target salient risk factors
B. are skills oriented
C. have follow-up
D. take into account the socioeconomic and cultural realities of the targeted communities
E. all of the above

51.8 The treatment for alcohol abuse in adolescents includes all of the following *except*

A. drug-specific counseling
B. self-help groups
C. relapse prevention programs
D. disulfiram (Antabuse) treatment
E. individual psychotherapy

51.9 Risk factors for the development of adolescent substance abuse include all of the following *except*

A. early onset of cigarette smoking
B. diminished parental supervision
C. high academic achievement
D. parental substance abuse
E. conduct disorder

51.10 Of adolescents who present to a pediatric trauma center, the number of cases that involve alcohol or drug use is approximately

    A. 10 percent
    B. 25 percent
    C. 30 percent
    D. 50 percent
    E. 80 percent

DIRECTIONS: These lettered headings are followed by a list of numbered phrases. For each numbered phrase, select the lettered heading most closely associated with it. Each lettered heading may be used once, more than once, or not at all.

Questions 51.11–51.15

    A. Substance abuse
    B. Substance dependence
    C. Substance intoxication
    D. Substance withdrawal

51.11 Only category in DSM-IV-TR used for caffeine

51.12 A maladaptive pattern of substance use causing impairment manifested as tolerance, withdrawal, and inability to decrease substance use

51.13 The development of a reversible syndrome causing behavioral or psychological changes caused by a substance

51.14 A maladaptive pattern of substance use causing impairment as manifested by diminished performance in school, legal problems, and continued use despite recurrent social and interpersonal problems

51.15 The development of a substance-specific syndrome due to the cessation of a substance that causes distress and impairment

---

ANSWERS

Adolescent Substance Abuse

51.1 The answer is B

Alcohol is the substance of choice for most adolescents. According to the University of Michigan Monitoring the Future 1996 Survey of high school students, 79.2 percent of 12th graders, 71.8 percent of 10th graders, and 55.3 percent of 8th graders report lifetime use. Although 26.8 percent of 8th graders reported ever having been drunk, by the 10th and 12th grades this percentage had risen to 48.5 and 61.8 percent, respectively. In terms of regular drinking, 30.2 percent of 12th graders, 24.0 percent of 10th graders, and 15.6 percent of 8th graders report having five or more drinks on a single occasion in the preceding 2 weeks.

From 1991 to 1996 the proportion of high school students reporting the use of any illicit drug in the past 12 months increased from 27 to 40 percent for 12th graders, from 20 to 38 percent for 10th graders, and from 11 to 24 percent for 8th graders. Marijuana accounted for much of this increase during the early 1990s. Almost 5 percent (4.9 percent) of 12th graders reported daily marijuana use, and 36 percent reported use during the past year. Among 8th graders, 18 percent reported marijuana use within the past year.

The annual prevalence in the use of a number of other substances also rose in the early 1990s. In 1996, 4 percent of 8th graders and 9 percent of 12th graders reported *lysergic acid diethylamide (LSD)* use in the preceding year. Annual prevalence rates for amphetamines were 9 percent for 8th graders, 12 percent for 10th graders, and 10 percent for 12th graders. In 1996, 2.8 percent of 12th graders reported the use of methamphetamine ("ice") and nearly 5 percent reported the use of *methylenedioxymethamphetamine (MDMA, "ecstasy")* during the past year. The annual prevalence of other substances remained low in 1996. Heroin was used by 1.6 percent of 8th graders and 1 percent of 12th graders; *cocaine* was used by 4.9 percent of 12th graders and 3 percent of 8th graders, while crack cocaine was used by 2.1 percent of 12th graders and 1.8 percent of 8th graders during the preceding year.

51.2 The answer is D

In general, *male adolescents use substances of all kinds more than females do (not equally).* Overall, white and Hispanic students are more likely (not less likely) than African-American students to report *lifetime alcohol use and heavy episodic use.* African-American students are less likely (not more likely) *to report both lifetime and current marijuana use.*

Few studies have examined the prevalence of substance-use disorders in general population samples. *Rates of lifetime alcohol abuse* or dependence range from 5.3 percent in 15 year olds to *30 percent in 17 to 19 year olds.* The lifetime prevalence of drug abuse or dependence ranges from 3.3 percent in 15 year olds to 9.7 percent in 17 to 19 year olds.

51.3 The answer is A

A number of psychiatric disorders are commonly associated with substance-use disorders in youths (Table 51.1). Many adolescents who use substances also display a variety of other deviant behaviors. It may be difficult to attribute dysfunction to a particular deviant behavior, such as substance use, rather than to other deviant behaviors, the entire syndrome of deviant behavior (i.e., conduct disorder), or other psychiatric disorders. *Conduct disorder* and constituent criteria such as aggression usually precede and accompany adolescent substance-use disorders. Clinical populations of adolescents with substance-use disorders show rates of conduct disorder ranging from 50 to almost 80 percent. Although *attention-deficit/hyperactivity disorder* is commonly noted in substance-using and substance-abusing youths, the observed association is likely due to the high level of comorbidity between conduct disorder and attention-deficit/hyperactivity disorder. Earlier onset of conduct problems and aggressive behavior, in addition to the presence

Table 51.1
Psychiatric Disorders Commonly Comorbid with Substance Use Disorders in Adolescents

Disruptive behavior disorders
    Conduct disorder
    Oppositional defiant disorder
    Attention-deficit/hyperactivity disorder
Mood disorders
    Dysthymic disorder
    Cyclothymic disorder
    Major depressive disorder
    Bipolar disorder
Anxiety disorders
    Posttraumatic stress disorder
    Social phobia
Bulimia nervosa
Schizophrenia

of attention-deficit/hyperactivity disorder, may increase the risk for later substance abuse.

Onset of mood disorders (including *anxiety disorders*), and especially *depressive disorders*, frequently precedes or follows the onset of substance use and substance-use disorders in adolescents. The point prevalence of depressive disorders in these studies ranged from 24 to over 50 percent.

51.4 The answer is E (all)

The literature supports substance-use disorders among adolescents as a risk factor for *suicidal* behavior, including *ideation, attempts,* and completed suicide. Possible mechanisms for this relationship include acute and chronic effects of psychoactive substances. Adolescent suicide victims are frequently using alcohol or other drugs at the time of suicide. Short-term substance use may produce transient but intense dysphoric states, disinhibition, impaired judgment, and increased level of impulsivity or may exacerbate preexisting psychopathology including depressive or anxiety disorders.

Aggressive behaviors are present in many adolescents with substance-use disorders. Consumption of such substances as alcohol, amphetamines, and phencyclidine (PCP) may increase the likelihood of subsequent aggressive behavior. The direct pharmacological effects resulting in aggression may be further exacerbated by the presence of preexisting psychopathology, the use of multiple agents simultaneously, and the frequent relative inexperience of the adolescent substance user.

A number of studies of clinical populations show high rates of anxiety disorders among youth with substance-use disorders. In clinical populations of adolescents with substance-use disorders, the prevalence of anxiety disorder ranged from 7 to over 40 percent. The order of appearance of comorbid anxiety and substance-use disorders appears to vary, depending on the specific anxiety disorder. Social phobia usually precedes abuse, while *panic* and *generalized anxiety disorder* may more often follow the onset of substance-use disorders. Adolescents with substance-use disorders often have a history of *posttraumatic stress disorder.* Bulimia nervosa is also common in adolescents with substance-use disorders. As suggested by studies showing language deficits in youth affected by or at high risk for sub-

stance-use disorders, *learning disorders* may also show an increased incidence of comorbidity. Multiple psychiatric disorders, both internalizing and externalizing types, are often noted in populations of adolescents with substance-use disorders.

51.5 The answer is E (all)

Alcoholism is a serious problem for 10 to 20 percent of the adolescent population. Furthermore, 97 percent of adolescents who are drug abusers also use alcohol. *Marijuana* has been called a gateway drug, since it is the most widely used illicit drug among high school students, and it is the *strongest predictor of future cocaine use.* Inhalants are surprisingly widely used among younger adolescents. More than 17 percent of high school students *in the 8th grade and above* have experimented with inhalants, including glue, aerosols, and gasoline. *The prevalence rate of cocaine use in adolescence* appears to be decreasing. *Children of alcoholics reportedly have a 25 percent chance* of also becoming alcoholics.

51.6 The answer is C

Psychoactive substances, by virtue of their pharmacological properties, affect the mood, thought processes, and sensory perception of their users. Adolescent substance users are more likely to be novices with minimal tolerance, and *they may experience more noxious or adverse reactions to substances* than more experienced adult substance users. Inexperienced adolescent substance users may not appreciate the extent of their impairment from use or intoxication.

Substance use by adolescents has a number of short-term consequences. Accidents and trauma, including those due to driving motor vehicles or riding bicycles while intoxicated, and drownings are common.

Research on the outcomes of adolescent substance-abuse treatment has lagged behind research on the predictors, course, and correlates of treatment outcome among adults. Unfortunately, data indicate that most adolescents return to some level of alcohol or other drug abuse following treatment. Despite these outcomes, studies have identified specific predictors of treatment outcome, including patient or adolescent characteristics, social support system variables, and program characteristics. Adolescents in substance-abuse treatment begin substance use at an earlier age, progress rapidly to the use of "hard" drugs, and usually use multiple drugs. Other clinical features of adolescents entering treatment often include high levels of coexisting psychopathology or early personality difficulties, deviant behavior, school difficulties including high levels of truancy, and family disruption and substance abuse. Several pretreatment characteristics predict completion of treatment by adolescents: more severe alcohol problems; greater use of drugs other than alcohol, marijuana, and tobacco; a higher level of internalizing problems; and lower self-esteem. Premorbid psychopathology, such as *conduct disorder, is negatively correlated* with treatment completion and future abstinence. Although factors such as severity of substance use may predict short-term treatment outcomes, most longer-term outcomes may depend on social and environmental factors. This is consistent with studies that suggest that *relapse in adolescents* is more often associated with social pressures to use rather than situations involving negative affect (not vice versa), as is usually found in adult relapse. Attendance at self-support or aftercare groups is associated with higher rates of abstinence and other measures of improved outcome than those in adolescents who did not attend such groups.

Despite a higher (not a lower) level of return to substance use among adolescents after treatment, abstinent teens may expect decreased interpersonal conflict, improved academic functioning, and increased involvement in social and occupational activities. Patterns of substance abuse among adolescents appear to become more stable between 6 and 12 months after treatment. Reviews of treatment outcome conclude that treatment can be effective and is certainly better than no treatment.

51.7 The answer is E (all)

Prevention efforts are based on various theoretical models of adolescent substance-use and -abuse development. Most prevention interventions are based on social learning models. If one can change what young persons are exposed to and what they learn from their environment, then behavioral changes will follow. These interventions include educational approaches, family-based treatment, and community-based projects. Educational approaches include three basic methods: (1) knowledge and attitude, (2) values and decision making, and (3) social competency or skills. Although prevention interventions that are educational, individually focused, family focused (e.g., parent training), and community focused (e.g., advocacy groups, media campaigns, and regulatory changes) are an increasing part of the total prevention effort, the variety of critical risk factors for the development of adolescent substance use and abuse suggests the targeting of multiple risk factors or influences as part of comprehensive prevention initiatives. The successful prevention programs appear to be those that *target salient risk factors,* are *skills oriented*, have sufficient intensity and duration, *include follow-up, and* respect the *socioeconomic and cultural realities* of the affected communities.

51.8 The answer is D

Treatment programs for alcoholic adolescents contain a number of basic components. *Disulfiram (Antabuse) medication* is not a current treatment of choice. Treatment components usually include some form of *individual psychotherapy*, a *self-help* group component, *drug-specific counseling*, and *relapse prevention* treatment. These may be combined in any of a number of inpatient or outpatient programs.

51.9 The answer is C

Risk factors for the development of alcohol or drug abuse include diminished *parental supervision, early onset of cigarette smoking*, an underlying *conduct disorder*, and *parental substance abuse*. *High academic achievement* is not a risk factor for substance abuse, but academic difficulties may increase risk.

51.10 The answer is C

Thirty percent of adolescents brought to a pediatric trauma center have evidence of involvement with drugs and alcohol. The four most common causes of death in young people between the ages of 15 and 24 years are motor vehicle accidents (37 percent), homicide (14 percent), suicide (12 percent), and other injuries or accidents (12 percent).

Answers 51.11–51.15

51.11 The answer is C

51.12 The answer is B

51.13 The answer is C

51.14 The answer is A

51.15 The answer is D

Substance dependence refers to a group of cognitive, behavioral, and sometimes physiological symptoms that accompany the continued use of a substance. There is a pattern of repeated self-administration that may result in *tolerance, withdrawal*, and compulsive drug taking. *Caffeine (caffeinism)* does not fall within any of the substance-use disorders except *intoxication*, according to DSM-IV-TR. Dependence requires the presence of at least three symptoms of the maladaptive pattern, all of which must occur within the same year. Substance abuse refers to a *maladaptive pattern of substance use* leading to a clinically significant amount of distress within a 12-month period. The impairment may take the form of decreased performance in school or work, or it may cause physical danger or legal problems. Substance intoxication is the *development of a reversible substance-specific syndrome* due to the use of the substance. Clinically significant maladaptive changes, behavioral or psychological, must be present. Substance withdrawal refers to a *substance-specific syndrome related to the cessation or reduction of a substance that* causes clinically significant distress or impairment.

52 ▲

Child Psychiatry: Additional Conditions That May Be a Focus of Clinical Attention

Borderline intellectual functioning, academic problem, childhood or adolescent antisocial behavior, and identity problem are conditions listed in the revised fourth edition of the *Diagnostic and Statistical Manual of Mental Disorders* (DSM-IV-TR) as ones that may be a focus of clinical attention but are not categorized as major disorders. They may be related to a major disorder in a number of ways.

Borderline intellectual functioning is defined in DSM-IV-TR as characteristic of a person with an IQ in the range of 71 to 84. It is diagnosed when difficulties related to the borderline intellectual functioning become the focus of clinical attention. Only about 6 to 7 percent of the population is found to have borderline IQ. The condition is included in DSM-IV-TR because the intellectual deficits may lead to impaired adaptive capacities. The intellectual deficits alone, separate from any emotional or physical traumas, can lead to severe emotional distress, which in turn can lead to circumstances warranting psychiatric intervention. This condition is coded on Axis II.

DSM-IV-TR states that the "differential diagnosis between Borderline Intellectual Functioning and Mental Retardation (an IQ of 70 or below) is especially difficult when the coexistence of certain mental disorders (e.g., Schizophrenia) is involved." The focus of treatment is generally on improving social skills and overall adaptive functioning. Many people with borderline intellectual functioning may be able to function quite well in certain areas and not so well in others, and it is often the goal of therapy to focus on and strengthen the person's capabilities.

In DSM-IV-TR, academic problem is defined either as a problem that is not caused by a mental disorder or, if caused by a mental disorder, as a problem still severe enough to warrant individual clinical attention. A child or adolescent is diagnosed with this condition if he or she is experiencing significant academic difficulties not attributable to a specific learning, communication, or other psychiatric disorder. A child or adolescent of normal intelligence without a specific mental or learning disorder who is doing poorly in school falls into this category. Academic problems have many contributing factors and may occur at any time during school years. Since school is the major occupation of children and adolescents, their general coping capacities are reflected in how well they negotiate the develop-

mental tasks and challenges presented by school. Children must learn to deal with separating from their parents, adjusting to a new environment, competition, intimacy, and various peer pressures. These tasks may be further complicated by such common factors as the presence of family conflict or shyness. Academic problems can arise when a child has significant problems dealing with any of these areas. A teacher's negative affective response to a child can trigger the appearance of an academic problem. Early efforts to resolve an academic problem are critical, as sustained problems can intensify and accumulate, leading to more severe difficulties.

DSM-IV-TR refers to child or adolescent antisocial behavior as isolated antisocial acts, not as a pattern of behavior. As with the other conditions described here, it is not caused by a more specific mental disorder, such as, in this case, a conduct or impulse-control disorder. This category may include lying, stealing, truancy, running away from home, staying out late at night, or even acts of violence. Sometimes a single act of aggression toward another child can be serious enough to necessitate attention on its own. Antisocial behavior in the general population has been estimated at 5 to 15 percent, with a somewhat lower rate among children and adolescents. The rates are described as higher in urban areas than in rural ones and as being reported more often in boys than in girls. Factors that have been associated with antisocial behavior in children and adolescents are low IQ, academic failure, low levels of adult supervision, parental criminality, and a history of physical abuse.

Identity problem in DSM-IV-TR is defined as an uncertainty about identity issues, such as sexual behavior and orientation, friendships, moral values, group loyalties, and overall life goals. The onset is most often in late adolescence, and the course is usually relatively brief (resolving by the mid-20s), given appropriate support and acceptance. The consolidation of identity is a normal development task, defined by Erik Erikson as the phase in adolescence of "identity vs. role diffusion," and, thus, various identity confusions can be normative. However, identity problem is defined when it causes significant enough distress that it leads a young person to seek professional help. It is not defined as a mental disorder in DSM-IV-TR, and as such is not usually associated with marked deterioration in school or social functioning, or with severe subjective distress. At times, however, what may seem initially to be an identity problem can turn out to be the prodromal manifestations of a true mental disorder, such as schizophrenia, borderline personality disorder, or a mood disorder. The causes of identity problems are numerous and multifactorial. The essential features of identity problem revolve around a young person attempting to figure out who she or he "really" is. A problem may develop if the adolescent is unable to integrate various conflicts into a coherent sense of self. Associated features may include moderate anxiety and depression related to the problem, self-doubt and uncertainty about the future, difficulties in making choices, or impulsive experiments in an attempt to establish an independent identity. Individual psychotherapy is the treatment of choice.

The student should study the questions and answers below for a useful review of these conditions.

HELPFUL HINTS

The student should be able to define the following terms.

- abulia
- academic failure
- achievement tests
- adaptive function
- adolescent turmoil
- comorbid disorders
- dysfunctional family
- Erik Erikson
- hyperactivity and impulsivity
- identity formation
- irreconcilable conflicts
- juvenile delinquent
- learning disorder
- mental retardation
- parental criminality
- performance anxiety
- physical abuse
- role diffusion
- sense of self
- sexual orientation
- substance use
- superego
- tutoring
- underachievement
- "V" code
- violation of rights

▲ QUESTIONS

DIRECTIONS: The incomplete statement below is followed by five suggested completions. Select the *one* that is *best*.

52.1 In evaluating possible identity problems in children, the following aspects of the child's relationships with friends should be considered:

A. number of friends
B. quality of friendships
C. behavioral and emotional difficulties of friends
D. all of the above
E. none of the above

DIRECTIONS: Each set of lettered headings below is followed by a list of numbered words or phrases. For each numbered word or phrase, select the *best* lettered heading. Each heading can be used once, more than once, or not at all.

Questions 52.2–52.4

A. Identity problem
B. Normal adolescence
C. Both
D. Neither

52.2 Deterioration in occupational, school, or social functioning

52.3 Subjective anxiety and confusion

52.4 Disturbances in thinking processes, such as flight of ideas or thought blockage

Questions 52.5–52.8

A. Academic problem
B. Childhood or adolescent antisocial behavior
C. Borderline intellectual functioning

52.5 Intelligence quotient (IQ) within the range of 71 to 84

52.6 Normal intelligence and no learning disorder or communication disorder but is failing in school

52.7 Covers many acts that violate the rights of others

52.8 Must be differentiated from conduct disorder

ANSWERS

Child Psychiatry: Additional Conditions That May Be a Focus of Clinical Attention

52.1 The answer is D (all)

The development of an identity has been the subject of much debate, and numerous efforts have been made to describe the process that leads to identity formation. Failure to negotiate an identity is described in the revised fourth edition of *Diagnostic and Statistical Manual of Mental Disorders* (DSM-IV-TR) as an identity problem in the section entitled "Other Conditions That May Be a Focus of Clinical Attention." As defined in DSM-IV-TR, the criteria for identity problem make it very difficult to use rigorous research methodology to clarify this condition's validity.

Over the past 4 decades the syndrome of identity confusion was described by Erik Erikson in his classic paper, "The Problem of Ego Identity." Erikson described a group of adolescents who failed in the negotiation of the transition between childhood and adulthood. Adolescents who experienced difficulties with the formation of an identity shared clinical features with individuals with borderline personality disorder. Identity formation has been described by Erikson as a central task of adolescence.

The concept of identity problem represents the DSM-IV-TR current nosology "when the focus of clinical attention is uncertainty about multiple issues relating to identity such as long-term goals, career choice, friendship patterns, sexual orientation and behavior, moral values, and group loyalties." Identity problems may appear as a feature of a variety of other psychopathologies during adolescence, such as mood disorders, borderline personality disorder, posttraumatic stress disorder, and schizophrenia.

In a recent review of over 80 empirical studies investigating the role of friends in child development, Andrew F. Newcomb and Catherine L. Bagwell present impressive evidence regarding the crucial part that friends play in forming a healthy identity, fostering a positive self-concept, and promoting healthy psychological functioning. In recent years, a number of studies have also demonstrated the existence of a strong positive correlation between healthy friendships and school success and effective problem-solving skills. Rejected children tend to fall into two groups: disruptive children with high levels of aggression and socially withdrawn children who make easy targets for their peers. The work of Susan Harter and her colleagues has demonstrated that in both childhood and adolescence, friends tend to be similar to one another in abilities and outlook. Rejected children tend to become friends with other rejected children, and aggressive children with other acting-out children. It is therefore not surprising that studies find that a major predictor of antisocial behavior is a situation in which an adolescent's peer network is composed of friends who smoke, drink, use drugs, or have a negative attitude toward education. Conversely, children who are attracted to friends with positive outlooks are more likely to develop positive school-related attitudes, career aspirations, and achievements.

In evaluating possible identity problems in children, the following aspects of the child's relationships with friends should be considered: (1) *the number of friends* (a consistent finding in the literature is that the amount of time the child spends with peers relative to that spent with family members increases from infancy through adolescence); (2) *the quality of friendships* (e.g., most girls show an increasing capacity for self-disclosure and intimacy in their friendships during the preadolescent years); and (3) *the behavioral and emotional difficulties of friends* (since friendships are a major contributor to a child's identity, values, and behavior, a child or adolescent who interacts mainly with behaviorally disordered children is at increased risk for a variety of emotional and academic difficulties).

Answers 52.2–52.4

52.2 The answer is A

52.3 The answer is C

52.4 The answer is D
Identity problem can be differentiated from the normal conflicts of adolescence. Normal adolescence is not generally associated with *deterioration in occupational, school, or social functioning.*

Normal adolescents may argue with their parents, but their relationship with them remains intact. Adjustment disorders by definition are secondary to a specific stressor and are time limited. Although precipitating stressors may often occur at the onset of an identity problem, concerns with identity issues, such as career choice, gender identity, and future plans, are far less prominent in the adjustment disorders.

Identity problem must be differentiated from identity concerns that may represent the prodromal manifestations of schizophrenia, schizoaffective disorder, schizophreniform disorder, and mood disorders. Psychotic symptoms, such as hallucinations and

delusions, or *disturbances in thinking processes, such as thought blockage,* tangentiality, *or flight of ideas*, are not present in identity problem or in normal adolescence. Adolescents who are struggling with identity issues may *have subjective anxiety and confusion*, as do virtually all normal adolescents at various times, which often makes the initial differential diagnosis difficult.

The most difficult differential diagnosis involves borderline personality disorder. Confusion regarding identity concerns may be present in both conditions. In borderline personality disorder, the dramatic clinical picture includes a much more complex set of diagnostic criteria, such as chaotic, unstable sexual and interpersonal relationships, alternating idealization and devaluation, intense anger, self-destructive behaviors, and chronic dysphoria. Borderline personality disorder does not resolve in several months to a year but generally persists throughout adulthood, often with significant morbidity and mortality.

Answers 52.5–52.8

52.5 The answer is C

52.6 The answer is A

52.7 The answer is B

52.8 The answer is B
Borderline intellectual functioning is defined by the presence of an *intelligence quotient (IQ) within the range of 71 to 84.* According to the revised fourth edition of *Diagnostic and Statistical Manual of Mental Disorders* (DSM-IV-TR), a diagnosis of borderline intellectual functioning is made when issues pertaining to that level of cognition become the focus of clinical attention.

In DSM-IV-TR, *academic problem* is a condition that is not due to a mental disorder, such as a learning disorder or a communication disorder, or, if it is due to a mental disorder, it is severe enough to warrant independent clinical attention. Thus, a child or an adolescent who has *normal intelligence and no learning disorder or communication disorder* but is failing in school or doing poorly falls into this category.

Childhood and adolescent antisocial behavior covers many acts that violate the rights of others, including overt acts of aggression and violence and such covert acts as lying, stealing, truancy, and running away from home. However, it *must be differentiated from conduct disorder.* The DSM-IV-TR criteria for conduct disorder require a repetitive pattern of at least three antisocial behaviors over at least 6 months. Childhood or adolescent antisocial behavior consists of isolated events that do not constitute a mental disorder but do become the focus of clinical attention.

Some consider isolated antisocial behavior an inevitable part of growing up. Through minor transgressions, at first within families and then outside in the real world, children gradually learn about societal rules and limitations. Although more serious instances of antisocial behavior are viewed as delinquent, they are also relatively commonplace, especially during adolescence. Up to one-quarter of youth are apprehended by police and convicted of crimes, and the incidence of self-reported antisocial behavior is much greater than police arrests.

The relationship of antisocial behavior to psychopathology is complex. Not all antisocial behavior is psychopathological and therefore does not require treatment. Although most forms of juvenile antisocial behavior do not progress to criminality, it is quite difficult to distinguish youths with a good prognosis from those who will end up in the justice system and perpetrate severe transgressions. To help in this task, a careful delineation of normative risk-taking behavior and isolated antisocial behavior from syndromal clustering of behavior problems is necessary. Antisocial behavior must also be differentiated from more serious psychopathology, as behavioral disturbances are frequent accompaniments of many psychiatric disorders in children and adolescents, especially in boys. As there appears to be a fairly consistent progression from certain antisocial behaviors to more severe forms of psychopathology, antisocial behavior that comes to the attention of the clinician should be regarded as a marker or risk factor for more severe problems, such as oppositional defiant disorder, conduct disorder, and antisocial personality disorder.

53 ▲

Psychiatric Treatment of Children and Adolescents

As with adults, a combination of therapeutic interventions is often used to treat children and adolescents, ranging from different types of psychotherapy to medications. Clinicians must have a working knowledge of a variety of psychotherapeutic techniques as well as of pharmacokinetics and pharmacology. Treatment approaches with children and adolescents may include cognitive-behavioral, psychoanalytic, family, group, residential, hospital and day treatment, and biological therapies. All treatments must reflect an understanding of children's developmental levels, the differences between childhood and adult pharmacokinetics, and a sensitivity to families and environments in which the child lives. Child therapists may be called on to act as advocates for their patients in various settings, and may be asked to make recommendations that affect various aspects of a child's life.

In individual psychotherapy, psychodynamic approaches are sometimes mixed with supportive and behavioral management techniques. Individual therapy frequently is associated with family therapy, group therapy, and, when indicated, pharmacotherapy. The goal of therapy is to help develop good coping and conflict-resolution skills in children who are having trouble achieving or resolving developmental tasks that can lead to difficulties fulfilling later developmental capacities. Underlying child psychotherapy is the premise that a child will normally mature along a predictable, basically orderly, developmental path. The overriding focus on a developmental context is the primary feature that distinguishes child and adolescent therapies from adult ones. Child therapists must be knowledgeable about age-appropriate motor behaviors and emotional responses, about psychosexual development, about sociocultural, epigenetic phenomena, about the sequence of intellectual evolution, and about sequences of moral development.

Differences between children and adults with regard to therapy include the fact that children usually do not seek treatment on their own, and often begin treatment involuntarily. A child may initially view the therapist as a negative parental agent. Children are more likely than adults to externalize conflicts and to see problem resolution only in the manipulation of external environmental forces. Children may have a limited capacity for self-observation, and they may require a degree of physical stamina on the part of the therapist that is not required in the treatment of adults. Environmental pressures on therapists, such as family, school, or other factors, are usually greater in therapeutic work with children than with adults. Therapy, by and large, is more active and directed with children than it is with adults, and may involve more advising, directing, or educating than occurs in adult work. Psychotherapy with children

must involve parents to varying degrees. This can range from the entire therapeutic effort being directed toward the parents to the parents only being involved in paying the fees and bringing the child to the office. The issue of confidentiality is often dealt with differently in the treatment of children and adolescents than in adult treatment, and the matter takes on greater meaning as the child grows older. Often, what children do and say in psychotherapy becomes common knowledge to their parents, and this can be a major concern, particularly for adolescents. These issues must be openly discussed with patients and parents. The use of play and of playrooms as therapeutic modalities is clearly a key difference between the treatment of children and adults.

An evaluation for the use of medication in children must include a thorough physical examination, an assessment of the child's caregivers' abilities to monitor medication compliance and risks, and a rigorous diagnostic evaluation. Often, the success of drug trials hinges on the physician being available on a daily basis, especially at the beginning. An understanding of childhood pharmacokinetics is essential. Children, compared to adults, have greater hepatic capacity, more glomerular filtration, and less fatty tissue. Thus, many drugs are eliminated more quickly in children than in adults, are less often stored in fat, and have shorter half-lives. The goals of pediatric psychopharmacology include decreasing maladaptive behaviors and increasing adaptive functioning in academic and social settings. Cognitive dulling must be avoided. Indications for the use of medications in children and adolescents include behavioral and emotional problems associated with mental retardation, learning disorders, autistic disorder, attention-deficit/hyperactivity disorder, conduct disorder, Tourette's disorder, enuresis, separation anxiety disorder, schizophrenia, mood and anxiety disorders, obsessive-compulsive disorder, eating disorders, and sleep disorders. Clinicians must be aware of the indications, side effects, and risk to benefit ratios associated with each of the medications used in treatment of children and adolescents. Electroconvulsive therapy (ECT) is not indicated in childhood or adolescence.

The use of tricyclic drugs has decreased with the advent of the selective serotonin reuptake inhibitors (SSRIs), especially with reports of cardiotoxicity leading to the deaths of children who were taking desipramine (Norpramin) as part of a treatment for attention-deficit/hyperactivity disorder. Fluoxetine (Prozac), sertraline (Zoloft), paroxetine (Paxil), fluvoxamine (Luvox), and nefazodone (Serzone) are being used relatively frequently with children and adolescents. Bupropion (Wellbutrin) is also now commonly used in the treatment of depressive and attention-deficit/hyperactivity disorders. The management of severe aggression, disruptive behavior, and attention-deficit/hyperactivity disorders remains a challenge. The newer antipsychotics, such as risperidone (Risperdal) and olanzapine (Zyprexa), have enabled a wider range of patients to access neuroleptic treatment when required. Haloperidol (Haldol) is still a mainstay in the treatment of such conditions as Tourette's disorder and severe aggression, and lithium has also been used in the treatment of both mood disorders as well as aggression.

The student should study the questions and answers below for a useful review of these treatments.

HELPFUL HINTS

These terms should be known and defined by the student.

- acting out
- action-oriented defenses
- activity group therapy
- ADHD
- anticonvulsants
- atypical puberty
- autistic disorder
- behavioral contracting
- bell-and-pad conditioning
- biological therapies
- cardiovascular effects
- child guidance clinics
- child psychoanalysis
- classical and operant conditioning
- cognitive therapy
- combined therapy
- communication disorders
- compliance
- conduct disorder
- confidentiality
- conflict-resolution skills
- depressive equivalents
- developmental fluidity
- developmental lines
- developmental orientation
- dietary manipulation
- ECT
- enuresis
- externalization
- family systems theory
- filial therapy
- group living
- group selection criteria
- group therapy
- growth suppression
- haloperidol (Haldol)
- hospital treatment
- interview techniques
- learning-behavioral theories
- lithium
- liver to body-weight ratio
- MAOIs
- masked depression
- milieu therapy
- modeling theory
- mood disorders
- obsessive-compulsive disorder
- parent groups
- parental attitudes
- pharmacokinetics
- play group therapy
- playroom
- psychoanalytic theories
- psychoanalytically oriented therapy
- puberty and adolescence (differentiation)
- regression
- relationship therapy
- remedial and educational psychotherapy
- renal clearance
- residential and day treatment
- risk to benefit–ratio analysis
- same-sex groups
- schizophrenia
- self-observation
- sequential psychosocial capacities
- sleep terror disorder
- substance abuse
- suicide
- supportive therapy
- sympathomimetics
- tardive dyskinesia
- therapeutic interventions
- therapeutic playroom
- Tourette's disorder
- tricyclic drugs
- violence

▲ QUESTIONS

DIRECTIONS: Each of the questions or incomplete statements below is followed by five suggested responses or completions. Select the *one* that is *best* in each case.

53.1 Cognitive-behavioral therapy is useful in the treatment of which of the following disorders or situations?

A. Conduct disorder
B. Adolescent depression in the context of group therapy
C. Obsessive-compulsive disorder
D. Socially rejected children
E. All of the above

53.2 In attention-deficit/hyperactivity disorder

A. exclusive treatment with psychostimulant medication is, on the whole, maximally effective in older children and adolescents.
B. stimulant medication usually affects the full range of symptoms of children with the disorder.
C. for the most part, treatment with stimulants alone significantly improves the outcome for children with oppositional and aggressive behavior, academic underachievement, and poor peer relationships.
D. child and parent aggression are among the best predictors of poor outcome.
E. all of the above

53.3 Parent–child conflict is a risk factor for

A. depression
B. poor treatment outcome
C. relapse after treatment
D. cognitive distortions that negatively bias perceptions
E. all of the above

53.4 Groups for preschool children typically

    A. are homogeneous

    B. include children with the same diagnosis

    C. include eight to ten children

    D. utilize multiple therapists

    E. are not offered in combination with family therapy

53.5 The systems approach to family therapy

    A. places more emphasis on the meaning of a child's symptoms for the larger family than on the child's specific symptoms

    B. maintains that all things are interdependent and nothing changes without everything else changing

    C. sees symptoms as serving a purpose for the family system

    D. views each family member as acting in a way that opposes symptomatic improvement in the presenting patient

    E. all of the above

53.6 With regard to adverse effects of medications in children and adolescents

    A. tardive dyskinesia has not been observed in this age group

    B. withdrawal dyskinesias do occur in this age group

    C. anticholinergic and cardiovascular effects are rarely seen in this age group

    D. there is less risk for adverse effects in this age group than in adults

    E. none of the above

53.7 The developmental pathway that describes a continuity from the child's capacity to play to the adult's capacity to work is associated with the thinking of

    A. Sigmund Freud

    B. Anna Freud

    C. Melanie Klein

    D. Donald Winnicott

    E. Margaret Mahler

53.8 Integrating psychodynamic psychotherapy with other treatment modalities involves which of the following principles?

    A. Even developmentally or biologically based disorders are understood by a child in unique ways.

    B. The complexity of most psychiatric disorders and the inherent limits of any one approach warrant the use of combinations of modalities of treatment.

    C. The various modalities of treatment are organized through a basic psychodynamic understanding.

    D. How various treatment modalities interact is monitored through shifts in the material presented by the patient.

    E. All of the above

DIRECTIONS: Each set of lettered headings below is followed by a list of numbered statements. For each numbered statement, select the *best* lettered heading. Each heading can be used once, more than once, or not at all.

Questions 53.9–53.15

    A. Interpersonal, cognitive, and/or psychodynamic therapy plus fluoxetine (Prozac)

    B. Response prevention plus paroxetine (Paxil)

    C. Social skills group plus methylphenidate (Ritalin)

    D. Desmopressin (DDAVP) nasal spray

    E. Family therapy

    F. Partial hospital plus risperidone (Risperdal)

    G. Inpatient unit with psychodynamic, family, and behavioral interventions

53.9 A 12-year-old boy performs 3 hours of daily compulsive hand washing and has extreme difficulty getting to school because of contamination fears

53.10 A 10-year-old girl became oppositional and defiant shortly after her mother remarried a man with three children

53.11 A 15-year-old girl has lost 25 percent of her body weight and cannot control her purging behaviors

53.12 A 17-year-old girl has recently been discharged from an inpatient unit after a suicide attempt and severe depression

53.13 A 14-year-old girl has not been in school for several weeks because her derogatory auditory hallucinations have been bothering her; she is not suicidal

53.14 An 8-year-old boy will not attend sleep-over parties because of his bedwetting

53.15 A 7-year-old boy is about to be suspended from school because of his inability to sit in his seat and stay on task as well as his provocative behavior toward his classmates

ANSWERS

Psychiatric Treatment of Children and Adolescents

53.1 The answer is E (all)

Cognitive-behavioral therapy is probably the most extensively used therapy today for the treatment of all psychological problems, especially in children ages 9 years and above because of their increased ability to verbalize problems. It is used both for group and individual therapy. Following are some examples of the application of cognitive-behavioral therapy to various childhood disorders.

Children with *conduct disorders* may be impulsive, oppositional, defiant, and angry. Assessment sessions delineate the problem to be addressed. The way the child approaches the situation and his or her thought process is evaluated, and based on this evaluation, therapist and child construct an agenda for systematic therapy. The child is then taught to use a step-by-step approach to solving problems. Problem-solving–skills training involves having children make statements about themselves concerning a problem and guiding them to a more appropriate solution. Dysfunctional thought processes are examined, and the therapist helps children to generate alternate solutions to problems, focus on goals, see the consequences related to their behavior, and recognize the causes of other people's behavior (and become less sensitive to it). This technique may be adapted to accommodate children aged 4 years to young adults. The treatment uses structured tasks such as games, academic activities, and other age-appropriate tools. The therapist plays an active role by making verbal statements and applying the sequence of statements to a particular problem while encouraging the child to use the skills. Modeling follows, with practice and role playing. Punishment or withdrawal of privileges may be applied whenever necessary.

Peter Lewinsohn and his colleagues developed the *"Adolescents* Coping *with Depression* Course," which consists of 16 2-hour sessions conducted over an 8-week period for *groups* of up to ten adolescents. It includes a psychoeducational component that aims to destigmatize the problem, to emphasize skills training to promote control over one's mood, and to enhance the adolescents' ability to cope with problematic situations. The group activities include role playing. Social skills training is distributed throughout the therapy to facilitate and enhance communication by teaching conversational techniques, planning social activities, and developing strategies for making friends. Sessions are designed to increase pleasant activities, based on the assumption that depressed adolescents have few positive reinforcements in their lives. Relaxation training is provided to enhance enjoyability and performance in social situations. Focus on changing depressogenic cognitions is provided by identifying, challenging, and changing negative thoughts and irrational beliefs. Six sessions involve teaching communication skills focusing on the acquisition of positive behaviors, such as paraphrasing to verify the message, active responding, and appropriate eye contact. Adolescents are also taught negotiating and problem-solving techniques such as defining the problem without criticism, brainstorming alternative solutions, evaluating and mutually agreeing on a solution, and specifying the agreement with the inclusion of positive and negative consequences.

John March and his colleagues developed the cognitive-behavioral treatment called "How I Ran OCD Off My Land."

This treatment uses a variety of techniques including exposure, response prevention, extinction, anxiety-management training, reinforcement, modeling and shaping, habit reversal, individual therapy, group psychotherapy, and family therapy. After the assessment, the first session is devoted to educating the child about *obsessive-compulsive disorder* and categorizing it in the neurobehavioral framework, that is, equating obsessive-compulsive disorder with a medical illness and detailing the treatment. In the second session the aim is to make the disorder the target of treatment. The child is asked to give obsessive-compulsive disorder a disparaging nickname, so it becomes the enemy and allows the child to "boss back" the disorder. In addition, the use of story metaphors allows development of a therapeutic relationship and treatment monitoring through the use of informal symptom diaries. The third session is dedicated to mapping the disorder—that is, describing specific obsessions, compulsions, triggers, avoidance behaviors, and consequences. Sessions 4 to 16 deal with anxiety-management training and exposure and response prevention. Anxiety-management training includes relaxation, diaphragmatic breathing, and constructive self-talk. Exposure involves therapist-assisted imaginal and in vivo exposure. Finally, response prevention consists of exercises coupled with weekly homework. Parents are trained to ally with the child to "boss back" obsessive-compulsive disorder.

With regard to *socially rejected children*, Fred Frankel and his colleagues developed the 12-session cognitive-behavioral treatment called "Parent Assisted Social Skills Training." First the child's social network is examined, taking into consideration the natural environment, family, school, and neighborhood to develop an integrated approach to treatment. Children are seen in groups to learn the rules of peer etiquette. They are also offered training skills to expand their peer networks, while parents and children are taught how to work together to promote more successful play dates and how to improve the child's competence with nonaggressive responses to teasing and conflict with other children and adults. Coached play begins in session 2, in which coaches do not participate in activities but observe the children's play. They only intervene to dispense reinforcements (verbal and token) and, if necessary, a 2-minute time-out for misbehavior. Child socialization homework begins in session 1, with the aim of setting in place the mechanics of an appropriate telephone call. First, children phone someone from the group, then they call children outside the group. Also, children may bring a toy from home, so they may engage other children in play. Didactic presentations are made to parents to (1) inform them of their part in helping their child gain peer acceptance; (2) ensure that the parents adhere to their assigned roles in the child's socialization homework; and (3) provide supportive feedback for the principles being taught. Table 53.1 lists some of the techniques of cognitive-behavioral therapy.

53.2 The answer is D

Cognitive-behavior therapy targeting disruptive behaviors in children with attention-deficit/hyperactivity disorder has wider empirical support than any other area. It also provides a heuristically valuable example of how cognitive-behavioral therapy and medication can and should be combined.

Table 53.1
Techniques of Cognitive-Behavioral Therapy

Term	Definition	Examples
Cognitive restructuring	Actively altering maladaptive thought patterns and replacing these negative thoughts with more constructive adaptive cognitions and beliefs	Challenging aberrant risk appraisal in the patient with panic disorder, or helplessness in the patient with depression
Contrived exposure	Exposure in which the patient seeks out and confronts anxiety-provoking situations or triggers	Intentionally touching a "contaminated" toilet seat
Differential reinforcement of appropriate behavior	Attending to and positively rewarding appropriate behavior, especially when incompatible with inappropriate behavior	Praising (and maybe paying) the child with obsessive-compulsive disorder who has contamination fears and washes the dinner dishes in a nonritualized fashion
Exposure	The exposure principle states that anxiety will decrease after prolonged contact with the phobic stimulus in the absence of real threat; exposure may be contrived (sought-out contact with feared stimuli) or uncontrived (unavoidable contact with feared stimuli)	A patient with fear of heights goes up a ladder; the first time it is scary; the tenth time it is boring
Extinction	By convention, extinction is usually defined as the elimination of problem behaviors through removal of parental positive reinforcement; technically, extinction often means removing the negative reinforcement effect of the problem behavior so that it no longer persists	Refusal to reassure the anxious patient. Refusal by the mother to cave in to the oppositional child's tantruming by withdrawing a command
Generalization training	Moving the methods and success of problem-focused interventions to targets not specifically addressed in treatment	Exposure and response prevention for all toilets and sinks in the universe
Negative reinforcement	Self-reinforcing purposeful removal of an aversive stimulus; termination of an aversive stimulus, which when stopped, increases or stamps in the behavior that removed the aversive stimulus	Compulsions in obsessive-compulsive disorder provide short-term relief of obsessional anxiety via negative reinforcement blocking the negative reinforcement property of rituals is the job of response prevention
Positive reinforcement	Imposition of a pleasurable stimulus to increase a desirable behavior	Praise after successfully obeying a command
Prompting, guiding, and shaping	External commands and suggestions that increasingly direct the child toward more adaptive behavior that is then reinforced; typically, shaping procedures are rapidly faded in preference to generalization training	Gradually encouraging and helping the social phobic youngster to talk in class and with other children
Punishment	Imposition of an aversive stimulus to decrease an undesirable behavior	"Time out" because of unacceptable behavior or overcorrection (e.g., extra chores to make restitution for aggressive behavior)
Relapse prevention	Interventions designed to anticipate triggers for reemergence of symptoms; practicing skillful coping in advance	Imaginal exposure to a contamination fear followed by cognitive therapy and response prevention to resist the incursion of obsessive-compulsive disorder
Response cost	Removal of positive reinforcer as a consequence of undesirable behavior	Loss of points in a token economy
Response prevention	The response prevention principle states that adequate exposure is only possible in the absence of rituals or compulsions	Not doing an obsessive-compulsive disorder ritual (e.g., washing) after either contrived or uncontrived exposure (e.g., touching a toilet seat)
Restructure the environment	Changes in setting or stimuli that decrease problem behaviors, facilitate adaptive behavior, or both	Seating the child with attention-deficit hyperactivity disorder toward the front of the classroom
Stimulus hierarchy	A list of phobic stimuli ranked from least to most difficult to resist using fear thermometer rating scores	Unique list of obsessive-compulsive disorder specific contamination fears ranked by fear thermometer score; an individual patient may have one or more hierarchies, depending on the complexity of the disorder (e.g., a particular patient may have separate hierarchies for contamination fears and for touching and repeating rituals)
Token economy	A systematic set of contingencies that involve earning objects or symbols consequent on behaviors, which are then exchanged for meaningful positive reinforcers	A "star chart" linked to rewards that are meaningful to the child

First, *exclusive treatment with psychostimulant medication is effective, but may not be maximally effective* for attention-deficit/hyperactivity disorder, especially in older children or adolescents. Many children will experience reduced symptoms that nevertheless persist at clinically significant levels. Although many children improve substantially with pharmaco-therapy, many do not achieve full normalization with stimulant treatments alone, even at very high dosages. More children may achieve normalization with combination treatment.

Second, *stimulant medication may not affect (rather than usually affect) the full range of symptoms of children* with attention-deficit/hyperactivity disorder and other comorbid conditions. Although the primary symptoms of the syndrome (i.e., attention, impulsivity, and activity level) may be greatly improved, *stimulant medication effects on* other primary or comorbid characteristics of the syndrome (e.g., *oppositional and aggressive behavior, academic underachievement, and poor peer relationships) are often insufficient.* Because these conditions (along with family dysfunction) are robust predictors of poor long-term outcome for children with attention-deficit/hyperactivity disorder, treatment with stimulants alone may not significantly improve the outcome for these children. Research suggests the great relevance of the secondary problems of aggressive behavior (and the coercive family process associated with aggression), academic underachievement and associated school behavioral problems, and peer relationships to intervention in attention-deficit/hyperactivity disorder. These arenas are most amenable to psychosocial treatments. Moreover, psychosocial treatments may be the only interventions available for the minority of children with attention-deficit/hyperactivity disorder who do not respond to stimulants, who experience intolerable adverse effects, or whose parents reject the use of medication.

A final limitation of stimulant monotherapy involves its applicability to home behavior problems. Many pharmacotherapists limit the use of stimulants to school hours during the 9 months of the academic year to avoid appetite suppression, sleep disruption, and other unwanted effects. This leaves parents on their own to manage impulsive, oppositional, and disruptive behavior in the afternoons and evenings, weekends, and summers. When no other treatment is provided, parents frequently become coercive, hostile, and overly punitive, which may exacerbate the child's behavior problems. *Child and parent aggression are among the best predictors of poor outcome.* For all of these reasons, cognitive-behavioral therapy continues to be used and evaluated, alone and in combination with stimulant medication.

Psychosocial treatment for attention-deficit/hyperactivity disorder optimally involves a behavioral-therapy approach that focuses on the child, the parents, and the school. Intervention with parents typically uses parent training designed to teach parents skills and techniques for managing disruptive, impulsive, and oppositional behaviors in the home and in the community. Intervention in the school involves direct consultation with teachers about establishing behavior-management systems in the classroom. In addition, systems that tie the school and home together in a direct, cooperative effort are being used increasingly to improve school behavior and academic performance. Innovative treatment programs can be tailored to the individual child.

53.3 The answer is E (all)
At any one time, approximately 1 in 20 children and adolescents suffers from major depressive disorder, and rates of depression rise dramatically in adolescents, especially in girls. While the economic burden of depression in youths is uncertain, the human cost is considerable, especially with teenage suicide. The empirical literature shows more support for problem-specific psychotherapies, especially cognitive-behavioral therapy, than for medication management of pediatric depressive disorders. In particular, several controlled trials have demonstrated that individual or group cognitive-behavioral psychotherapy is effective for depressed youth, and some investigators now deem cognitive-behavioral therapy the treatment of choice.

Like other cognitive-behavioral treatment packages, cognitive-behavioral therapy for depression in youth is a skills-based treatment, in this case centered around the assumption that depression is either caused or maintained by inadequate social-cognitive skills for coping with stress. Personality is an interactive multidirectional system of behaviors, cognitions, and emotions, and depression is manifested in each of these three personality components. However, cognitive-behavioral therapy for depression assumes that symptom change is most likely to occur when interventions modify patterns of behavior or cognition, with emotion following. Among the behavioral and cognitive skills deficits that may characterize depressed youths are low involvement in pleasant activities, poor problem-solving and assertion skills, *cognitive distortions that negatively bias perceptions,* negative automatic thoughts, negative views of self and future, and failure to attribute positive outcomes to internal, stable, or global causes. Thus, the therapist must establish a working alliance with adolescents and help them learn new ways of behaving or thinking that will in turn reduce severity of depression and risk of relapse.

Most cognitive-behavioral treatment packages for depressed youths share two salient characteristics: (1) both overview, or require, skills-building sessions and modular, or optional, sessions for specific problems and (2) integration of parent and family sessions with individual cognitive-behavioral therapy. Treatment is generally designed to improve the teenager's problem-solving ability when faced with a stressful situation (e.g., parent–child conflict, role transitions, and grief reactions or peer problems). The required aspects of treatment include psychoeducation about depression and its causes, goal setting with the adolescent, and basic problem-solving skills. Modules chosen jointly by therapist and adolescent then address the specific skills deficits of the teenager. *Parent–child conflict is a risk factor for depression, cognitive distortions, poor treatment outcome, and relapse after treatment,* which justifies including a parental component in cognitive-behavioral therapy. Preliminary evidence suggests that parent and child treatment may be somewhat more effective than treatment directed at the teenager alone. Parents are taught contingency management procedures along with alternative, effective methods for parenting and creating a more positive family environment. Moreover, family interactions are targeted directly to shape and reinforce effective communication and interactions and to increase pleasant activities and positive affect.

53.4 The answer is D
Groups for preschool children are *typically heterogeneous (not homogeneous) and include children with different (not the same) diagnoses.* (In the homogeneous groups, children with a common problem [e.g., a chronic illness or parental divorce] share a psy-

choeducational and supportive group experience.) Preschool groups are structured around toys, play, artwork, and other age-appropriate activities. *These groups, for the most part, include only three to five (not eight to ten) same-sex children.* Because of the children's short attention span, time and space are important considerations, particularly with hyperactive, overanxious, and aggressive children. Groups should not last more than 45 to 60 minutes, including time for a snack. A medium-sized room with appropriate furniture for the age will help provide good boundaries and a therapeutic climate. It is recommended that play and artwork materials be stored away until group time. *The use of multiple therapists,* highly recommended for child and adolescent groups, is particularly indicated in the treatment of emotionally disturbed preschoolers. These children have acquired, at best, a basic repertoire of social skills, while emotional regulation is just beginning. As they do in individual therapy, children in a therapy group reenact their behavioral and emotional conflicts, which can become a serious management issue. At least two therapists are needed to maintain clear and firm limits in a consistent structure and to model prosocial behaviors and the development of new masteries. Several authors recommend a male-female co-therapy team as the ideal configuration. This is not always possible, and co-therapy teams may be of the same sex, including a senior clinician with a trainee or two trainees, frequently from different disciplines. Young children's limited verbal and social skills, emotional lability, impulsiveness, and out-of-control behaviors can be most challenging, even to the experienced clinician. Availability of consultation and supervision is essential for a successful group therapy program.

With younger children, therapists typically initiate each session's activities around educational and therapeutic themes. Using a warm, supportive approach, therapists engage children in play activities with puppets, toys, and art materials. The therapists' knowledge of patients' individual and family histories permits using the group context for further identification and understanding of children's conflicted behaviors and interactions. Mutual story-telling techniques can provide children with corrective models that introduce constructive, prosocial options and new achievements. Emphasis is placed on understanding the children's disturbed behaviors in light of their individual and family histories. Children soon reenact earlier experiences in the group, mostly through play and interpersonal behaviors. Interpretations should be kept at a minimum. Therapists' interventions are aimed at providing corrective emotional experiences that help children reach greater social and emotional mastery. *Most frequently these groups are offered in combination with family therapy* or parents' groups that tend to be largely supportive and psychoeducational. Close participation of the family in children's groups greatly facilitates the therapeutic engagement and progress. It also empowers parents by helping them become more competent in their role.

53.5 The answer is E (all)

The systems approach, a departure from so-called linear theories, uses cybernetics and general systems theory. Cybernetics holds that systems maintain an equilibrium, whereas in systems theory, all living systems are characterized by tension between homeostasis and change. All things are interdependent and *nothing changes without everything else changing accordingly.* In this view, *symptoms are* not seen as residing within the child but as

serving a purpose for the whole family system. These symptoms provide systemic survival, or continuity, and maintain homeostasis. *Each family member is presumed to act in a way that opposes symptomatic improvement in the presenting patient.* Most family-systems theorists maintain this perspective, and therapeutic interventions attempt to counteract the hypothetical process. For example, one must destabilize the family system to promote change. The formulation for a systems-oriented clinician has less to do with the symptoms residing within a child than with the meaning such symptoms have for the family. Problem-maintaining sequences are observed, and these processes are interrupted. Schools of family therapy seen as systems therapy include strategic and structural schools.

53.6 The answer is B

Despite their medication-handling efficiency, *children and adolescents are no less at risk than adults* and perhaps are more at risk in some cases for development of adverse effects. This has both physiological and practical significance: the clinician must know the adverse-effect profiles of all medications being prescribed as well as how to manage adverse effects if they arise. In addition, children and adolescents can be particularly sensitive about their bodies and how they work and often get quite frightened or suspicious if a sudden change or dysfunction occurs during pharmacotherapy. Such feelings can interfere with compliance and optimal outcome.

Many of the adverse effects of antipsychotic drugs, antidepressant agents, and lithium seen in adult patients can be observed in children and adolescents. Of particular concern are the *anticholinergic and cardiovascular effects* of the tricyclic drugs and the extrapyramidal adverse effects of the neuroleptics, including dyskinesias. *Withdrawal dyskinesias* seem *more frequent* than tardive dyskinesia in young children, but *tardive dyskinesia has been observed* in this age group.

In general, the best therapy for adverse effects is prevention. It is usually best to start with a low dosage and titrate upward in a stepwise fashion. Use of the lowest possible maintenance dosages in the therapeutic range can minimize adverse effects. Monotherapy is most often preferable. However, targeted combined pharmacotherapy may be necessary in children with multiple comorbid disorders. Judicious use of two or more agents in combination should not precede careful, systematic trials of single agents from two or more classes of medication, as indicated by the clinical situation. Table 53.2 lists a number of adverse medication effects.

53.7 The answer is B

Child psychotherapy begins with *Sigmund Freud's* case of Little Hans, a 5-year-old phobic boy. Published in 1909, it was the first description of the psychotherapeutic treatment of a child. The therapy in this case was actually rendered by Hans' father, who reported to Freud and received guidance from him. Significant interest in the mental and emotional lives of children was generated by Freud's theories of psychosexual development, which posited that symptoms in adulthood could be traced to conflicts arising at earlier stages of development. Sandor Ferenczi was one of the first to attempt to analyze children, but he quickly became frustrated with the endeavor, finding that children only wanted to play. Hermione Hug-Hellmuth published the first report of actual play therapy with children, suggesting that play and drawings were valid modes of communication.

Table 53.2
Adverse Effects and Their Management in Children and Adolescents

Drug Category	Common Adverse Effects	Clinical Management
Antipsychotics (dopamine receptor antagonists and serotonin-dopamine antagonists)	**Short term**	
	Autonomic nervous system	
	Dry mouth	In general, lower dosage if possible or switch drug if persistent, child may equilibrate after several weeks
	Urinary retention	Bethanechol (Urecholine) only if severe and persistent
	Constipation	Dioctyl sodium sulfosuccinate (Colace) tablets or bisacodyl (Dulcolax) suppositories
	Orthostatic hypotension	Avoid sudden postural changes; dosage reduction if severe
	Extrapyramidal	
	Acute dystonia	Diphenhydramine (Benadryl) or benztropine (Cogentin) intramuscularly, then switch to oral form
	Parkinsonism	Anticholinergic or antiparkinsonian medication p.r.n.
	Akathisia	Lower dosage; sometimes an anticholinergic agent can help
	Other	
	Hypersensitivity or rash	Discontinue use
	Drowsiness	Child usually becomes tolerant; if persistent switch to less sedating class
	Photosensitivity	Avoid sun exposure
	LFTs	May not have clinical significance; follow-up indicated
	Blood dyscrasias	
	Long term	
	Weight gain	Lower dosage; consider switch to another class
	Dyskinesias (tardive and withdrawal)	Prevention is best; use lowest possible dose for maintenance
Psychosympathomimetics stimulants	**Short term**	
	Anorexia, nausea, abdominal pain	Reduce dose; give most of dosage in the AM; consider switch
	Insomnia	Move PM dose to earlier in the day; reduce dosage then reintroduce
	Dysphoria	Consider another stimulant if persistent or tricyclic drug
	Long term	
	Weight loss	Supplement diet, institute drug holidays or change drug
	Tics	Discontinue, if stimulant is effective consider rechallenge; consider tricyclic drug
Tricyclic drugs	Autonomic nervous system	See antipsychotic agents
	Cardiovascular (blood pressure, HR, PR, T-wave changes, ↑ QTc, and arrhythmias)	Monitor ECGs serially; most changes have little clinical significance in healthy child
	CNS (seizures)	Discontinue medication gradually, EEG; may need anticonvulsant
Anxiolytics and sedative-hypnotic agents		
Antihistamines	Oversedation	Decrease total dosage; administer most at bedtime
	Rash	Discontinue medication
Benzodiazepines	Disinhibition	Discontinue medication
	Cognitive decrements	Reduce dosage or discontinue
Lithium	Gastrointestinal: nausea, vomiting, abdominal pain, diarrhea, metallic taste	Consider dose reduction if persistent
	CNS: tremor, memory lapses, fatigue	Consider dose reduction if persistent
	Endocrine: goiter	Discontinue medication and follow with laboratory studies
	Renal: polyuria/polydipsia	Monitor BUN, creatinine, electrolytes, and urinalysis on a regular basis (every 2–3 months)
	Hematological: leukocytosis	Monitor; may not be of clinical significance

LFTs, liver function tests; TCA, tricyclic antidepressant; ECG, electrocardiogram; CNS, central nervous system; EEG, electroencephalogram; BUN, blood urea nitrogen.

However, two analysts, *Anna Freud* and *Melanie Klein*, developed the field of child psychoanalysis. While they worked in different ways, they undertook the analyses of many children and spurred the work of many others. Klein understood play to be the actual equivalent of adult free association. She was interested in the earliest object relations; the importance of unconscious fantasies at each stage of development; the role of primitive defenses such as projection, projective identification, and omnipotent control; the process of early identifications; and the role of envy and guilt in these early relationships. Freud looked at play from a psychoanalytic perspective and learned about the child from play but did not view play as a substitute for free association. Her work concerned the development of the ego, the evolution of defenses, and the developmental pathway of various ego functions. In one example of a developmental pathway, she described a *continuity from the child's capacity to play to the adult's capacity to work.*

There were several other major early contributors to the field. *Donald Winnicott*, a psychoanalyst and pediatrician, emphasized the importance of the mother–infant relationship. His understanding of the transitional object, for instance, as playing a role in the child's ability to separate from the maternal figure, instilled a new appreciation of the meaning of commonly observed childhood behaviors. *Margaret Mahler* observed mother–toddler interactions in a more systematized way and described the evolution of early object relations from the perspective of separation and individuation. Winnicott's and Mahler's ideas have had great impact on the issues dealt with in children's psychotherapy. August Aichorn first extended the work to delinquent adolescents. Finally, the work of Jean Piaget focused on children's cognitive development, and this subsequently influenced the practice of psychotherapy.

53.8 The answer is E (all)

Owen Lewis presented integrated psychodynamic psychotherapy, an approach to dynamic psychotherapy based on four clinical principles. The first of these, the dual purposes of psychotherapy, holds that psychotherapy proceeds in two sometimes contradictory directions. Psychotherapy must function as a specific treatment for a specific disorder in a child at a specific developmental stage. With these parameters, specific techniques are used to treat the condition. On the other hand, psychotherapy also functions as an open-ended exploration of the unconscious factors that may have a role in the child's problems. Even if the *disorder* is developmentally or biologically based, it *will be understood and incorporated by the child in unique and individualized ways* that must be elucidated. These factors cannot be known in advance and are discovered in the course of psychotherapy.

The second principle, the use of all modalities of treatment, follows from the first. The complexity of most psychiatric disorders and the *inherent limits of any one approach warrant the use of any combination of modalities of treatment.* While certain approaches (e.g., classical psychoanalytic treatment) had been seen as incompatible with other modalities of treatment, integrated psychodynamic psychotherapy finds a positive synergistic interaction between modalities. Integrating treatment approaches requires innovation in order to create the best comprehensive treatment plan for a given child. The *various modalities* of treatment (e.g., behavioral, cognitive, familial, psychopharmacologic, and educational) are *organized through a basic psychodynamic understanding.*

The third principle involves tracking the psychodynamic process. *How these various modalities interact is monitored through shifts in the material presented by the patient.* Does alleviating an anxiety symptom through a behavioral intervention make the patient more or less interested in pursuing the symptom's cause? Do the effects of an antidepressant make a patient more or less able to talk about troubles? Intervention by intervention, session by session, the flow of material is watched. The therapist also notes positive interventions that quickly yield negative results. If the dynamic meaning of change is not appreciated, the patient will resist change.

The fourth principle holds that psychotherapy proceeds through the therapeutic relationship. In this interpersonal perspective, all therapy is ultimately organized by the relationship with the therapist, and without that relationship, there is no therapy. While transference is a necessary component of this relationship, patients are also bound by their developmental capacity for relatedness. This capacity is determined not only by developmental stage, but also by the patient's accumulated experience. A therapist who offers a child help with anxiety symptoms through a relaxation technique can simultaneously and symbolically expose a deficit in care by a parent (transference) and provide new opportunities for care (new identifications). From this point of view, the therapist must equally note transferences and the patient's resistance to these transferences as well as the real relationship and the patient's resistance to this.

Change, for the child, comes from a variety of sources. Specific behavioral techniques will shape behavior. Family interventions can modify parenting approaches. School consultations can help create an environment for children that is more conducive to their learning and social environment. All these interventions, which may or may not be accepted by the child, are processed through the therapeutic relationship and color that relationship in ways that have dynamic meaning. While classic interpretation may be used, interpretation per se often formulates for the child change that has already occurred. This change ultimately evolves from the new emotional, cognitive, and interpersonal integrations achieved within the therapeutic relationship.

Answers 53.9–53.15

53.9   **The answer is B**

53.10   **The answer is E**

53.11   **The answer is G**

53.12   **The answer is A**

53.13   **The answer is F**

53.14   **The answer is D**

53.15   **The answer is C**

The majority of children who present for psychiatric treatment are brought in by family members who are concerned about their functioning or who have followed up on suggestions from teachers or pediatricians. Often, children do not express a desire for treatment, nor do they understand the degree to which they have caused others concern. Occasionally, an adolescent will ask a parent for help, but more often distress is manifested through troubled behaviors. To synthesize a useful treatment approach, it is generally necessary to understand the views of both the child and the parents. In most cases, treatment consists of multiple modalities through which to manipulate the child's environment positively as well as to influence the behaviors and feelings of the child. The brief vignettes that follow exemplify the combined approach to addressing children's and adolescents' psychological needs.

A boy of 12 years who presents with impairment due to compulsive hand washing and obsessions regarding fears of becoming contaminated is a candidate for both medication and a behavioral intervention. *Paroxetine (Paxil)* is a selective serotonin reuptake inhibitor (SSRI) that is being investigated as a medication of choice for obsessive-compulsive symptoms. The SSRI class of medications (*fluoxetine [Prozac]*, sertraline [Zoloft], paroxetine [Paxil], and fluvoxamine [Luvox]) is known to have antiobsessional effects. The *response prevention technique* is a behavioral intervention that serves to diminish the hand-washing behavior by challenging the child to tolerate the feared situation (that his hands are contaminated and require washing). In this way, the child learns that the exposure to the feared situation does not in fact have the feared negative effects, and anxiety gradually diminishes.

A 10-year-old girl who responds to a new family constellation with oppositional and defiant behaviors is expressing her discomfort about a major change in the family's functioning. *Family therapy* is a useful modality to begin with, in order to understand the triggers, responses, and meanings of these behaviors to the family and to the child. It is likely that when the child is given a forum in which to express her discomfort, her oppositional behaviors will diminish.

A 15-year-old girl who has lost 25 percent of her body weight and cannot control her purging behaviors generally *requires an inpatient setting* in which to initiate treatment, to establish refeeding, and to observe her continuously to prevent vomiting. Given the complex effects of starvation, a malnourished adolescent is not a good candidate for outpatient treatment. The treatment approaches for the restricting and purging type of anorexia nervosa are multimodal. A *behavioral* component is necessary to systematically address nutritional needs and to prevent behaviors that further increase malnutrition; a *family* approach is needed to probe the family's role in the disorder; and a *psychodynamic* approach is beneficial in order to work with the adolescent regarding the meaning of, and psychological forces driving, the disorder. Medications are some-

times used to treat concurrent anxiety and depression and to ameliorate bingeing and purging.

A 17-year-old girl who has been discharged from an inpatient unit presumably is stable, not posing an imminent danger to herself, and is ready to engage in outpatient treatment. There is evidence from at least one double-blind, placebo-controlled study that *fluoxetine* is efficacious in the treatment of major depression in adolescents. Given the far-reaching ramifications of a major depression and a suicide attempt and the longevity of lingering depressive constructs and symptoms, *psychotherapy* (i.e., *interpersonal, cognitive,* and/or *psychodynamic*) *is indicated.* Interpersonal psychotherapy, a mode of individual therapy that has been used in adults and adolescents, is aimed at improving interpersonal skills, as this is identified as pivotal in modifying depressive thoughts and feelings. The therapy addresses decreasing social isolation and is supportive around issues of furthering positive relationships.

A 14-year-old girl who has recently stopped attending school because of an increase in auditory hallucinations is in a crisis. Since she is not suicidal, she may not need the containment of an inpatient unit, but she could be a candidate for a *partial hospital program*, in which she can receive daily monitoring of *antipsychotic* and *antidepressant medication*, as well as receive daily support from staff. School refusal in an adolescent is usually a sign of severe psychopathology and requires immediate evaluation and intervention.

Enuresis (in the 8-year-old boy) is much more common in boys than in girls, and it may cause social awkwardness and psychological stress for children who still have this condition in the mid-elementary years. Approximately 7 percent of 5 year olds have enuresis on a regular basis, and about 3 percent of 10 year olds have it. *Desmopressin (DDAVP)* nasal spray has been effective in some children with enuresis, and it can be used on an occasional basis if it is not needed every night.

A 7-year-old boy who cannot stay on task and who is hyperactive and socially provocative is exhibiting typical symptoms of attention-deficit/hyperactivity disorder. The main treatment for the core symptoms of this disorder is a stimulant medication such as *methylphenidate (Ritalin)*. Most children with ADHD have social difficulties and many are eventually rejected by peers. Thus, it is often beneficial to include *social skills groups* as an additional therapeutic intervention.

54 ▲

Forensic Issues in Child Psychiatry

Child and adolescent psychiatrists must be particularly concerned with the forensic issues of consent, confidentiality, and professional responsibility, and these issues are dealt with in the context of the potentially conflicting rights of children, parents, and general society. For instance, in 1980 the American Academy of Child and Adolescent Psychiatry's Code of Ethics stated that breaches and limits of confidentiality can occur in the face of child abuse, maltreatment, or for purposes of appropriate education. Although not legally necessary with a child or adolescent, consent for disclosure should be obtained when possible. Child and adolescent psychiatrists often face the conflict of having to weigh the potential benefits and harm in divulging to a child's parents confidential information obtained from the child. Among adolescents, this information may include drug or alcohol abuse, unsafe sexual practices, or dangerous behavior. The issues are complex and are not always easily resolved. Clinicians must always be aware of their patients' vulnerabilities and of the importance of maintaining a therapeutic bond as well as of the need to maintain patient safety.

Child and adolescent psychiatrists must frequently confront child custody issues. At the turn of the century, the "tender-years" doctrine became the standard for determining child custody and it supported custody decisions in the mother's favor in most cases. The "best interest of the child" doctrine has replaced the tender-years standard and expands considerations of the optimal parent. As such, in difficult and unclear cases, psychological expert testimony has become more widely accepted as an integral part of child custody decisions. Psychiatric evaluators are expected to try to determine the best interests of the child while keeping in mind, among other issues, the wishes of the parents and child; relationships with significant others in the child's life; the psychiatric and physical health of all involved; the level of conflict or potential danger to the child under the care of either parent; and the child's social and academic adjustment. A psychiatric evaluator is an advocate for the best interest of the child. The child custody evaluation is not confidential and the evaluator may be called to testify in court.

Juvenile offenders are dealt with in a separate juvenile court system whose mandate is to rehabilitate, not to punish. Unlike adult court, guilt or innocence is determined solely by a judge, not a jury. Delinquent acts refer to ordinary crimes committed by juveniles, and status offenses refer to behaviors that would not be criminal if committed by adults. On occasion, youths who may have committed more serious crimes are turned over to adult criminal courts. Psychiatrists may be called at any point in the juvenile justice process to provide expert opinion and recommendations, including whether psychiatric treatment would be indicated. Court decisions may be based, in part, on the psychiatrist's evaluation of the juvenile's psychiatric history and current mental status.

Students should study the questions and answers below for a useful review of basic issues.

HELPFUL HINTS

These terms should be known and defined by the student.

- ▶ adjudicated delinquent
- ▶ adjudication
- ▶ "best interests of the child"
- ▶ breach of confidentiality
- ▶ child custody evaluation
- ▶ confidentiality
- ▶ delinquent act
- ▶ disposition
- ▶ intake
- ▶ joint custody
- ▶ juvenile court
- ▶ mediation
- ▶ proof beyond a reasonable doubt
- ▶ rehabilitation
- ▶ status offenses
- ▶ "tender-years" doctrine
- ▶ waiver of confidentiality

▲ QUESTIONS

DIRECTIONS: The incomplete statement below is followed by five suggested responses or completions. Select the *one* that is *best*.

54.1 Breach of confidentiality by a psychiatrist is required in all of the following situations *except*

   A. a suicidal adolescent patient
   B. a homicidal adolescent patient
   C. disclosure of sexual abuse by a patient
   D. a child custody evaluation
   E. drug or alcohol use by an adolescent patient

DIRECTIONS: Each set of lettered headings below is followed by a list of numbered statements. For each numbered statement, select

   A. if the item is associated with *A only*
   B. if the item is associated with *B only*
   C. if the item is associated with *both A and B*
   D. if the item is associated with *neither A nor B*

Questions 54.2–54.7

   A. Juvenile court system
   B. Adult court system
   C. Both
   D. Neither

An alleged perpetrator has the following rights:

54.2 Legal counsel, Fifth Amendment privilege, and notice of charges
54.3 Pretrial hearing, trial, sentencing
54.4 Trial by jury
54.5 Intake, adjudication, disposition
54.6 Disposition right after confession
54.7 Trial only by judge, without a jury

Questions 54.8–54.10

   A. "Tender-years" doctrine
   B. "Best interest of the child" doctrine
   C. Both
   D. Neither

54.8 Young children are usually better off with their mothers
54.9 Current law in the United States
54.10 There may be a situation in which custody should reside with a nonparent

Questions 54.11–54.14

   A. "In re Gault" case
   B. "In re Winship" case
   C. Both
   D. Neither

54.11 "Beyond a reasonable doubt"
54.12 The right to confront witnesses
54.13 All handicapped children should be provided a free and appropriate public education in the least restrictive environment
54.14 Reports of child abuse are mandatory in all states

ANSWERS

Forensic Issues in Child Psychiatry

54.1 The answer is E
Breaches of confidentiality occur in situations of danger to the life of a patient or information disclosure leading the clinician to believe that the patient poses a danger to the life of another. Patients who are *suicidal or homicidal* and cases of *sexual abuse* automatically require breach of confidentiality. *Child custody* evaluations are also exempt from confidentiality (this is established through a written waiver of confidentiality at the beginning of a custody evaluation). Disclosure by an adolescent patient of *use of drugs or alcohol* does not necessarily fall into the category of required breach of confidentiality. The specific nature, situation, and type of drug and alcohol use allow the clinician to determine whether such behaviors constitute an imminent danger to the life of the patient. If so, the clinician is obligated to override the confidentiality.

Answers 54.2–54.7

54.2 The answer is C

54.3 The answer is B

54.4 The answer is B

54.5 The answer is A

54.6 The answer is A

54.7 The answer is A
Both the juvenile court and the adult court system must conform to the same rights of due process. These include the right to *notice of charges*, the *right to legal counsel*, the *Fifth Amendment privilege* against self-incrimination, and the right to confront witnesses. The adult court system uses the following process: the *pretrial hearing*, *trial*, and *sentencing*. The juvenile court, however, has a different procedure in that there is *intake, adjudication*, and *disposition*. If a juvenile defendant makes a *confession*, disposition may proceed without the trial. The adult court system uses *jury* decision making in its trials, or trials held by a judge without a jury. In the juvenile court all trials are decided by a judge.

Answers 54.8–54.10

54.8 The answer is A

54.9 The answer is B

54.10 The answer is B
Child custody disputes throughout recorded history have reflected a society's view of the child in the family. The practice of courts becoming involved in such private family affairs is fairly recent. The history of this issue traces movement from seeing children as essentially owned by their father to considerations of what is in their best interests. Judicial decisions have been informed by various presumptions, such as "the tender years" and "the best interests of the child." The *"tender-years" presumption* existed well into the 20th century. It held that *young children* (from birth to about age 7) *were usually better off with their mothers*, who were generally assumed to be better skilled in nurturing and raising their offspring. This presumption was replaced in the last third of the 20th century by *"the best interest of the child" doctrine, which is the current law in the United States*. This presumption holds that the focus of a child custody case should be the child and courts ought not lean toward one parent or the other strictly on the basis of sex. *Fur-*

thermore, there may be situations in which custody should reside with a nonparent rather than a parent, if that represents the best interests of the child.

Answers 54.11–54.14

54.11 The answer is B

54.12 The answer is A

54.13 The answer is D

54.14 The answer is D

Knowledge of the juvenile court system and its strengths and weaknesses is essential for the forensic child psychiatrist working in this area. Likewise, the clinician must appreciate the indications for waiver hearings and the grounds for judicial determination that a minor be tried as an adult. Although the juvenile court system operated for decades as supposedly child oriented and protective, the United States Supreme Court, in the landmark case *"In re Gault,"* determined that the system sometimes did not accord juveniles rights equal to those of adults. This decision held that in delinquency cases, juveniles must be accorded basic due process rights: the right to notice of charges, the right to legal counsel, the Fifth Amendment privilege against self-incrimination, and *the right to confront witnesses.* Another important Supreme Court case, *"In re Winship,"* held that the standard *"beyond a reasonable doubt"* must be followed in delinquency hearings.

Child and adolescent psychiatrists may be involved in forensic evaluations outside the more common venues of the family or criminal court. For example, they may be called upon to make certain recommendations for a student with special needs under the landmark Education for All Handicapped Children Act of 1975. This law requires that *all handicapped children,* regardless of the severity of their condition, be provided a free and appropriate public education in the least restrictive environment. Handicapped children are defined as those who are mentally retarded, learning disabled, physically disabled, or emotionally disturbed. A treating or evaluating child psychiatrist may be asked to testify at various hearings required under the law. Knowledge of the law's implications as well as of the particular child will be critical to performing a proper evaluation.

Most child and adolescent therapists spell out the limits of confidentiality to the families they are working with at the outset of therapy and also clarify how communications with parents are to be handled; further, they need to discuss the limits of confidentiality with respect to insurance plans. Additional limitations to confidentiality include behaviors harmful to self or others. When disclosures need to be made to parents, the patient may be given the option of telling them himself or herself or of discussing it with parents and therapist together. Other exceptions to confidentiality include laws on *reporting child abuse,* which are *mandatory in all states.* A physician who fails to report suspicion of abuse may be liable for civil as well as criminal sanctions. If an abuse report needs to be filed, parents should be so informed. In some states physicians may have a duty to protect third parties under *Tarasoff I* and *Tarasoff II* (i.e., the 1976 and 1982 rulings of the California Supreme Court in the two cases of *Tarasoff v. Regents of University of California*).

55

Geriatric Psychiatry

The population of people over 65 years of age has grown nearly 90 percent in the United States since 1960, while the total population has only grown 39 percent. Life expectancy has increased from 47 years in 1900 to nearly 76 years in 1996, and the "oldest old" people (those at least 85 years of age) are the fastest growing group of the 65-and-over age population. The first certification examination in geriatric psychiatry was given in 1991, and today the field is the most rapidly expanding in psychiatry. Geriatric psychiatry requires a special knowledge, because older people may have coexisting medical disorders and disabilities, may take many medications with potentially troubling side effects, and may have cognitive impairments. The National Institute of Mental Health's Epidemiologic Catchment Area (ECA) program has found that the most common mental disorders of old age are depressive disorders, cognitive disorders, phobias, and alcohol-use disorders. Elderly people may be more vulnerable to drug-induced psychiatric symptoms such as confusion, agitation, psychosis, and mood impairments. Older people have a higher risk for suicide, with almost 20 percent of suicides being committed by people over 65 years of age. Age itself is not considered a risk factor for depressive disorders, but losing a spouse or having a chronic medical condition, both more common in the elderly than in younger people, are associated with increased vulnerability.

Predisposing psychosocial risk factors for mental disorders in the elderly include many losses, such as those of social roles, autonomy and independence, family and friends, health, and finances. There is a high prevalence of cognitive disorders in older people, ranging from what are considered minor age-related memory impairments, termed benign senescent forgetfulness, to full-blown dementias, such as Alzheimer's disease. Dementia is the second most common cause of disability in people over 65 years of age, after arthritis. In the United States, about 5 percent of people over 65 years of age have severe dementia, and about 15 percent have mild dementia. Over the age of 80 years, about 20 percent have severe dementia.

Before initiating psychopharmacological treatment in an older person, a thorough medical evaluation is required. Adults over 65 years of age use the greatest number of medications of any age group. Physiological changes occur as people age, necessitating alterations of drug treatment in the elderly. These changes may include decreased renal clearance, decreased ability to metabolize drugs, and impaired drug absorption. Changes in the ratio of lean to fat body mass affect drug distribution, and as a result a drug's action may be prolonged in the elderly. A general rule in the pharmacological treatment of older people is to use the lowest possible effective dose to minimize side effects. Clinicians need to be aware of the indications, pharmacodynamics and kinetics, and interactions with other drugs of all medications prescribed.

The student should study the questions and answers below for a useful review of these issues in this field.

HELPFUL HINTS

Each of the following terms relating to geriatric issues should be defined.

- ▶ adaptational capacity
- ▶ advocacy
- ▶ agedness
- ▶ agitation and aggression
- ▶ akathisia
- ▶ alcohol- and other substance-use disorders
- ▶ Alzheimer's disease
- ▶ anoxic confusion
- ▶ anxiety disorder
- ▶ benign senescent forgetfulness
- ▶ benzodiazepines
- ▶ cerebral anoxia
- ▶ code of ethics
- ▶ cognitive functioning
- ▶ consent for disclosure of information
- ▶ conversion disorder
- ▶ delirium
- ▶ dementia
- ▶ dementing disorder
- ▶ depression
- ▶ developmental phases
- ▶ diabetes
- ▶ disorders of awareness
- ▶ drug blood level
- ▶ elder abuse
- ▶ emphysema
- ▶ expert testimony
- ▶ fluoxetine (Prozac)
- ▶ FSH
- ▶ Geriatric Depression Scale
- ▶ hepatic failure
- ▶ hypochondriasis
- ▶ hypomanic disorder
- ▶ ideational paucity
- ▶ insomnia
- ▶ L-dopa (Larodopa)
- ▶ late-onset schizophrenia
- ▶ LH
- ▶ lithium
- ▶ loss of mastery
- ▶ manic disorder
- ▶ MMSE (Mini-Mental Status Examination)
- ▶ mood disorder
- ▶ neurosis
- ▶ norepinephrine
- ▶ nutritional deficiencies
- ▶ obsessive-compulsive disorder
- ▶ organic mental disorder
- ▶ orientation
- ▶ overt behavior
- ▶ paradoxical reaction
- ▶ paraphrenia
- ▶ presbyopia
- ▶ psychopharmacology
- ▶ psychotropic danger
- ▶ ranitidine (Zantac)
- ▶ remotivation techniques
- ▶ ritualistic behavior
- ▶ role of anxiety
- ▶ sensorium
- ▶ sexual history
- ▶ trazodone (Desyrel)
- ▶ uremia

▲ QUESTIONS

DIRECTIONS: Each of the questions or incomplete statements below is followed by five suggested responses or completions. Select the *one* that is *best* in each case.

55.1 Elderly persons taking antipsychotics are especially susceptible to the following side effects *except*

A. tardive dyskinesia
B. akathisia
C. a toxic confusional state
D. paresthesias
E. dry mouth

55.2 Abnormalities of cognitive functioning in the aged are most often due to

A. depressive disturbances
B. schizophrenia
C. medication
D. cerebral dysfunctioning or deterioration
E. hypochondriasis

55.3 Which of the following statements about the biology of aging is *false*?

A. Each cell of the body has a genetically determined life span.
B. The optic lens thins.
C. The T-cell response to antigens is altered.
D. A decrease in melanin occurs.
E. Brain weight decreases.

55.4 Changes in the ratio of lean to fat body mass affect the distribution of all of the following *except*

A. imipramine (Toframil)
B. diazepam (Valium)
C. chlorpromazine (Thorazine)
D. lithium (Eskalith)
E. fluoxetine (Prozac)

55.5 Which of the following statements about learning and memory in the elderly is *false*?

A. Complete learning of new material still occurs.
B. On multiple choice tests, recognition of correct answers persists.
C. Simple recall remains intact.
D. IQ remains stable until age 80 years.
E. Memory-encoding ability diminishes.

55.6 In the physical assessment of the aged, which of the following statements is *false*?

A. Toxins of bacterial origin are common.
B. The most common metabolic intoxication causing mental symptoms is uremia.
C. Cerebral anoxia often precipitates mental syndromes.
D. Severe vitamin deficiencies are common.
E. Nutritional deficiencies may cause mental symptoms.

55.7 Which of the following statements about the pharmacological treatment of the elderly is *false*?

A. The elderly use more medications than any other age group.
B. Some 25 percent of prescriptions are for those over age 65 years.
C. In the United States, 250,000 people a year are hospitalized because of adverse reactions to medications.
D. About 25 percent of hypnotics dispensed in the United States each year are to those over age 65 years.
E. About 70 percent of the elderly use over-the-counter (OTC) medications.

55.8 The annual incidence of dementia of the Alzheimer's type for men and women 70 to 74 years of age is about

A. 0.5 percent
B. 1.0 percent
C. 5.0 percent
D. 10.0 percent
E. 15.0 percent

55.9 All of the following risk factors for dementia of the Alzheimer's type are regarded as confirmed *except*

A. apolipoprotein E genotype
B. Down's syndrome
C. family history
D. aluminum
E. age

55.10 Possible protective factors against dementia include

A. antiinflammatory drugs
B. estrogen replacement therapy
C. red wine
D. education
E. all of the above

55.11 Sleep changes associated with normal aging include

A. reduction in stage 4 sleep
B. increased fragmentation of sleep
C. reduction in REM sleep
D. disruption of the circadian sleep–wake rhythm
E. all of the above

55.12 In older patients, fluoxetine has been associated with

A. problematic weight loss
B. syndrome of inappropriate antidiuretic hormone secretion (SIADH)
C. agitation
D. parkinsonism
E. all of the above

55.13 Medications available for prescription in the United States that are indicated for treating cognitive impairment currently include

A. cholinergic agonists
B. selegiline (Eldepryl)
C. vitamin E
D. cholinesterase inhibitors
E. all of the above

55.14 Antidepressants considered unsuitable for use in elderly patients include

A. desipramine (Norpramin)
B. amitriptyline (Elavil)
C. tranylcypromine (Parnate)
D. venlafaxine (Effexor)
E. all of the above

ANSWERS

Geriatric Psychiatry

55.1 The answer is D

Paresthesias, which are spontaneous tingling sensations, are not typically a side effect of antipsychotics. Elderly persons, particularly if they have organic brain disease, are especially susceptible to the side effects of antipsychotics, which include *dry mouth, tardive dyskinesia, akathisia,* and a *toxic confusional state.* Tardive dyskinesia is characterized by disfiguring and involuntary buccal and lingual masticatory movements; akathisia is a restlessness marked by a compelling need for constant motion. Choreiform body movements, which are spasmodic and involuntary movements of the limbs and the face, and rhythmic extension and flexion movements of the fingers may also be noticeable. Examination of the patient's protruded tongue for fine tremors and vermicular (worm-like) movements is a useful diagnostic procedure. A toxic confusional state, also called a central anticholinergic syndrome, is characterized by a marked disturbance in short-term memory, impaired attention, disorientation, anxiety, visual and auditory hallucinations, increased psychotic thinking, and peripheral anticholinergic side effects.

55.2 The answer is D

Abnormalities of cognitive functioning in the elderly are most often due to some *cerebral dysfunctioning or deterioration,* although they may also be the result of *depressive disturbances, schizophrenia,* or the effects of *medication.* In many instances, intellectual difficulties are not obvious, and a searching evaluation is necessary to detect them. The elderly are sensitive to the effects of medication; in some instances, cognitive impairment may result from overmedication. *Hypochondriasis,* the fear that one has a disease or preoccupation with one's health, is not the cause of an abnormality of cognitive functioning.

55.3 The answer is B

As a person ages, *the optic lens thickens (not thins)* in association with an inability to accommodate (presbyopia), and hearing loss is progressive, particularly at the high frequencies. The process of aging, known as senescence, results from a complex interaction of genetic, metabolic, hormonal, immunological, and structural factors acting on molecular, cellular, histological, and organ levels. The most commonly held theory is that *each cell of the body has a genetically determined life span* during which replication occurs a limited number of times before the cell dies. One study found 50 such replications in human cells. Structural changes in cells take place with age. In the central

nervous system (CNS), for example, age-related cell changes occur in neurons, which show signs of degeneration.

Changes in the structure of deoxyribonucleic acid (DNA) and ribonucleic acid (RNA) are also found in aging cells; the cause has been attributed to genotypic programing, x-rays, chemicals, and food products, among others. Aging probably has no single cause. All areas of the body are affected to some degree, and changes vary from person to person.

A progressive decline in many bodily functions includes a *decrease in melanin* and decreases in cardiac output and stroke volume, glomerular filtration rate, oxygen consumption, cerebral blood flow, and vital capacity. Many immune mechanisms are altered, with *impaired T-cell response to antigens* and an increase in the formation of autoimmune antibodies. These altered immune responses probably play a role in aged persons' susceptibility to infection and possibly even to neoplastic disease. Some neoplasms, most notably cancers of the colon, prostate, stomach, and skin, show a steadily increasing incidence with age.

Variable changes in endocrine function are seen. For example, postmenopausal estrogen levels decrease, producing breast tissue involution and vaginal epithelial atrophy. Testosterone levels begin to decline in the sixth decade; however, follicle-stimulating hormone and luteinizing hormone increase. In the central nervous system, there is a *decrease in brain weight,* ventricular enlargement, and neuronal loss of approximately 50,000 a day, with some reduction in cerebral blood flow and oxygenation.

55.4 The answer is D

Lithium, a hydrophilic drug, is excreted by the kidneys. The elderly person's decrease in renal clearance may cause an accumulation of lithium.

As a person ages, the ratio of lean to fat body mass changes. With normal aging, lean body mass decreases, and body fat increases. Because of that and because of decreases in plasma volume, total body water, and total plasma, the volume of distribution (V_d) for lipophilic drugs is increased. Increases in the V_d of the lipophilic drugs *imipramine, diazepam, chlorpromazine,* and *fluoxetine* may reduce their efficacy if the drugs are given in single or as-needed doses. The increased V_d also contributes to drug accumulation.

55.5 The answer is C

In the elderly, *simple recall* becomes difficult (*does not remain intact*) and *memory-encoding ability diminishes.* Those functions decline with age. However, many cognitive abilities are retained in old age. Although the elderly take longer than young persons to learn new material, *complete learning of new material still occurs.* Old adults maintain their verbal abilities, and their *IQs remain stable until approximately age 80 years. On multiple-choice tests, recognition of correct answers persists.*

55.6 The answer is D

Severe vitamin deficiencies in the aged are *rare (rather than common).* However, a number of conditions and deficiencies are typical and should be considered in the physical assessment of the aged. *Toxins of bacterial origin* and metabolic origins are common in old age. Bacterial toxins usually originate in occult or inconspicuous foci of infection, such as suspected pneumonic conditions and urinary infections. In the aged, the most common metabolic intoxication causing mental symptoms is *uremia,* which is an excess of urea and other nitrogenous waste products in the blood. Mild diabetes, hepatic failure, and gout are also known to cause mental symptoms in the aged and may easily be missed unless they are actively investigated. Alcohol and drug misuse may cause many mental disturbances in late life, but these abuses, with their characteristic effects, are usually determined by taking a history.

Cerebral anoxia often precipitates mental symptoms as a result of cardiac insufficiency or emphysema. Anoxic confusion may follow surgery, a cardiac infarct, gastrointestinal bleeding, or occlusion or stenosis of the carotid arteries. *Nutritional deficiencies may cause mental symptoms* or may be a symptom of a mental disorder.

55.7 The answer is D

Psychotropic drugs are among those most commonly prescribed for the elderly; *40 percent (not 25 percent) of all hypnotics* dispensed in the United States each year are to those over age 65 years. *The elderly use more medications than any other age group.* Indeed, *25 percent of all prescriptions are written for those over age 65 years.* Many old persons have adverse drug reactions, as evidenced by the fact that, *in the United States, 250,000 people a year are hospitalized because of adverse medication reactions.* The physician must remember that about *70 percent of the elderly use over-the-counter* (OTC) *medications.* These preparations can interact with prescribed drugs and lead to dangerous side effects. The physician should include the use of OTC medications when taking a patient's drug history.

55.8 The answer is D

There are many fewer studies of the incidence than of the prevalence of dementia, but enough exist to allow some estimate of age-specific rates in the community. As an approximate guide, for dementia of all types the incidence is about one new case per year for every 100 persons aged 65 years and over. What is clear is that the age-specific incidence of both dementia of the Alzheimer's type and vascular dementia rises steeply from the 60s. It is uncertain whether this continues to extreme old age, reaches a plateau, or even decreases in those who survive until then. Data from the Framingham study suggest that the *annual incidence of dementia of the Alzheimer's type is about 10 percent for men and women aged 70 to 74 years.*

55.9 The answer is D

The power of individual case-control studies of dementia of the Alzheimer's type has been greatly enhanced by an initiative undertaken by the European Consortium on Dementia (EURO-DEM) established by the European community. They carried out a collaborative reanalysis of 11 case-controlled studies, six from the United States and one each from Australia, Finland, Italy, Japan, and the Netherlands. That analysis revealed risk factors that had hitherto been only speculative. From this and other sources, only four risk factors can now be regarded as confirmed.

Age. As for dementia in general, the incidence rises steeply with age, making it the strongest of all risk factors.

Family History. Having a parent or sibling with dementia of the Alzheimer's type increases the risk of developing the disease about 3.5 times. The risk is greater for relatives of early-onset patients than later-onset patients. In interpreting the epidemiological data for individual patients, however, the clinician needs to emphasize that the risk conferred by a positive family history depends on how long that person lives. Those who do not reach old age have a low risk. Even for relatives who live to age 90 years, the probability that they themselves will develop the disease is only about 50 percent.

Apolipoprotein E Genotype. The much rarer, early-onset dementia of the Alzheimer's type is caused by single genes, such as a mutation of the amyloid precursor gene on chromosome 21 or the presenilin genes on chromosomes 1 and 14. But in most cases of dementia of the Alzheimer's type, onset is not until the 70s or 80s. In this group, of much greater public health importance, there are multiple genetic and environmental influences. One of the most exciting discoveries is that the apolipoprotein E ε4 allele on chromosome 19 affects the risk of developing the disease. The ε4 allele of this gene increases risk, and the ε2 allele may reduce it. Although early research with clinical samples showed a very strong relationship between apolipoprotein E ε4 genotype and dementia of the Alzheimer's type, more recent studies with general population samples show a weaker relationship. Currently, much interest exists in preliminary findings that a combination of having the ε4 allele and being infected with the herpes simplex type 1 virus confers a very high risk. It is now clear that although all individuals with the ε4 allele are at increased risk, even homozygotes can live to age 90 years with only a 50 percent chance of developing a dementia. An interesting proposal is that the apolipoprotein E genotype predicts when (not whether) a person is predisposed to develop this dementia. These epidemiological findings may in time lead to the development of pharmacological methods to slow the deposition of β-amyloid.

Down's Syndrome. Persons with Down's syndrome may develop the brain changes of dementia of the Alzheimer's type before age 40 years. This is believed to be related to their having an extra copy of the amyloid precursor gene on chromosome 21.

Because aluminum, known to be neurotoxic, occurs in neuritic plaques, evidence has been sought for an association between exposure to this metal and the development of dementia of the Alzheimer's type. Aluminum is ingested in food, drinking water, antacids, and toothpaste. It is used in kitchen utensils and it is applied to the body in antiperspirants. The widespread use of aluminum as a flocculent in water supplies has led to public concern, although drinking water provides only a tiny percentage of dietary aluminum. The amount absorbed depends on its bioavailability, and considerable uncertainty exists about its subsequent deposition in the brain. From the epidemiological evidence, involvement of aluminum from drinking water or other sources in causing dementia of the Alzheimer's type remains unproven.

55.10 The answer is E (all)

A recurrent finding in field surveys is that rates for dementia and cognitive impairment are higher in elderly persons who have had little *education*. This may be partly due to bias in ascertainment, whereby the tests are done better by persons who are more literate. While such bias may be present in the detection of mild impairment in surveys, it is much less likely to influence the diagnosis of a fully developed dementia. There may indeed be a true gradient in the incidence of dementia, including dementia of the Alzheimer's type, across educational levels. In this way, lack of education could be seen as an exposure that may confer increased risk. One interpretation is that education may delay the point at which a developing dementia becomes clinically manifest. In interpreting results of a large survey in Shanghai, the authors raised the possibility that having no education may lower brain reserve, allowing the earlier appearance of symptoms of dementia. It is also possible that education is a proxy for other beneficial factors, as in diet or lifestyle. But a recent longitudinal study of American nuns suggests that education and intelligence may actually protect against the neuropathological processes in dementia of the Alzheimer's type. This means that exposure to education in childhood may conceivably have some protective effect many decades later.

Since an inverse association between rheumatoid arthritis and dementia of the Alzheimer's type was first observed, over 20 publications have examined the possibility that persons who have taken steroids, aspirin, or other nonsteroidal *antiinflammatory drugs* (NSAIDs) over long periods have a lower risk of dementia or have slower cognitive decline in late life. Some of these studies have reported a protective effect, but many have deficient designs, and there may be publication bias (i.e., papers with negative evidence for such an effect are less likely to be submitted and accepted for publication). Yet comprehensive and balanced information on the topic is needed. The most recent information is that antiinflammatory drugs probably do prevent or attenuate the symptoms of dementia of the Alzheimer's type. This effect is biologically plausible in terms of the action of these drugs to inhibit the immune and chronic inflammatory pathology suspected to apply in dementia of the Alzheimer's type. But it is premature for physicians to prescribe antiinflammatory drugs for dementia of the Alzheimer's type before their effect is established in a randomized controlled trial and the findings balanced with their risks.

Case-controlled studies suggest possible protection against dementia of the Alzheimer's type afforded to women who take *estrogen*. But since these women also tend to be better educated and to differ in other lifestyle factors, this finding could be misleading. The use of estrogen replacement therapy is currently controversial.

A large population-based prospective study in France has found evidence that *moderate consumption of red wine* protects against the onset of dementia. The work was conducted in Bordeaux, France.

55.11 The answer is E (all)

Age-related changes in the amount and pattern of the various stages of sleep and wakefulness are well described. Elderly people spend more time in bed and less time asleep and are more easily aroused from sleep than are young people. The most striking changes include a *reduction in slow-wave sleep (particularly stage 4 sleep)*, increased nighttime wakefulness, and *increased fragmentation of sleep* by periods of wakefulness. Less striking age *reductions in rapid eye movement (REM) sleep* and total nighttime sleep also occur. The age-related impairments in sleep depth and maintenance seem to be accompanied by an age-related increase in sensitivity to environmental stimuli that disturb sleep; for example, elderly people are more easily aroused from nighttime sleep by auditory stimuli than are young people.

Many age-related changes in sleep patterns suggest that aging may *disrupt the circadian sleep–wake rhythm*. Increased nighttime wakefulness in elderly persons is mirrored by more daytime fatigue, more daytime napping, and a greater likelihood of falling asleep during the day. Advancing age has also been associated with a tendency to fall asleep and awaken earlier than in earlier years, and older people are less tolerant of phase shifts of the sleep–wake schedule, such as those caused by shift work and transmeridian flight (jet lag). Because these changes are also observed in healthy seniors, they are attributed to normal, age-related neuronal alterations in brain areas controlling sleep physiology rather than to pathological processes.

55.12 The answer is E (all)

In addition to problems that can be anticipated, the fact that most of the data on a new drug's effects were obtained in younger patients means that unexpected adverse effects are not infrequent in older patients. For example, fluoxetine has been associated with *problematic weight loss* in older patients and with the *syndrome of inappropriate antidiuretic hormone secretion (SIADH)*. While SIADH is a rare adverse effect of many psychotropic medications, including tricyclic drugs and all SSRIs, most reports of antidepressant-induced SIADH have involved patients older than 65 years and have implicated fluoxetine. In an analysis of 760 reports of hyponatremia associated with SSRIs, the median time to onset of the hyponatremia was 13 days (range, 3 to 120 days). In older patients, fluoxetine has also been associated with insomnia, nervousness, delirium, apathy, *agitation*, and *parkinsonism* or worsening of motor disability in patients suffering from idiopathic parkinsonism. Although all of these unanticipated effects have now been reported with other SSRIs, it is not possible, at present, to determine the differential geriatric adverse-effect profile of the more recently introduced medications, given the much longer and more extensive use of fluoxetine in the United States and the lack of comparative trials.

55.13 The answer is D

So-called antidementia drugs are, by definition, medications intended to improve cognitive function in patients with dementia. The term has regulatory significance with the U.S. Food and Drug Administration (FDA), since it differentiates these medications from cognition enhancers, medications that might be expected to improve cognition without reference to a particular illness. Worldwide, a broad range of putative cognition-enhancing agents are available for prescription, including piracetam derivatives, ergoloid mesylates (Hydergine), *cholinesterase inhibitors, cholinergic agonists*, and *selegiline (Eldepryl)*; antioxidants; vitamins; food supplements; so-called nutriceuticals; and various plant derivatives, including extracts of *Ginkgo biloba*. In the United States the latter four groups of the products are regulated by the FDA only with respect to apparent safety and inappropriate advertising claims; efficacy for the conditions being treated need not be addressed.

The medications available for prescription in the United States that are indicated for treating cognitive impairment currently include only ergoloid mesylates and the *cholinesterase inhibitors* tacrine (Cognex), donepezil (Aricept), and rivastigmine (ENA 713, Exelon, Novartis). The three cholinesterase inhibitors are specifically indicated for dementia of the Alzheimer's type. Results of clinical trials performed throughout the world, however, suggest that other medications available in the United States might have efficacy in patients with Alzheimer's disease, including selegiline, various estrogen preparations, *vitamin E,* and antiinflammatories.

55.14 The answer is B

Antidepressants with particular relevance to elderly adults include the secondary amine tricyclic drugs, such as nortriptyline (Aventyl, Pamelor) and *desipramine (Norpramin)*; the selective serotonin reuptake inhibitors (SSRIs), including citalopram (Celexa), fluoxetine (Prozac), fluvoxamine (Luvox), paroxetine (Paxil), and sertraline (Zoloft); the monoamine oxidase inhibitors (MAOIs), such as phenelzine (Nardil) and *tranylcypromine (Parnate)*; and miscellaneous agents, including bupropion (Wellbutrin), trazodone (Desyrel), nefazodone (Serzone), and *venlafaxine (Effexor). Agents considered unsuitable for use in elderly adults because of significant adverse effects include amitriptyline (Elavil),* imipramine (Tofranil), and clomipramine (Anafranil). The amount of information available from controlled clinical trials in elderly adults is relatively meager; hence, drug recommendations are extrapolated from small numbers of older patients (mostly under age 75 years) or from younger and middle-aged adults.

56

Palliative Medicine and End-of-Life Care

Physicians are trained to diagnose and manage illness but are often ill-prepared for the dying patient who has reached a point where no treatment will prevent the inevitable. Unfortunately, many physicians may experience dying patients as reminders of their own limitations, or even as personal failures, and thus avoid or withdraw from them. Medical training tends to focus almost exclusively on control or elimination of disease, often at the expense of the care and comfort of the person dying. The primary role of caring for dying patients must be the provision of ongoing compassionate support, so that the person and the family do not feel abandoned. Being able to be tactfully honest with patients may be one of the physician's greatest tools.

This support may include the recognition, acknowledgement, and vigorous control of pain. Effective pain management is critical, and physicians must use narcotics as liberally as they are needed and tolerated. This aspect of care is difficult for many doctors, who have been trained to use narcotics sparingly, if at all, out of fear of creating addictions, and who may also have become desensitized to or skeptical of expressions of pain in their patients.

The hospice movement began in the early 1960s, largely in response to perceived inadequacies in traditional and hospital-based approaches with respect to the dying patient. A hospice is a place (it may be an institution or home) where a multidisciplinary team provides round-the-clock coverage to the terminal patient and includes the control of pain as a primary goal. Narcotics are provided without fear of addiction. Hospice care's essential goal is to allow dying patients and their families to conduct their final interactions with as much dignity and control as possible.

A living will is a legal document in which patients provide instructions to their doctors about what life-support measures they will and will not accept. The American Medical Association (AMA) states that doctors can withhold all life-support treatment, including food and water, from patients in irreversible comas, as long as the diagnosis is confirmed adequately. In these cases, a physician does not intentionally cause the person's death (euthanasia) but rather, in consultation with the patient's family or guardian, lets the patient die. Euthanasia, or physician-assisted suicide, is defined as the doctor's deliberate act to kill a patient by directly administering a lethal dose of some drug or other agent. The ethical issues surrounding euthanasia are profound.

The student should study the questions and answers below for a useful review of this field.

HELPFUL HINTS

The student should know and define the following terms.

- advance directives
- DNI
- DNR
- end-of-life symptoms
- euthanasia (active, passive, involuntary, voluntary)
- health care proxies
- hospice
- hydromorphone
- living wills
- maintenance versus prn analgesics
- mercy killing
- morphine
- neonatal and child end-of-life decisions
- neuropathic pain
- opioids
- pain suppression pathways
- palliative versus curative treatment
- Patients Self-Determination Act
- physician-assisted suicide
- psychogenic pain
- psychotoxicity
- somatic pain
- Uniform Rights of the Terminally Ill Act
- visceral pain

▲ QUESTIONS

DIRECTIONS: Each of the questions or incomplete statements below is followed by five suggested responses or completions. Select the *one* that is *best* in each case.

56.1 Of the following drugs, the *least* likely to cause psychotoxicity is

A. morphine
B. levorphanol (Levo-Dromoran)
C. methadone (Dolophine)
D. hydromorphone (Dilaudid)
E. none of the above

56.2 Maintenance analgesia when compared to as-needed administration

    A. decreases drug efficiency

    B. increases patient anxiety

    C. slows pain control

    D. decreases well-informed staffs' complaints about drug-seeking behavior

    E. does not require extra doses for breakthrough

56.3 Advance directives

    A. are legally binding in all 50 states

    B. include living wills

    C. include health care proxies

    D. include DNR and DNI

    E. all of the above

56.4 With regard to neonatal end-of-life decisions

    A. there are clear-cut criteria as to which patients should receive intensive care and which should receive palliative care

    B. the American Academy of Pediatrics permits non-treatment decisions when the infant is irreversibly comatose or when treatment would only prolong the process of dying

    C. rarely do physicians have to be concerned about legal actions regardless of position taken

    D. there is a consensus among neonatologists about when to terminate newborn life

    E. none of the above

56.5 With regard to child end-of-life care

    A. cancer is the second most common cause of death in children

    B. children require less support than adults in coping with death

    C. on average, a child views death as permanent by age 7

    D. assurances about *terminal illness*'s being made pain free and physically comfortable are less important for children than adults

    E. none of the above

56.6 In hospice care

    A. around-the-clock pain control with opioids is an essential component

    B. a patient must be physician-certified as having 6 months or fewer to live

    C. medicare guidelines emphasize home care

    D. patients indicate that they agree to receive palliative rather than curative treatment

    E. all of the above

DIRECTIONS: Each group of questions below consists of lettered headings followed by a list of numbered words or statements. For each numbered word or statement, select the *one* lettered heading that is most closely associated with it. Each lettered heading may be selected once, more than once, or not at all.

Questions 56.7–56.10

    A. Somatic pain

    B. Visceral pain

    C. Neuropathic pain

    D. Psychogenic pain

    E. None of the above

56.7 Increasingly rare as a pure phenomenon in cancer patients

56.8 Usually constant, deep, rarely localized

56.9 Usually constant, aching, well localized

56.10 Burning dysesthetic pain

Questions 56.11–56.16

    A. Delusions

    B. Fatigue or weakness

    C. Dysphagia

    D. Incontinence

    E. Dyspnea or cough

56.11 Occurs in 80 percent of terminal lung cancer patients

56.12 May follow pelvic radiation

56.13 Common in end-state multiple sclerosis

56.14 Most common occurrence in terminal illness

56.15 Occurs in the majority of all terminal patients

56.16 Opioids may be of use

Questions 56.17–56.18

    A. Uniform Rights of the Terminally Ill Act

    B. Patients Self-Determination Act

    C. Both

    D. Neither

56.17 Authorizes an adult to control the decisions regarding the administration of life-sustaining treatment

56.18 Requires that all health care facilities provide patients with written information about the right to refuse treatment

Questions 56.19–56.26

    A. Euthanasia

    B. Physician-assisted suicide

    C. Both

    D. Neither

56.19 Mercy killing

56.20 Physician withholds artificial life-sustaining measures

56.21 Physician deliberately intends to kill a patient to alleviate or prevent suffering

56.22 Imparting of information or means that enable a person to take his or her own life

56.23 Palliative care designed to alleviate the suffering of a dying patient

56.24 Legal in states of Washington and California

56.25 Opposed by the American Medical Association (AMA) and the American Psychiatric Association (APA)

56.26 Adequate pain control may dramatically decrease the demand

---

ANSWERS

Palliative Medicine and End-of-Life Care

56.1 The answer is D

Opioids commonly cause delirium and hallucinosis. A frequent mechanism of psychotoxicity is the accumulation of drugs or metabolites whose duration of analgesia is shorter than their plasma half-lives (*morphine, levorphanol [Levo-Dromoran],* and *methadone [Dolophine]*). Use of drugs like *hydromorphone (Dilaudid),* with half-lives closer to their analgesic duration, can relieve the problem without loss of pain control. Cross-tolerance is incomplete between opiates; hence, several may be tried in any patient, with the dosage lowered when switching drugs.   lists opioid analgesics.

56.2 The answer is D

The importance of maintenance analgesia administration in terminal patients as opposed to as-needed administration cannot be overemphasized. *It improves (not slows) pain control, increases (not decreases) drug efficiency, and relieves (not increases) patient anxiety.* As-needed orders do not provide the immediate response of patient-controlled analgesia and allow pain to increase while waiting for the drug to be given. While it *decreases well-informed staffs' complaints about drug-seeking behavior,* it perversely sets up the patient for complaints made by staff members who are poorly informed as to proper palliative care. Even on maintenance treatment, *extra doses should be available for breakthrough pain,* and their repeated use should signal the need for raising the maintenance dose.

56.3 The answer is E (all)

Advance directives are wishes and choices about medical intervention when the patient's condition is considered to be terminal. *Advance directives are legally binding in all 50 states.* There are three types:

1. ***Living Will.*** A patient who is mentally competent gives specific instructions that doctors must follow when he or she is unable to communicate with them because of illness. They may include rejection of (1) feeding tubes, (2) artificial airways, or (3) any other measures to prolong life.

Table 56.1
Opioid Analgesics for Management of Pain

Drug and Equianalgesic Dose Relative Potency	Dose (mg IM or oral)	Plasma Half-Life (hr)[a]	Starting Oral Dose[b] (mg)	Available Commercial Preparations
Morphine	10 IM 60 oral	3–4	30–60	Oral: tablet, liquid, slow-release tablet Rectal: 5–30 mg Injectable: sc, IM, IV, epidural, intrathecal
Hydromorphone	1.5 IM 7.5 oral	2–3	2–18	Oral: tablets: 1, 2, 4 mg Injectable: sc, IM, IV 2 mg/mL, 3 mg/mL, and 10 mg/mL
Methadone	10 IM 20 oral	12–24	5–10	Oral: tablets, liquid Injectable: sc, IM, IV
Levorphanol	2 IM 4 oral	12–16	2–4	Oral: tablets Injectable: sc, IM, IV
Oxymorphone	1 IM	2–3	NA	Rectal: 10 mg Injectable: sc, IM, IV
Heroin	5 IM 60 oral	3–4	NA	NA
Meperidine	75 IM 300 oral	3–4 (normeperidine 12–16)	75	Oral: tablets Injectable: sc, IM, IV
Codeine	130 oral 200 oral	3–4	60	Oral: tablets and combination with acetylsalicylic acid, acetaminophen, liquid
Oxycodone[c]	15 oral 30 oral	—	5	Oral: tablets, liquid, oral formulation in combination with acetaminophen (tablet and liquid) and aspirin (tablet)

[a]The time of peak analgesia in nontolerant patients ranges from 1/2 hour to 1 hour, and the duration from 4 to 6 hours. The peak analgesic effect is delayed, and the duration is prolonged after oral administration.
[b]Recommended starting IM doses; the optimal dose for each patient is determined by titration, and the maximal dose is limited by adverse effects.
[c]A long-acting sustained-release form of oxycodone (Oxycontin) has been abused by drug addicts and its use has been criticized because of this; however, it is a very useful preparation available in 10-, 20-, 40-, and 160-mg doses that need to be taken once every 12 hours. It is used as a maintenance therapy for severe persistent pain.
Adapted from Foley K. Management of cancer pain. In: DeVita VT, Hellman S, Rosenberg SA, eds. *Cancer: Principles and Practice of Oncology.* 4th ed. Philadelphia: JB Lippincott; 1993:936.

2. **Health Care Proxy.** Also known as durable power of attorney, the health care proxy gives another person the power to make medical decisions if the patient is unable to do so. That person, also known as the surrogate, is empowered to make all decisions about terminal care based upon what he or she thinks the patient would have wanted.

3. **DNR and DNI.** These are orders that prohibit doctors from attempting to resuscitate—do not resuscitate (DNR)—or intubate—do not intubate (DNI)—the patient who is in extremis. DNR and DNI orders are made by the patient who is competent to do so. They can be made part of the living will or expressed by the health care proxy.

56.4 The answer is B

Advances in reproductive medicine have increased the number of infants born prematurely as well as the number of multiple births. With these advances the need for life-sustaining methods of care has increased and decisions about when to use palliative care have become more complex and controversial. Some bioethicists believe that withholding life-sustaining interventions is appropriate under certain circumstances; others hold that life-sustaining methods should not be used at all. An extensive study of attitudes among neonatologists about end-of-life decisions found *no consensus about if and when to terminate newborn life.* Most decisions to forgo life-sustaining procedures for newborns, if made at all, concern those whose death is imminent. Even if their future quality of life is determined to be bleak, a majority of physicians feel that some life is better than no life at all. Those physicians who support withholding intensive care consider the following quality of life issues: (1) extent of bodily damage (e.g., severe neurological impairment), (2) the burden that a disabled child will be for the family, and (3) the ability of the child to derive some pleasure from existence (e.g., having an awareness of being alive, being able to form relationships).

The American Academy of Pediatrics permits decisions not to treat newborns when the infant is irreversibly comatose or when treatment would be futile and only prolong the process of dying. These standards do not permit the parents to have any input into the decision-making process. In a well-publicized case in England in 2000, it was decided to surgically separate conjoined twins knowing that one would die as a result of the procedure and in spite of the objections of the parents, who believed that nature should take its course even if that led to the death of both infants.

Neonatal end-of-life decisions remain in a state of limbo. *There are no clear-cut criteria* as to which patients should receive intensive care and which should receive palliative care. *In all cases (not rarely) doctors are concerned about legal actions,* regardless of which position they take.

56.5 The answer is A

After accidents, *cancer is the second most common cause of death in children.* While many childhood cancers are treatable, palliative care is necessary for those that are not. *Children often require more (not less) support than adults in coping with death. On the average, a child does not view death as permanent until the age of about 10 (not age 7);* prior to that, death is viewed as a sleep or separation. Therefore, children should be told only what they can understand; if they are capable, they should be involved in the decision-making process about treatment plans. *Assurance about terminal illness's being made pain free and physically comfortable* is as (not less) important for children as for adults.

56.6 The answer is E (all)

Around-the-clock pain control with opioids is an essential component of hospice management. In 1983 Medicare began reimbursing hospice care. *Medicare guidelines emphasize home care,* with benefits provided for a broad spectrum of physician, nursing, psychosocial, and spiritual services at home or, if necessary, in a hospital or nursing home. *To be eligible, the patient must be physician-certified as having 6 months or fewer to live.* By electing hospice care *patients* indicate that they *agree to receive palliative rather than curative treatment.* Many hospice programs are hospital-based, sometimes in separate units and sometimes in the form of hospice beds interspersed throughout the facility. Other program models include free-standing hospices, hospital-affiliated hospices, nursing-home hospice care, and home care. Nursing homes are the site of death for many elderly patients with incurable chronic illness, yet dying nursing-home residents have limited access to palliative and hospice care. For example, in 1997 only 13 percent of hospice enrollees were in nursing homes, while 87 percent were in private homes, and 70 percent of nursing homes had no hospice patients.

Answers 56.7–56.10

56.7 The answer is D

56.8 The answer is B

56.9 The answer is A

56.10 The answer is C

Dying patients are subject to several different kinds of pain, summarized in . The distinctions are important because they call for different treatment strategies; *somatic (usually constant, aching, and well localized)* and *visceral (usually constant, deep, and rarely localized) pain,* are more responsive to opiates, while *neuropathic (burning dysesthetic*

Table 56.2
Types of Pain

Nociceptive pain	
Somatic pain	Usually but not always constant, aching, gnawing, and well localized; e.g., bone metastases
Visceral pain	Usually but not always constant, deep, squeezing, poorly localized, with possible cutaneous referral; e.g., pleural effusion leading to (1) deep chest pain, (2) diaphragmatic irritation referred to shoulder
Neuropathic pain	Burning dysesthetic pain with shock-like paroxysms associated with direct damage to peripheral receptors, afferent fibers, or CNS, leading to loss of central inhibitory modulation and spontaneous firing; e.g., phantom limb pain; can involve sympathetic somatic afferents
Psychogenic pain	Variable characteristics, secondary to psychological factors in the absence of medical factors; vanishingly rare as a pure phenomenon in cancer patients but often an additional factor in the presence of organic pain

Courtesy of Marguerite S. Lederberg, M.D., and Jimmie C. Holland, M.D.

Table 56.3
Neurophysiology of Nociceptive Pain

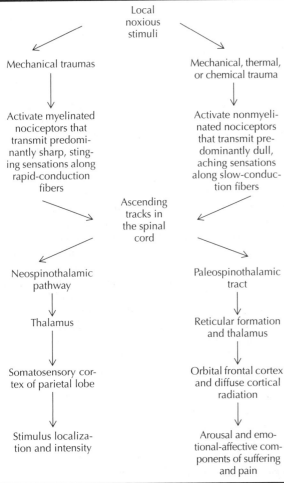

Courtesy of Marguerite S. Lederberg, M.D., and Jimmie C. Holland, M.D.

Table 56.4
Endogenous Pain Suppression Pathways

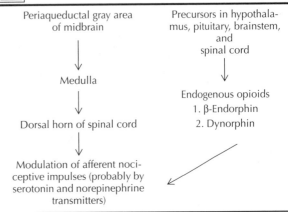

Courtesy of Marguerite S. Lederberg, M.D., and Jimmie C. Holland, M.D.

may not be as real to them.   lists common end-of-life symptoms. A comprehensive approach to palliation involves attending to end-of-life symptoms as well as to pain. Sources of distress include psychiatric symptoms (e.g., severe anxiety) and physical symptoms (e.g., nausea). *Dyspnea or cough* can occur in 80 percent of terminal lung cancer patients and may be responsive to opioid treatment. *Incontinence* not uncommonly follows pelvic radiation. *Dysphagia* is common in end-state multiple sclerosis, while *fatigue or weakness* is the most common occurrence in all terminal illness. Psychiatric symptoms are frequent in terminal patients, in particular *delusions* of various types.

Answers 56.17–56.18

56.17 The answer is A

56.18 The answer is B
The *Uniform Rights of the Terminally Ill Act*, drafted by the National Conference on Uniform State Laws, was approved and recommended for enactment in all states. The act *authorizes an adult to control the decisions regarding the administration of life-sustaining treatment* by executing a declaration instructing a physician to withhold or to withdraw life-sustaining treatment if the person is in a terminal condition and is unable to participate in medical treatment decisions. In 1991, the Federal *Patients Self-Determination Act* became law in the United States, requiring that all health care facilities (1) *provide each patient admitted to a hospital with written information about the right to refuse treatment,* (2) ask about advance directives, and (3) keep written records of whether the patient has an advance directive or has designated a health care proxy.

Answers 56.19–56.26

56.19 The answer is A

56.20 The answer is A

56.21 The answer is A

56.22 The answer is B

56.23 The answer is D

pain) and sympathetically maintained pain respond better to adjuvant medication. Most advanced cancer patients, for example, have more than one kind of pain *(psychogenic pain, for example, has become increasingly rare)* and require complex treatment regimens.   and   outline the neurophysiology of pain and pain suppression pathways.

Answers 56.11–56.16

56.11 The answer is E

56.12 The answer is D

56.13 The answer is C

56.14 The answer is B

56.15 The answer is A

56.16 The answer is E
Symptom management is an area of high priority in palliative care. Patients are often more concerned about the day-to-day distress of their symptoms than they are about their impending death, which

Table 56.5
Common End-of-Life Symptoms/Signs

Symptom/Sign	Comments
Delusions	Occur in 90% of all terminal patients; can be reversed if cause is treatable, e.g., pain, medication; respond to antipsychotic medication
Fatigue or weakness	Most common occurrence in terminal illness; psychostimulants can be used for short-term relief
Dysphagia	Common in neurological disease end states, e.g., multiple sclerosis, amyotrophic lateral sclerosis
Incontinence	May follow pelvic radiation, which can produce fistulas; use indwelling or condom catheter
Dyspnea or cough	Produces severe anxiety with fear of suffocation; occurs in 80% of terminal lung cancer patients; opioids, bronchodilators of use
Nausea or vomiting	Adverse effect of radiation and chemotherapy; antiemetics, e.g., metoclopramide, prochlorperazine, of use; marijuana cigarettes of use in selected patients
Anorexia	All terminal disease states are associated with cachexia secondary to anorexia and dehydration; feeding tubes do not prevent aspiration
Loss of skin integrity	Decubiti most common on weight-bearing areas, e.g., hips, sacrum, outer ankle; important to turn body frequently; elbow and hip pads of use
Anxiety or depression	Psychological factors, e.g., fear of death, abandonment; physiological factors, e.g., pain, hypoxia; antianxiety and antidepressant medication of use; opioids have strong antianxiety effects

From Mitka M. Suggestions for help when the end is near. *JAMA* 2000; 284:2441; adapted from National Coalition on Health Care (NCHC) and the Institute for Health Care Improvement (IHI). *Promises to Keep: Changing the Way We Provide Care at the End of Life,* release, October 12, 2000. With permission.

56.24 The answer is D

56.25 The answer is C

56.26 The answer is C
Euthanasia is defined as a physician's deliberate act to cause a patient's death by directly administering a lethal dose of medication or another agent. Because such patients are deemed by the treating physician to be hopelessly ill or injured, euthanasia has been called *mercy killing.*

On the basis of the doctor's action and the patient's condition, several types of euthanasia have been described: *active euthanasia,* in which *a physician deliberately intends to kill a patient to alleviate or prevent uncontrollable suffering; passive euthanasia,* in which *a physician withholds artificial life-sustaining measures; voluntary euthanasia,* in which the person who is to die is competent to give consent and does so; *and involuntary euthanasia,* in which the person who is to die is incompetent or incapable of giving consent.

Suicide is a deliberate taking of a person's own life. *Assisted suicide* is the *imparting of information or means that enable such an act* to take place. When the assistance is provided by a physician, the suicide is physician assisted. Assisted suicide and euthanasia should not be confused with *palliative care designed to alleviate the suffering of dying patients.* Palliative care includes giving pain relief and emotional, social, and spiritual support, as well as psychiatric care, if indicated. The intent of palliative care is to relieve pain and suffering, not to end a patient's life, even though death may result from palliative care.

In a survey of physicians in Oregon (the only U.S. state at the time of this writing where assisted suicide is legal), 5 percent of 2,649 physicians reported that they had received one or more requests for lethal prescriptions between late 1997 and early 1999. Most patients in question had cancer and a life expectancy of less than 6 months.

In the United States, physician-assisted suicide and euthanasia have been consistently *opposed by the American Psychiatric Association (APA),* the American Medical Association (AMA), the American Nurses Association, the National Legal Center for the disabled, and the Roman Catholic Church. Support, comfort, respect for patient autonomy, good communication, and *adequate pain control may dramatically decrease the demand for euthanasia and assisted suicide.* In certain carefully defined circumstances, it is humane to recognize that death is certain and suffering is great. Nevertheless, societal risks of involving physicians in medical interventions to cause patients' deaths are too great to condone active euthanasia or physician-assisted suicide.

57 ◮

Forensic Psychiatry

The word forensic (from the Latin "forum") means "belonging to, or suitable for, the courts or public discussion." Forensic psychiatry deals with mental disorders as they intersect the legal and court systems, and as such, forensic psychiatrists have a very different relationship to their patients than do other psychiatrists. Their primary goal is to obtain information from the patient that will then be shared with various other people, often in open court. Confidentiality essentially does not exist between psychiatrist and patient, and there is no doctor–patient relationship aimed at improving emotional or behavioral functioning. Forensic psychiatry is generally concerned with such legal matters as competency, criminal responsibility, and malpractice litigation.

Psychiatrists can act as either witnesses of fact or expert witnesses. As a witness of fact, a psychiatrist is acting as an ordinary witness, someone who has observed something and is being called to describe it in open court. This can include simply reading portions of a medical record into the legal record, but does not include expressing opinions or reporting others' statements. An expert witness is one who is accepted by the court and by advocates of both sides of the case as qualified to perform expert functions, and whose qualifications may include education, publications, and board certifications. Expert witnesses may render opinions, for example, that a patient meets the legal criteria for a guardian appointment. Psychiatrists often act as expert witnesses and may be hired by the defense or prosecution to provide opinions. This may lead to the common situation in which two psychiatrists representing two different sides provide diametrically opposed opinions about the case under dispute. The result can be confusion both on the parts of juries and the public about the value of psychiatric testimony, as well as cynicism and disillusionment. Many experts in forensic psychiatry believe that this problem could be minimized if the testifying psychiatrists were appointed by, and reported only to, the court.

Students should be familiar with the different issues (and terms) associated with forensic psychiatry. These include privilege and confidentiality, involuntary hospitalization and treatment, right to treatment, least restrictive alternatives, seclusion and restraints, informed consent, competency, criminal responsibility, malpractice, and worker's compensation. Among the important historical terms associated with criminal responsibility are the M'Naghten rule, irresistible impulse, Durham rule, and the model penal code. All of these should be familiar to clinicians and students.

The student should study the questions and answers below for a useful review of all of these topics.

▲ QUESTIONS

DIRECTIONS: Each of the questions or incomplete statements below is followed by five suggested responses or completions. Select the *one* that is *best* in each case.

57.1 The most frequent issue involving lawsuits against psychiatrists is

A. suicide
B. improper use of restraints
C. sexual involvement
D. drug reactions
E. violence

57.2 Involuntary termination of treatment of a patient by a therapist

A. may result in a malpractice claim of abandonment
B. cannot be done during a patient emergency
C. requires careful documentation
D. should include transfer of services to others
E. all of the above

57.3 Pick the *one* best answer regarding *Dusky v United States.*

A. Harmless mental patients cannot be confined against their wills without treatment if they can survive outside.
B. An involuntary patient who is not receiving treatment has a constitutional right to be discharged.
C. A test of competence was approved to see if a criminal defendant can rationally consult with a lawyer and has a factual (and rational) understanding of the proceedings against him or her.
D. Civilly committed persons have a constitutional right to adequate treatment.
E. A clinician must notify the intended victim(s) when there is an imminent threat posed by his or her patient.

57.4 If an attending psychiatrist is sued for the actions of a first-year resident, the principle applied is

A. *mens rea*
B. *parens patriae*
C. *respondeat superior*
D. *habeas corpus*
E. *actus reus*

57.5 Confidential communications can be shared with which of the following *without* the patient's consent?

A. A medical or psychiatric consultant
B. The patient's family
C. The patient's attorney
D. The patient's previous therapist
E. An insurer of the patient

57.6 Product rule is concerned with

A. testimonial privilege
B. involuntary admission
C. criminal responsibility
D. competency to stand trial
E. all of the above

57.7 The Gault decision applies to

A. minors
B. *habeas corpus*
C. informed consent
D. battery
E. none of the above

57.8 Situations in which there is an obligation on the part of the physician to report to authorities information that may be confidential include

A. suspected child abuse
B. the case of a patient who will probably commit murder and can only be stopped by notification of police
C. the case of a patient who will probably commit suicide and can only be stopped by notification of police
D. the case of a patient who has potentially life-threatening responsibilities (for example, airline pilot) and who shows marked impairment of judgment
E. all of the above

57.9 Of the following, which is the *least* common cause of malpractice claims against psychiatrists by patients?

A. suicide attempts
B. improper use of restraints
C. failure to treat psychosis
D. sexual involvement
E. substance dependence

57.10 To reduce the risk of malpractice, preventive approaches include

A. documenting good care
B. providing only the kind of care the psychiatrist is qualified to deliver
C. acquiring informed consent
D. obtaining a second opinion
E. all of the above

DIRECTIONS: Each group of questions below consists of lettered headings followed by a list of numbered phrases or statements. For each numbered phrase or statement, select the *one* lettered heading that is most closely associated with it. Each lettered heading may be selected once, more than once, or not at all.

Questions 57.11–57.15

A. *Rouse v Cameron*
B. *Wyatt v Stickney*
C. *O'Connor v Donaldson*
D. *The Myth of Mental Illness*
E. None of the above

57.11 Harmless mental patients cannot be confined against their wills.
57.12 Standards were established for staffing, nutrition, physical facilities, and treatment.
57.13 The purpose of involuntary hospitalization is treatment.
57.14 A patient who is not receiving treatment has a constitutional right to be discharged.
57.15 All forced confinements because of mental illness are unjust.

Questions 57.16–57.20

    A. Irresistible impulse
    B. M'Naghten rule
    C. Model penal code
    D. Durham rule
    E. Diminished capacity

57.16 Known commonly as the right-wrong test

57.17 A person charged with a criminal offense is not responsible for an act if the act was committed under circumstances that the person was unable to resist because of mental disease

57.18 An accused is not criminally responsible if his or her unlawful act was the product of mental disease or mental defect

57.19 As a result of mental disease or defect, the defendant lacked substantial capacity either to appreciate the criminality of his or her conduct or to conform the conduct to the requirement of the law

57.20 The defendant suffered some impairment (usually but not always because of mental illness) sufficient to interfere with the ability to formulate a specific element of the particular crime charged

Questions 57.21–57.25

    A. *Ramon v Farr*
    B. *Clites v State*
    C. *Redmond v Jaffe*
    D. *Youngberg v Romeo*
    E. ALI (American Law Institute) test

57.21 A person is not responsible for criminal conduct if he or she has a mental disease and lacks substantial capacity to either appreciate the wrongfulness of the conduct or to conform his or her conduct to the requirements of the law

57.22 Allegations of negligence involving tardive dyskinesia

57.23 The acceptability of restraint or seclusion for the purpose of training

57.24 Confidentiality

57.25 Drug inserts alone do not set the standard of care

Questions 57.26–57.30

    A. *Mens rea*
    B. *Actus reus*
    C. Both
    D. Neither

57.26 The level of intent to commit a criminal act

57.27 Conduct associated with committing a criminal act

57.28 Diminished capacity

57.29 Necessary for conviction of a crime

57.30 Automatism defense

Questions 57.31–57.35

    A. Testimonial privilege
    B. Patient-litigant exception
    C. Both
    D. Neither

57.31 The patient retains the right to prevent confidential material from being exposed in court

57.32 Insulates certain information from disclosure in court

57.33 Child abuse reporting

57.34 Civil commitment proceedings

57.35 Worker's compensation cases

Questions 57.36–57.39

    A. Indications for seclusion and restraint
    B. Contraindications to seclusion and restraint

57.36 Patient voluntarily requests

57.37 Prevent significant disruption to treatment program

57.38 Part of ongoing behavior therapy

57.39 For punishment

ANSWERS

Forensic Psychiatry

57.1 The answer is A

Suicide and suicide attempts are the most frequent causes for lawsuits against psychiatrists; 50 percent of suicides lead to malpractice actions by relatives. The greatest degree of supervision (inpatient setting) is associated with the most culpability. The *use of restraints, drug reactions*, and *patients committing violence* are all potential causes of malpractice that can be forestalled with proper documentation of clinical decision making and informed consent. *Sexual involvement* with a patient is both illegal and unethical.

57.2 The answer is E (all)

A potential pitfall of involuntary discharge or termination is the *charge of abandonment*. Malpractice litigation is often associated with situations in which there are bad feelings and a bad outcome. Consultation and *careful documentation* are important safeguards. Charges of abandonment can be avoided by referring the patient to another hospital or therapist. Some *authorities recommend giving a patient three names* of therapists, clinics, or hospitals. *A patient's treatment cannot be terminated while in a state of emergency.* The emergency must be resolved (for example, by hospitalization in cases of dangerousness) before treatment can be terminated and the patient transferred.

57.3 The answer is C

The Supreme Court, in *Dusky v United States* (1960), approved a test of competence that seeks to *ascertain whether a criminal defendant "has sufficient present ability to consult with his lawyer* with a reasonable degree of rational understanding and whether he has a rational as well as factual understanding of the proceedings against him." According to the 1976 case of *O'Connor v Donaldson*, the Supreme Court ruled that *harmless mental patients cannot be confined against their wills without treatment* if they can survive outside. In 1966, the District of Columbia Court of Appeals ruled in *Rouse v Cameron* that an involuntary inpatient who is not receiving treatment has a constitutional *right to be discharged*. According to this decision, the purpose of involuntary hospitalization is treatment.

In *Wyatt v Stickney* (1971), it was decided that civilly committed patients have a constitutional right to receive *adequate treatment*. In Tarasoff I (the case of *Tarasoff v Regents of the University of California* in 1974), it was ruled that *a psychotherapist or physician who has reason to believe that a patient may injure or kill someone must notify* the potential victim, the patient's relatives or friends, or the authorities.

57.4 The answer is C

Respondeat superior is a Latin phrase meaning "let the master answer for the deed of the servant." A person high in the chain of command is responsible for the actions of those under his or her supervision. Some psychiatrists carry vicarious liability insurance, which protects them against liability for actions against clinicians they supervise directly or indirectly. Psychiatrists should remove themselves from situations in which they bear responsibility for clinicians whom they cannot control. *Mens rea* and *actus reus* are concepts that apply to criminal law. A criminal act has two components: (1) voluntary conduct (*actus reus*) and (2) evil intent (*mens rea*). The insanity defense deals with these principles in that there cannot be evil intent when an offender's mental status deprives him or her of the capacity for rational intent.

Parens patriae is the doctrine that allows the state to intervene and act as surrogate parent for those who are unable to care for themselves or may harm themselves. This principle originally referred to a monarch's duty to protect the people (literally meaning "father of his country"). In U.S. common law, this doctrine refers to paternalism in which the state acts for people who are mentally ill and for minors. A writ of *habeas corpus* (literally, "you must have the body") is a legal procedure that asks a court to decide whether a patient has been hospitalized without due process of law. A writ of *habeas corpus* may be proclaimed by those who believe they have been illegally deprived of liberty.

57.5 The answer is A

Confidentiality pertains to the premise that all information imparted to the physician by the patient should be held secret. However, sharing information with other staff members treating the patient, clinical supervisors, and *a medical or psychiatric consultant* does not require the patient's permission. Sharing patient information with the *patient's family*, the *patient's attorney*, the *patient's previous therapist*, or *an insurer of the patient* does require the patient's permission. Courts may compel disclosure of confidential material (*subpoena duces tecum*). In emergencies, limited information may be released, but after the emergency, the clinician should inform the patient.

57.6 The answer is C

In 1954, in the case of *Durham v United States*, a decision was made by Judge David Bazelon, a pioneering jurist in forensic psychiatry in the District of Columbia Court of Appeals, that resulted in the *product rule of criminal responsibility*. An accused is not criminally responsible if his or her unlawful act was the product of mental disease or defect. Judge Bazelon stated that the purpose of the rule was to get good and complete psychiatric testimony. He sought to break the criminal law out of the theoretical straitjacket of the M'Naghten test.

Testimonial privilege is the right to maintain secrecy or confidentiality in the face of a subpoena. The privilege belongs to the patient, not to the physician, and it is waivable by the patient. *Involuntary admission* involves the question of whether or not the patient is a danger to self or others, such as in the suicidal or homicidal patient. Because those individuals do not recognize their need for hospital care, application for admission to a hospital may be made by a relative or friend and is involuntary. *Competency to stand trial* refers to defendants being able to comprehend the nature and the object of the proceedings against them in order to consult with counsel as well as to assist in preparing the defense.

57.7 The answer is A

The Gault decision applies to minors, those under the care of a parent or guardian and usually under age 18. In the case of minors, the parent or guardian is the person legally empowered to give consent to medical treatment. However, most states by statute list specific diseases or conditions that a minor may consent to have treated, such as venereal diseases, pregnancy, substance-related disorders, and contagious diseases. In an emergency, a physician may treat a minor without parental consent. The trend is to adopt the mature minor rule, allowing minors to consent to treatment under ordinary circumstances. As a result of the Gault decision, the juvenile must now be represented by counsel, be able to confront witnesses, and be given proper notice of any charges. Emancipated minors have the rights of adults when it can be demonstrated that they are living as adults with control over their own lives.

A writ of *habeas corpus* may be proclaimed on behalf of anyone who claims he or she is being deprived of liberty illegally. The legal procedure asks a court to decide whether hospitalization has been accomplished without due process of the law, and the petition must be heard by a court at once, regardless of the manner or form in which it is filed. Hospitals are obligated to submit those petitions to the court immediately. *Informed consent* is knowledge of the risks and alternatives of a treatment method and formal acceptance of treatment.

Under classical tort (a tort is a wrongful act) theory, an intentional touching to which one has given no consent is a *battery*. Thus, the administration of electroconvulsive therapy or chemotherapy, although it may be therapeutic, is a battery when done without consent. Indeed, any unauthorized touching outside of conventional social intercourse constitutes a battery. It is an offense to the dignity of the person, an invasion of the right of self-determination, for which punitive and actual damages may be imposed.

57.8 The answer is E (all)

In some situations—such as *suspected child abuse*—the physician must report to the authorities, as specifically required by law. According to the American Psychiatric Association (APA), confidentiality may be broken when the patient will *probably commit murder* and the act can only be stopped by notification of police, when the patient will *probably commit suicide* and the act can only be stopped by notification of police, or when a patient who has *potentially life-threatening responsibilities* (for example, an airline pilot) shows marked impairment of judgment.

57.9 The answer is D

Sexual involvement with patients accounts for 6 percent of malpractice claims against psychiatrists and is the *least common cause of malpractice litigation*. This fact does not, however, minimize its importance as a problem. (It should be noted that the short statute of limitations for this particular offense may well discourage patients from pursuing litigation because they have not had sufficient time to reach a point of emotional readiness.) Sexual intimacy with a patient is both illegal and unethical. There are also serious legal and ethical questions about a psychotherapist's dating or marrying a patient even after discharging the patient from therapy. Most psychiatrists believe in the adage "Once a patient, always a patient."

For other malpractice claims, the following figures are given: *failure to manage suicide attempts*, 21 percent; *improper use of restraints*, 7 percent; and *failure to treat psychosis*, 14 percent. *Substance dependence* accounts for about 10 percent of claims and refers to the patient's having developed a substance-related disorder as a result of a psychiatrist's not monitoring carefully the prescribing of potentially addicting drugs.

57.10 The answer is E (all)

Although it is impossible to eliminate malpractice, some preventive approaches have been invaluable in clinical practice. The *documentation of good care* is a strong deterrent to liability. Such documentation should include the decision-making process, the clinician's rationale for treatment, and an evaluation of costs and benefits. *Psychiatrists should provide only the kind of care that they are qualified to deliver.* They should never overload their practices or overstretch their abilities, and they should take reasonable care of themselves. The *informed consent* process refers to a discussion between doctor and patient of the treatment proposed, the side effects of drugs, and the uncertainty of psychiatric practice. Such a dialogue helps prevent a liability suit. A consultation affords protection against liability because it allows the clinician to obtain information about his or her peer group's standard of practice. It also provides *a second opinion*, enabling the clinician to submit his or her judgment to the scrutiny of a peer. The clinician who takes the trouble to obtain a consultation in a difficult and complex case is unlikely to be viewed by a jury as careless and negligent. The patient's acceptance of the proposed treatment should be documented.

Answers 57.11–57.15

57.11 The answer is C

57.12 The answer is B

57.13 The answer is A

57.14 The answer is A

57.15 The answer is D

Various landmark legal cases have affected psychiatry and the law over the years. In the 1976 case of *O'Connor v Donaldson*, the U.S. Supreme Court ruled that *harmless mental patients cannot be confined against their will* without treatment if they can survive outside. According to the Court, a finding of mental illness alone cannot justify a state's confining persons in a hospital against their will; such patients must be considered dangerous to themselves or others before they are confined.

In 1971, in *Wyatt v Stickney* in Alabama Federal District Court, it was decided that persons civilly committed to a mental institution have a constitutional right to receive adequate care, and *standards were established for staffing, nutrition, physical facilities, and treatment.* In 1966, the District of Columbia Court of Appeals in *Rouse v Cameron* ruled that *the purpose of involuntary hospitalization is treatment* and that *a patient who is not receiving treatment has a constitutional right to be discharged* from the hospital.

In *The Myth of Mental Illness*, Thomas Szasz argued that the various psychiatric diagnoses are totally devoid of significance and that therefore *all forced confinements because of mental illness are unjust.* Szasz contended that psychiatrists have no place in the courts of law.

Answers 57.16–57.20

57.16 The answer is B

57.17 The answer is A

57.18 The answer is D

57.19 The answer is C

57.20 The answer is E

The precedent for determining legal responsibility was established in the British courts in 1843. The *M'Naghten rule* is known commonly as the right-wrong test because the alleged perpetrator is not guilty, by reason of insanity, if he or she is unable to tell right from wrong due to a mental disease. In 1922, jurists in England reexamined the M'Naghten rule and suggested broadening the concept of insanity in criminal cases to include the concept of the *irresistible impulse*—that is, a person charged with a criminal offense is not responsible for an act if the act was committed under circumstances that the person was unable to resist because of mental disease. To most psychiatrists the law is unsatisfactory because it covers only a small group of those who are mentally ill. However, it was used successfully in Virginia in the 1994 case of *Virginia v Bobbitt*, in which the defendant was acquitted of malicious wounding. The wife had cut off her husband's penis after apparently enduring a prolonged period of sexual, physical, and emotional abuse.

In 1954 in the case of *Durham v United States*, a decision resulted in the product rule of criminal responsibility, or the *Durham rule,* which states that an accused is not criminally responsible if his or her unlawful act was the product of mental disease or mental defect. Judge Bazelon stated that the purpose of the rule was to get good and complete psychiatric testimony. In 1972, the Court of Appeals for the District of Columbia in *United States v Brawner* discarded the rule in favor of the American Law Institute's 1962 model penal code test of criminal responsibility.

In its *model penal code*, the American Law Institute (ALI) recommended the following test of criminal responsibility: (1) Persons are not responsible for criminal conduct if at the time of such conduct, as the result of mental disease or defect, they lacked substantial capacity either to appreciate the criminality of their conduct or to conform their conduct to the requirement of the law, and (2) the term "mental disease or defect" in this test does not include an abnormality manifested only by repeated criminal or otherwise antisocial conduct.

Other attempts at reform have included the defense of *diminished capacity*, which is based on the claim that the defendant suffered some impairment (usually but not always because of mental illness) sufficient to interfere with the ability to formulate a specific element of the particular crime charged. Hence, the defense finds its most common use with so-called specific-intent crimes, such as first-degree murder.

Answers 57.21–57.25

57.21 The answer is E

57.22 The answer is B

57.23 The answer is D

57.24 The answer is C

57.25 The answer is A

The ALI (American Law Institute) test has two parts: a person is not responsible for criminal conduct if at the time of such conduct, as a result of mental disease or defect, he or she lacks substantial capacity either (1) to appreciate the criminality (wrongfulness) of his or her conduct or (2) to conform his or her conduct to the requirements of law. As used in this context, the term mental disease or defect does not include an abnormality manifested only by repeated criminal or otherwise antisocial conduct.

Thus, the ALI test contains both a cognitive and a volitional prong. Both John Hinckley, Jr., and Jeffrey Dahmer were tried under the ALI test. For example, Dahmer had struggled hard against his aberrant sexual impulses in the 7 years that elapsed between his first and second killings. However, the fact that Dahmer could plan his murders and systematically dispose of the bodies convinced the jury that he was able to control his behavior. All the testimony bolstered the notion that like most serial killers, Dahmer knew what he was doing and knew right from wrong. Finally, the jury did not accept the defense that Dahmer suffered from a mental illness to the degree that it had disabled his thinking or behavioral controls.

Allegations of negligence involving tardive dyskinesia are based on a failure to evaluate a patient properly, a failure to obtain informed consent, a negligent diagnosis of the patient's condition, and a failure to monitor.

Most of the above-noted allegations of negligence were claimed in the landmark case *Clites v State*. The plaintiff was a mentally retarded man who was institutionalized from age 11 and treated with major tranquilizers from age 18 to 23. The plaintiff's family sued, claiming that the defendants negligently prescribed medication, did not inform the patient of the possibility of developing tardive dyskinesia, and failed to monitor and subsequently treat the patient for the adverse effects of the drugs. The jury found for the plaintiff and awarded damages in the amount of $760,165. This award was affirmed on appeal.

The appellate court ruled that the defendants were negligent and deviated from the standards of "the industry." Among the "deviations" the court noted were the failure to conduct regular physical examinations and laboratory tests, the failure to intervene at the first signs of tardive dyskinesia, the inappropriate use of multiple medications at the same time, the

use of drugs for convenience (e.g., "behavior management") rather than for therapy, and the failure to obtain the plaintiff's informed consent.

The acceptability of restraint or seclusion for the purposes of training was recognized by the Supreme Court in *Youngberg v Romeo*, which challenged the treatment practices at the Pennhurst State School and Hospital in Pennsylvania. The Court held that patients could not be restrained except to ensure their safety or, in certain undefined circumstances, "to provide needed training." Although recognizing that the defendant had a liberty interest in safety and freedom from bodily restraint, the Court noted that these interests were not absolute nor in conflict with the need to provide training. The Court also held that decisions made by appropriate professionals regarding restraining the patient would be presumed correct. Psychiatrists and other mental health professionals have lauded the decision because the Court recognized that professionals are better able than courts to determine the needs of patients, including deciding when restraint is appropriate.

Confidentiality refers to the right of a patient to have communications spoken or written in confidence to a psychiatrist kept undisclosed to outside parties without authorization. Four general sources provide the bases for recognizing and safeguarding patient confidences. First, all 50 states and the District of Columbia have acknowledged this right of protection by creating some form of confidentiality provisions in either professional licensure laws or confidentiality and privilege statutes. In 1996, the United States Supreme Court (in *Redmond v Jaffe*) ruled that communications between psychotherapist and patient are confidential and need not be disclosed in federal trials. The second source, with the longest tradition, comprises the ethical codes of the various mental health professions. Third, common law has long recognized an attorney–client privilege; developing case law has established similar protection for physicians and psychotherapists. Fourth, the right of confidentiality may be subsumed under the right of privacy.

Most courts now follow the ruling in *Ramon v Farr*—that is, that drug inserts alone do not set the standard of care. They are only one factor to be considered, in addition to previous personal experience, the scientific literature, expert testimony, approvals in other countries, and other pertinent factors. The PDA, the *Physicians' Desk Reference*, or any other reference source cannot substitute for the psychiatrist's clinical judgment. A substantial body of scientific literature that justifies the clinician's treatment is vastly more persuasive. Similarly, in managed care settings, psychiatrists must vigorously resist efforts to restrict their choice of drugs by predetermined, limited formularies, nor should the choice of generic or proprietary drugs or drug dosages be dictated by others. The treating psychiatrist must determine the specific drug to be prescribed according to the clinical needs of the patient.

Answers 57.26–57.30

57.26 The answer is A

57.27 The answer is B

57.28 The answer is A

57.29 The answer is C

57.30 The answer is D

Under the common law, the basic elements of a crime are (1) the mental state or *level of intent to commit the act* (known as the *mens rea* or guilty mind), (2) the act itself or *conduct associated with committing the crime* (known as *actus reus* or guilty act), and (3) a concurrence in time between the guilty act and the guilty state of mind. The state must prove beyond a reasonable doubt that the defendant committed the criminal act with the requisite intent in order to convict a person of a particular crime. The law recognizes shades of mental impairment that can affect *mens rea*, but not necessarily to the extent of completely nullifying it. The concept of *diminished capacity* was developed for these situations.

Diminished capacity allows the defendant to introduce medical and psychological evidence that relates directly to the *mens rea* for the crime charged, without having to assert a defense of insanity. For example, in the crime of assault with the intent to kill, psychiatric testimony may be permitted to address whether the offender acted with the purpose of committing homicide at the time of the assault. When a defendant's *mens rea* for the crime charged is not supported by clinical evidence, the defendant is acquitted only of that charge. The diminished capacity defense does not lead to total exculpation of criminal responsibility nor to automatic commitment to a mental institution.

The automatism (or unconscious) defense recognizes that some criminal acts may be committed involuntarily. Automatism, defined as "having performed in a state of mental unconsciousness or dissociation without full awareness," is applied to actions or conduct occurring "without will, purpose, or reasoned intention."

For conviction for a crime, a criminal state of mind (*mens rea*) must be accompanied by the commission of a prohibited act (*actus reus*). The physical act must be conscious and volitional. Statutory and common law in most jurisdictions specifically excludes from the *actus reus* a reflex or convulsion, a bodily movement occurring during unconsciousness or sleep, acts during hypnosis or resulting from hypnotic suggestion, and a bodily movement that is not conscious and voluntary.

The classic, though rare, example of an automatism is the person who commits an offense while sleepwalking. Courts have held that such individuals do not have conscious control of their physical actions and therefore act involuntarily. This defense exists for persons committing a crime during a state of unconsciousness caused by a concussion following a head injury, involuntary ingestion of drugs or alcohol, hypoxia or hypoglycemia, or epileptic seizures.

There are clear limitations to the automatism defense. The automatism defense is not available if the person was aware of the condition prior to the offense and failed to take reasonable steps to prevent the crime. If, for example, a defendant with a known history of poorly controlled epileptic seizures loses control of a car during a seizure and kills another person, that defendant cannot assert the defense of automatism.

Answers 57.31–57.35

57.31 The answer is A

57.32 The answer is A

57.33 The answer is D

57.34 The answer is D

57.35 The answer is B

Testimonial privilege, a statutorily created rule of evidence, permits the holder of the privilege (e.g., the patient) to exercise the right to prevent the person to whom confidential information was given (e.g., the psychiatrist) from disclosing it in a judicial proceeding. *The patient—not the psychiatrist—holds the privilege that controls the release of confidential information.* It is called testimonial privilege because it applies only to the judicial setting. Privilege statutes represent the most common recognition by the state of the importance of protecting information provided by a patient to a psychotherapist. This recognition departs from the essential truth-finding purpose of the American system of justice by *insulating certain information from disclosure in court*. This protection is justified by the special need for privacy in the doctor–patient relationship that outweighs the quest for an accurate outcome in court.

Privilege statutes cover most of the mental health professions. Cases have been successfully litigated in which the broader physician–patient category was applied to the psychotherapist in the absence of an applicable statute.

Privilege statutes also specify numerous exceptions to testimonial privilege. The most common exceptions include *child abuse reporting, civil commitment proceedings*, court-ordered examinations, competency proceedings, and cases in which a patient's mental state is in question as part of litigation. This last exception, known as the *patient-litigant exception*, commonly occurs in will contests*, workers' compensation cases,* child custody disputes, personal injury litigation, and malpractice actions.

Answers 57.36–57.39

57.36 The answer is A

57.37 The answer is A

57.38 The answer is A

57.39 The answer is B

Most states have enacted statutes that regulate the use of restraints, often specifying the circumstances in which restraints can be used—usually when a risk of harm to self or danger to others is imminent. Statutory regulation of the use of seclusion is much less common. About one-half of states have laws governing seclusion. Most states with laws regarding seclusion and restraint require some type of documentation of the usage. A number of courts and state statutes outline certain due-process procedures that must be followed before restraint or seclusion can be used for nonclinically indicated, disciplinary purposes. These include some form of notice, a hearing, and involvement of an impartial decision-maker.

The APA Task Force on the Psychiatric Uses of Seclusion and Restraint has developed guidelines for the appropriate use of seclusion and restraints, and the Joint Commission on Accreditation of Healthcare Organizations (JCAHO) has promulgated guidelines for hospitals regarding seclusion and

Table 57.1
Indications for Seclusion and Restraint

1. Prevent clear, imminent harm to the patient or others
2. *Prevent significant disruption to treatment program* or physical surroundings
3. Assist in treatment as *part of ongoing behavior therapy*
4. Decrease sensory overstimulation*a*
5. At *patient's voluntary reasonable request*

*a*Seclusion only.
Reprinted with permission from Simon RI. *Concise Guide to Psychiatry and the Law for Clinicians.* 2nd ed. Washington, DC: American Psychiatric Press; 1998.

Table 57.2
Contraindications to Seclusion and Restraint

1. Extremely unstable medical and psychiatric conditions
2. Delirious or demented patients unable to tolerate decreased stimulation
3. Overtly suicidal patients
4. Patients with severe drug reactions, overdoses, or requiring close monitoring of drug dosages
5. *For punishment* or convenience of staff

restraint requirements. Professional opinion concerning the clinical uses of physical restraints and seclusion varies considerably among psychiatrists. Seclusion can be justified on both clinical and legal grounds for a variety of uses, unless precluded by state freedom from restraint and seclusion statutes.

Seclusion and restraint raise complex psychiatric legal issues and *have both indications and contraindications* (Tables 57.1 and 57.2). Further, seclusion and restraint have become increasingly regulated over the past decade.

Legal challenges to the use of restraints and seclusion have been brought on behalf of institutionalized mentally ill and mentally retarded persons. Typically, these lawsuits do not stand alone but are part of a challenge to a wide range of alleged abuses.

Generally, courts hold, or consent decrees provide, that restraints and seclusion be implemented only when a patient creates a risk of harm to self or others and no less-restrictive alternative is available. Additional restrictions include the following:

1. Restraint and seclusion can only be implemented by a written order from an appropriate medical official.
2. Orders are to be confined to specific, time-limited periods.
3. A patient's condition must be reviewed regularly and documented.
4. Any extension of an original order must be reviewed and reauthorized.

58

Ethics in Psychiatry

Psychiatrists routinely confront basic ethical issues, in particular through the imposing of involuntary treatments on patients against their wills. These issues highlight the profound ethical dilemmas between autonomy and beneficence that psychiatrists and their patients deal with continually. In other words, it is the potential—and common—conflict between the right of patients to self-determination and the duty of psychiatrists to act in the best interest of their patients. Beneficence refers to "the duty to do no harm," and autonomy to a patient's right to choose. It is easy to see how in psychiatry these concepts can be highly complex, leading to conflicting interpretations and opinions about appropriate care. Psychiatry has a less-than-illustrious history with regard to adequately safeguarding the rights of mentally ill patients, and this history has led to an extensive involvement of the legal system in all aspects of psychiatric involuntary care and decision making.

Major ethical theories underlie most of the ethical questions routinely faced by psychiatrists, and clinicians need to be aware of how these theories conceptualize the issues. These theories include utilitarian theory, which postulates that a fundamental obligation in decision making is to produce the greatest possible benefit to the greatest number of people. Utilitarian theory is most often the basis of large societal decisions about the allocation of services and resources. Autonomy theory postulates that the doctor–patient relationship is one between two equal parties, and that patients are self-governing, with a fundamental right to self-determination in medical and psychiatric decision making. Truth telling, confidentiality, informed consent, the right to refuse treatment, the right to die, limitations on the right of psychiatrists to involuntarily treat and hospitalize people, and sexual contact with patients are all examples of ethical concerns addressed by ethical theory.

The student should study the questions and answers below for a useful review of this topic.

▲ QUESTIONS

DIRECTIONS: Each of the questions or incomplete statements below is followed by five suggested responses or completions. Select the *one* that is *best* in each case.

58.1 Choose the *one* best answer about *Cruzan v Missouri Board of Health.*

A. All patients hold the right to have life support withdrawn.
B. Early-stage fetuses have no legal standing.
C. Only conscious patients can have life-sustaining treatment withdrawn.
D. All competent patients can refuse medical care.
E. None of the above

58.2 Confidentiality

A. is maintained under the principles of patient autonomy
B. may be broken under the principle of distributive justice
C. may be broken under the principle of beneficence
D. was an issue in the *Tarasoff* decision
E. all of the above

58.3 In the *Tarasoff* case

A. The principle of beneficence outweighed the principle of justice.

B. The principle of beneficence outweighed the principle of nonmaleficence.

C. The principle of justice outweighed the principle of nonmaleficence.

D. The principle of nonmaleficence outweighed the principle of justice.

E. None of the above

58.4 *Tarasoff II*

A. requires that therapists report a patient's fantasies of homicide

B. reinforces that a therapist has only the duty to warn

C. expands on the earlier ruling to include the duty to protect

D. states that usually the patient must be a danger both to a person and property

E. none of the above

58.5 The most pervasive ethical conflict in psychiatry is between

A. autonomy and beneficence

B. autonomy and justice

C. justice and nonmaleficence

D. beneficence and justice

E. beneficence and nonmaleficence

58.6 Possible ethical transgressions that psychiatrists may commit fall into which of the following categories?

A. Sexual boundary violations

B. Nonsexual boundary violations

C. Violations of confidentiality

D. Mistreatment of the patient (e.g., incompetence)

E. All of the above

58.7 Sexual activity in the context of psychiatric treatment is considered acceptable if

A. the sexual activity is consensual

B. the sexual activity is with a patient's family member and not the patient

C. the sexual activity is with a former (not current) patient

D. the psychiatrist in question obtains a consultation with a more experienced colleague

E. none of the above

DIRECTIONS: These lettered headings are followed by a list of numbered phrases. For each numbered phrase, select the *one* lettered heading most associated with it. Each lettered heading may be used once, more than once, or not at all.

Questions 58.8–58.11

A. Utilitarian theory

B. Paternalism

C. Autonomy theory

58.8 The basis for making decisions about the allocation of society's resources for treatment and medical research

58.9 The traditional model of the physician–patient relationship

58.10 The physician's duty of beneficence

58.11 The right to informed consent

DIRECTIONS: For each numbered question below, answer whether or not the situation described is ethical by selecting the appropriate lettered heading.

Questions 58.12–58.15

A. Yes

B. No

58.12 Confidentiality must be maintained after the death of a patient

58.13 The psychiatrist can make a determination of suicide as a result of mental illness for insurance purposes solely from reading the patient's records

58.14 Dating a patient 1 year after discharge is ethical

58.15 The psychiatrist may divulge information about the patient if the patient desires

DIRECTIONS: Each group of lettered headings below is followed by a list of numbered phrases. For each numbered phrase, select

A. if the item is associated with *A only*

B. if the item is associated with *B only*

C. if the item is associated with *both A and B*

D. if the item is associated with *neither A nor B*

Questions 58.16–58.20

A. Ethical dilemma

B. Ethical conflict

C. Both

D. Neither

58.16 Preserving patient confidentiality versus protecting endangered third parties

58.17 Patient–therapist sexual relations

58.18 Choice between two ethically legitimate alternatives

58.19 Compromise of an ethical principle, usually because of self-interest

58.20 American Psychiatric Association (APA) may expel or suspend members from the organization

ANSWERS

Ethics in Psychiatry

58.1 The answer is D

In *Cruzan v Missouri Board of Health*, the U.S. Supreme Court upheld *the right of a competent person* to have "a constitutionally protected liberty interest *in refusing* unwanted *medical treatment.*" *The Court applied this principle to all patients, conscious or unconscious, who have made their wishes clearly known,* whether or not they ever regain consciousness. *Life support can be refused or withdrawn provided that the patient made his or her wishes known.* The *legal standing of fetuses relates to Roe v Wade,* not *Cruzan v Missouri.* Cruzan applies to both conscious and unconscious patients, provided that the latter have already made their wishes known. The U.S. Supreme Court permits each state to decide the standards it wishes to apply when asked to withhold or withdraw treatment from a person in a persistent vegetative state who has not previously stated his or her wishes on the subject.

58.2 The answer is E (all)

Therapist–patient confidentiality is a broad right. Under normal conditions, *patient autonomy* mandates maintenance of confidentiality. The principle of *distributive justice* means that all members of society are allocated an equal share of public safety. Under this principle, confidentiality can be broken to protect members of society from harm. *The Tarasoff decision* mandates that third parties must be notified and protected when a therapist believes a patient to be an immediate threat to the third party. Confidentiality may be broken in certain circumstances by a physician's beneficent action. *Beneficence* is a feature of paternalism in which physicians act in the best interest of a patient. A therapist calling the authorities to hospitalize a suicidal patient is an example of a legal and beneficent breach of confidentiality.

58.3 The answer is E (none)

The Tarasoff case is an example of the legal system's attempt to solve a social problem—the need to safeguard life—by creating an ethical dilemma for the psychiatrist. This case, which began as a civil lawsuit, ended up with the California Supreme Court ruling that a psychotherapist has a duty to warn and protect a potential victim of a potentially dangerous patient. *The court proclaimed that the principles of justice and nonmaleficence outweighed the principle of beneficence.* Most states have agreed with the Tarasoff court and have enacted laws requiring psychotherapists to warn potential victims or to warn the police when an identified person is threatened.

Nonmaleficence is the duty of the psychiatrist to avoid either inflicting physical and emotional harm on the patient or increasing the risk of such harm. That principle is captured by *primum non nocere,* "first, do no harm."

Like the principles of autonomy, nonmaleficence, and beneficence, the principle of justice in psychiatry does not operate in a vacuum but is responsive to the ever-changing social, political, religious, and legal mores of the moment.

Does establishment of a therapist–patient relationship oblige the therapist to care for the safety of not only the patient but also others? This issue was raised in 1976 in the case of *Tarasoff v Regents of University of California* (now known as *Tarasoff I*). In

this case, Prosenjit Poddar, a student and voluntary outpatient at the mental health clinic of the University of California, told his therapist that he intended to kill a student readily identified as Tatiana Tarasoff. Realizing the seriousness of the intention, the therapist, with concurrence of a colleague, concluded that Poddar should be committed for observation under a 72-hour emergency psychiatric detention provision of the California commitment law. The therapist notified the campus police both orally and in writing that Poddar was dangerous and should be committed.

Concerned about the breach of confidentiality, the therapist's supervisor vetoed the recommendation and ordered all records relating to Poddar's treatment destroyed. At the same time, the campus police temporarily detained Poddar but released him on his assurance that he would "stay away from that girl." Poddar stopped going to the clinic when he learned from the police about his therapist's recommendation to commit him. Two months later, he carried out his threat to kill Tatiana. The young woman's parents then sued the university for negligence.

The California Supreme Court deliberated the case for the unprecedented time of about 14 months and ruled that a physician or a psychotherapist who has reason to believe that a patient may injure or kill someone must notify the potential victim, the victim's relatives or friends, or the authorities.

58.4 The answer is C

The *Tarasoff I* ruling *does not require that therapists report a patient's fantasies of homicide;* instead, it requires therapists to report an intended homicide; further, it is the therapist's duty to exercise good judgment.

In 1982, the California Supreme Court issued a second ruling in the case of *Tarasoff v Regents of University of California (now known as Tarasoff II), which broadened (rather than merely reinforced) its earlier ruling, the duty to warn, to include the duty to protect.*

The *Tarasoff II* ruling has stimulated intense debates in the medicolegal field. Lawyers, judges, and expert witnesses argue the definition of protection, the nature of the relationship between the therapist and the patient, and the balance between public safety and individual privacy. Clinicians argue that the duty to protect hinders treatment because a patient may not trust a doctor if confidentiality is not maintained. Furthermore, because it is not easy to determine whether a patient is dangerous enough to justify long-term incarceration, unnecessary involuntary hospitalization may occur because of a therapist's defensive practices.

As a result of such heated debates in the field since 1976, the state courts have not made a uniform interpretation of the *Tarasoff II* ruling (the duty to protect). Generally, clinicians should note whether a specific identifiable victim seems to be in imminent and probable danger from the threat of an action contemplated by a mentally ill patient; the harm, in addition to being imminent, should be potentially serious or severe. *Usually the patient must be a danger to another person, not to property,* and the therapist should take clinically reasonable actions.

In a few cases (none successful so far) claims have already been advanced that a *Tarasoff*-like duty applies to potential infection of partners with human immunodeficiency virus (HIV) by patients under mental health treatment. The breach of confidentiality in *Tarasoff* cases is justified only by the threat of violence. Laws vary confusingly by jurisdiction. Perhaps the ideal solution is to persuade patients to make the disclosure to and report the matter to public health authorities.

58.5 The answer is A

Which one of the four core ethical principles—*autonomy, nonmaleficence, beneficence,* and *justice*—dominates depends on the particular situation. On the one hand, respect for patient autonomy is salient when psychosurgery is proposed, but the principle of social justice may be in force in deciding who receives an expensive new medication that is scarce. The most pervasive ethical conflict in psychiatry and in medicine as a whole is that between autonomy, the right of patients to self-determination, and beneficence, the duty of physicians to act in the best interest of their patients.

The principle of patient autonomy is of central importance and, conceptually, is in many ways coextensive with the legal concept of competence. A patient makes an autonomous choice by giving informed consent when that choice is (1) intentional, (2) free of undue outside influence, and (3) made with rational understanding. Usually, when patients respond to a choice by saying "yes," the desire to comply is assumed. However, that assumption may not be valid with a highly confused patient.

The principle of beneficence—to prevent or remove harm and promote well-being—was the primary driving principle of medical and psychiatric practice throughout history until the rise of consumerism and other factors in the late 1960s. The expression of the principle is paternalism, use of the psychiatrist's judgment as to what course of action is best for the patient or the research subject.

58.6 The answer is E (all)

Most professional organizations and many business groups have codes of ethics. Such codes reflect a consensus about the general standards of appropriate professional conduct. The American Medical Association's (AMA) *Principles of Medical Ethics*, the American Psychiatric Association's (APA) *The Principles*, and the American College of Physicians *Ethics Manual* articulate ideal standards of practice and professional virtues of practitioners.

The 1995 edition of *The Principles* provides a useful and comprehensive example of an ethics code geared to the psychiatric profession. The manual covers a broad array of psychiatric ethical issues, from fee splitting and sex with former patients to psychiatrists' participation in executions, all of which are unethical. Another useful manual is the 1995 edition of the *Opinions of the Ethics Committee on the Principles of Medical Ethics with Annotations Especially Applicable to Psychiatry*. This manual, developed by APA Ethics Committee members and consultants, provides answers to commonly asked ethical questions.

The Principles, if carefully read, will suggest to the student and practitioner certain behaviors that are expected of an ethical psychiatrist and certain behaviors deemed by the profession to be unethical and unacceptable. The APA and its district branches have a carefully worked out set of procedures to be followed if a member of that organization is accused of violating the ethical principles. While these procedures are not perfect, they seem to have served the profession well for more than 20 years. Further, they are changed in response to changes in federal and state laws and the oversights that have become apparent.

From a practical point of view, the transgressions that psychiatrists most frequently commit fall into a few categories, and certain activities may fit in more than one category:

1. *sexual boundary violations*
2. *nonsexual boundary violations*
3. *violations of confidentiality*
4. *mistreatment of the patient* (incompetence, double agentry)
5. illegal activities (insurance, billing, insider stock trading)

58.7 The answer is E (none)

Sexual activity with a current or former patient is unethical—a black-and-white matter. The rest is commentary.

By far the most publicized ethical transgressions of psychiatrists involve sexual activity with a patient or a former patient. A variety of defenses have been advanced by psychiatrists accused of such activity; yet it should be obvious what a sexual activity is, what a patient is, and what a former patient is.

The Principles is quite clear on the subject. *Sexual activity with a current or former patient is unethical.* Glen Gabbard has studied a great many psychotherapists who have gotten into trouble because of sexual involvement with patients. He categorized them into some interesting groups including psychotic disorders, predatory psychopathy and paraphilias, lovesickness, and masochistic surrender.

Clearly, with such different types of psychotherapists involved in sexual activity with patients, no one pattern of behavior can provide a danger signal. Yet, if one studies complaints brought to professional societies, a rather distinctive pattern does emerge, the slippery slope of smaller violations leading to greater violations.

A male therapist is treating a female patient who may have some borderline personality traits. During a particularly emotional session, the doctor holds the patient's hand or puts his arm around her shoulder to comfort her. Perhaps there is even a hug; later, another emotional session and another hug, this time a bit longer. Soon each session ends with a hug, and maybe a kiss on the cheek. Later, the patient calls the doctor in the evening, sobbing. The doctor makes a house call; more hugs, more kisses. A suicide gesture is often catalytic. This scenario can get quite complicated and involved but it is not uncommon. At this point the situation is, without question, a psychiatric emergency. The doctor must obtain an immediate *consultation from an experienced colleague.* Unfortunately, this option is rarely taken. Whether due to embarrassment, fear of criticism from the community, denial, or an unwarranted sense of omnipotence, the scenarios usually progress down the slippery slope, and sexual activity replaces treatment.

An argument occasionally put forward is that the *sexual activity is consensual*—that is, it takes place between two autonomous adults, and consequently they should be able to do as they please. Yet even a rudimentary knowledge of dynamic psychiatry reveals that the two adults are virtually never autonomous. Powerful, unconscious forces are at work in all doctor–patient relationships. The patient does not have to lie on a couch five times a week to develop transference. Transference occurs in every encounter with a therapist. Even the brief medication-management visit produces transference (and countertransference). *Sexual activity with a former patient* is also unacceptable. *The Principles* is quite clear in Section 2.1.

Although not spelled out in *The Principles*, sexual activity with a patient's family member is also unethical. This is most important when the psychiatrist is treating a child or adolescent. Most training programs in child and adolescent psychiatry emphasize that the parents are patients too, and that the ethical and legal proscriptions apply to parents (or parent surrogates) as well as to the child. Nevertheless, some psychiatrists ignore this ethical violation.

Answers 58.8–58.11

58.8 The answer is A

58.9 The answer is B

58.10 The answer is B

58.11 The answer is C

Utilitarian theory holds that our fundamental obligation when making decisions is to try to produce the greatest possible happiness for the greatest number of people. Sometimes the choices available are dismal. In that case, one should act in ways that produce the least pain. Utilitarian theory is still used as *the basis for making decisions about the allocation of society's resources* for treatment and medical research.

Paternalism may be defined as a system in which someone acts for another's benefit without that person's consent. The requirement that health care practitioners be licensed is an example of state paternalism. *Individual paternalism* was *the traditional model of the physician–patient relationship*. In this model the physician is supposed to treat the patient as a caring parent would treat a child. The parent is assumed to know what is best for the child and has no obligation to ask the child for permission to perform actions that may benefit the child. *The physician's duty of beneficence*, the principle of doing good and avoiding harm, is a *paternalistic principle*. The physician is presumed to have knowledge that the patient may not understand or in certain instances is better off not knowing.

Autonomy theory presumes that the normal adult patient has the ability and the right to make rational and responsible decisions. The patient is self-governing (autonomous) and has rights to self-determination. The relationship between physician and patient is perceived as a relationship between two responsible adults. The patient's right to refuse treatment, *the right to informed consent*, and the assumption of competence are examples of the person's right to self-determination.

Answers 58.12–58.15

58.12 The answer is A (yes)

58.13 The answer is A (yes)

58.14 The answer is B (no)

58.15 The answer is A (yes)

Ethically, confidences survive a patient's death. Exceptions include proper legal compulsions and protecting others from imminent harm.

It is *ethical to make a diagnosis of suicide secondary to mental illness* on the basis of reviewing the patient's records. Sometimes called a psychological autopsy, interviews with friends, family, and others who knew the deceased may also be useful.

Proponents of the view "Once a patient, always a patient" insist that any involvement with an ex-patient—even a date or one that leads to marriage—should be prohibited. They maintain that a transferential reaction always exists between the patient and the therapist and that it prevents a rational decision about their emotional or sexual union. Some psychiatrists maintain that a reasonable time should elapse before any such liaison. The length to the "reasonable" period remains controversial: Some have suggested 2 years, not 1 year.

The *Principles of Medical Ethics with Annotations Especially Applicable to Psychiatry*, however, states: "*Sexual activity with a* current or *former patient is unethical.*"

The patient has the right (known as privilege) of insisting *that information about his or her case be divulged* to those who request it. Psychiatrists are allowed to contest that right if they believe that the patient will be harmed by revealing such information. Psychiatrists may stipulate that a report sent to a third party not be shown to the patient; however, in complex cases proper disposition of records may have to be adjudicated.

Answers 58.16–58.20

58.16 The answer is A

58.17 The answer is B

58.18 The answer is A

58.19 The answer is B

58.20 The answer is B

The term "ethics" is usually reserved for the moral principles restricted to certain groups, such as those in a profession. That role-bound morality can consist of internal or external standards of ethical conduct. For the psychiatric profession, *The Principles of Medical Ethics with Annotations Especially for Psychiatry*, developed by the American Psychiatric Association (APA), is an example of an internal standard used by the profession's major organization to regulate the behavior of its members. Judicial, legislative, or executive bodies may impose external standards as well.

Distinguishing between an ethical dilemma and an ethical violation or conflict is important. One is faced with an *ethical dilemma when asked to choose between two ethically legitimate alternatives,* such as *preserving patient confidentiality or protecting endangered third parties.* An *ethical conflict* involves the *compromise of an ethical principle, usually because of self-interest,* such as *patient–therapist sexual relations.*

For ethical violations the *APA may expel members* from the organization *or*, for less severe violations, *suspend membership for a time.* During that time a member may be required to undergo supervision or extra training. For still less severe violations a member may be reprimanded or admonished, with no effect on membership status. Expulsion or suspension from the APA is publicly reported. Further, such actions must be reported to the National Practitioners Data Bank.

59 ▲

Public and Hospital Psychiatry

Public psychiatry refers to the treatment of mentally ill people in the community and reflects the profound changes in the approach to the treatment of the chronically mentally ill since the 1960s. Chronic psychiatric patients are no longer institutionalized for lengthy periods of time but are now much more often hospitalized only briefly, under specific legal restrictions, and then managed in community mental health centers. Generally, all aspects of care, from hospitalization to case management, day treatment, and other supportive living arrangements, fall in the public domain and are government funded. Implicit in this description is the fact that public mental health is a total system of care, not a single service. Prevention is a part of public psychiatry, with the goal of decreasing the onset, duration, and ongoing disabilities of psychiatric illness. Unfortunately, a number of the chronically mentally ill have fallen through the cracks of deinstitutionalization, and their numbers are evident in the problem of the homeless mentally ill visible particularly in large urban areas. Public psychiatry faces the dilemma of trying to provide services to extremely vulnerable people with multiple needs, in a time of tight federal, state, and local budgets.

The student should study the questions and answers below for a useful review of this topic.

HELPFUL HINTS

The student should be able to define and categorize the signs and symptoms and other terms listed below.

- ▶ case management
- ▶ chronic mental illness
- ▶ community mental health
- ▶ conservatorship
- ▶ consultations
- ▶ deinstitutionalization
- ▶ evaluation and research
- ▶ family issues
- ▶ federal regulations
- ▶ homeless mentally ill
- ▶ hospital treatment programs
- ▶ indications for hospitalization
- ▶ intensive care managers
- ▶ least-restrictive alternative
- ▶ long-term care
- ▶ National Alliance for the Mentally Ill (NAMI)
- ▶ National Mental Health Association (NMHA)
- ▶ outreach programs
- ▶ partial hospitalization
- ▶ prevention (primary, secondary, tertiary)
- ▶ prison psychiatric issues
- ▶ psychiatric nursing
- ▶ public psychiatry
- ▶ rehabilitation
- ▶ services
- ▶ single-room occupancy residences
- ▶ therapeutic community
- ▶ token economy
- ▶ transinstitutionalization

▲ QUESTIONS

DIRECTIONS: Each of the incomplete statements below is followed by five suggested responses or completions. Select the *one* that is *best* in each case.

59.1 True statements about public psychiatry include

    A. It encompasses all federal, state, and local mental health service systems.

    B. Services may be provided directly by civil servants or contracted by government to either nonprofit or for-profit agencies.

    C. The essential feature is that all services are the responsibility of government and are provided to those who don't have the means to provide their own care.

    D. The present idea of public psychiatry was largely shaped by federal regulations passed in the 1960s.

    E. All of the above

59.2 The Community Mental Health Centers Act

    A. was passed under the leadership of President Jimmy Carter in the 1970s

    B. provided funds for the construction of community mental health centers without specified catchment areas

    C. stipulated that each center must provide five basic psychiatric services, including emergency services and inpatient care

    D. does not require the provision of drug-abuse services

    E. none of the above

59.3 True statements about the concept of "least-restrictive alternatives" include

    A. Patients' rights advocates argue that this is the least crucial principle in the treatment of the mentally ill.

    B. Clinicians rarely feel that the principle can be compromised in the intent of therapeutic efficacy.

    C. It refers to the practice of involuntary hospitalization in the case of suicidal ideation.

    D. It is not accepted by most mental health practitioners.

    E. None of the above

59.4 The goal of preventative psychiatry is to decrease the

    A. onset (incidence) of mental disorders

    B. duration (prevalence) of mental disorders

    C. residual disability of mental disorders

    D. chronicity of mental disorders

    E. all of the above

DIRECTIONS: The following group of questions consists of lettered headings followed by a list of numbered phrases. For each numbered phrase, select the *one* lettered heading that is most closely associated with it. Each lettered heading may be selected once, more than once, or not at all.

Questions 59.5–59.10

    A. Primary prevention
    B. Secondary prevention
    C. Tertiary prevention

59.5 Reduces incidence
59.6 Reduces risk factors
59.7 "Debriefing" group programs for disaster survivors
59.8 Shortens duration of a condition
59.9 Reduces prevalence of residual disabilities
59.10 Rehabilitation

DIRECTIONS: Each of the questions or incomplete statements below is followed by five suggested responses or completions. Select the *one* that is *best* in each case.

59.11 True statements about homeless mentally ill persons include

    A. The percentage of homeless people estimated to be mentally ill is approximately 10 percent.
    B. Comorbid substance abuse in the homeless mentally ill is relatively low.
    C. Most suffer from schizophrenia or schizoaffective disorder.
    D. Uniformity in diagnosis and functional performance is the rule.
    E. None of the above

59.12 Medical conditions associated with the homeless mentally ill include

    A. cellulitis
    B. tuberculosis
    C. anemia
    D. lice infestation
    E. all of the above

59.13 Outpatient commitment programs (OCP)

    A. are mandated by a judge
    B. are the same as conservatorships
    C. cannot mandate medication treatment
    D. do not involve case managers
    E. have shown a high rate of noncompliance

59.14 The therapeutic community model of in-patient hospitalization

    A. is most effective in units that treat a large number of psychotic patients
    B. was originally designed for patients with primary mood disorders
    C. looks at the hospital unit as a social system
    D. emphasizes hospital hierarchy in unit decision making
    E. is derived from experimental psychology and principles of operant conditioning

---

ANSWERS

Public and Hospital Psychiatry

59.1 The answer is E (all)

Public psychiatry encompasses all mental health service systems that are primarily sponsored and funded by governments—federal, state, and local. It is no longer appropriate to conceptualize hospital and community services as separate treatment systems: They are integral components of the spectrum of services essential to any public mental health treatment system. All aspects of care, from hospitalization, case management, and crisis intervention to day treatment and supportive living arrangements, are the province of public psychiatry. *Services may be provided directly by civil servants or contracted by government* to either nonprofit or for-profit agencies. *The essential feature is that all services are the responsibility of government* and are offered to those who do not have the means to provide for their own care.

    The present idea of public psychiatry was largely shaped by federal regulations passed in the 1960s to offer persons who were mentally ill financial support in their communities and to establish community mental health centers. Rather than isolat-ing persons with mental disorders for long periods in state hospitals, legislators thought it preferable to treat these persons in the community and to hospitalize them only briefly and under certain restrictions.

59.2 The answer is C

In 1963 (not the 1970s), under the leadership of President John F. Kennedy (not Jimmy Carter), Congress passed the Community Mental Health Centers Act, which provided funds for the construction of community mental health centers with specified catchment areas (geographical regions with a population of 75,000 to 200,000). *Each community health center must provide five basic psychiatric services: inpatient care, emergency services* (on a 24-hour basis), community consultation, day care (including partial hospitalization programs, halfway houses, aftercare services, and a broad range of outpatient services), and research and education. *In 1975, Congress added the requirements of services* for children and older persons, prehospitalization, screening, follow-up services for those who have been hospitalized, transitional housing, and alcoholism and *drug-abuse services to the community centers' responsibilities.* By the early 1980s, the community mental health center movement had strongly influenced mental health services, the practice of psychiatry, and the other mental health professions.

59.3 The answer is E (none)

The well-accepted concept of least-restrictive alternatives means that *mentally ill persons should be treated in settings that interfere least with their civil rights and freedom* to participate in society. Patients should not be hospitalized (especially against their wills in locked facilities) if their illnesses can be treated in a more open setting. *("Least-restrictive alternatives" does not relate to involuntary hospitalization.)* Most states now have legislation protecting the rights of patients, and treatment in the least restrictive setting is usually one of those rights.

How far the concept of least-restrictive care should be carried remains controversial. *Patients' rights advocates argue that this is the overriding (not the least crucial) principle,* even if the therapeutic potential of the least-restrictive facility is seriously compromised. *Clinicians argue that therapeutic efficacy is the greatest concern* and that the least-restrictive principle can be compromised in the interest of better treatment. One must consider carefully whether any restriction on a patient is for the convenience of the psychiatrist and staff or for the protection of the patient.

59.4 The answer is E (all)

The disabilities associated with chronic mental illness are major social, economic, and public health problems. In the United States, these disabilities afflict more than 3 million persons; they are costly and create suffering for those affected, their families, and society. Although the term *chronic mental illness* has traditionally been associated with older patients who have a long history of mental hospitalization, it has been broadened to include young adults with repeated episodes of mental disorders. Many of these persons have never been hospitalized, but their ability to lead productive lives in the community is severely impaired. Psychiatric rehabilitation addresses the medical, psychiatric, and social needs of persons who are persistently mentally ill.

Preventative psychiatry is part of public psychiatry. *The goal of prevention is to decrease the onset (incidence), duration (prevalence), and residual disability of mental disorders.* The prevention of mental disorders is based on public health principles and is divided into primary, secondary, and tertiary prevention.

Answers 59.5–59.10

59.5 The answer is A

59.6 The answer is A

59.7 The answer is A

59.8 The answer is B

59.9 The answer is C

59.10 The answer is C

The goal *of primary prevention* is to prevent the onset of a disease or disorder and thereby reduce its incidence (the ratio of new cases to the population in a specific period). This goal is reached by eliminating causative agents, *reducing risk factors,* enhancing host resistance, and interfering with disease transmission. *The "debriefing" group programs* for victims of the World Trade Center and Pentagon terrorist attacks that occurred on September 11, 2001 are examples of specific techniques used to prevent posttraumatic stress disorder.

Secondary prevention is defined as the early identification and prompt treatment of an illness or disorder, with the goal of reducing the prevalence (the proportion of existing cases in the population at risk at a specified time) of the condition by *shortening its duration.* Crisis intervention and public education are components of secondary prevention. In psychiatry, secondary prevention targets children who are emotionally ill for early intervention.

The goal of tertiary prevention is to reduce the prevalence of residual defects and disabilities caused by an illness or a disorder. In the case of mental disorders, tertiary prevention enables those with chronic mental illness to reach the highest feasible level of functioning. Tertiary prevention, or *rehabilitation,* in psychiatry nearly always addresses patients suffering from the most severe and debilitating illnesses (e.g., schizophrenia), the most severe affective disorders, and the most disabling personality disorders.

59.11 The answer is E (none)

The homeless mentally ill population continues to grow; one major survey found a 7 percent rise in urban homeless persons who are mentally ill over a 19-month period, with a concurrent decline in the number of shelter beds.

An average of 33 percent (not 10 percent) of homeless persons are mentally ill. The percentage ranges from 15 percent of homeless persons in Kansas City, Missouri, to 70 percent of homeless single adults in Boston. *On average, 45 percent (not a relatively low percentage) of homeless mentally ill persons are also dependent on alcohol or other substances.* The estimated percentage of these persons with dual diagnoses ranges from 23 percent in Philadelphia to more than 60 percent in several other major cities. There was a 9 percent rise in the number of dually diagnosed homeless persons during a recent 19-month period, with a concurrent increase in the average length of time of homelessness for those who are homeless and mentally ill.

Like those who are chronically mentally ill, *homeless mentally ill persons are a heterogeneous population, with no uniformity in diagnosis,* demographics, *functional performance,* or residential history.

59.12 The answer is E (all)

In one group of homeless mentally ill patients studied, close to one-third had concomitant physical illnesses that were secondary to alcohol dependence. The patients suffered from significant medical problems, including *anemia, lice infestation,* nutritional deficiencies (B_{12}, folate, and iron deficiencies), *cellulitis, and evidence of exposure to, and an increased incidence of, tuberculosis.*

59.13 The answer is A

In 1993, a program was begun at Bellevue Hospital Center to provide involuntary outpatient treatment of mentally ill persons, the goals of which are to help patients live and function in the community and to avoid relapse resulting in rehospitalization. *Involuntary outpatient treatment is mandated by a judge,* and patients report to the clinic for medication, individual or group therapy, psychosocial therapy, and vocational training. In addition, living arrangements are made for the patient and *a case manager is assigned. The court may order medication if the patient cannot make a treatment decision.* All court-mandated outpatient commitment procedures are made after the patient is evaluated by a psychiatrist. *Noncompliance is minimal (not at a high rate)* because of close supervision and the patient's preference for outpatient commitment procedures over involuntary hospitalization.

An alternative to (not the same as) outpatient commitment, conservatorship is used in many states. Conservators—usually not part of the treatment system and often family members—are given responsibility for the patients' well-being and varying amounts of authority over their lives, up to and including the ability to place them in locked facilities if their conditions demand such placement.

59.14 The answer is C
The therapeutic community model was originally introduced in England, conceived by T. F. Main and popularized by Maxwell Jones. This model *looks at the hospital unit as a social system.*

It seeks to optimize the patient's healthy functioning in a setting that *levels (rather than emphasizes) the hierarchy of the hospital* and involves patients in decision making in the unit. It places responsibility on the patients to serve as agents of change, with a significant role in the rehabilitation of other patients on the unit. This model depends upon older patients transmitting to newer patients the norms, skills, and values essential for meaningful participation in the therapeutic community. *Jones' treatment program was primarily designed for patients with personality disorders (rather than mood disorders).* Therapeutic community approaches are *more difficult to implement (not most effective) in units that treat a large number* of psychotically disturbed patients because groups may be overstimulating to them.

The token-economy model applies principles derived from experimental psychology and operant conditioning, with token rewards used as positive reinforcement for desired behaviors. These programs are used with more regressed, lower-functioning, chronically ill patients. As the patients receive rewards for preferred, adaptive behavior, they can exchange the tokens for desired privileges and activities.

Appendix A ◢

Case Studies

MARK S.

Mark S., a 40-year-old man, comes for a psychiatric consultation at the urging of his family because of worsening depression, auditory hallucinations, and motor disturbances. Eight months ago he noticed slurring of speech and the onset of uncontrollable, mild jerking movements of his head and upper body. Over the next month his slurred speech and jerky movements became slightly more pronounced and he began to have trouble walking. He experienced difficulty with bathing, cooking, and cleaning, and became more isolated, seldom leaving his home. Four months ago he started hearing voices. At first he thought a radio had been left on but later had conversations with the voices. He knew that other people would think it strange if he were seen talking to himself, and he became even more reclusive. For the past 2 months he has been depressed, with crying spells, poor sleep, and a 10-pound weight loss. He has recurrent thoughts of hanging himself, but insists he would not act on these thoughts.

He has no previous psychiatric or medical history. His mother, maternal uncle, and maternal grandmother died of Huntington's disease. Mark has been divorced for 3 years and now rarely sees his wife and two children. He lives alone in a cabin in the woods and has infrequent contact with friends or family. He experimented with drugs in college, using cocaine, LSD, and marijuana, but has not used any drugs for 15 years. He does not drink alcohol.

On examination his speech is slurred but intelligible. His mood is sad and he appears downcast and tearful. He avoids making eye contact. He is alert and oriented. He registers three out of three objects but can remember only two out of three after 5 minutes. Calculations, fund of knowledge, and abstract reasoning are unimpaired. He agrees to the psychiatrist's recommendation of hospitalization for stabilization and further evaluation.

1. What is his risk for Huntington's disease?

   A. 1 percent
   B. 10 percent
   C. 25 percent
   D. 50 percent
   E. 100 percent

2. Which of the following tests is most likely to confirm a diagnosis of Huntington's disease?

   A. electroencephalogram (EEG)
   B. head CT scan
   C. brain magnetic resonance imaging (MRI)
   D. brain biopsy
   E. genetic analysis

3. Appropriate treatment for Huntington's disease is most likely to include which of the following medications?

   A. L-Dopa (Larodopa)
   B. Haloperidol (Haldol)
   C. Benztropine (Cogentin)
   D. Tacrine (Cognex)
   E. Dantrolene (Dantrum)

Answers: 1,D; 2,E; 3,B

Discussion

Huntington's disease is an autosomal dominant genetic disorder. Having one parent with the disease means a risk of 50 percent to the child. The family history and the characteristic clinical course of choreoathetoid movement abnormalities coupled with mood disturbances and psychotic symptoms strongly suggest the disorder. The diagnosis is confirmed on genetic analysis by identification of the Huntington's gene.

Huntington's disease is a subcortical dementia. Typically, as is the case with this man, the movement abnormalities are more prominent than cognitive dysfunction. As the disease progresses, dementia becomes complete. The underlying pathology is degeneration of cholinergic and GABAergic neurons, especially in the pathways involving the basal ganglia. The result is an excess of dopamine transmission, which is normally inhibited by GABA. Accordingly, the mainstay of treatment is with an antipsychotic drug that decreases dopamine transmission. Dopamine agonists and anticholinergic drugs will aggravate the condition. There are no definitive treatments. Medication helps to control symptoms but does not halt the progression of the disease, which inevitably results in death.

HENRY D.

Henry D., a 30-year-old man, is brought to a psychiatric emergency room by police after he disrobed completely in a major intersection in the center of the city. He states that he took off his clothes in order to prove his faith in God. He heard God's voice say "strip" and understood the command as a test of his faith that God would protect him from the consequences of the act. He reports no recent change in sleep or appetite.

Henry was diagnosed with ADHD as a child. He was treated with methylphenidate, which improved concentration but did not improve his overall school performance. He had difficulty getting along with others and was seen as a loner. He started college but dropped out after a year and a half because of difficulties with his studies. He sought treatment for depression at the age of 19 and received fluoxetine in addition to individual psychotherapy. He seemed to respond well to both. He was hospitalized for the first time when he was 20 years old. He reported hearing God's voice and believed that his actions were being monitored in order to test his faith. A year later he was rehospitalized for disrobing in a train station. At the time of that admission his speech was pressured, his mood was euphoric, and he was emotionally labile. He had not slept for more than 30 hours, but was still remarkably energetic. A year later he made a suicide attempt by jumping naked from the upper balcony of a church onto the pews below. He sustained a fractured pelvis and a ruptured spleen, which was subsequently removed.

Henry has a history of heavy marijuana use and glue sniffing during adolescence, but he denies using illicit drugs for the past 12 years. On admission he describes his mood as "neutral" and his expression appears blank. He speaks in a monotone voice and occasionally stops mid-sentence without continuing. He is alert and oriented. Concentration is impaired.

1. Which of the following is the most likely diagnosis?

    A. Schizophrenia
    B. Bipolar disorder
    C. Adult ADHD
    D. Schizoaffective disorder
    E. Exhibitionism

2. Initial pharmacotherapy with which of the following medications is most appropriate?

    A. Alprazolam (Xanax)
    B. Olanzapine (Zyprexa)
    C. Methylphenidate (Brevital)
    D. Phenelzine (Nardil)
    E. Depo-provera

3. Long-term maintenance pharmacotherapy is most likely to include which of the following medications?

    A. Valproate (Depakene)
    B. Diazepam (Valium)
    C. Buspirone (Buspar)
    D. Bupropion (Wellbutrin)
    E. Dextroamphetamine (Dexedrine)

Answers: 1,D; 2,B; 3,A

Discussion

Henry has a chronic, recurrent illness with both mood and psychotic symptoms. The diagnosis will depend on the relative prominence of each and whether they always occur together. The mood symptoms in the past have been prominent enough to require treatment, even in the absence of psychotic symptoms. He was treated for depression at age 19 and then for symptoms of mania a year later. These episodes cannot be explained on the basis of schizophrenia, in which episodes of mood symptoms—if they occur at all—are always brief relative to the total duration of illness. The current episode includes psychotic symptoms (hallucinations, delusions) with no discernible disturbance of mood. In bipolar disorder, psychotic symptoms would occur only during periods of mood disturbance. Adult ADHD would present with difficulty concentrating but not with

psychotic symptoms. His disrobing in public does not sound as though it is sexually driven, but rather occurs in response to his delusional beliefs and auditory hallucinations, and therefore would not qualify for the diagnosis of exhibitionism. There is not enough information presented in the case to determine whether or not formal diagnostic criteria for schizoaffective disorder have been met: a period of mood symptoms plus psychotic symptoms and, *during the same period of illness*, a 2-week history of psychotic symptoms without mood symptoms. Nevertheless, schizoaffective disorder remains the best choice. (It should be noted that suicidality is seen in multiple psychiatric disorders and, although associated with depression, is diagnostically nonspecific. High rates of suicide are also seen in schizophrenia, bipolar disorder, and other conditions.)

Treatment should be initiated with an antipsychotic medication. Resolution of hallucinations and delusions will make it easier to evaluate the underlying disorder. Antipsychotics have the advantage of working relatively quickly—usually within a few days. Mood stabilizers and antidepressants take longer to work and, in the end, may or may not be indicated. For the long-term control of schizoaffective disorder, a mood stabilizer such as lithium or valproate is usually the mainstay of pharmacotherapy. An antipsychotic, and sometimes an antidepressant, may be used adjunctively, depending upon the particular symptoms.

LOUISE M.

Louise M., a 32-year-old woman, is hospitalized following an altercation in a restaurant in which she assaulted another woman, apparently without provocation. Louise said that the other woman was staring at her with a look full of jealousy. She tried to ignore the woman, but eventually found her stares so upsetting that she went to the woman's table to say something. She denies that she hit her, only that there was a sharp exchange of words. Louise believes the jealousy was motivated by her being the mother of a famous rock star's baby. She believes she became pregnant a year ago when the rock star visited her at a psychiatric state hospital where she had been hospitalized for 3 months. She states that she carried the man's baby to full term and that she had a normal vaginal delivery, although she is unable to name the hospital where the delivery occurred. The infant is now in a "baby home." She reports that she retains full custody and the rock star visits when his schedule permits. She mentions the names of several other celebrities with whom she claims to be on intimate terms.

Louise was discharged from the state hospital 6 months ago and was being followed at a local clinic. She was prescribed olanzapine, 20 mg, but because of sedation and weight gain, she had stopped taking the medication several weeks before. She has not experienced any changes in sleep or appetite.

She was first hospitalized at the age of 14. Since that time she has had a total of ten hospitalizations at different city and state psychiatric hospitals for periods of 2 months to a year. She has been treated with chlorpromazine, fluphenazine, lithium, valproate, fluoxetine, and venlafaxine. She does not believe she needs any medication, and states that her many hospitalizations were for a "rest." She denies ever having had hallucinations, suicidal thoughts or actions, or periods of depression or of decreased need for sleep with excess energy.

Louise was a top student until her first hospitalization at the age of 14. She finished high school by taking an extra year, with grades of mostly Cs and Ds. She has been on disability since age 20 and has no significant work history. Despite the impressive list of famous people with whom she claims to be close friends, she is unable to give the name or phone number of a single personal contact. She claims to have received a Ph.D. in psychology through private tutoring by famous Ivy League professors who visited her during her many hospitalizations.

Louise has no significant medical history. She takes no medication other than olanzapine. She denies alcohol or illicit drug use. The physical examination reveals mild obesity with a blood pressure of 140/90. A random glucose is 150. All other routine admission labs are within normal limits.

On mental status examination she appears cheerful, personable, and forthright. She offers to shake the examiner's hand and maintains good eye contact throughout the interview. Her speech is clear and not pressured. She smiles and laughs appropriately. She is alert and oriented; cognitive functions are intact.

1. Which of the following is the most appropriate diagnosis for this woman?

    A. Delusional disorder
    B. Bipolar disorder
    C. Narcissistic personality disorder
    D. Histrionic personality disorder
    E. Schizophrenia

2. Which of the following is the best treatment approach at this point?

    A. Continue the current dose of olanzapine alone.
    B. Stop olanzapine and withhold other medication.
    C. Stop olanzapine and start haloperidol.
    D. Continue the current dose of olanzapine and start lithium.
    E. Increase the dose of olanzapine.

3. Which of the following therapies is most likely to be beneficial?

    A. Psychodynamic psychotherapy
    B. Interpersonal psychotherapy
    C. Cognitive psychotherapy
    D. Psychosocial rehabilitation
    E. Dialectical behavioral therapy

Answers: 1,A; 2,C; 3,D

Discussion

The long, chronic course of Louise's illness, the multiple relapses and hospitalizations, and the gradual impairment in her ability to function independently all raise the suspicion of schizophrenia, but there is not enough in her history to justify that diagnosis. She claims never to have had hallucinations, does not appear to have a formal thought disorder or emotional blunting, and, despite her assault of a restaurant patron, does not have a history of disorganized behavior. Indeed the only clear psychopathological symptom is her delusion of involvement with famous people. The belief is nonbizarre—that is, something that could happen in everyday life. Her assertion that she is the mother of a rock star's baby is plausible enough that taken by itself, it is not clearly delusional.

Earning her Ph.D. through tutoring by famous Ivy League professors during her hospitalizations is almost certainly delusional, and although wildly implausible, is still nonbizarre. With prominent nonbizarre delusions and no other psychotic symptoms, the most appropriate diagnosis is delusional disorder. The elements of grandiosity are similar to those seen in bipolar disorder, but there are none of the mood or behavioral symptoms that would be needed for that diagnosis. Narcissistic personality disorder describes a person who demands praise and attention and who is insensitive to the needs of others (perhaps to compensate for deep-seated feelings of inadequacy). Histrionic personality disorder describes a person who is dramatic, flamboyant, and flirtatious and who strives to be the center of attention. Neither personality disorder would include delusions sustained over several years.

Delusional disorders are notoriously difficult to treat. They often do not respond—or do not respond fully—to antipsychotic medication. Nevertheless, in the absence of better treatments, antipsychotic therapy should be attempted. Louise has had multiple trials of several different antipsychotics. She does not believe she needs medication, and she stopped olanzapine because of weight gain and sedation. For these reasons and because her glucose is elevated, it is not a good idea simply to continue with higher doses of olanzapine, which can cause diabetes mellitus. A better approach, although by no means one that is guaranteed to work, is to switch to another antipsychotic such as haloperidol. Alternative strategies would combine antipsychotics or combine an antipsychotic with a mood stabilizer.

In addition to her delusions, Louise is suffering from the effects of a chronic relapsing illness and multiple hospitalizations. Although the mental status examination describes her as personable and outgoing, she is friendless and out of work. Psychosocial rehabilitation may help her develop a life that is more productive and satisfying, and may help her become better integrated into a community of others. Social isolation is one of the risk factors for delusional disorder. Increasing her social involvement may help diminish the intensity of her symptoms. Psychodynamic psychotherapy can be effective but must be started very early in the course of the disorder, before the patient is likely to incorporate the therapist into his or her delusional belief.

MARSHALL D.

Marshall D., a 35-year-old police officer, comes to his internist with the complaint that he is unable to sleep at night. For the past 6 months he has had trouble falling asleep and staying asleep. These difficulties have been worsening, and he feels less and less able to function on the job. A year ago he was involved in a "buy and bust" operation in which he shot and killed a man who had pulled a gun and fired at him. He was honored for heroism by the police commissioner and mayor of the city in a ceremony at which he was given the department's highest medal for valor. In the months following the shooting, he had trouble concentrating and on occasion would break into tears for no reason that he could discern. He requested and received a transfer to a desk job in another precinct. However, he was still required to perform overtime street duty in uniform with his gun for crowd control at parades and public demonstrations. In the weeks before having to do such street duty, he felt anxious, suffered diarrhea, and was unable to eat much. The night before each assignment he did not sleep more than 1 or 2 hours. Over the last 6 months he has begun to have nightmares about the shooting. He describes being constantly on edge and refuses to drive past the site of the shooting. He is again having crying spells.

Marshall graduated from college before joining the police department. Before his recent transfer he had a good relationship with his partner, but few friends. He has never been married but has dated a series of women, none for longer than 8 months. He drinks every evening and often to the point of intoxication on the weekend. For the past month he has seen no friends or family and has stayed in his apartment with the blinds closed and the curtains drawn when he is not at work. The internist recommends a referral to a psychiatrist but Marshall refuses, saying that if he acquires any psychiatric history, his gun will be taken away and he will lose all chance for future promotions.

1. Which of the following is the most likely diagnosis?

    A. Adjustment disorder with depressed mood
    B. Alcohol-induced mood disorder
    C. Acute stress disorder
    D. Posttraumatic stress disorder
    E. Major depression

2. Which of the following is the most appropriate next step for the internist?

    A. Report the consultation to Marshall's commanding officer.
    B. Insist that Marshall see a psychiatrist.
    C. Inquire about suicide.
    D. Offer to see Marshall for weekly therapy.
    E. Initiate fluoxetine therapy.

3. The lifetime prevalence of the disorder diagnosed in Marshall among adults in the United States is

    A. 10 percent
    B. 25 percent
    C. 50 percent
    D. 75 percent
    E. 90 percent

Answers: 1,D; 2,C; 3,A

Discussion

Marshall's symptoms meet criteria for a diagnosis of posttraumatic stress disorder (PTSD). He describes symptoms of both arousal and avoidance. He is reexperiencing the trauma of the shooting through nightmares, has trouble sleeping, feels anxious, avoids going to the scene of the shooting, and requested a transfer out of his old precinct. Despite these efforts he is experiencing marked mood and anxiety symptoms. It is now more than a month after the traumatic event, and, accordingly, a diagnosis of an acute stress disorder is no longer accurate. There is not enough information provided in the history and mental status examination to determine whether or not a diagnosis of a major depressive episode is also warranted. If so, it would coexist with a diagnosis of posttraumatic stress disorder.

A striking feature of the case as presented is the lack of any information about current suicidal thoughts or past suicide attempts. The situation is one of considerable risk: He is emotionally distressed, socially isolated, drinking heavily, and has ready access to a gun. He feels unable to accept psychiatric help out of fear that his job would be in jeopardy, even though his work—in particular the special assignments—is a major source of ongoing stress. Fluoxetine may well be indicated, but any benefit is likely to be delayed for 2 or more weeks, and Marshall is at immediate high risk. Similarly, it may or may not be appropriate, depending on his or her training and experience, for the internist to offer weekly therapy sessions, but a solid suicide assessment must still come first. If there is no threat to another person, the internist is under no legal obligation to report this consultation to anyone; he or she is bound by ethical constraints to maintain confidentiality. (If Marshall made a credible threat against a third person, then the internist does have a legal obligation to notify that person.) If Marshall discloses suicidal thoughts or plans, the internist's response will be based on assessment of the risk and his or her relationship with his or her patient. The safest intervention, of course, would be psychiatric hospitalization, even if it had to be against the patient's will. An alternative would be to contract for safety and work closely with Marshall in the days ahead.

The lifetime prevalence for PTSD in adults in the United States is about 10 percent. Of people who experience a severe trauma, the number who go on to suffer a posttraumatic stress disorder is variable and may range up to 50 percent. The characteristics separating those who do from those who don't remain obscure. Possibilities that have been suggested include preexisting psychopathology, personality make-up, previous exposure to traumatic events, and drug and alcohol use. The severity of the trauma is also significant, with the highest rates associated with rape, military combat, and survivors of torture.

CHARLES N.

Charles N., a 69-year-old man, is brought for a psychiatric evaluation after he was arrested by police for breaking into a neighbor's house. Charles had been in his typical state of good health until he woke up at 4 AM feeling unusually well-rested and full of energy. He decided to complete several projects he had been putting off, including reorganizing his personal insurance. As he was working through his papers he began to dwell on the idea that his neighbor—with whom he had no financial dealings—was involved in massive insurance fraud. He became convinced that he had an obligation to find and report evidence of the fraud. Later, when he knew his neighbor would be at work, he broke a window with a stone, let himself in, and began going through papers and files in the man's home office. He heard the house burglar alarm go off and knew that police would arrive shortly, but decided to work as quickly as possible. When they came he offered no resistance. Except for the previous night, he reported no change in sleep, appetite, or mood. He is taking no medications and does not use illicit drugs. He drinks moderately at social events, usually one or two drinks a month. He has no previous psychiatric history and his medical history is benign. His physical examination is unremarkable. On mental status examination his speech is pressured and his mood expansive. He is irritable, labile, and difficult to interrupt. He denies hallucinations. He is alert and oriented.

Charles had a long, profitable, and illustrious career as an investment banker. He retired 2 years ago and is active in a number of community projects. He is married with two children and three grandchildren. He and his wife have a large circle of friends, and they see their children and grandchildren often. He plays tennis three times a week and is a voracious reader.

The neighbor declines to press charges and Charles is admitted to a psychiatric hospital. His blood pressure is 125/75, heart rate 70, and temperature 37°C. His physical examination is unremarkable. Urine toxicology is negative and routine laboratory studies are within normal limits. He is treated with olanzapine, 20 mg, at night. He sleeps for 12 hours and when he wakes no longer feels euphoric or full of energy. He remembers clearly the events of yesterday but cannot imagine why he thought his neighbor was involved in insurance fraud or why he felt it so imperative that he find evidence.

Over the next week, the olanzapine is tapered off and lithium therapy begun, tapering up to a dose of 1,200 mg/day, which gives him a lithium blood level of 1.1 mEq/L. He remains symptom-free and is discharged to the care of a private psychiatrist who maintains the lithium at 1,200 mg. Over the next 6 months Charles complains of sluggishness, tremor, incoordination, and weight gain. He has difficulty with his tennis game and eventually stops playing. He complains of these problems to his psychiatrist but is told that he must keep taking the lithium. After another 3 months, Charles unilaterally decreases the dose of lithium to 600 mg/day. Side effects diminish but do not disappear. He seeks a second opinion from another psychiatrist recommended by his internist. With Charles's consent, the consulting psychiatrist speaks with the treating psychiatrist to review the history.

1. Which of the following is the most appropriate diagnosis?

    A. Bipolar I disorder
    B. Bipolar II disorder
    C. Adjustment disorder with disturbance of conduct
    D. Delusional disorder
    E. Brief psychotic episode

2. Without medication, what is the risk of recurrence following a single manic episode?

    A. 10 percent
    B. 25 percent
    C. 50 percent
    D. 75 percent
    E. 90 percent

3. Which of the following is the most appropriate recommendation for the consulting psychiatrist to make?

    A. Stop lithium.
    B. Stop lithium and add valproate.
    C. Continue lithium at 600 mg/day and check the blood level.
    D. Increase lithium back to 1,200 mg/day and check the blood level.
    E. Continue lithium at 600 mg/day and add valproate.

Answers: 1,A; 2,E; 3,C

Discussion:

The clinical circumstances of this case are unusual: the sudden eruption of destructive psychiatric symptoms and their quick resolution in a high-functioning older man with no psychiatric history who appears to be physically healthy. The symptoms—

increased energy, pressured speech, euphoric mood and irritability, and the delusion about his neighbor—are all consistent with a manic episode. According to DSM-IV-TR criteria, the diagnosis of a manic episode requires symptoms to be present for a week *unless* hospitalization is required, in which case there is no minimum required time period. Accordingly, Charles meets criteria for the diagnosis of a manic episode, and a single manic episode justifies a diagnosis of bipolar I disorder. (In bipolar II disorder, there is a history of major depressive episodes and hypomanic episodes, but never full manic episodes.) Diagnosing bipolar I carries significant and potentially serious long-term consequences. Because the risk of relapse without medication after a single manic episode is 90 percent, such an episode often leads to long-term management with a mood stabilizer. The 90 percent relapse rate, however, must be understood in context. It represents an average of individuals studied who span a spectrum of ages of onset and seriousness of condition. It includes people who are diagnosed early and who subsequently have long, chronic, relapsing illnesses, with or without medication. For the very fact that Charles' circumstances are so unusual, there simply are no good data to predict his risk of relapse. The acute onset of symptoms in a previously healthy older person raises the suspicion of an underlying medical or drug-related cause, but there is nothing else in the information presented to support either of those possibilities. Whatever the source of Charles' 1-day manic episode, long-term therapy with 1,200 mg/day of lithium is excessive. Maintenance therapy is usually managed at a lower dose and blood level than those required for acute treatment, and the intensity of the side effects he experienced originally suggests that the dose is too high. Each of the three main mood stabilizers currently used—lithium, valproate, and carbamazepine—is associated with troublesome side effects and toxicities. It is unwise for the consultant to recommend major changes until he or she understands the situation more fully. The best approach would be to continue the lithium at its current reduced dose and check the blood level. There is no reason to consider adding or switching to valproate. Without first finding out the current blood level, and in the absence of continuing symptoms, increasing the dose of lithium is not justified. A reasonable long-term goal is discontinuation of medication. This will most safely be accomplished in the context of a trusting doctor–patient relationship, in which possible early symptoms will be reported and evaluated.

ALBERT G.

Albert G., a 36-year-old man, is admitted to a psychiatric unit after having been brought to the emergency department by police. As he was walking past a hotel in the central part of the city, he saw a man and woman standing on the sidewalk about to take a photograph of a building across the street. Thinking that they were going to take his picture, he grabbed the camera, smashed it on the ground, and pulled out all the film. He explained his actions by saying the photograph would be used to control him and that it is illegal to take another person's photograph.

Albert has a history of multiple hospitalizations dating back to age 14. During the hospitalizations his symptoms have been well-controlled with a variety of typical and atypical antipsychotic medications. Once discharged he begins drinking four to five beers a day, neglects getting prescriptions refilled, and stops medication when his supply runs out. He made two prior suicide attempts, both by hanging, in which he suffered no serious medical sequelae. He reports numerous blackouts from drinking, but he has never had seizures or DTs. He does not use illicit drugs.

Albert dropped out of high school in the 11th grade. He worked a number of short-term, unskilled jobs before going on public assistance at age 21. He lives alone, is estranged from his family, and has no friends. On examination, Albert is lying motionless. He makes good eye contact and says, "I'm trying not to move." He fears that if he moves he may die. He currently hears voices saying, "Be good," "Get the dog," and "He's the one." He also sees shapes, which he describes as colored letters dancing in front of his eyes. He talks about being monitored by hidden cameras and microphones everywhere he goes in the city. He is alert and oriented. He can recall three out of three objects after 5 minutes. Concentration is impaired.

1. Which of the following is the most likely diagnosis?

    A. Schizophrenia, catatonic type
    B. Schizophrenia, undifferentiated type
    C. Schizophrenia, paranoid type
    D. Delusional disorder
    E. Schizoaffective disorder

2. Which of the following interventions is most likely to prevent relapse?

    A. Vocational rehabilitation
    B. Increased socialization
    C. Use of a long-term depot antipsychotic
    D. Alcohol counseling
    E. Use of an atypical antipsychotic

Answers: 1,B; 2,D

Discussion

Albert has a long-standing illness characterized by periods of hallucinations and delusions. He is socially isolated and not working. The most likely diagnosis is schizophrenia. There is no description of current or past mood symptoms that would make a diagnosis of schizoaffective disorder reasonable, and the presence of prominent hallucinations is inconsistent with a diagnosis of delusional disorder. The designation of the subtype of schizophrenia is based on the current episode. Although Albert's attempt not to move superficially resembles catatonia, his openly discussing with the examiner his reasons for remaining still is most uncharacteristic of the catatonic subtype. The continued presence of delusions and auditory and visual hallucinations makes the diagnosis of an undifferentiated subtype more appropriate.

Albert is lucky in having a good response to many different antipsychotics. There is no reason to suppose that an atypical agent will help him more than conventional antipsychotics. His multiple relapses result from his failure to fill prescriptions because of his drinking, and a long-acting depot medication is not likely to disturb that pattern. It is probable that he would get an injection, start drinking, and not go for his next injection. Alcohol counseling is, therefore, of the greatest importance in giving him some stability and freedom from the ongoing cycle of relapse and rehospitalization. Vocational counseling and increased socialization may help, but only if his drinking is brought under control.

JAMES K.

James K., a 4-year-old boy, is referred for a psychiatric evaluation at the suggestion of his preschool teacher, who noticed unusual interactions with other children. He is an only child who started preschool 4 months ago. He seldom plays with other children, preferring to play with a specific toy truck or toy dog. He spends much of the morning with the toy, moving it back and forth in a repetitive pattern. If he is unable to find the toy, or if another child is playing with it, he sits on the floor and wails until it is found and given to him. On the occasions when he approaches another child, it is in a blunt, verbose way, devoid of give-and-take, and other children tend to avoid him. The teacher never observes reciprocal interactions, and James never seems to catch on to what is happening in games. He approaches adults in a similar blunt, one-sided manner.

James was the product of a full-term vaginal delivery without complications. His mother describes him as a fussy baby who did not like being held. She and his father cannot remember James smiling as a baby or ever wanting to play peek-a-boo, despite their efforts to engage him. He talked before he walked and was speaking two to three word sentences by age 2. Because of his early and rich vocabulary, his parents assumed that he was probably gifted. He achieved bowel control at 3 years and bladder control at 4 years, with the exception of occasional nighttime accidents. He is able to dress and bathe himself with minimal help. He enjoys looking at pictures in his parents' art books and tends to return to the same pages again and again. His parents say that James's play at home is similar to what his teacher describes at school. He almost never initiates an activity or engages in reciprocal play. They assumed that his preference for being left alone was due to his superior intelligence. He sleeps and eats well. They have never observed or heard anything that would lead them to believe that James was experiencing hallucinations.

On examination James is found to be at the 30th percentile for height and weight for his age. He is well-developed and there are no facial abnormalities. His vocabulary is above average for his age, and he talks freely but without engaging in back-and-forth conversation. He avoids eye contact with the examiner and tends not to respond to questions or commands. When he is allowed to choose a toy, he selects a truck and spends several minutes spinning one of the wheels backward and forward.

1. Which of the following is the most likely diagnosis?

    A. Fetal alcohol syndrome
    B. Autistic disorder
    C. Down's syndrome
    D. Childhood schizophrenia
    E. Asperger's disorder

2. What is the most likely cause of James's difficulties?

    A. Neurodevelopmental abnormalities
    B. Maternal neglect
    C. Autosomal recessive inheritance
    D. Lead poisoning
    E. Chromosomal nondisjunction

3. Which of the following interventions is most likely to be helpful?

   A. Risperidone therapy
   B. Psychodynamic play therapy
   C. Social skills training
   D. Methylphenidate therapy
   E. Interpersonal psychotherapy

Answers: 1,E; 2,A; 3,C

Discussion

Fetal alcohol syndrome and Down's syndrome include characteristic facial and other features that James does not have. In addition, he does not appear to be impaired cognitively: He is able to function at a level of independence (dressing, bathing) appropriate to his age. Schizophrenia in children can be difficult to diagnose because of their limitations in describing inner experiences and the sometime difficulty in distinguishing normal childhood fantasy from hallucinations and delusions. However, unlike James, children who have schizophrenia almost always develop symptoms after a period of normal childhood development. James's unwillingness to be held, failure to make eye contact, and lack of pleasure in playing peek-a-boo all suggest impaired social interactions from very early on. These are core feature of both autistic disorder and Asperger's disorder. The difference between them is that language is impaired in autistic disorder and normal in Asperger's disorder. James's language is normal or perhaps even a little advanced. The experience of his parents is not uncommon among parents and teachers of children with Asperger's disorder, for whom good language skills may mask the social deficits. James is lucky in having a teacher astute enough to recognize the limitations behind his verbosity.

The etiology of Asperger's disorder (as with autism) is unknown. There is no evidence that it is caused by parental neglect or any other pattern of parenting. There is a slight familial trend to the disorder—the prevalence among first- and second-degree relatives is greater than the prevalence for the population at large—but whether or not this represents a genetic factor is not established. There is a growing consensus among clinicians and researchers that both autism and Asperger's disorder are the result of neurodevelopmental abnormalities, but no specific neuroanatomic or neurofunctional deficit has been identified.

There is no definitive treatment for Asperger's disorder. Pharmacotherapy will not treat the underlying disorder but may be helpful for ancillary symptoms such as aggression or depression. Psychodynamic and interpersonal psychotherapy are inappropriate because of the problems with social understanding and empathy. Therapy that focuses on social and communications skills, problem solving, and deriving strategies for dealing with novel situations has the greatest likelihood of being helpful. In addition, many adults with Asperger's disorder benefit from self-support groups in which they can meet and learn from other people with similar disabilities.

SHARON R.

Sharon R., a 24-year-old woman, is brought for a psychiatric consultation by her mother who complains of bizarre behavior. One month ago Sharon was fired from her job at a local bookstore because of frequently arriving late and not performing her duties adequately. She states that she fell in love with another employee and tried to get his attention and spend time with him, even though he seemed uninterested. Over the past 3 months she increased her use of alcohol and marijuana to three beers a day and two to three joints per day. Her mother reports a 2-week history of increased energy, eating little, talking a great deal, and interrupting others frequently. A week ago Sharon reported that her former work colleagues were plotting against her and attempting to control her by broadcasting thoughts into her brain. She did not sleep the last 2 nights. Sharon has no significant psychiatric or medical history. She takes no medications.

Physical examination reveals a blood pressure of 135/75, heart rate of 84, and a temperature of 37°C. Her conjunctivae are pink and her pupils are equal, 3 mm and reactive to light. Deep tendon reflexes are normal throughout. Urine toxicology reveals the presence of cannabinoids. On mental status testing, her mood is euphoric, her speech is pressured, and she is emotionally labile and irritable. Her thinking is illogical and disorganized. She denies hallucinations. She is alert and oriented to person, place, and time. Immediate recall and recent and remote memory are intact. Throughout the interview she is preoccupied by thoughts of the co-worker with whom she has fallen in love.

Sharon is admitted to a psychiatric unit and treatment is initiated with haloperidol, 10 mg/day, which is increased to 20 mg/day on day 5 because of continued agitation. On day 6 she becomes withdrawn and uncommunicative. She is diffusely rigid with a temperature of 39°C. Her white blood count is 14,300 and her CPK 2,100. Several blood cultures are negative.

1. Which of the following is the most likely diagnosis at the time of admission?

   A. Schizophrenia
   B. Delusional disorder, erotomanic type
   C. Marijuana-induced psychotic disorder
   D. Bipolar disorder
   E. Schizoaffective disorder, bipolar type

2. Which of the following is the most likely explanation for her behavior on day 6?

   A. Worsening psychosis
   B. Anticholinergic delirium
   C. Neuroleptic malignant syndrome
   D. Marijuana-induced delirium
   E. Occult infection

3. Which of the following pharmacologic approaches is most appropriate on day 6?

   A. Increase dose of haloperidol
   B. Stop haloperidol and add risperidone
   C. Stop haloperidol, add bromocriptine, and seek medical consultation
   D. Continue the same dose of haloperidol and add risperidone
   E. Continue the same dose of haloperidol and add benztropine

Answers: 1,D; 2,C; 3,C

Discussion

The diagnosis of bipolar disorder best fits the history and symptoms, but it is by no means certain. She presents with a 1-month history of impaired judgment and erratic behavior followed by increased energy, pressured speech, mood lability, and decreased need for sleep, all of which indicate a manic episode. The emergence of paranoid delusions is also consistent with mania, and a single manic episode, with or without major depressive episodes, qualifies for a diagnosis of bipolar disorder. That diagnosis can only be made, however, if it is believed that the symptoms are not the result of a general medical condition or substance use. We know that she has been using increased amounts of marijuana and alcohol, and that she is probably intoxicated with marijuana at the time of admission. Heavy marijuana use in some individuals can cause a psychotic state with paranoid delusions and hallucinations. There are some features, however, that are inconsistent with a purely marijuana-induced state, which more typically presents with decreased talkativeness and long response latency than with the pressured speech seen here. In addition, increased energy and activity, and decreased need for sleep, are much more likely in bipolar disorder than in a marijuana psychosis. The delusional belief of her thoughts being controlled by an outside force is strikingly similar to delusions of control that are so often seen in schizophrenia, but the prominent mood symptoms and time course (1 month) preclude that diagnosis. The diagnosis of schizoaffective disorder would require a 2-week period of psychotic symptoms without prominent mood symptoms, which is not the case here. An erotomanic delusional belief is that the patient is loved by another (often famous) person, not as is the case here, that the patient herself is preoccupied with being in love with someone else.

The events of days 5 and 6 almost certainly represent the emergence of a neuroleptic malignant syndrome (NMS), an idiosyncratic response to antipsychotics (especially high-potency, typical agents) characterized by fever, rigidity, and obtundation. The clinical diagnosis is confirmed, with the typical findings of leukocytosis and greatly increased CPK. Anticholinergic delirium includes fever but not the rigidity or laboratory findings. In addition, patients with an anticholinergic delirium are more likely to be agitated than withdrawn. Neuroleptic malignant syndrome is a life-threatening medical emergency. All medications must be stopped; switching to an atypical agent such as risperidone will not help her. Appropriate treatment—in addition to life support, maintaining fluid and electrolyte balance, and decreasing her fever—is with bromocriptine, a centrally acting dopamine agonist that presumably works by reversing the effects of the antipsychotic-caused dopamine blockade. The treatment of NMS commonly combines bromocriptine with dantrolene, a peripheral muscle relaxant. Consultation with the medical service is crucial, as the treatment may be complex.

ALEX C.

Alex C., a 35-year-old man, is referred from prison for a psychiatric evaluation because of exposing his genitals and masturbating in front of female corrections officers. He has been arrested for public masturbation and as a repeat offender is being held in jail prior to his first court hearing. He acknowledges the behavior and explains that he thought it would be sexually exciting to the officers and that they might want to have sex with him.

As an adolescent, Alex had numerous sexual encounters with other adolescents, with prepubertal children, and with adults of both sexes. He began going to pornographic movie theaters in his late teens, where he would always masturbate and, on occasion, have an anonymous sexual encounter with a stranger. During his 20s, he began masturbating in public with the belief that it would lead to sex with strangers. However, on those rare occasions when his exposure did lead to a proposition for sexual favors, he became frightened and ran away. He discovered that squeezing the urethra at the head of his penis would help delay orgasm, and he used the technique to prolong masturbation. When he learned (erroneously) that this would cause retrograde ejaculation into the bladder, he began to eat his own semen and drink his urine, variously describing the reasons for so doing as "saving sperm" or "as a perfect source of protein." He acknowledged that the practice does not literally save sperm and that most people would think it bizarre.

Alex had two psychiatric hospitalizations 8 and 12 years ago, each for hallucinations and paranoid delusions in the context of crack cocaine use. He insists that he has never had hallucinations when he was not using cocaine. He has used no illicit drugs for the past 5 years, but he drinks one or two beers each night and once or twice a month he will drink to the point of being unsteady on his feet and slurring his words. He has five prior arrests for public indecency but until now has never served time in jail. Alex has never married and denies ever having had a long-term romantic relationship. He graduated from high school and works the late-night shift at a local convenience store.

1. Which of the following is the most likely Axis I diagnosis?

   A. Social phobia
   B. Exhibitionism
   C. Schizophrenia
   D. Obsessive-compulsive disorder
   E. Sexual aversion disorder

2. Which of the following is the most likely Axis II diagnosis?

   A. Antisocial personality disorder
   B. Borderline personality disorder
   C. Obsessive-compulsive personality disorder
   D. Histrionic personality disorder
   E. Schizotypal personality disorder

3. Without treatment, which of the following is the most likely long-term course for Alex's Axis I condition?

   A. Gradual decrease in symptomatic behavior
   B. Progressive functional deterioration
   C. Development of a recurrent psychotic disorder
   D. Progression to pedophilia
   E. Progressive cognitive deterioration

Answers: 1,B; 2,E; 3,B

Discussion

At first glance the diagnosis for Alex seems fairly straightforward. He has a long history of public exposure and masturbation that has continued despite repeated arrests and, astoundingly, even while he was in jail. The absence of any long-term romantic relationships adds to the impression that exposing himself and publicly masturbating is his preferred method of sexual expression, all of which leads to a diagnosis of exhibitionism, one of the sexual paraphilias. An intriguing question, however, is whether

Alex also has an underlying psychotic disorder. He has been hospitalized twice in the past with hallucinations and delusions, but he insists that they occurred only when he used crack cocaine. The behavior of eating his own semen and drinking his urine is, as he recognizes, profoundly bizarre. It does not, however, seem to be driven by any delusional belief, and without further information, it is difficult to conclude that it is not just bizarre but psychotic. Because of impaired judgment and disinhibition, people with schizophrenia or other cognitive or psychotic disorders may have isolated episodes of unusual sexual behavior. Alex, however, has a pattern of numerous, repeated episodes of public exposure over many years, despite a number of arrests.

Because personality disorder diagnoses are intended to describe deeply ingrained, maladaptive fixed habits over an individual's lifetime, it is always difficult to make an Axis II diagnosis based on a short case history. Nevertheless the features attributed to Alex are most consistent with a diagnosis of schizotypal personality disorder, most remarkably his social isolation and his strange beliefs and behavior, which fall short of being psychotic. Antisocial personality disorder describes a broader pattern of systematically violating the rights of others than just repeated public exposure. Borderline personality disorder implies intense, chaotic relationships, not the absence of relationships. Individuals with the diagnosis of histrionic personality disorder often have a quality of promiscuous flirtatiousness but without the extraordinary lack of judgment, violation of the law, and compulsiveness described here. There is no evidence that exhibitionism progresses to another paraphilia or other Axis I disorder. However, a poor prognosis is associated with an earlier age of onset, a high frequency of acts, no guilt or shame, substance abuse, a lack of a history of coitus, and referral from a legal authority, all present in this case.

EMILY R.

Emily R., a 24-year-old woman, is brought to an emergency room by her father with a chief complaint, "I have bugs all over my body and in my hair. They're making me weaker." Two weeks earlier, the apartment Emily shares with a roommate flooded after a pipe burst. Following the flood, the apartment was infested with insects. At one point, Emily had insects crawling in an open wound on her arm. The apartment was cleaned and fumigated, but Emily persisted in believing bugs were everywhere. She washed herself with alcohol several times a day and avoided seeing friends and family because of her fear that the infestation would spread to others. She believed that a cocoon was being spread over her body and that insects were crawling over her internal organs. She spent most of the last 3 days immersed in a bathtub of water. Her roommate became alarmed and called her father, who brought her to the emergency room. She denies sleep or appetite changes, and has not experienced auditory or visual hallucinations.

Emily had a history of outpatient treatment for anorexia nervosa and a major depressive episode. When she was 16 she became withdrawn, tearful, preoccupied with death, had difficulty sleeping, and lost 10 pounds. She was treated with individual psychotherapy and citalopram pharmacotherapy. All symptoms of depression resolved within a month and she had no recurrence. When she was 19, coinciding with a brief modeling career, she began a severe diet, exercised intensively, and lost 25 pounds. Her menses ceased for 6 months. She resumed psychotherapy but not medication. Her modeling career ended abruptly when the agency representing her went out of business. She began a romantic relationship and went back to school. Gradually, she lost interest in dieting, her weight stabilized, and menses returned. She experimented with cocaine around that time, but claims not to have used illicit drugs for over 4 years. She drinks no more than one or two glasses of wine a week. She has been working as an administrative assistant for a recording studio and was going to work regularly and working without difficulties until the day of the flood and the infestation. She has not returned to work since.

Her blood pressure is 115/75, HR 70, and temperature 37°C. She weighs 125 pounds and is 5 feet 6 inches tall. Physical examination is unremarkable. Routine laboratory studies, including liver function tests, are within normal limits. A urine toxicology screen is negative. She appears apprehensive. She describes feeling bugs crawling on her skin and she believes that insects have entered her body and are slowly enveloping her in a cocoon. She denies auditory hallucinations. Her thoughts are logical and goal-directed. She is alert and oriented.

1. Which of the following is the most likely diagnosis?
   A. Schizophrenia
   B. Cocaine-induced psychotic disorder
   C. Major depression with psychotic symptoms
   D. Delusional disorder
   E. Brief psychotic episode

2. Intoxication with which of the following drugs is most likely to present with formication?
   A. Marijuana
   B. Amphetamine
   C. Heroin
   D. Alcohol
   E. LSD

Answers: 1,E; 2,B

Discussion

Emily's symptoms do not appear to be caused by a recurrence of either of the two disorders for which she had previously been treated. Although the delusions in psychotic depression are often somatic, there are no disturbances in appetite, sleep, or mood to suggest that diagnosis. Anorexia nervosa does not include psychotic symptoms (although there is some debate about whether the characteristic disturbance of body image—seeing oneself as fat rather than emaciated—should be considered delusional). More important, she is at normal weight, and a diagnosis of anorexia is not correct. The history and mental status examination strongly suggest that she has both delusions and tactile hallucinations of insects crawling on her skin. More focused questioning would help to clarify this point. Delusional disorders do not include prominent hallucinations, and the delusional belief must be nonbizarre—that is, something that could happen in everyday life. The belief of body infestation is arguably nonbizarre, but the beliefs that insects are crawling inside her and that she is being wrapped in a cocoon are bizarre by any measure. Schizophrenia requires the presence of symptoms for 6 months. Her psychotic symptoms have been present for only 2 weeks and are best described, at least provisionally, as a brief psychotic episode. By definition, in a brief psychotic episode symptoms are present for more than a day but less than a month. She was working well and was symptom-free up until the time of the flood and the real invasion of insects in the apartment. It appears that those events triggered the brief psychotic episode, but this can only be an item of conjecture and is unlikely to affect treatment.

It is essential to rule out a medical or drug-related cause. We are not given information about her current medical history, but her unremarkable physical examination and normal laboratory studies make a medical cause less likely.

Formication—tactile hallucinations of insects crawling on the skin—are associated with CNS stimulant intoxication or CNS sedative withdrawal, especially delirium tremens. The negative urine toxicology does not rule out a drug-related cause, since symptoms will sometimes persist after a drug has been cleared, and since in a withdrawal state it is expected that the toxicology will be negative. More important in ruling out a drug cause for her symptoms are the normal vital signs, normal physical examination, and the fact that she is alert and oriented. Marijuana intoxication can cause psychotic symptoms, although more likely paranoid delusions and auditory and visual hallucinations than tactile hallucinations, and the signs of marijuana intoxication usually show up in the physical examination: tachycardia, high blood pressure, and injected conjunctivae. Visual hallucinations and illusions are characteristic of LSD intoxication. Opioid intoxication does not generally include any psychotic symptoms.

HARRIET J.

Harriet J., a 30-year-old woman, is referred for psychiatric evaluation by her internist after her fourth request for mammography in 6 months. Two years ago a close friend died of breast cancer. Since that time she has been preoccupied with the possibility that she also has the disease. She examines herself several times a day and when she finds something that seems unusual she goes to her doctor for medical evaluation. Initially, the doctor's reassurance was enough to convince her that her fears were exaggerated. However, over the past year she has required a mammogram to prove to herself that she does not have cancer. Each time when the mammography is reported to be normal, she is momentarily relieved but within several days starts to doubt the accuracy of the test and suspect that she does have undetected cancer. There are periods in which she is so convinced that she becomes despondent and is unable to do normal work around the house. She has started to neglect her 3-year-old son because of painful thoughts that he will be left motherless. She now spends several hours a day searching the internet for information on breast cancer or in breast cancer support chat rooms.

She is married to a successful architect, and by mutual agreement she quit her job as a financial analyst 3 years ago in order to spend full time at home with her son. She is friends with several

of the mothers in her son's play group and occasionally sees colleagues from her former office. Despite her concerns, her health is good. Her most recent physical examination was unremarkable except for small bruises over both breasts that were the result of repeated self-examination. She drinks an occasional glass of wine with meals. She smoked marijuana in college but has not used any illicit drugs for 6 years.

On psychiatric examination she appears mildly anxious. She describes herself as being at her wits' end, saying that the fear of cancer is ruining her life. She acknowledges that the fear is greatly exaggerated but she feels powerless to control it. She denies ever having had hallucinations. She is alert, oriented, her memory is good, and concentration is mildly impaired.

1. Which of the following is the most likely diagnosis?

   A. Obsessive-compulsive disorder
   B. Major depressive disorder with psychotic features
   C. Delusional disorder
   D. Hypochondriasis
   E. Body dysmorphic disorder

2. Pharmacotherapy with which of the following is most appropriate?

   A. Fluoxetine (Prozac)
   B. Halopendol (Haldol)
   C. Lithium (Eskalith)
   D. Diazepam (Valium)
   E. Zolpidem (Ambien)

3. The usual age of onset for this condition is

   A. Childhood
   B. Adolescence
   C. Early adulthood
   D. Middle age
   E. Old age

4. Which of the following is the most likely outcome without treatment?

   A. Complete recovery
   B. Chronic waxing and waning of symptoms
   C. Development of cognitive impairment
   D. Development of physical impairment
   E. Development of psychotic symptoms

Answers: 1,D; 2,A; 3,C; 4,B

Discussion

It is important early on in the assessment of any psychiatric patient to determine whether or not she has psychotic symptoms. This woman presents with the recurrent false belief that she has breast cancer; it is disrupting her life and causing considerable distress. The belief is probably not delusional, however, because she is able to be reassured, at least momentarily, and she recognizes that the fear is exaggerated. A delusion is, by definition, fixed and impervious to outside evidence that contradicts the belief. Accordingly, it is most unlikely that she is suffering a delusional disorder or a major depressive disorder with psychotic symptoms. Obsessive-compulsive disorder is a serious consideration: She has both obsessive, intrusive, and unwanted thoughts, and compulsive-like behavior in her self-examinations and time spent on the internet. However, DSM-IV-TR does not permit a diagnosis of OCD if the symptoms are limited to health concerns. Body dysmorphic disorder describes concerns about appearance, not underlying disease. The appropriate diagnosis is hypochondriasis. Intriguingly, some researchers are now speculating that hypochondriasis is part of an OCD spectrum of disorders. Although it has historically been regarded as difficult to treat, there are now data showing good response to selective serotonin reuptake inhibitors in doses similar to those used to treat OCD—typically higher than doses to treat depression alone. The onset of hypochondriasis can be at any age but is commonly in the young adult years of the 20s to early 30s. It sometimes follows a serious medical illness or, as was true for Harriet, the illness or death of a close friend. The usual course of hypochondriasis is chronic, with symptoms waxing and waning over the years, often worsening during periods of stress. There are several features in Harriet's case to suggest the prognosis may be brighter. The onset of symptoms was acute, there is no clear secondary gain, and there is nothing in the case description to suggest that she suffers from a personality disorder, all of which are associated with a better prognosis. There is no specific psychotherapy for hypochondriasis. Cognitive-behavioral therapy is helpful to some individuals. It is worth noting that her cancer fears began not only in the context of a friend's illness and death, but also of a dramatic change in life circumstances. She left a job that required considerable training and skills, that provided constant interaction with other smart, educated adults, in order to stay home alone with the demands of a young baby. Consideration should be given to a psychotherapy that would help her explore her feelings, motivations, and reactions to this important decision.

MARIAN W.

Marian W., a 44-year-old woman, is brought by police to an emergency room after she attempted to mace EMS workers in her apartment. Following her mother's death 5 years ago, Marian started to receive spiritual messages from her mother. The messages took the form of intuitions and were never voices or visions. Two weeks ago they changed from the usual kind, humorous, and supportive messages she had been receiving to frightening descriptions of family happenings. Based on these intuitions, she became convinced that her mother's brother had sexually abused her—Marian—when she was a child. One week earlier, she had gone to confront her uncle and demand that he apologize. He is now 93 years old and wheelchair-bound. She described at length to him and his wife the sexual abuse she believed she suffered, and added that he had murdered her mother in order to keep her from revealing the abuse. In reality her mother had died of uterine cancer. Her uncle's wife demanded that she leave the apartment and then phoned Marian's sister to describe what happened. Over the next several days Marian tried to rally the support of family members against her uncle, but no one would take her allegations seriously. On the day of admission she called her sister and in an agitated voice claimed that she could no longer bear not being believed about the abuse and that she planned to jump from the window of her 15th floor apartment. When her sister arrived 30 minutes later accompa-

nied by EMS workers, Marian screamed that they had been sent by her uncle to kill her. She ran to the kitchen and returned with a can of mace, which she sprayed on them. The police arrived shortly after.

Marian had a depressive episode 8 years ago shortly after receiving treatment for Lyme disease. She saw a psychiatrist who prescribed phenelzine. She felt that the medication helped her but stopped taking it after 5 weeks because she found the dietary restrictions too cumbersome. She has not had any further episodes of depression or other mood symptoms. Her sleep and appetite have been stable for years.

The diagnosis of Stage I Lyme disease followed a weekend spent at a boyfriend's house in the country. She was treated with tetracycline, doxycycline, and erythromycin. She appeared to have recovered 2 years later without heart or CNS involvement. Three years ago she experienced malaise, myalgia, and arthralgias. Titers showed that she once again had Stage I Lyme disease. She was treated with erythromycin and remained symptom-free. Marian works as an executive assistant in a major financial institution. She continued working until the day of admission. She drinks one or two alcoholic drinks per month and she uses no illicit drugs. Two weeks ago she began using Kava on the advice of a friend to help her relax after work. Physical examination is unremarkable. Routine laboratory studies are within normal limits and Lyme titers are negative. Mental status testing reveals the fixed belief that her uncle abused her, murdered her mother, and sent the EMS workers to assassinate her. She has had no hallucinations. Her thinking is logical and goal directed.

1. Which of the following is the most likely diagnosis?

    A. Schizophrenia
    B. Brief psychotic episode
    C. Psychosis secondary to Lyme disease
    D. Delusional disorder
    E. Psychosis secondary to Kava use

2. Which of the following treatments is the most appropriate?

    A. Risperidone therapy
    B. Psychodynamic psychotherapy
    C. Sertraline therapy
    D. Family therapy
    E. Clonazepam therapy

3. Which of the following symptoms is most suggestive of a psychotic disorder due to substance use or a general medical condition?

    A. Nonbizarre delusions
    B. Hallucinations without delusions
    C. Visual hallucinations
    D. Delusions without hallucinations
    E. Hallucinations in more than one modality

Answers: 1,B; 2,A; 3,B

Discussion

The abrupt onset of psychotic symptoms in a previously healthy middle-aged adult raises immediate concerns about medical or drug-related causes. Lyme disease is known to cause a variety of neuropsychiatric symptoms ranging from mild mood disturbances to psychotic symptoms. Marian's Lyme disease titers on admission were negative, but titers can be unreliable; a negative titer does not absolutely rule out the presence of Lyme disease. More important is the fact that she was diagnosed only with Stage I disease, which seems to have been adequately treated with antibiotics. There is no evidence of CNS involvement, and it is unlikely that Lyme disease is the cause of her current delusions. Her symptoms began at the same time she started using Kava. Kava is an herbal anxiolytic made from the bark of a shrub found on islands in the South Pacific. There are no reports of Kava causing psychotic symptoms. Long-term use can cause liver damage, but Marian has been using it for only 2 weeks.

Schizophrenia and schizophreniform disorder include similar symptoms but differ in their time courses. In schizophreniform disorder, symptoms are present for more than a month but less than 6 months. Both disorders require more than a single psychotic symptom to establish the diagnosis. The most appropriate diagnosis in this case is a brief psychotic episode. Her delusions about her uncle have been present for less than a month. If she remains symptomatic into the future, the diagnosis will convert to delusional disorder.

Antipsychotic medications work for almost all psychotic symptoms, including many cases in which there is an underlying medical or drug-related cause. Psychodynamic psychotherapy is contraindicated for psychotic patients. Family therapy can help a family deal with a member who has a psychotic illness, but it will not resolve the illness itself. Antidepressants and antianxiety medication may be used as adjuncts to the antipsychotic, which should be the primary treatment.

The type of hallucination—whether auditory or visual—has no clear diagnostic significance. Both are common in schizophrenia as well as medical and drug states. Hallucinations in more than one modality also occur often enough not to be diagnostically discriminating.

Nonbizarre delusions without hallucinations—as are found in this case—are the defining feature of delusional disorder. It is not common however, for people with a psychiatric disorder to have hallucinations without delusions. Ninety percent of individuals diagnosed with a primary psychiatric disorder who have hallucinations also have delusions.

JACOB M.

Jacob M., a 19-year-old man, is hospitalized after being brought by his mother to an emergency room complaining that he "freaked out." Yesterday he was arrested for shoplifting CDs in a neighborhood store. He was placed in a holding cell overnight and released to his mother's custody the next morning. He then went with his mother to the spot where he had parked and locked his bicycle and discovered that the bike had been stolen overnight. Jacob became enraged, shouted obscenities, pushed over several trash containers, and threatened to kill himself by running into the passing traffic.

Jacob had two prior hospitalizations. The first, at age 16, followed an explosive outburst at home, when he threw a chair and several dishes at his mother. The hospital record notes that he was experiencing auditory hallucinations at the time. He was treated with risperidone and discharged after 2 weeks. He discontinued medication after discharge and did not keep follow-up appoint-

ments. He was hospitalized for a second time at the age of 18. He had jumped off a bridge and was seen by a passing policeman, who rescued him and called an ambulance. Jacob sustained only minor soft-tissue injuries, and he insisted the jump was not a suicide attempt but that he just wanted to go swimming, despite the fact that he was fully clothed. He was hospitalized on a psychiatric unit and again the hospital record states that he was experiencing auditory hallucinations. He was treated with risperidone. He demanded that he be released and, after a court hearing, was discharged against medical advice. He stopped medication and there was no further psychiatric follow-up.

Jacob is an only child. His father and mother are both artists who teach part time at a local community college. All developmental milestones were on time or early. He was a bright and quick learner. He played soccer in the 7th and 8th grades, and, although never very gregarious, he did have two close friends with whom he spent much time. During his freshman year of high school he received all As. During his sophomore year he received mostly Cs and by junior year his grades had deteriorated to Ds and Fs. He finished his junior year but did not go back to school and he never graduated. Over the next 6 months, he stopped seeing his friends and began spending most of his time alone in his room, on his computer, or reading about religion and philosophy. He claims to have used no illicit drugs or alcohol for the last 2 years. He had tried marijuana with one of his friends but he became extremely agitated and paranoid. The experience was so unpleasant that he did not use it again. He had gotten drunk in his early teens, but as he became more isolated, he stopped drinking altogether. His medical history is unremarkable.

Jacob's parents seem unconcerned about his condition. They are aware that he dropped out of high school and is now admitted to a psychiatric unit, but they do not know how he has been spending his time from day to day. They are disturbed by his disruptions at home, and they ask that residential placement be arranged when Jacob is discharged.

On admission Jacob is cooperative. He appears vacant with little emotional expression. There is not much spontaneous speech, and he answers questions with one- or two-word answers. He denies visual or auditory hallucinations and insists that the old hospital records are wrong in saying that he ever had auditory hallucinations. He denies any past or present suicidal thoughts. He is alert and oriented, and his memory is good. A physical examination is unremarkable. Routine laboratory studies on admission are normal; a urine toxicology screen is negative.

1. Which of the following is the most likely diagnosis?

   A. Schizophrenia
   B. Drug-induced psychotic disorder
   C. Psychotic disorder due to a general medical condition
   D. Adjustment disorder with disturbance of conduct
   E. Schizotypal personality disorder

2. Which of the following investigations is most likely to help with diagnosis and management?

   A. Head computed tomography (CT) scan
   B. Brain magnetic resonance image (MRI)
   C. Thyroid function tests
   D. Neuropsychological testing
   E. Electroencephalogram

3. Which of the following features is most associated with a better prognosis in Jacob's disorder?

    A. Social isolation
    B. Early age of onset
    C. Marked emotional features
    D. Never being married
    E. Male sex

4. In addition to medication, which of the following therapies is most likely to be of benefit?

    A. Psychoanalytic psychotherapy
    B. Cognitive-behavioral therapy
    C. Psychoeducation
    D. Dialectical behavioral therapy
    E. Social skills training

Answers: 1,A; 2,D; 3,C; 4,C

Discussion

There is not enough information to make a definitive diagnosis, but the clinical symptoms and course suggest schizophrenia. The prodrome to a first psychotic episode in schizophrenia is typically characterized by declining school performance, social isolation, and emotional flattening, all of which are true for Jacob. He claims that he has not been using drugs or alcohol, and his urine toxicology screen is negative. However, people are not always forthcoming about drug use, and a negative toxicology screen does not rule out a drug-related condition. More importantly, the chronicity, and the absence of any cognitive impairment, physical findings, or laboratory abnormalities, make a disorder secondary to either drug use or a general medical condition much less likely. It is plausible that his angry outburst prompting admission was related to the stress of being in jail, but it is difficult to explain the entire clinical course as an adjustment disorder.

Whatever the final diagnosis, it is clear that something bad has been happening to Jacob and that it is getting worse. Getting more information may help with the diagnosis and should be a top priority. It is unlikely that neuroimaging studies such as a CT or PET scan or an EEG will be helpful. The length of his disturbance—at least 3 years—and the absence of physical or cognitive findings significantly decrease the possibility of neurological disease. Similarly, there is nothing in the history or physical examination to raise suspicion about an endocrinopathy. More information is needed. Jacob is currently saying very little, and what he does say about the past is not always convincing (jumping from a bridge to go swimming). His denials of auditory hallucinations may or may not be accurate. Neuropsychological testing can be helpful in a number of ways. It will not give us a diagnosis, but it will help us to understand the major issues with which he is preoccupied and the extent to which his thinking is disorganized, and will help clarify whether he is experiencing psychotic symptoms. It will more clearly reveal mood or cognitive disturbances that have not been identified by the history or mental status examination.

Prognosis in schizophrenia is not invariably grim. Some individuals do much better than others. A better prognosis is associated with late onset, social connectedness, being married, and being female. Strong emotional features are also associated with a better prognosis. However, the studies on which that observation is based are increasingly being called into question because of the possibility that their subjects included individuals with psychotic mood disturbances who were misdiagnosed as having schizophrenia.

A troubling feature of this case is the level of disengagement by Jacob's parents. It isn't clear whether it is in response to his difficulties or a cause of his difficulties (or merely coincidental), but the pervasive denial and neglect on their parts (and Jacob's) is a serious hindrance to effective treatment. This is best approached through psychoeducation for both Jacob and his parents. His behavior, including the violent outburst, can be explained as symptoms of a treatable psychiatric disorder and the need for medication compliance underscored. Different patterns of family interactions that exacerbate or reduce symptoms can be discussed, and the need for long-term follow-up and their collaboration with his treatment emphasized. Jacob is still young. The best chance he has for a satisfying, productive future lies in early, consistent, and sustained treatment.

MARGARET R.

Margaret R., a 59-year-old woman, requests a psychiatric consultation because of feelings of depression for the last 3 months. Three months ago her husband of 35 years announced that he was no longer certain he wanted to remain married. He was not romantically involved with anyone else, but he felt he was reaching the age that would be his last chance for independence. He moved into an apartment of his own several miles from the large family home where Margaret remains. Since that time she has had frequent crying spells every day, has felt hopeless, and has begun to think that she might be better off dead. She was troubled with frequent, recurring, nighttime wakenings during the first month after her husband left, but her sleep is now normal and restorative. She has had no change in appetite, and her weight remains the same. She runs a successful design firm, and although she did not go into the office for the first 2 weeks, she has since resumed work, and the business is doing quite well. With the exception of two single women friends, she feels uncomfortable getting together with old friends she used to see with her husband. She turns down most social invitations.

Margaret keeps two horses at their country house and goes riding most weekends. She describes being on horseback as the one time she can clear her mind of all that has happened and feel some of the joy she felt before. She has no prior psychiatric history. She and her husband started marital counseling twice before, once 5 years ago and then last year. The counseling was started at her insistence because of what she felt to be a growing distance between her and her husband, but each time he stopped going after only a few sessions.

She drinks one or two glasses of wine each night but does not use any illicit drugs. She takes no medications and has no known medical problems. Margaret has a 34-year-old son and a 31-year-old daughter who both live out of state. She has not told them about the separation but realizes that she cannot keep it from them much longer. She feels ashamed and is worried about their reactions.

1. Which of the following is the most likely diagnosis?

    A. Major depressive disorder
    B. Dysthymia
    C. Adjustment disorder with depressed mood
    D. Acute stress disorder
    E. Posttraumatic stress disorder

2. Which of the following is the most appropriate recommendation for Margaret?

   A. diazepam therapy
   B. amitriptyline therapy
   C. marital therapy
   D. buspirone therapy
   E. individual psychotherapy

Answers: 1,C; 2,E

Discussion

It seems clear from the history that Margaret's depressed mood is in response to her husband's leaving. Her symptoms began at that time and she has no previous psychiatric history. Dysthymia, in which depressive symptoms must be present for 2 years or longer, is not a consideration. Both acute stress disorder and posttraumatic stress disorder occur in response to a psychosocial stressor, but the stressor must be extreme and there must be symptoms of arousal or avoidance of circumstances associated with the trauma. Neither of these is true for Margaret.

A major depressive episode can certainly occur in response to an unhappy or stressful event. However, the clinical information given does not justify a diagnosis of major depression for Margaret. She has a depressed mood, hopelessness, and passive thoughts of suicide, but these do not meet DSM-IV-TR criteria, which would require additional symptoms such as insomnia, anorexia, and weight loss, trouble concentrating or other cognitive symptoms, or fatigue. A depressed mood in response to a stressful or upsetting circumstance that does not meet criteria for major depression is, by definition, an adjustment disorder with depressed mood. That is the most appropriate diagnosis in this case.

The best treatment recommendation is individual psychotherapy—especially one that uses both exploratory and supportive interventions. Such a therapy would draw on her previous experiences in handling distressing situations in order to enlarge her circle of supportive friends and to be able to discuss the situation with her children. It would allow her to articulate and examine the multiple and possibly conflicting emotions she is experiencing, which, in addition to depression, could very likely include anger and humiliation. Marital therapy did not work twice in the past. There is no reason to think it would work better this time around, particularly without some expression of interest in counseling from her estranged husband. Anxiety is not prominent, sleep is untroubled, and work is for the most part unimpaired. The use of an anxiolytic, whether buspirone or diazepam, is not indicated. Many psychiatrists would recommend an antidepressant in addition to psychotherapy. However, a tricyclic such as amitriptyline would almost certainly not be a drug of first choice because of its side effects and potential toxicities. Selective serotonin reuptake inhibitors, such as fluoxetine or citalopram, have relatively benign side-effect profiles and are often therapeutic, even when the mood disturbance is minor.

Appendix B △

Objective Examinations in Psychiatry

There is a wide variety of objective multiple-choice question formats. They range from case histories followed by a series of questions relating to diagnosis, laboratory findings, treatment complications, and prognosis to the most widely used form, known as the one-best-response type, wherein a question or incomplete statement is followed by four or five suggested answers or completions, with the examinee being directed to select the one best answer. The multiple-choice questions are described as objective because the correct response is predetermined by a group of experts who compose the items, eliminating the observer bias seen in ratings of essay questions. The responses are entered on an answer sheet, which is scored by machine, giving a high degree of reliability. Two basic item types are used with the greatest frequency, one-best-response type (type A) and matching type (type B), which are detailed in Table B.1.

The case history or situation type of item consists of an introductory statement that may be an abbreviated history, with or without the results of the physical examination or laboratory tests, followed by a series of questions, usually of the A type. In similar fashion, charts, electroencephalograms, pictures of gross or microscopic slides, or even patients' graphs may be presented, again followed by the one-best-response type or matching type.

Present testing procedures using objective multiple-choice items are highly effective in regard to reliability and validity in measuring the examinee's knowledge and its application. Experienced test constructors are able to develop items based on a given content and to word the answers in a neutral fashion. Thus, correct and incorrect responses are similar in style, length, and phrasing. However, no matter how well constructed a test is, with a high degree of reliability and validity for a large group of examinees, it is subject to inaccuracies about individual testees. Some examinees underscore, and others overscore, depending on their experience and test-taking skills, known as testmanship. In the final analysis, there is no substitute for knowledge, understanding, and clinical competence when a physician is being evaluated. However, some suggestions and clues inevitably appear in the most carefully composed and edited multiple-choice test. To improve one's testmanship, one should consider the following:

1. There is no penalty for a wrong response in the objective-type multiple-choice question. The testee has a 20 percent chance of guessing correctly when there are five options. Therefore, no question should be left unanswered.

2. In medicine it is rare for anything to be universally correct or wrong. Thus, options that imply "always" or "never" are more likely to be incorrect than otherwise.

3. Especially in psychiatry, many words are often needed to include the exceptions or qualifications in a correct statement. Thus, the longest option is likely to be the correct response. Test constructors who are also aware of this fact often try to lengthen the shorter incorrect responses by adding unnecessary phrases, but that tactic can readily be detected by experienced test takers.

4. The use of a word like "possibly," or "may," or "sometimes" in an option often suggests a true statement, whereas choices with universal negative or positive statements tend to be false.

5. Each distractor that can be ruled out increases the percentage chance of guessing correctly. In a five-choice situation, being able to discard three options increases the percentage from 20 percent to 50 percent and enables the examinee to focus on only the two remaining choices.

6. With questions in which one cannot rule out any of the distractors and these suggestions do not apply, the testee should always select the same lettered option. The examination constructors try to distribute the correct answers among the five options. In some tests the middle, or C, response is correct more often than the others.

Examinations are constructed for the most part by persons from the cultural background in which the test originates. Therefore, those who have been trained abroad and whose native languages are not English are often slower in reading the items and have less time to reflect on the options.

A significant contribution to the evaluation of clinical competence is the development of patient management–problem tests. Those tests try to simulate an actual clinical situation, with emphasis on a functional problem-solving, patient-oriented approach. From thousands of reported examples of outstandingly good or poor clinical performance, test designers defined the major areas of performance, such as history taking, physical examination, use of diagnostic procedures, laboratory tests, treatment, judgment, and continuing care. Armed with that information, the test designers evolved a type of test known as programmed testing. The test provides feedback of information to the examinee, who can use these data in the solution of additional problems about the same patient.

The format starts with general patient information, which gives historical data. The section may be followed by a summary

Table B.1
Types of Items Used in Multiple-Choice Questions

Type A:
One-best-response type

Each item consists of an introductory statement or question, known as the stem, followed by four or five suggested responses. The incorrect options are known as distractors, as differentiated from the correct response. Some of the distractors may be true in part, but the one *best* response of those offered must be selected to receive full credit.

DIRECTIONS: Each of the statements or questions below is followed by five suggested responses or completions. Select the one that is *best* in each case.

1. A 2-year-old boy occasionally plays with his older sister's doll, imitating her activities. This implies
   A. pathological problems with sibling rivalry
   B. undue identification with his mother
   C. future problems with heterosexual orientation
   D. development of problems with gender identity
   E. natural exploration of his environment

2. Children in the fourth grade in urban area schools who cannot read are most commonly
   A. isolated from peers
   B. mentally retarded
   C. culturally disadvantaged
   D. brain damaged
   E. handicapped by a major perceptual deficiency

(Annotations: Stem; Distractors; Correct Response — grouped as Choices or Options)

Type B:
Matching type

DIRECTIONS: Each group of questions consists of five lettered headings, followed by a list of numbered words or phrases. For each numbered word or statement, select the one lettered heading or component that is most closely associated with it.

Questions 3–8
A. Mood disorder
B. Psychotic disorder
C. Chromosomal abnormality
D. Cognitive disorder
E. None of the above

	Correct responses
3. Delusional disorder	B
4. Conversion disorder	E
5. Down's syndrome	C
6. Bipolar I disorder	A
7. Obsessive-compulsive disorder	E
8. Wernicke's syndrome	D

The use of "None of the above" in a type A or B question often makes the item more difficult and tends to lower the percentage of candidates giving correct responses. It should also be noted that the same response may be used more than once.

Type C:

A modified form of the matching type (type C) is also used. It necessitates the ability to compare and contrast two entities, such as diagnostic procedures, treatment modalities, or causes. The association is on an all-or-none basis. For instance, even if a treatment is only occasionally used or associated with a given disorder, it is to be included as a correct response.

DIRECTIONS: Each set of lettered headings below is followed by a list of numbered words or phrases. For each of the numbered words or phrases select

A. if the item is associated with *A only*
B. if the item is associated with *B only*
C. if the item is associated with *both A and B*
D. if the item is associated with *neither A nor B*

Questions 9–13
A. Down's syndrome (mongolism)
B. Tuberous sclerosis (epiloia)
C. Both
D. Neither

	Correct responses
9. Mental deficiency	C
10. Nodular type of skin rash	B
11. Higher than chance association with leukemia	A
12. Chromosomal nondisjunction	A
13. Specific disorder of amino acid metabolism	D

Adapted from Small SM. Role of examinations in psychiatry. In: Kaplan HI, Sadock BJ, eds. *Comprehensive Textbook of Psychiatry.* 6th ed. Baltimore: Williams & Wilkins; 1995:2734.

of the physical examination and positive elements in the psychiatric status. Then the testees are presented with a series of problems, each with a variable number of options. If the examinees select an option, they receive the results of the laboratory test they requested, the patients' reaction to the medication they ordered, or just a confirmation of the order. The examinees may select as few or as many options as befits good clinical judgment. The testees lose both credit and informational feedback if they do not select an important and necessary option. They may also lose credit by selecting unnecessary or dangerous options.

Having completed problem 1 about a patient, the testee is usually given some additional follow-up information, and the procedure is repeated for problems 2, 3, and so on. An oversimplified and much abbreviated example is as follows:

A young college student has been hyperactive, has slept poorly, and has lost weight during the past month. He has been known to use cannabis and possibly other substances on many occasions. Last night he became excited, thought he was going insane, and complained of a rapid pounding sensation over his heart. He was taken to the emergency room by his roommate. No history of prior psychiatric difficulty was obtained. Physical examination reveals a temperature of 99.5°F, pulse rate of 108 per minute, respiration rate of 22 per minute, and a blood pressure of 142/80 mm Hg. His pupils are dilated but react to light, his mouth is dry, and the rest of the examination is noncontributory except for a generalized hyperreflexia. On psychiatric examination he is irritable, restless, and very suspicious. He states that people are after him and wish to harm him. He is well oriented.

1. At this time you would

   A. order morphine sulfate, 30 mg, intramuscularly
   B. inquire about drug usage
   C. order an electrocardiogram
   D. tell the patient that no one wants to harm him and that it is all his imagination
   E. arrange for hospitalization plus many additional options

Of the choices given, the feedback on B could be "Roommate states patient was taking amphetamines." D feedback: "Patient becomes excited and refuses to answer questions." E feedback: "Arrangements made."

2. The following morning, after a restless sleep, the patient continues to express fears of being harmed. You would now order

   F. chlorpromazine, 100 mg, three times daily
   G. urine screen for drugs
   H. projective psychological tests
   I. imipramine, 50 mg, four times daily and other options

The feedback on F might be "Patient quieter after a few hours." G feedback: "Ordered." H feedback: "Patient uncooperative." I feedback: "Order noted."

Although programmed testing differs from the real-life situation—in which the physician has to originate his orders or recommendations, rather than selecting them from a given set of options—it does simulate the clinical situation to a great extent. Examinees like this type of test and readily appreciate its clinical significance and relevance.

Various modifications of patient management problems have been introduced. It seems that the format, coupled with other forms of testing, is a favorable development in approaching the goal of a standardized, reliable, and valid means of evaluating some major components of clinical competence.

New methods of testing using computer-based systems for objective evaluation of clinical competence are being developed and tested. They are useful in patient management problems because they provide extensive and instantaneous feedback. They also provide contemporaneous scoring, so the testee knows the result of the test upon completion.

The National Board of Medical Examiners (NBME) has been exploring the use of interactive computerized clinical simulations (CBX) in the evaluation of clinical competence. Each CBX case is an interactive dynamic patient simulation. The student or physician interacting with CBX is presented with a brief description of the condition, circumstances, and chief complaints of the simulated patient. The CBX physician is then expected to diagnose, treat, and monitor the patient's condition as it changes over time and in response to treatment. As the case unfolds, patient information is provided only through uncued requests by the CBX physician for tests, therapies, procedures, or physical examination.

Index

Note: Page numbers followed by *f* indicate figures; numbers followed by *t* indicate tables.